2015

the calorie carb and fat bible 2015

Juliette Kellow BSc RD, Lyndel Costain BSc RD & Laurence Beeken

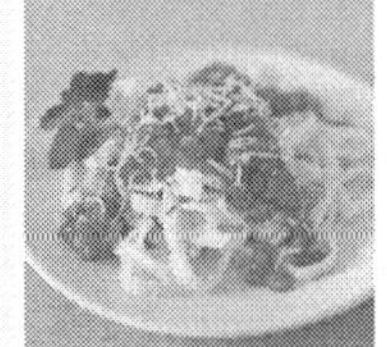
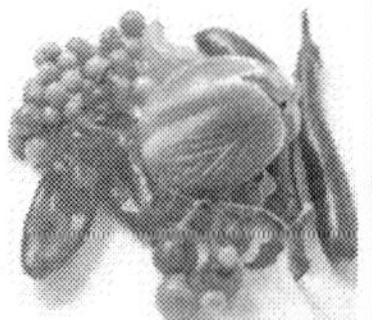
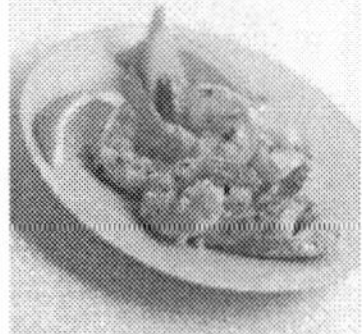
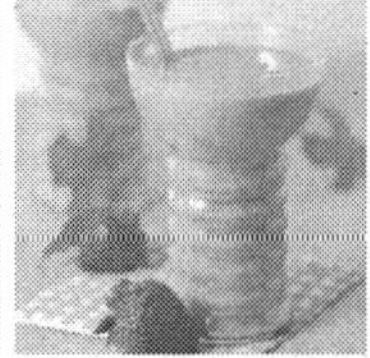
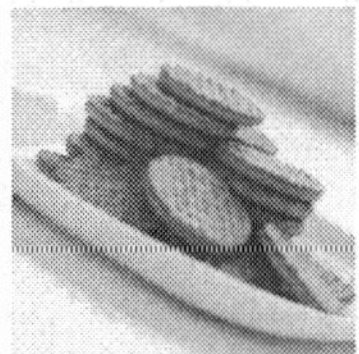
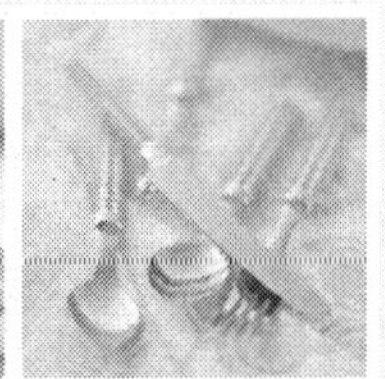

The UK's Most Comprehensive Calorie Counter

The Calorie, Carb & Fat Bible 2015

Published by:
Weight Loss Resources Ltd
2C Flag Business Exchange
Vicarage Farm Road
Peterborough
PE1 5TX.

Tel: 01733 345592
www.weightlossresources.co.uk

Companies and other organisations wishing to make bulk purchases of the Calorie, Carb and Fat Bible should contact their local bookstore or Weight Loss Resources direct.

ISBN 978-1-904512-14-1

Authors: Lyndel Costain BSc RD
Juliette Kellow BSc RD
Laurence Beeken, Weight Loss Resources

Database Editor: Laurence Beeken

Design and Layout: Joanne Putney

Printed and bound by:
Bookprintinguk.com, Peterborough, PE2 9BF

Contents

Losing weight – the easy way

Juliette Kellow BSc RD

CHINESE TAKEAWAYS, curries, chocolate, chips and a glass of wine! Imagine being told the best diet to help you lose weight includes all these foods and more. It sounds too good to be true, doesn't it? But the truth is, these are exactly the types of foods you can still enjoy if you opt to lose weight by counting calories.

But you'd be forgiven for not knowing you can still eat all your favourite foods *and* lose weight. In recent years, endless trendy diets that cut carbs, boost protein intake or skip entire groups of foods, have helped to make dieting a complicated business. Added to this, an increasing number of celebrities and so-called nutrition experts have helped mislead us into thinking that dieting is all about restriction and denial. Is it any wonder then that most of us have been left feeling downright confused and miserable about what we should and shouldn't be eating to shift those pounds?

Dieting doesn't have to be complicated or an unhappy experience. In fact, there's really only one word you need to remember if you want to shift those pounds healthily and still eat all your favourite foods. And that's CALORIE!

It's calories that count

When it comes to losing weight, there's no getting away from the fact that it's calories that count. Ask any qualified nutrition expert or dietitian for advice on how to fight the flab and you'll receive the same reply: quite simply you need to create a calorie deficit or shortfall. In other words, you need to take in fewer calories than you use up so that your body has to draw on its fat stores to provide it with the energy it needs to function properly. The result: you start losing fat and the pounds start to drop off!

Fortunately, it couldn't be easier to create this calorie deficit. Regardless of your age, weight, sex, genetic make up, lifestyle or eating habits, losing weight is as simple as reducing your daily calorie intake slightly by modifying your diet and using up a few more calories by being slightly more active each day.

Better still, it's a complete myth that you need to change your eating and exercise habits dramatically. You'll notice I've said you need to reduce your calorie intake 'slightly' and be 'slightly' more active. It really is just LITTLE differences between the amount of calories we take in and the amount we use up that make BIG differences to our waistline over time. For example, you only need to consume one can of cola more than you need each day to gain a stone in a year. It's no wonder then that people say excess weight tends to 'creep up on them'.

10 simple food swaps you can make every day *(and won't even notice!)*

Make these simple swaps every day and in just 4 weeks you'll lose 7lb!

SWAP THIS...	FOR THIS...	SAVE...
300ml full-fat milk *(195 calories)*	300ml skimmed milk *(100 calories)*	*95 calories*
1tsp butter *(35 calories)*	1tsp low-fat spread *(20 calories)*	*15 calories*
1tbsp vegetable oil *(100 calories)*	10 sprays of a spray oil *(10 calories)*	*90 calories*
1tsp sugar *(16 calories)*	Artificial sweetener *(2 calories)*	*14 calories*
1tbsp mayonnaise *(105 calories)*	1tbsp fat-free dressing *(10 calories)*	*95 calories*
Regular sandwich *(600 calories)*	Low-fat sandwich *(350 calories)*	*250 calories*
Can of cola *(135 calories)*	Can of diet cola *(1 calorie)*	*134 calories*
Large (50g) packet of crisps *(250 calories)*	Small (25g) packet of crisps *(125 calories)*	*125 calories*
1 chocolate digestive *(85 calories)*	1 small chocolate chip cookie *(55 calories)*	*30 calories*
1 slice thick-cut wholemeal bread *(95 calories)*	1 slice medium-cut wholemeal bread *(75 calories)*	*20 calories*
	TOTAL CALORIE SAVING:	***868 calories***

The good news is the reverse is also true. You only need to swap that daily can of cola for the diet version or a glass of sparking water and you'll lose a stone in a year – it really is as easy as that!

Of course, most people don't want to wait a year to shift a stone. But there's more good news. To lose 1lb of fat each week you need to create a calorie deficit of just 500 calories a day. That might sound like a lot, but you can achieve this by simply swapping a croissant for a wholemeal fruit scone, a regular sandwich for a low-fat variety, a glass of dry white wine for a gin and slimline tonic and using low-fat spread on two slices of toast instead of butter. It is also important to become more active and increase your level of exercise. Losing 1lb a week, amounts to a stone in 14 weeks, or just under 4 stone in a year!

Taking control of calories

By now you've seen it really is calories that count when it comes to shifting those pounds. So it should be no surprise that a calorie-controlled diet is the only guaranteed way to help you shift those pounds – and that's a scientific fact! But better still, a calorie-controlled diet is one of the few that allows you to include anything, whether it's pizza, wine or chocolate. A healthy diet means including a wide range of foods *(see 'Healthy Eating Made Easy' page 32)*.

And that's where this book can really help. Gone are the days when it was virtually impossible to obtain information about the calorie contents of foods. This book provides calorie information for more than 22,000 different branded and unbranded foods so that counting calories has never been easier.

The benefits of counting calories

- *It's guaranteed to help you lose weight providing you stick to your daily calorie allowance*
- *You can include favourite foods*
- *No foods are banned*
- *It's a great way to lose weight slowly and steadily*
- *Nutrition experts agree that it's a proven way to lose weight*

Calorie counting made easy

Forget weird and wacky science, complicated diet rules and endless lists of foods to fill up on or avoid every day! Counting calories to lose weight couldn't be easier. Quite simply, you set yourself a daily calorie allowance to help you lose between ½-2lb (¼-1kg) a week and then add up the calories of everything you eat and drink each day, making sure you don't go over your limit.

To prevent hunger from kicking in, it's best to spread your daily calorie allowance evenly throughout the day, allowing a certain amount of calories for breakfast, lunch, dinner and one or two snacks. For example, if you are allowed 1,500 calories a day, you could have 300 calories for breakfast, 400 calories for lunch, 500 calories for dinner and two snacks or treats of 150 calories each. You'll find more detailed information on p26-31 (Your step-by-step guide to using this book and shifting those pounds).

QUESTION

What affects the calorie content of a food?

ANSWER:

Fat, protein, carbohydrate and alcohol all provide the body with calories, but in varying amounts:

- *1g fat provides 9 calories*
- *1g alcohol provides 7 calories*
- *1g protein provides 4 calories*
- *1g carbohydrate provides 3.75 calories*

The calorie content of a food depends on the amount of fat, protein and carbohydrate it contains. Because fat provides more than twice as many calories as an equal quantity of protein or carbohydrate, in general, foods that are high in fat tend to contain more calories. This explains why 100g of chips (189 calories) contains more than twice as many calories as 100g of boiled potato (72 calories).

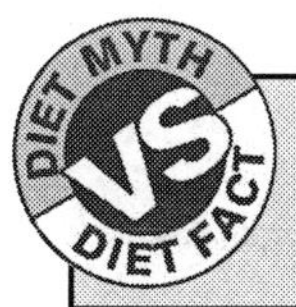

DIET MYTH:
Food eaten late at night stops you losing weight

DIET FACT:
It's not eating in the evening that stops you losing weight. It's consuming too many calories throughout the day that will be your dieting downfall! Providing you stick to your daily calorie allowance you'll lose weight, regardless of when you consume those calories. Nevertheless, it's a good idea to spread your calorie allowance throughout the day to prevent hunger from kicking in, which leaves you reaching for high-calorie snack foods.

Eat for good health

While calories might be the buzz word when it comes to shifting those pounds, it's nevertheless important to make sure your diet is healthy, balanced and contains all the nutrients you need for good health. Yes, you can still lose weight by eating nothing but, for example, chocolate, crisps and biscuits providing you stick to your calorie allowance. But you'll never find a nutrition expert or dietitian recommending this. And there are plenty of good reasons why.

To start with, an unbalanced diet is likely to be lacking in essential nutrients such as protein, vitamins, minerals and fibre, in the long term putting you at risk of nutritional deficiencies. Secondly, research proves that filling up on foods that are high in fat and/or salt and sugar can lead to many different health problems. But most importantly, when it comes to losing weight, it's almost impossible to stick to a daily calorie allowance if you're only eating high-calorie foods.

Filling up on lower-calorie foods also means you'll be able to eat far more with the result that you're not constantly left feeling unsatisfied. For example, six chocolates from a selection box contain around 300 calories, a lot of fat and sugar, few nutrients – and are eaten in just six mouthfuls! For 300 calories, you could have a grilled skinless chicken breast (packed with protein and zinc), a large salad with fat-free dressing (a great source of fibre, vitamins and minerals), a slice of wholemeal bread with low-fat spread (rich in fibre and B vitamins) and a satsuma (an excellent source of vitamin C). That's a lot more food that will take you a lot more time to eat! Not convinced? Then put six chocolates on one plate, and the chicken, salad, bread and fruit on another!

Bottom line: while slightly reducing your calorie intake is the key to losing weight, you'll be healthier and far more likely to keep those pounds off if you do it by eating a healthy diet *(see 'Healthy Eating Made Easy' page 32)*.

Eight steps to a healthy diet

1. *Base your meals on starchy foods.*
2. *Eat lots of fruit and vegetables.*
3. *Eat more fish.*
4. *Cut down on saturated fat and sugar.*
5. *Try to eat less salt - no more than 6g a day.*
6. *Get active and try to be a healthy weight.*
7. *Drink plenty of water.*
8. *Don't skip breakfast.*

SOURCE: www.nhs.uk/Livewell/Goodfood/Pages/eatwell-plate.aspx

Fat facts

Generally speaking, opting for foods that are low in fat can help slash your calorie intake considerably, for example, swapping full-fat milk for skimmed, switching from butter to a low-fat spread, not frying food in oil and chopping the fat off meat and poultry. But don't be fooled into believing that all foods described as 'low-fat' or 'fat-free' are automatically low in calories or calorie-free. In fact, some low-fat products may actually be higher in calories than standard products, thanks to them containing extra sugars and thickeners to boost the flavour and texture. The solution: always check the calorie content of low-fat foods, especially for things like cakes, biscuits, crisps, ice creams and ready meals. You might be surprised to find there's little difference in the calorie content when compared to the standard product.

Uncovering fat claims on food labels

Many products may lure you into believing they're a great choice if you're trying to cut fat, but you need to read between the lines on the labels if you want to be sure you're making the best choice. Here's the lowdown on what to look for:

LOW FAT	by law the food must contain less than 3g of fat per 100g for solids. These foods are generally a good choice if you're trying to lose weight.
REDUCED FAT	by law the food must contain 25 percent less fat than a similar standard product. This doesn't mean the product is low-fat (or low-calorie) though! For example, reduced-fat cheese may still contain 14g fat per 100g.
FAT FREE	the food must contain no more than 0.5g of fat per 100g or 100ml. Foods labelled as Virtually Fat Free must contain less than 0.3g fat per 100g. These foods are generally a good choice if you're trying to lose weight.
LESS THAN 8% FAT	this means the product contains less than 8g fat per 100g. It's only foods labelled 'less than 3% fat' that are a true low-fat choice.
X% FAT FREE	claims expressed as X% Fat Free shall be prohibited.
LIGHT OR LITE	claims stating a product is 'light' or 'lite' follows the same conditions as those set for the term 'reduced'.

10 easy ways to slash fat (and calories)

1. Eat fewer fried foods – grill, boil, bake, poach, steam, roast without added fat or microwave instead.
2. Don't add butter, lard, margarine or oil to food during preparation or cooking.
3. Use spreads sparingly. Butter and margarine contain the same amount of calories and fat – only low fat spreads contain less.
4. Choose boiled or jacket potatoes instead of chips or roast potatoes.
5. Cut off all visible fat from meat and remove the skin from chicken before cooking.
6. Don't eat too many fatty meat products such as sausages, burgers, pies and pastry products.
7. Use semi-skimmed or skimmed milk instead of full-fat milk.
8. Try low-fat or reduced-fat varieties of cheese such as reduced-fat Cheddar, low-fat soft cheese or cottage cheese.
9. Eat fewer high-fat foods such as crisps, chocolates, cakes, pastries and biscuits.
10. Don't add cream to puddings, sauces or coffee.

Getting Ready for Weight Loss Success

Lyndel Costain BSc RD

THIS BOOK not only provides tools to help you understand more about what you eat and how active you are, but guidance on how to use this information to develop a weight loss plan to suit your needs. Getting in the right frame of mind will also be a key part of your weight control journey, especially if you've lost weight before, only to watch the pounds pile back on.

The fact is that most people who want to lose weight know what to do. But often there is something that keeps stopping them from keeping up healthier habits. The same may be true for you. So what's going on? For many it's a lack of readiness. When the next diet comes along with its tempting promises it's so easy to just jump on board. But if you have struggled with your weight for a while, will that diet actually help you to recognise and change the thoughts and actions that have stopped you shifting the pounds for good?

Check out your attitude to weight loss programmes

Before starting any new weight loss programme, including the Weight Loss Resources approach, ask yourself:

Am I starting out thinking that I like myself as a person right now?	(YES or NO)
OR I feel I can only like myself once I lose weight?	(YES or NO)
Do I want to stop overeating, but at the same time find myself justifying it – in other words I want to be able to eat what I want, but with no consequences?	(YES or NO)
Do I believe that I need to take long-term responsibility for my weight?	(YES or NO)
OR Am I relying on 'it' (the diet) to do it for me?	(YES or NO)

Keep these questions, and your replies, in mind as you read through this chapter.

Next Steps

You may have already assessed the healthiness of your weight using the BMI guide on page 37. If not, why not do it now, remembering that the tools are a guide only. The important thing is to consider a weight at which you are healthy and comfortable – and which is realistic for the life you lead *(see opposite - What is a healthy weight?).*

The next step is to have a long hard think about why you want to lose weight. Consider all the possible benefits, not just those related to how you look. Psychologists have found that if we focus only on appearance we are less likely to succeed in the long-term. This is because it so often reflects low self-esteem or self-worth – which can sabotage success – as it saps confidence and keeps us stuck in destructive thought patterns. Identifying key motivations other than simply how you look - such as health and other aspects of physical and emotional well being - is like saying that you're an OK person right now, and worth making changes for. Making healthy lifestyle choices also has the knock on effect of boosting self-esteem further.

Write down your reasons for wanting to lose weight in your Personal Plan *(see page 42)* – so you can refer back to them. This can be especially helpful when the going gets tough. It may help to think of it in terms of what your weight is stopping you from doing now. Here's some examples: to feel more confident; so I can play more comfortably with my kids; my healthier diet will give me more energy; to improve my fertility.

What is a Healthy Weight?

With all the 'thin is beautiful' messages in the media it can be easy to get a distorted view about whether your weight is healthy or not. However, as the BMI charts suggest, there is no single 'ideal' weight for anybody. Research also shows that modest amounts of weight loss can be very beneficial to health and are easier to keep off. Therefore, health professionals now encourage us to aim for a weight loss of 5-10%. The ideal rate of weight loss is no more than 1-2 pounds (0.5-1kg) per week – so averaging a pound a week is great, and realistic progress.

The health benefits of modest weight loss include:

- *Reduced risk of developing heart disease, stroke and certain cancers*
- *Reduced risk of developing diabetes and helping to manage diabetes*
- *Improvements in blood pressure*
- *Improvements in mobility, back pain and joint pain*
- *Improvements with fertility problems and polycystic ovarian syndrome*
- *Less breathlessness and sleep/snoring problems*
- *Increased self esteem and control over eating*
- *Feeling fitter and have more energy*

Are You Really Ready to Lose Weight?

When you think of losing weight, it's easy just to think of what weight you'd like to get to. But weight loss only happens as a result of making changes to your usual eating and activity patterns – which allow you to consume fewer calories than you burn *(see 'It's calories that count' page 5)*.

So here comes the next big question. Are you really ready to do it? Have you thought about the implications of your decision? If you have lost weight in the past, and put it all back on - have you thought about why that was? And how confident do you feel about being successful this time?

To help you answer these questions, try these short exercises.

Where would you place yourself on the following scales?

Importance

How important is it to you, to make the changes that will allow you to lose weight?

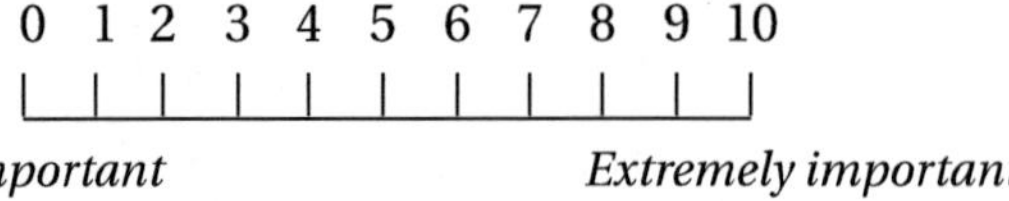

Not at all important *Extremely important*

If you ranked yourself over half way along the scale then move on to the next question. If you were half way or less along the scale, you may not be mentally ready to make the required changes to lose weight. To further explore this, go to *'The Pros and Cons of Weight Loss' (page 17)*.

Confidence

How confident are you in your ability to make the changes that will allow you to lose weight?

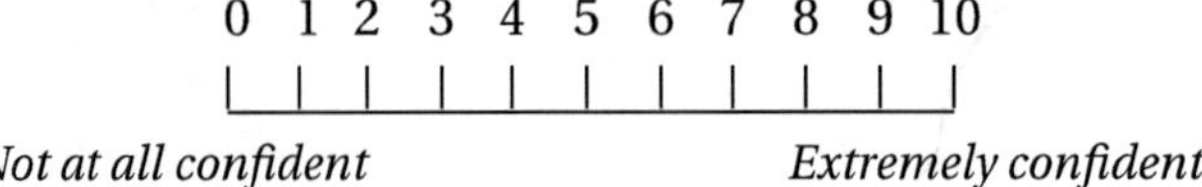

Not at all confident *Extremely confident*

Now ask yourself (regarding your confidence ratings):

1. Why did I place myself here?
2. What is stopping me moving further up the scale (if anything)?
3. What things, information, support would help me move further up the scale? (if not near 10)

If you aren't sure about answers to question 3, then keep reading for some pointers.

The Pros and Cons of Weight Loss

Making lifestyle changes to lose weight is simpler if there are lots of clear benefits or pros, for example, clothes fit again, more energy, helps back pain - but there will also be associated downsides or cons. For example, some may feel it interferes with their social life, or don't have the time to plan meals or check food labels. Or overeating can help, if only temporarily, as a way of coping with unwanted feelings. Being overweight allows some people to feel strong and assertive, or to control their partner's jealousy. So in these cases there are downsides to losing weight, even if the person says they are desperate to do it.

If you are aware of the possible downsides, as well as the pros, you will be better prepared to deal with potential conflicts. Understanding what could be (or were with past weight loss efforts) barriers to success gives you the chance to address them. This boosts confidence in your ability to succeed this time, which in turn maintains your motivation.

Have a go at weighing up the pros and cons using the charts below and on page 18. Some examples are included. If you decide that the pros outweigh the cons, then great. You can also use the cons as potential barriers to plan strategies for *(see page 42)*. If you find it's the other way around, this may not be the best time to actively lose weight. Try the exercise again in a month or so.

Making Lifestyle Changes to Lose Weight Now

CONS *e.g. Must limit eating out, take aways*	**PROS** *e.g. Feel more energetic, slimmer*

Not Making Changes Now – how would I feel in 6 months time?

PROS *e.g. Haven't had to worry about failing; Still able to eat take aways a lot*	**CONS** *e.g. Probably gained more weight; Back pain may be worse*

To change your weight, first change your mind

To lose weight you may already have a list of things to change, such as eating more fruit and veg, calculating your daily calorie intake, going for a walk each morning or buying low fat options. Others could also give you tips to try. But knowing what to do isn't the same as feeling motivated or able to do it. To be effective, you have to believe the changes are relevant, do-able and worth it.

What you think, affects how you feel, and in turn the actions you take.

Self-efficacy

In fact, research is telling us that one of the most important factors that influences weight loss success are your feelings of 'self-efficacy'. Self-efficacy is a term used in psychology to describe a person's belief that any action they take will have an effect on the outcome. It reflects our inner expectation that what we do will lead to the results we want. Not surprisingly, high levels of self-efficacy can enhance motivation, and allow us to deal better with uncertainty and conflict, and recovery from setbacks. But low levels, can reduce our motivation. We fear that whatever we do will not bring about our desired goal. This can lead self-defeating thoughts or 'self-talk', which make it hard to deal with set-backs, meaning we are more likely to give up. Here's some examples.

Examples: Low self-efficacy

'No matter how carefully I diet, I don't lose weight . . .'

'I have eaten that chocolate and as usual blown my diet, so I may as well give up now.'

'I had a rich dessert – I have no willpower to say no. I can't stand not being able to eat what I want.'

If you have a strong sense of self-efficacy, your mindset and 'self-talk' will be more like:

Examples: High self-efficacy

'I know from previous weight loss programmes, that if I stay focussed on what I am doing I do lose weight. I have always expected to lose too much too quickly which frustrates me. I know that I will lose weight if I keep making the right changes, and this time it is important to me.'

'The chocolate bar won't ruin my diet, but if I think it has and keep on eating, then my negative self-talk will. So I will get back on track.'

'I don't like having to eat differently from others, but losing weight is very important to me, so I ***can*** *stand it. After all, the world won't stop if I say no to dessert, and I will feel great afterwards. If I think about it, I am not hungry so would just feel bloated and guilty if I ate it.'*

Willpower is a Skill

Many people feel that they just need plenty of willpower or a good telling off to lose weight. But willpower isn't something you have or you don't have. Willpower is a skill. Like the dessert example on page 19, it's a sign that you've made a conscious choice to do something, because you believe the benefits outweigh any downsides. In reality everything we do is preceded by a thought. This includes everything we eat. It just may not seem like it because our actions often feel automatic *(see 'Look out for trigger eating' page 21).*

When it comes to weight loss, developing a range of skills – including choosing a lower calorie diet, coping with negative self-talk and managing things that don't go to plan - will boost your sense of self-efficacy to make the changes you want. This is especially important because we live in such a weight-promoting environment.

Our weight-promoting environment

We are constantly surrounded by tempting food, stresses that can trigger comfort eating and labour-saving devices that make it easy not to be physically active. In other words, the environment we live in makes it easy to gain weight, unless we stop and think about the food choices we make and how much exercise we do. In fact, to stay a healthy weight/maintain our weight, just about all of us need to make conscious lifestyle choices everyday. This isn't 'dieting' but just part of taking care of ourselves in the environment we live in.

It is also true that some people find it more of a challenge than others to manage their weight, thanks to genetic differences in factors such as appetite control, spontaneous activity level and emotional responses to food – rather than metabolic rate, as is often believed. The good news is that with a healthy diet and active lifestyle a healthier weight can still be achieved. But do talk to your doctor if you feel you need additional support.

Coping with Common Slimming Saboteurs

Lyndel Costain BSc RD

Look out for 'trigger' eating

Much of the overeating we do or cravings we have are actually down to unconscious, habitual, responses to a variety of triggers. These triggers can be external, such as the sight or smell of food, or internal and emotion-led, such as a response to stress, anger, boredom or emptiness. Your food diary (see page 43) helps you to recognise 'trigger' or 'non-hungry' eating which gives you the chance to think twice before you eat (see below).

Get some support

A big part of your success will be having someone to support you. It could be a friend, partner, health professional, health club or website. Let them know how they can help you most.

Make lapses your ally

Don't let a lapse throw you off course. You can't be, nor need to be perfect all the time. Doing well 80-90% of the time is great progress. Lapses are a normal part of change. Rather than feel you have failed and give up, look at what you can learn from a difficult day or week and use it to find helpful solutions for the future.

Understand why you eat

When I ask people what prompts them to eat, hunger usually comes down near the bottom of their list of reasons. Some people struggle to remember or appreciate what true hunger feels like. We are lucky that we have plenty of food to eat in our society. But its constant presence makes it harder to control what we eat, especially if it brings us comfort or joy.

If you ever find yourself in the fridge even though you've recently eaten, then you know hunger isn't the reason but some other trigger. The urge to eat can be so automatic that you feel you lack willpower or are out of control. But it is in fact a learned or conditioned response. A bit like Pavlov's dogs. He rang a bell every time he fed them, and from then on, whenever they heard the bell ring they were 'conditioned' to salivate in anticipation of food.

Because this 'non-hungry' eating is learned, you can reprogramme your response to the situations or feelings that trigger it. The first step is to identify when these urges strike. When you find yourself eating when you aren't hungry ask yourself 'why do I want to eat, what am I feeling?' If you aren't sure think back to what was happening before you ate. Then ask yourself if there is another way you can feel better without food. Or you could chat to your urge to eat in a friendly way, telling it that you don't want to give into it, you have a planned meal coming soon, and it's merely a learned response. Whatever strategy you choose, the more often you break into your urges to eat, the weaker their hold becomes.

Practise positive self-talk

Self-talk may be positive and constructive (like your guardian angel) or negative and irrational (like having a destructive devil on your shoulder).

If you've had on-off battles with your weight over the years, it's highly likely that the 'devil' is there more often. 'All or nothing' self-talk for example, 'I ate a "bad food" so have broken my diet', can make you feel like a failure which, can then trigger you into the action of overeating and/or totally giving up *(see 'Diet-binge cycle' page 23)*. One of the most powerful things about it is that the last thoughts we have are what stays in our mind. So if we think 'I still look fat' or 'I will never be slim', these feelings stay with us.

To change your self-talk for the better, the trick is to first recognise it's happening (keeping a diary really helps, *see Keep a Food Diary, page 29*). Then turn it around into a positive version of the same events *(see Self-efficacy, page 18)* where the resulting action was to feel good and stay on track. Reshaping negative self-talk helps you to boost your self-esteem and feelings of self-efficacy, and with it change your self-definition - from someone who can't 'lose weight' or 'do this or that', to someone 'who can'. And when you believe you can...

The Diet – Binge Cycle

If this cycle looks familiar, use positive self-talk, and a more flexible dietary approach, to help you break free.

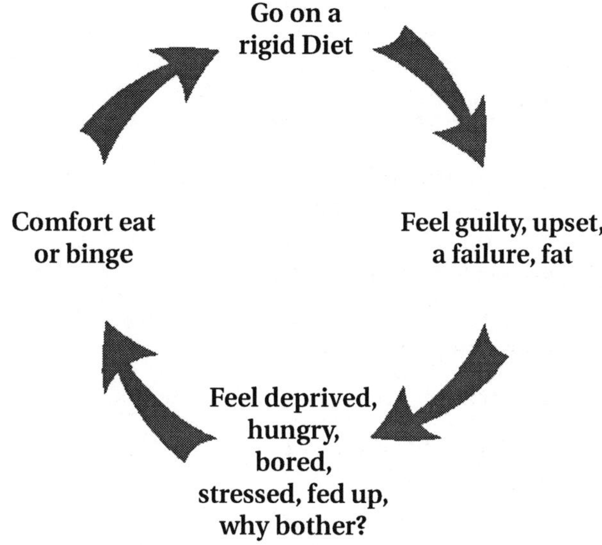

Really choose what you want to eat

This skill is like your personal brake. It also helps you to manage 'trigger/non-hungry' eating and weaken its hold. It legalises food and stops you feeling deprived. It helps you to regularly remind yourself why you are making changes to your eating habits, which keeps motivation high. But it doesn't just happen. Like all skills it requires practise. Sometimes it will work well for you, other times it won't – but overall it will help. Basically, ask yourself if you really want to eat that food in front of you. This becomes the prompt for you to make a conscious choice, weighing up the pros and cons or consequences of making that choice, and feeling free to have it, reject it or just eat some. Remembering all the while that you can eat this food another time if you want to.

Action Planning

Successful people don't just wait for things to happen. They believe in themselves, plan ahead, take action and then refine their plan until it gets, and keeps on getting the results they want. Successful slimmers use a very similar approach. They don't rely on quick-fixes or magic formulas, but glean information from reliable sources to develop a plan or approach that suits their needs, tastes and lifestyle. Thinking of weight management as a lifelong project, which has a weight loss phase and a weight maintenance phase, is also a route to success.

When the Going Gets Tough - Staying on Track

If things start to go off track, don't panic. Learning new habits takes time. And life is never straightforward so there will be times when it all seems too much, or negative 'self- talk' creeps in to try and drag you back into old ways. So if the going gets tough:

- Value what you've achieved so far, rather than only focus on what you plan to do.
- Look back at your reasons to lose weight and refer to the list often.
- Don't expect to change too much, too quickly. Take things a step at a time.
- Accept difficulties as part of the learning and skill building process.
- Enjoy a non-food reward for achieving your goals (including maintaining your weight).
- Use recipes and meal ideas to keep things interesting.
- Talk to your supporters and get plenty of encouragement. This is really vital!

Strategies of Successful Slimmers

Thanks to research conducted by large studies such as the US National Weight Control Registry and the German Lean Habits Study, we now know more about what works best for people who have lost weight and successfully kept it off. So be inspired!

The key elements of success are to:

- Believe that you can control your weight and the changes involved are really worth it.
- Stay realistic and value what you have achieved rather than dwell on a weight you 'dream' of being.
- Be more active – plan ways to fit activity into your daily life – aim for 1 hour of walking daily.
- Plan ahead for regular meals and snacks, starting with breakfast.
- Choose a balanced, low-fat diet with plenty of fruit and vegetables *(see Healthy Eating Made Easy, page 32)*.
- Watch portion size and limit fast food.
- Sit down to eat and take time over meals, paying attention to what you are eating.
- Have a flexible approach – plan in and enjoy some favourite foods without guilt.
- Recognise and address 'all or nothing' thinking and other negative 'self-talk'.
- Keep making conscious choices.
- Learn to confront problems rather than eat, drink, sleep or wish they would go away.
- Enlist ongoing help and support from family, friends, professionals or websites.
- Regularly (at least once a week but not more than once daily) check your weight.
- Take action before your weight increases by more than 4-5lb (2kg).
- Accept that your weight management skills need to be kept up long-term.
- Take heart from successful slimmers, who say that it gets easier over time.

Your step-by-step guide to using this book and shifting those pounds

Juliette Kellow BSc RD and Rebecca Walton

1. Find your healthy weight

Use the weight charts, body mass index table and information on pages 36-43 to determine the right weight for you. Then set yourself a weight to aim for. Research shows it really helps if you make losing 10% of your weight your first overall target. It also brings important health benefits too *(see 'What is a Healthy Weight?' page 15)*. You can break this down into smaller manageable steps, for example, 3kg/6.5lbs at a time. If 10% is too much, then go for a 5% loss – this has important health benefits too. In fact, just keeping your weight stable is a great achievement these days, because of our weight-promoting environment *(see page 20)*.

Waist Management

In addition to BMI, another important way to assess your weight is by measuring your waist just above belly button level. It is especially useful for men as they tend to carry more excess weight around their bellies, but women should test it out too. Having excess weight around your middle (known as being 'apple-shaped') increases your risk of heart disease and type 2 diabetes. A simple way to stay aware of your waist is according to how well, or otherwise, skirts and trousers fit. Talk to your doctor about any weight and health concerns.

WAIST MEASUREMENT

	Increased Health Risk	High Risk to Health
Women	32-35in (81-88cm)	more than 35in (88cm)
Men	37-40in (94-102cm)	more than 40in (102cm)

2. Set a realistic time scale

With today's hectic lifestyles, everything tends to happen at breakneck speed, so it's no wonder that when it comes to losing weight, most of us want to shift those pounds in an instant. But it's probably taken years to accumulate that extra weight, with the result that it's unrealistic to expect to lose the excess in just a few weeks! Instead, prepare yourself to lose weight slowly and steadily. It's far healthier to lose weight like this. But better still, research shows you'll be far more likely to maintain your new, lower weight.

If you only have a small amount of weight to lose, aim for a weight loss of around 1lb (½kg) a week. But if you have more than 2 stone (28kg) to lose, you may prefer to aim for 2lb (1kg) each week. Remember though, it's better to keep going at 1lb (½kg) a week than to give up because trying to lose 2lb (1kg) a week is making you miserable! The following words may help you to keep your goal in perspective:

'Never give up on a goal because of the time it will take to achieve it – the time will pass anyway.'

Weight Fluctuations

Weight typically fluctuates on a day to day basis. You know that shock/horror feeling when you weigh yourself in the morning then later in the day, or after a meal out, and it looks like youve gained pounds in hours! But this is due to fluid not fat changes. Real changes in body fat can only happen more gradually (remember, to gain 1lb you need to eat 3500 calories more than you usually do). Don't be confused either by seemingly very rapid weight loss in the first week or so.

When calorie intake is initially cut back, the body's carbohydrate stores in the liver and muscles (known as glycogen) are used up. Glycogen is stored with three times its weight in water, meaning that rapid losses of 4.5- 6.6lb (2 -3 kg) are possible. These stores can be just as rapidly refilled if normal eating is resumed. True weight loss happens more gradually and this book helps you to lose weight at the steady and healthy rate of no more than 1-2 lbs per week.

3. Calculate your calorie allowance

Use the calorie tables on pages 39-40 to find out how many calories you need each day to maintain your current weight. Then use the table below to discover the amount of calories you need to subtract from this amount every day to lose weight at your chosen rate. For example, a 35 year-old woman who is moderately active and weighs 12 stone (76kg) needs 2,188 calories a day to keep her weight steady. If she wants to lose ½lb (¼kg) a week, she needs 250 calories less each day, giving her a daily calorie allowance of 1,938 calories. If she wants to lose 1lb (½kg) a week, she needs 500 calories less each day, giving her a daily calorie allowance of 1,688 calories, and so on.

TO LOSE...	Cut your daily calorie intake by	In three months you could lose...	In six months you could lose...	In one year you could lose...
½lb a week	250	6.5lb	13lb	1st 12lb
1lb a week	500	13lb	1st 12lb	3st 10lb
1½lb a week	750	1st 5.5lb	2st 11lb	5st 8lb
2lb a week	1,000	1st 12lb	3st 10lb	7st 6lb

TO LOSE...	Cut your daily calorie intake by	In three months you could lose...	In six months you could lose...	In one year you could lose...
¼kg a week	250	3.25kg	6.5kg	13kg
½kg a week	500	6.5kg	13kg	26kg
¾kg a week	750	9.75kg	19.5kg	39kg
1kg a week	1,000	13kg	26kg	52kg

4. Keep a food diary

Writing down what you eat and drink and any thoughts linked to that eating helps you become more aware of your eating habits. Recognising what is going on helps you feel in control and is a powerful way to start planning change. Keeping a food diary before you start to change your eating habits will also help you identify opportunities for cutting calories by substituting one food for another, cutting portion sizes of high-calorie foods or eating certain foods less often. Simply write down every single item you eat or drink during the day and use this book to calculate the calories of each item. Then after a few days of eating normally, introduce some changes to your diet to achieve your daily calorie allowance. Remember to spread your daily calorie allowance fairly evenly throughout the day to prevent hunger. You'll find a template for a daily food and exercise diary on page 43. Try to use it as carefully as you can as research shows that people who do, do best.

Top Tip

If you only fill in your main food diary once a day, keep a pen and notepad with you to write down all those little extras you eat or drink during the day – that chocolate you ate in the office, the sliver of cheese you had while cooking dinner and the few chips you pinched from your husband's plate, for example! It's easy to forget the little things if they're not written down, but they can make the difference between success and failure.

QUESTION: Why are heavier people allowed more calories than those who have smaller amounts of weight to lose?

ANSWER: This confuses a lot of people but is easily explained. Someone who is 3 stone overweight, for example, is carrying the equivalent of 42 small packets of butter with them everywhere they go – up and down the stairs, to the local shops, into the kitchen. Obviously, it takes a lot more energy simply to move around when you're carrying that extra weight. As a consequence, the heavier you are, the more calories you need just to keep your weight steady. In turn, this means you'll lose weight on a higher calorie allowance. However, as you lose weight, you'll need to lower your calorie allowance slightly as you have less weight to carry around.

5. Control your portions

As well as making some smart food swaps to cut calories, it's likely you'll also need to reduce your serving sizes for some foods to help shift those pounds. Even 'healthy' foods such as brown rice, wholemeal bread, chicken, fish and low-fat dairy products contain calories so you may need to limit the amount you eat. When you first start out, weigh portions of foods like rice, pasta, cereal, cheese, butter, oil, meat, fish, and chicken rather than completing your food diary with a 'guesstimated' weight! That way you can calculate the calorie content accurately. Don't forget that drinks contain calories too, alcohol, milk, juices and sugary drinks all count.

6. Measure your success

Research has found that regular weight checks do help. Weighing yourself helps you assess how your eating and exercise habits affect your body weight. The important thing is to use the information in a positive way – to assess your progress - rather than as a stick to beat yourself up with. Remember that weight can fluctuate by a kilogram in a day, for example, due to fluid changes, premenstrually, after a big meal out, so weigh yourself at the same time of day and look at the trend over a week or two.

People who successfully lose weight and keep it off, also tend to continue weighing themselves at least once a week, and often daily (but not in an obsessive way), because they say it helps them stay 'on track'. Probably because they use it as an early warning system. People who weigh themselves regularly (or regularly try on a tight fitting item of clothing) will notice quickly if they have gained a couple of kilograms and can take action to stop gaining more. Checking your weight less often can mean that you might discover one day that you gained 6kg. That can be pretty discouraging, and it might trigger you to just give up.

TOP TIP

Top Tip

Don't just focus on what the bathroom scales say either – keep a record of your vital statistics, too. Many people find it doubly encouraging to see the inches dropping off, as well as the pounds!

7. Stay motivated

Each time you lose half a stone, or reach your own small goal – celebrate! Treat yourself to a little luxury – something new to wear, a little pampering or some other (non-food) treat. It also helps replace the comfort you once got from food and allows you to take care of yourself in other ways. Trying on an item of clothing that used to be tight can also help to keep you feeling motivated. Make sure you keep in touch with your supporters, and if the going gets tough take another look at the *'Coping with Common Slimming Saboteurs' section on page 21*. Once you've reviewed how well you've done, use this book to set yourself a new daily calorie allowance based on your new weight to help you lose the next half stone *(see point 3 - page 28 - Calculate your calorie allowance)*.

8. Keep it off

What you do to stay slim is just as important as what you did to get slim. Quite simply, if you return to your old ways, you are likely to return to your old weight. The great thing about calorie counting is that you will learn so much about what you eat, and make so many important changes to your eating and drinking habits, that you'll probably find it difficult to go back to your old ways – and won't want to anyway. It's still a good idea to weigh yourself at least once a week to keep a check on your weight. The key is to deal with any extra pounds immediately, rather than waiting until you have a stone to lose *(see page 30)*. Simply go back to counting calories for as long as it takes to shift those pounds and enjoy the new slim you. Page 25 has more information about how successful slimmers keep it off.

QUESTION: **Do I need to stick to exactly the same number of calories each day or is it OK to have a lower calorie intake during the week and slightly more at the weekend?**

ANSWER: The key to losing weight is to take in fewer calories than you need for as long as it takes to reach your target, aiming for a loss of no more than 2lb (1kg) a week. In general, most nutrition experts recommend a daily calorie allowance. However, it's just as valid to use other periods of time such as weeks. If you prefer, simply multiply your daily allowance by seven to work out a weekly calorie allowance and then allocate more calories to some days than others. For example, a daily allowance of 1,500 calories is equivalent to 10,500 calories a week. This means you could have 1,300 calories a day during the week and 2,000 calories a day on Saturday and Sunday.

Healthy Eating Made Easy

Juliette Kellow BSc RD

GONE ARE THE DAYS when a healthy diet meant surviving on bird seed, rabbit food and carrot juice! The new approach to eating healthily means we're positively encouraged to eat a wide range of foods, including some of our favourites – it's just a question of making sure we don't eat high fat, high sugar or highly processed foods too often.

Eating a healthy diet, together with taking regular exercise and not smoking, has huge benefits to our health, both in the short and long term. As well as helping us to lose or maintain our weight, a healthy diet can boost energy levels, keep our immune system strong and give us healthy skin, nails and hair. Meanwhile, eating well throughout life also means we're far less likely to suffer from health problems such as constipation, anaemia and tooth decay or set ourselves up for serious conditions in later life such as obesity, heart disease, stroke, diabetes, cancer or osteoporosis.

Fortunately, it couldn't be easier to eat a balanced diet. To start with, no single food provides all the calories and nutrients we need to stay healthy, so it's important to eat a variety of foods. Meanwhile, most nutrition experts also agree that mealtimes should be a pleasure rather than a penance. This means it's fine to eat small amounts of our favourite treats from time to time.

To help people eat healthily, the Food Standards Agency recommends eating plenty of different foods from four main groups of foods and limiting the amount we eat from a smaller fifth group. Ultimately, we should eat more fruit, vegetables, starchy, fibre-rich foods and fresh products, and fewer fatty, sugary, salty and processed foods.

The following guidelines are all based on the healthy eating guidelines recommended by the Food Standards Agency.

Bread, other cereals and potatoes

Eat these foods at each meal. They also make good snacks.

Foods in this group include bread, breakfast cereals, potatoes, rice, pasta, noodles, yams, oats and grains. Go for high-fibre varieties where available, such as wholegrain cereals, wholemeal bread and brown rice. These foods should fill roughly a third of your plate at mealtimes.

TYPICAL SERVING SIZES

- *2 slices bread in a sandwich or with a meal*
- *a tennis ball sized serving of pasta, potato, rice, noodles or couscous*
- *a bowl of porridge*
- *around 40g of breakfast cereal*

Fruit and vegetables

Eat at least five portions every day.

Foods in this group include all fruits and vegetables, including fresh, frozen, canned and dried products, and unsweetened fruit juice. Choose canned fruit in juice rather than syrup and go for veg canned in water without added salt or sugar.

TYPICAL PORTION SIZES

- *a piece of fruit eg: apple, banana, pear*
- *2 small fruits eg: satsumas, plums, apricots*
- *a bowl of fruit salad, canned or stewed fruit*
- *a small glass of unsweetened fruit juice*
- *a cereal bowl of salad*
- *3tbsp vegetables*

Milk and dairy foods

Eat two or three servings a day.

Foods in this group include milk, cheese, yoghurt and fromage frais. Choose low-fat varieties where available such as skimmed milk, reduced-fat cheese and fat-free yoghurt.

TYPICAL SERVING SIZES

- *200ml milk*
- *a small pot of yoghurt or fromage frais*
- *a small matchbox-sized piece of cheese*

Meat, fish and alternatives

Eat two servings a day

Foods in this group include meat, poultry, fish, eggs, beans, nuts and seeds. Choose low-fat varieties where available such as extra-lean minced beef and skinless chicken and don't add extra fat or salt.

TYPICAL SERVING SIZES

- *a piece of meat, chicken or fish the size of a deck of cards*
- *1-2 eggs*
- *3 heaped tablespoons of beans*
- *a small handful of nuts or seeds*

TOP TIP

Healthy Eating on a plate

A simple way to serve up both balance and healthy proportions is to fill one half of your plate with salad or vegetables and divide the other half between protein-rich meat, chicken, fish, eggs or beans, and healthy carbs (potatoes, rice, pasta, pulses, bread or noodles).

Fatty and sugary foods

Eat only small amounts of these foods

Foods in this group include oils, spreading fats, cream, mayonnaise, oily salad dressings, cakes, biscuits, puddings, crisps, savoury snacks, sugar, preserves, confectionery and sugary soft drinks.

TYPICAL SERVING SIZES:

- *a small packet of sweets or a small bar of chocolate*
- *a small slice of cake*
- *a couple of small biscuits*
- *1 level tbsp mayo, salad dressing or olive oil*
- *a small packet of crisps*

Useful Tools

Body Mass Index

The Body Mass Index (BMI) is the internationally accepted way of assessing how healthy our weight is. It is calculated using an individual's height and weight. Use the Body Mass Index Chart to look up your BMI, and use the table below to see what range you fall into.

BMI Under 18.5	*Underweight*
BMI 18.5-25	*Healthy*
BMI 25-30	*Overweight*
BMI 30-40	*Obese*
BMI Over 40	*Severely Obese*

This is what different BMI ranges mean.

- **Underweight:** you probably need to gain weight for your health's sake. Talk to your doctor if you have any concerns, or if you feel frightened about gaining weight.
- **Healthy weight:** you are a healthy weight, so aim to stay in this range (note that most people in this range tend to have a BMI between 20-25).
- **Overweight:** aim to lose some weight for your health's sake, or at least prevent further weight gain.
- **Obese:** your health is at risk and losing weight will benefit your health.
- **Severely obese:** your health is definitely at risk. You should visit your doctor for a health check. Losing weight will improve your health.

Please note that BMI is not as accurate for athletes or very muscular people (muscle weighs more than fat), as it can push them into a higher BMI category despite having a healthy level of body fat. It is also not accurate for women who are pregnant or breastfeeding, or people who are frail.

Body Mass Index Table

WEIGHT IN STONES / LBS	HEIGHT IN FEET / INCHES														
	4'6	**4'8**	**4'10**	**5'0**	**5'2**	**5'4**	**5'6**	**5'8**	**5'10**	**6'0**	**6'2**	**6'4**	**6'6**	**6'8**	**6'10**
6st 7	22.0	20.5	19.1	17.8	16.7	15.7	14.7	13.9	13.1	12.4	11.7	11.1	10.6	10.0	9.5
7st 0	23.7	22.1	20.6	19.2	18.0	16.9	15.9	15.0	14.1	13.3	12.6	12.0	11.4	10.8	10.3
7st 7	25.4	23.6	22.0	20.6	19.3	18.1	17.0	16.0	15.1	14.3	13.5	12.8	12.2	11.6	11.0
8st 0	27.1	25.2	23.5	22.0	20.6	19.3	18.1	17.1	16.1	15.2	14.4	13.7	13.0	12.3	11.8
8st 7	28.8	26.8	25.0	23.3	21.8	20.5	19.3	18.2	17.1	16.2	15.3	14.5	13.8	13.1	12.5
9st 0	30.5	28.4	26.4	24.7	23.1	21.7	20.4	19.2	18.1	17.2	16.2	15.4	14.6	13.9	13.2
9st 7	32.2	29.9	27.9	26.1	24.4	22.9	21.5	20.3	19.2	18.1	17.1	16.2	15.4	14.7	14.0
10st 0	33.9	31.5	29.4	27.4	25.7	24.1	22.7	21.4	20.2	19.1	18.0	17.1	16.2	15.4	14.7
10st 7	35.6	33.1	30.8	28.8	27.0	25.3	23.8	22.4	21.2	20.0	18.9	18.0	17.0	16.2	15.4
11st 0	37.3	34.7	32.3	30.2	28.3	26.5	24.9	23.5	22.2	21.0	19.8	18.8	17.9	17.0	16.2
11st 7	39.0	36.2	33.8	31.6	29.6	27.7	26.1	24.6	23.2	21.9	20.7	19.7	18.7	17.8	16.9
12st 0	40.7	37.8	35.2	32.9	30.8	28.9	27.2	25.6	24.2	22.9	21.6	20.5	19.5	18.5	17.6
12st 7	42.3	39.4	36.7	34.3	32.1	30.1	28.3	26.7	25.2	23.8	22.5	21.4	20.3	19.3	18.4
13st 0	44.0	41.0	38.2	35.7	33.4	31.4	29.5	27.8	26.2	24.8	23.5	22.2	21.1	20.1	19.1
13st 7	45.7	42.5	39.6	37.0	34.7	32.6	30.6	28.8	27.2	25.7	24.4	23.1	21.9	20.8	19.8
14st 0	47.4	44.1	41.1	38.4	36.0	33.8	31.7	29.9	28.2	26.7	25.3	23.9	22.7	21.6	20.6
14st 7	49.1	45.7	42.6	39.8	37.3	35.0	32.9	31.0	29.2	27.6	26.2	24.8	23.5	22.4	21.3
15st 0	50.8	47.3	44.0	41.2	38.5	36.2	34.0	32.0	30.2	28.6	27.1	25.7	24.4	23.2	22.0
15st 7	52.5	48.8	45.5	42.5	39.8	37.4	35.2	33.1	31.2	29.5	28.0	26.5	25.2	23.9	22.8
16st 0	54.2	50.4	47.0	43.9	41.1	38.6	36.3	34.2	32.3	30.5	28.9	27.4	26.0	24.7	23.5
16st 7	55.9	52.0	48.5	45.3	42.4	39.8	37.4	35.2	33.3	31.4	29.8	28.2	26.8	25.5	24.2
17st 0	57.6	53.6	49.9	46.6	43.7	41.0	38.6	36.3	34.3	32.4	30.7	29.1	27.6	26.2	25.0
17st 7	59.3	55.1	51.4	48.0	45.0	42.2	39.7	37.4	35.3	33.3	31.6	29.9	28.4	27.0	25.7
18st 0	61.0	56.7	52.9	49.4	46.3	43.4	40.8	38.5	36.3	34.3	32.5	30.8	29.2	27.8	26.4
18st 7	62.7	58.3	54.3	50.8	47.5	44.6	42.0	39.5	37.3	35.3	33.4	31.6	30.0	28.6	27.2
19st 0	64.4	59.9	55.8	52.1	48.8	45.8	43.1	40.6	38.3	36.2	34.3	32.5	30.8	29.3	27.9
19st 7	66.1	61.4	57.3	53.5	50.1	47.0	44.2	41.7	39.3	37.2	35.2	33.3	31.7	30.1	28.6
20st 0	67.8	63.0	58.7	54.9	51.4	48.2	45.4	42.7	40.3	38.1	36.1	34.2	32.5	30.9	29.4
20st 7	69.4	64.6	60.2	56.3	52.7	49.4	46.5	43.8	41.3	39.1	37.0	35.1	33.3	31.6	30.1
21st 0	71.1	66.2	61.7	57.6	54.0	50.6	47.6	44.9	42.3	40.0	37.9	35.9	34.1	32.4	30.9
21st 7	72.8	67.7	63.1	59.0	55.3	51.9	48.8	45.9	43.3	41.0	38.8	36.8	34.9	33.2	31.6
22st 0	74.5	69.3	64.6	60.4	56.5	53.1	49.9	47.0	44.4	41.9	39.7	37.6	35.7	34.0	32.3
22st 7	76.2	70.9	66.1	61.7	57.8	54.3	51.0	48.1	45.4	42.9	40.6	38.5	36.5	34.7	33.1
23st 0	77.9	72.5	67.5	63.1	59.1	55.5	52.2	49.1	46.4	43.8	41.5	39.3	37.3	35.5	33.8
23st 7	79.6	74.0	69.0	64.5	60.4	56.7	53.3	50.2	47.4	44.8	42.4	40.2	38.2	36.3	34.5
24st 0	81.3	75.6	70.5	65.9	61.7	57.9	54.4	51.3	48.4	45.7	43.3	41.0	39.0	37.0	35.3
24st 7	83.0	77.2	71.9	67.2	63.0	59.1	55.6	52.3	49.4	46.7	44.2	41.9	39.8	37.8	36.0
25st 0	84.7	78.8	73.4	68.6	64.2	60.3	56.7	53.4	50.4	47.6	45.1	42.8	40.6	38.6	36.7
25st 7	86.4	80.3	74.9	70.0	65.5	61.5	57.8	54.5	51.4	48.6	46.0	43.6	41.4	39.4	37.5
26st 0	88.1	81.9	76.3	71.3	66.8	62.7	59.0	55.5	52.4	49.5	46.9	44.5	42.2	40.1	38.2
26st 7	89.8	83.5	77.8	72.7	68.1	63.9	60.1	56.6	53.4	50.5	47.8	45.3	43.0	40.9	38.9
27st 0	91.5	85.1	79.3	74.1	69.4	65.1	61.2	57.7	54.4	51.5	48.7	46.2	43.8	41.7	39.7
27st 7	93.2	86.6	80.8	75.5	70.7	66.3	62.4	58.7	55.4	52.4	49.6	47.0	44.7	42.4	40.4
28st 0	94.9	88.2	82.2	76.8	72.0	67.5	63.5	59.8	56.4	53.4	50.5	47.9	45.5	43.2	41.1
28st 7	96.5	89.8	83.7	78.2	73.2	68.7	64.6	60.9	57.5	54.3	51.4	48.7	46.3	44.0	41.9
29st 0	98.2	91.4	85.2	79.6	74.5	69.9	65.8	62.0	58.5	55.3	52.3	49.6	47.1	44.8	42.6
29st 7	99.9	92.9	86.6	80.9	75.8	71.1	66.9	63.0	59.5	56.2	53.2	50.5	47.9	45.5	43.3

Weight Chart

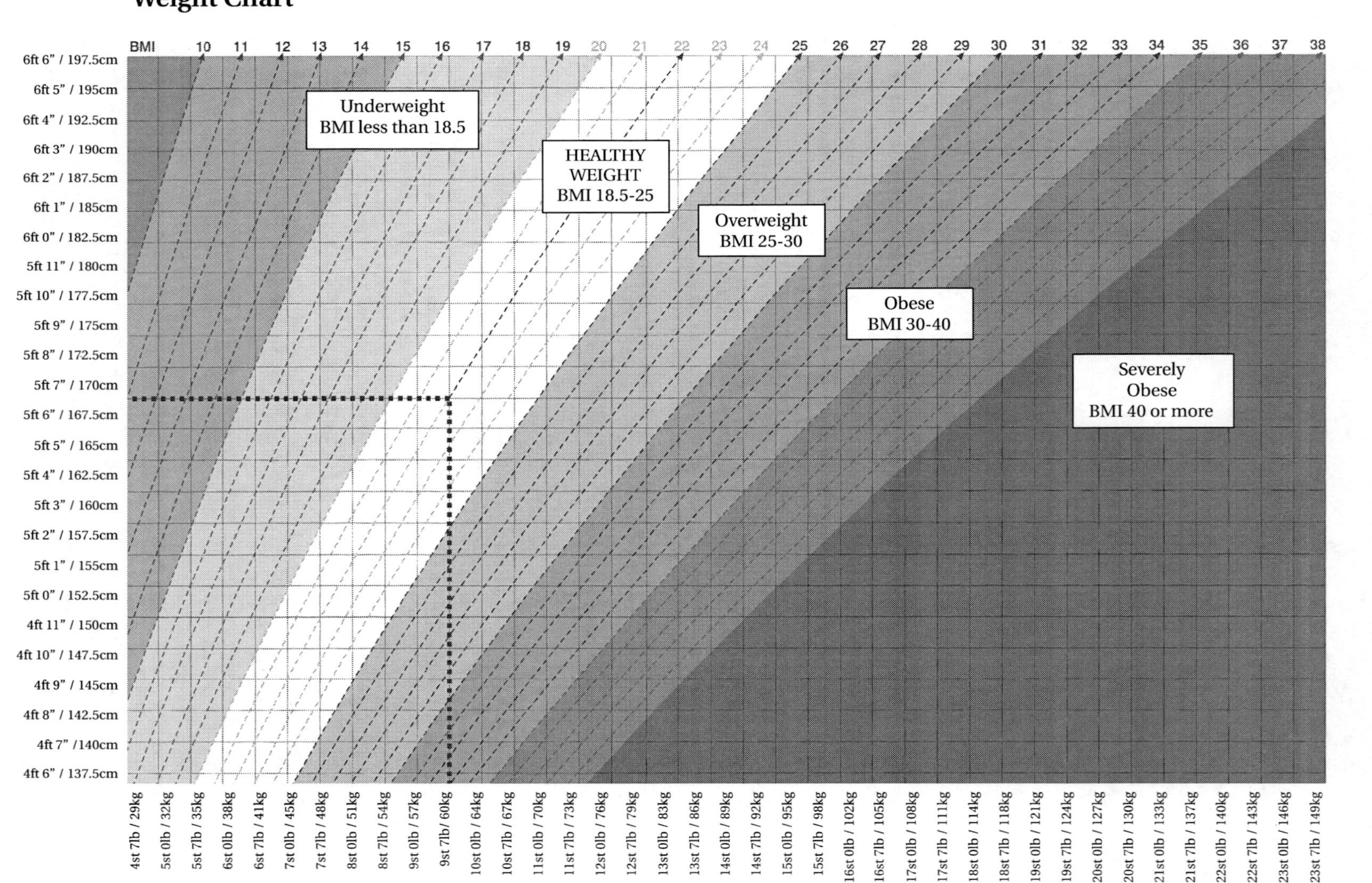

Calories Required to Maintain Weight
Adult Females

ACTIVITY LEVEL / AGE

WEIGHT IN STONES / LBS	VERY SEDENTARY			MODERATELY SEDENTARY			MODERATELY ACTIVE			VERY ACTIVE		
	<30	30-60	60+	<30	30-60	60+	<30	30-60	60+	<30	30-60	60+
7st 7	1425	1473	1304	1544	1596	1412	1781	1841	1630	2138	2210	1956
8st 0	1481	1504	1338	1605	1629	1450	1852	1880	1673	2222	2256	2008
8st 7	1537	1535	1373	1666	1663	1487	1922	1919	1716	2306	2302	2059
9st 0	1594	1566	1407	1726	1696	1524	1992	1957	1759	2391	2349	2111
9st 7	1650	1596	1442	1787	1729	1562	2062	1996	1802	2475	2395	2163
10st 0	1706	1627	1476	1848	1763	1599	2133	2034	1845	2559	2441	2214
10st 7	1762	1658	1511	1909	1796	1637	2203	2073	1888	2644	2487	2266
11st 0	1819	1689	1545	1970	1830	1674	2273	2111	1931	2728	2534	2318
11st 7	1875	1720	1580	2031	1863	1711	2344	2150	1975	2813	2580	2370
12st 0	1931	1751	1614	2092	1897	1749	2414	2188	2018	2897	2626	2421
12st 7	1987	1781	1648	2153	1930	1786	2484	2227	2061	2981	2672	2473
13st 0	2044	1812	1683	2214	1963	1823	2555	2266	2104	3066	2719	2525
13st 7	2100	1843	1717	2275	1997	1861	2625	2304	2147	3150	2765	2576
14st 0	2156	1874	1752	2336	2030	1898	2695	2343	2190	3234	2811	2628
14st 7	2212	1905	1786	2397	2064	1935	2766	2381	2233	3319	2858	2680
15st 0	2269	1936	1821	2458	2097	1973	2836	2420	2276	3403	2904	2732
15st 7	2325	1967	1855	2519	2130	2010	2906	2458	2319	3488	2950	2783
16st 0	2381	1997	1890	2580	2164	2047	2976	2497	2362	3572	2996	2835
16st 7	2437	2028	1924	2640	2197	2085	3047	2535	2405	3656	3043	2887
17st 0	2494	2059	1959	2701	2231	2122	3117	2574	2449	3741	3089	2938
17st 7	2550	2090	1993	2762	2264	2159	3187	2613	2492	3825	3135	2990
18st 0	2606	2121	2028	2823	2298	2197	3258	2651	2535	3909	3181	3042
18st 7	2662	2152	2062	2884	2331	2234	3328	2690	2578	3994	3228	3093
19st 0	2719	2182	2097	2945	2364	2271	3398	2728	2621	4078	3274	3145
19st 7	2775	2213	2131	3006	2398	2309	3469	2767	2664	4162	3320	3197
20st 0	2831	2244	2166	3067	2431	2346	3539	2805	2707	4247	3366	3249
20st 7	2887	2275	2200	3128	2465	2383	3609	2844	2750	4331	3413	3300
21st 0	2944	2306	2235	3189	2498	2421	3680	2882	2793	4416	3459	3352
21st 7	3000	2337	2269	3250	2531	2458	3750	2921	2836	4500	3505	3404
22st 0	3056	2368	2303	3311	2565	2495	3820	2960	2879	4584	3552	3455
22st 7	3112	2398	2338	3372	2598	2533	3890	2998	2923	4669	3598	3507
23st 0	3169	2429	2372	3433	2632	2570	3961	3037	2966	4753	3644	3559
23st 7	3225	2460	2407	3494	2665	2608	4031	3075	3009	4837	3690	3611
24st 0	3281	2491	2441	3554	2699	2645	4101	3114	3052	4922	3737	3662
24st 7	3337	2522	2476	3615	2732	2682	4172	3152	3095	5006	3783	3714
25st 0	3394	2553	2510	3676	2765	2720	4242	3191	3138	5091	3829	3766
25st 7	3450	2583	2545	3737	2799	2757	4312	3229	3181	5175	3875	3817
26st 0	3506	2614	2579	3798	2832	2794	4383	3268	3224	5259	3922	3869
26st 7	3562	2645	2614	3859	2866	2832	4453	3307	3267	5344	3968	3921
27st 0	3618	2676	2648	3920	2899	2869	4523	3345	3310	5428	4014	3973
27st 7	3675	2707	2683	3981	2932	2906	4594	3384	3353	5512	4060	4024
28st 0	3731	2738	2717	4042	2966	2944	4664	3422	3397	5597	4107	4076
28st 7	3787	2768	2752	4103	2999	2981	4734	3461	3440	5681	4153	4128

Calories Required to Maintain Weight
Adult Males

ACTIVITY LEVEL / AGE

WEIGHT IN STONES / LBS	VERY SEDENTARY			MODERATELY SEDENTARY			MODERATELY ACTIVE			VERY ACTIVE		
	<30	30-60	60+	<30	30-60	60+	<30	30-60	60+	<30	30-60	60+
9st 0	1856	1827	1502	2010	1979	1627	2320	2284	1878	2784	2741	2254
9st 7	1913	1871	1547	2072	2026	1676	2391	2338	1933	2870	2806	2320
10st 0	1970	1914	1591	2134	2074	1724	2463	2393	1989	2955	2871	2387
10st 7	2027	1958	1636	2196	2121	1772	2534	2447	2045	3041	2937	2454
11st 0	2084	2001	1680	2258	2168	1820	2605	2502	2100	3127	3002	2520
11st 7	2141	2045	1724	2320	2215	1868	2677	2556	2156	3212	3067	2587
12st 0	2199	2088	1769	2382	2262	1916	2748	2611	2211	3298	3133	2654
12st 7	2256	2132	1813	2444	2310	1965	2820	2665	2267	3384	3198	2720
13st 0	2313	2175	1858	2506	2357	2013	2891	2719	2322	3470	3263	2787
13st 7	2370	2219	1902	2568	2404	2061	2963	2774	2378	3555	3329	2854
14st 0	2427	2262	1947	2630	2451	2109	3034	2828	2434	3641	3394	2920
14st 7	2484	2306	1991	2691	2498	2157	3106	2883	2489	3727	3459	2987
15st 0	2542	2350	2036	2753	2545	2205	3177	2937	2545	3813	3525	3054
15st 7	2599	2393	2080	2815	2593	2253	3248	2992	2600	3898	3590	3120
16st 0	2656	2437	2125	2877	2640	2302	3320	3046	2656	3984	3655	3187
16st 7	2713	2480	2169	2939	2687	2350	3391	3100	2711	4070	3721	3254
17st 0	2770	2524	2213	3001	2734	2398	3463	3155	2767	4155	3786	3320
17st 7	2827	2567	2258	3063	2781	2446	3534	3209	2823	4241	3851	3387
18st 0	2884	2611	2302	3125	2828	2494	3606	3264	2878	4327	3917	3454
18st 7	2942	2654	2347	3187	2876	2542	3677	3318	2934	4413	3982	3520
19st 0	2999	2698	2391	3249	2923	2591	3749	3373	2989	4498	4047	3587
19st 7	3056	2741	2436	3311	2970	2639	3820	3427	3045	4584	4112	3654
20st 0	3113	2785	2480	3373	3017	2687	3891	3481	3100	4670	4178	3721
20st 7	3170	2829	2525	3434	3064	2735	3963	3536	3156	4756	4243	3787
21st 0	3227	2872	2569	3496	3112	2783	4034	3590	3211	4841	4308	3854
21st 7	3285	2916	2614	3558	3159	2831	4106	3645	3267	4927	4374	3921
22st 0	3342	2959	2658	3620	3206	2880	4177	3699	3323	5013	4439	3987
22st 7	3399	3003	2702	3682	3253	2928	4249	3754	3378	5098	4504	4054
23st 0	3456	3046	2747	3744	3300	2976	4320	3808	3434	5184	4570	4121
23st 7	3513	3090	2791	3806	3347	3024	4392	3862	3489	5270	4635	4187
24st 0	3570	3133	2836	3868	3395	3072	4463	3917	3545	5356	4700	4254
24st 7	3627	3177	2880	3930	3442	3120	4534	3971	3600	5441	4766	4321
25st 0	3685	3220	2925	3992	3489	3168	4606	4026	3656	5527	4831	4387
25st 7	3742	3264	2969	4054	3536	3217	4677	4080	3712	5613	4896	4454
26st 0	3799	3308	3014	4116	3583	3265	4749	4135	3767	5699	4962	4521
26st 7	3856	3351	3058	4177	3630	3313	4820	4189	3823	5784	5027	4587
27st 0	3913	3395	3103	4239	3678	3361	4892	4243	3878	5870	5092	4654
27st 7	3970	3438	3147	4301	3725	3409	4963	4298	3934	5956	5158	4721
28st 0	4028	3482	3191	4363	3772	3457	5035	4352	3989	6042	5223	4787
28st 7	4085	3525	3236	4425	3819	3506	5106	4407	4045	6127	5288	4854
29st 0	4142	3569	3280	4487	3866	3554	5177	4461	4101	6213	5354	4921
29st 7	4199	3612	3325	4549	3913	3602	5249	4516	4156	6299	5419	4987
30st 0	4256	3656	3369	4611	3961	3650	5320	4570	4212	6384	5484	5054

Calories Burned in Exercise

This table shows the approximate number of extra* calories that would be burned in a five minute period of exercise activity.

ACTIVITY	CALORIES BURNED IN 5 MINUTES
Aerobics, Low Impact	*25*
Badminton, Recreational	*17*
Cross Trainer	*30*
Cycling, Recreational, 5mph	*17*
Dancing, Modern, Moderate	*13*
Fencing	*24*
Gardening, Weeding	*19*
Hill Walking, Up and Down, Recreational	*22*
Jogging	*30*
Kick Boxing	*30*
Netball Playing	*23*
Rebounding	*18*
Roller Skating	*30*
Rowing Machine, Moderate	*30*
Running, 7.5mph	*48*

ACTIVITY	CALORIES BURNED IN 5 MINUTES
Situps, Continuous	*17*
Skiing, Moderate	*30*
Skipping, Moderate	*30*
Squash Playing	*39*
Tennis Playing, Recreational	*26*
Toning Exercises	*17*
Trampolining	*17*
Volleyball, Recreational	*10*
Walking, Uphill, 15% Gradient, Moderate	*43*
Walking Up and Down Stairs, Moderate	*34*
Walking, 4mph	*24*
Weight Training, Moderate	*12*
Yoga	*13*

*Extra calories are those in addition to your normal daily calorie needs.

My Personal Plan

Date:

Body Mass Index:

Weight:

Waist Measurement:

Height:

Body Fat % (if known)

10% Weight Loss Goal:

Current weight	16stone (224lb)	100kg
- 10% weight	1stone 8½lb (22½lb)	10kg
= 10% loss goal	14stone 5½lb (201½lb)	90kg

My smaller weight targets on the way to achieving my 10% goal will be:

Reasons why I want to lose weight:

Changes I will make to help me lose weight:

Diet:

Activity:

Potential saboteurs or barriers will be:

Ways I will overcome these:

My supporters will be:

I will monitor my progress by:

I will reward my progress with:

In the short term:

In the long term:

Food and Exercise Diary

Date: / /

Daily Calorie Allowance: [ ] **A**

Food/Drink Consumed	Serving Size	Calories

Total calories consumed [ ] **B**

Exercise/Activity	No. mins	Calories

Calories used in exercise [ ] **C**

Calorie balance [ ] **D**

You are aiming for your Calorie Balance (Box D) to be as close to zero as possible - ie. you consume the number of calories you need.

Your Daily Calorie Allowance (Box A) should be set to lose ½-2lb (¼-1kg) a week, or maintain weight, depending on your goals.

Daily Calorie Allowance (A) *plus* Extra Calories used in Exercise (C) *minus* Total Calories Consumed (B) *equals* Calorie Balance (D)

A + C - B = D

You can also write down any comments or thoughts related to your eating if you want to.

Food Information

Nutritional Information

CALORIE AND FAT values are given per serving, plus calorie and nutrition values per 100g of product. This makes it easy to compare the proportions of fat, protein, carbohydrate and fibre in each food.

The values given are for uncooked, unprepared foods unless otherwise stated. Values are also for only the edible portion of the food unless otherwise stated. ie - weighed with bone.

Finding Foods

The Calorie, Carb & Fat Bible has an Eating Out section which is arranged alphabetically by brand. In the General Foods and Drinks A-Z most foods are grouped together by type, and then put in to alphabetical order. This makes it easy to compare different brands, and will help you to find lower calorie and/or fat alternatives where they are available.

This format also makes it easier to locate foods. Foods are categorised by their main characteristics so, for example, if it is bread, ciabatta or white sliced, you'll find it under "Bread".

Basic ingredients are highlighted to make them easier to find at a glance. You'll find all unbranded foods in bold - making the index easier to use, whether it's just an apple or all the components of a home cooked stew.

There are, however, some foods which are not so easy to categorise, especially combination foods like ready meals. The following pointers will help you to find your way around the book until you get to know it a little better.

FILLED ROLLS AND SANDWICHES - Bagels, baguettes, etc which are filled are listed as "Bagels (filled)" etc. Sandwiches are under "Sandwiches".

CURRIES - Popular types of curry, like Balti or Jalfrezi, are listed under their individual types. Unspecified or lesser known types are listed under their main ingredient.

BURGERS - All burgers, including chicken-type sandwiches from fast-food outlets, are listed under "Burgers". CHIPS & FRIES - Are listed separately, depending on the name of the particular brand. All other types of potato are listed under "Potatoes".

SWEETS & CHOCOLATES - Well-known brands, eg. Aero, Mars Bar, are listed under their brand names. Others are listed under "Chocolate" (for bars) and "Chocolates" (for individual sweets).

READY MEALS - Popular types of dishes are listed under their type, eg. "Chow Mein", "Casserole", "Hot Pot", etc. Others are listed by their main ingredient, eg. "Chicken With", "Chicken In", etc.

EATING OUT & FAST FOODS - By popular demand this edition has the major eating out and fast food brands listed separately, at the back of the book. They are alphabetised first by brand, then follow using the same format as the rest of the book.

Serving Sizes

Many ready-meal type foods are given with calories for the full pack size, so that an individual serving can be worked out by estimating the proportion of the pack that has been consumed. For example, if you have eaten a quarter of a packaged pasta dish, divide the calorie value given for the whole pack by 4 to determine the number of calories you have consumed. Where serving sizes are not appropriate, or unknown, values are given per 1oz/28g. Serving sizes vary greatly from person to person and, if you are trying to lose weight, it's very important to be accurate – especially with foods that are very high in calories such as those that contain a fair amount of fat, sugar, cream, cheese, alcohol etc.

Food Data

Nutrition information for basic average foods has been compiled by the Weight Loss Resources food data team using many sources of information to calculate the most accurate values possible. Some nutrition information for non-branded food records is from The Composition of Foods 6th Edition (2002). Reproduced under licence from The Controller of Her Majesty's Stationary Office. Where basic data is present for ordinary foodstuffs such as 'raw carrots'; branded records are not included.

Nutrition information for branded goods is from details supplied by retailers and manufacturers, and researched by Weight Loss Resources staff. The Calorie Carb & Fat Bible contains data for over 1400 UK brands, including major supermarkets and fast food outlets.

The publishers gratefully acknowledge all the manufacturers and retailers who have provided information on their products. All product names, trademarks or registered trademarks belong to their respective owners and are used only for the purpose of identifying products.

Calorie & nutrition data for all food and drink items are typical values.

Caution

The information in The Calorie, Carb and Fat Bible is intended as an aid to weight loss and weight maintenance, and is not medical advice. If you suffer from, or think you may suffer from a medical condition you should consult your doctor before starting a weight loss and/or exercise regime. If you start exercising after a period of relative inactivity, you should start slowly and consult your doctor if you experience pain, distress or other symptoms.

Weights, Measures & Abbreviations

ABBREVIATIONS	
kcal	*kilocalories / calories*
prot	*protein*
carb	*carbohydrate*
sm	*small*
med	*medium*
av	*average*
reg	*regular*
lge	*large*
tsp	*teaspoon*
tbsp	*tablespoon*
dtsp	*dessertspoon*
gf	*gluten free*

BRAND ABBREVIATIONS USED	
ASDA	
Good for You	*GFY*
Chosen by You	*CBY*
MARKS & SPENCER	*M & S*
Count on Us	*COU*
MORRISONS	
Better For You	*BFY*
SAINSBURY'S	
Be Good to Yourself	*BGTY*
Way to Five	*WTF*
Taste the Difference	*TTD*
TESCO	
Healthy Eating	*HE*
Healthy Living	*HL*
Light Choices	*LC*
WAITROSE	
Perfectly Balanced	*PB*

	Measure INFO/WEIGHT	per Measure KCAL	FAT	Nutrition Values per 100g / 100ml KCAL	PROT	CARB	FAT	FIBRE
ABALONE								
Cooked, Fried, Weighed without Shells	1 Serving/85g	161	5.8	189	19.6	11.0	6.8	0.0
Raw, Weighed without Shells	1 Serving/85g	89	0.6	105	17.1	6.0	0.8	0.0
ABSINTHE								
Average	***1 Shot/35ml***	***127***	***0.0***	***363***	***0.0***	***38.8***	***0.0***	***0.0***
ACKEE								
Canned, Drained, Average	***1oz/28g***	***43***	***4.3***	***151***	***2.9***	***0.8***	***15.2***	***0.0***
ADVOCAAT								
Average	***1 Shot/35ml***	***91***	***2.2***	***260***	***4.7***	***28.4***	***6.3***	***0.0***
AERO								
Honeycomb, Nestle*	1 Serving/40g	199	10.0	497	5.9	62.2	25.0	0.0
Milk, Giant, Bar, Nestle*	1 Bar/125g	674	38.6	539	6.6	57.7	30.9	2.2
Milk, Medium, Bar, Nestle*	1 Bar/43g	232	13.3	539	6.6	57.7	30.9	2.2
Milk, Snacksize, Bar, Nestle*	1 Bar/21g	110	6.5	537	6.6	55.9	31.9	2.2
Milk, Standard, Bar, Nestle*	1 Bar/31g	165	9.6	531	6.3	56.9	30.9	0.8
Minis, Nestle*	1 Bar/11g	57	3.2	518	6.8	58.1	28.7	0.8
Mint, Bubbles, Aero, Nestle*	1 Bubble/3g	16	0.9	538	5.4	60.5	30.1	1.4
Mint, Nestle*	1 Bar/41g	221	12.3	538	5.1	61.5	29.9	0.9
Mint, Snack Size, Nestle*	1 Bar/21g	112	6.7	548	7.7	55.3	32.8	0.9
Mint, Standard, Aero, Nestle*	1 Bar/43g	233	13.2	542	5.2	60.5	30.8	0.9
Orange, Bubbles, Aero, Nestle*	1 Bubble/3g	16	0.9	538	5.4	60.5	30.0	1.4
Orange, Nestle*	6 Squares/22g	119	6.8	542	5.1	60.7	30.7	0.9
ALFALFA SPROUTS								
Raw, Average	1 Serving/33g	8	0.3	24	3.0	3.0	0.9	3.0
ALLSPICE								
Ground, Schwartz*	1 Tsp/3g	11	0.1	358	6.1	74.3	4.0	0.0
ALMONDS								
Blanched, Average	***1 Serving/100g***	***617***	***54.3***	***617***	***25.1***	***6.9***	***54.3***	***8.1***
Candied, Sugared	1 Serving/100g	458	16.3	458	8.4	69.2	16.3	2.2
Flaked, Average	***1oz/28g***	***172***	***15.2***	***613***	***24.9***	***6.5***	***54.3***	***7.6***
Flaked, Toasted, Average	***1oz/28g***	***176***	***15.8***	***629***	***24.6***	***5.8***	***56.4***	***7.5***
Ground, Average	***1 Serving/10g***	***62***	***5.6***	***625***	***24.0***	***6.6***	***55.8***	***7.4***
Marcona, Average	***1 Serving/100g***	***608***	***53.7***	***608***	***22.1***	***13.0***	***53.7***	***9.7***
Toasted, Average	***1oz/28g***	***178***	***15.8***	***634***	***25.0***	***6.6***	***56.4***	***6.6***
Whole, Average	***1 Serving/20g***	***122***	***11.0***	***612***	***23.4***	***21.2***	***54.8***	***8.4***
Yoghurt Coated, Holland & Barrett*	1 Pack/100g	536	37.0	536	10.9	45.3	37.0	2.8
ALOO TIKKI								
Average	1 Serving/25g	48	2.0	191	4.5	25.2	8.0	3.5
AMARANTH								
Grain, Cooked	1 Serving/100g	102	2.0	102	4.0	19.0	2.0	2.0
ANCHOVIES								
Fillets, Flat, John West*	1 Can/50g	113	7.0	226	25.0	0.1	14.0	0.0
in Oil, Canned, Drained	1 Anchovy/4g	8	0.5	195	23.4	0.0	11.3	0.0
Marinated, Sainsbury's*	¼ Pot/44g	78	4.0	177	22.0	2.0	9.0	0.1
Salted, Finest, Tesco*	1 Serving/10g	9	0.2	93	18.2	0.0	2.2	0.0
White, Flat, Tesco*	1 Serving/100g	130	3.2	130	22.9	1.5	3.2	0.0
ANGEL DELIGHT								
Banana Flavour, Kraft*	1 Sachet/59g	280	12.3	474	2.3	69.3	20.9	0.3
Banana Toffee Flavour, No Added Sugar, Kraft*	1 Sachet/59g	292	15.6	495	4.8	58.5	26.5	0.0
Butterscotch Flavour, No Added Sugar, Kraft*	1 Sachet/47g	226	11.3	480	4.5	61.0	24.0	0.0
Chocolate Flavour, Kraft*	1 Sachet/67g	305	12.1	455	3.7	69.5	18.0	0.4
Raspberry Flavour, No Added Sugar, Kraft*	1 Sachet/59g	292	15.3	495	4.8	59.5	26.0	0.0
Strawberry Flavour, No Added Sugar, Kraft*	1 Sachet/47g	230	12.5	490	4.8	59.0	26.5	0.0
Toffee Flavour, Kraft*	1 Sachet/59g	283	12.4	480	2.6	70.0	21.0	0.0

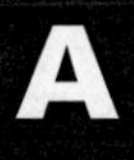

	Measure INFO/WEIGHT	per Measure KCAL	FAT	Nutrition Values per 100g / 100ml KCAL	PROT	CARB	FAT	FIBRE
ANGEL DELIGHT								
Vanilla Ice Cream Flavour, No Added Sugar, Kraft*	1 Sachet/59g	295	15.9	500	4.8	59.5	27.0	0.0
ANGEL HAIR								
Pasta, Dry	1 Serving/50g	181	1.1	362	12.4	73.6	2.2	4.4
ANTIPASTO								
Artichoke, Sainsbury's*	1 Serving/50g	68	6.2	135	2.0	3.6	12.5	2.3
Coppa, from Selection Platter, TTD, Sainsbury's*	1 Serving/100g	255	17.1	255	25.2	0.1	17.1	0.0
Felino, from Selection Platter, TTD, Sainsbury's*	1 Serving/100g	349	24.9	349	31.1	0.1	24.9	0.0
Mixed, Misto Cotto, Arrosto Erbe, Waitrose*	1 Slice/9g	11	0.4	129	22.2	0.0	4.4	0.0
Mushroom, Mixed, Sainsbury's*	¼ Jar/72g	70	6.5	97	2.7	1.4	9.0	3.7
Parma, Salami Milano, Bresaola, Finest, Tesco*	¼ Pack/30g	104	7.9	345	26.4	0.5	26.3	0.0
Parma Ham, from Selection Platter, TTD, Sainsbury's*	1 Serving/100g	236	12.9	236	29.9	0.1	12.9	0.0
Pepper, Mixed, Sainsbury's*	½ Jar/140g	48	1.8	34	1.3	4.2	1.3	3.5
Pepper, Roasted, Drained, Tesco*	1 Jar/170g	128	9.4	75	0.9	5.5	5.5	4.1
Seafood, Drained, Sainsbury's*	½ Jar/84g	150	9.7	178	14.3	4.1	11.6	1.4
Sun Dried Tomato, Sainsbury's*	¼ Jar/70g	275	25.0	393	4.5	13.4	35.7	6.2
APPLES								
Bites, Average	1 Pack/118g	58	0.1	49	0.3	11.6	0.1	2.2
Braeburn, Average	***1 Apple/123g***	***58***	***0.1***	***47***	***0.4***	***11.4***	***0.1***	***2.0***
Cape, Tesco*	1 Apple/100g	50	0.1	50	0.4	11.8	0.1	1.8
Cooking, Baked with Sugar, Flesh Only, Average	***1 Serving/140g***	***104***	***0.1***	***74***	***0.5***	***19.2***	***0.1***	***1.7***
Cooking, Raw, Peeled, Average	***1oz/28g***	***10***	***0.0***	***35***	***0.3***	***8.9***	***0.1***	***1.6***
Cooking, Stewed with Sugar, Average	***1 Serving/140g***	***104***	***0.1***	***74***	***0.3***	***19.1***	***0.1***	***1.2***
Cooking, Stewed without Sugar, Average	***1 Serving/140g***	***46***	***0.1***	***33***	***0.3***	***8.1***	***0.1***	***1.5***
Cox, English, Average	***1 Apple/108g***	***52***	***0.1***	***48***	***0.4***	***11.3***	***0.1***	***2.0***
Discovery, Average	***1 Apple/182g***	***82***	***0.9***	***45***	***0.4***	***10.6***	***0.5***	***1.0***
Dried, Average	***1 Pack/250g***	***537***	***0.7***	***215***	***0.8***	***52.8***	***0.3***	***5.9***
Empire, Average	***1 Apple/120g***	***58***	***0.1***	***48***	***0.4***	***11.8***	***0.1***	***2.0***
Fuji, Average	1 Apple/132g	64	0.1	48	0.4	11.8	0.1	1.8
Gala, Average	***1 Apple/152g***	***73***	***0.2***	***48***	***0.4***	***11.6***	***0.1***	***1.6***
Golden Delicious, Average	***1 Med/102g***	***48***	***0.2***	***48***	***0.4***	***11.2***	***0.2***	***1.8***
Granny Smith, Average	***1 Sm/125g***	***62***	***0.1***	***50***	***0.4***	***11.9***	***0.1***	***2.0***
Green, Raw, Average	***1 Med/182g***	***86***	***0.2***	***48***	***0.4***	***11.3***	***0.1***	***1.8***
Mackintosh, Red, Average	***1 Apple/165g***	***81***	***0.5***	***49***	***0.2***	***12.8***	***0.3***	***1.8***
Pink Lady, Average	***1 Apple/125g***	***62***	***0.1***	***50***	***0.4***	***11.7***	***0.1***	***2.1***
Sliced, Average	***1oz/28g***	***14***	***0.0***	***49***	***0.4***	***11.6***	***0.1***	***1.8***
APPLETISER*								
Juice Drink, Sparkling, Appletiser, Coca-Cola*	1 Glass/200ml	94	0.0	47	0.0	11.0	0.0	0.4
APRICOTS								
Bite Size, Dried, Stoned, Ready to Eat, Whitworths*	1 Pack/36g	76	0.1	210	1.6	46.7	0.3	6.6
Canned, in Syrup, Average	***1oz/28g***	***18***	***0.0***	***63***	***0.4***	***16.1***	***0.1***	***0.9***
Dried, Average	***1 Apricot/10g***	***17***	***0.1***	***171***	***3.6***	***37.4***	***0.5***	***6.3***
Dried, Soft, Average	***1 Serving/50g***	***104***	***0.2***	***208***	***2.4***	***48.5***	***0.4***	***5.2***
Halves, in Fruit Juice, Average	***1 Can/221g***	***87***	***0.1***	***40***	***0.5***	***9.2***	***0.1***	***1.0***
Raw, Flesh Only, Average	***1 Apricot/37g***	***19***	***0.2***	***52***	***1.5***	***12.0***	***0.4***	***2.2***
Raw, Weighed with Stone, Average	***1 Apricot/40g***	***19***	***0.2***	***48***	***1.4***	***11.1***	***0.4***	***2.0***
Ready to Eat, Dried, Organic, Love Life, Waitrose*	1 Serving/40g	97	0.2	243	3.4	55.3	0.5	7.3
ARCHERS*								
Aqua, Peach, Archers*	1 Bottle/275ml	206	0.0	75	0.3	7.7	0.0	0.0
Peach (Calculated Estimate), Archers*	1 Shot/35ml	91	0.0	260	0.0	0.0	0.0	0.0
Vea, Wildberry, Schnapps, Archers*	1 Bottle/275ml	124	0.0	45	0.0	5.8	0.0	0.0
ARTICHOKE								
Chargrilled, in Olive Oil, Cooks Ingredients, Waitrose*	1 Serving/40g	52	4.9	129	1.7	2.7	12.3	2.7
Chargrilled, Italian, Drained, Sainsbury's*	1/3 Tub/43g	40	2.7	92	3.1	2.8	6.1	6.5

	Measure	per Measure		Nutrition Values per 100g / 100ml				
	INFO/WEIGHT	KCAL	FAT	KCAL	PROT	CARB	FAT	FIBRE
ARTICHOKE								
Fresh, Raw, Average	***1oz/28g***	***13***	***0.0***	***47***	***3.3***	***10.5***	***0.2***	***5.4***
Hearts, Canned, Drained, Average	***½ Can/117g***	***35***	***0.1***	***30***	***1.9***	***5.4***	***0.0***	***2.2***
Hearts, Marinated & Grilled, Waitrose*	1 Serving/50g	57	5.0	114	3.0	3.0	10.0	3.0
Hearts, Sliced with Extra Virgin Olive Oil, Waitrose*	1 Serving/40g	24	1.6	59	1.3	4.4	4.0	7.0
ASAFOETIDA								
Powder, Schwartz*	1 Tbsp/0.7g	2	0.0	271	6.5	56.2	2.2	0.0
ASPARAGUS								
Boiled, in Salted Water, Average	***5 Spears/125g***	***32***	***1.0***	***26***	***3.4***	***1.4***	***0.8***	***1.4***
Canned, Average	***1 Can/250g***	***48***	***0.5***	***19***	***2.3***	***2.0***	***0.2***	***1.6***
Spears, Frozen, Asda*	1 Serving/80g	23	0.6	29	3.4	1.4	0.8	1.4
Tips, Sainsbury's*	1 Pack/125g	36	0.8	29	2.9	2.0	0.6	2.1
Trimmed, Raw, Average	***1 Serving/80g***	***20***	***0.4***	***24***	***2.9***	***1.9***	***0.6***	***1.7***
ASPIRE*								
Cranberry Flavoured Soft Drink, Aspire*	1 Can/250ml	12	0.0	5	0.0	1.1	0.0	0.0
AUBERGINE								
Baby, Tesco*	1 Aubergine/50g	8	0.2	15	0.9	2.2	0.4	2.3
Baked Topped, M & S*	1 Serving/150g	165	11.6	110	2.4	7.4	7.7	0.9
Fried, Average	***1oz/28g***	***85***	***8.9***	***302***	***1.2***	***2.8***	***31.9***	***2.3***
Marinated & Grilled, Waitrose*	½ Pack/100g	106	10.0	106	1.0	3.0	10.0	2.0
Parmigiana, M & S*	1 Pack/350g	332	18.6	95	4.6	7.6	5.3	1.1
Raw, Fresh, Average	***1 Sm/250g***	***38***	***1.0***	***15***	***0.9***	***2.2***	***0.4***	***2.0***
AVOCADO								
Flesh Only, Average	***1 Med/145g***	***276***	***28.3***	***190***	***1.9***	***1.9***	***19.5***	***3.4***
Raw, Weighed with Stone	1 Avocado/201g	324	30.8	161	2.0	7.4	15.3	5.0

B

	Measure INFO/WEIGHT	per Measure KCAL	FAT	Nutrition Values per 100g / 100ml KCAL	PROT	CARB	FAT	FIBRE
BACARDI*								
& Diet Cola, Bacardi*	1 Bottle/275ml	85	0.0	31	0.0	1.0	0.0	0.0
37.5% Volume, Bacardi*	***1 Shot/35ml***	***72***	***0.0***	***207***	***0.0***	***0.0***	***0.0***	***0.0***
40% Volume, Bacardi*	***1 Shot/35ml***	***78***	***0.0***	***222***	***0.0***	***0.0***	***0.0***	***0.0***
Breezer, Cranberry, Bacardi*	1 Bottle/275ml	154	0.0	56	0.0	7.1	0.0	0.0
Breezer, Half Sugar, Bacardi*	1 Bottle/275ml	122	0.0	44	0.0	0.0	0.0	0.0
Breezer, Lemon, Diet, Bacardi*	1 Bottle/275ml	96	0.0	35	0.0	1.2	0.0	0.0
Breezer, Orange, Bacardi*	1 Bottle/275ml	179	0.0	65	0.0	8.2	0.0	0.0
Breezer, Orange, Diet, Bacardi*	1 Bottle/275ml	80	0.0	29	0.0	0.0	0.0	0.0
BACON								
Back, Dry Cured, Average	***1 Rasher/31g***	***77***	***4.7***	***250***	***28.1***	***0.3***	***15.1***	***0.3***
Back, Dry Fried or Grilled, Average	***1 Rasher/25g***	***72***	***5.4***	***287***	***23.2***	***0.0***	***21.6***	***0.0***
Back, Lean, Average	***1 Rasher/33g***	***57***	***4.0***	***174***	***16.3***	***0.1***	***12.0***	***0.5***
Back, Smoked, Average	***1 Rasher/25g***	***66***	***5.0***	***265***	***20.9***	***0.0***	***19.9***	***0.0***
Back, Smoked, Lean, Average	***1 Rasher/25g***	***41***	***1.2***	***163***	***28.2***	***1.1***	***5.0***	***0.2***
Back, Smoked, Rindless, Average	***1 Rasher/25g***	***60***	***4.3***	***241***	***21.0***	***0.1***	***17.4***	***0.0***
Back, Tendersweet, Average	***1 Rasher/25g***	***63***	***3.6***	***250***	***29.8***	***0.4***	***14.4***	***0.0***
Back, Unsmoked, Average	***1 Rasher/32g***	***78***	***5.5***	***243***	***21.3***	***0.4***	***17.3***	***0.0***
Back, Unsmoked, Rindless, Average	***1 Rasher/23g***	***56***	***3.9***	***241***	***22.5***	***0.0***	***16.9***	***0.0***
Chops, Average	***1oz/28g***	***62***	***4.2***	***222***	***22.3***	***0.0***	***14.8***	***0.0***
Collar Joint, Lean & Fat, Boiled	***1oz/28g***	***91***	***7.6***	***325***	***20.4***	***0.0***	***27.0***	***0.0***
Collar Joint, Lean & Fat, Raw	***1oz/28g***	***89***	***8.1***	***319***	***14.6***	***0.0***	***28.9***	***0.0***
Collar Joint, Lean Only, Boiled	***1oz/28g***	***53***	***2.7***	***191***	***26.0***	***0.0***	***9.7***	***0.0***
Cooking, Pieces, Smart Price, Asda*	1 Serving/100g	215	22.0	215	23.0	0.0	22.0	0.0
Fat Only, Cooked, Average	***1oz/28g***	***194***	***20.4***	***692***	***9.3***	***0.0***	***72.8***	***0.0***
Fat Only, Raw, Average	***1oz/28g***	***209***	***22.7***	***747***	***4.8***	***0.0***	***80.9***	***0.0***
Gammon Rasher, Lean Only, Grilled	***1oz/28g***	***48***	***1.5***	***172***	***31.4***	***0.0***	***5.2***	***0.0***
Lardons, Smoked, Sainsbury's*	1 Serving/200g	476	30.8	238	21.4	0.1	15.4	0.1
Lean, Average	***1 Rasher/33g***	***47***	***2.2***	***142***	***19.6***	***0.9***	***6.7***	***0.2***
Lean Only, Fried, Average	***1 Rasher/25g***	***83***	***5.6***	***332***	***32.8***	***0.0***	***22.3***	***0.0***
Lean Only, Grilled, Average	***1 Rasher/25g***	***73***	***4.7***	***292***	***30.5***	***0.0***	***18.9***	***0.0***
Loin Steaks, Grilled, Average	***1 Serving/120g***	***229***	***11.6***	***191***	***25.9***	***0.0***	***9.7***	***0.0***
Medallions, Average	***1 Rasher/18g***	***27***	***0.6***	***151***	***29.4***	***0.9***	***3.3***	***0.1***
Middle, Fried	***1 Rasher/40g***	***140***	***11.4***	***350***	***23.4***	***0.0***	***28.5***	***0.0***
Middle, Grilled	***1 Rasher/40g***	***123***	***9.2***	***307***	***24.8***	***0.0***	***23.1***	***0.0***
Middle, Raw	***1 Rasher/43g***	***104***	***8.6***	***241***	***15.2***	***0.0***	***20.0***	***0.0***
Rashers, Lean Only, Trimmed, Average	1 Rasher/20g	24	0.8	119	20.6	0.0	4.0	0.0
Rindless, Average	***1 Rasher/20g***	***30***	***1.7***	***150***	***18.5***	***0.0***	***8.5***	***0.0***
Smoked, Average	***1 Rasher/28g***	***46***	***2.1***	***166***	***24.8***	***0.2***	***7.4***	***0.0***
Smoked, Crispy, Cooked, Average	***1 Serving/10g***	***46***	***2.7***	***460***	***53.0***	***2.1***	***26.9***	***0.0***
Smoked, Rindless, Average	***1 Rasher/20g***	***21***	***0.6***	***106***	***19.8***	***0.0***	***3.0***	***0.0***
Streaky, Average	***1oz/28g***	***76***	***5.9***	***270***	***20.0***	***0.0***	***21.0***	***0.0***
Streaky, Cooked, Average	***1 Rasher/20g***	***68***	***5.6***	***342***	***22.4***	***0.3***	***27.8***	***0.0***
BACON BITS								
Average	***1oz/28g***	***75***	***5.9***	***268***	***18.6***	***0.7***	***21.2***	***0.1***
BACON VEGETARIAN								
Rashers	***1 Rasher/16g***	***33***	***1.7***	***206***	***19.5***	***8.6***	***10.4***	***2.8***
Rashers, Cheatin', The Redwood Co*	1 Rasher/16g	32	1.2	196	25.9	7.3	7.3	0.5
Rashers, Tesco*	1 Rasher/20g	41	2.2	203	22.5	3.3	11.1	3.9
Realeat*	1 Rasher/19g	49	1.1	260	27.0	25.0	5.8	1.6
Streaky Style Rashers, Tesco*	1 Rasher/8g	17	0.8	215	23.7	5.0	10.6	2.2
Strips, Morningstar Farms*	1 Strip/8g	30	2.3	375	12.5	12.5	28.1	6.2
BAGEL								
Bacon, & Soft Cheese, Boots*	1 Serving/148g	481	25.2	325	12.0	31.0	17.0	2.2

	Measure INFO/WEIGHT	per Measure KCAL	FAT	Nutrition Values per 100g / 100ml KCAL	PROT	CARB	FAT	FIBRE
BAGEL								
Cream Cheese, M & S*	1 Bagel/23g	79	4.9	352	7.8	31.0	21.8	1.8
Ham, & Pesto, COU, M & S*	1 Pack/173g	260	2.4	150	11.1	23.5	1.4	1.7
Salmon, Smoked, & Cream Cheese, M & S*	1 Bagel185g	480	18.8	260	12.3	29.5	10.2	1.9
Tuna, & Salad, BGTY, Sainsbury's*	1 Bagel/170g	325	7.1	191	10.4	26.0	4.2	1.0
Turkey, & Cranberry, Bagelmania*	1 Pack/198g	325	7.3	164	9.0	24.5	3.7	1.1
Turkey, Pastrami & American Mustard, Shapers, Boots*	1 Bagel/146g	296	5.0	203	11.0	32.0	3.4	1.4
BAGUETTE								
All Day Breakfast, Darwins Deli*	1 Serving/184g	498	21.5	271	13.4	31.9	11.7	0.0
Beef, & Horseradish, Freshly Prepared, M & S*	1 Baguette/274g	795	31.0	290	12.1	37.2	11.3	2.0
Brie, Tomato & Rocket, Freshly Prepared, M & S*	1 Baguette/219g	570	21.7	260	10.3	33.2	9.9	1.9
Cheese, Mixed, & Spring Onion, Asda*	1 Pack/190g	629	34.8	331	9.5	32.1	18.3	1.3
Cheese, Tomato, & Basil, Asda*	¼ Baguette/42g	138	5.9	329	10.0	40.8	14.0	1.3
Cheese & Ham, Average	1 Baguette/203g	593	20.8	292	14.0	35.9	10.3	1.4
Cheese & Pickle, Fullfillers*	1 Baguette/280g	767	31.1	274	11.9	35.5	11.1	0.0
Cheese & Tomato, Tesco*	1 Baguette/108g	243	8.3	225	9.7	29.3	7.7	1.8
Chicken, Honey & Mustard, BGTY, Sainsbury's*	1 Pack/187g	340	3.7	182	11.0	30.0	2.0	0.0
Chicken, Oakham, Fresh, M & S*	1 Baguette/225g	450	10.8	200	12.4	26.7	4.8	1.5
Chicken & Mayonnaise, Asda*	1 Pack/190g	407	16.5	214	9.7	30.5	8.7	1.3
Chicken & Salad, Asda*	1 Serving/158g	326	9.5	206	9.0	29.0	6.0	2.1
Chicken & Salad, Shapers, Boots*	1 Baguette/132g	222	2.6	168	11.0	27.0	2.0	1.5
Chicken & Stuffing, Hot, Sainsbury's*	1 Baguette/227g	543	16.3	239	13.7	29.6	7.2	0.0
Chicken Tikka, Asda*	1 Pack/190g	439	17.9	231	10.4	32.8	9.4	1.3
Egg, Bacon & Tomato, Freshly Prepared, M & S*	1 Baguette/182g	455	17.3	250	12.9	28.0	9.5	1.7
Egg & Tomato, Oldfields*	1 Pack/198g	416	15.0	210	8.7	27.0	7.6	0.0
Ham & Salad, with Mustard Mayonnaise, Sainsbury's*	1 Baguette/100g	412	15.9	412	17.6	49.6	15.9	0.1
Ham & Turkey, Asda*	1 Baguette/360g	774	18.4	215	11.6	30.7	5.1	1.3
Mozzarella, Tomato, & Pesto, Darwins Deli*	1 Serving/210g	531	20.4	253	11.7	29.7	9.7	0.0
Prawn, French, Shell*	1 Baguette/63g	171	7.2	272	9.7	32.4	11.5	0.0
Prawn Mayonnaise, Asda*	1 Pack/190g	399	9.3	210	9.1	32.5	4.9	1.3
Salmon, Smoked, & Egg, Freshly Prepared	1 Baguette/178g	455	17.3	255	13.7	28.4	9.7	1.6
Steak & Onion, Snack 'n' Go, Sainsbury's*	1 Baguette/177g	398	8.8	225	14.3	30.6	5.0	2.2
Tuna, Crunch, Shapers, Boots*	1 Pack/138g	315	4.8	228	14.0	35.0	3.5	3.1
Tuna, Melt, Sainsbury's*	1 Serving/204g	373	8.0	183	11.3	25.8	3.9	0.0
BAILEYS*								
Glide, Baileys*	1 Serving/200ml	212	2.4	106	0.0	18.0	1.2	0.0
Irish Cream, Original, Baileys*	***1 Serving/50ml***	***164***	***6.5***	***327***	***3.0***	***25.0***	***13.0***	***0.0***
BAKE								
Aubergine & Mozzarella, Finest, Tesco*	1 Pack/400g	288	13.6	72	3.6	6.7	3.4	2.6
Aubergine & Spinach, BGTY, Sainsbury's*	1 Pack/360g	148	6.5	41	2.2	4.0	1.8	1.3
Bean & Pasta, Asda*	1 Pack/450g	598	22.5	133	5.0	17.0	5.0	1.7
Bolognese, Mini Classics, Co-Op*	1 Pack/300g	345	13.2	115	5.8	12.5	4.4	2.1
Broccoli & Cheese, Asda*	1 Bake/132g	269	15.4	204	5.3	19.3	11.7	2.5
Cheese & Spinach, Tesco*	1 Bake/140g	269	10.9	192	4.5	26.0	7.8	1.4
Chicken, Bacon & Potato, British Classics, Tesco*	½ Pack/375g	435	16.5	116	7.0	12.2	4.4	1.4
Chicken, Tomato, & Mascarpone, HL, Tesco*	1 Serving/400g	468	10.8	117	7.6	15.5	2.7	0.8
Chicken & Mushroom, COU, M & S*	1 Serving/360g	324	8.3	90	7.3	10.3	2.3	1.1
Chicken Arrabiatta, M & S*	1 Pack/450g	540	13.5	120	7.6	16.0	3.0	2.0
Chicken Spiralli, M & S*	1 Serving/400g	400	15.2	100	7.9	9.1	3.8	1.1
Cod & Prawn, COU, M & S*	1 Pack/400g	320	8.0	80	6.5	8.8	2.0	1.0
Corned Beef, 379, Wiltshire Farm Foods*	1 Bake/290g	322	11.2	111	3.8	15.2	3.9	2.1
Courgette & Tomato, Cauldron Foods*	1 Pack/285g	593	37.0	208	10.0	17.0	13.0	6.4
Fish, Haddock, Average	1 Serving/400g	312	9.2	78	6.4	8.0	2.3	0.9
Fish, with Carrots & Peas, Light & Easy, Youngs*	1 Pack/240g	168	4.1	70	8.3	5.4	1.7	1.4

	Measure INFO/WEIGHT	per Measure KCAL	FAT	Nutrition Values per 100g / 100ml KCAL	PROT	CARB	FAT	FIBRE
BAKE								
Fish & Vegetable, Youngs*	1 Serving/375g	446	23.6	119	5.6	10.0	6.3	1.3
Lentil, Spiced, Vegetarian, TTD, Sainsbury's*	1 Bake/132g	245	8.4	186	4.8	27.3	6.4	4.2
Mushroom, Cauldron Foods*	1 Serving/100g	164	12.0	164	6.0	15.0	12.0	6.0
Mushroom, Leek & Cheddar, Chosen By You, Asda*	½ Pack/199g	181	8.8	91	3.7	8.1	4.4	1.9
Mushroom, Leek & Spinach, Cumberland, Sainsbury's*	1 Pack/450g	518	24.3	115	3.6	12.9	5.4	1.2
Penne Bolognese, BGTY, Sainsbury's*	1 Pack/400g	492	10.8	123	7.0	17.7	2.7	1.3
Potato, Cheese, & Bacon, Homepride*	1 Serving/210g	277	26.2	132	1.6	3.2	12.5	0.0
Potato, Cheese, & Onion, Tesco*	1 Pack/400g	376	19.6	94	2.4	10.0	4.9	1.0
Potato, Leek & Gruyere, M & S*	½ Pack/200g	240	15.4	120	2.2	10.3	7.7	1.4
Potato, Mushroom & Leek, M & S*	1 Serving/225g	225	13.3	100	3.5	10.0	5.9	2.0
Potato & Vegetable, Co-Op*	1 Bake/340g	425	27.2	125	4.0	11.0	8.0	1.0
Salmon & Broccoli, Youngs*	1 Bake/375g	409	19.1	109	6.3	9.6	5.1	1.3
Salmon & Broccoli 329, Oakhouse Foods Ltd*	1 Meal/400g	624	44.4	156	5.0	9.1	11.1	0.6
Salmon & Prawn, M & S*	1 Bake/329g	460	31.2	140	7.4	6.6	9.5	0.7
Vegetable, Multigrain, Grassington's Food Co*	1 Bake/106g	148	3.6	140	4.9	22.4	3.4	5.0
BAKING POWDER								
Average	***1 Tsp/2g***	***3***	***0.0***	***163***	***5.2***	***37.8***	***0.0***	***0.0***
BAKLAVA								
Average	2 Pieces/50g	239	14.2	478	8.0	47.4	28.4	2.8
BALTI								
Chick Pea, & Spinach, Cauldron Foods*	1 Pack/400g	356	8.0	89	2.3	15.5	2.0	1.0
Chicken, & Mushroom, Tesco*	1 Serving/350g	326	10.5	93	12.3	4.2	3.0	0.7
Chicken, & Rice, M & S*	1 Pack/400g	380	6.0	95	6.9	14.1	1.5	1.2
Chicken, M & S*	½ Pack/175g	245	15.2	140	13.0	2.0	8.7	1.7
Chicken, Sainsbury's*	½ Pack/200g	222	11.2	111	11.6	3.6	5.6	1.3
Chicken, Takeaway, Sainsbury's*	1 Pack/400g	404	18.0	101	10.4	4.8	4.5	1.4
Chicken, with Garlic & Coriander Naan, Frozen, Patak's*	1 Pack/375g	431	18.8	115	6.3	11.1	5.0	1.1
Chicken, with Naan Bread, Sharwood's*	1 Pack/375g	529	23.2	141	7.3	14.1	6.2	2.2
Chicken, with Pilau Rice, Asda*	1 Pack/504g	625	24.7	124	5.0	15.0	4.9	1.2
Chicken, with Pilau Rice & Naan Bread, Tesco*	1 Meal/550g	660	19.8	120	6.1	15.5	3.6	1.4
Chicken Tikka, & Wedges, HL, Tesco*	1 Pack/450g	392	9.9	87	6.0	10.7	2.2	1.3
Lamb, Bhuna, Tesco*	1 Pack/400g	360	14.8	90	9.2	4.8	3.7	1.1
Vegetable, Average	1 Serving/200g	182	8.3	91	1.9	11.3	4.1	1.7
Vegetable, GFY, Asda*	1 Pack/450g	324	4.0	72	1.9	14.0	0.9	1.5
Vegetable, Indian Meal for 2, Finest, Tesco*	½ Pack/150g	144	10.8	96	1.6	6.1	7.2	2.9
BAMBOO SHOOTS								
Canned, Average	***1 Sm Can/120g***	***11***	***0.2***	***9***	***1.1***	***0.9***	***0.1***	***0.9***
Canned in Water, Drained, Kingfisher*	1 Can/120g	14	0.2	12	1.5	0.7	0.2	1.4
BANANA								
Raw, Flesh Only, Average	***1 Med/100g***	***95***	***0.3***	***95***	***1.2***	***20.9***	***0.3***	***4.2***
Raw, Weighed with Skin, Average	***1 Med/152g***	***144***	***0.5***	***95***	***1.2***	***20.9***	***0.3***	***4.2***
BANANA CHIPS								
Average	***1oz/28g***	***143***	***8.8***	***511***	***1.0***	***59.9***	***31.4***	***1.7***
BANGERS & MASH								
Asda*	1 Pack/400g	636	28.0	159	9.0	15.0	7.0	1.6
Co-Op*	1 Pack/300g	375	18.0	125	4.0	13.0	6.0	0.8
BARS								
All Bran, Apple, Kellogg's*	1 Bar/40g	158	7.6	395	8.0	48.0	19.0	5.0
All Bran, Honey & Oat, Kellogg's*	1 Bar/27g	99	2.2	366	6.0	67.0	8.0	12.0
Am, Breakfast Muffin, Apple & Sultana, McVitie's*	1 Bar/45g	168	7.5	373	4.4	54.9	16.7	1.6
Am, Cereal, Apple, McVitie's*	1 Bar/40g	160	5.4	400	4.3	65.4	13.5	3.1
Am, Cereal, Apricot, McVitie's*	1 Bar/30g	146	6.2	486	6.5	68.8	20.5	0.5
Am, Cereal, Berry, McVitie's*	1 Bar/30g	146	6.2	486	6.5	68.8	20.5	0.5

	Measure	per Measure		Nutrition Values per 100g / 100ml				
	INFO/WEIGHT	KCAL	FAT	KCAL	PROT	CARB	FAT	FIBRE
BARS								
Am, Cereal, Fruit & Nut, McVitie's*	1 Bar/35g	167	7.5	477	6.6	64.9	21.4	3.4
Am, Cereal, Grapefruit, McVitie's*	1 Bar/35g	136	3.3	389	5.1	70.9	9.4	3.1
Am, Cereal, Raisin & Nut, McVitie's*	1 Bar/35g	148	5.8	422	6.4	62.1	16.4	2.4
Am, Cereal, Strawberry, McVitie's*	1 Bar/35g	138	3.5	395	5.7	70.5	10.1	2.7
Am, Granola, Almond, Raisin & Cranberry, McVitie's*	1 Bar/35g	133	4.0	380	7.1	62.9	11.4	4.0
Apple, Fruit Bake, Go Ahead, McVitie's*	1 Bar/35g	124	2.5	354	2.7	73.8	7.2	1.2
Apple, Geobar, Traidcraft*	1 Bar/35g	132	3.1	376	5.3	69.0	8.8	3.5
Apple, Granola, McVitie's*	1 Bar/35g	128	3.4	366	6.6	63.1	9.7	4.3
Apple & Blackberry, Fruit Bakes, Go Ahead, McVitie's*	1 Bar/35g	131	3.0	374	3.5	71.8	8.5	3.9
Apple & Cinnamon, Chewy, GFY, Asda*	1 Bar/27g	95	0.7	351	6.0	76.0	2.6	3.5
Apple & Raisin, Dorset Cereals*	1 Bar/30g	109	1.1	363	4.0	78.3	3.7	5.3
Apple & Raspberry, Chewy & Crisp, Tesco*	1 Bar/27g	123	5.3	456	3.4	66.8	19.5	2.8
Apple Pie, Nak'd*	1 Bar/68g	221	5.9	325	6.8	57.2	8.7	7.4
Apricot, Dried Fruit, Sunsweet*	1 Bar/33g	96	0.0	292	3.6	72.5	0.1	0.0
Apricot & Almond, Yoghurt Coated, Eat Natural*	1 Bar/35g	162	9.3	471	7.5	39.7	27.0	5.0
Apricot & Orange, Diet Chef Ltd*	1 Bar/25g	97	1.8	388	4.3	75.2	7.0	2.4
Apricot & Peach, Multigrain, BGTY, Sainsbury's*	1 Bar/25g	70	0.6	282	6.6	58.2	2.5	23.1
Baked Apple Pie, Weight Watchers*	1 Bar/27g	76	0.4	283	4.4	55.7	1.5	14.7
Banana, Mango & Brazil, Cereal, Dove's Farm*	1 Bar/40g	196	4.6	490	6.5	63.3	11.5	5.3
Banoffee, Weight Watchers*	1 Bar/18g	68	0.9	379	6.3	77.0	5.1	3.0
Berry Delight, GF, Nak'd*	1 Bar/35g	135	5.2	385	9.0	52.0	15.0	6.0
Berry Snack, Diet Chef Ltd*	1 Bar/27g	96	2.2	356	7.2	64.0	8.2	5.5
Black Forest, Weight Watchers*	1 Bar/23g	94	2.0	408	3.9	78.4	8.8	1.4
Blackcurrant & Raspberry, Diet Chef Ltd*	1 Bar/25g	98	1.8	392	3.7	75.5	7.4	3.3
Blue Riband, 99 Calories, Nestle*	1 Bar/19g	99	4.7	513	5.5	66.5	24.6	2.0
Blue Riband, Double Choc, Nestle*	1 Bar/22g	113	5.6	513	4.8	66.4	25.3	1.1
Blueberry, Fruit & Grain, Asda*	1 Bar/37g	124	2.6	335	4.1	64.0	7.0	3.9
Blueberry, Nupo*	1 Bar/29g	99	2.9	343	10.8	41.5	10.0	25.4
Blueberry, Weight Watchers*	1 Bar/25g	91	1.8	365	4.5	74.9	7.4	2.2
Breakfast, Apple Crisp, Morning Start, Atkins*	1 Bar/37g	145	7.9	392	29.2	25.4	21.4	13.8
Breakfast, Blueberry, Free From, Sainsbury's*	1 Bar/35g	163	7.8	467	3.8	62.6	22.4	0.2
Breakfast, Cherry, Oats & More, Nestle*	1 Bar/30g	109	2.0	363	6.0	70.2	6.5	3.6
Breakfast, Chocolate Chip, Crisp, Morning Start, Atkins*	1 Bar/37g	137	7.0	370	31.8	22.5	18.8	15.0
Breakfast, Vitality, Fruit & Fibre, Asda*	1 Bar/29g	113	2.9	390	6.0	69.0	10.0	4.1
Breakfast, with Cranberries, Asda*	1 Bar/28g	105	1.4	376	6.0	77.0	4.9	3.0
Caramel, Nut Chew, Endulge, Atkins*	1 Bar/34g	130	2.7	382	5.0	17.0	8.0	6.0
Caramel Crisp, Go Ahead, McVitie's*	1 Bar/33g	141	4.0	428	4.8	75.1	12.0	0.8
Caramel Crunch, Go Ahead, McVitie's*	1 Bar/24g	106	3.3	440	4.7	76.6	13.8	0.8
Caramel Nougat, Soft, Shapers, Boots*	1 Bar/25g	86	2.5	343	2.9	60.4	10.0	0.6
Cereal, & Milk, Nesquik, Nestle*	1 Bar/25g	108	3.7	433	6.2	68.5	14.9	1.0
Cereal, 3 Berries & Cherries, Dorset Cereals*	1 Bar/35g	127	1.7	363	5.7	73.9	4.9	5.2
Cereal, 3 Fruit, Nuts & Seeds, Dorset Cereals*	1 Bar/35g	136	3.6	389	7.4	66.6	10.3	6.2
Cereal, Apple, Chewy, BGTY, Sainsbury's*	1 Bar/25g	85	0.5	340	4.8	76.0	2.0	2.0
Cereal, Apple & Blackberry with Yoghurt, Alpen*	1 Bar/29g	117	3.1	404	5.4	71.8	10.6	5.0
Cereal, Apple & Cinnamon, Fruit 'n' Grain, Asda*	1 Bar/37g	131	2.6	353	4.5	68.0	7.0	2.9
Cereal, Apple & Raisin, Harvest, Quaker Oats*	1 Bar/22g	87	2.5	396	5.0	70.0	11.5	4.0
Cereal, Apple & Raspberry, Chewy & Crisp, Tesco*	1 Bar/27g	123	5.3	456	3.3	66.7	19.6	3.0
Cereal, Apple & Sultana, Light, Alpen*	1 Bar/20g	63	0.7	330	4.1	59.4	3.6	21.7
Cereal, Apricot & Yoghurt, Shapers, Boots*	1 Bar/27g	99	1.5	366	3.7	75.0	5.7	3.3
Cereal, Banana, Value, Tesco*	1 Bar/21g	80	1.6	387	6.0	73.9	7.5	3.7
Cereal, Banoffee, COU, M & S*	1 Bar/20g	75	0.4	375	4.5	82.5	2.0	2.5
Cereal, Benefit, with Fruit, Aldi*	1 Bar/27g	108	2.3	401	5.8	75.2	8.6	1.9
Cereal, Blackcurrant & Apple, GFY, Asda*	1 Bar/25g	72	0.6	287	7.0	59.0	2.6	22.0

	Measure INFO/WEIGHT	per Measure KCAL	FAT	Nutrition Values per 100g / 100ml KCAL	PROT	CARB	FAT	FIBRE
BARS								
Cereal, Cheerios & Milk Bar, Nestle*	1 Bar/22g	92	3.0	416	7.6	66.1	13.5	2.0
Cereal, Chewy, BGTY, Sainsbury's*	1 Bar/25g	85	0.5	342	4.9	75.8	2.1	1.9
Cereal, Choc Chip, Brunch, Cadbury*	1 Bar/35g	156	6.2	445	6.0	64.0	17.6	4.1
Cereal, Choc Chip, White, Chewy, Harvest Morn, Aldi*	1 Bar/22g	88	2.0	400	5.9	71.8	9.1	2.7
Cereal, Chocolate, Dark, with Ginger, Weight Watchers*	1 Bar/22g	82	1.5	371	4.5	67.1	6.8	11.9
Cereal, Chocolate, Geobar, Traidcraft*	1 Bar/32g	130	2.7	407	4.3	78.5	8.4	0.0
Cereal, Chocolate, Milk, Double, Special K, Kellogg's*	1 Bar/20g	79	1.8	396	9.0	66.0	9.0	10.0
Cereal, Chocolate, Milk, Oaty, Weetabix*	1 Bar/23g	80	1.5	342	6.9	51.7	6.5	24.3
Cereal, Chocolate, Milk, Weetos, Weetabix*	1 Bar/20g	88	2.9	440	5.9	70.9	14.7	1.6
Cereal, Chocolate, Oats & More, Nestle*	1 Bar/30g	118	3.2	395	6.8	68.3	10.5	3.4
Cereal, Chocolate, White, Oaty, Weetabix*	1 Bar/23g	78	1.4	341	6.4	52.4	6.3	24.3
Cereal, Chocolate & Fudge, Light, Alpen*	1 Bar/18g	62	1.2	344	4.9	55.4	6.5	22.0
Cereal, Chocolate & Orange, Light, Alpen*	1 Bar/21g	71	1.2	339	4.8	56.0	5.5	23.1
Cereal, Chocolate Chip, Special K, Kellogg's*	1 Bar/21g	84	1.5	401	9.0	76.0	7.0	1.5
Cereal, Cinnamon Grahams, Nestle*	1 Bar/25g	106	3.7	426	7.2	66.2	14.7	1.9
Cereal, Cranberry, Raisin & Nut, Shapers, Boots*	1 Bar/35g	140	4.4	400	7.1	65.7	12.6	3.7
Cereal, Cranberry & Orange, Brunch, Cadbury*	1 Bar/35g	154	5.6	440	5.9	67.7	15.9	0.0
Cereal, Cranberry & Orange, Weight Watchers*	1 Bar/28g	102	1.1	365	4.5	77.6	4.1	2.3
Cereal, Fruit, Average	1 Bar/34g	130	3.9	382	5.9	64.7	11.5	6.5
Cereal, Fruit & Nut, Alpen*	1 Bar/28g	109	2.3	390	5.8	73.0	8.3	2.9
Cereal, Fruits, Citrus, Light, Alpen*	1 Bar/21g	59	0.9	283	5.6	55.9	4.1	22.4
Cereal, Frusli, Apricot, Absolutely, Jordans*	1 Bar/33g	120	3.3	365	5.0	63.8	10.0	6.3
Cereal, Frusli, Blueberry, Jordans*	1 Bar/30g	113	2.1	375	5.2	70.2	7.1	4.9
Cereal, Frusli, Cranberry & Apple, Jordans*	1 Bar/30g	113	2.1	376	5.1	75.6	7.1	5.0
Cereal, Ginger, Perfectly Balanced, Waitrose*	1 Bar/26g	90	0.5	352	4.0	79.2	2.1	3.0
Cereal, Ginger & Raisin, BGTY, Sainsbury's*	1 Bar/40g	91	1.1	228	2.0	48.5	2.8	0.0
Cereal, Golden Grahams, Nestle*	1 Bar/25g	106	3.4	425	6.5	68.8	13.7	0.0
Cereal, Hazelnut, Brunch, Cadbury*	1 Bar/35g	160	7.4	460	7.0	60.5	21.4	2.2
Cereal, Hazelnut, Roast, Organic, Jordans*	1 Bar/33g	150	7.2	455	8.0	56.7	21.8	7.8
Cereal, Hazelnut & Pistachio, Go Ahead, McVitie's*	1 Bar/30g	117	3.4	389	4.8	66.5	11.5	2.5
Cereal, Marmite*	1 Bar/25g	93	2.0	372	18.5	56.2	8.1	6.0
Cereal, Mixed Berry, Go Ahead, McVitie's*	1 Bar/35g	134	2.2	383	4.6	77.1	6.3	3.1
Cereal, Multigrain, Maple, Balance, BGTY, Sainsbury's*	1 Bar/27g	75	0.8	276	6.4	56.2	2.8	25.5
Cereal, Multigrain, Peach & Apricot, BGTY, Sainsbury's*	1 Bar/28g	77	0.6	274	6.4	57.0	2.3	24.2
Cereal, Nutty, Free From, Sainsbury's*	1 Bar/25g	114	5.0	454	6.8	61.8	20.0	2.3
Cereal, Oaty, Strawberry, Weetabix*	1 Bar/23g	69	1.4	299	6.2	54.7	6.1	24.5
Cereal, Pink Grapefruit, Chewy, BGTY, Sainsbury's*	1 Bar/25g	86	0.5	345	5.0	76.5	2.1	2.4
Cereal, Pomegranate, with Prebiotic, GFY, Asda*	1 Bar/22g	76	0.6	345	6.2	69.3	2.8	13.4
Cereal, Raisin & Apricot, Weight Watchers*	1 Bar/28g	100	1.3	358	6.8	72.2	4.6	3.2
Cereal, Raisin & Coconut, Value, Tesco*	1 Bar/21g	84	2.4	400	5.5	67.2	11.6	5.0
Cereal, Redberry & Chocolate, Sveltesse, Nestle*	1 Bar/25g	97	2.5	389	5.4	69.2	9.9	6.8
Cereal, Strawberry, Fitness, Nestle*	1 Bar/24g	89	1.6	378	4.9	73.8	7.0	4.1
Cereal, Strawberry, Fruit 'n' Grain, Asda*	1 Bar/37g	126	2.6	340	4.2	65.0	7.0	4.5
Cereal, Sultana & Apple, Sainsbury's*	1 Bar/27g	101	1.4	374	6.7	75.3	5.1	4.3
Cereal, Sultana & Honey, Jordans*	1 Bar/36g	130	3.0	361	6.0	65.9	8.2	9.2
Cereal, Toffee Apple, Chewy, Eat Smart, Morrisons*	1 Bar/25g	88	0.7	354	4.0	78.3	2.8	2.9
Cereal, Very Berry, Weight Watchers*	1 Bar/27g	92	2.7	340	6.6	42.6	9.9	26.8
Chocolate, & Orange, Crispy, Shapers, Boots*	1 Bar/22g	94	2.6	425	3.6	77.0	12.0	0.8
Chocolate, & Raisin, Shapers, Boots*	1 Bar/30g	99	2.0	331	5.4	55.0	6.8	5.0
Chocolate, & Toffee, Free From, Sainsbury's*	1 Bar/30g	139	5.4	465	4.8	71.0	18.0	0.8
Chocolate, Coffee & Nougat, Shapers, Boots*	1 Bar/24g	99	2.6	414	3.4	75.0	11.0	0.4
Chocolate, Crisp, Weight Watchers*	1 Bar/25g	92	2.6	369	5.4	75.1	10.2	0.8
Chocolate, Dark, Chewy Delight, Special K, Kellogg's*	1 Bar/24g	97	3.4	404	4.5	57.0	14.0	17.0

	Measure	per Measure		Nutrition Values per 100g / 100ml				
	INFO/WEIGHT	KCAL	FAT	KCAL	PROT	CARB	FAT	FIBRE
BARS								
Chocolate, Decadence, Atkins*	1 Bar/60g	227	12.2	378	27.1	30.7	20.4	11.6
Chocolate, Double, Caramel, Crunch, Atkins*	1 Bar/44g	160	9.0	364	22.7	50.0	20.4	25.0
Chocolate, Fruit & Nut, M & S*	1 Bar/50g	235	12.0	470	6.5	57.1	24.1	2.5
Chocolate, Milk, Chewy Delight, Special K, Kellogg's*	1 Bar/24g	95	3.1	397	5.0	57.0	13.0	17.0
Chocolate, Milk, Crispy, Endulge, Atkins*	1 Bar/30g	141	9.6	469	13.0	48.0	32.0	2.0
Chocolate, Polar, Sainsbury's*	1 Bar/25g	133	7.2	533	5.5	63.0	28.6	1.2
Chocolate, Soya, Dairy Free, Free From, Sainsbury's*	1 Bar/50g	274	17.5	548	10.8	47.5	35.0	4.3
Chocolate Brownie, Average	1 Bar/68g	240	4.0	353	14.7	60.3	5.9	8.8
Chocolate Caramel, Weight Watchers*	1 Bar/20g	80	2.5	400	5.0	70.0	12.5	0.0
Chocolate Chip, Snack, Diet Chef Ltd*	1 Bar/27g	99	2.7	367	5.8	63.6	9.9	4.5
Chocolate Cookie Dough, Meal, Slim Fast*	1 Bar/56g	220	5.0	393	14.3	64.3	8.9	3.6
Chocolate Creme, Endulge, Atkins*	1 Bar/14g	70	4.8	504	12.5	38.6	34.3	2.5
Chocolate Crisp, Weight Watchers*	1 Bar/25g	94	2.6	378	4.8	66.8	10.2	1.6
Club, Biscuit, Chocolate, Milk, Jacob's*	1 Biscuit/24g	123	6.3	511	5.8	62.6	26.4	2.0
Club, Biscuit, Fruit, Jacob's*	1 Biscuit/25g	124	6.2	496	5.6	62.2	25.0	2.3
Club, Biscuit, Mint, Jacob's*	1 Biscuit/24g	124	6.5	517	5.6	62.5	27.2	1.7
Club, Biscuit, Orange, Jacob's*	1 Biscuit/23g	117	6.1	509	5.7	61.8	26.5	2.3
Cocoa Delight, GF, Nak'd*	1 Bar/35g	135	5.3	386	9.4	49.8	15.1	7.0
Cocoa Loco, Wildly Different, Nak'd*	1 Bar/30g	100	3.0	332	8.0	65.0	10.0	7.0
Cocoa Mint, GF, Raw, Wholefood, Nak'd*	1 Bar/35g	135	5.2	386	9.0	49.0	15.0	7.0
Cocoa Orange, GF, Nak'd*	1 Bar/35g	145	7.0	415	11.0	45.0	20.0	6.0
Coconut Whip, Weight Watchers*	1 Bar/20g	81	2.8	404	2.4	70.6	14.1	1.5
Cookie, Oreo, Nabisco*	1 Bar/35g	180	10.2	514	2.0	66.0	29.0	0.0
Creme Brulee, Wonka*	2 Pieces/20g	111	6.5	555	5.7	59.1	32.6	1.1
Creme Brulee Chocolate, M & S*	1 Bar/36g	178	10.5	495	4.4	54.0	29.2	0.4
Crunchy Nut, Kellogg's*	1 Bar/30g	119	1.5	397	6.0	82.0	5.0	2.5
Digestive, Chocolate, Milk, McVitie's*	1 Bar/23g	118	5.8	511	6.6	64.6	25.1	1.9
Digestive, Chocolate, Milk, Tesco*	1 Bar/19g	96	4.9	506	6.8	61.6	25.8	2.4
Digestive, Chocolate, Milk, Value, Tesco*	1 Bar/19g	96	4.9	505	6.6	61.8	25.8	3.0
Echo, Fox's*	1 Bar/25g	126	6.6	513	7.1	60.7	26.7	2.3
Echo, Mint, Fox's*	1 Bar/25g	130	6.6	518	7.9	60.7	26.6	1.6
Frosties, & Milk, Kellogg's*	1 Bar/25g	102	2.8	408	7.0	71.0	11.0	1.0
Frosties, Chocolate, Kellogg's*	1 Bar/25g	103	3.0	412	6.0	72.0	12.0	1.6
Frosties, Snack Bar, Kellogg's*	1 Bar/25g	104	2.8	414	7.0	72.0	11.0	1.0
Fruit, Nut & Seed Bars, The Village Bakery*	1 Bar/25g	93	1.6	373	5.7	73.7	6.2	0.1
Fruit & Fibre, Whole Grain, Sainsbury's*	1 Bar/27g	109	3.0	405	6.2	70.1	11.1	3.8
Fruit & Grain, Apple, Aldi*	1 Bar/37g	129	3.0	349	4.2	65.0	8.0	4.5
Fruit & Nut, Eat Natural*	1 Bar/50g	223	11.2	446	11.6	49.8	22.3	5.3
Fruit & Nut, Ginger Snap, Larabar*	1 Bar/51g	220	14.0	431	9.8	47.1	27.4	9.8
Fruit & Nut, Multigrain, Jordans*	1 Bar/40g	164	6.5	410	7.0	59.1	16.2	5.7
Fruit & Nut, Organic, Eat Natural*	1 Bar/50g	244	15.3	488	10.2	42.9	30.6	0.0
Fruit 'n' Fibre, Kellogg's*	1 Bar/25g	95	2.2	380	5.0	71.0	9.0	5.0
Fruit 'n' Fibre Bakes with Sultanas, Kellogg's*	1 Bar/40g	146	5.2	365	4.5	58.0	13.0	9.0
Ginger Bread, Nak'd*	1 Bar/35g	158	10.8	450	10.0	35.0	31.0	9.0
Golden Syrup, Morning, Oat So Simple, Quaker Oats*	1 Bar/35g	142	3.5	407	8.2	67.6	10.0	6.8
Granola, Almond & Raisin, McVitie's*	1 Bar/35g	133	4.0	380	7.0	62.9	11.3	4.1
Granola, Crunchy, Oats & Chocolate, Nature Valley*	2 Bars/42g	195	8.3	464	8.3	59.8	19.8	7.1
Granola, Crunchy, Roasted Almond, Nature Valley*	1 Bar/42g	193	7.6	459	8.1	65.6	18.2	3.7
Granola, Maple Syrup, Twin Pack, Tesco*	2 Bars/42g	204	9.4	485	6.0	64.7	22.3	4.1
Granola, Oats & Hazlenuts, Nature Valley*	2 Bars/42g	195	8.4	465	8.4	58.9	20.1	7.5
Granola, Peanut Butter, Advantage, Atkins*	1 Bar/48g	210	11.0	438	29.2	39.6	22.9	10.4
Granola, Peanut Butter, Quaker Oats*	1 Bar/28g	110	3.5	393	7.1	64.3	12.5	3.6
Harvest Cheweee, Apple & Raisin, Quaker Oats*	1 Bar/22g	89	2.6	405	5.5	68.0	12.0	3.0

	Measure INFO/WEIGHT	per Measure KCAL	FAT	Nutrition Values per 100g / 100ml KCAL	PROT	CARB	FAT	FIBRE
BARS								
Harvest Cheweee, Choc Chip, Quaker Oats*	1 Bar/22g	95	3.5	430	5.5	68.0	16.0	3.5
Harvest Cheweee, Chocolate Chip, White, Quaker Oats*	1 Bar/22g	94	3.4	425	6.0	67.0	15.5	3.5
Harvest Cheweee, Toffee, Quaker Oats*	1 Bar/22g	94	3.3	427	5.0	68.0	15.0	3.0
Honey, Natural, Trail Mix, Kallo*	1 Bar/40g	196	13.3	490	15.7	40.9	33.2	5.7
Honey Nut, Special K, Special K, Kellogg's*	1 Bar/22g	90	2.0	409	9.1	72.7	9.1	13.6
Honeycomb, Club, Jacob's*	1 Bar/23g	116	6.0	512	5.7	61.9	26.3	2.3
Mint, Double Take, Sainsbury's*	1 Bar/20g	107	6.2	534	7.2	56.9	30.8	1.3
Muesli, Apricot & Almond, Carmen's*	1 Bar/45g	190	8.2	423	10.4	50.6	18.2	7.4
Muesli, Cherry & Milk, Sirius*	1 Bar/25g	104	2.8	417	7.2	71.3	11.4	3.9
Muesli, Special, Jordans*	1 Bar/40g	152	4.8	379	6.0	61.6	12.1	5.8
Muffin, Cadbury*	1 Bar/68g	274	17.3	403	5.6	38.0	25.4	0.0
Multigrain, Apple & Sultana, Jordans*	1 Bar/40g	141	2.5	353	4.4	70.0	6.2	4.8
Multigrain, Cranberry & Raspberry, Jordans*	1 Bar/37g	135	2.4	364	4.8	71.3	6.6	4.8
Multigrain, Fruit & Nut, Jordans*	1 Bar/40g	164	6.5	410	7.0	59.1	16.2	5.7
Nougat, Cool Mint, & Dark Chocolate, Shapers, Boots*	1 Bar/23g	83	3.2	362	2.6	70.0	14.0	1.1
Nougat, Summer Strawberry, Shapers, Boots*	1 Bar/23g	83	3.0	361	2.7	73.0	13.0	0.6
Nutri-Grain, Apple, Kellogg's*	1 Bar/37g	131	3.3	355	4.0	67.0	9.0	4.0
Nutri-Grain, Apple, Soft & Fruity, Kellogg's*	1 Bar/37g	133	3.0	359	4.0	70.3	8.1	4.0
Nutri-Grain, Blackberry & Apple, Kellogg's*	1 Bar/37g	131	3.3	355	4.0	67.0	9.0	4.0
Nutri-Grain, Blueberry, Soft & Fruity, Kellogg's*	1 Bar/37g	133	3.0	359	4.0	70.3	8.1	4.0
Nutri-Grain, Cherry, Kellogg's*	1 Bar/37g	129	3.0	348	4.0	67.0	8.0	4.0
Nutri-Grain, Chocolate, Kellogg's*	1 Bar/37g	136	3.7	367	4.5	66.0	10.0	4.0
Nutri-Grain, Chocolate Chip, Chewy, Kellogg's*	1 Bar/25g	103	3.0	413	4.5	73.0	12.0	2.5
Nutri-Grain, Elevenses, Choc Chip Bakes, Kellogg's*	1 Bar/45g	179	5.8	397	4.0	66.0	13.0	2.0
Nutri-Grain, Elevenses, Ginger Bakes, Kellogg's*	1 Bar/45g	168	4.0	373	5.0	68.0	9.0	3.0
Nutri-Grain, Elevenses, Raisin Bakes, Kellogg's*	1 Bar/45g	168	4.0	374	4.5	68.0	9.0	2.5
Nutri-Grain, Honey Oat & Raisin, Chewy, Kellogg's*	1 Bar/25g	98	2.0	393	3.5	78.0	8.0	2.5
Nutri-Grain, Oat & Raisin, Soft Oaties, Kellogg's*	1 Bar/40g	173	6.4	432	6.0	66.0	16.0	3.5
Nutri-Grain, Oat Bakes, Cherry, Kellogg's*	1 Bar/50g	204	7.0	408	4.5	66.0	14.0	2.5
Nutri-Grain, Oat Bakes, Totally Oaty, Kellogg's*	1 Bar/50g	206	7.5	411	5.0	64.0	15.0	3.0
Nutri-Grain, Raspberry, Kellogg's*	1 Bar/37g	131	3.3	355	4.0	67.0	9.0	4.0
Nutri-Grain, Strawberry, Kellogg's*	1 Bar/37g	133	3.0	359	3.5	69.0	8.0	3.5
Nutri-Grain, Strawberry, Soft & Fruity, Kellogg's*	1 Bar/37g	133	3.0	359	4.0	70.3	8.1	4.0
Oat, Original, with Golden Syrup, Quaker Oats*	1 Bar/38g	139	3.6	366	7.1	64.5	9.5	7.9
Oat, Quaker Oats*	1 Bar/38g	137	3.4	360	6.8	64.5	8.8	8.0
Oaty, Strawberry Crusher, Weetabix*	1 Bar/23g	79	1.4	345	6.1	55.2	6.1	22.2
Optivita, Berry Oat, Kellogg's*	1 Bar/28g	101	2.0	360	7.0	68.0	7.0	9.0
Orange Crunch, Go Ahead, McVitie's*	1 Bar/23g	99	2.9	430	4.1	78.0	12.8	0.8
Original, Crunchy, Honey & Almond, Jordans*	1 Bar/30g	139	6.8	463	8.3	56.7	22.7	6.7
Original, Muesli, Diet Chef Ltd*	1 Bar/50g	199	6.9	398	6.1	59.0	13.8	6.4
Peach, Apricot & Almond, Altu*	1 Bar/40g	158	4.6	395	7.9	65.2	11.4	4.3
Peach & Apricot, Special K, Kellogg's*	1 Bar/21g	80	1.3	383	8.0	75.0	6.0	2.5
Peanut, & Oat, Trek, Nak'd*	1 Bar/68g	239	7.5	352	16.0	49.0	11.0	7.0
Peanut, Raisin & Chocolate, Weight Watchers*	1 Bar/25g	97	2.8	388	7.6	60.0	11.2	12.8
Peanut & Caramel Whip, Weight Watchers*	1 Bar/20g	76	2.7	381	4.4	73.7	13.7	1.2
Pear & Ginger, Fruit Break, Lyme Regis Foods*	1 Bar/42g	160	8.8	381	2.7	45.4	20.9	9.9
Pecan Apricot & Peach, M & S*	1 Bar/50g	255	17.8	510	9.3	38.2	35.5	4.9
Pecan Pie, GF, Nak'd*	1 Bar/35g	156	10.8	447	8.0	36.0	31.0	9.0
Pecan Pie, Larabar*	1 Bar/45g	200	14.0	444	6.7	48.9	31.1	8.9
Penguin, Bigstix, McVitie's*	1 Biscuit/13g	64	3.2	508	6.4	62.8	25.7	2.6
Penguin, Biscuit, Chocolate, Mint, McVitie's*	1 Bar/25g	133	6.9	531	5.4	65.0	27.7	1.5
Penguin, Biscuit, Chocolate, Orange, McVitie's*	1 Bar/25g	133	6.9	531	5.4	65.0	27.7	1.5
Penguin, Biscuit, Chocolate, Original, McVitie's*	1 Bar/20g	106	5.6	515	5.1	61.4	27.1	2.4

	Measure INFO/WEIGHT	per Measure KCAL	per Measure FAT	Nutrition Values per 100g / 100ml KCAL	PROT	CARB	FAT	FIBRE
BARS								
Penguin, Chukka, McVitie's*	1 Bar/28g	135	6.1	481	6.1	65.1	21.8	0.0
Protein, Chocolate & Banana, MuleBar*	1 Bar/65g	254	5.8	390	21.0	56.0	9.0	2.0
Protein, Chocolate Chewy Crisp, Pro-Bar Xs*	1 Bar/70g	239	4.6	341	44.0	6.0	6.5	12.0
Protein, Chocolate Date, MuleBar*	1 Bar/65g	261	6.5	401	20.0	58.0	10.0	2.0
Protein, Flapjack, Oat Crunch, Natural Balance Foods*	1 Bar/56g	249	12.9	444	18.0	43.0	23.0	3.0
Protein, Fudge Cookies & Cream, McVitie's*	1 Bar/100g	230	4.5	230	14.0	33.0	4.5	1.0
Protein, Muscle To Go, Balance*	¼ Bar/22g	70	1.4	316	38.9	8.8	6.5	12.3
Protein, Peanut Blast, Natural Energy, Ball, Bounce*	1 Ball/49g	210	8.0	429	28.6	38.8	16.3	4.1
Protein, Peanut Chewy Crisp, Chemical Protein Pro-Xs*	1 Bar/70g	243	5.2	347	42.9	5.5	7.5	12.5
Protein, Premium, Ball, Bounce*	1 Ball/49g	209	9.0	426	30.6	40.8	18.4	2.0
Protein, Vanilla, Low Carb, Protein Plus, Power Bar*	1 Bar/35g	131	7.4	373	16.0	21.5	21.0	26.5
Protein, Whey, Sculptress, Maxitone*	1 Bar/60g	203	5.6	339	33.9	30.6	9.3	8.5
Protein Pack, X-Treme with White Chocolate, Inkospor*	1 Bar/35g	136	3.5	388	32.0	43.0	10.0	0.3
Raisin & Hazelnut, Weight Watchers*	1 Bar/24g	95	2.4	396	5.0	71.2	10.0	2.9
Raisin & Oatmeal, Breakfast Snack, Tesco*	1 Bar/38g	133	4.4	355	5.6	56.8	11.7	2.8
Raspberry, Baked, Asda*	1 Bar/27g	104	2.1	385	3.4	74.2	7.6	1.8
Rice Krispies, & Milk, Kellogg's*	1 Bar/20g	83	2.4	416	7.0	71.0	12.0	0.3
Rice Krispies, Snack, Kellogg's*	1 Bar/20g	83	2.0	415	7.0	70.0	10.0	0.5
Rich Toffee, Weight Watchers*	1 Bar/26g	83	2.8	319	3.6	52.3	10.6	0.8
Rocky Road, Rice Krispies Squares, Kellogg's*	1 Square/34g	143	3.7	420	4.0	76.0	11.0	1.5
Special K, Chocolate Chip, Kellogg's*	1 Bar/22g	90	1.6	401	9.0	76.0	7.0	1.5
Special K, Fruits of the Forest, Kellogg's*	1 Bar/22g	87	1.8	397	8.0	74.0	8.0	2.5
Special K, Mint Chocolate, Bliss, Special K, Kellogg's*	1 Bar/22g	88	2.2	401	4.5	74.0	10.0	3.5
Special K, Red Berry, Kellogg's*	1 Bar/23g	90	1.2	383	8.0	77.0	5.0	2.0
Strawberry, Breakfast, Carb Control, Tesco*	1 Bar/37g	144	8.6	389	7.0	40.5	23.2	4.0
Strawberry, Fruit Bakes, Go Ahead, McVitie's*	1 Bar/35g	131	3.0	375	3.5	72.0	8.5	4.0
Strawberry, Morning Shine, Atkins*	1 Bar/37g	145	8.0	392	28.9	24.9	21.6	14.1
Strawberry, Shapers, Boots*	1 Bar/22g	75	2.4	343	2.5	77.0	11.0	0.9
Toffee, Slim Fast*	1 Bar/39g	122	3.3	314	19.7	47.1	8.5	5.6
Toffee & Banana, Weight Watchers*	1 Bar/18g	67	0.7	372	6.1	77.2	3.9	1.7
Totally Chocolatey, Rice Krispies Squares, Kellogg's*	1 Bar/36g	156	5.3	439	4.5	72.0	15.0	1.5
Tracker, Breakfast, Banana, Mars*	1 Bar/37g	176	8.4	476	4.7	63.3	22.6	9.4
Tracker, Breakfast, Lemon, Mars*	1 Bar/26g	124	5.8	477	4.6	64.3	22.4	0.0
Tracker, Chocolate Chip, Mars*	1 Bar/37g	178	8.7	480	6.8	58.0	23.6	3.8
Tracker, Forest Fruits, Mars*	1 Bar/26g	123	5.8	474	4.6	64.1	22.2	0.0
Tracker, Roasted Nut, Mars*	1 Bar/26g	127	6.6	489	8.1	55.0	25.3	4.9
Tracker, Strawberry, Mars*	1 Bar/26g	118	4.8	452	4.2	63.2	18.4	2.9
Tracker, Yoghurt, Mars*	1 Bar/27g	133	6.3	491	6.3	64.2	23.2	0.0
Triple Dazzle, Wonka*	1 Bar/39g	195	10.0	504	5.9	61.9	25.9	0.0
Vanilla Caramel, Eurodiet*	1 Bar/45g	162	5.5	360	31.7	24.5	12.3	11.1
Wafer, Chocolate Flavour Crisp, Carbolite*	1 Bar/25g	120	8.7	482	8.5	52.3	34.8	2.0
BASA								
Tempura, Fillets, Northern Catch*	1 Fillet/160g	248	11.0	155	17.5	7.9	6.9	1.9
BASIL								
Dried, Ground	***1 Tsp/1g***	***4***	***0.1***	***251***	***14.4***	***43.2***	***4.0***	***0.0***
Fresh, Average	***1 Tbsp/5g***	***2***	***0.0***	***40***	***3.1***	***5.1***	***0.8***	***0.0***
BASKETS								
Brandy Snap, Askeys*	1 Basket/20g	98	4.3	490	1.9	72.7	21.3	0.0
BATTER MIX								
for Yorkshire Puddings, Baked, Aunt Bessie's*	1 Pudding/13g	48	1.1	356	9.8	34.0	8.1	2.3
for Yorkshire Puddings & Pancakes, Morrisons*	1 Pudding/30g	43	0.8	143	6.4	23.1	2.8	4.1
for Yorkshire Puddings & Pancakes, Tesco*	1 Serving/17g	34	0.3	200	2.3	43.3	1.5	2.5
Green's*	1 Bag/125g	296	9.0	237	8.7	34.3	7.2	0.0

B

	Measure INFO/WEIGHT	per Measure KCAL	FAT	Nutrition Values per 100g / 100ml KCAL	PROT	CARB	FAT	FIBRE
BATTER MIX								
Pancake, Buttermilk, Krusteaz*	3 Pancakes/16g	57	0.8	352	11.3	66.0	4.7	3.4
Pancake, Sainsbury's*	1 Pancake/63g	96	1.1	152	6.5	27.4	1.8	3.1
BAY LEAVES								
Dried, Average	***1 Tsp/0.6g***	***2***	***0.1***	***313***	***7.6***	***48.6***	***8.4***	***0.0***
BEAN SPROUTS								
Mung, Canned, Drained, Average	***1 Serving/90g***	***9***	***0.1***	***10***	***1.6***	***0.8***	***0.1***	***0.7***
Mung, Raw, Average	***1oz/28g***	***9***	***0.1***	***31***	***2.9***	***4.0***	***0.5***	***1.5***
Mung, Stir-Fried in Blended Oil, Average	***1 Serving/90g***	***65***	***5.5***	***72***	***1.9***	***2.5***	***6.1***	***0.9***
Raw, Average	***1 Serving/150g***	***55***	***2.6***	***37***	***2.2***	***3.2***	***1.8***	***1.2***
BEANFEAST								
Bolognese Style, Dry, Batchelors*	1 Pack/120g	362	6.7	302	23.9	39.0	5.6	13.5
Mexican Chilli, Batchelors*	1 Serving/65g	203	3.2	312	24.3	42.7	4.9	13.6
BEANS								
Aduki, Cooked in Unsalted Water, Average	***1 Tbsp/30g***	***37***	***0.1***	***123***	***9.3***	***22.5***	***0.2***	***5.5***
Aduki, Dried, Raw	***1 Tbsp/30g***	***82***	***0.2***	***272***	***19.9***	***50.1***	***0.5***	***11.1***
Adzuki, Dry, Love Life, Waitrose*	1 Serving/100g	340	0.5	340	19.9	62.9	0.5	12.7
Adzuki, in Water, Canned, Drained, Tesco*	½ Can/118g	118	0.5	100	6.5	13.6	0.4	6.5
Baked, & Jumbo Sausages, Asda*	1 Can/405g	486	17.0	120	6.9	11.2	4.2	5.0
Baked, & Pork Sausages, Sainsbury's*	1 Serving/210g	248	9.2	118	5.7	13.9	4.4	3.4
Baked, & Pork Sausages, Tesco*	½ Can/210g	231	5.7	110	5.5	15.6	2.7	3.0
Baked, & Sausage, Asda*	½ Can/203g	211	4.0	104	6.7	13.0	2.0	3.5
Baked, & Sausages, Meatfree, Sainsbury's*	1 Can/420g	500	16.8	119	8.0	12.6	4.0	2.7
Baked, & Vegetarian Sausages, Asda*	½ Can/210g	204	4.0	97	7.4	12.5	1.9	8.4
Baked, Barbecue, Beanz, Heinz*	1 Can/390g	343	0.8	88	4.9	14.6	0.2	3.8
Baked, Chilli, in Tomato & Chilli Sauce, Fiery, Heinz*	1 Serving/100g	91	0.3	91	4.9	15.1	0.3	3.8
Baked, Curried, Average	***½ Can/210g***	***203***	***1.9***	***96***	***4.8***	***17.2***	***0.9***	***3.6***
Baked, Curry, Beanz, Heinz*	1 Can/200g	218	3.2	109	4.8	17.0	1.6	4.0
Baked, Eat Smart, Morrisons*	1 Can/420g	294	1.7	70	5.3	11.4	0.4	5.6
Baked, Five, in Tomato Sauce, Heinz*	1 Can/415g	361	0.8	87	5.4	13.6	0.2	4.3
Baked, HL, Tesco*	1 Can/420g	315	2.1	75	4.3	12.1	0.5	3.8
Baked, in Barbeque Sauce, Tesco*	1 Can/220g	198	1.3	90	5.0	13.6	0.6	5.2
Baked, in Tomato Sauce, Average	***1 Can/400g***	***318***	***1.6***	***80***	***4.6***	***13.9***	***0.4***	***3.7***
Baked, in Tomato Sauce, Beanz, Heinz*	½ Can/208g	162	0.4	78	4.7	12.9	0.2	3.7
Baked, in Tomato Sauce, Corale, Aldi*	½ Can/220g	200	0.9	91	5.2	14.4	0.4	4.3
Baked, in Tomato Sauce, Organic, Beanz, Heinz*	1 Can/415g	336	0.8	81	4.8	12.9	0.2	3.8
Baked, in Tomato Sauce, Reduced Sugar & Salt	***½ Can/210g***	***159***	***0.7***	***76***	***4.6***	***13.6***	***0.3***	***3.8***
Baked, in Tomato Sauce, Snap Pot, Beanz, Heinz*	1 Pot/200g	157	0.4	78	4.7	12.9	0.2	3.7
Baked, Jalfrezi, Mean, Beanz, Heinz*	1 Serving/195g	135	2.5	69	4.5	9.8	1.3	3.6
Baked, Mexican, Mean, Beanz, Heinz*	½ Can/208g	158	1.0	76	5.0	12.9	0.5	4.0
Baked, Sweet Chilli, Mean, Beanz, Heinz*	½ Can/195g	142	0.6	73	4.5	13.0	0.3	3.6
Baked, Tikka, Mean, Beanz, Heinz*	1 Serving/195g	172	5.9	88	4.8	10.6	3.0	3.5
Baked, Virtually Fat Free, Heinz*	½ Can/207g	164	0.4	79	4.7	12.9	0.2	3.7
Baked, with Chicken Nuggets, Beanz, Heinz*	1 Can/200g	210	6.3	105	6.8	12.4	3.2	3.2
Baked, with Hidden Veg, Beanz, Heinz*	½ Can/208g	156	0.6	75	4.7	13.5	0.3	4.1
Baked, with HP Sauce, Beanz, Heinz*	½ Can/208g	158	0.6	76	4.8	13.7	0.3	3.9
Baked, with Lea & Perrins Sauce, Beanz, Heinz*	1 Can/415g	303	0.8	73	4.8	13.1	0.2	3.8
Baked, with Sausages, Branston, Crosse & Blackwell*	½ Can/202g	233	6.5	115	6.9	12.2	3.2	5.0
Baked, with Spicy Meatballs, Beanz, Heinz*	1 Can/400g	372	9.6	93	5.8	12.0	2.4	2.9
Baked, with Steak Chunks, Beanz, Heinz*	1 Can/415g	344	1.7	83	6.8	12.9	0.4	3.6
Baked, with Vegetable Sausages, Beanz, Heinz*	1 Sm Can/200g	210	7.2	105	6.0	12.2	3.6	2.9
Black, Cooked, Average	***1 Cup/172g***	***227***	***0.9***	***132***	***8.8***	***23.7***	***0.5***	***8.7***
Black, Dried, Average	***1 Serving/100g***	***341***	***1.4***	***341***	***21.6***	***62.4***	***1.4***	***15.2***
Blackeye, Canned, Average	***1 Can/172g***	***206***	***1.3***	***120***	***8.4***	***19.8***	***0.8***	***3.3***

	Measure INFO/WEIGHT	per Measure KCAL	FAT	Nutrition Values per 100g / 100ml KCAL	PROT	CARB	FAT	FIBRE
BEANS								
Blackeye, Dried, Raw	***1oz/28g***	***87***	***0.4***	***311***	***23.5***	***54.1***	***1.6***	***8.2***
Borlotti, Canned, Average	***1oz/28g***	***29***	***0.1***	***103***	***7.6***	***16.9***	***0.5***	***4.7***
Borlotti, Dried, Raw, Average	***1 Serving/100g***	***335***	***1.2***	***335***	***23.0***	***60.0***	***1.2***	***24.7***
Broad, Canned, Drained, Average	***1 Can/195g***	***136***	***1.1***	***70***	***6.9***	***9.2***	***0.6***	***6.8***
Broad, Crispy, Wasabi Flavoured, Khao Shong*	1 Serving/30g	116	3.0	386	17.0	57.0	10.0	7.0
Broad, Dried, Raw, Average	***1oz/28g***	***69***	***0.6***	***245***	***26.1***	***32.5***	***2.1***	***27.6***
Broad, Frozen, Average	1 Serving/80g	63	0.6	79	7.6	10.8	0.7	5.3
Broad, Weighed with Pod, Raw, Average	***1oz/28g***	***17***	***0.3***	***59***	***5.7***	***7.2***	***1.0***	***6.1***
Butter, Canned, Drained, Average	***1oz/28g***	***24***	***0.1***	***86***	***6.3***	***13.5***	***0.5***	***4.6***
Butter, Dried, Boiled, Average	***1oz/28g***	***30***	***0.2***	***106***	***7.2***	***18.6***	***0.6***	***5.2***
Butter, Dried, Raw, Average	***1oz/28g***	***81***	***0.5***	***290***	***19.1***	***52.9***	***1.7***	***16.0***
Cannellini, Canned, Average	***1 Can/400g***	***375***	***2.1***	***94***	***7.2***	***15.0***	***0.5***	***5.7***
Cannellini, Dried, Tesco*	1 Serving/32g	83	0.3	260	24.8	37.4	0.8	20.9
Cannellini, with Chorizo & Red Peppers, Morrisons*	½ Pack/100g	155	10.0	155	6.9	9.2	10.0	2.8
Chilli, Canned, Average	***1 Can/420g***	***381***	***3.1***	***91***	***5.2***	***15.8***	***0.7***	***4.4***
Curried, Mixed, Morrisons*	1 Can/420g	420	16.4	100	4.2	12.1	3.9	5.6
Dwarf, Sainsbury's*	1oz/28g	7	0.1	24	1.9	3.1	0.5	2.2
Edamame, Sainsbury's*	1 Serving/150g	212	9.6	141	12.3	6.8	6.4	4.2
Fajita Beanz, Heinz*	½ Can/196g	155	1.6	79	4.0	11.7	0.8	4.5
Flageolet, Canned, Average	***1 Can/265g***	***235***	***1.6***	***89***	***6.8***	***14.0***	***0.6***	***3.5***
Flageolet, Dried, Love Life, Waitrose*	1 Serving/50g	125	3.1	250	30.4	19.8	6.2	40.4
French, Boiled, Average	***1 Serving/150g***	***38***	***0.0***	***25***	***2.3***	***3.8***	***0.0***	***3.7***
French, Canned, Average	***1oz/28g***	***6***	***0.1***	***22***	***1.6***	***3.5***	***0.3***	***2.5***
French, Raw	***1oz/28g***	***7***	***0.1***	***24***	***1.9***	***3.2***	***0.5***	***2.2***
Green, Cut, Average	***1oz/28g***	***7***	***0.1***	***24***	***1.7***	***3.6***	***0.2***	***2.7***
Green, Extra Fine, in Salted Water, Lidl*	1 Serving/220g	37	0.4	17	1.3	2.5	0.2	3.5
Green, Fine, Average	***1 Serving/75g***	***18***	***0.3***	***24***	***1.8***	***3.2***	***0.4***	***2.9***
Green, Sliced, Average	***1oz/28g***	***6***	***0.1***	***23***	***1.9***	***3.5***	***0.2***	***2.1***
Green, Sliced, Frozen, Average	***1 Serving/50g***	***13***	***0.0***	***26***	***1.8***	***4.4***	***0.1***	***4.1***
Green, Very Fine, Field Fresh, Birds Eye*	1 Serving/80g	20	0.4	25	1.8	2.9	0.5	2.4
Green, Whole, Average	***1oz/28g***	***6***	***0.1***	***22***	***1.6***	***3.0***	***0.4***	***1.7***
Haricot, Canned, Average	1 Can/400g	77	0.5	77	6.2	10.7	0.5	5.9
Haricot, Dried, Boiled in Unsalted Water	***1oz/28g***	***27***	***0.1***	***95***	***6.6***	***17.2***	***0.5***	***6.1***
Haricot, Dried, Raw	***1oz/28g***	***80***	***0.4***	***286***	***21.4***	***49.7***	***1.6***	***17.0***
Haricot, in Water, Canned, Drained, Tesco*	½ Can/118g	75	0.6	64	5.7	9.0	0.5	7.8
Kidney, Red, Canned, Drained, Average	***½ Can/120g***	***117***	***0.7***	***98***	***7.6***	***21.2***	***0.6***	***5.7***
Kidney, Red, Dried, Boiled in Unsalted Water	***1oz/28g***	***29***	***0.1***	***103***	***8.4***	***17.4***	***0.5***	***6.7***
Kidney, Red, Dried, Raw	***1oz/28g***	***74***	***0.4***	***266***	***22.1***	***44.1***	***1.4***	***15.7***
Kidney, Red, in Chilli Sauce, Sainsbury's*	1 Can/420g	365	1.7	87	5.3	15.6	0.4	4.5
Kidney, Red, in Chilli Sauce, Waitrose*	½ Can/201g	175	0.8	87	5.5	15.3	0.4	3.2
Kidney, Red, Value, Tesco*	1 Serving/65g	60	0.4	93	6.9	15.0	0.6	6.2
Kidney, White, Dry, Raw, Unico*	½ Cup/80g	270	0.9	338	22.5	61.2	1.1	21.2
Mixed, Canned, Average	***1 Can/300g***	***300***	***3.5***	***100***	***6.8***	***15.6***	***1.2***	***4.1***
Mixed, Spicy, Average	***1 Serving/140g***	***108***	***0.7***	***78***	***4.8***	***13.4***	***0.5***	***3.9***
Mixed, with Lentils, Waitrose*	1 Pack/300g	399	21.9	133	5.1	11.6	7.3	3.1
Mixed, with Passata, Tesco*	1 Can/300g	237	2.1	79	6.0	12.1	0.7	3.9
Mung, Whole, Dried, Boiled in Unsalted Water	***1oz/28g***	***25***	***0.1***	***91***	***7.6***	***15.3***	***0.4***	***3.0***
Mung, Whole, Dried, Raw	***1oz/28g***	***78***	***0.3***	***279***	***23.9***	***46.3***	***1.1***	***10.0***
Pinto, Dried, Boiled in Unsalted Water	***1oz/28g***	***38***	***0.2***	***137***	***8.9***	***23.9***	***0.7***	***0.0***
Pinto, Dried, Raw	***1oz/28g***	***92***	***0.4***	***327***	***21.1***	***57.1***	***1.6***	***14.0***
Refried, Average	***1 Serving/215g***	***162***	***1.5***	***76***	***4.6***	***12.7***	***0.7***	***1.8***
Runner, Average	***1 Serving/80g***	***16***	***0.3***	***20***	***1.4***	***2.8***	***0.4***	***2.2***
Soya, Dried, Average	***1oz/28g***	***104***	***5.1***	***370***	***34.2***	***15.4***	***18.3***	***19.6***

	Measure INFO/WEIGHT	per Measure KCAL	FAT	Nutrition Values per 100g / 100ml KCAL	PROT	CARB	FAT	FIBRE
BEANS								
Soya, Dried, Boiled in Unsalted Water	***1oz/28g***	***39***	***2.0***	***141***	***14.0***	***5.1***	***7.3***	***6.1***
Soya, Frozen, Birds Eye*	1 Serving/80g	98	5.1	123	12.4	4.0	6.4	4.2
Soya, in Water, Salt Added, Sainsbury's*	1 Serving/100g	102	7.3	102	4.0	5.1	7.3	6.1
Soya, Shelled, Frozen, Raw, Average	***1 Serving/80g***	***99***	***4.3***	***124***	***12.2***	***6.9***	***5.3***	***4.4***
Tuscan Beanz, Heinz*	½ Can/195g	178	3.3	91	4.9	12.0	1.7	4.1
White, Campo Largo, Lidl*	½ Jar/200g	180	1.0	90	7.1	11.2	0.5	0.0
BEEF								
Brisket, Boiled, Lean	1 Serving/100g	225	11.0	225	31.4	0.0	11.0	0.0
Brisket, Boiled, Lean & Fat	1 Serving/100g	268	17.4	268	27.8	0.0	17.4	0.0
Brisket, Braised, Lean	1 Serving/100g	280	17.4	280	29.0	0.0	17.4	0.0
Brisket, Raw, Lean	***1oz/28g***	***39***	***1.7***	***139***	***21.1***	***0.0***	***6.1***	***0.0***
Brisket, Raw, Lean & Fat	***1oz/28g***	***61***	***4.5***	***218***	***18.4***	***0.0***	***16.0***	***0.0***
Cooked, Sliced, From Supermarket, Average	***1 Slice/35g***	***47***	***1.2***	***135***	***23.6***	***2.0***	***3.5***	***0.5***
Diced, British, Extra Special, Asda*	1 Pack/250g	461	11.2	184	33.9	1.7	4.5	0.1
Diced, British, Fresh, Value, Tesco*	1 Serving/125g	175	7.8	140	20.8	0.0	6.2	0.0
Diced, for Casserole, Lean, Average	***1oz/28g***	***35***	***1.1***	***126***	***23.0***	***0.0***	***3.8***	***0.0***
Diced, Traditional, TTD, Sainsbury's*	1 Serving/100g	136	5.1	136	22.5	0.0	5.1	0.0
Escalope, Healthy Range, Average	***1 Serving/170g***	***233***	***6.7***	***137***	***24.2***	***1.2***	***4.0***	***0.4***
Flank, Pot-Roasted, Lean	***1oz/28g***	***71***	***3.9***	***253***	***31.8***	***0.0***	***14.0***	***0.0***
Flank, Pot-Roasted, Lean & Fat	***1oz/28g***	***87***	***6.2***	***309***	***27.1***	***0.0***	***22.3***	***0.0***
Flank, Raw, Lean	***1oz/28g***	***49***	***2.6***	***175***	***22.7***	***0.0***	***9.3***	***0.0***
Flank, Raw, Lean & Fat	***1oz/28g***	***74***	***5.8***	***266***	***19.7***	***0.0***	***20.8***	***0.0***
Fore Rib, Lean & Fat, Average	***1oz/28g***	***40***	***1.8***	***144***	***21.7***	***0.0***	***6.2***	***0.2***
Fore Rib, Raw, Lean	***1oz/28g***	***41***	***1.8***	***145***	***21.5***	***0.0***	***6.5***	***0.0***
Fore Rib, Roasted, Lean	***1oz/28g***	***66***	***3.2***	***236***	***33.3***	***0.0***	***11.4***	***0.0***
Fore Rib, Roasted, Lean & Fat	***1oz/28g***	***84***	***5.7***	***300***	***29.1***	***0.0***	***20.4***	***0.0***
Grill Steak, Average	***1 Steak/170g***	***501***	***39.5***	***295***	***19.3***	***2.1***	***23.2***	***0.1***
Grill Steak, Peppered, Average	***1 Serving/172g***	***419***	***24.4***	***244***	***23.6***	***5.2***	***14.2***	***0.3***
Joint, for Roasting, Average	***1oz/28g***	***38***	***1.0***	***134***	***24.5***	***1.4***	***3.4***	***0.2***
Joint, Sirloin, Roasted, Lean	***1oz/28g***	***53***	***1.8***	***188***	***32.4***	***0.0***	***6.5***	***0.0***
Joint, Sirloin, Roasted, Lean & Fat	***1oz/28g***	***65***	***3.5***	***233***	***29.8***	***0.0***	***12.6***	***0.0***
Mince, Cooked, Average	***1 Serving/75g***	***214***	***15.3***	***286***	***24.0***	***0.0***	***20.3***	***0.0***
Mince, Extra Lean, Raw, Average	***1 Serving/100g***	***124***	***5.0***	***124***	***21.2***	***0.1***	***5.0***	***0.0***
Mince, Extra Lean, Stewed	***1oz/28g***	***50***	***2.4***	***177***	***24.7***	***0.0***	***8.7***	***0.0***
Mince, Lean, Raw, Average	***1oz/28g***	***48***	***2.8***	***172***	***20.8***	***0.0***	***10.0***	***0.1***
Mince, Raw, Average	***1oz/28g***	***68***	***5.1***	***242***	***19.6***	***0.2***	***18.1***	***0.0***
Mince, Raw, Frozen, Average	***1 Serving/100g***	***176***	***10.0***	***176***	***20.4***	***0.0***	***10.0***	***0.0***
Mince, Steak, Extra Lean, Average	***1oz/28g***	***37***	***1.6***	***131***	***20.5***	***0.4***	***5.6***	***0.0***
Mince, Steak, Raw, Average	***1 Serving/125g***	***318***	***25.0***	***254***	***17.2***	***0.0***	***20.0***	***0.0***
Mince, Stewed	***1oz/28g***	***59***	***3.8***	***209***	***21.8***	***0.0***	***13.5***	***0.0***
Peppered, Sliced, Average	***1 Slice/20g***	***26***	***1.1***	***129***	***18.2***	***1.3***	***5.6***	***1.0***
Roast, Sliced, Average	***1 Slice/35g***	***48***	***1.3***	***136***	***26.1***	***0.4***	***3.6***	***0.2***
Salt, Average	***1 Serving/70g***	***80***	***1.7***	***114***	***21.7***	***1.0***	***2.5***	***0.1***
Salted, Dried, Raw	***1oz/28g***	***70***	***0.4***	***250***	***55.4***	***0.0***	***1.5***	***0.0***
Silverside, Pot-Roasted, Lean	***1oz/28g***	***54***	***1.8***	***193***	***34.0***	***0.0***	***6.3***	***0.0***
Silverside, Pot-Roasted, Lean & Fat	***1oz/28g***	***69***	***3.8***	***247***	***31.0***	***0.0***	***13.7***	***0.0***
Silverside, Raw, Lean	***1oz/28g***	***38***	***1.2***	***134***	***23.8***	***0.0***	***4.3***	***0.0***
Silverside, Raw, Lean & Fat	***1oz/28g***	***60***	***4.1***	***215***	***20.4***	***0.0***	***14.8***	***0.0***
Silverside, Salted, Boiled, Lean	***1oz/28g***	***52***	***1.9***	***184***	***30.4***	***0.0***	***6.9***	***0.0***
Silverside, Salted, Boiled, Lean & Fat	***1oz/28g***	***63***	***3.5***	***224***	***27.9***	***0.0***	***12.5***	***0.0***
Silverside, Salted, Raw, Lean	***1oz/28g***	***39***	***2.0***	***140***	***19.2***	***0.0***	***7.0***	***0.0***
Silverside, Salted, Raw, Lean & Fat	***1oz/28g***	***64***	***5.0***	***227***	***16.3***	***0.0***	***18.0***	***0.0***
Steak, Braising, Braised, Lean	***1oz/28g***	***63***	***2.7***	***225***	***34.4***	***0.0***	***9.7***	***0.0***

	Measure INFO/WEIGHT	per Measure KCAL	FAT	Nutrition Values per 100g / 100ml KCAL	PROT	CARB	FAT	FIBRE
BEEF								
Steak, Braising, Braised, Lean & Fat	***1oz/28g***	***69***	***3.6***	***246***	***32.9***	***0.0***	***12.7***	***0.0***
Steak, Braising, Lean, Raw, Average	***1oz/28g***	***40***	***1.4***	***144***	***24.8***	***0.0***	***5.0***	***0.0***
Steak, Braising, Raw, Lean & Fat	***1oz/28g***	***45***	***2.4***	***160***	***20.7***	***0.0***	***8.6***	***0.0***
Steak, Economy, Average	***1oz/28g***	***53***	***2.4***	***190***	***26.9***	***1.2***	***8.7***	***0.4***
Steak, Fillet, Cooked, Average	***1oz/28g***	***54***	***2.4***	***191***	***28.6***	***0.0***	***8.5***	***0.0***
Steak, Fillet, Lean, Average	***1oz/28g***	***42***	***2.0***	***150***	***21.0***	***0.0***	***7.3***	***0.0***
Steak, Fillet, Lean, Cooked, Average	***1oz/28g***	***52***	***2.2***	***186***	***28.6***	***0.0***	***8.0***	***0.0***
Steak, Frying, Average	***1 Steak/110g***	***128***	***2.7***	***116***	***23.7***	***0.0***	***2.5***	***0.0***
Steak, Rump, Cooked, Average	***1oz/28g***	***69***	***4.0***	***246***	***29.1***	***0.5***	***14.1***	***0.0***
Steak, Rump, Grilled, Rare, Lean	***1 Steak/227g***	***381***	***15.6***	***168***	***26.5***	***0.0***	***6.9***	***0.0***
Steak, Rump, Lean, Cooked, Average	***1oz/28g***	***50***	***1.7***	***179***	***31.0***	***0.0***	***6.1***	***0.0***
Steak, Rump, Raw, Lean, Average	***1 Steak/175g***	***219***	***7.2***	***125***	***22.0***	***0.0***	***4.1***	***0.0***
Steak, Rump, Raw, Lean & Fat	***1oz/28g***	***49***	***2.8***	***174***	***20.7***	***0.0***	***10.1***	***0.0***
Steak, Sirloin, Fried, Rare, Lean	***1oz/28g***	***53***	***2.3***	***189***	***28.8***	***0.0***	***8.2***	***0.0***
Steak, Sirloin, Fried, Rare, Lean & Fat	***1oz/28g***	***65***	***3.9***	***233***	***26.8***	***0.0***	***14.0***	***0.0***
Steak, Sirloin, Grilled, Medium-Rare, Lean	***1oz/28g***	***49***	***2.2***	***176***	***26.6***	***0.0***	***7.7***	***0.0***
Steak, Sirloin, Grilled, Medium-Rare, Lean & Fat	***1oz/28g***	***60***	***3.5***	***213***	***24.8***	***0.0***	***12.6***	***0.0***
Steak, Sirloin, Grilled, Rare, Lean	***1oz/28g***	***46***	***1.9***	***166***	***26.4***	***0.0***	***6.7***	***0.0***
Steak, Sirloin, Grilled, Rare, Lean & Fat	***1oz/28g***	***60***	***3.6***	***216***	***25.1***	***0.0***	***12.8***	***0.0***
Steak, Sirloin, Grilled, Well-Done, Lean	***1oz/28g***	***63***	***2.8***	***225***	***33.9***	***0.0***	***9.9***	***0.0***
Steak, Sirloin, Grilled, Well-Done, Lean & Fat	***1oz/28g***	***72***	***4.0***	***257***	***31.8***	***0.0***	***14.4***	***0.0***
Steak, Sirloin, Raw, Lean, Average	***1 Steak/150g***	***202***	***6.8***	***135***	***23.5***	***0.0***	***4.5***	***0.0***
Steak, Sirloin, Raw, Lean & Fat	***1oz/28g***	***56***	***3.6***	***201***	***21.6***	***0.0***	***12.7***	***0.0***
Stewed Steak, Average	***1 Serving/220g***	***258***	***10.1***	***117***	***15.8***	***3.3***	***4.6***	***0.0***
Stewing Steak, Lean & Fat, Raw, Average	***1 Serving/100g***	***136***	***4.3***	***136***	***24.2***	***0.1***	***4.3***	***0.1***
Stewing Steak, Raw, Lean	***1oz/28g***	***34***	***1.0***	***122***	***22.6***	***0.0***	***3.5***	***0.0***
Stewing Steak, Stewed, Lean	***1oz/28g***	***52***	***1.8***	***185***	***32.0***	***0.0***	***6.3***	***0.0***
Stewing Steak, Stewed, Lean & Fat	***1oz/28g***	***57***	***2.7***	***203***	***29.2***	***0.0***	***9.6***	***0.0***
Stir Fry Strips, Raw, Average	***1 Serving/125g***	***149***	***3.8***	***119***	***23.0***	***0.0***	***3.0***	***0.2***
Topside, Lean & Fat, Raw, Average	***1oz/28g***	***55***	***3.6***	***198***	***20.4***	***0.0***	***12.9***	***0.0***
Topside, Raw, Lean	***1oz/28g***	***32***	***0.8***	***116***	***23.0***	***0.0***	***2.7***	***0.0***
BEEF &								
Beer, Princes*	½ Can/205g	215	6.2	105	14.0	5.5	3.0	0.0
Black Bean, Sizzling, Oriental Express*	1 Pack/400g	420	8.4	105	7.2	14.0	2.1	2.1
Black Bean, with Rice, Weight Watchers*	1 Pack/320g	288	4.2	90	5.0	14.6	1.3	0.1
Chips, Steak, HE, Tesco*	1 Pack/450g	472	12.2	105	6.3	13.8	2.7	0.5
Mashed Potato, Braised, Sainsbury's*	1 Pack/434g	425	14.3	98	7.6	9.4	3.3	0.8
Onions, Minced, Asda*	½ Can/196g	314	19.6	160	13.0	4.6	10.0	0.1
Potatoes, Minced, LC, Tesco*	1 Pack/450g	400	9.5	80	4.3	10.3	1.9	2.3
Yorkshire Pudding, Minced, Sainsbury's*	1 Pack/350g	374	11.9	107	8.4	10.7	3.4	1.1
BEEF BOURGUIGNON								
Extra Special, Asda*	1 Serving/300g	279	11.0	93	9.3	5.7	3.7	0.7
Finest, Tesco*	½ Pack/300g	247	7.8	82	9.9	4.8	2.6	0.5
BEEF BRAISED								
& Gravy, My Fit Lifestyle, Tesco*	1 Pack/375g	263	3.8	70	6.2	8.8	1.0	0.9
& New Potatoes, GFY, Asda*	1 Pack/448g	242	6.3	54	8.1	2.2	1.4	3.1
Steak, & Cabbage, COU, M & S*	1 Pack/380g	323	9.9	85	8.3	6.7	2.6	1.9
Steak, & Carrots, Mini Favourites, M & S*	1 Serving/200g	140	5.0	70	8.0	4.2	2.5	1.3
Steak, & Mash, GFY, Asda*	1 Pack/400g	260	3.2	65	3.4	11.0	0.8	0.7
Steak, & Mash, HL, Tesco*	1 Pack/450g	418	12.2	93	7.0	10.2	2.7	0.7
Steak, & Red Wine, Veg Mash, HL, Tesco*	1 Pack/500g	360	13.5	72	5.1	6.9	2.7	1.2
Steak & Mash, Tastes of Home, M Kitchen, Morrisons*	1 Meal/250g	209	6.0	87	6.4	9.1	2.5	1.1
Tender, Pub Specials, Birds Eye*	1 Pack/450g	243	3.6	54	5.5	6.1	0.8	1.8

	Measure INFO/WEIGHT	per Measure KCAL	FAT	Nutrition Values per 100g / 100ml KCAL	PROT	CARB	FAT	FIBRE
BEEF CANTONESE								
Sainsbury's*	½ Pack/175g	200	2.3	114	5.5	20.1	1.3	0.5
BEEF CHASSEUR								
& Potato Mash, BGTY, Sainsbury's*	1 Pack/450g	387	10.8	86	7.8	8.4	2.4	1.3
BEEF CHILLI								
Crispy, Cantonese, Chilled, Sainsbury's*	1 Pack/250g	682	38.8	273	11.4	22.1	15.5	1.9
Crispy, Tesco*	1 Pack/250g	472	17.2	189	10.8	21.0	6.9	0.5
Sweet, Asda*	1 Pack/400g	356	3.6	89	7.8	12.3	0.9	1.9
BEEF DINNER								
Roast, Iceland*	1 Serving/340g	354	12.6	104	8.5	9.1	3.7	1.6
Roast, Sainsbury's*	1 Pack/400g	356	6.8	89	6.5	12.0	1.7	1.9
Roast, with Trimmings	1 Dinner/840g	1310	63.0	156	6.1	17.7	7.5	2.3
BEEF IN								
Ale, Diet Chef Ltd*	1 Meal/300g	201	3.6	67	8.2	6.0	1.2	2.1
Ale, with Mushrooms, BGTY, Sainsbury's*	1 Pack/251g	193	3.8	77	10.2	5.6	1.5	0.4
Ale Gravy, Chunky, Birds Eye*	1 Pack/340g	272	6.8	80	7.4	8.3	2.0	1.5
Au Poivre, Medallions, Skinny Chef, All About Weight*	1 Meal/280g	230	3.1	82	8.4	8.2	1.1	2.9
Black Bean, with Egg Noodles, M & S*	1 Pack/400g	460	6.0	115	8.6	16.7	1.5	1.8
Black Bean Sauce, Chinese, Tesco*	1 Pack/400g	396	12.4	99	9.1	8.7	3.1	0.5
Black Bean Sauce, Chosen By You, Asda*	1 Pack/450g	378	14.0	84	6.3	7.4	3.1	0.7
Black Pepper Sauce, & Egg Fried Rice, Tesco*	1 Pack/451g	622	24.8	138	7.0	15.2	5.5	1.2
Black Velvet Porter, Diet Chef Ltd*	1 Meal/300g	201	3.6	67	8.2	6.0	1.2	2.1
Black Velvet Porter, with Potatoes, Look What We Found*	1 Pack/300g	201	3.6	67	8.2	6.0	1.2	2.1
Gravy, Madeira & Mushroom, Sliced, Finest, Tesco*	1 Pack/400g	536	24.8	134	15.2	4.3	6.2	1.0
Gravy, Roast, Birds Eye*	1 Pack/227g	177	3.9	78	13.4	2.2	1.7	0.0
Gravy, Sliced, Iceland*	1 Pack/200g	172	3.2	86	12.1	5.9	1.6	0.3
Gravy, Sliced, Sainsbury's*	1 Serving/125g	100	2.2	80	13.5	2.6	1.8	0.2
Gravy, Sliced, Tesco*	1 Serving/200g	152	4.2	76	11.3	3.1	2.1	0.2
Oriental Sauce, Lean Cuisine, Findus*	1 Pack/350g	420	8.8	120	4.5	20.0	2.5	1.5
Oyster Sauce, Asda*	1 Serving/100g	82	4.0	82	7.0	4.4	4.0	1.7
Peppercorn Sauce, Creamy, Steak, Tesco*	1 Steak/150g	189	8.2	126	16.5	2.6	5.5	0.1
Red Wine, 117, Oakhouse Foods Ltd*	1 Meal/380g	403	17.1	106	7.7	8.1	4.5	1.5
Red Wine, Burgundy, GFY, Asda*	1 Pack/405g	348	8.1	86	8.0	9.0	2.0	1.1
Red Wine Sauce, Milson's Kitchen, Aldi*	1 Pack/400g	256	6.0	64	5.6	9.6	1.5	2.1
Red Wine Sauce, Simply Bistro, Aldi*	1 Pack/400g	316	6.0	79	5.6	9.2	1.5	2.1
BEEF TERIYAKI								
Incredibly Tender, Charlie Bigham's*	½ Pack/300g	477	26.7	159	5.0	10.9	8.9	0.9
with Noodles, BGTY, Sainsbury's*	1 Pack/400g	320	4.0	80	7.7	10.1	1.0	1.0
BEEF WELLINGTON								
Average	1 Serving/200g	530	33.3	265	12.4	17.0	16.6	1.0
Extra Special, Asda*	1 Serving/218g	605	37.1	277	11.0	20.0	17.0	0.9
Finest, Tesco*	1/3 Pack/216g	525	33.9	243	13.0	12.3	15.7	1.5
BEEF WITH								
Black Bean Sauce, Chilli, Sainsbury's*	1 Pack/300g	336	14.4	112	8.7	8.6	4.8	1.0
Black Bean Sauce, Rice Bowl, Uncle Ben's*	1 Pack/350g	368	4.9	105	5.6	17.4	1.4	0.0
Diane Sauce, Rump Steak, Tesco*	1 Steak/165g	182	8.1	110	15.1	1.1	4.9	0.3
Horseradish Dressing, Slow Cooked, HL, Tesco*	1 Pack/356g	285	10.3	80	5.4	7.5	2.9	1.4
Onion & Gravy, Minced, Princes*	1 Serving/200g	342	24.4	171	9.9	5.5	12.2	0.0
Onions & Gravy, Minced, Tesco*	1 Can/198g	224	10.1	113	14.0	2.8	5.1	0.8
Oyster Sauce, Ooodles of Noodles, Oriental Express*	1 Pack/425g	378	5.5	89	4.9	14.2	1.3	1.5
Peppercorn Crusted, Pink, Easy, Steak, Waitrose*	1 Steak/125g	195	6.6	156	18.4	8.6	5.3	1.1
Peppercorn Sauce, Rib Eye Joint, Sainsbury's*	1 Serving/181g	299	12.7	165	22.2	3.4	7.0	0.1
Peppercorn Sauce, Steak, Just Cook, Sainsbury's*	½ Pack/128g	174	7.3	136	17.7	3.4	5.7	1.2
Shiraz Wine Sauce, Pot Roast, Finest, Tesco*	1 Pack/350g	350	9.1	100	14.1	5.1	2.6	0.9

	Measure INFO/WEIGHT	per Measure KCAL	FAT	Nutrition Values per 100g / 100ml KCAL	PROT	CARB	FAT	FIBRE
BEEF WITH								
Vegetables, Tesco*	1 Pot/300g	102	3.0	34	2.9	3.3	1.0	1.1
Vegetables & Gravy, Minced, Birds Eye*	1 Pack/178g	155	6.1	87	9.1	5.1	3.4	0.6
BEER								
Ale, Bottled, Old Speckled Hen*	1 Bottle/330ml	124	0.3	38	0.2	1.8	0.1	0.2
Ale, Brown, Bottled, Average	***1 Bottle/330ml***	***99***	***0.0***	***30***	***0.3***	***3.0***	***0.0***	***0.0***
Ale, Gingerbeard, Wychwood, Marstons PLC*	1 Bottle/500ml	304	0.0	61	0.3	3.0	0.0	0.0
Ale, Goliath, Wychwood, Marstons PLC*	1 Bottle/500ml	192	0.0	38	0.4	2.8	0.0	0.0
Ale, Hopping Hare, Hall & Woodhouse Ltd*	1 Bottle/500ml	188	0.0	38	0.4	3.0	0.0	0.0
Ale, Old Peculiar, Theakstons*	1 Serving/500ml	250	0.0	50	0.0	4.6	0.0	0.0
Ale, Old Speckled Hen*	1 Pint/568ml	185	0.6	32	0.2	1.6	0.1	0.2
Ale, Pale, IPA, Greene King*	1 Pint/568ml	157	0.1	28	0.2	1.6	0.0	0.1
Ale, Pale, Sierra Nevada*	1 Bottle/350g	175	0.0	50	0.4	4.0	0.0	0.0
Ale, Scarecrow, Wychwood, Marstons PLC*	1 Bottle/500ml	214	0.0	43	0.4	4.3	0.0	0.0
Ale, Wychcraft, Wychwood, Marstons PLC*	1 Bottle/500ml	210	0.0	42	0.3	4.2	0.0	0.0
Bitter, Average	***1 Can/440ml***	***141***	***0.0***	***32***	***0.3***	***2.3***	***0.0***	***0.0***
Bitter, Cask, Draught, London Pride, Fullers*	1 Pint/568ml	201	0.0	35	0.0	0.0	0.0	0.0
Bitter, Draught, Average	***1 Pint/568ml***	***182***	***0.0***	***32***	***0.3***	***2.3***	***0.0***	***0.0***
Bitter, Keg, Average	***1 Pint/568ml***	***176***	***0.0***	***31***	***0.3***	***2.3***	***0.0***	***0.0***
Bitter, Low Alcohol, Average	***1 Pint/568ml***	***74***	***0.0***	***13***	***0.2***	***2.1***	***0.0***	***0.0***
Bitter, Original, Tetley's*	1 Can/440ml	140	0.0	32	0.2	4.6	0.0	0.0
Bitter, Strong, Broadside, Adnams*	1 Bottle/500ml	285	0.0	57	0.0	0.0	0.0	0.0
Bitter, Victoria, Carlton United Breweries*	1 Bottle/375ml	142	0.0	38	0.0	2.9	0.0	0.0
Especial, Modelo*	1 Bottle/355ml	145	0.0	41	0.0	1.1	0.0	0.0
Guinness*, Draught	***1 Can/440ml***	***158***	***0.2***	***36***	***0.3***	***3.0***	***0.0***	***0.0***
Guinness*, Stout	***1 Pint/568ml***	***205***	***0.0***	***36***	***0.3***	***3.0***	***0.0***	***0.0***
Guinness* Extra Stout, Bottled	***1 Bottle/500ml***	***215***	***0.0***	***43***	***4.0***	***0.0***	***0.0***	***0.0***
Honey Dew, Ale, Fullers*	1 Bottle/500ml	232	0.0	46	0.0	4.6	0.0	0.0
Kilkenny, Diageo*	1 Pint/568ml	210	0.0	37	0.3	3.0	0.0	0.0
Low Calorie, Low Carb, Cobra*	1 Bottle/330ml	96	0.0	29	0.1	1.3	0.0	0.0
Mild, Draught, Average	***1 Pint/568ml***	***136***	***0.0***	***24***	***0.2***	***1.6***	***0.0***	***0.0***
Non Alcoholic, Cobra*	1 Bottle/330ml	79	0.0	24	0.8	2.0	0.0	0.0
Oak Aged, Innis & Gunn*	1 Bottle/330ml	120	0.0	36	0.0	3.6	0.0	0.0
Raspberry, Framboise, Lindemans*	1 Serving/355ml	185	0.0	52	0.0	8.8	0.0	0.0
Resolution, Low Carb, Marstons PLC*	1 Glass/250ml	78	0.2	31	0.3	0.6	0.1	0.0
Stout, Mackeson	***1 Pint/568ml***	***205***	***0.0***	***36***	***0.4***	***4.6***	***0.0***	***0.0***
Ultra, Michelob*	1 Bottle/275ml	88	0.0	32	0.0	0.9	0.0	0.0
Weissbier, Alcohol Free, Erdinger*	1 Bottle/500ml	125	0.0	25	0.4	5.3	0.0	0.0
Wheat, Tesco*	1 Bottle/500ml	155	0.0	31	0.5	0.4	0.0	0.0
BEETROOT								
Baby, Pickled, Average	***1 Beetroot/13g***	***5***	***0.0***	***37***	***1.7***	***7.2***	***0.1***	***1.2***
Bunched, TTD, Sainsbury's*	1 Serving/100g	38	0.1	38	1.7	7.6	0.1	0.2
Cocktail, TTD, Sainsbury's*	½ Pack/100g	87	0.1	87	0.9	20.7	0.1	1.5
Cooked, Boiled, Drained, Average	***1 Serving/100g***	***44***	***0.2***	***44***	***1.7***	***10.0***	***0.2***	***2.0***
Crinkle Cut, Drained, Baxters*	1 Slice/10g	3	0.0	26	1.2	5.1	0.1	1.2
Pickled, in Sweet Vinegar, Average	***1oz/28g***	***16***	***0.0***	***57***	***1.2***	***12.8***	***0.1***	***1.5***
Pickled, in Vinegar, Average	***1 Serving/50g***	***19***	***0.0***	***37***	***1.6***	***7.5***	***0.1***	***1.2***
Raw, Unprepared, Average	***1oz/28g***	***9***	***0.0***	***32***	***1.6***	***6.0***	***0.1***	***1.8***
Rosebud, M & S*	½ Pack/90g	45	0.3	50	1.9	8.9	0.3	3.2
BHAJI								
Aubergine & Potato, Fried in Vegetable Oil, Average	1oz/28g	36	2.5	130	2.0	12.0	8.8	1.7
Cabbage & Pea, Fried in Vegetable Oil, Average	1oz/28g	50	4.1	178	3.3	9.2	14.7	3.4
Cauliflower, Fried in Vegetable Oil, Average	1oz/28g	60	5.7	214	4.0	4.0	20.5	2.0
Cauliflower, from 8 Snack Pack, Takeaway, Tesco*	1 Bhaji/18g	30	1.1	170	7.1	20.6	6.3	4.7

	Measure INFO/WEIGHT	per Measure KCAL	per Measure FAT	KCAL	PROT	CARB	FAT	FIBRE
				Nutrition Values per 100g / 100ml				
BHAJI								
Mushroom, Fried in Vegetable Oil, Average	1oz/28g	46	4.5	166	1.7	4.4	16.1	1.3
Okra, Bangladeshi, Fried in Butter Ghee, Average	1oz/28g	27	1.8	95	2.5	7.6	6.4	3.2
Onion, Asda*	1 Bhaji/49g	96	4.9	196	6.0	20.0	10.0	2.0
Onion, Indian Meal for One, Tesco*	1 Bhaji/100g	204	7.3	204	5.5	29.2	7.3	1.3
Onion, Indian Starter Selection, M & S*	1 Bhaji/22g	65	5.1	295	5.7	15.8	23.3	2.8
Onion, Mini, Asda*	1 Bhaji/35g	63	2.8	179	4.8	22.0	8.0	4.4
Onion, Mini, Snack Selection, Sainsbury's*	1 Bhaji/22g	49	3.4	226	4.1	17.4	15.5	3.5
Onion, Sainsbury's*	1 Bhaji/38g	93	5.1	245	6.5	24.7	13.4	6.4
Onion, Tesco*	1 Bhaji/47g	85	4.9	181	5.7	16.2	10.4	4.3
Onion, Waitrose*	1 Bhaji/45g	124	9.4	276	4.7	17.5	20.8	2.5
Onion, with Tomato & Chilli Dip, M & S*	1 Bhaji/54g	111	6.3	205	4.1	21.1	11.7	3.6
Potato, Onion & Mushroom, Fried, Average	1oz/28g	58	4.9	208	2.0	12.0	17.5	1.5
Potato, Spinach & Cauliflower, Fried, Average	1oz/28g	47	4.2	169	2.2	7.1	15.1	1.4
Potato & Onion, Fried in Vegetable Oil, Average	1oz/28g	45	2.8	160	2.1	16.6	10.1	1.6
Spinach, Fried in Vegetable Oil, Average	1oz/28g	23	1.9	83	3.3	2.6	6.8	2.4
Spinach & Potato, Fried in Vegetable Oil, Average	1oz/28g	53	3.9	191	3.7	13.4	14.1	2.3
Turnip & Onion, Fried in Vegetable Oil, Average	1oz/28g	36	3.1	128	1.3	7.1	10.9	2.2
Vegetable, Fried in Vegetable Oil, Average	1oz/28g	59	5.2	212	2.1	10.1	18.5	2.4
BHUNA								
Chicken, & Rice, Sainsbury's*	1 Pack/501g	696	31.5	139	7.3	13.3	6.3	1.5
Chicken, Curry, Tesco*	1 Serving/300g	396	22.8	132	11.4	4.5	7.6	0.5
Chicken, Hyderabadi, Sainsbury's*	1 Pack/400g	472	20.8	118	12.6	5.2	5.2	1.3
Chicken, Indian Takeaway, Tesco*	1 Pack/350g	438	27.6	125	8.3	4.6	7.9	2.2
Chicken, with Naan Bread, Sharwood's*	1 Pack/375g	465	19.1	124	6.8	12.8	5.1	2.8
Chicken, with Rice, Ready Meal, Average	1 Pack/350g	444	20.8	127	9.4	8.9	5.9	1.4
Chicken Tikka, Tesco*	1 Pack/350g	438	23.4	125	11.3	5.0	6.7	0.9
King Prawn, Chosen By You, Asda*	1 Pack/375g	296	17.2	79	4.4	4.3	4.6	1.4
King Prawn, M & S*	1 Pack/350g	262	13.3	75	6.7	3.3	3.8	1.5
King Prawn, Morrisons*	1 Pack/350g	301	20.6	86	6.5	1.8	5.9	0.5
Lamb, & Rice, Sainsbury's*	1 Pack/500g	619	26.5	124	7.4	11.6	5.3	2.0
Prawn, Co-Op*	1 Pack/400g	300	16.0	75	3.0	6.0	4.0	1.0
BIERWURST								
Average	***1 Slice/10g***	***25***	***2.1***	***252***	***14.4***	***1.0***	***21.2***	***0.0***
BILBERRIES								
Fresh, Raw	***1oz/28g***	***8***	***0.1***	***30***	***0.6***	***6.9***	***0.2***	***1.8***
BILTONG								
Average	***1 Serving/25g***	***64***	***1.0***	***256***	***50.0***	***0.0***	***4.0***	***0.0***
BIRYANI								
Chicken, COU, M & S*	1 Pack/400g	360	8.4	90	6.9	10.8	2.1	1.9
Chicken, Easy Steam, HL, Tesco*	1 Pack/400g	424	7.2	106	7.0	15.5	1.8	0.6
Chicken, LC, Tesco*	1 Serving/450g	495	10.4	110	7.0	15.0	2.3	3.4
Chicken, Ready Meal, Average	1 Pack/400g	521	17.1	130	7.5	15.2	4.3	1.6
Chicken, Ready Meal, Healthy Range, Average	1 Pack/400g	369	5.5	92	7.4	12.6	1.4	0.9
Chicken Tikka, & Lentil Pilau, Fuller Longer, M & S*	1 Pack/400g	440	11.6	110	9.5	12.0	2.9	2.3
Chicken Tikka, BGTY, Sainsbury's*	1 Pack/400g	316	3.8	84	6.8	10.7	1.0	2.9
Chicken Tikka, Ready Meal, Average	1 Pack/400g	460	11.5	115	7.3	14.8	2.9	1.5
Lamb, Average	1 Serving/200g	390	19.4	195	7.3	20.9	9.7	0.0
Lamb, HL, Tesco*	1 Pack/400g	560	17.6	140	5.1	19.0	4.4	3.1
Lamb, Ready Meal, Average	1 Pack/400g	535	18.9	134	6.0	16.6	4.7	2.2
Seafood, M & S*	1 Pack/450g	619	25.7	138	7.1	14.4	5.7	1.7
Vegetable, & Rice, Sainsbury's*	½ Pack/125g	229	5.0	183	4.4	32.4	4.0	0.7
Vegetable, HL, Tesco*	1 Pack/450g	454	9.4	101	2.7	17.9	2.1	1.6
Vegetable, Sainsbury's*	1 Serving/225g	328	17.8	146	2.4	16.3	7.9	1.1

	Measure INFO/WEIGHT	per Measure KCAL	per Measure FAT	Nutrition Values per 100g / 100ml KCAL	PROT	CARB	FAT	FIBRE
BIRYANI								
Vegetable, Tikka, Vegelicious, Tesco*	1 Pack/340g	340	10.5	100	4.6	11.4	3.1	3.0
Vegetable, Waitrose*	1 Pack/450g	521	19.8	116	2.4	14.9	4.4	3.6
BISCUITS								
Abbey Crunch, McVitie's*	1 Biscuit/9g	43	1.6	477	6.0	72.8	17.9	2.5
Abernethy, Simmers*	1 Biscuit/12g	61	2.7	490	5.7	69.2	21.9	0.0
Aero, Nestle*	1 Bar/19g	99	5.5	534	6.4	59.4	29.4	2.1
Aero, Orange, Aero, Nestle*	1 Biscuit/19g	101	5.6	534	6.0	60.6	29.3	1.7
After Eight, Nestle*	1 Biscuit/5g	26	1.4	525	6.5	62.6	27.7	1.5
All Butter, Tesco*	1 Biscuit/9g	44	2.1	486	6.3	63.5	23.0	1.9
Almond, Artisan Bakery, Extra Special, Asda*	1 Biscuit/19g	103	6.1	548	7.9	54.3	32.3	4.2
Almond Thins, Continental, Tesco*	1 Biscuit/3g	15	0.5	450	6.7	72.8	14.7	3.1
Almond Thins, Morrisons*	1 Biscuit/4g	16	0.5	450	6.7	72.8	14.7	3.1
Almond Thins, Sainsbury's*	1 Biscuit/3g	13	0.3	430	7.0	80.3	9.0	1.0
Almond Thins, TTD, Sainsbury's*	1 Biscuit/4g	16	0.5	450	6.7	72.8	14.7	3.1
Amaretti, Doria*	1 Biscuit/4g	17	0.3	433	6.0	84.8	7.8	0.0
Amaretti, M & S*	1 Biscuit/6g	30	1.1	480	9.6	71.3	17.2	3.8
Amaretti, Sainsbury's*	1 Biscuit/6g	27	0.7	450	6.5	80.5	11.3	1.1
Anzac, Bitesmart*	1 Biscuit/20g	84	4.6	420	5.1	46.8	23.0	0.0
Apricot, Low Fat, M & S*	1 Biscuit/23g	79	1.0	343	6.1	69.6	4.4	7.8
Arrowroot, Thin, Crawfords*	1 Biscuit/7g	35	1.2	450	6.9	71.4	15.2	2.8
Assortment, Mini, M & S*	1 Biscuit/3g	12	0.6	480	6.1	63.9	22.5	2.8
Berry GI, Diet Chef Ltd*	1 Biscuit/20g	87	3.2	435	7.0	65.2	16.1	7.2
Bisc & Bounty, Master Foods*	1 Bar/25g	132	8.2	526	4.8	52.3	33.0	0.0
Bisc & M&M's, Master Foods*	1 Biscuit/17g	90	5.0	527	5.8	59.2	29.6	0.0
Bisc & Mars, Master Foods*	1 Bar/27g	141	7.7	523	5.3	61.4	28.5	0.0
Bisc & Twix, Master Foods*	1 Bar/27g	140	7.6	520	5.2	61.1	28.3	0.0
Blueberry, Biscuit Moments, Special K, Kellogg's*	2 Biscuits/25g	99	2.3	394	4.5	73.0	9.0	1.5
Blueberry & Vanilla, Oaty, Weight Watchers*	1 Biscuit/19g	86	3.3	452	7.3	62.1	17.6	8.0
BN, Chocolate Flavour, McVitie's*	1 Biscuit/18g	83	3.0	460	6.6	71.0	16.7	2.6
BN, Strawberry Flavour, McVitie's*	1 Biscuit/18g	71	1.2	395	5.6	78.0	6.8	0.0
BN, Vanilla Flavour, McVitie's*	1 Biscuit/18g	85	3.0	470	5.9	74.0	16.6	1.2
Bourbon, Average	1 Biscuit/13g	63	2.8	488	5.7	68.2	21.3	2.1
Bourbon, Gluten & Wheat Free, Lovemore*	1 Biscuit/15g	70	2.9	469	4.1	67.9	19.1	4.7
Bourbon, Trufree*	1 Biscuit/13g	61	2.8	486	7.5	62.6	22.6	1.1
Bournville, Cadbury*	1 Biscuit/16g	85	5.0	520	6.0	54.9	30.7	1.4
Brandy Snaps, Average	1 Biscuit/15g	69	2.2	460	2.7	79.8	14.4	0.5
Breakfast, Average	4 Biscuits/56g	249	8.8	445	11.8	61.7	15.7	7.0
Breakfast, Cranberry, Belvita, Nabisco*	1 Biscuits/13g	55	1.7	435	8.3	67.5	13.7	5.7
Breakfast, Forest Fruits, Belvita, Nabisco*	1 Biscuit/13g	60	2.1	460	8.5	67.0	16.0	5.3
Breakfast, Honey & Nuts, Belvita, Nabisco*	1 Biscuit/13g	58	2.1	464	8.0	68.0	17.0	3.5
Breakfast, Honey & Yoghurt Crunch, Belvita, Nabisco*	2 Biscuits/51g	230	8.6	455	7.6	66.0	17.0	4.0
Breakfast, Milk & Cereals, Belvita, Nabisco*	1 Biscuit/13g	56	1.9	445	8.7	69.0	15.0	3.6
Breakfast, Muesli, Belvita, Nabisco*	1 Biscuit/13g	59	2.1	455	8.2	67.0	16.0	4.1
Breakfast, Original, All Bran, Kellogg's*	1 Pack/40g	176	8.0	440	8.0	49.0	20.0	16.0
Breakfast, Strawberry & Yoghurt, Belvita, Nabisco*	1 Biscuit/25g	113	3.8	445	6.9	70.0	15.0	4.3
Breakfast, Yoghurt Crunch, Belvita, Nabisco*	2 Biscuits/50g	230	8.6	455	7.6	66.0	17.0	4.0
Butter, Chocolate, Dark, Momento, Aldi*	1 Biscuit/14g	69	3.2	491	6.2	63.5	22.6	4.2
Butter, Crinkle Crunch, Fox's*	1 Biscuit/11g	50	1.9	460	5.8	69.8	17.5	2.4
Cafe Noir, McVitie's*	1 Biscuit/9g	39	0.5	420	4.5	87.0	5.5	1.1
Cantuccini, with Almonds, Average	1 Biscotti/30g	130	5.0	433	10.0	60.0	16.7	3.3
Cheese Melts, Carr's*	1 Biscuit/4g	20	0.9	483	11.2	57.0	22.5	3.9
Cheese Sandwich, Ritz*	1 Biscuit/9g	50	2.8	530	9.5	55.0	30.2	2.0
Cheese Savouries, Sainsbury's*	1 Serving/50g	268	15.3	536	11.6	53.3	30.6	2.5

	Measure INFO/WEIGHT	per Measure KCAL	FAT	Nutrition Values per 100g / 100ml KCAL	PROT	CARB	FAT	FIBRE
BISCUITS								
Choc Chip, Double, Trufree*	1 Biscuit/11g	58	3.0	523	3.0	67.0	27.0	1.8
Choc Chip, Paterson's*	1 Biscuit/17g	79	3.6	474	5.6	64.0	21.6	3.1
Chocahoops, Cadbury*	1 Biscuit/13g	65	3.4	510	5.8	62.7	26.4	0.0
Chockas, Original, Fox's*	1 Biscuit/24g	85	1.0	355	1.1	10.4	4.2	0.4
Choco Leibniz, Dark Chocolate, Bahlsen*	1 Biscuit/14g	69	3.6	493	6.8	59.0	26.0	5.1
Choco Leibniz, Milk, Bahlsen*	1 Biscuit/14g	72	3.6	515	7.9	63.4	25.5	2.4
Choco Leibniz, Orange Flavour, Bahlsen*	1 Biscuit/14g	70	3.7	504	7.9	58.5	26.4	0.0
Chocolate, & Coconut, Duchy Originals*	1 Biscuit/13g	68	4.3	543	6.3	52.1	34.4	2.6
Chocolate, & Hazelnut, Quirks, McVitie's*	1 Biscuit/13g	66	3.6	511	5.0	58.4	28.0	2.6
Chocolate, Breakaway, Nestle*	1 Bar/19g	99	4.9	509	6.0	62.7	25.2	3.7
Chocolate, Double, Quirks, McVitie's*	1 Biscuit/13g	66	3.6	505	5.0	57.2	27.8	3.2
Chocolate, Milk, Ace, McVitie's*	1 Biscuit/24g	122	5.9	510	6.1	66.2	24.5	1.6
Chocolate, Quirks, McVitie's*	1 Biscuit/13g	66	3.6	509	5.0	58.7	27.7	2.5
Chocolate Break, Plain Chocolate, Tesco*	1 Biscuit/21g	112	6.1	535	6.7	61.2	29.2	3.8
Chocolate Chip & Peanut, Trufree*	1 Biscuit/11g	55	2.6	496	4.0	66.0	24.0	2.0
Chocolate Chip GI, Diet Chef Ltd*	1 Pack/20g	90	3.6	450	7.4	64.4	17.9	6.4
Chocolate Fingers, Average	1 Biscuit/6g	31	1.6	514	6.7	61.4	26.8	1.5
Chocolate Fingers, Caramel, Cadbury*	1 Finger/8g	39	1.9	490	5.8	63.2	23.8	0.0
Chocolate Fingers, Milk, Cadbury*	1 Biscuit/6g	31	1.6	515	6.8	60.8	27.1	1.7
Chocolate Fingers, Milk, Extra Crunchy, Cadbury*	1 Biscuit/5g	25	1.2	505	6.6	66.2	23.6	0.0
Chocolate Fingers, Plain, Cadbury*	1 Biscuit/6g	30	1.6	508	6.2	60.6	26.8	0.0
Chocolate Fingers, Plain, Mint, Tesco*	2 Fingers/22g	115	6.0	525	6.3	61.8	27.6	2.3
Chocolate Florentine, M & S*	1 Serving/39g	195	9.7	500	7.4	64.5	24.9	1.7
Chocolate Ginger, Organic, Duchy Originals*	1 Biscuit/12g	64	3.6	518	4.6	59.7	29.0	2.1
Chocolate Ginger, Thorntons*	1 Biscuit/19g	96	5.3	512	5.9	58.2	28.4	0.0
Chocolate Nibbles, High Lights, Cadbury*	1 Pack/16g	75	2.6	465	6.2	73.4	16.1	1.7
Chocolate Seville, Thorntons*	1 Biscuit/19g	97	5.3	512	5.7	59.0	28.1	0.0
Chocolate Teddy, Arnotts*	1 Biscuit/17g	80	3.2	478	6.6	69.3	19.2	2.0
Chocolate Toffee, Crunch, Moments, McVitie's*	1 Biscuit/17g	89	4.7	520	5.6	62.3	27.6	1.7
Chocolate Viennese, Fox's*	1 Biscuit/16g	85	4.9	530	6.7	56.6	30.7	1.7
Christmas Shapes, Assorted, Sainsbury's*	1 Biscuit/15g	77	4.3	525	5.2	59.0	29.8	1.7
Classic, Creams, Fox's*	1 Biscuit/14g	72	3.6	516	4.4	65.2	25.8	1.7
Classic, Milk Chocolate, Fox's*	1 Biscuit/13g	67	3.1	517	6.1	64.9	24.0	1.6
Coconut, Ring, Average	1 Biscuit/9g	44	2.0	490	6.1	67.4	21.8	2.6
Coconut Crinkles, Fox's*	1 Biscuit/11g	53	2.5	487	5.2	63.8	22.6	3.7
Cranberry, & Pumpkin Seed, BGTY, Sainsbury's*	1 Biscuit/17g	68	2.8	410	7.2	56.6	17.1	13.9
Cranberry, & Sunflower Seed, Oaty, Weight Watchers*	1 Biscuit/19g	87	3.7	457	7.9	58.0	19.3	10.0
Crinkles, Classics, Milk Chocolate, Fox's*	1 Biscuit/14g	67	3.1	487	5.7	65.2	22.7	2.7
Crispy Fruit Slices, Apple, Sultana, Go Ahead, McVitie's*	1 Slice/13g	50	0.9	388	5.4	74.0	7.1	2.9
Crispy Fruit Slices, Forest Fruit, Go Ahead, McVitie's*	1 Biscuit/13g	49	0.9	380	5.4	73.7	7.0	3.0
Crunchers, Salted, Savoury, Crackers, Sainsbury's*	1 Cracker/5g	22	1.0	448	6.1	59.4	20.4	1.4
Crunchie, Cadbury*	1 Biscuit/13g	64	3.1	495	4.8	65.7	23.6	0.9
Custard Cream, Gluten & Wheat Free, Lovemore*	1 Biscuit/15g	71	2.5	475	0.0	33.0	16.8	0.0
Custard Creams, 25% Less Fat, Sainsbury's*	1 Biscuit/13g	59	2.2	469	5.8	72.7	17.3	1.3
Custard Creams, Asda*	1 Biscuit/12g	59	2.7	495	5.0	67.0	23.0	2.0
Custard Creams, Crawfords*	1 Biscuit/11g	57	2.7	517	5.9	69.2	24.1	1.5
Custard Creams, Jacob's*	1 Biscuit/16g	77	3.3	481	5.3	68.0	20.9	1.6
Custard Creams, Sainsbury's*	1 Biscuit/13g	67	3.0	514	5.5	70.4	23.4	1.6
Custard Creams, Trufree*	1 Biscuit/12g	60	2.8	504	8.7	65.0	23.0	1.0
Digestive, 25% Less Fat, Asda*	1 Biscuit/16g	73	2.6	455	7.3	69.8	16.3	2.6
Digestive, BGTY, Sainsbury's*	1 Biscuit/15g	70	2.6	468	7.4	71.0	17.2	3.8
Digestive, Caramels, Milk Chocolate, McVitie's*	1 Biscuit/17g	81	3.7	478	5.6	65.1	21.7	2.3
Digestive, Caramels, Plain Chocolate, McVitie's*	1 Biscuit/17g	82	3.8	481	5.7	65.5	22.1	2.1

	Measure	per Measure		Nutrition Values per 100g / 100ml				
	INFO/WEIGHT	KCAL	FAT	KCAL	PROT	CARB	FAT	FIBRE
BISCUITS								
Digestive, Chocolate	1 Biscuit/17g	84	4.1	493	6.8	66.5	24.1	2.2
Digestive, Chocolate, Dark, McVitie's*	1 Biscuit/17g	83	4.1	495	6.0	60.8	24.2	4.2
Digestive, Chocolate, Double, Mcvitie's*	1 Biscuit/17g	83	4.1	497	6.5	60.9	24.3	3.6
Digestive, Chocolate, Milk, 25% Less Fat, Tesco*	1 Biscuit/17g	79	3.0	466	7.4	69.0	17.8	2.6
Digestive, Chocolate, Milk, 25% Reduced Fat, McVitie's*	1 Biscuit/17g	78	2.9	459	7.2	68.6	17.3	3.2
Digestive, Chocolate, Milk, Cadbury*	1 Biscuit/16g	80	3.8	490	7.4	61.3	23.3	3.9
Digestive, Chocolate, Milk, GFY, Asda*	1 Biscuit/17g	78	2.9	457	7.0	69.0	17.0	3.2
Digestive, Chocolate, Milk, Homewheat, McVitie's*	1 Biscuit/17g	83	4.1	486	6.0	61.5	24.0	4.0
Digestive, Chocolate, Milk, McVitie's*	1 Biscuit/17g	84	4.0	488	6.7	62.7	23.4	2.9
Digestive, Chocolate, Milk, Mini, McVitie's*	1 Bag/25g	124	6.2	496	6.6	61.9	24.7	2.9
Digestive, Chocolate, Milk, Mint, McVitie's*	1 Biscuit/17g	81	3.9	487	6.7	62.6	23.4	2.9
Digestive, Chocolate, Milk, Trufree*	1 Biscuit/12g	63	3.0	521	4.0	70.0	25.0	2.0
Digestive, Chocolate, Plain, Tesco*	1 Biscuit/17g	85	4.1	499	6.2	63.5	24.4	2.8
Digestive, Chocolate Chip, Asda*	1 Biscuit/14g	68	3.2	491	6.0	65.0	23.0	2.9
Digestive, Cracker Selection, Tesco*	1 Biscuit/12g	56	2.3	464	7.1	65.2	19.4	4.3
Digestive, Crawfords*	1 Biscuit/12g	58	2.4	484	7.1	68.8	20.0	3.4
Digestive, Creams, McVitie's*	1 Biscuit/12g	60	2.8	502	5.6	68.2	23.0	2.1
Digestive, Economy, Sainsbury's*	1 Biscuit/13g	65	3.0	498	6.8	66.3	22.8	3.3
Digestive, Finger, Reduced Fat, Sainsbury's*	1 Finger/8g	39	1.8	482	6.8	63.6	22.2	3.2
Digestive, Fingers, Morrisons*	1 Finger/8g	39	1.8	482	6.8	63.6	22.2	3.2
Digestive, GFY, Asda*	1 Biscuit/14g	65	2.4	461	6.0	71.0	17.0	3.6
Digestive, Gluten & Wheat Free, Lovemore*	1 Biscuit/15g	55	2.7	378	3.4	49.3	18.5	18.4
Digestive, High Fibre, Reduced Sugar, M & S*	1 Biscuit/13g	60	2.8	460	6.5	59.3	21.7	9.4
Digestive, Hovis*	1 Biscuit/6g	27	1.1	447	10.2	60.0	18.5	4.4
Digestive, Jacob's*	1 Biscuit/14g	67	3.0	479	6.6	65.7	21.1	3.4
Digestive, Lemon & Ginger, McVitie's*	1 Biscuit/15g	72	3.1	480	6.7	66.7	20.7	2.7
Digestive, Light, McVitie's*	1 Biscuit/15g	66	2.1	444	7.3	69.5	14.4	3.6
Digestive, McVitie's*	1 Biscuit/15g	70	3.2	470	7.2	62.7	21.5	3.6
Digestive, Munch Bites, McVitie's*	1 Pack/40g	205	10.2	512	6.5	64.5	25.5	2.0
Digestive, Oat, Nairn's*	1 Biscuit/11g	50	2.0	437	12.0	57.8	17.5	7.8
Digestive, Oat, TTD, Sainsbury's*	1 Biscuit/13g	56	2.3	448	9.8	56.4	18.5	8.5
Digestive, Oat, Weight Watchers*	1 Biscuit/11g	50	2.1	457	6.0	66.3	18.6	6.9
Digestive, Organic, Sainsbury's*	1 Biscuit/12g	60	2.9	483	6.6	60.9	23.7	5.8
Digestive, Organic, Tesco*	1 Biscuit/13g	60	2.7	464	7.7	66.3	20.8	4.6
Digestive, Plain, Average	1 Biscuit/14g	67	2.9	480	7.1	65.6	20.5	3.5
Digestive, Reduced Fat, M & S*	1 Biscuit/16g	75	2.7	480	7.2	73.3	17.5	3.4
Digestive, Reduced Fat, McVitie's*	1 Biscuit/15g	70	2.4	467	7.1	72.8	16.3	3.4
Digestive, Reduced Fat, Tesco*	1 Biscuit/16g	70	2.6	453	7.0	69.1	16.6	3.4
Digestive, Sweetmeal, Asda*	1 Biscuit/14g	68	3.1	499	7.0	66.0	23.0	3.5
Digestive, Sweetmeal, Sainsbury's*	1 Biscuit/14g	72	3.3	498	6.0	66.4	23.1	3.3
Digestive, Trufree*	1 Biscuit/10g	48	2.2	485	6.1	62.4	22.1	6.2
Digestive, Whole Wheat, Organic, Dove's Farm*	1 Biscuit/13g	56	2.4	446	5.9	61.6	19.5	7.8
Digestive, with Wheatgerm, Hovis*	1 Biscuit/12g	37	2.2	306	6.2	66.8	18.5	5.8
Fig Roll, Tesco*	1 Biscuit/19g	70	1.6	375	4.0	69.3	8.8	3.1
Figfuls, Go Ahead, McVitie's*	1 Biscuit/15g	54	0.7	355	4.2	76.8	4.6	2.9
First Class, Bahlsen*	1 Serving/125g	711	45.2	569	7.5	53.4	36.2	0.0
Florentines, Sainsbury's*	1 Florentine/8g	40	2.5	506	10.0	47.2	30.8	7.0
Fruit Bake, Organic, Tesco*	1 Biscuit/12g	53	2.1	453	7.5	65.1	18.1	5.6
Fruit Jambos, Rowntree's*	1 Biscuit/11g	47	1.4	435	4.7	73.6	13.4	1.7
Fruit Shortcake, McVitie's*	1 Biscuit/8g	37	1.6	464	5.7	65.1	20.1	2.7
Fruit Shortcake, Sainsbury's*	1 Biscuit/8g	39	1.6	483	5.9	69.6	20.1	2.1
Fruit Shortcake, Tesco*	1 Biscuit/9g	43	1.7	473	5.8	70.1	18.8	1.9
Galettes, Bonne Maman*	1 Serving/90g	460	22.5	511	6.0	65.7	25.0	0.0

	Measure INFO/WEIGHT	per Measure KCAL	FAT	Nutrition Values per 100g / 100ml KCAL	PROT	CARB	FAT	FIBRE
BISCUITS								
Garibaldi, Asda*	1 Biscuit/10g	39	0.9	375	4.7	68.5	9.1	2.2
Garibaldi, Sainsbury's*	1 Biscuit/9g	35	1.0	389	5.7	67.1	10.9	3.3
Ginger, Traditional, Fox's*	1 Biscuit/8g	33	1.0	404	4.4	70.1	11.7	1.4
Ginger Crinkle, Sainsbury's*	1 Biscuit/11g	53	2.5	486	6.2	63.8	22.9	2.9
Ginger Crinkle Crunch, Fox's*	1 Biscuit/12g	50	1.4	435	4.7	75.3	12.5	1.6
Ginger Crunch Creams, Fox's*	1 Biscuit/14g	73	3.7	518	4.6	64.8	26.7	0.0
Ginger Nuts, Chocolate, Milk, McVitie's*	1 Biscuit/14g	68	2.8	489	5.8	71.8	19.9	1.5
Ginger Nuts, McVitie's*	1 Biscuit/10g	47	1.7	459	5.5	71.1	16.6	2.3
Ginger Snap, Fox's*	1 Biscuit/8g	35	1.0	443	4.6	77.1	12.8	1.5
Ginger Snap, Less Than 10% Fat, Sainsbury's*	1 Biscuit/12g	51	1.1	424	6.5	78.9	9.1	1.9
Ginger Snap, Sainsbury's*	1 Biscuit/11g	47	1.6	445	5.3	73.0	14.7	2.2
Ginger Thins, Asda*	1 Biscuit/5g	23	0.8	462	6.0	73.0	16.0	1.9
Gingernut	1 Biscuit/11g	50	1.7	456	5.6	79.1	15.2	1.4
Golden Crunch, Bronte*	1 Biscuit/15g	69	3.3	474	5.1	62.5	22.6	0.0
Golden Crunch, Go Ahead, McVitie's*	1 Biscuit/9g	38	0.9	419	7.7	75.2	9.7	2.1
Golden Crunch, Paterson's*	1 Biscuit/15g	69	3.3	474	5.1	62.5	22.6	4.8
Golden Crunch Creams, Fox's*	1 Biscuit/15g	75	3.8	515	4.7	64.8	26.3	1.2
Golden Shortie, Jacob's*	1 Biscuit/11g	54	2.6	492	6.0	64.9	23.2	0.0
Golden Syrup, McVitie's*	1 Biscuit/12g	63	3.0	508	5.1	67.3	24.2	2.2
Happy Faces, Jacob's*	1 Biscuit/16g	78	3.6	485	4.8	66.1	22.3	1.6
Hobnobs, Chocolate, Milk, McVitie's*	1 Biscuit/19g	92	4.5	479	6.8	60.7	23.3	4.5
Hobnobs, Chocolate, Milk, Mini, McVitie's*	1 Pack/25g	121	5.9	483	6.6	61.3	23.5	4.4
Hobnobs, Chocolate, Plain, McVitie's*	1 Biscuit/16g	81	3.9	498	6.7	63.3	24.3	4.2
Hobnobs, Chocolate Creams, McVitie's*	1 Biscuit/12g	60	3.1	503	6.7	60.3	26.1	4.0
Hobnobs, Light, 25% Reduced Fat, McVitie's*	1 Biscuit/14g	62	2.3	435	8.1	64.6	16.1	6.2
Hobnobs, McVitie's*	1 Biscuit/15g	72	3.2	473	7.0	61.8	20.7	5.4
Hobnobs, Vanilla Creams, McVitie's*	1 Biscuit/12g	60	3.0	501	6.1	62.3	25.2	3.6
Honeycomb Nibbles, High Lights, Cadbury*	1 Bag/16g	75	2.6	465	6.2	73.4	16.2	1.8
Iced Gems, Jacob's*	1 Serving/30g	118	0.9	393	5.0	86.3	3.1	2.0
Jaffa Cakes, Asda*	1 Cake/12g	43	1.0	368	4.7	67.5	8.8	1.9
Jaffa Cakes, Basics, Sainsbury's*	1 Jaffa Cake/11g	43	1.0	377	4.5	69.5	9.0	2.0
Jaffa Cakes, Blackcurrant, McVitie's*	1 Cake/12g	45	1.0	371	4.8	69.7	8.1	2.3
Jaffa Cakes, Chocolate, Dark, M & S*	1 Cake/11g	45	1.5	395	3.7	64.9	13.2	2.8
Jaffa Cakes, Chocolate, Dark, Mini, M & S*	1 Cake/5g	20	0.8	410	3.9	62.8	15.8	1.9
Jaffa Cakes, Free From, Asda*	1 Cake/12g	42	0.9	340	5.8	62.6	7.4	8.0
Jaffa Cakes, Lemon & Lime, McVitie's*	1 Cake/12g	45	1.0	370	4.7	69.5	8.1	2.1
Jaffa Cakes, Lunch Box, McVitie's*	1 Cake/7g	26	0.6	395	4.2	74.3	9.0	1.4
Jaffa Cakes, McVitie's*	1 Cake/12g	45	1.0	374	4.8	70.6	8.0	2.1
Jaffa Cakes, Mini, Bags, McVitie's*	1 Cake/5g	20	0.7	396	4.2	65.0	13.1	3.5
Jaffa Cakes, Mini, Orange Pods, McVitie's*	1 Cake/40g	150	3.4	380	4.3	71.2	8.7	3.5
Jam Creams, Jacob's*	1 Biscuit/15g	75	3.4	486	5.0	67.4	21.8	1.6
Jam Rings, Crawfords*	1 Biscuit/12g	56	2.1	470	5.5	73.0	17.2	1.9
Jam Sandwich Creams, M & S*	1 Biscuit/17g	80	3.7	485	5.7	64.5	22.6	1.8
Jam Sandwich Creams, Sainsbury's*	1 Biscuit/16g	77	3.4	486	5.0	67.0	21.8	1.6
Jammie Dodgers, Minis, Lunchbox, Burton's*	1 Pack/20g	90	2.9	452	5.5	72.7	14.7	2.5
Jammie Dodgers, Original, Burton's*	1 Biscuit/19g	83	3.0	437	5.1	69.5	15.9	1.9
Lebkuchen, Sainsbury's*	1 Biscuit/10g	39	0.8	400	5.7	76.1	8.0	1.3
Lemon, All Butter, Half Coated, Finest, Tesco*	1 Biscuit/17g	84	4.5	505	5.6	60.4	26.9	3.6
Lemon Butter, Thins, Sainsbury's*	1 Biscuit/13g	65	3.5	515	5.3	60.7	27.9	2.2
Lemon Curd Sandwich, Fox's*	1 Biscuit/14g	69	3.3	494	4.7	66.2	23.4	1.3
Lemon Puff, Jacob's*	1 Biscuit/13g	69	4.1	533	4.3	58.8	31.2	2.8
Lemon Thins, Sainsbury's*	1 Biscuit/10g	47	1.7	468	5.6	72.3	17.3	1.7
Lincoln, McVitie's*	1 Biscuit/8g	41	1.9	514	6.3	69.0	23.6	2.0

	Measure INFO/WEIGHT	per Measure KCAL	FAT	Nutrition Values per 100g / 100ml KCAL	PROT	CARB	FAT	FIBRE
BISCUITS								
Lincoln, Sainsbury's*	1 Biscuit/8g	40	1.7	479	7.2	66.1	20.6	2.1
Malted Milk, Average	1 Biscuit/9g	42	1.9	490	7.0	65.6	22.2	1.8
Malted Milk, Chocolate, Milk, Asda*	1 Biscuit/11g	56	2.8	509	7.0	64.0	25.0	1.7
Malted Milk, Chocolate, Tesco*	1 Biscuit/10g	52	2.5	500	6.7	64.4	24.0	1.9
Maple Leaf, M & S*	1 Biscuit/13g	50	1.9	395	5.1	59.8	14.8	2.0
Marie, Crawfords*	1 Biscuit/7g	33	1.1	475	7.5	76.3	15.5	2.3
Melts, Sesame, with Chive, Carr's*	1 Biscuit/5g	23	1.2	498	8.2	57.4	26.2	3.5
Mikado, Jacob's*	1 Biscuit/13g	53	1.6	397	4.2	67.7	12.1	2.5
Mint, Chocolate, Plain, Tesco*	1 Biscuit/25g	136	7.5	538	5.1	63.0	29.5	1.7
Mint, Viscount*	1 Biscuit/13g	73	3.8	552	5.1	60.6	28.8	1.3
Morning Coffee, Asda*	1 Biscuit/5g	22	0.7	455	8.0	72.0	15.0	2.4
Morning Coffee, Tesco*	1 Biscuit/5g	22	0.7	450	7.6	72.3	14.5	2.4
Nice, Average	1 Biscuit/8g	36	1.6	484	6.3	67.3	21.0	2.5
Nice, Belmont, Aldi*	1 Biscuit/8g	39	1.6	489	6.2	68.9	20.4	2.3
Nice, Cream, Tesco*	1 Serving/13g	65	3.1	510	4.9	67.0	24.0	2.0
Nice, Fox's*	1 Biscuit/9g	39	1.7	450	6.3	62.4	19.4	5.0
Nice, Jacob's*	1 Biscuit/7g	33	1.3	471	6.1	68.5	19.2	1.8
Oat, Fruit & Spice, Nairn's*	1 Biscuit/10g	43	1.5	425	7.8	65.3	14.7	7.6
Oat, Mixed Berries, Nairn's*	1 Biscuit/10g	43	1.5	427	7.5	64.8	15.3	7.1
Oat, Santiveri*	1 Biscuit/5g	23	0.9	428	10.0	58.8	17.0	7.0
Oat, Stem Ginger, Nairn's*	1 Biscuit/10g	43	1.5	434	8.8	65.6	15.2	6.1
Oat & Chocolate Chip, Cadbury*	1 Biscuit/17g	80	3.9	485	6.9	60.2	23.9	4.2
Oat & Raisin, Organic, United Biscuits*	1oz/28g	129	6.4	460	5.6	62.2	22.8	2.8
Oat & Wholemeal, Crawfords*	1 Biscuit/14g	67	3.0	482	7.7	64.2	21.6	4.8
Oat Bites, Caramelised Onion, Diet Chef Ltd*	1 Pack/23g	99	3.9	430	7.5	64.2	16.8	6.0
Oat Bites, Cheese, Diet Chef Ltd*	1 Pack/23g	99	3.6	430	15.0	57.4	15.8	4.9
Oat Bites, Chilli, Diet Chef Ltd*	1 Pack/23g	128	3.1	556	8.1	68.4	13.3	7.2
Oat Crumbles, Border*	1 Biscuit/15g	66	3.1	443	5.3	58.9	20.7	1.8
Oat Crunch, M & S*	1 Biscuit/14g	65	2.7	450	7.8	62.0	18.7	6.1
Oat Crunch, Weight Watchers*	1 Biscuit/12g	52	2.1	448	7.4	65.2	17.8	6.1
Oaten, Organic, Duchy Originals*	1 Biscuit/16g	71	2.7	441	9.8	62.3	16.9	5.3
Oaties, Oatland, Tesco*	1 Biscuit/15g	70	3.1	470	6.5	64.9	20.5	4.5
Oatmeal, Asda*	1 Biscuit/12g	54	2.5	470	6.0	62.0	22.0	6.0
Oatmeal Crunch, Jacob's*	1 Biscuit/8g	37	1.5	458	6.8	65.9	18.6	3.6
Oaty Thins, Rude Health*	1 Thin/6g	23	0.3	380	11.5	68.5	4.7	8.7
Party Rings, Iced, Fox's*	1 Biscuit/6g	29	0.9	459	5.1	75.8	15.0	0.0
Peanut Butter, American Style, Sainsbury's*	1 Biscuit/13g	63	2.9	504	5.2	68.7	23.1	2.2
Peanut Butter, Cups, Mini, Hershey*	1 Cup/8g	44	2.4	564	10.3	56.4	30.8	2.6
Petit Beurre, Stella Artois*	1 Biscuit/6g	26	0.9	440	9.0	73.0	15.0	0.0
Pink Wafers, Crawfords*	1 Biscuit/7g	36	1.9	521	2.5	68.6	26.5	1.1
Pink Wafers, Sainsbury's*	1 Biscuit/8g	36	1.8	486	4.6	64.2	23.4	1.7
Puffin, Chocolate, Asda*	1 Biscuit/25g	133	7.2	533	5.0	63.0	29.0	1.2
Puffin, Orange, Asda*	1 Biscuit/25g	133	7.3	529	5.0	62.0	29.0	2.2
Redcurrant Puffs, Eat Well, M & S*	1 Biscuit/7g	32	1.4	470	5.6	67.7	19.8	2.0
Rich Tea, Average	1 Biscuit/10g	45	1.5	451	6.8	72.8	14.5	2.5
Rich Tea, BGTY, Sainsbury's*	1 Biscuit/10g	43	1.1	430	7.8	75.9	10.6	2.4
Rich Tea, Chocolate, Milk, Sainsbury's*	1 Biscuit/13g	66	3.0	504	6.3	68.5	22.7	2.1
Rich Tea, Chocolate, Plain, Sainsbury's*	1 Biscuit/13g	65	3.0	497	6.6	66.0	23.0	2.6
Rich Tea, Chocolate Covered, Milk, Cadbury*	1 Biscuit/12g	60	2.6	490	6.6	67.6	21.4	0.0
Rich Tea, Classic, McVitie's*	1 Biscuit/8g	38	1.3	453	7.1	71.2	15.5	2.9
Rich Tea, Finger, Essential, Waitrose*	1 Biscuit/5g	22	0.7	450	7.2	72.5	14.3	3.0
Rich Tea, Finger, Tesco*	1 Finger/5g	23	0.7	451	7.4	72.9	14.4	2.3
Rich Tea, Light, McVitie's*	1 Biscuit/8g	36	0.9	436	7.6	75.3	10.7	3.1

	Measure INFO/WEIGHT	per Measure KCAL	FAT	Nutrition Values per 100g / 100ml KCAL	PROT	CARB	FAT	FIBRE
BISCUITS								
Rich Tea, Low Fat, M & S*	1 Biscuit/9g	40	1.0	435	8.3	76.7	10.5	2.4
Rocky, Chocolate, Fox's*	1 Biscuit/21g	106	5.4	505	5.7	62.4	25.7	2.4
Rocky, Chocolate & Caramel, Fox's*	1 Biscuit/21g	107	4.1	507	6.9	60.3	19.3	15.5
Rocky, Funki Fudge, Fox's*	1 Biscuit/24g	125	6.6	520	6.9	60.3	27.7	1.1
Rocky, Rounds, Caramel, Fox's*	1 Biscuit/15g	72	3.4	480	6.2	62.3	22.9	1.1
Rocky, Rounds, Chocolate, Fox's*	1 Biscuit/6g	31	1.7	517	7.2	58.5	28.3	1.6
Rolo, Nestle*	1 Biscuit/18g	95	4.7	507	4.4	64.2	25.2	0.6
Rosemary & Raisin, M & S*	1 Biscuit/7g	35	1.7	490	5.1	62.5	24.1	1.8
Rosemary & Thyme, Savoury, Weight Watchers*	1 Biscuit/8g	34	1.5	419	8.1	55.0	18.8	13.1
Savoury, Gluten, Wheat & Dairy Free, Sainsbury's*	1 Biscuit/17g	77	2.9	467	11.7	65.1	17.7	2.4
Savoury, Organic, M & S*	1 Biscuit/7g	28	1.0	395	7.0	58.4	14.6	8.7
Shortcake, Average	1 Biscuit/11g	55	3.0	501	6.3	66.1	27.1	2.1
Shortcake, Caramel, Average	1 Biscuit/37g	183	10.5	494	4.8	54.7	28.3	0.8
Shortcake, Caramel, Mr Kipling*	1 Biscuit/36g	182	10.4	506	4.2	57.6	28.8	1.3
Shortcake, Crawfords*	1 Biscuit/10g	52	2.5	504	6.2	63.5	24.4	2.6
Shortcake, Dutch, M & S*	1 Biscuit/17g	90	5.1	540	5.4	59.0	30.8	2.5
Shortcake, Fruit, Crawfords*	1 Biscuit/8g	34	1.5	419	5.4	55.9	19.3	2.4
Shortcake, Jacob's*	1 Biscuit/10g	48	2.2	485	6.7	65.6	21.8	2.0
Shortcake, Mini Pack, Paterson's*	1 Biscuit/17g	82	4.2	490	5.5	60.8	25.0	3.2
Shortcake, Organic, Waitrose*	1 Biscuit/13g	64	3.2	495	5.8	63.0	24.4	1.8
Shortcake, Ring, Creations, Fox's*	1 Biscuit/20g	105	5.6	515	7.8	59.1	27.4	1.0
Shortcake, Rounds, Value, Tesco*	1 Biscuit/22g	120	7.0	540	5.5	58.8	31.4	2.1
Shortcake, Snack, Cadbury*	2 Biscuits/15g	70	3.7	475	7.0	54.5	25.0	1.7
Shorties, Cadbury*	1 Biscuit/15g	77	3.6	511	6.5	67.3	24.0	0.0
Shorties, Fruit, Value, Tesco*	1 Serving/10g	46	1.7	457	5.7	69.3	17.4	3.0
Shorties, Rich Highland, Tesco*	1 Biscuit/10g	48	2.2	485	6.1	65.3	21.7	2.6
Shorties, Sainsbury's*	1 Biscuit/10g	50	2.2	500	6.4	69.8	21.8	2.0
Signature Collection, Cadbury*	1 Biscuit/15g	80	4.4	530	6.2	60.1	29.5	0.0
Spiced, Whole Wheat, Prodia*	1 Biscuit/5g	17	1.0	339	7.1	41.4	19.4	8.5
Sports, Fox's*	1 Biscuit/9g	41	1.7	483	6.7	67.0	20.0	2.0
Stem Ginger, Brakes*	1 Biscuit/13g	62	3.1	495	5.6	62.6	24.7	0.0
Vanilla, Ser*	1 Biscuit/4g	14	0.3	408	8.5	77.0	8.2	3.0
Viennese, Bronte*	1 Biscuit/25g	106	6.2	424	4.4	45.6	24.8	0.0
Viennese, Chocolate, Melts, Fox's*	1 Biscuit/12g	64	3.4	526	6.1	60.5	28.3	2.4
Viennese, Jaffa, M & S*	1 Biscuit/17g	80	3.7	465	5.9	61.1	21.7	0.9
Viennese, Mini Pack, Paterson's*	1 Biscuit/20g	106	6.2	527	5.4	67.1	30.8	1.6
Viennese, Raspberry & Cream, Melts, Fox's*	1 Biscuit/16g	84	4.5	521	4.0	62.1	28.1	1.7
Viennese Creams, Raspberry, M & S*	1 Biscuit/17g	90	4.9	520	4.6	60.4	28.6	1.3
Viennese Creams, Strawberry, M & S*	1 Biscuit/17g	80	3.7	485	6.4	63.0	22.2	1.7
Viennese Finger, Mr Kipling*	1 Finger/32g	167	10.2	523	4.3	54.9	31.8	0.0
Viennese Whirl, Chocolate, Border*	1 Biscuit/19g	96	4.3	512	6.5	61.9	23.2	0.0
Viennese Whirl, Fox's*	1 Biscuit/25g	130	7.0	518	6.7	60.1	27.8	0.0
Wafer, Vanilla, Loacker*	1 Pack/45g	231	12.6	514	7.5	58.0	28.0	0.0
Water, Average	1 Biscuit/6g	24	0.7	440	10.8	75.8	12.5	3.1
Water, High Bake, Jacob's*	1 Biscuit/5g	22	0.4	414	10.5	76.4	7.4	3.0
Water, Table, Large, Carr's*	1 Biscuit/8g	31	0.6	408	9.9	73.1	7.5	4.1
Water, Table, Small, Carr's*	1 Biscuit/3g	14	0.3	406	10.1	80.0	7.6	4.2
Yorkie, Nestle*	1 Biscuit/25g	128	6.7	510	6.7	60.4	26.8	1.3
BISON								
Raw	***1oz/28g***	***31***	***0.5***	***109***	***21.6***	***0.0***	***1.8***	***0.0***
BITTER LEMON								
Fever-Tree*	1 Glass/200ml	77	0.0	38	0.0	9.2	0.0	0.0
Low Calorie, Tesco*	1 Glass/200ml	6	0.2	3	0.1	0.3	0.1	0.1

	Measure INFO/WEIGHT	per Measure KCAL	FAT	Nutrition Values per 100g / 100ml KCAL	PROT	CARB	FAT	FIBRE
BITTER LEMON								
Sainsbury's*	1 Glass/250ml	45	0.2	18	0.1	4.4	0.1	0.1
Schweppes*	1 Glass/250ml	85	0.0	34	0.0	8.2	0.0	0.0
BLACK GRAM								
Urad Gram, Dried, Raw	***1oz/28g***	***77***	***0.4***	***275***	***24.9***	***40.8***	***1.4***	***0.0***
BLACK PUDDING								
Average, Uncooked	***1 Serving/40g***	***101***	***6.0***	***252***	***10.2***	***19.0***	***14.9***	***0.6***
Slices, Grilled, Asda*	1 Slice/36g	150	10.7	417	13.3	23.2	29.7	1.9
VLH Kitchens	1 Serving/40g	105	39.0	262	11.0	20.3	15.6	0.4
BLACKBERRIES								
Fresh, Raw, Average	***1oz/28g***	***7***	***0.1***	***25***	***0.9***	***5.1***	***0.2***	***3.1***
Frozen, Average	1 Serving/80g	37	0.1	46	0.9	9.6	0.2	2.9
in Fruit Juice, Average	***½ Can/145g***	***52***	***0.3***	***36***	***0.6***	***7.9***	***0.2***	***1.3***
BLACKCURRANTS								
Dried, Graze*	1 Pack/30g	95	0.3	317	3.3	79.0	1.0	0.0
Fresh, Raw, Fresh	***1 Serving/80g***	***22***	***0.0***	***28***	***0.9***	***6.6***	***0.0***	***3.6***
in Fruit Juice, Average	***1 Serving/30g***	***11***	***0.0***	***38***	***0.6***	***8.6***	***0.2***	***2.4***
Stewed with Sugar	***1oz/28g***	***16***	***0.0***	***58***	***0.7***	***15.0***	***0.0***	***2.8***
Stewed without Sugar	***1oz/28g***	***7***	***0.0***	***24***	***0.8***	***5.6***	***0.0***	***3.1***
BLINIS								
Cocktail, M & S*	½ Pack/81g	154	1.9	190	6.3	35.9	2.3	2.0
Sausage, Cocktail, Waitrose*	1 Blini/16g	30	0.4	190	6.3	35.9	2.3	2.0
Smoked Salmon, M & S*	1oz/28g	67	3.6	240	11.9	18.9	13.0	1.8
BLUEBERRIES								
Chocolate Covered, Waitrose*	1 Serving/25g	120	5.6	481	4.0	65.6	22.4	3.0
Dried, Whitworths*	1 Pack/75g	226	0.1	301	0.9	74.2	0.1	11.4
Dried & Sweetened, Sainsbury's*	1oz/28g	77	0.2	275	1.7	65.7	0.6	11.7
Fresh, Raw, Average	30 Berries/50g	29	0.2	57	0.8	14.5	0.3	2.4
Frozen, Average	1 Serving/80g	41	0.2	51	0.6	13.8	0.2	4.4
Organic, Tesco*	1 Punnet/150g	102	0.4	68	0.7	14.5	0.3	2.4
BOAR								
Wild, Raw, Average	***1 Serving/200g***	***244***	***6.7***	***122***	***21.5***	***0.0***	***3.3***	***0.0***
BOILED SWEETS								
Average	1 Sweet/7g	21	0.0	327	0.0	87.1	0.0	0.0
Cough Sweets, Fundays, Bassett's*	1oz/28g	107	0.0	383	0.0	94.9	0.0	0.0
Lockets, Mars*	1 Pack/43g	165	0.0	383	0.0	95.8	0.0	0.0
Mentho-Lyptus, Cherry, Sugar Free, Hall's*	1 Lozenge/4g	8	0.0	234	0.0	62.4	0.0	0.0
Mentho-Lyptus, Extra Strong, Hall's*	1 Lozenge/4g	14	0.0	389	0.0	96.9	0.0	0.0
Soothers, Blackcurrant, Hall's*	1 Lozenge/5g	16	0.0	365	0.0	91.4	0.0	0.0
Soothers, Cherry, Hall's*	1 Pack/45g	165	0.0	365	0.0	91.3	0.0	0.0
Soothers, Strawberry Flavour, Hall's*	1 Sweet/5g	19	0.0	385	0.0	96.0	0.0	0.0
BOLOGNESE								
Al Forno, Charlie Bigham's*	½ Pack/325g	514	27.0	158	7.8	11.8	8.3	0.8
Al Forno, Weight Watchers*	1 Pack/354g	312	6.7	88	6.6	10.3	1.9	1.8
Beef, 2 Minute Meals, Sainsbury's*	1 Pack/200g	144	7.2	72	4.2	5.6	3.6	1.8
Beef, Asda*	1 Pack/392g	412	19.6	105	8.0	7.0	5.0	0.0
Beef, Diet Chef Ltd*	1 Serving/300g	246	6.9	82	7.7	7.6	2.3	3.4
Meatless, Granose*	1 Pack/400g	400	16.0	100	8.0	8.0	4.0	0.0
Penne, Heinz*	1 Pack/300g	213	2.7	71	3.8	11.8	0.9	0.6
Shells, Italiana, Weight Watchers*	1 Can/395g	280	5.1	71	5.2	9.6	1.3	0.7
Tagliatelle, Weight Watchers*	1 Serving/300g	300	5.4	100	5.5	15.4	1.8	0.1
Vegetarian, M & S*	1 Pack/360g	360	12.6	100	4.5	12.5	3.5	2.1
Vegetarian, Vegelicious, Tesco*	1 Pack/400g	420	10.8	105	4.6	14.9	2.7	2.0

	Measure INFO/WEIGHT	per Measure KCAL	FAT	Nutrition Values per 100g / 100ml KCAL	PROT	CARB	FAT	FIBRE
BOMBAY MIX								
Average	1oz/28g	141	9.2	503	18.8	35.1	32.9	6.2
Suma*	½ Pack/125g	595	35.6	476	13.6	41.2	28.5	10.1
BON BONS								
Bassett's*	1 Sweet/7g	28	0.5	417	1.1	85.4	7.5	0.0
BOOST								
Bar, Cadbury*	1 Bar/61g	305	17.0	510	5.8	57.0	28.5	0.9
Treat Size, Cadbury*	1 Bar/24g	130	7.4	535	5.3	59.6	30.5	0.0
with Glucose, Cadbury*	1 Bar/61g	315	17.8	521	5.6	58.0	29.4	4.0
with Glucose & Guarana, Cadbury*	1 Bar/61g	314	18.0	515	5.5	56.7	29.5	0.0
BOUILLABAISSE								
Average	1 Serving/400g	556	38.8	139	11.2	2.0	9.7	0.4
BOUILLON								
Beef, Benedicta*	1 fl oz/30ml	22	0.2	73	7.5	9.5	0.5	0.0
Chicken, Benedicta*	1 fl oz/30ml	22	0.9	75	4.0	8.0	3.0	5.6
Powder, Miso, Marigold*	1 Tsp/5g	12	0.5	248	7.0	34.0	9.3	1.4
Powder, Swiss Vegetable, Green Tub, Marigold*	1 Tsp/5g	12	0.4	243	10.5	29.4	8.1	0.7
Vegetable, Benedicta*	1 fl oz/30ml	30	0.1	101	7.5	17.0	0.3	0.0
BOUNTY								
Dark, Mars*	1 Funsize/29g	142	8.0	488	3.7	55.7	27.6	0.0
Milk, Mars*	1 Funsize/29g	137	7.4	471	3.7	56.4	25.6	0.0
BOUQUET GARNI								
Handtied, Fresh, Asda*	1 Bunch/2g	11	0.2	455	8.3	69.4	7.9	31.6
BOURNVITA*								
Powder, Made Up with Semi-Skimmed Milk	1 Mug/227ml	132	3.6	58	3.5	7.8	1.6	0.0
Powder, Made Up with Whole Milk	1 Mug/227ml	173	8.6	76	3.4	7.6	3.8	0.0
BOVRIL*								
Beef Extract, Drink, Made Up with Water, Bovril*	1 Serving/12g	22	0.1	184	38.9	4.6	1.2	0.0
Chicken Savoury Drink, Bovril*	1 Serving/13g	16	0.2	129	9.7	19.4	1.4	2.1
BRANDY								
37.5% Volume, Average	***1 Shot/35ml***	***72***	***0.0***	***207***	***0.0***	***0.0***	***0.0***	***0.0***
40% Volume, Average	***1 Shot/35ml***	***78***	***0.0***	***224***	***0.0***	***0.0***	***0.0***	***0.0***
Cherry, Average	***1 Shot/35ml***	***89***	***0.0***	***255***	***0.0***	***32.6***	***0.0***	***0.0***
BRAZIL NUTS								
Average	***6 Whole/20g***	***136***	***13.7***	***682***	***15.3***	***2.8***	***68.4***	***5.4***
Chocolate, Milk, Tesco*	1 Nut/8g	47	3.5	585	9.9	38.0	43.7	1.9
BREAD								
50/50, Wholemeal & White, Medium Sliced, Kingsmill*	1 Slice/40g	94	0.9	235	9.9	41.2	2.3	4.9
Bagel, 4 Everything, Finest, Tesco*	1 Bagel/100g	268	1.8	268	11.1	51.9	1.8	2.5
Bagel, Blueberry, Sara Lee*	1 Bagel/104g	290	1.5	279	9.6	58.6	1.4	1.9
Bagel, Cinnamon & Raisin, New York Bagel Co*	1 Bagel/90g	231	1.0	257	10.1	49.9	1.1	3.6
Bagel, Cranberry & Orange, New York Bakery Co*	1 Bagel/90g	246	2.3	273	9.6	51.0	2.5	3.9
Bagel, Fruit & Fibre, Kingsmill*	1 Bagel/85g	225	1.2	265	9.8	50.8	1.4	5.2
Bagel, Fruit & Spice, Sainsbury's*	1 Bagel/85g	234	1.8	275	9.7	54.3	2.1	3.8
Bagel, Granary, Bagel Factory*	1 Bagel/100g	288	2.1	288	11.9	57.4	2.1	4.5
Bagel, Multi Seed, New York Bagel Co*	1 Bagel/90g	244	4.3	271	12.4	41.6	4.8	5.8
Bagel, Multigrain, Sainsbury's*	1 Bagel/113g	293	3.5	259	10.0	49.6	3.1	2.0
Bagel, Onion, New York Bagel Co*	1 Bagel/85g	222	1.6	261	10.6	50.4	1.9	3.1
Bagel, Onion, Red, & Chive, New York Bakery Co.*	1 Bagel/90g	225	1.2	250	10.4	47.2	1.3	3.8
Bagel, Onion & Poppy Seed, Average	1 Bagel/85g	225	2.8	264	9.0	50.5	3.3	3.2
Bagel, Original, Organic, New York Bagel Co*	1 Bagel/85g	220	1.2	259	9.3	52.2	1.4	4.1
Bagel, Plain, Average	***1 Bagel/78g***	***202***	***1.5***	***259***	***10.1***	***50.4***	***1.9***	***3.1***
Bagel, Plain, Free From, Tesco*	1 Bagel/80g	215	5.5	270	3.4	47.7	6.9	4.7
Bagel, Plain, GFY, Asda*	1 Bagel/84g	218	1.8	259	10.0	50.0	2.1	1.8

	Measure INFO/WEIGHT	per Measure KCAL	FAT	Nutrition Values per 100g / 100ml KCAL	PROT	CARB	FAT	FIBRE
BREAD								
Bagel, Plain, New York Bagel Co*	1 Bagel/90g	230	1.7	255	9.1	50.4	1.9	2.9
Bagel, Plain, Organic, Tesco*	1 Bagel/85g	216	2.3	254	9.0	48.4	2.7	3.6
Bagel, Poppy Seed, New York Bagel Co*	1 Bagel/85g	233	2.4	274	11.4	50.8	2.8	3.2
Bagel, Rye, Bagel Factory*	1 Bagel/85g	279	1.3	329	14.5	64.3	1.6	6.2
Bagel, Sesame, M & S*	1 Bagel/87g	240	2.8	275	10.2	51.2	3.2	2.1
Bagel, Sesame, New York Bagel Co*	1 Bagel/85g	226	2.6	266	10.3	49.2	3.1	4.0
Bagel, Sesame Seed, Essential, Waitrose*	1 Bagel/85g	243	2.7	286	9.6	54.6	3.2	3.6
Bagel, Sesame Seed, GFY, Asda*	1 Bagel/84g	227	2.1	271	11.0	51.0	2.5	2.6
Bagel, Soda, Round, Genesis Crafty*	1 Bagel/135g	307	5.3	227	6.9	41.3	3.9	2.9
Bagel, White, Original, Weight Watchers*	1 Bagel/67g	158	0.5	236	9.5	42.4	0.8	10.7
Bagel, Wholemeal, Average	1 Bagel/90g	235	2.7	261	12.7	44.6	3.0	7.7
Bagel, Wholemeal, Multiseed, M & S*	1 Bagel/84g	215	5.6	255	13.1	35.4	6.6	8.3
Bagel, Wholemeal, New York Bagel Co*	1 Bagel/90g	223	2.1	248	11.4	41.5	2.3	7.5
Baguette, Crusty Brown, M & S*	½ Loaf/71g	160	1.1	225	9.8	42.7	1.6	6.3
Baguette, Granary, Average	1 Serving/100g	250	2.8	250	20.0	46.0	2.8	6.0
Baguette, Part Baked, Half, Tesco*	½ Baguette/75g	180	0.9	240	7.8	49.5	1.2	3.4
Baguette, Sourdough, la Brea Bakery*	1 Serving/60g	160	0.4	266	8.8	56.1	0.7	1.8
Baguette, White, Half, Crusty, M & S*	1 Baguette/162g	420	1.8	260	8.4	53.5	1.1	2.3
Baguette, White, Ready to Bake, Asda*	1 Serving/60g	168	1.1	280	10.0	56.0	1.8	2.6
Baps, Brown, Large, Asda*	1 Bap/58g	140	0.9	242	10.0	47.0	1.6	0.0
Baps, Brown, Malted Grain, Large, Tesco*	1 Bap/93g	228	3.1	245	9.9	42.7	3.3	5.3
Baps, Cheese Top, Sainsbury's*	1 Bap/75g	218	6.4	291	12.1	41.6	8.5	2.0
Baps, Floured, M & S*	1 Bap/60g	168	3.7	280	11.5	46.8	6.2	2.0
Baps, Malted, Large, Co-Op*	1 Bap/85g	208	2.6	245	10.2	44.3	3.1	5.0
Baps, Multigrain, Tesco*	1 Bap/98g	238	3.1	244	8.7	45.1	3.2	1.9
Baps, White, Average	1 Bap/65g	167	2.3	257	9.5	47.0	3.5	1.9
Baps, White, Giant, Sainsbury's*	1 Bap/86g	235	3.2	273	8.3	51.7	3.7	3.4
Baps, White, Sandwich, Kingsmill*	1 Bap/80g	209	3.2	261	10.1	46.2	4.0	2.2
Baps, White, Sliced, Large, Asda*	1 Bap/58g	148	1.0	255	10.0	50.0	1.7	0.0
Baps, White, Soft, Floured, M & S*	1 Bap/61g	175	3.4	285	11.5	46.6	5.5	2.8
Baps, White, Warburton's*	1 Bap/57g	144	2.5	252	9.8	43.4	4.3	2.7
Baps, Wholemeal, Tesco*	1 Bap/46g	104	2.4	227	9.6	41.4	5.3	5.6
Baps, Wholemeal, Village Green*	1 Bap/65g	151	2.3	232	10.0	40.0	3.5	3.8
Baps, Wholemeal, Waitrose*	1 Bap/63g	148	3.3	235	11.0	35.9	5.3	7.7
Best of Both, Farmhouse, Hovis*	1 Slice/44g	99	1.4	226	9.5	40.0	3.1	4.9
Best of Both, Thick Sliced, Hovis*	1 Slice/50g	113	0.9	224	9.0	40.4	1.8	5.0
Bloomer, COU, M & S*	1 Slice/33g	78	0.5	235	9.5	45.5	1.5	3.6
Bloomer, Multiseed, Average	1 Slice/50g	120	2.4	240	11.8	37.2	4.9	7.7
Bloomer, Soft Grain, M & S*	1 Slice/34g	80	0.5	235	9.5	45.5	1.5	3.6
Bloomer, White, Sliced, Waitrose*	1 Slice/50g	130	0.9	259	8.5	52.1	1.8	2.6
Bloomer, Wholemeal, Organic, M & S*	1 Slice/50g	110	2.1	220	10.2	35.5	4.2	6.4
Brown, Danish, Sliced, Weight Watchers*	1 Slice/20g	48	0.4	233	9.9	40.7	1.8	7.6
Brown, Danish, Weight Watchers*	1 Slice/20g	47	0.4	235	9.8	40.7	2.0	7.4
Brown, GF, Genius*	1 Slice/35g	97	4.7	277	6.7	42.2	13.3	9.5
Brown, Gluten & Wheat Free, Sliced	1 Slice/25g	56	1.3	224	3.4	41.0	5.2	9.4
Brown, Good Health, Warburton's*	1 Slice/35g	79	1.0	226	10.3	39.6	2.9	7.2
Brown, High Fibre, Ormo*	1 Slice/24g	57	0.6	239	9.2	42.9	2.6	7.5
Brown, Kingsmill Gold, Seeds & Oats, Kingsmill*	1 Slice/45g	126	4.4	280	12.2	35.6	9.8	4.9
Brown, Malted, Average	1 Slice/25g	60	0.6	242	9.4	45.5	2.4	4.2
Brown, Medium Sliced, Average	***1 Slice/34g***	***74***	***0.7***	***218***	***8.5***	***44.3***	***2.0***	***3.5***
Brown, Medium Sliced, Premium, Warburton's*	1 Slice/24g	59	0.9	249	10.5	43.2	3.7	4.3
Brown, Mixed Grain, Original, Vogel*	1 Slice/45g	102	0.6	227	9.8	47.1	1.2	6.4
Brown, Multi Grain, Wheat Free, GF	1 Slice/33g	76	1.7	229	5.1	40.8	5.1	5.6

B

	Measure INFO/WEIGHT	per Measure KCAL	FAT	Nutrition Values per 100g / 100ml KCAL	PROT	CARB	FAT	FIBRE
BREAD								
Brown, Sandwich Bread, GF, Udi's*	1 Slice/37g	79	1.1	216	5.2	39.2	2.9	6.3
Brown, Seeded Batch, Large Loaf, 800g, Warburton's*	1 Slice/46g	132	4.1	288	12.3	39.7	8.9	6.0
Brown, Sliced, by Brennans, Weight Watchers*	1 Slice/20g	51	0.4	257	9.5	45.4	2.1	6.8
Brown, Sliced, Free From, Tesco*	1 Slice/45g	121	3.7	268	5.4	43.2	8.2	3.6
Brown, Soda, M & S*	1 Slice/40g	92	1.4	229	9.2	43.6	3.6	4.9
Brown, Sunflower & Barley, Vogel*	1 Slice/42g	100	1.9	239	9.4	40.3	4.5	6.7
Brown, Thick, Warburton's*	1 Slice/38g	80	0.7	211	9.4	39.2	1.8	6.2
Brown, Toasted, Average	***1 Slice/24g***	***65***	***0.5***	***272***	***10.4***	***56.5***	***2.1***	***4.5***
Brown, Toastie, Thick Sliced, Kingsmill*	1 Slice/44g	101	1.4	230	9.5	40.5	3.3	4.7
Brown, Very Dark, Albert Heijn*	1 Slice/35g	84	1.4	240	12.0	35.0	4.0	7.4
Brown, Wholemeal, Healthy Choice, Warburton's*	1 Slice/40g	98	1.0	244	10.4	40.7	2.5	6.5
Buns, Burger, American Style, Sainsbury's*	1 Bun/50g	131	2.1	261	10.5	45.6	4.1	3.6
Buns, Burger, Giant, Sainsbury's*	1 Bun/95g	249	4.9	262	8.7	45.2	5.2	2.9
Buns, Burger, Sesame, American Style, Sainsbury's*	1 Bun/60g	162	3.8	270	7.3	46.2	6.3	2.2
Buns, White, Stay Fresh, Tesco*	1 Bun/56g	152	3.7	271	7.5	45.5	6.6	0.0
Challah, Average	***1 Slice/50g***	***143***	***3.6***	***286***	***8.9***	***53.6***	***7.1***	***3.6***
Cheese, Onion & Garlic, Tear & Share, Waitrose*	¼ Bread/112g	326	14.6	290	9.4	33.9	13.0	2.1
Cheese, Onion Mustard Seed, Cluster, Sainsbury's*	1 Cluster/100g	276	8.1	276	10.0	40.6	8.1	3.1
Cheese, Tear & Share, Tesco*	¼ Loaf/73g	225	7.8	310	8.8	44.0	10.7	0.8
Cheese & Garlic, Pizza Style, Sainsbury's*	¼ Bread/63g	199	8.1	318	10.7	39.7	13.0	2.2
Cheese & Garlic, Stonebaked, Morrisons*	¼ Bread/69g	228	9.9	331	10.9	39.5	14.4	1.9
Cheese & Onion, Tear & Share, Sainsbury's*	¼ Bread/71g	202	6.6	285	9.8	40.6	9.3	1.9
Cheese & Onion, Toastie, Warburton's*	1 Slice/42g	120	5.8	286	7.5	33.1	13.7	0.0
Cheese & Tomato, Tear & Share, Sainsbury's*	¼ Bread/72g	211	9.5	293	8.0	35.7	13.2	1.5
Cholla, Average	***1/10 Loaf/154g***	***421***	***14.3***	***274***	***6.9***	***40.8***	***9.3***	***1.0***
Ciabatta, Black Olive, Part Baked, Sainsbury's*	¼ Ciabatta/67g	172	2.5	257	8.8	46.8	3.8	2.4
Ciabatta, Finest, Tesco*	1/6 Ciabatta/45g	124	2.7	275	10.4	44.8	5.9	2.7
Ciabatta, Gluten & Wheat Free, Average	1 Slice/55g	136	1.6	248	2.0	52.4	2.9	4.2
Ciabatta, Green Olive, Tesco*	¼ Ciabatta/70g	155	3.1	222	7.4	38.2	4.4	1.9
Ciabatta, Half, M & S*	1 Ciabatta/135g	354	5.5	262	10.3	48.1	4.1	2.1
Ciabatta, Half, Organic, Sainsbury's*	½ Ciabatta/63g	152	0.6	241	9.1	48.7	1.0	2.3
Ciabatta, Half, Part Baked, TTD, Sainsbury's*	¼ Pack/67g	173	3.3	257	8.6	44.6	4.9	3.5
Ciabatta, Italian Style, Waitrose*	1 Ciabatta/89g	231	1.2	260	10.7	51.2	1.4	2.2
Ciabatta, Olive & Rosemary, Mini, Tesco*	1 Pack/75g	319	8.2	425	17.8	63.0	10.9	3.6
Ciabatta, Plain, Tesco*	¼ Ciabatta/73g	174	2.8	240	9.8	41.5	3.9	2.4
Ciabatta, Ready to Bake, M & S*	1 Serving/150g	393	6.2	262	10.3	48.1	4.1	2.1
Ciabatta, Spicy Topped, Finest, Tesco*	1 Serving/73g	163	4.0	223	9.2	34.0	5.5	1.7
Ciabatta, Sun Dried Tomato & Basil, Tesco*	¼ Ciabatta/75g	193	4.3	257	8.9	42.4	5.7	2.4
Ciabatta, Sweet Pepper, HE, Tesco*	1 Serving/50g	135	1.4	270	11.8	49.5	2.7	2.8
Ciabatta, Tomato & Basil, GFY, Asda*	1 Serving/55g	143	1.2	260	9.0	51.0	2.2	0.0
Ciabatta, Tomato & Mozzarella, Iceland*	1 Ciabatta/150g	374	15.2	249	10.0	29.6	10.1	3.3
Ciabatta, TTD, Sainsbury's*	¼ Pack/68g	185	4.0	274	10.4	44.8	5.9	2.7
Cottage Loaf, Stonebaked, Asda*	1 Serving/67g	155	0.9	232	10.0	45.0	1.3	3.2
Farl, Irish Soda, Irwin's Bakery*	1 Farl/150g	334	5.1	223	4.0	44.0	3.4	2.3
Focaccia, Onion & Herb, Tesco*	½ Pack/190g	547	23.8	288	8.7	35.2	12.5	3.7
Focaccia, Roast Cherry Tomato & Olive, GFY, Asda*	½ Pack/148g	350	6.0	237	9.0	41.0	4.1	2.8
Focaccia, Roasted Onion & Cheese, M & S*	1 Serving/89g	240	4.1	270	10.4	45.7	4.6	2.8
French	1½" Slice/45g	110	0.0	244	8.9	53.3	0.0	2.2
French, Sliced, Parisian*	2 Slices/39g	100	1.0	256	5.1	48.7	2.6	0.0
French Stick, Average	***1 Serving/60g***	***147***	***0.2***	***245***	***8.7***	***52.2***	***0.4***	***2.1***
Fruit, Continental, Schneider Brot*	1 Slice/65g	198	3.5	305	5.4	57.0	5.4	0.0
Fruit, Raisin Swirl, Sun-Maid*	1 Slice/33g	95	1.9	287	8.3	50.4	5.8	2.6
Fruit Loaf, Apple, M & S*	1 Slice/39g	100	0.6	255	8.5	51.9	1.5	3.3

B

	Measure INFO/WEIGHT	per Measure KCAL	per Measure FAT	Nutrition Values per 100g / 100ml KCAL	PROT	CARB	FAT	FIBRE
BREAD								
Fruit Loaf, Apple & Cinnamon, Soreen*	1 Serving/10g	31	0.4	307	6.9	60.5	4.2	0.0
Fruit Loaf, Banana, Lunchbox, Soreen*	1 Bar/30g	100	1.3	332	8.2	63.3	4.4	2.9
Fruit Loaf, Banana, Soreen*	1 Slice/25g	78	1.0	313	6.6	61.2	4.1	2.6
Fruit Loaf, Cinnamon & Raisin, Soreen*	1/8 Loaf/25g	77	1.0	308	7.7	54.1	4.0	4.1
Fruit Loaf, Fresh, Free From, Sainsbury's*	1 Slice/33g	93	2.5	279	3.2	45.5	7.5	8.1
Fruit Loaf, Fruity Five, Snack Pack, Soreen*	1 Pack/61g	200	5.5	329	7.1	54.9	9.0	2.7
Fruit Loaf, Luxury, Christmas, Soreen*	1 Serving/28g	85	0.6	303	4.5	66.6	2.1	0.0
Fruit Loaf, Mixed Berry, Weight Watchers*	1 Slice/34g	79	0.9	231	7.6	44.3	2.6	7.7
Fruit Loaf, Mother's Pride*	1 Slice/36g	92	1.0	256	8.2	49.3	2.9	2.6
Fruit Loaf, Plum, Lincolnshire, Soreen*	1 Slice/25g	65	0.8	261	8.4	49.3	3.4	2.1
Fruit Loaf, Sliced, Asda*	1 Serving/33g	89	1.2	269	8.0	51.0	3.7	2.9
Fruit Loaf, Sultana & Cherry, Sainsbury's*	1 Slice/50g	178	6.1	357	2.7	59.0	12.2	1.7
Fruit Loaf, Toasted, Cafe Instore, Asda*	1 Slice/33g	89	1.2	269	8.0	51.0	3.7	2.9
Garlic, & Cheese, Tesco*	1 Serving/143g	490	24.0	343	9.4	38.5	16.8	2.0
Garlic, & Herb, Giant Feast, Sainsbury's*	1 Serving/50g	158	6.4	317	8.0	42.1	12.9	2.6
Garlic, & Herb, Tear & Share, Tesco*	1 Serving/73g	218	9.2	300	6.3	40.0	12.7	1.7
Garlic, & Tomato, Pizza, Italiano, Tesco*	½ Bread/140g	405	15.1	289	7.5	40.5	10.8	2.5
Garlic, 25% Less Fat, Sainsbury's*	½ Baguette/85g	268	11.9	315	7.8	39.4	14.0	3.1
Garlic, 30% Less Fat, Morrisons*	1 Serving/80g	231	7.4	289	7.9	43.8	9.2	2.7
Garlic, Average	1 Serving/100g	327	13.8	327	8.1	43.7	13.8	1.4
Garlic, Baguette, Average	1 Slice/20g	66	2.8	330	7.8	43.1	14.2	1.8
Garlic, Baguette, Extra Strong, Italiano, Tesco*	¼ Baguette/53g	178	8.7	340	7.9	39.8	16.6	2.8
Garlic, Baguette, Frozen, GFY, Asda*	¼ Baguette/48g	132	4.3	277	7.0	42.0	9.0	2.7
Garlic, Baguette, GFY, Asda*	¼ Baguette/43g	106	2.7	249	8.1	39.9	6.3	2.1
Garlic, Baguette, Good Choice, Iceland*	1/3 Baguette/54g	158	4.6	292	8.7	45.1	8.5	2.9
Garlic, Baguette, Italiano, Tesco*	¼ Baguette/53g	186	9.9	355	6.9	39.2	18.8	2.4
Garlic, Baguette, LC, Tesco*	¼ Baguette/52g	130	2.9	250	7.0	42.2	5.5	2.4
Garlic, Baguette, Mediterranean Herb, Tesco*	¼ Baguette/54g	181	8.8	335	6.9	40.3	16.3	2.3
Garlic, Baguette, Organic, Tesco*	1 Serving/60g	192	8.1	320	8.5	41.1	13.5	2.5
Garlic, Baguette, Reduced Fat, Average	¼ Baguette/40g	102	2.6	256	7.9	41.6	6.4	2.6
Garlic, Baguette, Slices, Tesco*	1 Serving/60g	187	9.2	312	9.8	33.8	15.3	1.7
Garlic, Baguette, White, Homebake, Tesco*	1/3 Baguette/55g	160	5.5	290	7.0	43.1	10.0	1.9
Garlic, Ciabatta, & Herb Butter, Sainsbury's*	½ Ciabatta/105g	345	16.3	329	8.5	38.8	15.5	0.0
Garlic, Ciabatta, BGTY, Sainsbury's*	½ Ciabatta/105g	306	13.0	291	8.7	36.2	12.4	2.7
Garlic, Ciabatta, Finest, Tesco*	1 Serving/65g	205	8.9	316	8.1	40.1	13.7	2.4
Garlic, Ciabatta, Hand Stretched, Sainsbury's*	¼ Pack/75g	244	10.6	325	8.4	41.0	14.1	2.9
Garlic, Ciabatta, Italiano, Tesco*	1 Ciabatta/65g	211	9.4	324	7.7	40.9	14.4	2.2
Garlic, Ciabatta, TTD, Sainsbury's*	1 Serving/67g	199	8.1	298	8.3	38.7	12.2	3.1
Garlic, Ciabatta, with Herbs, Weight Watchers*	1 Pack/88g	216	3.5	245	9.2	43.0	4.0	2.9
Garlic, Finest, Tesco*	¼ Loaf/60g	187	7.9	311	7.7	40.3	13.2	1.8
Garlic, Flatbread, BGTY, Sainsbury's*	¼ Bread/56g	177	5.7	316	9.6	46.6	10.1	2.7
Garlic, Flatbread, Tesco*	1 Serving/83g	249	8.6	302	6.7	45.3	10.4	3.0
Garlic, Focaccia, & Herb, Italian Style, Morrisons*	1/6 Focaccia/76g	259	10.9	341	8.5	44.7	14.3	2.5
Garlic, Focaccia, & Onion, GFY, Asda*	¼ Focaccia/55g	150	2.2	272	12.0	47.0	4.0	0.0
Garlic, Focaccia, & Rosemary, Sainsbury's*	¼ Focaccia/75g	219	7.4	292	8.0	43.0	9.8	2.8
Garlic, Foccacia, & Rosemary, Tesco*	¼ Loaf/73g	193	4.9	266	9.0	42.1	6.8	3.7
Garlic, GFY, Asda*	1 Slice/31g	108	1.4	350	12.0	65.0	4.5	4.0
Garlic, Organic, Waitrose*	1 Baguette/170g	536	23.3	315	8.7	39.1	13.7	1.8
Garlic, Reduced Fat, Waitrose*	1 Pack/170g	551	18.7	324	6.9	49.4	11.0	0.9
Garlic, Slices, 50 % Less Fat, Asda*	1 Slice/29g	75	1.1	262	7.9	47.1	3.9	3.2
Garlic, Slices, Asda*	1 Slice/27g	88	3.3	328	8.0	46.2	12.4	2.8
Garlic, Slices, BGTY, Sainsbury's*	1 Slice/27g	82	2.2	305	9.4	48.9	8.0	2.9
Garlic, Slices, Chilled, Sainsbury's*	1 Pack/368g	1369	60.0	372	9.1	47.3	16.3	3.2

	Measure INFO/WEIGHT	per Measure KCAL	FAT	Nutrition Values per 100g / 100ml KCAL	PROT	CARB	FAT	FIBRE
BREAD								
Garlic, Slices, HL, Tesco*	1 Slice/52g	131	2.2	251	8.6	44.6	4.2	2.6
Garlic, Slices, Italian, Chilled, Tesco*	1 Slice/27g	110	6.0	415	6.2	46.8	22.4	2.7
Garlic, Slices, LC, Tesco*	1 Slice/30g	75	1.7	250	7.3	42.3	5.7	2.9
Garlic, Stonebaked, M & S*	1 Loaf/85g	264	10.1	310	9.3	41.4	11.9	3.1
Garlic, to Share, M & S*	¼ Loaf/82g	230	10.7	280	6.5	33.2	13.0	1.3
Garlic, with Cheese, Asda*	1 Slice/34g	130	6.1	382	11.0	44.0	18.0	0.0
Garlic & Cheese, Slices, Tesco*	1 Slice/31g	118	5.2	380	11.7	43.9	16.8	2.0
Garlic & Gruyere, Fougasse, TTD, Sainsbury's*	¼ Bread/76g	219	6.8	288	9.5	42.6	8.9	2.9
Garlic & Herb, Ciabatta, GFY, Asda*	¼ Ciabatta/60g	137	1.4	230	8.8	43.2	2.4	1.0
Garlic & Herb, Tear & Share, Chosen By You, Asda*	¼ Portion/63g	185	6.7	295	9.2	39.0	10.7	2.7
Granary, Average	***1 Slice/35g***	***85***	***1.0***	***242***	***9.8***	***44.0***	***2.8***	***4.8***
Granary, Country, Multiseeded, Hovis*	1 Slice/44g	96	1.3	218	11.1	37.0	2.9	6.5
Granary, Malted, Medium Brown, Asda*	1 Slice/35g	81	0.9	231	9.0	43.0	2.6	3.3
Granary, Oatmeal, Hovis*	1 Slice/44g	104	0.9	236	9.2	45.3	2.1	3.1
Granary, Original, All Sizes, Hovis*	1 Slice/33g	85	0.8	256	10.6	46.4	2.4	3.7
Granary, Seeded, Sunflower, Hovis*	1 Slice/44g	119	2.5	271	10.1	44.9	5.7	2.9
Granary, White, Hovis*	1 Slice/44g	102	1.5	233	9.7	40.8	3.5	5.6
Granary, White, Seeded, Medium Sliced, Hovis*	1 Slice/44g	109	1.8	248	10.9	41.7	4.2	3.8
Granary, Wholemeal, Average	1 Slice/35g	80	0.9	228	10.8	38.4	2.6	6.6
Granary, Wholemeal, Hovis*	1 Slice/44g	104	1.1	237	10.6	39.8	2.4	6.8
Granary, Wholemeal, Seeded, Medium Sliced, Hovis*	1 Slice/44g	104	1.1	237	10.6	39.8	2.4	6.8
Half Wheat Rye, The Polish Bakery, Tesco*	1 Slice/44g	140	0.7	319	8.0	38.3	1.7	0.0
Hi Bran, M & S*	1 Slice/26g	55	0.8	210	12.6	32.5	3.0	6.3
Hi Fibre, Seed, Lifefibre*	1 Slice/35g	109	3.5	313	12.5	43.6	10.1	2.7
High Bran, M & S*	1 Slice/26g	60	0.8	230	13.4	34.2	3.0	7.4
Juvela*	1 Slice/25g	60	0.8	240	3.3	50.0	3.0	1.7
Khobez, Flatbread, White, Dina Foods Ltd*	1 Bread/56g	158	0.6	282	10.5	57.5	1.1	3.0
Malt Loaf, Chocolatey, Soreen*	1/8 Loaf/28g	95	1.7	344	8.0	58.7	6.3	5.1
Malt Loaf, Family, Asda*	1 Serving/20g	54	0.3	270	8.0	56.0	1.5	5.0
Malt Loaf, Fruited, Sliced, Weight Watchers*	1 Slice/23g	68	0.4	294	8.9	60.2	1.9	3.6
Malt Loaf, Fruited, Weight Watchers*	1 Serving/23g	68	0.4	294	8.9	60.2	1.9	3.6
Malt Loaf, Organic, Tesco*	1 Slice/28g	82	0.6	292	7.2	61.2	2.0	2.3
Malt Loaf, Sticky, M & S*	1 Slice/16g	47	0.4	295	6.9	64.9	2.3	3.1
Malt Loaf, Weight Watchers*	1 Slice/23g	68	0.4	294	8.9	60.2	1.9	3.6
Malted, Brown, Slice, BGTY, Sainsbury's*	1 Slice/22g	53	0.6	239	12.1	41.4	2.8	5.8
Malted, Brown, Thick Sliced, Organic, Tesco*	1 Slice/44g	111	0.9	249	8.9	48.8	2.0	3.5
Malted, Crusty, Sainsbury's*	1 Slice/42g	109	1.4	259	8.6	48.6	3.3	4.4
Malted, Danish, Sliced, Weight Watchers*	1 Slice/20g	51	0.3	249	11.8	45.1	1.5	4.2
Malted, Danish, Weight Watchers*	1 Slice/20g	49	0.3	241	12.3	44.5	1.7	4.3
Malted, Farmhouse, Morrisons*	1 Serving/40g	94	0.7	235	9.1	45.6	1.8	4.7
Malted, Grain, Co-Op*	1 Slice/43g	99	0.9	230	8.0	46.0	2.0	3.0
Malted, Grain, Good As Gold, Kingsmill*	1 Slice/47g	114	1.2	243	9.5	45.4	2.6	4.2
Malted, Oat, Duchy Originals*	1 Serving/80g	195	3.0	244	8.8	43.6	3.8	3.7
Malted, Sunblest*	1 Serving/45g	115	1.0	256	9.9	49.1	2.2	3.8
Malted, Wheatgrain, Roberts Bakery*	1 Slice/30g	80	1.0	265	11.0	48.0	3.3	3.6
Malted & Seeded, Batch, Organic, Waitrose*	1 Slice/50g	118	2.0	236	10.9	39.5	3.9	6.2
Mediterranean Style, M & S*	1/6 Loaf/48g	150	5.3	315	10.9	42.5	11.1	1.2
Milk Roll, Warburton's*	1 Slice/18g	46	0.5	253	11.0	45.1	2.7	2.7
Mixed Seed, Organic, Duchy Originals*	1 Slice/43g	114	3.4	269	10.9	39.1	8.1	5.3
Multi Seeded Loaf, Gluten & Wheat Free, Lovemore*	1 Serving/35g	102	4.3	291	0.0	3.0	12.3	0.0
Multigrain, Batch, Finest, Tesco*	1 Slice/50g	117	1.4	235	10.8	40.4	2.9	5.5
Multigrain, Brennans*	1 Slice/40g	110	1.3	275	8.8	48.0	3.3	6.3
Multigrain, Brown, Farmhouse Baker's, M & S*	1 Slice/51g	115	2.8	225	13.0	31.2	5.4	5.1

	Measure INFO/WEIGHT	per Measure KCAL	FAT	Nutrition Values per 100g / 100ml KCAL	PROT	CARB	FAT	FIBRE
BREAD								
Multigrain, Crusty, Finest, Tesco*	1 Slice/40g	98	1.4	245	9.0	44.7	3.4	5.0
Multigrain, GF, Sainsbury's*	1 Slice/17g	39	0.8	229	5.1	40.8	5.0	5.6
Multigrain, Sliced, Fresh & Easy*	1 Slice/40g	110	1.0	275	10.0	52.5	2.5	5.0
Multigrain, Soft Batch, Sainsbury's*	1 Slice/44g	106	2.9	242	11.3	34.5	6.5	5.6
Multigrain, Sunblest*	1 Slice/30g	76	0.8	254	9.0	47.0	2.5	4.5
Multigrain, Tesco*	1 Slice/31g	66	1.0	214	11.1	36.8	3.2	8.9
Multiseed, Farmhouse, Finest, Tesco*	1 Slice/50g	135	3.8	270	12.5	37.0	7.7	5.8
Multiseed, Low GI, Percy Ingle*	1 Slice/35g	99	3.1	283	0.0	0.0	8.9	6.0
Multiseed Farmhouse Batch, Finest, Tesco*	1 Slice/44g	108	1.9	245	9.9	40.4	4.4	7.5
Naan, Average	***1 Naan/130g***	***344***	***5.6***	***264***	***8.3***	***48.5***	***4.3***	***2.0***
Naan, Chilli & Mango, Finest, Tesco*	½ Naan/90g	230	5.1	255	8.4	41.9	5.7	3.2
Naan, Fresh, BGTY, Sainsbury's*	1 Serving/150g	368	4.6	245	9.4	44.9	3.1	2.2
Naan, Garlic & Coriander, Free From, Tesco*	1 Naan/90g	215	6.0	240	5.1	38.7	6.7	4.9
Naan, Garlic & Coriander, Fresh, Sharwood's*	1oz/28g	71	0.9	252	7.7	47.8	3.3	2.2
Naan, Garlic & Coriander, Large, TTD, Sainsbury's*	¼ Pack/70g	194	3.8	277	9.4	47.7	5.4	2.2
Naan, Garlic & Coriander, M & S*	1 Naan/150g	375	2.1	250	9.8	50.1	1.4	2.0
Naan, Garlic & Coriander, Mild, Patak's*	1 Naan/140g	452	15.1	323	9.0	47.5	10.8	0.0
Naan, Garlic & Coriander, Mini, Sainsbury's*	1 Naan/50g	140	2.0	280	8.2	51.2	4.1	2.6
Naan, Garlic & Coriander, Mini, Sharwood's*	1 Naan/40g	114	3.0	285	7.5	45.5	7.5	3.4
Naan, Garlic & Coriander, Mini, Weight Watchers*	1 Naan/40g	100	1.0	250	9.3	47.6	2.5	4.2
Naan, Garlic & Coriander, Sainsbury's*	1 Serving/130g	373	10.0	287	8.7	45.8	7.7	2.4
Naan, Garlic & Coriander, Weight Watchers*	1 Naan/60g	155	2.6	259	8.9	46.0	4.3	3.4
Naan, Indian Meal for One, BGTY, Sainsbury's*	1 Serving/45g	115	1.9	257	10.3	44.2	4.3	2.1
Naan, Indian Meal for Two, Sainsbury's*	1 Naan//125g	357	9.3	285	8.7	45.9	7.4	1.9
Naan, Long Life, Sharwood's*	1oz/28g	72	1.4	258	7.3	45.8	5.1	2.0
Naan, Onion & Mint, M & S*	½ Naan/135g	351	11.7	260	8.9	35.8	8.7	2.5
Naan, Onion Bhaji, M & S*	1 Naan/140g	400	17.0	285	9.5	34.2	12.1	2.0
Naan, Onion Bhaji, Sharwood's*	1 Pack/130g	378	9.9	291	7.3	48.4	7.6	2.2
Naan, Peshwari, Apple & Coconut, Mini, Sharwood's*	1 Naan/40g	112	2.7	281	6.9	46.6	6.7	3.1
Naan, Peshwari, Fresh, Sharwood's*	1oz/28g	67	1.4	240	6.8	41.9	5.0	2.5
Naan, Peshwari, Long Life, Sharwood's*	1oz/28g	71	1.8	252	6.2	42.0	6.6	2.6
Naan, Peshwari, M & S*	1 Serving/127g	394	12.8	310	9.2	45.8	10.1	1.9
Naan, Peshwari, Sainsbury's*	1 Naan/166g	511	18.3	308	7.1	45.1	11.0	4.7
Naan, Peshwari, Sharwood's*	1 Naan/130g	334	6.9	257	7.2	45.1	5.3	2.5
Naan, Peshwari, TTD, Sainsbury's*	1 Serving/80g	247	10.1	309	6.3	42.5	12.6	4.4
Naan, Plain, Average	1 Naan/160g	437	10.5	273	8.0	45.7	6.5	2.1
Naan, Plain, GFY, Asda*	1 Naan/130g	307	2.7	236	8.4	45.9	2.1	2.4
Naan, Plain, Large, TTD, Sainsbury's*	¼ Pack/70g	202	4.1	288	9.5	49.3	5.9	2.5
Naan, Plain, Mini, Asda*	1 Naan/58g	156	2.7	269	8.0	49.0	4.6	2.3
Naan, Plain, Mini, BGTY, Sainsbury's*	1 Naan/50g	113	1.1	226	8.2	43.2	2.2	3.3
Naan, Plain, Mini, Fresh, Sharwood's*	1oz/28g	70	0.9	251	7.3	48.0	3.3	2.0
Naan, Plain, Mini, Weight Watchers*	1 Naan/44g	108	1.1	245	9.1	46.5	2.5	4.9
Naan, Plain, Sharwood's*	1 Naan/120g	326	8.9	272	8.5	42.9	7.4	2.4
Naan, Tandoori, Sharwood's*	1 Naan/130g	330	6.5	254	7.3	45.0	5.0	2.0
Naan, Tandoori Baked, Waitrose*	1 Naan/140g	372	4.3	266	9.8	49.6	3.1	2.9
Oatmeal, Farmhouse, Extra Special, Asda*	1 Slice/44g	102	1.1	231	11.0	41.0	2.6	6.0
Oatmeal, Loaf, Greggs*	1 Serving/80g	190	2.0	238	10.0	38.8	2.5	0.0
Olive, Oval, la Brea Bakery*	1 Serving/100g	249	3.8	249	7.0	46.4	3.8	2.7
Olive, Waitrose*	1 Slice/28g	86	3.0	306	9.0	43.6	10.6	2.0
Pave, Mixed Olive, Waitrose*	1oz/28g	59	0.5	209	6.3	41.6	1.9	2.6
Pave, Sun Dried Tomato, Waitrose*	1oz/28g	76	0.4	271	10.8	53.4	1.6	3.3
Pave, Walnut, Sainsbury's*	1 Serving/50g	140	4.8	280	9.0	40.0	9.5	3.5
Pea, Artisan*	1 Slice/50g	102	1.2	204	9.5	31.8	2.4	9.4

	Measure INFO/WEIGHT	per Measure KCAL	FAT	Nutrition Values per 100g / 100ml KCAL	PROT	CARB	FAT	FIBRE
BREAD								
Petit Pain, Homebake, Mini, Tesco*	1 Roll/50g	120	0.6	240	7.8	48.5	1.2	3.4
Petit Pain, Organic, Tesco*	1 Roll/100g	235	0.8	235	7.8	49.1	0.8	1.2
Petit Pain, Part Bake, Weight Watchers*	1 Roll/50g	111	0.4	223	6.8	43.5	0.9	6.8
Petits Pain, Mini, Homebake, Tesco*	1 Roll/45g	110	0.6	245	7.8	49.7	1.3	2.5
Petits Pain, White, Ready to Bake, Sainsbury's*	1 Roll/50g	122	0.7	242	7.8	49.7	1.3	2.8
Pitta, Brown, Organic, Waitrose*	1 Pitta/60g	137	0.8	228	6.4	47.5	1.4	6.6
Pitta, Free From, Sainsbury's*	1 Pitta/65g	164	2.5	252	4.1	50.0	3.9	2.9
Pitta, Garlic, Morrisons*	1 Pitta/60g	149	1.1	249	9.7	51.1	1.8	0.0
Pitta, Garlic, Pride Valley*	1 Pitta/63g	157	1.1	249	9.7	51.1	1.8	2.7
Pitta, Garlic, Sainsbury's*	1 Pitta/60g	153	0.6	255	9.5	52.0	1.0	2.5
Pitta, Garlic & Coriander, Asda*	1 Pitta/55g	116	0.5	212	7.0	44.0	0.9	1.8
Pitta, Garlic & Herb, Tesco*	1 Pitta/60g	134	1.2	223	9.6	44.6	2.0	3.0
Pitta, Mexican, Santa Maria*	1 Pitta/66g	165	0.7	250	7.5	52.0	1.0	0.0
Pitta, Multi Seed & Cereal, The Food Doctor*	1 Pitta/70g	157	1.9	224	10.1	39.9	2.7	10.2
Pitta, Pockets, Pride Valley*	1 Pitta/63g	151	0.6	239	9.3	48.4	0.9	3.2
Pitta, Pockets, Sainsbury's*	1 Pitta/75g	188	0.8	250	8.5	52.0	1.0	3.5
Pitta, Seeded, HL, Tesco*	1 Pitta/60g	153	3.6	255	10.8	39.4	6.0	12.8
Pitta, Sesame, Sainsbury's*	1 Pitta/59g	156	1.4	264	9.8	50.8	2.4	3.1
Pitta, Tex Mex Style, Mini, Morrisons*	1 Pitta/18g	43	0.2	240	9.2	48.7	0.9	3.3
Pitta, White, Average	***1 Pitta/75g***	***191***	***1.1***	***255***	***9.2***	***50.8***	***1.5***	***2.7***
Pitta, White, Free From, Tesco*	1 Pitta/55g	140	1.2	255	6.5	52.6	2.1	5.5
Pitta, White, Greek Style, Asda*	1 Pitta/50g	126	1.0	253	8.0	51.0	1.9	0.0
Pitta, White, Mini, Sainsbury's*	1 Pitta/20g	54	0.2	268	8.8	54.6	1.2	2.0
Pitta, White, Organic, Sainsbury's*	1 Pitta/59g	150	0.6	254	10.3	50.7	1.1	2.5
Pitta, White, Soft, Sandwich, Warburton's*	½ Pitta/36g	81	0.9	228	9.8	41.4	2.6	1.8
Pitta, White, Speciality Breads, Waitrose*	1 Pitta/60g	149	0.7	249	10.3	49.3	1.2	3.5
Pitta, White, Weight Watchers*	1 Pitta/45g	106	0.3	238	8.7	45.9	0.7	6.7
Pitta, White Picnic, Waitrose*	1 Pitta/30g	75	0.4	249	10.3	49.3	1.2	3.5
Pitta, Wholemeal, Acropolis, Lidl*	1 Pitta/57g	136	0.9	238	12.0	44.0	1.6	6.0
Pitta, Wholemeal, Average	***1 Pitta/64g***	***154***	***1.1***	***241***	***11.0***	***45.8***	***1.7***	***6.4***
Pitta, Wholemeal, Healthy Eating, Co-Op*	1 Pitta/63g	135	1.3	215	12.0	37.0	2.0	9.0
Pitta, Wholemeal, Hollyland Bakery*	1 Pitta/20g	48	0.3	242	13.1	43.7	1.6	6.0
Pitta, Wholemeal, Mini, M & S*	1 Pitta/18g	44	0.4	247	10.3	45.8	2.5	5.6
Pitta, Wholemeal, Mini, Organic, Newbury Phillips*	1 Pitta/100g	144	1.7	144	10.3	50.8	1.7	6.4
Pitta, Wholemeal, Mini, Sainsbury's*	1 Pitta/30g	69	0.5	231	10.0	43.8	1.7	6.2
Pitta, Wholemeal, So Organic, Sainsbury's*	1 Pitta/60g	140	1.0	233	9.8	44.8	1.6	8.1
Pitta, Wholemeal, Weight Watchers*	1 Pitta/46g	106	0.6	229	8.7	44.5	1.2	7.6
Pitta, Wholemeal, with Extra Virgin Olive Oil, Tesco*	1 Pitta/60g	135	1.6	225	8.3	41.5	2.6	5.5
Potato & Rosemary, M & S*	1 Serving/40g	108	2.7	270	9.4	42.2	6.8	2.3
Potato Farls, Irish, Rankin Selection, Irwin's Bakery*	1 Farl/60g	110	2.2	184	2.3	34.4	3.6	2.5
Potato Farls, M & S*	1 Farl/55g	79	0.2	144	4.2	33.8	0.4	4.7
Potato Farls, Sunblest*	1 Farl/100g	156	0.9	156	3.8	33.2	0.9	1.9
Pumpernickel, Organic, Bavarian Pumpernickel*	1 Slice/50g	90	0.5	180	6.0	38.0	1.0	10.0
Pumpernickel, Rye, Kelderman*	1 Slice/50g	92	0.5	185	6.0	38.0	1.0	0.0
Rolls, 3 Seeded, Sandwich, Warburton's*	1 Roll/77g	242	6.7	314	13.3	41.2	8.7	6.0
Rolls, American Style Deli, Tesco*	1 Roll/65g	162	2.2	249	7.8	46.8	3.4	1.6
Rolls, Batched Sandwich, Warburton's*	1 Roll/60g	148	2.5	246	9.6	42.7	4.1	0.0
Rolls, Best of Both, Hovis*	1 Roll/62g	148	2.9	239	9.8	39.7	4.6	5.0
Rolls, Brioche, Average	1 Roll/49g	177	6.9	361	8.8	50.1	14.1	1.5
Rolls, Brioche, Brialys*	1 Roll/35g	121	3.9	347	8.8	52.8	11.2	1.5
Rolls, Brioche, Butter, Tesco*	1 Roll/35g	124	4.0	355	8.8	53.3	11.4	2.0
Rolls, Brioche, Continental Classics*	1 Roll/35g	122	3.3	349	8.2	58.3	9.3	0.0
Rolls, Brioche, Finest, Tesco*	1 Roll/52g	207	11.6	398	10.8	38.3	22.4	2.0

	Measure INFO/WEIGHT	per Measure KCAL	FAT	Nutrition Values per 100g / 100ml KCAL	PROT	CARB	FAT	FIBRE
BREAD								
Rolls, Brioche, La Boulangere, Lidl*	1 Roll/35g	122	3.6	350	8.2	55.5	10.2	1.8
Rolls, Brioche, Plain Chocolate Chip, Sainsbury's*	1 Roll/35g	131	5.6	374	8.5	49.0	16.0	5.9
Rolls, Brown, Carb Control, Tesco*	1 Roll/45g	98	2.7	218	20.5	20.7	5.9	10.7
Rolls, Brown, Crusty	***1 Roll/50g***	***128***	***1.4***	***255***	***10.3***	***50.4***	***2.8***	***3.5***
Rolls, Brown, Free From, Tesco*	1 Roll/65g	174	5.3	268	5.4	43.2	8.2	3.6
Rolls, Brown, M & S*	1 Roll/105g	242	6.4	230	9.2	37.3	6.1	4.4
Rolls, Brown, Malted Grain, Tesco*	1 Roll/58g	144	1.9	248	8.7	46.2	3.2	1.9
Rolls, Brown, Mini, M & S*	1 Roll/33g	80	2.5	245	9.8	35.5	7.6	3.8
Rolls, Brown, Old Fashioned, Waitrose*	1 Roll/63g	152	2.6	241	9.6	41.3	4.1	4.7
Rolls, Brown, Seeded, Organic, Sainsbury's*	1 Roll/70g	166	3.2	237	9.9	39.1	4.6	6.5
Rolls, Brown, Snack, Allinson*	1 Roll/44g	119	2.9	270	10.8	41.6	6.7	5.6
Rolls, Brown, Soft, Average	1 Roll/50g	134	1.9	268	10.0	51.8	3.8	3.5
Rolls, Brown, Soft, Organic, Sainsbury's*	1 Roll/70g	166	3.2	237	9.9	39.1	4.6	6.6
Rolls, Brown, Square, M & S*	1 Roll/105g	242	6.4	230	9.2	37.3	6.1	4.4
Rolls, Cheese Topped, Sandwich Rolls, Warburton's*	1 Roll/62g	168	4.0	270	12.1	40.7	6.5	2.6
Rolls, Cheese Topped, Village Green*	1 Roll/56g	159	4.1	284	13.1	41.2	7.4	4.8
Rolls, Ciabatta, Cheese Topped, Mini, Finest, Tesco*	1 Roll/30g	85	2.4	282	11.5	40.9	8.1	3.8
Rolls, Ciabatta, Garlic, Asda*	1 Roll/93g	333	16.7	358	9.0	40.0	18.0	2.3
Rolls, Ciabatta, M & S*	1 Roll/80g	210	3.3	262	10.3	48.1	4.1	2.1
Rolls, Ciabatta, Sun Dried Tomato, Mini, Finest, Tesco*	1 Roll/30g	79	1.9	262	8.7	42.3	6.4	2.6
Rolls, Ciabatta, Tesco*	1 Roll/80g	208	2.5	260	8.6	48.2	3.1	3.3
Rolls, Corn Topped, Greggs*	1 Roll/76g	190	2.5	250	9.9	44.7	3.3	0.0
Rolls, COU, M & S*	1 Roll/51g	120	1.2	235	9.8	44.0	2.3	3.4
Rolls, Country Grain, Mini, M & S*	1 Roll/31g	85	3.0	275	10.2	38.9	9.7	3.8
Rolls, Crusty, Booths*	1 Roll/50g	124	0.6	247	8.7	50.3	1.2	2.6
Rolls, Crusty, French, M & S*	1 Roll/65g	159	0.8	245	8.1	50.5	1.2	3.3
Rolls, Crusty, Part-Baked, Budgens*	1 Roll/50g	148	0.7	296	9.4	61.4	1.4	2.5
Rolls, Finger, White, Sainsbury's*	1 Roll/40g	96	1.0	240	9.0	45.2	2.6	3.2
Rolls, Focaccia, Tesco*	1 Roll/75g	226	7.0	302	8.7	45.6	9.4	3.8
Rolls, GF, Antoinette Savill*	1 Roll/70g	157	1.5	224	1.9	48.8	2.2	1.5
Rolls, Granary, Average	1 Roll/70g	176	2.7	251	9.6	45.2	3.9	3.3
Rolls, Granary, Bakers Premium, Tesco*	1 Roll/65g	158	0.8	243	9.9	47.8	1.3	2.3
Rolls, Granary, Original, Hovis*	1 Roll/70g	180	2.9	257	10.7	44.3	4.1	5.3
Rolls, Granary Malted Wheatgrain, Soft, M & S*	1 Roll/80g	208	3.1	260	9.3	47.2	3.9	2.3
Rolls, Green Olive, M & S*	1 Roll/75g	210	4.5	280	11.2	44.0	6.0	1.8
Rolls, Hot Dog, Sliced, Asda*	1 Roll/84g	197	2.8	234	7.0	44.0	3.3	0.0
Rolls, Hot Dog, Tesco*	1 Roll/85g	200	2.8	235	7.3	44.0	3.3	1.9
Rolls, Hot Dog, Warburton's*	1 Roll/60g	137	2.8	228	8.7	37.8	4.7	1.7
Rolls, Malted, Whole Grain Rolls, Batched, Soft, M & S*	1 Roll/80g	180	3.6	225	7.8	38.5	4.5	3.1
Rolls, Malted Grain, Sainsbury's*	1 Roll/68g	190	2.9	280	8.7	51.6	4.3	4.2
Rolls, Malted Grain, Soft, Weight Watchers*	1 Roll/57g	142	1.0	251	11.7	47.1	1.8	4.2
Rolls, Morning, Tesco*	1 Roll/48g	117	1.2	243	10.4	44.8	2.5	4.7
Rolls, Multi Seed, Free From, Tesco*	1 Roll/70g	214	8.3	305	5.4	44.2	11.8	6.3
Rolls, Multigrain, Torpedo, Sainsbury's*	1 Roll/112g	328	7.5	293	10.5	47.7	6.7	6.3
Rolls, Oatmeal, Co-Op*	1 Roll/70g	175	3.2	250	10.1	42.6	4.6	5.6
Rolls, Oatmeal, Ploughmans, GFY, Asda*	1 Roll/72g	181	3.2	252	10.0	43.0	4.4	3.9
Rolls, Oatmeal, Soft, M & S*	1 Roll/83g	224	3.9	270	12.3	43.4	4.7	3.4
Rolls, Oval Bite, Greggs*	1 Roll/79g	230	5.0	291	10.1	45.6	6.3	0.0
Rolls, Panini, White, Tesco*	1 Roll/75g	210	4.6	280	10.1	45.2	6.1	2.7
Rolls, Part Baked, Mini, Tesco*	1 Roll/50g	120	0.6	240	7.8	49.5	1.2	3.4
Rolls, Poppy Seed, Knot, Waitrose*	1 Roll/60g	169	3.2	282	10.3	48.3	5.3	2.2
Rolls, Rye, Toasting, Good & Hot*	1 Roll/65g	143	0.7	220	7.3	44.6	1.1	7.1
Rolls, Seed Sensations, Deli, Hovis*	1 Roll/70g	184	6.0	263	10.3	36.5	8.5	10.6

B

	Measure INFO/WEIGHT	per Measure KCAL	FAT	Nutrition Values per 100g / 100ml KCAL	PROT	CARB	FAT	FIBRE
BREAD								
Rolls, Seeded, Genius*	1 Roll/80g	228	9.0	285	6.6	32.8	11.2	13.0
Rolls, Seeded, Mixed Mini Loaf Pack, M & S*	1 Roll/76g	220	7.3	290	10.6	39.7	9.6	4.0
Rolls, Seeded, Oval Bite, Gregg's*	1 Roll/79g	220	4.5	278	10.1	44.3	5.7	0.0
Rolls, Seeded, Sandwich, Warburton's*	1 Roll/77g	242	6.7	314	13.3	41.2	8.7	6.0
Rolls, Snack, Mini, Tesco*	1 Roll/35g	95	2.1	271	19.0	43.0	6.0	4.0
Rolls, Submarine, Malted Grain, M & S*	1 Roll/109g	300	4.7	275	8.9	53.6	4.3	3.0
Rolls, Tiger, Crusty, Baked by Us, Morrisons*	1 Roll/63g	143	1.8	227	6.3	46.0	2.9	2.5
Rolls, White, 50/50, Soft, Kingsmill*	1 Roll/63g	154	2.4	245	9.3	41.2	3.8	4.4
Rolls, White, BGTY, Sainsbury's*	1 Roll/50g	114	0.5	227	9.1	45.3	1.0	3.0
Rolls, White, Cheese Topped, Sainsbury's*	1 Roll/75g	218	6.4	291	12.1	41.6	8.5	2.0
Rolls, White, Chunky, Hovis*	1 Roll/73g	173	2.4	237	9.4	41.7	3.3	2.5
Rolls, White, Ciabatta, GF, Dietary Specials*	1 Roll/50g	106	0.9	213	4.1	40.9	1.8	8.3
Rolls, White, Crusty, Average	***1 Roll/50g***	***140***	***1.2***	***280***	***10.9***	***57.6***	***2.3***	***1.5***
Rolls, White, Finger, Tesco*	1 Roll/68g	170	2.4	250	8.5	45.8	3.5	2.1
Rolls, White, Floured, Batch, Tesco*	1 Roll/76g	193	2.5	254	8.8	47.3	3.3	2.2
Rolls, White, Floured, Warburton's*	1 Roll/50g	124	1.9	247	9.8	43.3	3.8	2.7
Rolls, White, Floury, Batch, Sainsbury's*	1 Roll/68g	168	1.9	247	8.3	47.2	2.8	2.2
Rolls, White, Floury, Roberts Bakery*	1 Roll/63g	160	1.6	254	8.4	49.5	2.5	2.0
Rolls, White, Good Health, Warburton's*	1 Roll/54g	122	1.1	226	9.6	42.0	2.0	4.1
Rolls, White, Large, Sliced, Warburton's*	1 Roll/89g	230	4.0	258	10.1	44.4	4.5	2.7
Rolls, White, Low Price, Sainsbury's*	1 Roll/44g	107	0.7	243	8.9	48.2	1.6	2.1
Rolls, White, Morning, Co-Op*	1 Roll/47g	134	1.4	285	12.0	53.0	3.0	2.0
Rolls, White, Part Baked, Morrisons*	1 Roll/75g	227	1.0	303	9.6	63.0	1.4	2.6
Rolls, White, Ploughman's, Sainsbury's*	1 Roll/65g	185	2.5	285	8.6	54.1	3.8	2.3
Rolls, White, Premium, Brown Hill Bakery*	1 Roll/74g	206	2.2	279	11.0	51.5	3.0	2.3
Rolls, White, Premium, Hovis*	1 Roll/70g	180	3.1	257	9.5	44.8	4.4	3.0
Rolls, White, Sandwich, Large, Warburton's*	1 Roll/88g	224	3.5	254	10.2	44.3	4.0	2.5
Rolls, White, Sandwich, Regular, Warburton's*	1 Roll/58g	143	2.5	249	9.7	42.6	4.4	2.4
Rolls, White, Scottish, Tesco*	1 Roll/48g	117	1.2	243	10.4	44.8	2.5	4.7
Rolls, White, Seeded, Sainsbury's*	1 Roll/80g	217	4.7	271	10.9	43.4	5.9	4.8
Rolls, White, Seeded, Soft, M & S*	1 Roll/75g	214	4.3	285	11.7	46.2	5.7	2.8
Rolls, White, Snack, Sainsbury's*	1 Roll/67g	159	0.7	237	7.9	49.2	1.0	2.3
Rolls, White, Soft, Average	***1 Roll/45g***	***114***	***1.5***	***253***	***9.2***	***46.5***	***3.3***	***2.2***
Rolls, White, Soft, Dietary Specials*	1 Roll/75g	130	2.9	172	2.2	29.8	3.8	4.7
Rolls, White, Soft, Farmhouse, Warburton's*	1 Roll/59g	148	2.6	250	9.7	43.0	4.4	2.5
Rolls, White, Soft, Hovis*	1 Roll/70g	180	3.1	257	9.5	44.8	4.4	3.0
Rolls, White, Soft, Kingsmill*	1 Roll/62g	156	1.7	252	8.9	46.7	2.8	2.4
Rolls, White, Softgrain, GFY, Asda*	1 Roll/54g	128	1.0	237	9.0	46.0	1.9	2.9
Rolls, White, Submarine, M & S*	1 Roll/109g	300	5.4	275	11.0	47.0	5.0	1.0
Rolls, White, Tesco*	1 Roll/65g	180	2.5	277	8.7	52.0	3.8	2.7
Rolls, White, Warburton's*	1 Roll/57g	141	2.4	248	9.7	42.8	4.2	0.0
Rolls, White, Weight Watchers*	1 Roll/54g	135	1.0	251	11.7	47.1	1.8	4.2
Rolls, Wholemeal, Average	***1 Roll/45g***	***108***	***1.3***	***241***	***9.0***	***48.3***	***2.9***	***5.9***
Rolls, Wholemeal, COU, M & S*	1 Roll/110g	226	3.1	205	11.3	33.4	2.8	7.1
Rolls, Wholemeal, Floury Batch, Sainsbury's*	1 Roll/68g	152	2.3	223	9.9	37.8	3.4	6.5
Rolls, Wholemeal, Food Explorers, Waitrose*	1 Roll/32g	74	1.0	231	10.6	40.2	3.1	5.7
Rolls, Wholemeal, Golden, Hovis*	1 Roll/50g	112	2.0	223	10.5	36.5	3.9	6.8
Rolls, Wholemeal, HL, Tesco*	1 Roll/68g	155	1.4	230	10.4	41.3	2.1	6.6
Rolls, Wholemeal, Kingsmill*	1 Roll/68g	167	2.7	245	10.7	41.5	4.0	5.1
Rolls, Wholemeal, Milk, Warburton's*	1 Roll/22g	51	0.7	231	12.5	38.1	3.2	7.0
Rolls, Wholemeal, Mini, Assorted, Waitrose*	1 Roll/35g	86	2.1	244	9.7	37.9	6.0	7.3
Rolls, Wholemeal, Mini, Tesco*	1 Roll/34g	82	1.9	240	10.9	36.4	5.6	5.8
Rolls, Wholemeal, Oat Topped, Deli, Tesco*	1 Roll/65g	170	3.5	260	10.9	38.3	5.3	6.7

	Measure INFO/WEIGHT	per Measure KCAL	FAT	Nutrition Values per 100g / 100ml KCAL	PROT	CARB	FAT	FIBRE
BREAD								
Rolls, Wholemeal, Oat Topped, Tesco*	1 Roll/65g	166	2.9	255	11.3	42.2	4.5	5.1
Rolls, Wholemeal, Oatbran, HL, Tesco*	1 Roll/56g	115	1.4	205	11.4	33.6	2.5	7.4
Rolls, Wholemeal, Old Fashioned, Waitrose*	1 Roll/57g	135	2.7	236	11.1	37.2	4.8	6.6
Rolls, Wholemeal, Organic, Sainsbury's*	1 Roll/66g	152	1.8	230	10.7	41.0	2.7	6.6
Rolls, Wholemeal, Organic, Tesco*	1 Roll/65g	177	4.0	273	10.3	44.1	6.2	5.5
Rolls, Wholemeal, Ploughman's, Sainsbury's*	1 Roll/67g	153	2.1	229	10.7	39.3	3.2	8.6
Rolls, Wholemeal, Seeded, The Country Miller, Waitrose*	1 Roll/75g	190	7.7	255	13.6	26.9	10.3	7.6
Rolls, Wholemeal, Sliced, Hovis*	1 Roll/60g	150	3.5	250	10.6	38.7	5.9	6.8
Rolls, Wholemeal, Soft, Average	1 Roll/65g	151	2.7	233	10.8	37.3	4.1	6.3
Rolls, Wholemeal, Soft, Seeded, Sainsbury's*	1 Roll/75g	193	5.6	257	11.8	35.6	7.4	6.2
Rolls, Wholemeal, Submarine, Warburton's*	1 Roll/94g	231	4.1	246	10.9	40.6	4.4	6.3
Rolls, Wholemeal, Submarine, Wheatfield Bakery*	1 Roll/100g	230	3.4	230	10.4	39.0	3.4	6.2
Rolls, Wholemeal, Sunflower & Honey, Sainsbury's*	1 Roll/85g	225	4.3	265	9.2	45.4	5.1	4.5
Rolls, Wholemeal, Tasty, Great Everyday, Kingsmill*	1 Roll/68g	158	2.6	232	10.6	38.8	3.8	6.5
Rolls, Wholemeal, Warburton's*	1 Roll/58g	124	2.1	214	10.2	35.1	3.7	6.6
Rolls, Wholemeal & White, Kingsmill*	1 Roll/60g	151	2.5	251	9.5	43.7	4.2	3.5
Rolls, Wholemeal with Cracked Wheat, Allinson*	1 Roll/58g	134	2.3	231	11.0	38.0	3.9	7.0
Rolls, Wholewhite, Kingsmill*	1 Roll/63g	158	2.6	251	9.5	43.7	4.2	3.5
Rolls, Wholmeal, Deli, Tesco*	1 Roll/65g	156	3.1	240	9.0	40.2	4.8	5.7
Rye, Artisan Bread Organic*	1 Slice/50g	80	0.7	160	5.0	28.4	1.4	7.1
Rye, Average	***1 Slice/25g***	***55***	***0.4***	***219***	***8.3***	***45.8***	***1.7***	***4.4***
Rye, Baltic, Organic, The Village Bakery*	1oz/28g	68	0.4	243	8.0	50.3	1.4	2.9
Rye, Dark, Sliced, Trianon*	1 Slice/41g	74	0.6	180	6.5	35.0	1.5	0.0
Rye, German Style, Bolletje*	1 Slice/60g	114	1.2	190	6.0	35.0	2.0	9.5
Rye, German Style, Kelderman*	1 Slice/64g	122	1.3	190	6.0	35.0	2.0	9.5
Rye, German Style, Loaf, Bakery in Store, M & S*	2 Slices/50g	112	0.6	225	9.5	40.8	1.1	6.3
Rye, Light, Finest, Tesco*	1 Slice/20g	47	0.4	237	10.4	44.3	2.0	3.7
Rye, Organic, Waitrose*	1 Serving/100g	207	1.2	207	6.4	42.7	1.2	5.1
Rye, Organic with Coriander, Village Bakery*	1 Slice/30g	63	0.8	209	4.9	49.9	2.7	8.5
Rye, Swedish Style, Kelderman*	1 Slice/50g	92	1.6	185	7.2	31.5	3.2	4.3
Rye, Wheat Free, New York Deli, The Stamp Collection*	1 Slice/33g	61	0.5	184	6.6	43.6	1.4	7.3
Rye, Wholemeal with Sunflower Seeds, Organic, Biona*	1 Slice/72g	150	2.9	210	7.0	36.0	4.0	6.0
Sandwich Thins, White, Chosen By You, Asda*	1 Thin/55g	141	2.2	257	9.3	44.3	4.0	3.1
Seeded, Batch, Finest, Tesco*	1 Slice/65g	168	4.0	259	9.3	41.8	6.1	6.1
Seeded, Medium Sliced, Average	1 Slice/44g	116	2.9	262	11.3	38.6	6.5	5.6
Seeded, Rye, Loaf, la Brea Bakery*	1 Slice/55g	120	0.6	218	7.0	42.5	1.0	5.7
Seeded Batch, Toasted Seeds, 800g, Warburton's*	1 Slice/50g	137	3.7	270	11.4	35.1	7.3	10.2
Seeded Farmhouse, Organic, Cranks*	2 Slices/94g	232	3.5	247	10.1	39.9	3.7	6.9
Sesame Seed, la Brea Bakery*	1 Slice/35g	85	0.8	244	8.8	47.1	2.3	2.0
Seven Grain, Hearty, Golden Wonder*	1 Slice/38g	80	1.0	211	10.5	47.4	2.6	7.9
Soda	***1oz/28g***	***72***	***0.7***	***258***	***7.7***	***54.6***	***2.5***	***2.1***
Soda, Fruit, M & S*	1 Slice/40g	105	1.9	260	5.9	51.3	4.6	2.5
Soda, M & S*	1 Slice/40g	82	0.6	205	8.7	39.2	1.6	4.2
Soda Farls, M & S*	1 Farl/110g	267	3.0	243	9.6	50.1	2.7	2.3
Softgrain, Farmhouse, M & S*	1 Slice/25g	60	0.9	238	8.4	42.8	3.7	3.2
Softgrain, Medium Sliced, GFY, Asda*	1 Slice/35g	79	0.5	226	7.0	46.0	1.5	3.7
Softgrain, Mighty White*	1 Slice/36g	81	0.5	224	7.2	45.5	1.5	3.7
Sourdough, Average	1 Slice/50g	144	0.9	289	11.8	56.4	1.8	2.4
Soya & Linseed, Burgen*	1 Slice/44g	124	4.4	282	15.9	27.3	10.1	9.3
Soya & Linseed, Vogel*	1 Slice/42g	95	2.1	227	11.7	34.1	4.9	6.8
Spelt, with Raisins, Sprouted, Everfresh Bakery*	¼ Loaf/100g	230	1.9	230	9.2	43.9	1.9	6.6
Spelt & Seed, Sliced, Lifefibre*	1 Slice/42g	141	5.8	335	11.6	32.2	13.7	9.2
Sprouted Grain, Ezekiel*	1 Slice/34g	80	0.5	235	11.8	44.1	1.5	0.9

	Measure INFO/WEIGHT	per Measure KCAL	FAT	Nutrition Values per 100g / 100ml KCAL	PROT	CARB	FAT	FIBRE
BREAD								
Square Wraps, White, Warburton's*	1 Wrap/65g	159	2.9	245	12.5	38.6	4.5	2.2
Sunflower, Multi-Grain, Allinson*	1 Slice/47g	113	2.2	240	9.8	39.6	4.7	3.9
Sunflower & Honey, Organic, Cranks*	1 Slice/30g	64	0.9	215	11.6	37.2	3.0	8.3
Sunflower & Pumpkin Seed, Batched, Organic, Tesco*	1 Slice/30g	73	2.2	243	11.0	33.1	7.4	5.2
Sunflower & Pumpkin Seed, So Organic, Sainsbury's*	1 Slice/30g	76	1.6	254	11.4	40.0	5.4	12.9
Sunflower Seed, Bolletje, Delhaize*	1 Slice/44g	106	3.1	240	7.5	35.0	7.0	6.0
Sunflower Seed, Organic, Natural, Mestemacher*	1 Slice/75g	162	3.0	216	5.6	34.7	4.0	9.4
Tandoori Rustic Marble, Graze*	1 Punnet/36g	117	5.0	324	8.7	41.2	13.8	4.8
Tiger Loaf, Tesco*	1 Slice/40g	96	0.8	239	8.7	46.6	2.0	2.6
Toaster, White, Rathbones*	1 Slice/38g	92	0.5	243	9.1	48.6	1.3	2.3
Tomato & Chilli, BGTY, Sainsbury's*	¼ Bread/65g	155	3.1	238	11.9	36.9	4.7	2.8
Tomato & Garlic, Flatbread, Italian Style, Iceland*	1 Serving/75g	195	8.8	260	6.3	32.3	11.8	2.4
Tomato & Garlic, Flatbread, Sainsbury's*	1/3 Bread/73g	191	4.9	261	8.4	41.7	6.7	3.4
Tomato & Garlic, Italian Style, Morrisons*	½ Pack/155g	355	12.4	229	5.8	33.4	8.0	2.5
Tomato & Herb, Tear & Share, Tesco*	¼ Pack/73g	164	3.2	226	6.3	40.2	4.4	2.1
Veda Malt, St Michael*	1 Serving/45g	99	0.5	219	7.1	45.3	1.1	2.2
Walnut, Waitrose*	1/8 Loaf/50g	170	7.6	339	10.0	40.6	15.2	5.9
Wheat	***1 Slice/25g***	***65***	***1.0***	***260***	***9.1***	***47.2***	***4.1***	***4.3***
Wheat, Tasty, Kingsmill*	1 Serving/38g	84	1.3	221	10.1	37.6	3.4	6.8
Wheat Rye, Wholemeal, Goldaehren, Aldi*	1 Slice/30g	68	1.2	226	8.0	36.0	4.0	7.0
Wheaten, Big Slice	1 Slice/65g	139	1.7	214	7.5	40.2	2.6	3.6
Wheaten, Loaf, Sliced, Genesis*	1 Slice/40g	86	1.0	214	7.5	40.2	2.6	3.6
Wheaten, M & S*	1 Slice/33g	74	1.2	225	9.3	42.9	3.5	3.9
Wheaten, Sliced, Healthy, Irwin's Bakery*	1 Slice/40g	76	0.8	190	9.0	40.5	1.9	6.2
Wheatgerm, Hovis, Soft, Sliced, M & S*	1 Slice/23g	50	0.7	220	10.1	38.5	3.0	4.6
Wheatgrain, Robertson*	1 Slice/30g	90	1.2	300	9.3	57.3	4.0	4.0
White, Average	***1 Slice/40g***	***94***	***0.8***	***235***	***8.4***	***49.3***	***1.9***	***1.5***
White, Batch, Warburton's*	1 Slice/42g	98	0.9	233	9.8	43.6	2.1	2.7
White, Batch Loaf, Extra Special, Asda*	1 Slice/47g	109	0.9	233	9.0	45.0	1.9	2.2
White, Bloomer, Loaf, Greggs*	1 Serving/56g	138	1.0	247	10.2	46.2	1.7	3.0
White, Chopped Roasted Garlic, Loaf, la Brea Bakery*	1 Loaf/400g	1196	16.4	299	9.9	53.0	4.1	2.5
White, Classic, Medium Sliced, Hovis*	1 Slice/38g	91	0.9	240	11.4	40.3	2.3	2.5
White, Classic, Thick Sliced, Hovis*	1 Slice/50g	120	2.2	240	9.2	40.5	4.5	3.1
White, Commercially Prepared, Average	1oz/28g	74	0.9	266	7.6	50.6	3.3	2.4
White, Commercially Prepared, Toasted, Average	1oz/28g	82	1.1	293	9.0	54.4	4.0	2.5
White, COU, M & S*	1 Slice/26g	60	0.6	231	10.6	41.9	2.3	4.6
White, Country Maid*	1 Slice/33g	76	0.7	229	8.5	44.1	2.1	3.0
White, Crusty, Fresh, Finest, Tesco*	1 Slice/52g	130	1.0	250	8.6	48.5	1.9	2.4
White, Crusty, Gold, Kingsmill*	1 Slice/27g	70	0.8	258	9.4	48.5	2.9	2.7
White, Crusty, Hovis*	1 Slice/44g	103	1.0	233	8.8	44.3	2.2	2.1
White, Crusty, Sliced, Premium, Budgens*	1 Slice/50g	121	1.1	242	8.8	46.9	2.2	2.2
White, Crusty, Sliced Loaf, Tesco*	1 Slice/50g	116	1.0	233	7.4	46.0	2.1	2.0
White, Danish, Lighter, Warburton's*	1 Slice/26g	63	0.3	238	10.5	45.8	1.2	2.6
White, Danish, Medium Sliced, BFY, Morrisons*	1 Slice/17g	42	0.3	245	10.2	49.1	1.8	2.2
White, Danish, Medium Sliced, Tesco*	1 Slice/20g	47	0.3	234	9.4	45.4	1.7	3.3
White, Danish, Sliced, Weight Watchers*	1 Slice/21g	50	0.3	243	9.8	46.5	1.3	2.9
White, Danish, Soft & Light, Thick Cut, Asda*	1 Slice/26g	60	0.4	230	9.0	45.0	1.6	2.1
White, Extra Thick Sliced, Kingsmill*	1 Slice/58g	135	1.4	232	8.8	43.8	2.4	2.8
White, Farmhouse, Crusty, M & S*	1 Slice/34g	82	0.7	240	8.9	46.6	2.2	3.0
White, Farmhouse, Hovis*	1 Slice/44g	103	1.0	234	8.7	44.6	2.3	2.4
White, Farmhouse, Seeded, Waitrose*	1 Serving/75g	192	4.1	256	10.8	40.9	5.5	5.6
White, Fibre, Morrisons*	1 Slice/40g	96	0.7	240	8.0	48.4	1.7	0.3
White, Fried in Blended Oil	***1 Slice/28g***	***141***	***9.0***	***503***	***7.9***	***48.5***	***32.2***	***1.6***

	Measure INFO/WEIGHT	per Measure KCAL	FAT	Nutrition Values per 100g / 100ml KCAL	PROT	CARB	FAT	FIBRE
BREAD								
White, GF, Bakers Delight*	1 Serving/28g	64	2.4	227	1.9	35.5	8.6	1.0
White, Gluten & Wheat Free, Free From, Sainsbury's*	1 Slice/33g	75	2.8	227	1.9	35.5	8.6	1.0
White, Gold Seeded, Kingsmill*	1 Slice/44g	108	2.5	245	9.7	38.8	5.7	3.5
White, Golden, Square Cut, M & S*	1 Slice/40g	85	0.8	215	8.9	40.7	2.1	6.1
White, Good Health, Warburton's*	1 Slice/38g	84	0.7	220	9.4	41.6	1.8	4.1
White, Harvest Crust Premium, Ormo*	1 Slice/40g	92	0.6	229	9.4	47.4	1.5	2.7
White, Invisible Crust, Hovis*	1 Slice/40g	90	0.6	226	8.8	44.1	1.6	2.4
White, Loaf, Crusty, Premium, Warburton's*	1 Slice/31g	76	0.7	249	10.6	46.5	2.3	2.6
White, Low Carb, Sliced, Tesco*	1 Slice/16g	35	0.4	211	11.3	36.4	2.2	6.9
White, Medium, Round Top, Kingsmill*	1 Slice/42g	97	1.0	232	8.8	43.8	2.4	2.8
White, Medium Sliced, Average	1 Slice/39g	93	0.6	238	7.5	48.5	1.6	1.8
White, Medium Sliced, Brace's*	1 Slice/32g	75	0.4	235	9.5	46.6	1.2	2.6
White, Medium Sliced, Great Everyday, Kingsmill*	1 Slice/40g	93	0.8	232	9.0	44.6	2.0	2.7
White, Medium Sliced, Long Life, Asda*	1 Slice/36g	82	0.6	228	8.0	45.0	1.8	2.7
White, Medium Sliced, Mother's Pride*	1 Slice/36g	82	0.6	229	8.0	45.6	1.6	3.0
White, Medium Sliced, Stay Fresh, Tesco*	1 Slice/36g	88	0.7	250	8.9	47.7	2.0	2.9
White, Medium Sliced, Superlife, Morrisons*	1 Slice/30g	79	1.2	263	9.6	47.4	3.9	2.5
White, Medium Sliced, Warburton's*	1 Slice/40g	94	0.8	234	9.9	43.8	2.0	2.6
White, Medium Sliced, Weight Watchers*	1 Slice/12g	30	0.2	247	12.5	45.2	1.9	3.2
White, Medium VLH Kitchens	1 Serving/30g	72	6.3	241	8.4	49.3	1.9	1.5
White, Oatmeal, Allinson*	1 Slice/47g	111	1.4	237	9.0	43.5	3.0	2.7
White, Organic, Hovis*	1 Slice/44g	108	1.4	246	8.6	45.8	3.2	2.3
White, Organic, Waitrose*	1oz/28g	69	0.1	246	8.8	48.8	0.5	1.8
White, Plain, Scottish, Sunblest*	1 Slice/57g	133	1.5	233	10.1	42.3	2.6	2.8
White, Premium, M & S*	1 Slice/40g	95	0.8	235	8.5	45.8	1.9	2.7
White, Premium Farmhouse, Lidl*	1 Slice/44g	99	0.7	225	7.4	45.4	1.5	2.5
White, Sandwich, Kingsmill*	1 Slice/42g	97	1.0	232	8.8	43.8	2.4	2.8
White, Sandwich Thins, Warburton's*	1 Thin/42g	100	1.0	239	9.2	47.1	2.5	3.8
White, Scottish Plain, Mother's Pride*	1 Slice/50g	114	0.8	227	8.7	44.6	1.5	3.0
White, Seeded, Batch, Loaf, Truly Irresistible, Co-Op*	1 Slice/47g	129	3.4	275	11.6	41.1	7.2	4.3
White, Sliced, Roberts Bakery*	1 Slice/35g	87	0.7	249	10.0	48.0	2.1	2.5
White, Soft, Batch Loaf, Sliced, Tesco*	1 Slice/50g	116	1.0	233	7.5	46.1	2.1	2.1
White, Soft, Farmhouse, M & S*	1 Slice/25g	60	0.8	239	9.8	42.6	3.3	2.5
White, Soft, Gold, Kingsmill*	1 Slice/47g	112	1.5	239	8.2	44.5	3.1	2.7
White, Soft, Hovis*	1 Slice/40g	94	0.9	234	8.7	44.6	2.3	2.4
White, Soft, Milk Roll, Warburton's*	1 Slice/18g	46	0.5	251	10.8	45.3	3.0	2.8
White, Soft, Organic, Warburton's*	1 Slice/27g	61	0.8	228	9.7	44.6	3.0	2.6
White, Soft, Sliced, Hovis*	1 Thin Slice/25g	58	0.6	234	8.7	44.6	2.3	2.4
White, Softgrain, Sliced, Tesco*	1 Med Slice/36g	81	0.5	224	7.2	45.5	1.5	3.7
White, Sourdough, Country, Oval, la Brea Bakery*	1 Slice/60g	143	0.4	239	8.8	49.4	0.6	1.6
White, Square, Extra Thick Sliced, Hovis*	1 Slice/67g	155	1.3	231	8.5	44.7	2.0	2.6
White, Square, Medium Sliced, Hovis*	1 Slice/40g	92	0.8	231	8.5	44.7	2.0	2.6
White, Square, Thick Sliced, Hovis*	1 Slice/50g	116	1.0	231	8.5	44.7	2.0	2.6
White, Super Toastie, Warburton's*	1 Slice/57g	134	1.0	235	10.1	44.6	1.8	2.7
White, Superior English Quality, Thin Cut, Hovis*	1 Slice/73g	169	1.1	232	9.2	42.8	1.5	3.8
White, Thick, So Organic, Sainsbury's*	1 Slice/44g	102	1.0	231	8.2	44.6	2.2	3.1
White, Thick, Super Soft, M & S*	1 Slice/48g	115	1.2	240	8.7	45.3	2.6	2.5
White, Thick, Toastie, 800g Loaf, Warburton's*	1 Slice/47g	111	0.9	234	9.9	43.9	1.9	2.5
White, Thick Sliced, Bakers Gold, Asda*	1 Slice/44g	101	0.8	229	8.0	45.0	1.9	2.3
White, Thick Sliced, Brace's*	1 Slice/38g	90	0.5	235	9.5	46.6	1.2	2.6
White, Thick Sliced, Family Favourite*	1 Slice/37g	83	0.5	225	8.5	44.5	1.4	2.3
White, Thick Sliced, Fine Lady*	1 Slice/44g	113	0.5	254	7.8	53.1	1.2	2.3
White, Thick Sliced, Golden Sun*	1 Slice/44g	100	0.7	228	7.5	46.1	1.5	2.4

	Measure INFO/WEIGHT	per Measure KCAL	FAT	Nutrition Values per 100g / 100ml KCAL	PROT	CARB	FAT	FIBRE
BREAD								
White, Thick Sliced, Healthy, Warburton's*	1 Slice/38g	84	0.7	222	10.3	41.2	1.8	4.1
White, Thick Sliced, Organic, Tesco*	1 Slice/44g	108	0.9	245	8.5	46.8	2.1	3.1
White, Thick Sliced, Premium, Tesco*	1 Slice/44g	99	0.3	222	8.7	45.2	0.7	1.5
White, Thick Sliced, Square Cut, Asda*	1 Slice/44g	101	0.7	230	8.0	46.0	1.5	2.1
White, Thick Sliced, Staysoft, Rathbones*	1 Slice/38g	87	0.5	228	8.5	45.5	1.3	2.7
White, Thick Sliced, Sunblest*	1 Slice/40g	91	0.6	228	8.0	45.7	1.5	2.8
White, Thick Sliced, Super Toastie, Morrisons*	1 Slice/50g	128	1.5	257	8.7	48.9	3.0	2.1
White, Thick Sliced, Warburton's*	1 Slice/28g	65	0.6	233	9.8	43.6	2.1	2.7
White, Toast, Gamle Mølle*	1 Slice/32g	83	0.6	260	8.0	52.0	2.0	3.0
White, Toasted, Average	***1 Slice/33g***	***87***	***0.5***	***265***	***9.3***	***57.1***	***1.6***	***1.8***
White, Toastie, Thick, Love to Toast, Kingsmill*	1 Slice/50g	116	1.0	232	9.0	44.6	2.0	2.7
White, Toastie, Thick Cut, Hovis*	1 Slice/50g	115	1.0	230	8.5	44.8	2.0	2.5
White, Weight Watchers*	1 Serving/5g	12	0.1	246	12.3	45.1	1.6	3.3
White, Whole, Extra Thick, Kingsmill*	1 Slice/57g	130	1.4	228	9.0	42.3	2.5	4.0
White, Whole, Kingsmill*	1 Slice/38g	87	1.0	230	9.0	42.9	2.5	3.4
White, Wholesome, Loaf, Sainsbury's*	1 Serving/36g	81	0.7	224	9.4	42.5	1.8	4.4
White, Wholesome, Medium Sliced, Asda*	1 Slice/35g	78	0.9	223	7.0	43.0	2.6	5.0
White Loaf, Gluten & Wheat Free, Lovemore*	1 Serving/35g	111	3.8	316	0.0	3.4	10.9	0.0
Whole Grain, & Rye, Schneider Brot*	1 Slice/50g	98	0.6	197	5.9	36.6	1.2	8.2
Whole Grain, Batch, Finest, Tesco*	1 Slice/44g	112	1.2	254	9.8	47.7	2.7	4.2
Whole Grain, Brennans*	1 Slice/39g	79	0.6	203	9.0	40.0	1.5	4.9
Whole Grain, with Sunflower Seeds, Landgut*	1 Slice/83g	183	4.2	221	7.0	37.0	5.0	29.0
Whole Wheat, 100%, Soft, Farmhouse, Ocean Spray*	1 Slice/43g	110	2.0	256	11.6	44.2	4.7	7.0
Whole Wheat, 100%, Stoneground, Maxwell House*	1 Slice/27g	60	0.5	222	11.1	44.4	1.9	7.4
Whole Wheat, Harvest	1 Serving/42g	90	1.0	214	7.1	45.2	2.4	7.1
Whole Wheat, Nature's Own*	1 Slice/28g	66	1.0	236	14.3	39.3	3.6	10.7
Whole Wheat, Soft, Trader Joe's*	1 Slice/37g	70	1.0	189	10.8	37.8	2.7	5.4
Wholegrain, Average	1 Slice/44g	117	1.9	265	13.4	43.3	4.2	7.4
Wholegrain, Medium Sliced, Irish Pride*	1 Slice/38g	90	0.8	237	9.2	46.6	2.1	7.6
Wholegrain, Soft, M & S*	1 Slice/51g	115	2.8	225	13.0	31.2	5.4	8.2
Wholegrain, Toasted, Average	1 Slice/40g	117	1.9	288	14.5	47.1	4.6	8.1
Wholemeal, & Oat Flakes, Gold, Kingsmill*	1 Slice/47g	103	1.6	220	10.0	37.3	3.4	7.0
Wholemeal, 7 Seeded, Irwin's Bakery*	1 Slice/38g	90	2.0	237	9.5	33.4	5.2	9.4
Wholemeal, American Sandwich, Harry's*	1 Slice/43g	110	2.1	259	9.0	45.0	5.0	5.0
Wholemeal, Average	***1 Slice/40g***	***88***	***1.0***	***215***	***9.2***	***41.6***	***2.5***	***5.8***
Wholemeal, Baker`s Soft, Medium, Tesco*	1 Slice/40g	94	1.1	235	10.8	37.8	2.8	6.9
Wholemeal, Batch, Organic, Waitrose*	1 Slice/40g	88	1.0	219	10.0	38.8	2.6	7.2
Wholemeal, BGTY, Sainsbury's*	1 Slice/20g	41	0.2	207	12.6	36.8	1.0	7.3
Wholemeal, Brennans*	1 Slice/33g	78	1.4	236	11.2	38.4	4.2	7.7
Wholemeal, Brown, Medium Sliced, 400g, Hovis*	1 Slice/25g	55	0.7	221	10.0	37.8	2.8	6.8
Wholemeal, COU, M & S*	1 Slice/21g	45	0.5	213	13.6	33.7	2.6	7.0
Wholemeal, Crusty, Finest, Tesco*	1 Slice/50g	103	0.8	206	10.8	37.0	1.7	6.9
Wholemeal, Crusty, Kingsmill*	1 Slice/42g	104	1.8	247	11.2	41.1	4.2	7.0
Wholemeal, Danish, BFY, Morrisons*	1 Slice/17g	39	0.3	228	11.2	47.9	1.8	6.2
Wholemeal, Danish, Warburton's*	1 Slice/25g	57	0.6	229	13.3	38.5	2.4	7.2
Wholemeal, Farmhouse, Average	1 Slice/43g	94	1.4	219	10.7	36.2	3.3	7.3
Wholemeal, Farmhouse, Hovis*	1 Slice/44g	91	1.0	207	11.0	36.0	2.2	7.1
Wholemeal, Fresher for Longer, Sainsbury's*	1 Slice/44g	98	1.6	222	10.9	36.2	3.7	6.5
Wholemeal, GF, Sliced, Glutano*	1 Slice/56g	107	1.7	191	7.0	34.0	3.0	0.0
Wholemeal, Gold, Kingsmill*	1 Slice/44g	95	1.3	217	10.9	36.8	2.9	7.0
Wholemeal, Golden Crust, Ormo*	1 Slice/38g	83	0.8	218	10.4	36.1	2.0	7.0
Wholemeal, Golden Wheat, Kingsmill*	1 Slice/44g	97	1.3	221	10.9	37.8	2.9	6.0
Wholemeal, Light, Irish Pride*	1 Slice/28g	68	0.4	241	13.3	44.1	1.3	4.5

B

	Measure INFO/WEIGHT	per Measure KCAL	FAT	Nutrition Values per 100g / 100ml KCAL	PROT	CARB	FAT	FIBRE
BREAD								
Wholemeal, Little Brown Loaf, Unsliced, Hovis*	1 Slice/40g	86	1.1	216	10.0	37.8	2.7	6.8
Wholemeal, Loaf, Sliced, Medium, 800g, Hovis*	1 Slice/40g	88	1.1	221	10.0	37.8	2.7	6.8
Wholemeal, Loaf, Sliced, Thick, 800g, Hovis*	1 Slice/50g	115	1.4	229	10.0	37.8	2.7	6.8
Wholemeal, Longer Life, Medium Sliced, Sainsbury's*	1 Slice/35g	78	1.3	222	10.9	36.2	3.7	6.5
Wholemeal, Longer Life, Sainsbury's*	1 Slice/36g	85	1.2	237	10.7	41.0	3.4	6.2
Wholemeal, Longer Life, Thick Slice, Sainsbury's*	1 Slice/45g	101	1.6	224	10.6	37.4	3.6	5.9
Wholemeal, Medium, 800g Loaf, Warburton's*	1 Slice/40g	93	1.0	231	10.2	39.6	2.5	6.5
Wholemeal, Medium Sliced, Baked by Us, Morrisons*	1 Slice/32g	69	0.4	216	9.6	38.0	1.4	6.5
Wholemeal, Medium Sliced, Great Everyday, Kingsmill*	1 Slice/40g	91	1.5	227	10.5	37.7	3.8	6.2
Wholemeal, Medium Sliced, Little Big Loaf, Kingsmill*	1 Slice/39g	93	1.5	239	10.5	37.7	3.8	6.2
Wholemeal, Medium Sliced, M & S*	1 Slice/40g	80	1.2	200	10.5	32.7	3.1	6.7
Wholemeal, Medium Sliced, Organic, Tesco*	1 Slice/27g	55	0.7	209	9.2	37.2	2.8	6.0
Wholemeal, Medium Sliced, Premium, Tesco*	1 Slice/36g	71	0.2	196	9.8	37.8	0.6	7.2
Wholemeal, Medium Sliced, Roberts Bakery*	1 Slice/37g	86	0.6	233	10.9	38.1	1.5	6.6
Wholemeal, Medium Sliced, Sainsbury's*	1 Slice/36g	77	0.9	214	10.3	37.8	2.4	7.4
Wholemeal, Medium Sliced, The Village Bakery*	1 Slice/33g	69	0.7	209	9.8	38.0	2.0	6.0
Wholemeal, Medium Sliced, Waitrose*	1 Slice/36g	76	0.9	213	10.1	37.6	2.4	7.0
Wholemeal, Multi Seeded, TTD, Sainsbury's*	1 Slice/47g	110	3.4	234	11.7	30.7	7.2	8.1
Wholemeal, Multigrain, Sliced, Finest, Tesco*	1 Slice/50g	123	2.0	246	10.1	42.1	4.1	6.5
Wholemeal, Multigrain, Soft Batch, Sainsbury's*	1 Slice/44g	106	2.9	242	11.3	34.5	6.5	5.6
Wholemeal, Multiseed, Organic, Sainsbury's*	1 Slice/26g	75	2.5	289	13.8	36.6	9.7	6.0
Wholemeal, Oat Topped, TTD, Sainsbury's*	1 Slice/47g	109	1.3	232	10.0	38.5	2.8	0.3
Wholemeal, Organic, 400g Loaf, Warburton's*	1 Slice/28g	63	0.9	223	10.3	37.9	3.2	6.7
Wholemeal, Organic, Hovis*	1 Slice/44g	92	1.3	209	10.2	35.6	2.9	7.6
Wholemeal, Organic, Sliced, Harvestime*	1 Slice/44g	95	1.2	216	9.0	38.8	2.7	5.6
Wholemeal, Premium, Medium Slice, M & S*	1 Slice/33g	65	1.0	200	10.5	32.9	3.1	6.7
Wholemeal, Premium, Thick Slice, M & S*	1 Slice/50g	95	1.5	190	9.8	30.8	3.0	6.4
Wholemeal, Rathbones*	1 Slice/27g	57	0.5	211	9.4	39.2	1.8	7.1
Wholemeal, Rustic, Tin, Tesco*	1 Slice/37g	92	1.3	249	12.2	44.0	3.5	3.1
Wholemeal, Sandwich Loaf, Brennans*	1 Slice/40g	88	0.7	221	9.8	38.5	1.7	8.0
Wholemeal, Seed Sensation, Hovis*	1 Slice/44g	109	2.5	249	11.9	31.4	5.6	12.4
Wholemeal, Sliced, McCambridge*	1 Slice/38g	90	0.7	237	7.9	44.7	1.8	0.0
Wholemeal, Sliced, Medium, Tesco*	1 Slice/36g	79	0.8	220	11.0	39.1	2.2	6.6
Wholemeal, Small Loaf, Sliced, 400g, Hovis*	1 Slice/25g	57	0.7	229	10.0	37.8	2.7	6.8
Wholemeal, Soft Crusty, M & S*	1 Slice/25g	58	0.8	230	11.4	39.1	3.1	6.5
Wholemeal, Square Cut, Thick Sliced, Asda*	1 Slice/44g	91	1.0	208	10.0	37.0	2.2	6.0
Wholemeal, Stayfresh, Tesco*	1 Slice/36g	81	0.8	225	11.0	39.1	2.2	6.0
Wholemeal, Stoneground, 800g Loaf, Warburton's*	1 Slice/45g	95	1.2	210	10.4	35.8	2.6	6.8
Wholemeal, Stoneground, Organic, Waitrose*	1 Slice/25g	57	0.9	228	10.8	38.2	3.6	7.1
Wholemeal, Stoneground, Thick Sliced, Sainsbury's*	1 Slice/44g	92	0.8	210	10.2	37.9	1.9	7.8
Wholemeal, Supersoft, Eat Well, M & S*	1 Slice/33g	81	1.1	245	10.9	40.0	3.3	6.7
Wholemeal, Tasty, Medium, Kingsmill*	1 Slice/40g	96	1.5	239	10.5	37.7	3.8	6.2
Wholemeal, Thick Slice, Brennans*	1 Slice/27g	69	0.6	257	9.2	45.4	2.1	6.8
Wholemeal, Thick Sliced, Bakers Gold, Asda*	1 Slice/44g	99	1.4	225	12.0	37.0	3.2	6.0
Wholemeal, Thick Sliced, COU, M & S*	1 Slice/26g	56	0.7	215	13.6	33.7	2.6	7.0
Wholemeal, Thick Sliced, Great Everyday, Kingsmill*	1 Slice/44g	100	1.7	227	10.5	37.7	3.8	6.2
Wholemeal, Thick Sliced, Healthy Living, Co-Op*	1 Slice/44g	95	0.9	215	11.0	38.0	2.0	7.0
Wholemeal, Thick Sliced, Organic, Tesco*	1 Slice/44g	98	1.2	220	8.8	38.8	2.8	5.9
Wholemeal, Thick Sliced, Premium, Tesco*	1 Slice/44g	95	0.7	214	10.0	40.1	1.5	5.7
Wholemeal, Thick Sliced, Sainsbury's*	1 Slice/48g	102	1.2	213	10.1	37.4	2.6	8.5
Wholemeal, Thick Sliced, Stephenson's Bakery*	1 Slice/40g	84	0.8	209	10.7	37.3	1.9	6.2
Wholemeal, Thick Sliced, Tesco*	1 Slice/40g	96	1.1	240	9.5	40.9	2.7	6.8
Wholemeal, Thick Sliced, Waitrose*	1 Slice/44g	94	1.1	213	10.1	37.6	2.4	7.0

	Measure INFO/WEIGHT	per Measure KCAL	FAT	Nutrition Values per 100g / 100ml KCAL	PROT	CARB	FAT	FIBRE
BREAD								
Wholemeal, Thick Sliced, with Mustard Seed, Lozzas	1 Slice/26g	56	0.7	215	13.6	33.7	2.6	7.0
Wholemeal, Toasted, Average	***1 Slice/26g***	***58***	***0.6***	***224***	***8.6***	***42.3***	***2.2***	***5.8***
Wholemeal, Toastie, 800g Loaf, Warburton's*	1 Slice/45g	101	1.1	224	9.7	39.3	2.4	6.6
BREAD & BUTTER PUDDING								
5% Fat, M & S*	1 Pudding/237g	367	10.0	155	4.4	24.8	4.2	0.4
Average	1 Serving/250g	400	19.5	160	6.2	17.5	7.8	0.3
BGTY, Sainsbury's*	1 Serving/125g	126	2.9	101	6.3	13.4	2.3	5.4
Chilled, Chosen By You, Asda*	¼ Pack/125g	267	13.9	213	5.1	22.0	11.1	2.4
COU, M & S*	1 Pot/140g	161	2.8	115	6.1	18.4	2.0	0.8
Frozen, Chosen By You, Asda*	1 Serving/125g	275	10.2	220	5.5	30.4	8.2	1.4
GFY, Asda*	1 Serving/125g	152	2.0	122	7.0	20.0	1.6	1.3
Individual, M & S*	1 Pudding/130g	280	16.4	215	4.4	21.4	12.6	0.5
Low Fat, Individual, BGTY, Sainsbury's*	1 Pack/125g	125	2.9	100	6.3	13.4	2.3	5.4
Reduced Fat, Waitrose*	1 Serving/205g	299	5.3	146	7.4	23.3	2.6	2.0
Sticky Toffee, M & S*	1oz/28g	83	3.0	295	4.1	46.3	10.6	2.2
BREAD MIX								
Brown, Sunflower, Sainsbury's*	1 Serving/60g	151	3.7	251	10.0	38.9	6.1	4.0
Cheese & Onion, Dry Mix, Sainsbury's*	1 Serving/100g	311	2.8	311	11.9	59.5	2.8	2.6
Ciabatta, Italian, Sainsbury's*	1 Slice/45g	96	0.9	213	8.7	40.0	2.0	2.4
Ciabatta, Made Up with Water & Olive Oil, Wrights*	1 Slice/45g	113	1.8	251	10.0	43.6	4.0	1.8
Focaccia, Garlic & Herb, Asda*	1 Serving/125g	385	10.0	308	11.0	48.0	8.0	3.3
Mixed Grain, Sainsbury's*	1 Serving/45g	103	0.7	228	7.7	46.0	1.5	4.4
Multiseed, Baked, Sainsbury's*	1 Slice/44g	112	4.3	252	10.8	30.5	9.6	6.8
Parmesan & Sun Dried Tomato, Made Up, Wrights*	1 Slice/45g	103	0.6	229	9.3	46.0	1.3	2.4
Sun Dried Tomato & Parmesan, Italian, Sainsbury's*	1 Serving/100g	247	1.7	247	8.1	50.1	1.7	2.5
White, Crusty, Made Up, Tesco*	1 Slice/126g	316	2.3	251	9.4	49.3	1.8	2.5
White Loaf, Asda*	1 Slice/60g	150	0.9	250	10.0	49.0	1.5	3.1
Wholemeal, Hovis*	1 Serving/65g	148	3.1	227	10.0	35.8	4.8	6.8
Wholemeal, Made Up, M & S*	1 Loaf/600g	1410	14.4	235	11.0	42.0	2.4	5.3
BREADCRUMBS								
Average	***1oz/28g***	***98***	***0.5***	***350***	***10.8***	***74.8***	***1.9***	***2.6***
Cooks' Ingredients, Waitrose*	1 Serving/50g	174	0.7	349	9.8	74.6	1.4	3.2
Golden, Paxo*	1 Serving/70g	248	1.1	354	11.5	73.5	1.6	3.4
Rusk, GF, Dove's Farm*	1 Serving/100g	342	4.5	342	12.6	62.7	4.5	9.7
BREADFRUIT								
Raw	***1oz/28g***	***27***	***0.1***	***95***	***1.3***	***23.1***	***0.3***	***0.0***
BREADSTICKS								
Asda*	1 Serving/5g	21	0.4	412	12.0	73.0	8.0	2.9
Bruschetta, Olive & Rosemary, Graze*	1 Punnet/29g	138	7.5	480	13.4	53.0	26.0	4.1
Cheese, Italian, Tesco*	4 Breadsticks/21g	84	1.7	399	14.2	67.5	8.0	3.4
Chive & Onion Twists, Tesco*	3 Twists/24g	115	5.3	480	11.6	57.6	22.1	2.2
Farleys*	1 Serving/12g	50	0.7	414	14.0	76.5	5.8	1.1
Grissini, Italian, Sainsbury's*	1 Breadstick/5g	20	0.4	408	11.6	72.9	7.8	2.9
Grissini, Waitrose*	1 Breadstick/6g	25	0.4	397	12.0	72.5	6.2	3.1
Mini, Sainsbury's*	4 Breadsticks/5g	20	0.4	404	15.6	68.7	7.4	4.8
Mini, Wheat & GF, Tesco*	1 Breadstick/3g	11	0.3	414	4.0	72.1	12.2	2.2
Olive, Italian, Finest, Tesco*	1 Breadstick/40g	170	5.4	424	10.5	65.0	13.6	4.8
Olive Oil & Rosemary, Finest, Tesco*	2 Breadsticks/10g	42	1.2	427	13.9	64.4	12.6	4.1
Onion, M & S*	1 Breadstick/40g	166	5.6	415	12.6	59.6	14.1	4.8
Original, Italian, Tesco*	1 Breadstick/6g	23	0.4	410	11.6	72.9	7.8	2.9
Original, Organic, Kallo*	1 Breadstick/6g	24	0.5	393	11.8	69.5	7.6	4.7
Oven Baked, Mini, Quaker Oats*	1 Pack/35g	145	3.1	415	12.9	71.0	8.8	3.7
Perfectly Balanced, Waitrose*	1 Breadstick/5g	20	0.1	378	13.7	77.3	1.6	3.8

	Measure INFO/WEIGHT	per Measure KCAL	FAT	Nutrition Values per 100g / 100ml KCAL	PROT	CARB	FAT	FIBRE
BREADSTICKS								
Plain, Asda*	1 Breadstick/5g	21	0.4	412	12.0	73.0	8.0	2.9
Plain, You Count, Love Life, Waitrose*	1 Breadstick/5g	17	0.1	349	13.4	70.1	1.7	5.6
Rosemary, Asda*	1 Breadstick/7g	29	1.0	439	12.0	64.0	15.0	3.5
Salted, Asda*	1 Breadstick/8g	36	1.4	445	13.0	60.0	17.0	4.3
Sesame Seed Grissini, Sainsbury's*	1 Breadstick/5g	21	0.6	419	12.7	65.5	11.8	3.2
Thin, Healthy Eating, D'oro, Primo*	1 Breadstick/3g	11	0.2	400	10.0	75.0	6.5	1.1
Torrinesi, TTD, Sainsbury's*	1 Breadstick/3g	13	0.2	411	11.0	77.0	6.5	1.1
BREAKFAST CEREAL								
Advantage, Weetabix*	1 Serving/30g	105	0.7	350	10.2	72.0	2.4	9.0
All Bran, Apple Flavoured Crunch, Kellogg's*	1 Serving/45g	162	1.4	361	10.4	64.5	3.0	15.2
All Bran, Apricot Bites, Kellogg's*	1 Serving/45g	126	1.1	279	11.0	55.0	2.5	19.0
All Bran, Asda*	1 Serving/40g	110	1.4	276	15.0	46.0	3.5	27.0
All Bran, Bran Flakes, & Fruit, Kellogg's*	1 Serving/40g	143	2.4	358	8.0	68.0	6.0	9.0
All Bran, Bran Flakes, Chocolate, Kellogg's*	1 Serving/30g	106	1.8	354	10.0	65.0	6.0	13.0
All Bran, Bran Flakes, Kellogg's*	1 Serving/30g	107	0.6	356	11.0	66.0	2.0	15.0
All Bran, Fruit 'n' Fibre, Kellogg's*	1 Serving/30g	114	1.8	380	8.0	69.0	6.0	9.0
All Bran, Fruitful, Kellogg's*	1 Serving/40g	136	3.0	340	12.5	57.5	7.5	0.0
All Bran, Golden Crunch, Kellogg's*	1 Serving/45g	182	5.0	405	8.0	62.0	11.0	13.0
All Bran, High Fibre, Morrisons*	1 Serving/40g	109	1.4	272	14.8	45.5	3.5	27.0
All Bran, Original, High Fibre, Kellogg's*	1 Serving/40g	134	1.4	334	14.0	48.0	3.5	27.0
All Bran, Splitz, Kellogg's*	1 Serving/40g	130	0.8	325	9.0	69.0	2.0	9.0
All Bran, Strawberry Medley, Kellogg's*	1 Serving/55g	170	1.5	309	9.1	80.0	2.7	1.8
All Bran, Yoghurty Flakes, As Sold, Kellogg's*	1 Serving/30g	112	1.2	372	10.0	68.0	4.0	12.0
Almond, Low Carb, Atkins*	1 Serving/30g	100	1.5	333	50.0	26.7	5.0	0.0
Almond, Oats & More, Nestle*	1 Serving/30g	119	2.7	398	10.7	68.7	8.9	5.5
Almond, Pecan & Cashew Muesli, Kellogg's*	1 Serving/45g	188	6.3	418	11.0	62.0	14.0	8.0
Almond, Raisin & Pecan, Nature's Pleasure, Kellogg's*	1 Serving/45g	184	5.4	408	10.0	65.0	12.0	8.0
Alpen*, Crunchy Bran*	1 Serving/40g	120	1.9	299	11.8	52.3	4.7	24.8
Amaranth, Flakes, Organic, Gillian McKeith*	1 Serving/50g	198	2.0	396	10.0	80.0	4.0	3.0
Apple, Blackberry & Raspberry Flakes, GFY, Asda*	1 Serving/30g	103	0.5	344	9.0	73.0	1.8	11.0
Apple & Cinnamon, 7 Grain Granola, Rude Health*	1 Serving/45g	197	5.8	437	10.0	64.0	13.0	7.0
Apple & Cinnamon, Crisp, Sainsbury's*	1 Serving/50g	216	7.4	433	6.2	69.1	14.7	3.4
Apple & Cinnamon, Quaker Oats*	1 Sachet/38g	136	2.1	358	8.0	68.0	5.5	2.5
Apple & Cinnamon Flakes, M & S*	1 Serving/30g	111	0.6	370	6.0	82.7	1.9	3.4
Apricot Wheats, Whole Grain, Tesco*	1 Serving/40g	130	0.6	326	7.6	70.6	1.4	8.0
Balance, Sainsbury's*	1 Serving/30g	111	0.4	370	11.4	77.7	1.5	3.2
Banana, Papaya & Honey Oat, Crunchy, Waitrose*	1 Serving/40g	170	4.8	426	9.6	69.8	12.0	5.5
Banana & Toffee Crisp, Mornflake*	1 Serving/30g	133	4.8	443	5.7	68.8	16.1	5.4
Barley Flakes, Organic, Infinity Foods*	1 Serving/45g	140	0.8	311	10.0	57.0	1.8	4.0
Benefit Flakes, Aldi*	1 Serving/40g	148	0.6	370	11.4	77.7	1.5	3.2
Berry Crunchy, Sainsbury's*	1 Serving/30g	122	3.6	408	7.7	67.3	12.0	4.8
Berry Granola, Rude Health*	1 Serving/40g	178	6.4	446	10.0	61.0	16.0	7.0
Biscuit, Baked with Golden Syrup, Weetabix*	2 Biscuits/44g	158	0.8	363	10.3	72.0	1.9	8.2
Bitesize, Weetabix*	1 Serving/40g	135	0.8	338	11.5	68.4	2.0	10.0
Blackberry & Apple, Alpen*	1 Serving/40g	140	1.5	349	9.2	69.4	3.8	8.3
Blueberry Wheats, Tesco*	1 Serving/50g	165	0.8	330	7.5	71.6	1.5	8.5
Bran, Natural, Sainsbury's*	1 Serving/30g	64	1.5	212	14.7	27.0	5.0	36.0
Bran Flakes, Asda*	1 Serving/47g	157	1.5	333	11.0	65.0	3.2	14.0
Bran Flakes, Crunchy Nut, Sainsbury's*	1 Serving/40g	203	3.8	508	19.8	85.8	9.5	11.0
Bran Flakes, Harvest Home, Nestle*	1 Serving/30g	99	0.7	331	10.2	67.1	2.4	14.1
Bran Flakes, Honey Nut, Asda*	1 Serving/50g	180	2.2	360	10.0	70.0	4.4	11.0
Bran Flakes, Honey Nut, Sainsbury's*	1 Serving/40g	143	1.8	358	9.6	70.0	4.4	11.0
Bran Flakes, Kellogg's*	1 Serving/50g	163	1.0	326	10.0	67.0	2.0	15.0

	Measure INFO/WEIGHT	per Measure KCAL	FAT	Nutrition Values per 100g / 100ml KCAL	PROT	CARB	FAT	FIBRE
BREAKFAST CEREAL								
Bran Flakes, Organic, Sainsbury's*	1 Serving/30g	100	0.7	332	10.2	67.4	2.4	14.1
Bran Flakes, Sainsbury's*	1 Serving/30g	100	0.8	333	10.3	67.5	2.5	14.3
Bran Flakes, Sultana, Dry, Sainsbury's*	1 Serving/30g	98	0.6	325	8.3	68.6	1.9	12.1
Bran Flakes, Sultana Bran, Kellogg's*	1 Serving/40g	138	0.8	344	8.0	67.0	2.0	13.0
Bran Flakes, Wholegrain, Sainsbury's*	1 Serving/30g	110	0.6	365	10.5	69.4	2.0	13.8
Caribbean Crunch, Alpen*	1 Serving/40g	155	3.6	388	8.8	67.9	9.0	4.6
Cheerios, Chocolate, Dry, Nestle*	1 Serving/30g	115	1.0	384	8.0	73.4	3.5	2.2
Cheerios, Honey, Nestle*	1 Serving/50g	184	1.4	369	6.6	79.2	2.8	5.8
Cheerios, Honey Nut, Nestle*	1 Serving/30g	112	1.1	374	7.0	78.3	3.7	5.2
Cheerios, Nestle*	1 Serving/30g	114	1.1	381	8.6	74.5	3.8	7.1
Choc & Nut Crisp, Tesco*	1 Serving/40g	185	8.0	462	8.3	62.5	19.9	4.8
Choco Crackles, Morrisons*	1 Serving/30g	115	0.7	383	5.5	84.8	2.4	1.9
Choco Flakes, Kellogg's*	1 Serving/30g	114	0.9	380	5.0	84.0	3.0	2.5
Choco Flakes, Sainsbury's*	1 Serving/30g	111	0.2	370	5.5	85.4	0.7	3.0
Choco Flakes, Tesco*	1 Serving/30g	112	0.2	374	5.6	86.3	0.7	2.6
Choco Hoops, Aldi*	1 Serving/30g	116	1.4	385	7.0	79.1	4.5	0.0
Choco Snaps, Asda*	1 Serving/30g	115	0.7	382	5.0	85.0	2.4	1.9
Choco Snaps, Sainsbury's*	1 Serving/30g	115	0.7	383	5.5	84.8	2.4	1.9
Choco Squares, Asda*	1 Serving/30g	130	4.2	434	10.0	67.0	14.0	4.0
Chocolate, Granola, Diet Chef Ltd*	1 Serving/40g	195	11.5	488	10.7	45.0	28.7	13.0
Chocolate Cereal, Tesco*	1 Serving/40g	169	5.6	423	8.0	66.3	14.0	6.0
Chocolate Crisp, Minis, Weetabix*	1 Serving/36g	134	1.9	371	9.0	71.7	5.3	8.5
Chocolate Hoops, Average	1 Serving/30g	116	1.3	386	7.2	79.3	4.4	3.4
Chocolate Rice, Puffed, Average	1 Serving/30g	117	1.2	389	5.7	81.0	4.1	3.2
Chocolate Wheats, Kellogg's*	1 Serving/40g	148	3.6	369	10.0	62.0	9.0	12.0
Cinnamon, Puffins, Barbara's Bakery*	1 Serving/30g	100	1.0	333	6.7	86.7	3.3	20.0
Cinnamon Grahams, Nestle*	1 Serving/40g	164	3.9	411	4.7	76.1	9.8	4.2
Clusters, Nestle*	1 Serving/30g	111	1.4	371	9.3	72.6	4.8	7.4
Coco Pops, Crunchers, Kellogg's*	1 Serving/30g	114	1.0	380	7.0	81.0	3.5	3.0
Coco Pops, Kellogg's*	1 Serving/30g	116	0.8	387	5.0	85.0	2.5	2.0
Coco Pops, Mega Munchers, Kellogg's*	1 Serving/30g	112	0.8	375	8.0	80.0	2.5	4.5
Coco Snaps, Value, Tesco*	1 Serving/30g	117	0.7	390	7.0	84.1	2.4	2.4
Cocoa Rice, GF, Organic, Dove's Farm*	1 Serving/30g	114	0.4	379	5.0	85.0	1.5	2.8
Coconut & Wheat Flakes, Toasted, Dorset Cereals*	1 Serving/45g	171	3.6	381	8.2	54.0	8.0	8.0
Cookie Crunch, Nestle*	1 Serving/40g	154	1.1	385	4.6	85.3	2.8	1.8
Corn Flakes, Asda*	1 Serving/30g	111	0.2	370	7.0	84.0	0.7	3.0
Corn Flakes, Banana Crunch, Kellogg's*	1 Serving/40g	163	3.2	408	6.0	78.0	8.0	3.0
Corn Flakes, Co-Op*	1 Serving/30g	112	0.3	375	8.0	84.0	1.0	1.0
Corn Flakes, Crispy Nut, Asda*	1 Serving/30g	117	1.3	390	7.0	81.0	4.2	2.5
Corn Flakes, Harvest Home, Nestle*	1 Serving/25g	92	0.2	367	7.3	82.7	0.8	3.6
Corn Flakes, Hint of Honey, Kellogg's*	1 Serving/30g	113	0.2	377	6.0	87.0	0.6	2.5
Corn Flakes, Honey Nut, Average	1 Serving/30g	118	1.3	393	7.0	81.4	4.3	2.4
Corn Flakes, Honey Nut, Harvest Home, Nestle*	1 Serving/30g	118	1.3	392	7.4	81.1	4.2	2.5
Corn Flakes, Honey Nut & Cranberries, Sainsbury's*	1 Serving/40g	166	4.0	416	7.4	74.4	9.9	3.1
Corn Flakes, Kellogg's*	1 Serving/30g	113	0.3	378	7.0	84.0	0.9	3.0
Corn Flakes, Morrisons*	1 Serving/30g	111	0.2	371	7.3	83.8	0.7	3.0
Corn Flakes, Organic, Lima*	1 Serving/50g	178	0.5	355	8.3	77.7	1.0	6.4
Corn Flakes, Organic, Whole Earth*	1 Serving/40g	154	0.4	386	8.6	84.2	1.0	3.0
Corn Flakes, Sainsbury's*	1 Serving/25g	93	0.2	371	7.3	83.8	0.7	3.0
Corn Flakes, Tesco*	1 Serving/25g	93	0.2	371	7.3	83.8	0.7	3.0
Corn Flakes, with 125ml Semi Skimmed Milk, Kellogg's*	1 Serving/30g	170	2.5	567	20.0	106.7	8.3	3.0
Country Crisp, & Flakes, Red Berry, Jordans*	1 Serving/50g	204	5.8	407	7.1	68.5	11.6	7.3
Country Crisp, Four Nut Combo, Jordans*	1 Serving/50g	240	12.4	480	8.9	55.4	24.7	6.9

	Measure	per Measure		Nutrition Values per 100g / 100ml				
	INFO/WEIGHT	KCAL	FAT	KCAL	PROT	CARB	FAT	FIBRE
BREAKFAST CEREAL								
Country Crisp, Wild About Berries, Jordans*	1 Serving/50g	222	7.8	443	7.5	68.0	15.7	5.7
Country Crisp, with Real Raspberries, Jordans*	1 Serving/50g	214	7.9	429	7.5	64.1	15.8	7.1
Country Crisp, with Real Strawberries, Jordans*	1 Serving/50g	214	7.8	428	7.5	64.1	15.7	7.1
Cranberry Wheats, Tesco*	1 Serving/50g	160	0.8	320	7.6	72.0	1.5	8.0
Cranberry Wheats, Whole Grain, Sainsbury's*	1 Serving/50g	162	0.7	325	7.3	70.9	1.4	7.7
Crispy Minis, Strawberry, Weetabix*	1 Serving/40g	150	0.9	375	9.4	74.1	2.3	10.0
Crunchy Bran, Weetabix*	1 Serving/40g	140	1.4	350	11.9	57.6	3.6	20.0
Crunchy Choco, Crisp & Square, Tesco*	1 Serving/50g	212	7.0	423	8.0	66.3	14.0	6.0
Crunchy Chocolate, Carrefour*	1 Serving/40g	176	6.8	440	9.0	62.0	17.0	8.0
Crunchy Nut, Clusters, Honey & Nut, Kellogg's*	1 Serving/40g	161	2.0	402	6.0	82.0	5.0	2.5
Crunchy Nut, Clusters, Milk Chocolate Curls, Kellogg's*	1 Serving/40g	183	7.2	458	8.0	66.0	18.0	4.0
Crunchy Nut, Clusters, Summer Berries, Kellogg's*	1 Serving/40g	176	6.0	439	8.0	68.0	15.0	5.0
Crunchy Nut, Corn Flakes, Kellogg's*	1 Serving/30g	118	1.2	392	6.0	83.0	4.0	2.5
Crunchy Nut, Red, Kellogg's*	1 Serving/40g	138	0.8	346	10.0	72.0	2.0	9.0
Crunchy Oat, Co-Op*	1 Serving/50g	202	6.5	405	8.0	64.0	13.0	10.0
Crunchy Oat, Golden Sun*	1 Serving/50g	206	6.4	411	8.6	65.0	12.9	6.2
Crunchy Oat, with Raisins, Almonds & Fruit, Tesco*	1 Serving/50g	202	6.3	403	8.5	63.8	12.6	6.6
Crunchy Oat, with Tropical Fruits, Jordans*	1 Serving/75g	319	11.0	425	8.1	65.4	14.6	6.7
Crunchy Oat, with Tropical Fruits, Tesco*	1 Serving/35g	146	4.8	417	7.8	65.3	13.8	6.1
Crunchy Rice, & Wheat Flakes, Co-Op*	1 Serving/30g	111	0.6	370	11.0	78.0	2.0	3.0
Curiously Cinnamon, Nestle*	1 Serving/30g	124	3.0	412	4.9	75.9	9.9	4.1
Fibre 1, Nestle*	1 Serving/40g	107	1.0	267	10.8	50.2	2.6	30.5
Fibre Flakes, GF, Organic, Dove's Farm*	1 Serving/30g	105	0.4	351	7.1	69.7	1.5	15.0
Fitnesse & Fruits, Nestle*	1 Serving/40g	148	0.4	370	6.6	83.4	1.1	3.4
Flakes, 7 Cereal, De Halm*	1 Serving/40g	139	1.3	347	11.3	66.7	3.4	9.0
Four Berry Crisp, Organic, Jordans*	1 Serving/50g	221	7.9	442	7.7	67.1	15.8	5.4
Froot Loops, 30g, & 125ml Semi Skim Milk, Kellogg's*	1 Serving/30g	176	3.5	587	23.3	100.0	11.7	3.3
Frosted Flakes, Sainsbury's*	1 Serving/30g	114	0.2	381	4.9	88.0	0.6	2.0
Frosted Flakes, Tesco*	1 Serving/30g	112	0.1	374	4.9	87.8	0.4	2.4
Frosted Wheats, Kellogg's*	1 Serving/30g	104	0.6	346	10.0	72.0	2.0	9.0
Frosties, Caramel, Kellogg's*	1 Serving/30g	113	0.2	377	5.0	88.0	0.6	2.0
Frosties, Chocolate, Kellogg's*	1 Serving/40g	158	2.4	394	5.0	80.0	6.0	3.5
Frosties, Kellogg's*	1 Serving/30g	112	0.2	375	4.5	87.0	0.6	2.0
Frosties, Reduced Sugar, Kellogg's*	1 Serving/30g	111	0.2	369	6.0	85.0	0.6	2.5
Fruit, Nuts & Flakes, M & S*	1 Serving/30g	117	2.6	391	9.1	69.6	8.5	3.5
Fruit & Fibre, Asda*	1 Serving/40g	146	2.6	366	8.2	68.4	6.6	8.5
Fruit & Fibre, Flakes, Waitrose*	1 Serving/40g	143	2.5	357	8.2	67.2	6.2	9.9
Fruit & Fibre, Harvest Morn, Aldi*	1 Serving/30g	105	1.5	349	8.5	67.6	4.9	10.1
Fruit & Fibre, Lidl*	1 Serving/25g	91	1.2	363	8.8	70.9	4.9	8.0
Fruit & Fibre, Organic, Sainsbury's*	1 Serving/40g	147	1.6	367	10.0	72.4	4.1	7.8
Fruit & Fibre, Whole Grain, Sainsbury's*	1 Serving/30g	108	1.8	361	8.1	68.7	6.0	8.9
Fruit & Nut Crisp, Minis, Weetabix*	1 Serving/40g	144	1.8	359	9.3	70.0	4.6	8.9
Fruit 'n' Fibre, Kellogg's*	1 Serving/40g	152	2.4	380	8.0	69.0	6.0	9.0
Golden Balls, Asda*	1 Serving/30g	112	0.4	374	5.0	85.0	1.5	1.5
Golden Grahams, Nestle*	1 Serving/30g	112	0.9	375	6.0	81.0	3.0	3.4
Golden Honey Puffs, Tesco*	1 Serving/30g	115	0.4	382	6.6	86.3	1.2	3.0
Golden Nuggets, Nestle*	1 Serving/40g	152	0.3	381	6.2	87.4	0.7	1.5
Golden Puffs, Sainsbury's*	1 Serving/28g	107	0.3	383	6.6	86.3	1.2	3.0
Granola, Average	1 Serving/45g	194	8.7	430	17.5	48.8	19.4	16.8
Granola, Chocolate, Dorset Cereals*	1 Serving/40g	206	12.0	515	8.8	47.2	30.0	10.5
Granola, Honey, Dorset Cereals*	1 Serving/40g	194	10.2	484	12.6	51.2	25.4	5.6
Granola, Low Fat, Home Farm*	1 Serving/55g	180	3.0	328	7.3	69.0	5.4	9.0
Granola, Organic, Lizi's, The GoodCarb Food Company*	1 Serving/50g	246	14.0	493	11.3	48.6	28.1	7.4

	Measure INFO/WEIGHT	per Measure KCAL	FAT	Nutrition Values per 100g / 100ml KCAL	PROT	CARB	FAT	FIBRE
BREAKFAST CEREAL								
Granola, Original, Diet Chef Ltd*	1 Pack/50g	248	14.6	496	10.9	46.2	29.3	10.6
Granola, Original, Lizi's, The GoodCarb Food Company*	1 Serving/50g	248	14.6	496	10.9	46.2	29.3	10.6
Granola, Pink Apple & Cinnamon, Diet Chef Ltd*	1 Pack/40g	193	10.7	483	10.1	49.3	26.8	11.2
Granola, Quaker Oats*	1 Serving/48g	210	7.0	438	10.4	72.9	14.6	6.2
Granola, Quinoa, Organic, Perfekt*	1 Serving/40g	186	6.6	466	12.4	48.5	16.4	8.9
Granola, Summer Fruits, Pomegranate Infused, M & S*	1 Serving/50g	200	6.4	400	8.6	63.2	12.7	5.8
Granola, Superfoods, Jordans*	1 Serving/50g	208	6.7	415	9.0	64.7	13.4	8.6
Granola, Treacle & Pecan, Diet Chef Ltd*	1 Pack/40g	196	11.3	490	9.7	47.6	28.3	11.3
Grape Nuts, Kraft*	1 Serving/45g	158	0.9	350	10.9	81.9	2.0	11.9
Harvest Crunch, Nut, Quaker Oats*	1 Serving/40g	184	7.8	459	8.0	62.5	19.5	6.0
Harvest Crunch, Real Red Berries, Quaker Oats*	1 Serving/50g	224	8.5	447	7.0	66.0	17.0	4.5
Harvest Crunch, Soft Juicy Raisins, Quaker Oats*	1 Serving/50g	221	8.0	442	6.0	67.0	16.0	4.0
Hawaiian Crunch, Asda*	1 Serving/50g	224	7.6	448	8.0	69.6	15.3	7.0
Hawaiian Crunch, Mornflake*	1 Serving/60g	247	7.4	411	8.1	66.8	12.4	6.8
Hi-Fibre Bran, Tesco*	1 Serving/40g	110	1.4	275	14.7	45.5	3.5	27.0
High Bran, Chosen By You, Asda*	1 Serving/40g	136	1.5	341	13.6	49.5	3.8	27.1
High Fibre, Alpen*	1 Serving/45g	154	3.2	343	7.7	62.1	7.1	14.1
High Fibre Bran, Co-Op*	1 Serving/40g	110	1.6	275	15.0	46.0	4.0	27.0
High Fibre Bran, Sainsbury's*	1 Serving/40g	134	1.5	335	14.3	48.4	3.7	25.4
High Fibre Bran, Tesco*	1 Serving/40g	110	1.4	275	14.7	45.5	3.5	27.0
High Fibre Bran, Waitrose*	1 Serving/40g	112	1.5	281	14.4	47.2	3.8	26.0
Honey, Crisp Minis, Weetabix*	1 Serving/40g	150	0.8	375	9.5	75.0	2.0	9.2
Honey, Oats & More, Nestle*	1 Serving/30g	114	1.6	379	9.7	73.1	5.3	5.9
Honey & Nut Crisp, Mini, Weetabix*	1 Serving/40g	150	0.8	375	9.4	75.1	2.0	9.3
Honey Cheerios, 125ml Semi Skim Milk, Nestle*	1 Serving/30g	174	2.9	580	21.0	99.7	9.7	5.7
Honey Loops, Kellogg's*	1 Serving/30g	110	0.9	367	8.0	77.0	3.0	6.0
Honey Nut, & Flakes, M & S*	1 Serving/40g	164	3.5	411	9.8	73.4	8.7	2.6
Hooplas, Sainsbury's*	1 Serving/30g	112	1.1	375	6.5	78.6	3.8	4.6
Hoops, Multigrain, Average	1 Serving/30g	112	1.1	374	6.6	77.4	3.6	6.1
Hot Cereal, Flax O Meal*	1 Serving/40g	130	6.0	325	52.5	2.5	15.0	30.0
Just Right, Kellogg's*	1 Serving/40g	145	1.2	362	7.0	77.0	3.0	4.5
Kashi, Crunch, Seven Whole Grains, Original, Kellogg's*	1 Serving/40g	162	3.6	405	8.0	73.0	9.0	5.0
Kashi, Honey, Seven Whole Grains, Kellogg's*	1 Serving/30g	110	0.8	367	9.0	77.0	2.5	7.0
Kids, Original, Projects No1, Dorset Cereals*	1 Serving/30g	112	0.5	373	7.2	82.4	1.7	3.8
Krave, Chocolate & Hazelnut, Kellogg's*	1 Serving/30g	132	4.8	440	8.0	66.0	16.0	4.0
Lion, Nestle*	1 Serving/40g	166	3.1	415	7.2	76.9	7.7	4.3
Lion, with 125ml Semi Skimmed Milk, Nestle*	1 Serving/30g	185	4.4	617	21.7	97.3	14.7	4.3
Malted Wheaties, Asda*	1 Serving/50g	171	1.4	342	10.0	69.0	2.9	10.0
Malted Wheats, Waitrose*	1 Serving/32g	110	0.6	343	9.7	71.7	1.9	9.9
Malties, Sainsbury's*	1 Serving/40g	137	1.2	343	10.0	69.2	2.9	10.0
Malty Flakes, Peach Melba, Tesco*	1 Serving/30g	116	1.1	385	8.0	79.6	3.8	1.7
Malty Flakes, Tesco*	1 Serving/40g	148	0.6	371	11.0	78.4	1.5	4.3
Malty Flakes, with Raspberries, M & S*	1 Serving/40g	148	1.4	370	7.4	77.5	3.5	3.2
Malty Flakes, with Red Berries, Tesco*	1 Serving/30g	111	0.6	369	9.9	78.1	1.9	3.1
Maple & Pecan, Crisp, Asda*	1 Serving/30g	135	5.7	451	8.0	62.0	19.0	6.0
Maple & Pecan, Sainsbury's*	1 Serving/60g	318	13.2	530	13.3	69.7	22.0	5.3
Maple & Pecan Crisp, Tesco*	1 Serving/50g	215	7.6	430	10.5	62.5	15.2	10.2
Maple Frosted Flakes, Whole Earth*	1 Serving/30g	112	0.3	375	6.2	85.6	1.0	1.6
Muesli, Apricot, Traidcraft*	1 Serving/30g	103	1.8	344	8.0	68.0	6.0	5.0
Muesli, Base, Nature's Harvest*	1 Serving/50g	179	2.6	358	11.0	71.2	5.1	7.4
Muesli, Basics, Sainsbury's*	1 Serving/50g	178	2.6	355	11.2	61.5	5.1	9.2
Muesli, Berries & Cherries, Dorset Cereals*	1 Serving/70g	225	1.5	321	6.5	68.8	2.2	6.3
Muesli, Bircher, Love Life, Waitrose*	1 Serving/45g	153	3.5	341	8.8	57.7	7.7	6.8

	Measure INFO/WEIGHT	per Measure KCAL	FAT	Nutrition Values per 100g / 100ml KCAL	PROT	CARB	FAT	FIBRE
BREAKFAST CEREAL								
Muesli, Carb Control, Tesco*	1 Serving/35g	154	9.3	439	25.0	25.0	26.6	13.8
Muesli, COU, M & S*	1 Serving/60g	201	1.5	335	7.6	70.2	2.5	8.1
Muesli, Cranberry & Blueberry, Love Life, Waitrose*	1 Serving/50g	164	1.8	329	8.5	65.3	3.7	7.5
Muesli, Creamy Tropical Fruit, Finest, Tesco*	1 Serving/80g	283	4.5	354	7.2	68.8	5.6	6.9
Muesli, Crunchy, Organic, Sainsbury's*	1 Serving/40g	168	5.8	420	10.6	62.0	14.4	9.2
Muesli, Crunchy Bran, Diet Chef Ltd*	1 Serving/40g	164	3.8	409	8.1	68.4	9.5	8.9
Muesli, De Luxe, No Added Salt or Sugar, Sainsbury's*	1 Serving/40g	161	5.6	403	11.9	57.6	13.9	8.4
Muesli, Flahavans*	1 Serving/52g	187	2.8	360	10.4	72.1	5.3	5.5
Muesli, Fruit, 55%, Asda*	1 Serving/35g	111	1.0	318	6.0	67.0	2.9	7.0
Muesli, Fruit, GFY, Asda*	1 Serving/50g	152	0.9	304	8.0	64.0	1.8	10.0
Muesli, Fruit, Luxury, Weight Watchers*	1 Serving/40g	127	0.8	318	7.2	67.7	2.0	8.1
Muesli, Fruit, Nuts & Seeds, Dorset Cereals*	1 Serving/70g	265	8.0	379	10.6	58.4	11.4	6.1
Muesli, Fruit, Sainsbury's*	1 Serving/40g	132	1.8	330	8.1	64.3	4.5	9.6
Muesli, Fruit, Vitality*	1 Serving/30g	86	0.6	288	7.9	59.6	2.0	8.8
Muesli, Fruit, Waitrose*	1 Serving/30g	101	1.4	338	7.2	66.8	4.7	6.8
Muesli, Fruit & Nut, 55%, Asda*	1 Serving/40g	151	5.6	378	9.0	54.0	14.0	7.0
Muesli, Fruit & Nut, COU, M & S*	1 Serving/40g	128	1.1	320	7.4	74.5	2.8	7.4
Muesli, Fruit & Nut, Iceland*	1 Serving/30g	105	2.2	350	9.3	61.0	7.5	8.1
Muesli, Fruit & Nut, Jordans*	1 Serving/50g	180	4.7	361	8.0	61.2	9.4	7.5
Muesli, Fruit & Nut, Luxury, Lidl*	1 Serving/57g	205	5.6	360	8.0	60.0	9.8	7.5
Muesli, Fruit & Nut, Luxury, Waitrose*	1 Serving/40g	145	3.8	363	9.0	60.3	9.5	6.5
Muesli, Fruit & Nut, M & S*	1 Serving/40g	128	1.1	320	7.4	74.5	2.8	7.4
Muesli, Fruit & Nut, Organic, M & S*	1 Serving/50g	166	3.0	333	8.2	61.6	6.0	7.6
Muesli, Fruit & Nut, Sainsbury's*	1 Serving/30g	114	3.1	379	9.5	58.7	10.3	6.9
Muesli, Fruit & Nut, Traidcraft*	1 Serving/28g	100	2.2	358	10.0	63.0	8.0	6.0
Muesli, Fruit & Nut, Whole Wheat, Organic, Asda*	1 Serving/50g	172	3.5	343	10.0	60.0	7.0	7.0
Muesli, Fruit & Seeds, Organic, Pertwood Farm*	1 Serving/50g	164	3.4	328	11.4	55.5	6.7	12.6
Muesli, Fruit & Spice, Sainsbury's*	1 Serving/50g	184	3.4	368	7.4	69.4	6.8	7.7
Muesli, Fruit Sensation, M & S*	1 Serving/50g	158	1.5	315	6.0	66.0	3.0	7.4
Muesli, Fruity Fibre, Jordans*	1 Serving/50g	172	3.2	344	7.7	64.2	6.3	8.5
Muesli, Golden Sun*	1 Serving/40g	144	3.9	360	8.0	60.0	9.8	7.5
Muesli, High Fibre, Neal's Yard*	1 Serving/50g	182	1.0	364	7.6	72.7	1.9	12.9
Muesli, High Fibre, You Count, Love Life, Waitrose*	1 Serving/45g	155	1.3	344	7.7	67.4	2.9	8.8
Muesli, High Fruit, BGTY, Sainsbury's*	1 Serving/50g	164	1.0	328	6.7	71.0	1.9	6.6
Muesli, HL, Tesco*	1 Serving/40g	126	0.9	315	7.6	64.3	2.3	7.5
Muesli, Light & Crispy, Jordans*	1 Serving/50g	172	2.5	343	7.7	66.7	5.0	9.5
Muesli, Luxury, Diet Chef Ltd*	1 Pack/40g	166	4.7	414	10.6	61.0	11.8	10.9
Muesli, Luxury, Finest, Tesco*	1 Serving/50g	197	6.6	394	8.3	60.8	13.1	5.4
Muesli, Luxury, Jordans*	1 Serving/40g	154	5.0	384	9.6	58.4	12.5	8.2
Muesli, Luxury, Sainsbury's*	1 Serving/40g	144	4.3	359	8.5	57.1	10.7	7.7
Muesli, Luxury Fruit, Harvest Morn, Aldi*	1 Serving/50g	158	1.6	315	6.8	64.5	3.3	6.9
Muesli, Luxury Fruit, Perfectly Balanced, Waitrose*	1 Serving/50g	162	1.6	324	7.1	66.4	3.3	7.0
Muesli, Luxury Fruit, Sainsbury's*	1 Serving/50g	162	1.6	324	7.1	66.4	3.3	7.0
Muesli, Natural, No Added Sugar Or Salt, Jordans*	1 Serving/50g	210	4.1	420	16.0	70.4	8.2	8.4
Muesli, No Added Sugar, Waitrose*	1 Serving/40g	146	2.5	364	12.0	64.9	6.3	6.7
Muesli, No Added Sugar or Salt, Organic, Jordans*	1 Serving/50g	175	4.4	350	9.2	58.4	8.8	9.3
Muesli, Organic, Waitrose*	1 Serving/50g	188	0.8	375	10.3	59.6	1.6	8.3
Muesli, Original, Holland & Barrett*	1 Serving/30g	105	2.5	351	11.1	61.2	8.4	7.1
Muesli, Original, Sainsbury's*	1 Serving/60g	226	5.0	376	9.3	65.7	8.4	7.1
Muesli, Original, Simply, Hubbards*	1 Serving/50g	212	6.7	424	11.8	59.4	13.4	9.2
Muesli, Peach & Vanilla, Sainsbury's*	1 Serving/50g	162	2.6	324	7.6	61.4	5.3	7.6
Muesli, Really Nutty, Dorset Cereals*	1 Serving/70g	253	6.1	362	9.8	61.1	8.7	6.3
Muesli, Rich, Nature's Harvest*	1 Serving/40g	143	3.7	358	10.0	60.5	9.2	7.6

	Measure INFO/WEIGHT	per Measure KCAL	FAT	Nutrition Values per 100g / 100ml KCAL	PROT	CARB	FAT	FIBRE
BREAKFAST CEREAL								
Muesli, Simply Delicious, Dorset Cereals*	1 Serving/45g	160	3.3	356	9.9	58.1	7.4	8.9
Muesli, Simply Fruity, As Sold, Dorset Cereals*	1 Serving/45g	152	1.1	337	7.3	68.0	2.4	6.8
Muesli, Simply Sumptuous, Luxury Fruit, Lidl*	1 Serving/45g	154	1.5	343	6.5	68.7	3.3	6.2
Muesli, Special, Fruit, Jordans*	1 Serving/50g	162	1.4	323	6.6	68.0	2.7	8.4
Muesli, Special, Jordans*	1 Serving/50g	183	5.4	366	7.9	59.5	10.7	8.5
Muesli, Super Berry, Jordans*	1 Serving/50g	174	3.8	348	9.0	60.8	7.6	8.1
Muesli, Super High Fibre, Dorset Cereals*	1 Serving/70g	250	6.6	357	8.0	60.1	9.4	8.4
Muesli, Superfoods, Jordans*	1 Serving/50g	173	3.6	346	9.2	60.9	7.3	10.2
Muesli, Swiss Style, Aldi*	1 Serving/50g	180	3.2	359	9.8	65.3	6.5	8.3
Muesli, Swiss Style, Co-Op*	1 Serving/40g	148	2.4	370	11.0	67.0	6.0	6.0
Muesli, Swiss Style, No Added Sugar Or Salt, Asda*	1 Serving/50g	182	3.5	363	11.0	64.0	7.0	8.0
Muesli, Swiss Style, Organic, Whole Earth*	1 Serving/50g	172	3.6	344	9.2	60.8	7.1	11.3
Muesli, Swiss Style, Sainsbury's*	1 Serving/50g	180	2.9	361	9.2	68.1	5.8	7.1
Muesli, Swiss Style, with Fruit, Tesco*	1 Serving/40g	144	2.1	360	10.4	67.4	5.3	7.4
Muesli, The Ultimate, Organic, Rude Health*	1 Serving/50g	163	4.5	326	10.8	50.5	9.0	12.3
Muesli, Tropical, Sainsbury's*	1 Serving/50g	182	3.4	365	6.5	69.4	6.8	6.4
Muesli, Tropical, Tesco*	1 Serving/50g	173	2.4	346	7.8	68.2	4.7	9.1
Muesli, Tropical Fruit, Holland & Barrett*	1 Serving/60g	197	1.9	328	7.5	69.8	3.2	5.1
Muesli, Tropical Fruits, Jordans*	1 Serving/50g	164	1.4	329	6.9	68.7	2.9	7.1
Muesli, Twelve Fruit & Nut, Sainsbury's*	1 Serving/50g	166	2.4	332	8.1	64.2	4.7	7.8
Muesli, Unsweetened, M & S*	1 Serving/40g	129	1.1	322	8.1	68.0	2.7	9.4
Muesli, Whole Wheat, Co-Op*	1 Serving/40g	140	2.8	350	11.0	61.0	7.0	7.0
Muesli, Whole Wheat, No Added Sugar & Salt, Tesco*	1 Serving/40g	154	5.0	386	9.5	59.1	12.4	7.4
Muesli, Whole Wheat, Organic, Asda*	1 Serving/50g	197	3.0	394	10.0	75.0	6.0	9.0
Muesli, Wholewheat, Asda*	1 Serving/45g	150	3.5	333	8.0	57.9	7.7	9.7
Muesli, Wild-Berry, Amaranth, Allos*	1 Serving/40g	160	4.2	401	12.5	63.3	10.6	4.3
Muesli, with Berries, Swiss, Dry, Love Life, Waitrose*	1 Serving/45g	172	4.3	383	13.5	55.7	9.6	9.8
Multi Fruit & Flake, COU, M & S*	1 Serving/39g	142	0.4	365	6.5	81.8	1.1	4.0
Multigrain, Balanced Lifestyle, Aldi*	1 Serving/30g	108	0.7	360	7.5	77.1	2.4	4.5
Multigrain, Fitnesse, Nestle*	1 Serving/30g	109	0.4	363	8.0	79.8	1.3	5.1
Multigrain Boulders, Tesco*	1 Serving/30g	112	0.4	375	8.2	82.3	1.3	3.6
Nesquik, Chocolatey Corn & Rice, Nestle*	1 Serving/30g	114	1.2	380	7.2	79.1	3.9	5.1
Nice Morning, Kellogg's*	1 Portion/30g	107	0.6	356	10.0	67.0	2.0	15.0
Nutty Crunch, Alpen*	1 Serving/40g	159	4.5	398	10.7	63.6	11.2	6.5
Nutty Crunch, Deliciously, M & S*	1 Serving/50g	238	11.2	476	8.8	59.6	22.5	4.4
Oat, Crunchy, Sainsbury's*	1 Serving/50g	226	10.2	453	8.2	59.3	20.3	6.6
Oat, Raisin, Nut & Honey, Crunchy, Dry, Sainsbury's*	1 Serving/50g	201	7.0	402	8.5	60.2	14.1	7.6
Oat & Bran Flakes, Sainsbury's*	1 Serving/30g	97	1.7	324	12.2	56.0	5.7	17.7
Oat Bran, Crispies, Quaker Oats*	1 Serving/40g	153	2.6	383	11.0	69.0	6.5	9.0
Oat Crisp, Chocolate, Quaker Oats*	1 Serving/35g	135	3.9	385	10.2	57.5	11.1	12.4
Oat Crunchy, Blueberry & Cranberry, Waitrose*	1 Serving/60g	259	9.1	432	8.0	65.9	15.2	8.5
Oat Granola, Quaker Oats*	1 Serving/50g	206	4.4	411	8.6	73.0	8.8	5.2
Oat Krunchies, Quaker Oats*	1 Serving/30g	118	2.1	393	9.5	72.0	7.0	5.5
Oat Meal, Medium, Heart's Content, Mornflake*	1 Serving/30g	108	2.4	359	11.0	60.4	8.1	8.5
Oatbran, Original Pure, Mornflake*	1 Serving/30g	104	2.9	345	14.8	49.7	9.7	15.2
Oatbran, Very Berry, Flakes, Mornflake*	1 Serving/40g	149	2.0	372	11.7	63.8	5.1	12.0
Oatbran & Oatgerm, Prewett's*	1 Serving/30g	104	2.9	345	14.8	49.7	9.7	15.2
Oatbran 100%, Mornflake*	1 Serving/40g	146	3.8	364	13.4	47.3	9.4	18.2
Oatbran Flakes, Nature's Path*	1 Serving/30g	124	1.4	414	8.7	83.0	4.7	6.7
Oatbran Flakes, Original, Mornflake*	1 Serving/40g	149	2.1	372	11.9	63.2	5.2	12.4
Oatbran Sprinkles, Mornflake*	1 Serving/40g	146	3.8	364	13.4	47.3	9.4	18.2
Oatibix, Cranberry, Bites, Weetabix*	1 Serving/40g	155	3.2	388	9.4	63.5	8.0	11.9
Oatibix, Flakes, Weetabix*	1 Serving/50g	190	2.8	381	9.5	73.2	5.6	3.5

	Measure INFO/WEIGHT	per Measure KCAL	FAT	Nutrition Values per 100g / 100ml KCAL	PROT	CARB	FAT	FIBRE
BREAKFAST CEREAL								
Oatibix, Original, Bitesize, Weetabix*	1 Serving/36g	133	2.4	370	10.6	66.5	6.8	10.1
Oatibix, Weetabix*	2 Biscuits/48g	189	3.8	394	12.5	64.3	8.0	7.3
Oatiflakes, with Raisin, Cranberry & Apple, Weetabix*	1 Serving/40g	135	0.5	338	6.7	75.0	1.2	8.6
Oatmeal, Coarse, Prewett's*	1 Serving/40g	137	4.2	343	14.3	47.6	10.6	16.0
Oatmeal, Instant, Heart to Heart, Kashi*	1 Serving/43g	150	2.0	349	7.0	76.7	4.6	9.3
Oatmeal, Quick Oats, Dry, Quaker Oats*	1 Serving/30g	114	2.0	380	14.0	66.7	6.7	10.0
Oatmeal, Scottish, Hamlyns of Scotland*	1 Portion/40g	157	3.7	392	11.2	66.0	9.2	7.1
Oats, Apple Flavour, Instant, Hot, Waitrose*	1 Serving/36g	141	2.2	392	8.1	76.4	6.0	6.7
Oats, Ginger Bread, Bench Press, Instant, Oomf*	1 Pot/75g	296	3.4	395	28.3	57.1	4.5	6.7
Oats, Golden Syrup Flavour, Instant, Hot, Waitrose*	1 Serving/39g	153	2.3	393	7.8	77.4	5.8	6.0
Oats, Jumbo, Organic, Waitrose*	1 Serving/50g	180	4.0	361	11.0	61.1	8.1	7.8
Oats, Original, Instant, Hot, Waitrose*	1 Sachet/27g	97	2.2	359	11.0	60.4	8.1	8.5
Oats, Pure, Free From, Sainsbury's*	1 Serving/40g	164	3.2	410	14.9	64.0	8.0	11.0
Oats, Strawberry & Banana, Toasted, Crunch, White's*	1 Serving/40g	175	5.5	437	7.7	67.3	13.8	6.2
Oats, Superfast, Mornflake*	1 Serving/40g	144	3.2	359	11.0	60.4	8.1	8.5
Oats, Tesco*	1 Serving/40g	142	3.2	356	11.0	60.0	8.0	8.0
Oats, Wholegrain, Organic, Quaker Oats*	1 Serving/25g	89	2.0	356	11.0	60.0	8.0	9.0
Optimum Power, Nature's Path*	1 Serving/30g	109	2.0	363	15.3	60.0	6.7	12.6
Optivita, Berry Oat Crisp, Kellogg's*	1 Serving/30g	107	1.5	357	10.0	68.0	5.0	9.0
Organic, Weetabix*	2 Biscuits/38g	134	0.7	358	11.5	68.6	2.0	10.0
Original, Crunchy, Raisins & Almonds, Jordans*	1 Serving/50g	204	6.4	407	8.7	64.0	12.9	6.6
Original, Crunchy, Tropical Fruits, Jordans*	1 Serving/50g	212	7.2	423	8.1	65.1	14.5	6.7
Perfect Balance, Weight Watchers*	1 Serving/30g	90	0.5	300	7.8	63.3	1.7	15.6
Perfekt, Granola, Ultimate, Organic, GranoVita*	1 Serving/40g	190	6.6	474	13.3	40.6	16.4	11.8
Porage Oats, Old Fashioned, Dry, Scotts*	1 Serving/40g	142	3.2	355	11.0	60.0	8.0	9.0
Porage Oats, Original, Dry, Scotts*	1 Serving/40g	142	3.2	356	11.0	60.0	8.0	9.0
Porage Oats, Original, So-Easy, Dry, Scotts*	1 Serving/30g	109	2.6	364	11.0	60.0	8.5	9.0
Porage Oats, Syrup Swirl, So-Easy, Dry, Scotts*	1 Sachet/37g	135	2.2	366	8.0	70.0	6.0	6.5
Porridge, Apple, Sultana & Cinnamon, M & S*	1 Sachet/40g	144	3.0	360	10.3	62.3	7.5	8.6
Porridge, Apple & Cinnamon, Express, Dry, Sainsbury's*	1 Sachet/36g	138	2.1	383	8.6	70.3	5.9	7.2
Porridge, Apple & Raisin, Fruity, Dorset Cereals*	1 Serving/70g	233	3.4	333	9.7	62.7	4.8	8.9
Porridge, Apple & Raspberry, Seriously Oaty, Weetabix*	1 Serving/40g	142	2.4	354	8.3	63.7	6.0	7.8
Porridge, Banana, Ready Brek, Weetabix*	1 Serving/40g	146	2.6	365	8.9	68.0	6.4	6.7
Porridge, Berry Burst, Oat So Simple, Quaker Oats*	1 Serving/39g	144	2.3	370	8.0	70.0	6.0	6.5
Porridge, Blueberries, Cranberries, & Nuts, Alpen*	1 Sachet/40g	154	3.4	385	10.8	62.6	8.5	7.3
Porridge, Cherry & Almond, without Milk, Graze*	1 Punnet/48g	174	3.3	364	7.0	68.0	7.0	6.0
Porridge, Chocolate, Instant, Grasshopper*	1 Pot/60g	221	3.0	368	15.0	68.3	5.0	0.0
Porridge, Chocolate, Oatibix, Weetabix*	1 Pack/40g	149	3.9	372	9.9	61.3	9.7	6.2
Porridge, Chocolate, Ready Brek, Weetabix*	1 Serving/30g	114	2.4	380	10.0	63.6	8.0	7.0
Porridge, Cinnamon & Raisin, Instant, Grasshopper*	1 Pot/60g	208	2.0	346	13.3	68.3	3.3	0.0
Porridge, Cranberry & Raspberry, Fruity, Dorset Cereals*	1 Sachet/30g	99	1.8	330	10.2	58.7	6.0	12.3
Porridge, Date & Coconut, Love Life, Waitrose*	1 Serving/40g	156	4.0	390	9.7	60.8	9.9	9.8
Porridge, Fig & Blueberry, without Milk, Graze*	1 Punnet/45g	149	2.3	331	8.0	62.0	5.0	9.0
Porridge, Flakes, Organic, Barkat*	1 Serving/30g	109	0.9	362	8.5	74.1	3.0	0.0
Porridge, Free From, Sainsbury's*	1 Serving/50g	174	1.5	348	8.6	72.0	3.0	3.4
Porridge, Fruit & Nut, Fruity, Dorset Cereals*	1 Serving/70g	242	5.6	346	9.4	59.0	8.0	8.2
Porridge, Fruitful, Traditional, Hubbards*	1 Bowl/50g	180	3.8	360	13.4	51.6	7.7	13.3
Porridge, Golden Syrup, Oat So Simple, Quaker Oats*	1 Sachet/36g	137	2.2	380	8.4	68.7	6.2	6.8
Porridge, Hazelnut & Flame Raisin, without Milk, Graze*	1 Punnet/45g	178	6.3	397	9.0	56.0	14.0	7.0
Porridge, Honey, Country, Oat So Simple, Quaker Oats*	1 Serving/36g	134	2.3	373	8.5	69.0	6.5	6.0
Porridge, Honey, Golden, Oatibix, Weetabix*	1 Serving/40g	145	2.6	363	9.2	66.7	6.6	7.0
Porridge, Honey, Manuka, & Apricot, Vogel*	1 Packet/35g	122	1.0	349	10.1	66.3	2.9	7.1
Porridge, Mealpak, All About Weight*	1 Mealpak/42g	153	5.0	364	39.5	21.1	11.9	7.4

B

	Measure INFO/WEIGHT	per Measure KCAL	FAT	Nutrition Values per 100g / 100ml KCAL	PROT	CARB	FAT	FIBRE
BREAKFAST CEREAL								
Porridge, Mixed Berries, Fruity, Dorset Cereals*	1 Serving/70g	243	4.2	347	10.8	62.6	6.0	7.9
Porridge, Morning Glory, Rude Health*	1 Bowl/50g	176	4.1	351	12.2	57.1	8.2	12.4
Porridge, Multigrain, Jordans*	1 Serving/40g	134	2.2	335	10.4	60.9	5.5	10.0
Porridge, Oats, Dry, Smart Price, Asda*	1 Serving/50g	186	4.0	372	11.0	60.0	8.0	8.0
Porridge, Oats, GF, Pure, Hale & Hearty*	1 Bowl/30g	104	2.2	348	12.5	57.5	7.5	10.0
Porridge, Oats, Golden Syrup, Sainsbury's*	1 Sachet/39g	143	2.1	367	6.3	73.6	5.3	6.7
Porridge, Original, Diet Chef Ltd*	1 Sachet/40g	157	2.5	392	12.0	67.0	6.3	9.8
Porridge, Original, Dry, Oat So Simple, Quaker Oats*	1 Serving/27g	100	2.1	370	11.0	58.9	7.7	10.5
Porridge, Original, Express, Sachet, Sainsbury's*	1 Packet/27g	100	2.2	370	11.0	58.0	8.0	10.8
Porridge, Original, Oatibix, Weetabix*	1 Sachet/30g	104	2.5	347	12.5	55.6	8.3	10.1
Porridge, Original, Ready Brek, Weetabix*	1 Serving/40g	149	3.5	373	11.7	57.9	8.7	7.9
Porridge, Original, Simply, Sachet, Asda*	1 Sachet/27g	96	2.2	356	11.0	60.0	8.0	8.0
Porridge, Perfectly, Dorset Cereals*	1 Sachet/30g	107	2.5	356	11.8	58.2	8.4	11.0
Porridge, Plain, Instant, Quaker Oats*	1 Serving/34g	124	2.9	364	11.0	60.0	8.5	9.0
Porridge, Ready Made, COU, M & S*	1 Pot/200g	180	4.4	90	3.9	13.3	2.2	0.9
Porridge, Real Fruit, Raisin & Apple, Jordans*	1 Serving/40g	133	2.7	332	9.1	58.8	6.7	7.4
Porridge, Real Fruit, Sultana & Apricot, Jordans*	1 Sachet/40g	127	2.3	317	8.5	57.7	5.8	7.2
Porridge, Rice & Buckwheat, Free From, Sainsbury's*	1 Serving/50g	179	0.4	358	6.8	81.1	0.7	1.4
Porridge, Spelt, Sharpham Park*	1 Serving/50g	159	1.6	318	11.3	7.0	3.3	9.5
Porridge, Spiced Apple, Sultana, Oatibix, Weetabix*	1 Sachet/40g	138	2.3	345	9.7	65.4	5.7	8.5
Porridge, Strawberry, Diet Chef Ltd*	1 Serving/40g	159	3.1	398	11.2	65.9	7.7	10.6
Porridge, Superfoods, Jordans*	1 Serving/40g	145	3.6	362	10.4	59.8	9.0	8.3
Porridge, Take Heart, Quaker Oats*	1 Serving/32g	194	5.7	606	30.9	80.3	17.8	7.8
Porridge, Toffee, Oat So Simple, Quaker Oats*	1 Serving/30g	122	3.9	407	6.5	66.0	13.0	5.0
Porridge, Vanilla & Banana, Diet Chef Ltd*	1 Pack/40g	151	2.2	378	10.7	70.6	5.6	9.8
Porridge, Walnut & Pecan, without Milk, Graze*	1 Punnet/39g	162	6.6	419	8.0	57.0	17.0	6.0
Porridge Oats, & Bran, Co-Op*	1 Serving/40g	141	2.8	353	12.5	60.0	7.0	12.0
Porridge Oats, Blueberry, Paw Ridge, Quaker Oats*	1 Sachet/28g	107	2.0	376	9.7	64.4	7.0	8.1
Porridge Oats, Co-Op*	1 Serving/40g	144	3.2	360	12.0	61.0	8.0	9.0
Porridge Oats, Dry Weight, Value, Tesco*	1 Serving/50g	180	4.0	359	11.0	60.4	8.1	8.5
Porridge Oats, Honey Flavour, Paw Ridge, Quaker Oats*	1 Sachet/29g	103	2.0	361	9.6	64.7	7.0	7.9
Porridge Oats, Mornflake*	1 Serving/50g	180	4.0	359	11.0	60.4	8.1	8.5
Porridge Oats, Organic, Evernat*	1 Serving/40g	167	3.8	418	13.0	69.0	9.6	7.4
Porridge Oats, Organic, Tesco*	1 Serving/28g	100	2.3	358	11.0	60.4	8.1	8.5
Porridge Oats, Original, Dry, Quaker Oats*	1 Serving/45g	160	3.6	356	11.0	60.0	8.0	4.0
Porridge Oats, Original, Paw Ridge, Quaker Oats*	1 Sachet/25g	89	2.0	356	11.0	60.0	8.0	9.0
Porridge Oats, Rolled, Tesco*	1 Serving/50g	180	4.0	359	11.0	60.4	8.1	8.5
Puffed Rice, Average	1 Serving/30g	115	0.8	382	7.1	82.2	2.8	3.0
Puffed Rice, Honey, Organic, Kallo*	1 Serving/25g	98	0.9	392	5.0	85.0	3.5	2.1
Puffed Rice, Organic, Natural, Kallo*	1 Bowl/25g	92	0.5	370	7.0	81.0	2.0	3.0
Puffed Wheat, Quaker Oats*	1 Serving/15g	49	0.2	328	15.3	62.4	1.3	5.6
Puffed Wheat, Tesco*	1 Serving/28g	104	0.9	373	13.9	72.2	3.2	5.7
Raisin, Oats & More, Nestle*	1 Serving/30g	112	1.4	373	8.9	73.7	4.7	5.8
Raisin & Almond, Crunchy, Jordans*	1 Serving/56g	230	7.0	411	8.4	66.0	12.5	5.0
Raisin & Coconut, Crunchy, Organic, Jordans*	1 Serving/50g	206	6.8	412	8.4	64.2	13.5	7.1
Raisin Wheats, Kellogg's*	1 Serving/30g	99	0.6	330	9.0	70.0	2.0	8.0
Raisin Wheats, Sainsbury's*	1 Serving/50g	166	0.8	332	8.2	71.5	1.5	8.0
Raspberry Crisp, Mornflake*	1 Serving/50g	214	7.2	428	6.5	68.2	14.3	6.8
Red Berry, & Almond, Luxury Crunch, Jordans*	1 Serving/40g	176	7.4	441	8.2	60.5	18.5	6.6
Rice Krispies, Honey, Kellogg's*	1 Serving/30g	114	0.2	380	4.0	89.0	0.7	1.0
Rice Krispies, Kellogg's*	1 Serving/30g	115	0.3	383	6.0	87.0	1.0	1.0
Rice Krispies, Multi-Grain, Shapes, Kellogg's*	1 Serving/30g	111	0.8	370	8.0	77.0	2.5	8.0
Rice Pops, Organic, Dove's Farm*	1 Serving/30g	107	0.2	357	6.8	86.1	0.8	2.0

	Measure INFO/WEIGHT	per Measure KCAL	FAT	Nutrition Values per 100g / 100ml KCAL	PROT	CARB	FAT	FIBRE
BREAKFAST CEREAL								
Rice Pops, Sainsbury's*	1 Serving/25g	98	0.4	391	6.7	87.1	1.4	1.7
Rice Snaps, Asda*	1 Serving/28g	105	0.4	376	7.0	84.0	1.3	1.5
Rice Snaps, Harvest Home, Nestle*	1 Serving/25g	94	0.3	378	7.4	84.2	1.3	1.5
Ricicles, Kellogg's*	1 Serving/30g	114	0.2	381	4.5	89.0	0.8	0.8
Shredded Wheat, Average	2 Biscuits/45g	157	0.8	348	9.0	77.0	1.8	10.0
Shredded Wheat, Bitesize, Nestle*	1 Serving/40g	148	0.9	369	11.8	69.6	2.2	11.8
Shredded Wheat, Fruitful, No Added Salt, Nestle*	1 Serving/40g	142	2.0	354	8.3	68.7	5.1	8.9
Shredded Wheat, Honey Nut, Nestle*	1 Serving/40g	151	2.6	378	11.2	68.8	6.5	9.4
Shredded Wheat, Triple Berry, Nestle*	1 Serving/40g	138	0.8	344	10.6	70.6	2.1	11.1
Shreddies, Coco, Nestle*	1 Serving/45g	161	0.9	358	8.4	76.5	2.0	8.6
Shreddies, Coco Orange Flavoured, Nestle*	1 Serving/40g	150	0.8	374	8.5	76.2	2.0	8.6
Shreddies, Frosted, Kellogg's*	1 Serving/50g	162	0.9	323	0.7	78.5	1.8	4.7
Shreddies, Frosted, Nestle*	1 Serving/45g	164	0.7	365	7.4	80.7	1.5	6.4
Shreddies, Frosted, Variety Pack, Nestle*	1 Pack/45g	163	0.6	363	6.7	81.1	1.3	6.8
Shreddies, Honey, Nestle*	1 Serving/45g	169	0.7	375	8.2	78.1	1.5	8.1
Shreddies, Honey, with 125ml Skimmed Milk, Nestle*	1 Serving/40g	210	2.7	525	17.8	91.8	6.8	8.0
Shreddies, Malt Wheats, Tesco*	1 Serving/45g	169	0.9	375	10.3	73.8	2.0	8.2
Shreddies, Nestle*	1 Serving/45g	186	1.0	371	10.0	73.7	1.9	9.9
Special K, Bliss, Creamy Berry Crunch, Kellogg's*	1 Serving/30g	114	0.8	379	13.0	76.0	2.5	2.5
Special K, Bliss, Strawberry & Chocolate, Kellogg's*	1 Serving/30g	115	0.9	383	13.0	76.0	3.0	2.5
Special K, Choco, Kellogg's*	1 Serving/40g	160	2.8	400	14.0	70.0	7.0	3.5
Special K, Clusters, Honey, Kellogg's*	1 Serving/45g	175	1.4	389	9.0	80.0	3.0	3.5
Special K, Kellogg's*	1 Serving/30g	114	0.4	379	14.0	76.0	1.5	2.5
Special K, Oats & Honey, Kellogg's*	1 Serving/30g	114	0.9	381	9.0	77.0	3.0	5.0
Special K, Peach & Apricot, Kellogg's*	1 Serving/30g	112	0.3	373	14.0	77.0	1.0	2.5
Special K, Protein Plus, Kellogg's*	1 Serving/29g	100	3.0	345	34.5	31.0	10.3	17.2
Special K, Purple Berries, Kellogg's*	1 Serving/30g	112	0.3	374	13.0	77.0	1.0	3.5
Special K, Red Berries, Kellogg's*	1 Serving/30g	112	0.4	374	14.0	76.0	1.5	3.0
Special K, Yoghurty, Kellogg's*	1 Serving/30g	115	0.9	383	14.0	75.0	3.0	2.5
Start, Kellogg's*	1 Serving/30g	117	1.0	390	8.0	79.0	3.5	5.0
Strawberry, Alpen*	1 Serving/40g	144	1.9	359	9.4	69.5	4.8	7.9
Strawberry & Almond Crunch, M & S*	1 Serving/40g	186	7.4	465	8.0	66.0	18.6	4.9
Strawberry Crisp, Asda*	1 Serving/45g	194	7.0	431	8.1	64.7	15.5	5.9
Sugar Puffs, Quaker Oats*	1 Serving/30g	114	0.5	379	5.3	85.8	1.6	3.7
Sultana Bran, Co-Op*	1 Serving/40g	130	1.2	325	9.0	66.0	3.0	11.0
Sultana Bran, HL, Tesco*	1 Serving/30g	98	0.6	325	8.2	68.0	1.9	12.0
Sultana Bran, Morrisons*	1 Serving/30g	98	0.9	325	8.8	65.8	3.0	11.4
Sultana Bran, Sainsbury's*	1 Serving/30g	97	0.6	324	8.2	68.6	1.9	11.6
Sultana Bran, Waitrose*	1 Serving/30g	97	0.6	324	8.2	68.6	1.9	11.6
Vitality, Asda*	1 Serving/30g	111	0.4	370	11.0	78.0	1.5	3.2
Vitality, with Red Fruit, Asda*	1 Serving/30g	110	0.5	366	11.0	77.0	1.6	3.8
Vitality, with Tropical Fruit, Asda*	1 Serving/30g	112	1.5	373	9.0	73.0	5.0	4.9
Weet Bix, Oat Bran, Sanitarium*	2 Biscuits/40g	156	1.0	390	12.8	71.9	2.5	11.7
Weet Bix, Sanitarium*	2 Biscuits/30g	106	0.4	352	12.0	67.0	1.4	10.5
Weetabix, Banana, Weetabix*	1 Serving/44g	157	0.9	357	10.0	70.4	2.0	9.8
Weetabix, Chocolate, Weetabix*	2 Biscuits/45g	166	1.8	368	10.1	67.9	4.0	10.0
Weetabix*	1 Biscuit/19g	67	0.4	358	11.5	68.6	2.0	10.0
Weetaflakes, Weetabix*	1 Serving/30g	102	0.4	340	8.9	72.9	1.4	11.0
Weetaflakes, with Raisin, Cranberry & Apple, Weetabix*	1 Serving/40g	135	0.5	338	6.7	75.0	1.2	8.6
Weetos, Chocolate, Weetabix*	1 Serving/30g	113	1.5	378	8.4	75.1	4.9	5.8
Wheat Biscuits, Average	2 Biscuits/38g	130	0.8	347	11.7	68.4	2.2	9.9
Wheat Bisks, Banana, Mini, Asda*	1 Serving/50g	190	2.7	380	9.7	73.1	5.4	7.4
Wheat Bisks, Harvest Morn, Aldi*	2 Biscuits/38g	136	0.8	358	11.5	68.6	2.0	10.0

	Measure INFO/WEIGHT	per Measure KCAL	FAT	Nutrition Values per 100g / 100ml KCAL	PROT	CARB	FAT	FIBRE
BREAKFAST CEREAL								
Wheat Flakes, Alpen*	1 Serving/40g	140	1.0	350	10.2	72.0	2.4	9.0
Wheat Flakes, Malted, Toasted, Suma*	1 Serving/75g	260	1.4	346	10.3	72.0	1.9	10.4
Wheat Pillows, Wholegrain, Tesco*	1 Biscuit/45g	151	0.9	335	10.6	67.6	2.1	11.3
Wheats, Mini, Maple & Brown Sugar, Sainsbury's*	1 Serving/52g	99	0.5	190	4.0	44.0	1.0	5.0
Wheats, Mini, Sainsbury's*	1 Serving/45g	157	1.0	348	11.8	69.9	2.3	11.8
Wheats, Original, Frosted, Mini, Kellogg's*	21 Biscuits/54g	190	1.0	352	9.3	83.3	1.8	11.1
Wheats, Wholegrain, Apricot, Sainsbury's*	1 Serving/50g	160	0.8	320	7.9	71.6	1.5	8.2
Wholegrain, Minis, Weetabix*	1 Serving/40g	149	0.8	372	10.2	73.2	2.0	10.0
BRESAOLA								
Della Valtellina, Sainsbury's*	1 Slice/14g	23	0.4	163	34.7	0.1	2.6	0.1
Finest, Tesco*	1 Serving/35g	64	1.4	182	36.0	0.5	4.0	0.0
BROCCOLI								
& Cauliflower, Crowns, TTD, Sainsbury's*	1 Serving/100g	33	0.9	33	4.4	1.8	0.9	2.6
& Cauliflower, Floret Mix, Fresh, Tesco*	1 Serving/80g	27	0.7	34	3.9	2.5	0.9	2.7
& Cauliflower, Floret Mix, Iceland*	1 Serving/100g	26	0.7	26	2.6	2.2	0.7	2.4
& Petit Pois with Hollandaise Sauce, Asda*	½ Pack/150g	114	5.4	76	3.8	5.0	3.6	4.0
Bellaverde, TTD, Sainsbury's*	1 Serving/100g	33	0.9	33	4.4	1.8	0.9	2.6
Chinese, Kai Lan, Cooked	1 Serving/80g	18	0.6	22	1.4	3.8	0.7	2.5
Florets, Broccoliroosjes, Albert Heijn*	1 Serving/100g	27	0.7	27	3.0	0.8	0.7	3.0
Green, Boiled, Average	***1 Serving/80g***	***19***	***0.6***	***24***	***3.1***	***1.1***	***0.8***	***2.3***
Green, Raw, Average	***1 Serving/80g***	***25***	***0.7***	***31***	***3.9***	***1.7***	***0.9***	***2.6***
Purple Sprouting, Boiled, Average	***1 Serving/80g***	***15***	***0.5***	***19***	***2.1***	***1.3***	***0.6***	***2.3***
Purple Sprouting, Raw	***1oz/28g***	***10***	***0.3***	***35***	***3.9***	***2.6***	***1.1***	***3.5***
Steamed, Average	1 Serving/100g	24	0.8	24	3.1	1.1	0.8	2.3
Tenderstem, Ready Prepared, Raw, M & S*	1 Pack/200g	80	0.4	40	4.1	4.9	0.2	1.7
BROWNIES								
Average	1 Brownie/60g	243	10.1	405	4.6	0.0	16.8	0.0
Chocolate, Average	1 Serving/100g	446	22.3	446	5.9	55.6	22.3	2.2
Chocolate, Bites, Mini, Weight Watchers*	1 Brownie/9g	29	0.5	325	5.3	63.7	5.5	2.2
Chocolate, Cadbury*	1 Brownie/36g	145	5.7	403	6.1	59.7	15.8	0.0
Chocolate, Chewy, M & S*	1 Brownie/29g	130	6.0	455	6.5	59.8	21.1	2.0
Chocolate, Chunky, Belgian, M & S*	1 Brownie/55g	242	11.2	440	6.2	57.7	20.3	2.5
Chocolate, Frosted, Fiber Gourmet*	1 Serving/35g	90	0.4	257	5.2	88.6	1.0	34.3
Chocolate, Fudgy, M & S*	1 Brownie/87g	400	21.9	460	4.8	56.9	25.2	3.0
Chocolate, Mini Bites, Asda*	1 Brownie/15g	62	3.0	420	5.0	55.0	20.0	1.4
Chocolate, Sainsbury's*	1 Brownie/60g	265	13.6	442	4.6	55.0	22.6	1.6
Chocolate, Slices, M & S*	1 Brownie/36g	158	8.7	440	5.3	51.1	24.1	1.3
Chocolate, Tray Bake, Tesco*	1 Brownie/37g	155	6.8	420	5.5	57.1	18.4	5.7
Chocolate, Weight Watchers*	1 Brownie/47g	143	1.8	304	4.8	62.5	3.8	3.2
Chocolate, Wheat & GF, Mrs Crimble's*	1 Slice/48g	180	9.6	379	4.2	47.9	20.3	1.5
Chocolate & Pecan, Gu*	1 Brownie/40g	188	11.6	471	7.2	47.6	29.1	2.5
Praline, Mini, Finest, Tesco*	1 Brownie/12g	59	3.1	492	4.2	60.0	25.8	0.8
BRUSCHETTA								
Cheese & Tomato, Asda*	1 Bruschetta/38g	68	1.7	180	8.6	26.0	4.6	2.9
Pane Italia*	1 Serving/75g	367	18.8	489	12.4	53.6	25.1	1.4
Ploughman's Relish, Brunchetta, Golden Vale*	1 Pack/90g	261	15.5	290	14.2	20.2	17.2	1.6
Red Pepper & Onion, Brunchetta, Golden Vale*	1 Pack/90g	266	17.1	296	14.6	17.0	19.0	1.3
Soft Cheese & Cranberry, Brunchetta, Golden Vale*	1 Pack/95g	200	8.6	211	8.2	24.8	9.0	1.3
Toasted, Olive Oil & Sea Salt, Tesco*	1 Serving/30g	126	4.6	420	11.5	58.7	15.5	4.5
BRUSSELS SPROUTS								
& Sweet Chestnuts, Asda*	1 Serving/100g	73	1.7	73	3.1	11.0	1.7	4.2
Baby, Sainsbury's*	1 Serving/80g	34	1.1	42	3.5	3.9	1.4	4.1
Boiled, Average	***1 Serving/80g***	***28***	***1.0***	***35***	***3.1***	***3.2***	***1.3***	***3.5***

	Measure INFO/WEIGHT	per Measure KCAL	FAT	Nutrition Values per 100g / 100ml KCAL	PROT	CARB	FAT	FIBRE
BRUSSELS SPROUTS								
Button, & Chestnuts, Tesco*	1 Serving/100g	80	1.8	80	3.1	12.8	1.8	4.1
Button, Raw, Average	***1 Serving/80g***	***30***	***1.1***	***37***	***3.5***	***2.9***	***1.3***	***3.2***
Canned, Drained	***1oz/28g***	***8***	***0.3***	***28***	***2.6***	***2.4***	***1.0***	***2.6***
Frozen, Morrisons*	1 Serving/200g	70	2.6	35	3.5	2.5	1.3	4.3
Raw, Average	***1 Serving/80g***	***29***	***0.9***	***37***	***3.5***	***3.3***	***1.1***	***3.0***
Steamed, Average	1 Serving/100g	35	1.3	35	3.1	3.2	1.3	3.5
BUBBLE & SQUEAK								
Aunt Bessie's*	1 Serving/100g	145	7.1	145	2.7	17.5	7.1	1.3
Fried in Vegetable Oil	1oz/28g	35	2.5	124	1.4	9.8	9.1	1.5
Morrisons*	1 Serving/110g	168	9.6	153	2.2	16.3	8.7	0.7
Tesco*	½ Pack/325g	292	12.7	90	1.6	11.3	3.9	0.9
Waitrose*	½ Pack/225g	166	5.2	74	1.4	11.9	2.3	2.2
BUCKWHEAT								
Average	***1oz/28g***	***102***	***0.4***	***364***	***8.1***	***84.9***	***1.5***	***2.1***
BUFFALO								
Mince, Raw, Lean, Abel & Cole*	1 Serving/100g	95	0.7	95	21.7	0.4	0.7	0.0
BULGAR WHEAT								
Dry, Love Life, Waitrose*	1oz/28g	108	0.6	384	14.8	72.2	2.3	7.4
Dry Weight, Average	***1oz/28g***	***99***	***0.5***	***353***	***9.7***	***76.3***	***1.7***	***8.0***
BUNS								
Bath, M & S*	1 Bun/71g	217	5.7	305	8.3	49.8	8.0	1.9
Bath, Tesco*	1 Bun/80g	262	8.9	328	8.0	48.9	11.1	5.8
Belgian, Asda*	1 Bun/133g	464	19.9	350	4.8	49.0	15.0	2.2
Belgian, Co-Op*	1 Bun/118g	413	15.3	350	5.0	54.0	13.0	2.0
Belgian, Iced, Chosen By You, Asda*	1 Bun/115g	375	6.8	327	6.1	62.3	5.9	2.9
Belgian, Sainsbury's*	1 Bun/110g	398	11.3	362	6.1	61.3	10.3	1.9
Belgian, Tesco*	1 Bun/123g	438	15.7	356	5.2	54.9	12.8	2.2
Chelsea	1 Bun/78g	285	10.8	366	7.8	56.1	13.8	1.7
Choux, Caramel, Asda*	1 Bun/189g	745	51.0	394	4.3	33.5	27.0	1.3
Choux, Chocolate, Belgian, Sainsbury's*	1 Bun/90g	347	35.3	386	6.2	22.0	39.2	1.4
Choux, Custard, M & S*	1 Bun/85g	234	18.7	275	4.2	15.0	22.0	0.3
Choux, Fresh Cream, Tesco*	1 Bun/95g	340	23.7	358	4.9	28.5	24.9	0.9
Choux, M & S*	1 Bun/78g	247	17.3	317	5.4	25.6	22.2	0.3
Currant	1 Bun/60g	178	4.5	296	7.6	52.7	7.5	0.0
Currant, HE, Tesco*	1 Bun/62g	157	1.6	253	6.6	50.8	2.6	3.2
Fingers, Sticky, Iced, Chosen By You, Asda*	1 Finger/40g	132	2.4	330	7.1	62.0	5.9	2.7
Fruit, Waitrose*	1 Bun/54g	155	2.3	287	8.1	54.0	4.3	1.6
Hot Cross	1 Bun/50g	156	3.5	312	7.4	58.5	7.0	1.7
Hot Cross, 25% Reduced Fat, Asda*	1 Bun/61g	153	1.4	253	9.0	49.0	2.3	3.0
Hot Cross, Apple & Cinnamon, Large, Finest, Tesco*	1 Bun/117g	342	8.2	292	7.3	49.9	7.0	3.6
Hot Cross, Best of Both, Hovis*	1 Bun/65g	185	4.3	285	9.1	47.3	6.6	4.4
Hot Cross, BGTY, Sainsbury's*	1 Bun/70g	187	1.9	267	6.3	52.7	2.7	3.5
Hot Cross, Chocolate, Coles*	1 Bun/86g	296	9.0	344	7.0	53.4	10.5	0.0
Hot Cross, Chocolate, Mini, Sainsbury's*	1 Bun/39g	127	4.4	325	7.7	48.1	11.3	2.5
Hot Cross, Chocolate & Raisin, Mini, Tesco*	1 Bun/40g	127	4.4	318	8.1	47.0	10.9	2.8
Hot Cross, Classics, M & S*	1 Bun/65g	159	1.2	245	8.5	49.1	1.8	2.2
Hot Cross, Extra Spicy, M & S*	1 Bun/76g	175	1.4	230	8.6	44.1	1.9	4.2
Hot Cross, Finest, Tesco*	1 Bun/75g	210	4.0	280	7.8	49.5	5.4	2.8
Hot Cross, Golden Wholemeal, 3% Fat, M & S*	1 Bun/67g	144	1.5	215	8.9	39.6	2.2	6.7
Hot Cross, Golden Wholemeal, Sainsbury's*	1 Bun/65g	180	4.0	277	9.9	45.4	6.2	4.3
Hot Cross, HE, Tesco*	1 Bun/60g	155	1.5	258	8.6	50.3	2.5	2.6
Hot Cross, Less Than 3% Fat, M & S*	1 Bun/70g	175	1.3	250	8.1	49.8	1.8	2.2
Hot Cross, Lightly Fruited, M & S*	1 Bun/64g	165	3.4	260	8.1	45.1	5.4	4.7

	Measure INFO/WEIGHT	per Measure KCAL	per Measure FAT	Nutrition Values per 100g / 100ml KCAL	PROT	CARB	FAT	FIBRE
BUNS								
Hot Cross, Low Fat, Co-Op*	1 Bun/60g	156	1.8	260	9.0	50.0	3.0	3.0
Hot Cross, Luxury, M & S*	1 Bun/79g	201	3.2	255	8.6	46.2	4.0	2.1
Hot Cross, Mini, M & S*	1 Bun/41g	110	1.4	265	7.8	51.4	3.4	3.7
Hot Cross, Mini, Tesco*	1 Bun/36g	99	2.0	274	7.9	48.1	5.5	2.7
Hot Cross, Reduced Fat, GFY, Asda*	1 Bun/63g	156	1.6	248	8.4	47.9	2.5	3.7
Hot Cross, Reduced Fat, Waitrose*	1 Bun/67g	171	1.4	255	8.1	54.3	2.1	3.3
Hot Cross, TTD, Sainsbury's*	1 Bun/75g	200	4.2	267	7.2	47.0	5.6	3.8
Hot Cross, White, Kingsmill*	1 Bun/70g	186	2.4	266	8.7	48.0	3.5	3.6
Hot Cross, White, LC, Tesco*	1 Bun/70g	185	1.4	260	8.3	50.3	1.9	3.8
Hot Cross, Wholemeal, Asda*	1 Bun/70g	182	4.2	262	9.0	43.0	6.0	6.0
Hot Cross, Wholemeal, Organic, Tesco*	1 Bun/55g	140	2.7	254	7.6	44.8	4.9	4.5
Hot Cross, Wholemeal, Waitrose*	1 Bun/64g	177	4.3	276	8.8	45.2	6.7	4.9
Hot Cross, You Count, Love Life, Waitrose*	1 Bun/70g	195	3.2	278	6.8	51.5	4.5	2.3
Iced, Filled, with Raspberry Jam, M & S*	1 Bun/48g	155	3.2	320	6.4	58.9	6.6	1.9
Iced, Finger, Average	1 Bun/40g	130	3.1	325	7.2	57.0	7.7	2.3
Iced, Fingers, Coconut, Genesis Crafty*	1 Bun/64g	210	6.9	328	7.7	52.4	10.8	2.4
Iced, Lemon, Tesco*	1 Bun/48g	156	4.2	325	5.2	56.5	8.7	1.9
Iced, Spiced Fruit, M & S*	1 Bun/90g	270	3.3	300	7.0	60.3	3.7	1.5
Iced, Tesco*	1 Bun/35g	117	3.4	334	7.0	54.8	9.6	2.5
BURGERS								
American Style, Tesco*	1 Burger/125g	250	9.1	200	13.0	20.4	7.3	3.9
Beef, & Mature Cheddar, Asda*	1 Burger/80g	178	10.0	223	21.5	6.2	12.5	0.5
Beef, & Onion, Grilled, Asda*	1 Burger/81g	201	11.5	248	23.1	6.9	14.2	0.5
Beef, 100%, Average	1 Burger/52g	148	11.6	286	20.5	0.6	22.3	0.1
Beef, 100%, Birds Eye*	1 Burger/41g	120	10.2	292	17.3	0.0	24.8	0.0
Beef, 100%, Half Pounders, Sainsbury's*	1 Burger/148g	462	33.1	313	26.0	1.7	22.4	0.2
Beef, 100%, Mega, Birds Eye*	1 Burger/96g	280	23.8	293	17.3	0.0	24.9	0.0
Beef, 100%, Organic, Waitrose*	1 Burger/57g	140	9.6	247	23.6	0.0	16.9	0.0
Beef, 100%, Pure, Ross*	1 Burger/56g	128	9.6	229	17.1	1.4	17.1	0.0
Beef, 100%, Quarter Pounders, Aldi*	1 Burger/114g	320	23.3	282	24.3	0.1	20.5	1.3
Beef, 100%, Quarter Pounders, Ross*	1 Burger/74g	222	18.8	301	16.8	1.1	25.5	0.0
Beef, 100%, with Seasoning, No Onion, Birds Eye*	1 Burger/41g	134	11.9	326	16.1	0.2	29.0	0.0
Beef, 100%, without Onion, Sainsbury's*	1 Burger/43g	133	10.4	308	21.9	0.8	24.1	0.8
Beef, Aberdeen Angus, Asda*	1 Burger/112g	249	13.3	222	22.2	6.7	11.8	0.9
Beef, Aberdeen Angus, Fresh, Waitrose*	1 Burger/113g	269	21.0	238	16.4	1.2	18.6	0.0
Beef, Aberdeen Angus, Frozen, Waitrose*	1 Burger/57g	145	11.6	255	18.1	0.0	20.3	1.1
Beef, Aberdeen Angus, Gourmet, Finest, Tesco*	1 Burger/118g	225	13.4	190	18.9	2.0	11.3	1.0
Beef, Aberdeen Angus, M & S*	1 Burger/142g	298	18.9	210	18.3	4.1	13.3	0.1
Beef, Aberdeen Angus, Mega, Birds Eye*	1 Burger/101g	279	22.6	276	16.3	2.4	22.4	0.1
Beef, Aberdeen Angus, Virgin Trains*	1 Burger/240g	695	37.6	290	13.5	23.8	15.7	0.0
Beef, Asda*	1 Burger/114g	304	18.6	267	26.8	3.2	16.3	0.7
Beef, Barbecue, Tesco*	1 Burger/114g	295	22.7	260	15.6	3.5	20.0	0.5
Beef, BGTY, Sainsbury's*	1 Burger/110g	177	6.0	161	20.8	7.1	5.5	1.1
Beef, British, Grilled, Finest, Tesco*	1 Burger/95g	185	11.8	195	17.2	3.3	12.4	0.9
Beef, British, Organic, Waitrose*	1 Burger/85g	226	16.6	266	19.0	3.5	19.5	1.0
Beef, British, Waitrose*	1 Burger/113g	279	21.0	247	18.6	1.2	18.6	0.0
Beef, Chargrill, Tesco*	1 Burger/114g	246	18.4	217	17.0	0.8	16.2	2.5
Beef, Chargrilled, Giant, Farmfoods*	1 Burger/170g	352	21.8	207	17.3	5.6	12.8	1.2
Beef, Economy, Value, Tesco*	1 Burger/41g	105	5.9	255	21.6	8.5	14.5	0.3
Beef, Farmfoods*	1 Burger/50g	128	9.8	255	14.4	5.4	19.6	0.1
Beef, Filled with Gorgonzola, M & S*	1 Burger/167g	384	26.9	230	16.5	4.9	16.1	0.5
Beef, Flame Grilled, Dalepak*	1 Burger/44g	134	11.4	304	15.3	2.1	26.0	0.4
Beef, Mega, Birds Eye*	1 Burger/109g	300	25.1	275	14.3	2.7	23.0	0.3

	Measure INFO/WEIGHT	per Measure KCAL	FAT	Nutrition Values per 100g / 100ml KCAL	PROT	CARB	FAT	FIBRE
BURGERS								
Beef, Morrisons*	1 Burger/57g	169	14.3	298	12.3	5.5	25.2	0.6
Beef, New York Style, Grilled, Tesco*	1 Burger/35g	80	5.2	229	18.6	5.7	14.9	0.6
Beef, Organic, M & S*	1 Burger/110g	239	17.6	217	18.2	0.0	16.0	0.2
Beef, Original, & Best, Birds Eye*	1 Burger/46g	115	8.9	252	14.1	5.1	19.5	0.4
Beef, Original, with Onion, Grilled, Birds Eye*	1 Burger/38g	110	9.5	287	13.4	2.6	24.8	0.3
Beef, Quarter Pounders, BGTY, Sainsbury's*	1 Burger/114g	188	9.3	166	16.9	6.1	8.2	1.0
Beef, Quarter Pounders, Farmfoods*	1 Burger/113g	289	22.1	256	14.4	5.4	19.6	0.1
Beef, Quarter Pounders, Flame Grilled, Rustlers*	1 Burger/190g	557	28.7	293	14.9	24.3	15.1	0.0
Beef, Quarter Pounders, Flame Grilled, Tesco*	1 Burger/88g	246	20.4	280	13.1	4.8	23.2	0.8
Beef, Quarter Pounders, Morrisons*	1 Burger/114g	338	28.6	298	12.3	5.5	25.2	0.6
Beef, Quarter Pounders, Reduced Fat, Tesco*	1 Burger/95g	171	12.4	180	14.0	1.8	13.0	0.8
Beef, Quarter Pounders, Steak Country, Lidl*	1 Burger/68g	188	15.1	276	16.3	2.4	22.2	0.1
Beef, Quarter Pounders, Tesco*	1 Burger/113g	292	23.1	258	17.8	0.7	20.4	1.3
Beef, Quarter Pounders, with Onion, BGTY, Sainsbury's*	1 Burger/83g	171	7.8	205	26.6	3.8	9.3	0.9
Beef, Quarter Pounders, with Onion, Birds Eye*	1 Burger/114g	286	22.1	252	14.1	5.1	19.5	0.4
Beef, Quarter Pounders, with Onion, Cooked, Birds Eye*	1 Burger/100g	230	16.0	230	16.0	5.9	16.0	0.4
Beef, Quarter Pounders, with Onion, Sainsbury's*	1 Burger/113g	306	22.4	271	18.0	5.1	19.8	1.5
Beef, Sainsbury's*	1 Burger/57g	152	9.1	267	29.6	1.3	15.9	1.5
Beef, Scotch, Ultimate, TTD, Sainsbury's*	1 Burger/119g	265	15.8	223	25.3	0.5	13.3	1.0
Beef, Simply Seasoned, TTD, Sainsbury's*	1 Burger/110g	298	25.0	271	15.3	18.1	22.7	0.5
Beef, Steak, British, Cooked, TTD, Sainsbury's*	1 Burger/93g	191	11.9	205	21.0	1.5	12.8	0.5
Beef, Steak, Ultimate, TTD, Sainsbury's*	1 Burger/136g	355	24.1	261	25.3	0.1	17.7	0.5
Beef, Sun Dried Tomato, Grilled, Finest, Tesco*	1 Burger/99g	170	7.3	172	20.5	5.8	7.4	0.5
Beef, Super Sized, Big Bite, Birds Eye*	1 Burger/122g	320	25.2	262	13.1	6.0	20.6	1.0
Beef, with Cheese Melt, COOK!, M & S*	1 Burger/182g	400	28.9	220	17.9	1.3	15.9	1.2
Beef, with Fresh Garden Herbs, Raw, TTD, Sainsbury's*	1 Burger/142g	280	14.8	197	21.5	4.4	10.4	1.3
Beef, with Herbs, Finest, Tesco*	1 Burger/105g	200	11.8	190	17.3	4.5	11.2	0.7
Beef, with Jalapeno Chilli, Finest, Tesco*	1 Burger/205g	379	22.3	185	17.0	3.4	10.9	0.4
Beef, with Mediterranean Tomato & Basil, M & S*	1 Burger/169g	304	18.6	180	15.7	5.1	11.0	1.4
Beef, with Onion, Cooked, Ross*	1 Burger/41g	117	9.8	284	14.7	2.8	23.8	0.4
Beef, with Onion, Sainsbury's*	1 Burger/42g	102	6.2	243	20.7	6.9	14.8	1.0
Beef, with Potato Gratin, Weight Watchers*	1 Pack/400g	320	10.0	80	3.0	10.0	2.5	0.0
Cheeseburger	1 Serving/275g	706	29.0	257	13.7	25.6	10.6	1.8
Cheeseburger, American, Tesco*	1 Burger/275g	660	26.3	240	13.6	24.9	9.6	1.6
Cheeseburger, Micro Snack, Tesco*	1 Burger/115g	309	14.5	269	12.6	26.4	12.6	0.0
Cheeseburger, Smart Price, Asda*	1 Burger/150g	374	14.0	249	13.3	28.0	9.3	1.4
Cheeseburger, with Relish, American Style, Tesco*	1 Burger/61g	132	6.0	215	14.2	17.5	9.8	4.2
Cheeseburger, with Sesame Seed Bun, Tesco*	1 Burger/275g	644	32.2	234	12.2	20.1	11.7	2.0
Chicken, Average	1 Burger/46g	111	5.6	242	14.9	18.7	12.1	1.0
Chicken, Breaded, Value, Tesco*	1 Burger/57g	165	10.8	290	10.5	19.2	19.0	1.4
Chicken, Crispy Crumb, Farmfoods*	1 Burger/242g	707	45.5	292	10.5	20.2	18.8	1.1
Chicken, Crunch Crumb, Tesco*	1 Burger/57g	161	10.8	282	12.3	15.6	18.9	0.0
Chicken, Fillet, Weight After Cooking, Birds Eye*	1 Burger/90g	126	4.1	140	20.0	5.1	4.6	0.2
Chicken, Fresh, Non Coated, Waitrose*	1 Burger/100g	141	4.0	141	16.0	10.4	4.0	0.9
Chicken, Southern Fried, Sainsbury's*	1 Burger/52g	154	10.3	297	12.6	17.2	19.8	1.3
Chicken Cajun, Fillet, Birds Eye*	1 Pack/180g	275	8.8	153	21.5	5.8	4.9	0.3
Chicken Crunch & Fries, M & S*	1 Pack/425g	915	47.6	215	8.8	20.8	11.2	2.1
Chilli, Quarter Pounders, Asda*	1 Burger/88g	221	14.0	252	25.0	2.0	16.0	0.0
Chilli, Quarter Pounders, Farmfoods*	1 Burger/115g	285	23.3	248	13.5	2.9	20.3	0.9
Chilli, Quarter Pounders, Iceland*	1 Burger/84g	265	20.1	316	18.6	6.5	23.9	0.4
Classic, Eddie Rockets*	1 Burger/295g	620	35.0	210	10.8	14.9	11.9	0.0
Economy, Smart Price, Asda*	1 Burger/49g	142	10.2	293	14.0	12.0	21.0	1.1
Lamb, Minted, Average	1 Burger/56g	125	7.4	223	20.6	5.5	13.2	0.2

B

	Measure INFO/WEIGHT	per Measure KCAL	per Measure FAT	KCAL	PROT	CARB	FAT	FIBRE
				Nutrition Values per 100g / 100ml				
BURGERS								
Lamb, Quarter Pounders, Average	1 Burger/113g	283	19.3	250	17.4	5.2	17.1	0.8
Lamb, Quarter Pounders, Birds Eye*	1 Burger/112g	232	16.9	207	13.9	3.8	15.1	0.3
Lamb, Quarter Pounders, Minted, Asda*	1 Burger/114g	241	14.0	212	19.2	6.1	12.3	0.0
Lamb, Waitrose*	1 Burger/67g	99	4.7	148	15.7	5.4	7.0	0.9
Less Than 7% Fat, Sainsbury's*	1 Burger/102g	164	5.6	161	20.8	7.1	5.5	1.1
Low Fat, Iceland*	1 Burger/85g	148	4.1	174	27.8	5.0	4.8	1.1
Meat Free, Sainsbury's*	1 Burger/57g	86	2.8	151	22.0	4.4	5.0	3.4
Mushroom & Spinach, Cooked, Love Veg, Sainsbury's*	1 Burger/76g	192	11.0	254	5.2	22.7	14.6	5.6
Mushroom & Wensleydale Cheese, Cauldron Foods*	1 Burger/87g	156	9.6	179	9.0	11.0	11.0	4.0
Nacho, Chicken & Sweetcorn, Asda*	½ Pack/144g	249	13.0	173	14.0	9.0	9.0	2.3
Ostrich, Quarter Pounder, Oslinc*	1 Burger/113g	132	1.5	117	22.9	3.5	1.3	1.1
Pork, Free Range, Waitrose*	1 Burger/115g	306	19.9	266	19.3	7.7	17.3	1.0
Pork, Quarter Pounders, Birds Eye*	1 Burger/122g	292	23.2	239	13.9	3.2	19.0	0.2
Pork & Apple, Grilled, Finest, Tesco*	1 Burger/88g	251	18.4	285	14.3	9.6	20.9	1.2
Pork & Apple, Quarter Pounder, Grilled, Asda*	1 Burger/80g	147	6.4	184	23.9	4.1	8.0	0.5
Quarter Pounders, Big Country*	1 Burger/90g	271	20.8	301	22.1	1.8	23.1	0.0
Quarter Pounders, Chargrilled, BGTY, Sainsbury's*	1 Burger/114g	184	6.3	161	20.8	7.1	5.5	1.1
Quarter Pounders, Highlander*	1 Burger/114g	335	26.3	295	21.7	4.2	23.2	0.0
Quarter Pounders, Iceland*	1 Burger/83g	253	18.8	305	20.4	5.1	22.6	0.6
Salmon, Quarter Pounders, Morrisons*	1 Burger/110g	235	13.0	214	21.4	5.5	11.8	1.7
Salmon, Quarter Pounders, Tesco*	1 Burger/114g	145	2.7	128	15.9	10.6	2.4	1.2
Salmon, Tesco*	1 Burger/100g	101	3.0	101	18.2	0.3	3.0	0.0
Tuna, Quarter Pounders, Tesco*	1 Burger/114g	132	1.8	116	18.8	6.7	1.6	0.9
Tuna, Sainsbury's*	1 Serving/105g	194	10.3	185	20.8	3.4	9.8	1.2
Turkey, Cheeseburgers, Tesco*	1 Burger/105g	252	14.8	240	15.4	12.8	14.1	1.3
Turkey, Crispy Crumb, Bernard Matthews*	1 Burger/60g	158	9.5	263	12.6	17.5	15.8	1.8
Turkey, Grilled, Cranberry Foods Ltd*	1 Serving/100g	173	5.9	173	21.1	8.8	5.9	1.4
Turkey, Harvestland*	1 Burger/112g	179	9.0	160	23.0	1.0	8.0	0.0
Value, Farmfoods*	1 Burger/49g	138	10.8	282	11.4	9.6	22.1	0.9
Venison, & Sweet Onion, M & S*	1 Burger/142g	163	5.0	115	19.3	1.4	3.5	0.5
Venison, Finnebrougue Estate*	1 Burger/142g	170	7.0	120	19.9	4.2	4.9	0.5
Venison, Grilled, Extra Special, Asda*	2 Burgers/227g	331	8.2	146	21.5	5.3	3.6	3.2
Venison, TTD, Sainsbury's*	1 Burger/150g	224	6.3	149	20.4	6.5	4.2	3.2
BURGERS VEGETARIAN								
Bean, Tesco*	1 Burger/90g	192	10.9	213	4.4	21.6	12.1	5.0
Black Bean, Organic, Cauldron Foods*	1 Burger/88g	169	10.1	193	9.2	13.1	11.5	8.5
Cheese & Spring Onion, Tesco*	1 Burger/87g	178	10.3	204	4.4	20.0	11.8	3.2
Chilli, Cauldron Foods*	1 Burger/88g	148	8.1	169	11.5	8.5	9.3	3.3
Flame Grilled, Linda McCartney*	1 Burger/60g	104	3.1	174	17.9	13.8	5.2	3.3
Meat Free, Average	¼ Pounder/113g	195	8.8	172	17.5	7.9	7.8	3.0
Meat Free, Spicy, Bean & Nacho, Cooked, Asda*	1 Burger/113g	247	9.6	218	5.3	27.7	8.5	4.7
Mexican Style, Bean, Meat Free, Tesco*	1 Burger/94g	206	8.7	220	4.9	28.2	9.3	3.9
Mushroom, Cauldron Foods*	1 Burger/88g	125	5.5	143	5.5	16.1	6.3	2.6
Mushroom, Meat Free, Tesco*	1 Burger/87g	151	9.5	173	3.6	15.3	10.8	3.7
Mushroom, Organic, Cauldron Foods*	1 Burger/88g	136	7.3	156	7.1	18.2	8.3	2.3
Peri Peri, Frozen, Linda McCartney*	1 Burger/113g	251	9.7	222	20.8	14.7	8.6	4.1
Quarter Pounders, Average	1 Burger/113g	210	9.8	186	9.1	17.7	8.6	3.2
Quarter Pounders, Beef Style, Sainsbury's*	1 Burger/114g	216	10.8	190	20.0	6.0	9.5	2.5
Quarter Pounders, Linda McCartney*	1 Burger/114g	187	11.3	165	14.4	4.4	10.0	4.2
Savoury, Cauldron Foods*	1 Burger/88g	145	8.0	166	108.0	7.9	9.2	2.4
Spicy Bean, Average	1 Burger/56g	125	6.8	223	5.6	24.3	12.2	4.8
Spicy Bean, BGTY, Sainsbury's*	1 Burger/85g	123	2.3	145	6.9	23.3	2.7	3.1
Spicy Bean, Cauldron Foods*	1 Burger/88g	203	9.8	232	5.4	27.4	11.2	6.2

	Measure INFO/WEIGHT	per Measure KCAL	FAT	Nutrition Values per 100g / 100ml KCAL	PROT	CARB	FAT	FIBRE
BURGERS VEGETARIAN								
Spicy Bean, Linda McCartney*	1 Burger/85g	190	9.5	223	4.3	26.2	11.2	2.9
Spicy Bean, Quarter Pounder, Dalepak*	1 Burger/115g	237	12.5	206	4.6	22.3	10.9	2.6
Traditional, Fry's Special Vegetarian*	1 Burger/75g	175	9.0	233	19.2	13.0	12.0	0.2
Vegeburger, Linda McCartney*	1 Burger/50g	62	1.4	124	15.8	10.7	2.9	5.8
Vegeburger, Retail, Grilled	1oz/28g	55	3.1	196	16.6	8.0	11.1	4.2
Vegetable, Average	1 Burger/56g	100	4.5	179	4.4	22.4	8.0	2.3
Vegetable, Captains, Birds Eye*	1 Burger/48g	96	4.2	200	4.7	25.5	8.8	2.0
Vegetable, Organic, Goodlife*	1 Burger/67g	114	3.9	170	3.2	26.3	5.8	2.6
Vegetable, Quarter Pounders, Crunchy, Birds Eye*	1 Burger/114g	240	11.6	211	4.8	24.9	10.2	1.8
Vegetable, Quarter Pounders, Dalepak*	1 Burger/114g	227	9.6	200	4.8	26.3	8.5	1.8
BUTTER								
Brandy, Average	1 Serving/10g	56	3.8	556	0.2	46.2	38.4	0.1
Brandy, with Cognac, Sainsbury's*	1/8 Pot/25g	146	10.9	584	0.3	41.8	43.5	0.3
Clarified, Cook's Range, Lurpak*	1 Serving/100g	898	99.8	898	0.0	0.0	99.8	0.0
Coconut, Artisana*	2 Tbsp/32g	186	18.0	574	6.2	21.6	55.5	15.4
Creamery, Average	***1 Serving/10g***	***74***	***8.1***	***736***	***0.5***	***0.4***	***81.4***	***0.0***
Fresh, Average	***1 Thin Spread/7g***	***51***	***5.7***	***735***	***0.6***	***0.4***	***81.3***	***0.0***
Goats, St Helen's Farm*	1 Serving/10g	79	8.8	794	0.5	0.0	88.0	0.0
Granules, Butter Buds*	1 Tsp/1g	5	0.1	368	1.8	77.9	6.5	2.3
Jersey, TTD, Sainsbury's*	1 Thin Spread/7g	52	5.8	744	0.5	0.6	82.2	0.0
Reduced Fat, Fresh, Average	***1 Thin Spread/7g***	***26***	***2.8***	***368***	***2.3***	***1.2***	***39.4***	***0.2***
Salted, Average	***1 Thin Spread/7g***	***51***	***5.7***	***729***	***0.4***	***0.3***	***81.1***	***0.0***
Spreadable, Butterpak, Lighter, Tesco*	1 Serving/10g	54	5.6	545	0.5	0.5	56.0	0.0
Spreadable, Fresh, Average	***1 Thin Spread/7g***	***51***	***5.7***	***730***	***0.4***	***0.3***	***80.8***	***0.0***
Spreadable, Lighter, Norpak, Aldi*	1 Serving/10g	51	5.6	510	0.6	0.9	56.0	0.0
Spreadable, Lightest, Lurpak*	1oz/28g	106	11.2	377	3.3	0.9	40.0	0.0
Spreadable, Organic, Lighter, Yeo Valley*	1 Serving/12g	66	7.3	550	0.7	0.9	60.7	0.0
Spreadable, Reduced Fat, Average	***1 Thin Spread/7g***	***38***	***4.2***	***540***	***0.5***	***0.5***	***60.0***	***0.0***
Spreadable, Slightly Salted, Lurpak*	1 Serving/10g	72	8.0	724	0.5	0.6	80.0	0.0
with Crushed Garlic, Lurpak*	1 Serving/10g	70	7.5	700	1.0	4.0	75.0	0.0
BUTTERMILK								
Average	***1 Mug/400ml***	***177***	***1.3***	***44***	***4.2***	***5.9***	***0.3***	***0.0***
BUTTONS								
Chocolate, Giant, Dairy Milk, Cadbury*	1 Button/3g	15	0.9	525	7.7	56.7	29.9	0.7
Chocolate, Milk, Asda*	1 Bag/70g	368	21.0	526	7.0	57.0	30.0	1.5
Chocolate, Milk, M & S*	1 Pack/75g	375	19.0	500	8.6	59.8	25.3	1.9
Chocolate, Milk, Tesco*	1 Bag/70g	359	19.3	513	7.1	59.1	27.6	2.1
Chocolate, White, Cadbury*	1 Pack/32g	180	11.0	555	4.5	58.4	33.8	0.0
Chocolate, White, Co-Op*	½ Pack/35g	186	9.8	530	7.0	64.0	28.0	0.0
Chocolate, White, Milkybar, Nestle*	1 Bag/30g	164	9.5	546	7.5	58.1	31.6	0.0
Chocolate, White, Tesco*	1 Bag/70g	388	23.4	554	5.1	58.0	33.5	0.0

	Measure INFO/WEIGHT	per Measure KCAL	FAT	Nutrition Values per 100g / 100ml KCAL	PROT	CARB	FAT	FIBRE
CABBAGE								
& Leek, Crunchy Mix, Ready to Cook, Sainsbury's*	1 Serving/125g	34	0.6	27	1.9	3.7	0.5	2.6
& Leek, Ready Sliced, Sainsbury's*	1 Pack/240g	53	1.2	22	1.1	2.2	0.5	2.1
& Leek, Sliced, Tesco*	1/3 Pack/100g	32	0.6	32	2.1	3.4	0.6	2.6
Boiled, Average	***1 Serving/90g***	***14***	***0.3***	***15***	***1.0***	***2.2***	***0.3***	***1.7***
Creamed, Cooked, Sainsbury's*	½ Pack/150g	95	6.8	67	2.0	2.6	4.8	2.5
Greens, Trimmed, Average	***1oz/28g***	***8***	***0.1***	***28***	***2.9***	***3.0***	***0.5***	***3.4***
Medley, Washed, Ready to Cook, Tesco*	1 Pack/200g	60	1.2	30	2.3	3.7	0.6	2.8
Raw, Average	***1 Serving/100g***	***21***	***0.4***	***21***	***1.3***	***3.2***	***0.4***	***1.8***
Red, Average	***1 Serving/90g***	***19***	***0.2***	***21***	***1.0***	***3.7***	***0.3***	***2.2***
Red, Braised, with Red Wine, M & S*	½ Pack/150g	180	7.2	120	1.4	17.1	4.8	1.0
Red, Pickled, Average	***1 Serving/100g***	***26***	***0.2***	***26***	***0.9***	***4.6***	***0.2***	***1.6***
Red, Pickled, Oak Lane*	1 Serving/100g	46	0.1	46	1.0	8.6	0.1	2.6
Red, Spiced, Steamer, Sainsbury's*	½ Pack/150g	105	3.3	70	1.0	10.5	2.2	2.9
Red, with Apple, Frozen, Sainsbury's*	1 Serving/75g	38	0.0	50	1.8	10.8	0.0	2.2
Red, with Apples, Onions & Redcurrant Jelly, M & S*	½ Pack/150g	112	3.3	75	0.9	12.4	2.2	2.0
Red, with Bramley Apple, Aunt Bessie's*	1 Serving/125g	72	1.1	58	0.9	10.0	0.9	2.7
Red, with Bramley Apple, Braised, Sainsbury's*	½ Pack/150g	146	7.2	97	0.9	12.6	4.8	1.7
Savoy, Boiled in Salted Water, Average	***1 Serving/90g***	***15***	***0.4***	***17***	***1.1***	***2.2***	***0.5***	***2.0***
Savoy, Raw, Average	***1 Serving/90g***	***24***	***0.4***	***27***	***2.1***	***3.9***	***0.5***	***3.1***
Steamed, Average	1 Serving/100g	15	0.3	15	1.0	2.2	0.3	1.7
Sweetheart, Raw	1 Serving/100g	26	0.6	26	2.1	3.2	0.6	2.8
White, Raw, Average	***1oz/28g***	***8***	***0.1***	***27***	***1.4***	***5.0***	***0.2***	***2.1***
CAKE								
Action Man, Birthday, Memory Lane Cakes*	1/12 Cake/83g	322	13.6	388	3.0	57.0	16.4	0.8
Aero, Celebration, Mint, Nestle*	1 Slice/58g	232	11.8	400	4.0	49.7	20.3	1.7
Alabama Chocolate Fudge, Farmfoods*	1/6 Cake/61g	201	5.9	329	4.7	55.7	9.7	2.7
Almond Flavoured Rounds, Country Garden Cakes*	1 Cake/45g	183	6.7	403	4.3	62.4	14.7	2.3
Almond Slices, GFY, Asda*	1 Slice/25g	67	0.8	268	4.0	56.0	3.1	0.7
Almond Slices, Lyons*	1 Slice/27g	114	6.9	426	7.1	41.3	25.8	1.6
Almond Slices, Mr Kipling*	1 Slice/33g	131	4.6	403	6.3	63.4	14.0	2.0
Almond Slices, Sainsbury's*	1 Serving/27g	120	7.1	444	5.9	45.9	26.3	1.5
Almond Slices, Weight Watchers*	1 Slice/26g	95	2.6	365	5.2	63.8	9.9	2.4
Angel, Average	1 Slice/44g	175	7.9	397	4.2	54.9	17.9	0.8
Angel Layer, Tesco*	1 Serving/25g	101	4.3	403	4.5	57.4	17.3	0.9
Angel Slices, Mr Kipling*	1 Slice/34g	140	6.2	417	2.8	59.4	18.5	0.6
Angel Slices, Snap Packs, Mr Kipling*	1 Slice/34g	148	6.6	417	2.7	60.1	18.5	0.6
Apple, Home Style, M & S*	1 Cake/54g	189	7.9	350	5.3	49.4	14.7	1.5
Apple & Cinnamon, Mini Popcorn, M & S*	1 Serving/22g	84	0.2	380	5.8	87.4	1.0	2.2
Apple & Cinnamon, Oat Break, Go Ahead, McVitie's*	1 Serving/35g	122	2.3	349	5.2	67.2	6.6	2.6
Apple Bakes, Go Ahead, McVitie's*	1 Cake/35g	126	2.7	361	2.6	70.0	7.8	2.0
Apple Crumble, Bramley, & Blackberry, M & S*	1/8 Cake/56g	221	10.0	395	4.4	54.1	17.9	1.5
Apple Crumble, Slices, Weight Watchers*	1 Slice/26g	90	2.0	346	4.5	64.8	7.7	2.3
Apple Slice, Delightful, Mr Kipling*	1 Slice/29g	92	1.1	317	4.4	66.2	3.9	1.3
Apricot & Apple, Trimlyne*	1 Cake/50g	134	1.4	267	4.3	58.4	2.7	1.9
Bakewell, Lemon, Average	1 Cake/42g	173	6.4	411	3.7	64.6	15.2	1.3
Bakewell, The Handmade Flapjack Company*	1 Cake/75g	311	17.1	415	4.5	47.4	22.8	0.0
Bakewell, Tray Bake, Kate's Cakes Ltd*	1 Serving/100g	475	28.3	475	6.6	46.3	28.3	2.8
Bakewell Slice, Weight Watchers*	1 Slice/26g	84	0.6	324	3.7	71.0	2.4	2.0
Bakewell Slices, Mr Kipling*	1 Slice/36g	163	7.3	454	4.2	63.4	20.4	1.2
Banana, Iced, Waitrose*	1/6 Cake/55g	190	5.9	345	4.2	58.0	10.7	2.7
Banana, Organic, Loaf, Respect Organics*	¼ Pack/65g	254	13.6	391	3.9	48.6	21.0	1.5
Banana, The Handmade Flapjack Company*	1 Cake/75g	290	10.8	387	5.3	59.2	14.4	0.0
Banana Bread, Brilliant, Graze*	1 Cake/23g	72	3.6	312	5.2	40.4	15.6	3.0

	Measure INFO/WEIGHT	per Measure KCAL	FAT	Nutrition Values per 100g / 100ml KCAL	PROT	CARB	FAT	FIBRE
CAKE								
Banana Loaf, Waitrose*	1 Slice/70g	236	7.5	337	5.0	55.2	10.7	1.7
Banoffee Slices, Dessert Classics, Mr Kipling*	1 Slice/34g	140	6.2	414	2.9	59.0	18.4	0.6
Battenberg, Asda*	1 Slice/25g	104	3.0	418	6.0	71.1	12.2	0.8
Battenberg, Mini, Mr Kipling*	1 Cake/35g	144	3.8	410	4.6	76.2	11.0	1.3
Battenberg, Mr Kipling*	1 Serving/38g	161	4.6	421	5.0	73.3	12.0	1.6
Birthday, M & S*	1 Serving/60g	240	7.1	400	2.3	70.9	11.9	0.8
Birthday Present, Tesco*	1 Serving/79g	347	13.9	439	3.5	66.6	17.6	0.4
Bites, Caramel, Mr Kipling*	1 Cake/14g	68	3.8	492	5.9	55.3	27.4	0.8
Bites, Chocolate Roll, Mini, Tesco*	1 Bite/18g	78	3.6	435	6.0	58.0	19.8	1.9
Bites, Coconut, Sainsbury's*	1 Bite/80g	339	16.9	424	5.3	53.0	21.2	4.2
Butterfly, Mr Kipling*	1 Cake/29g	114	6.4	392	4.4	43.4	22.2	0.6
Buttons, Happy Birthday, Cadbury*	1 Slice/50g	235	13.6	470	4.1	52.8	27.1	0.0
Cappuccino, Kate's Cakes Ltd*	1 Serving/100g	415	19.0	415	3.8	56.5	19.0	1.1
Caramel, Milk Chocolate, Holly Lane*	1 Cake/25g	110	5.1	441	6.9	57.6	20.3	1.1
Caramel Crunchy, Devondale*	1 Cake/80g	359	19.2	449	2.9	56.3	24.0	1.3
Caramel Shortbread, Devondale*	1 Cake/75g	356	18.6	474	3.0	57.0	24.8	0.8
Caramel Shortbread, Tray Bake, Kate's Cakes Ltd*	1 Serving/100g	471	27.3	471	3.0	53.3	27.3	1.2
Caramel Shortcake Slices, McVitie's*	1 Slice/32g	146	7.7	463	4.3	56.5	24.4	1.6
Caramel Slice, M & S*	1 Slice/64g	304	16.1	475	4.9	60.4	25.2	2.6
Carrot, & Orange, Extra Special, Asda*	1/6 Cake/65g	240	11.7	369	4.7	47.0	18.0	0.9
Carrot, & Orange, Finest, Tesco*	1/8 Cake/50g	205	10.2	410	4.6	51.2	20.5	2.1
Carrot, & Orange, LC, Tesco*	1/6 Cake/63g	227	6.2	360	3.9	64.2	9.8	1.3
Carrot, & Orange, Waitrose*	1/6 Cake/47g	164	7.4	350	5.3	46.8	15.7	1.8
Carrot, & Orange Slices, GFY, Asda*	1 Serving/23g	77	0.6	334	3.4	74.0	2.7	1.0
Carrot, & Pecan, M & S*	1 Slice/90g	330	14.6	365	6.4	48.7	16.2	2.3
Carrot, & Walnut, Layered, Asda*	1 Serving/42g	172	8.0	409	4.6	55.0	19.0	1.0
Carrot, & Walnut, Mini Classics, Mr Kipling*	1 Cake/39g	172	9.8	440	4.5	48.6	25.2	1.0
Carrot, Average	1 Slice/56g	211	10.4	377	4.6	47.6	18.6	1.4
Carrot, Entenmann's*	1 Serving/40g	156	8.2	391	4.1	47.4	20.5	1.5
Carrot, Handmade, Delicious, Boots*	1 Slice/75g	292	13.5	389	4.1	53.0	18.0	1.4
Carrot, Iced, Tesco*	1 Serving/61g	246	12.0	404	3.1	53.7	19.6	1.6
Carrot, Kate's Cakes Ltd*	1 Serving/100g	405	21.4	405	4.1	47.1	21.4	2.6
Carrot, Mini, Weight Watchers*	1 Cake/31g	120	3.3	388	3.7	68.9	10.8	2.7
Carrot, Organic, Respect Organics*	1 Slice/45g	179	10.1	398	3.1	47.4	22.4	1.5
Carrot, Slices, Asda*	1 Slice/80g	302	13.2	377	3.4	53.8	16.5	1.7
Carrot, Slices, GFY, Asda*	1 Slice/28g	83	0.6	298	2.8	66.4	2.3	2.1
Carrot, Slices, Inspirations, Mr Kipling*	1 Slice/34g	139	6.3	411	3.5	57.7	18.5	1.3
Carrot, Slices, Less Than 3% Fat, BGTY, Sainsbury's*	1 Slice/30g	94	0.8	313	3.4	68.7	2.7	2.4
Carrot, Slices, Weight Watchers*	1 Slice/27g	84	0.2	311	2.8	73.0	0.8	0.9
Carrot, Square, Margaret's Country Kitchen*	1 Cake/80g	307	13.5	384	3.6	54.4	16.9	2.4
Carrot, The Handmade Flapjack Company*	1 Cake/75g	295	13.0	393	6.4	53.0	17.3	0.0
Carrot, Ultimate, Entenmann's*	1/8 Cake/64g	234	10.1	367	4.7	51.4	15.8	0.3
Carrot, Wedge, Tesco*	1 Pack/175g	532	27.6	304	3.9	36.6	15.8	1.5
Cherry, Asda*	1 Slice/37g	131	4.5	351	4.7	56.0	12.0	0.6
Cherry, Co-Op*	1/8 Cake/47g	190	8.5	405	4.0	57.0	18.0	0.8
Cherry, M & S*	1 Serving/75g	285	9.5	380	5.0	60.6	12.7	0.8
Cherry Bakewell, Co-Op*	1 Cake/47g	205	8.0	435	3.7	67.2	16.9	1.8
Cherry Bakewell, GF, Bakers Delight*	1 Cake/50g	211	8.2	422	2.9	66.1	16.3	0.4
Cherry Bakewell, Layer, Asda*	1/8 Cake/50g	210	11.0	420	4.4	51.0	22.0	0.6
Cherry Bakewell, M & S*	1 Cake/44g	185	7.8	420	4.5	61.7	17.7	1.0
Cherry Bakewell, Mini, Sainsbury's*	1 Cake/27g	101	3.3	370	3.4	62.2	12.0	0.4
Cherry Bakewell, Sainsbury's*	1 Cake/46g	200	8.1	436	3.1	66.3	17.6	1.4
Cherry Bakewell, Sara Lee*	1/5 Slice/70g	228	7.9	326	4.1	51.9	11.3	1.4

	Measure INFO/WEIGHT	per Measure KCAL	FAT	Nutrition Values per 100g / 100ml KCAL	PROT	CARB	FAT	FIBRE
CAKE								
Cherry Bakewell, Waitrose*	1 Cake/44g	184	8.5	419	3.8	57.4	19.3	2.1
Cherry Bakewell, Weight Watchers*	1oz/28g	102	2.8	365	3.6	65.4	9.9	3.6
Cherry Bakewells, Delightful, Mr Kipling*	1 Cake/45g	176	5.8	390	3.9	66.4	12.9	1.2
Cherry Bakewells, Mr Kipling*	1 Cake/45g	193	8.3	428	3.9	61.3	18.5	1.4
Chocolate	1oz/28g	128	7.4	456	7.4	50.4	26.4	1.7
Chocolate, & Brandy Butter, Entenmann's*	1 Serving/39g	144	6.7	374	3.4	53.5	17.5	2.8
Chocolate, & Caramel Tiffin Bites, Gu*	1 Tiffin/35g	168	9.9	480	3.8	51.9	28.3	2.8
Chocolate, & Madeira, Marble Loaf, M & S*	1/6 Cake/88g	380	20.4	430	5.0	50.0	23.1	1.0
Chocolate, & Orange Rolls, M & S*	1 Cake/60g	228	17.0	380	3.6	27.0	28.4	1.3
Chocolate, & Orange Slices, GFY, Asda*	1 Serving/30g	95	0.8	315	3.2	70.0	2.5	1.3
Chocolate, Belgian, Slices, Weight Watchers*	1 Slice/25g	86	2.4	344	6.5	57.6	9.8	2.9
Chocolate, Belgian, Waitrose*	1 Slice/47g	223	12.6	474	4.8	53.1	26.9	1.9
Chocolate, Birthday, Tesco*	1 Serving/54g	229	13.2	425	5.9	45.5	24.4	2.1
Chocolate, Caterpillar, Tesco*	1 Serving/53g	248	13.2	468	5.7	55.3	24.9	1.1
Chocolate, Champagne, Sainsbury's*	1 Serving/75g	304	12.2	405	2.5	62.4	16.2	0.5
Chocolate, Cup, Mini, Weight Watchers*	1 Cake/17g	72	3.6	422	6.1	52.0	21.1	1.8
Chocolate, Double Dream, Nestle*	1 Serving/150g	638	37.6	425	5.0	44.7	25.1	0.9
Chocolate, Fondants, Weight Watchers*	1 Cake/19g	70	2.3	368	6.1	59.0	12.0	3.2
Chocolate, Fudge, The Cake Shop*	1 Cake/37g	178	10.8	480	3.7	50.5	29.2	1.3
Chocolate, Happy Birthday, Tesco*	1 Serving/58g	241	13.2	415	4.7	46.9	22.7	2.9
Chocolate, Iced, Tesco*	1 Serving/40g	158	6.3	395	4.7	58.5	15.8	1.8
Chocolate, Loaf, Moist, McVitie's*	1 Slice/30g	119	6.1	398	4.8	49.0	20.3	1.9
Chocolate, Part of Tea Time Selection, Iceland*	1 Cake/31g	144	7.9	464	4.5	54.1	25.5	2.0
Chocolate, Party, Tesco*	1 Slice/62g	244	13.1	394	4.6	46.3	21.2	0.9
Chocolate, Sara Lee*	¼ Cake/88g	339	14.8	385	4.1	54.3	16.8	0.0
Chocolate, Smarties, Celebration, Large, Nestle*	1/16 Cake/71g	308	17.4	432	5.4	48.9	24.4	1.2
Chocolate, The Handmade Flapjack Company*	1 Cake/75g	303	16.2	404	12.5	39.8	21.6	0.0
Chocolate, Thorntons*	1 Serving/87g	408	25.1	469	5.2	47.1	28.8	0.6
Chocolate, Triple, Frozen, Majestic*	¼ Cake/58g	87	5.4	150	2.2	14.1	9.4	0.1
Chocolate, Triple Layer, Celebration, Tesco*	1/24 Cake/79g	345	18.8	430	5.0	47.7	23.4	2.8
Chocolate, White Button, Asda*	1 Cake/30g	117	6.3	390	5.0	44.0	21.0	2.0
Chocolate, with Butter Icing, Average	1oz/28g	135	8.3	481	5.7	50.9	29.7	0.0
Chocolate Box, Asda*	1 Serving/60g	263	13.8	439	5.0	53.0	23.0	0.7
Chocolate Brownie, Devondale*	1 Cake/60g	246	12.9	410	4.4	51.0	21.5	2.1
Chocolate Brownie, Fudge, Entenmann's*	1/8 Cake/55g	168	2.4	306	4.0	62.7	4.4	1.5
Chocolate Brownie, Gluten & Wheat Free, Lovemore*	1 Slice/36g	127	4.6	352	3.7	56.1	12.8	0.2
Chocolate Brownie, Tray Bake, Kate's Cakes Ltd*	1 Serving/100g	435	22.0	435	5.7	51.5	22.0	3.3
Chocolate Chip, Co-Op*	1/6 Cake/63g	275	16.9	440	5.0	44.0	27.0	0.5
Chocolate Chip, The Cake Shop*	1 Cake/35g	178	11.0	508	4.7	50.2	31.5	1.1
Chocolate Crunch, Tray Bake, Kate's Cakes Ltd*	1 Serving/80g	400	23.0	500	4.8	53.4	28.8	3.7
Chocolate Egg, Small, Tesco*	1 Cake/31g	132	6.3	425	5.4	57.2	20.2	1.7
Chocolate Flavour, Slices, GFY, Asda*	1 Slice/28g	71	0.7	257	4.3	54.0	2.6	1.4
Chocolate Flower Pot, M & S*	1 Serving/69g	295	13.2	430	3.8	60.8	19.3	1.5
Chocolate Fudge	1 Serving/110g	415	19.1	377	4.4	50.4	17.4	1.4
Chocolate Fudge, & Vanilla Cream, M & S*	1/6 Cake/69g	310	17.9	450	5.2	49.8	26.0	1.3
Chocolate Fudge, Classics, M & S*	1 Serving/71g	195	7.5	275	2.8	42.8	10.6	1.1
Chocolate Fudge, Entenmann's*	1 Serving/48g	173	7.2	361	4.4	51.8	15.1	0.9
Chocolate Fudge, Tray bake, Kate's Cakes Ltd*	1 Serving/100g	360	16.9	360	4.8	46.8	16.9	1.1
Chocolate Heaven, Extra Special, Asda*	1/6 Cake/66g	255	13.1	388	4.0	48.0	20.0	1.0
Chocolate Log, Fresh Cream, Finest, Tesco*	1 Slice/85g	301	15.4	354	4.5	43.2	18.1	1.4
Chocolate Slice, Go Ahead, McVitie's*	1 Slice/32g	94	2.6	293	4.5	49.4	8.2	1.9
Chocolate Slices, Mr Kipling*	1 Slice/33g	132	6.7	406	5.6	50.4	20.6	2.7
Chocolate Tiffin, Devondale*	1 Cake/100g	513	27.0	513	2.8	54.0	27.0	1.7

	Measure INFO/WEIGHT	per Measure KCAL	FAT	Nutrition Values per 100g / 100ml KCAL	PROT	CARB	FAT	FIBRE
CAKE								
Chocolate Truffle, Extra Special, Asda*	1 Serving/103g	402	26.8	390	5.0	34.0	26.0	1.8
Chocolate Truffle, Mini, Finest, Tesco*	1 Cake/28g	125	6.6	448	5.9	52.9	23.7	0.3
Chorley, Asda*	1 Cake/60g	269	12.6	449	6.0	59.0	21.0	2.2
Christmas, Connoisseur, M & S*	1 Slice/60g	216	5.5	360	4.1	64.7	9.2	3.3
Christmas, Iced, Slices, Tesco*	1 Slice/45g	168	4.4	369	2.9	67.6	9.6	1.2
Christmas, Knightsbridge*	1 Slice/50g	188	5.4	377	4.3	65.7	10.8	3.2
Christmas, Rich Fruit, All Iced, Sainsbury's*	1/16 Cake/85g	307	7.6	361	4.0	66.4	8.9	1.5
Christmas, Rich Fruit, Free From, Tesco*	1 Serving/100g	340	3.6	340	2.6	73.6	3.6	2.7
Christmas, Rich Fruit, Organic, Tesco*	1 Serving/76g	282	7.6	374	3.9	67.1	10.0	2.0
Christmas, Rich Fruit, Tesco*	1 Serving/75g	256	5.6	342	3.9	64.3	7.4	3.1
Christmas, Royal Iced, Waitrose*	1/6 Cake/75g	270	4.6	360	3.7	71.3	6.2	2.0
Christmas, Slice, Devondale*	1 Cake/70g	245	6.9	350	3.6	65.9	9.8	1.3
Christmas Pudding, Slices, Mr Kipling*	1 Slice/51g	173	3.6	339	3.6	62.1	7.1	1.3
Christmas Slices, Mr Kipling*	1 Slice/43g	157	3.8	363	2.9	67.5	8.8	0.9
Christmas Slices, Weight Watchers*	1 Slice/40g	136	2.6	339	4.4	66.0	6.4	3.0
Coconut	1 Slice/70g	304	16.7	434	6.7	51.2	23.8	2.5
Coconut & Raspberry, M & S*	1 Serving/52g	231	13.9	445	5.0	45.5	26.8	2.3
Coconut Delight, Burton's*	1 Cake/21g	89	3.5	424	4.0	63.0	16.9	2.0
Coconut Snowball, Bobby's*	1 Cake/18g	80	4.0	436	2.2	57.3	22.1	0.0
Coconut Snowballs, Tunnock's*	1 Cake/30g	134	6.2	446	4.2	56.7	20.8	3.6
Coconut Sponge, Memory Lane*	1/6 Cake/42g	172	7.5	406	4.1	57.1	17.6	1.5
Coconut Sponge, Mini Classics, Mr Kipling*	1 Cake/38g	155	8.7	409	3.7	47.0	22.9	0.9
Coffee, Entenmann's*	1 Serving/41g	159	7.1	388	4.0	54.7	17.3	0.6
Coffee, Iced, M & S*	1 Slice/33g	135	6.5	410	4.4	54.5	19.6	1.6
Coffee, Sponge Roll, M & S*	1/6 Roll/42g	160	7.4	385	3.1	53.1	17.8	1.4
Coffee, TTD, Sainsbury's*	1 Slice/68g	294	16.4	430	4.3	49.1	24.0	2.6
Coffee & Walnut, Mrs Beeton's*	1 Slice/54g	219	13.5	405	3.7	41.4	25.0	0.3
Colin the Caterpillar, M & S*	1 Slice/60g	234	12.8	390	5.3	57.2	21.3	1.3
Cornflake, Average	1 Cake/18g	83	3.7	464	5.2	64.6	20.4	2.0
Cornflake, Bobby's*	1/6 Cake/45g	207	9.2	461	3.9	65.5	20.4	0.0
Cranberry, Linda Kearns*	1 Serving/100g	265	14.2	265	12.0	29.9	14.2	5.2
Cream Oysters, M & S*	1 Cake/72g	227	15.3	315	3.6	27.5	21.2	3.0
Cream Slices, M & S*	1 Slice/80g	310	18.3	387	2.3	45.7	22.9	0.6
Date, Linda Kearns*	1 Serving/100g	269	16.8	269	12.7	24.4	16.8	4.4
Date & Walnut, Loaf, Sainsbury's*	1/10 Slice/40g	148	8.2	371	6.7	40.1	20.4	1.0
Date & Walnut, Slices, GFY, Asda*	1 Slice/22g	62	0.3	281	5.0	61.8	1.5	1.8
Date & Walnut, Slices, LC, Tesco*	1 Slice/25g	72	0.3	290	5.6	63.7	1.1	1.1
Date & Walnut, Slices, Weight Watchers*	1 Slice/27g	73	0.4	271	3.5	60.6	1.6	4.2
Date & Walnut, Trimlyne*	1 Slice/50g	134	2.4	269	5.7	53.8	4.9	1.8
D'oh Nuts, Asda*	1 Cake/50g	186	9.5	372	4.0	47.0	19.0	0.0
Eccles, All Butter, M & S*	1 Cake/86g	345	14.8	400	4.5	57.4	17.2	3.2
Eccles, Fresh Baked	1 Cake/45g	171	7.6	381	4.3	56.3	17.0	1.5
Eccles, Weight Watchers*	1 Cake/48g	190	7.9	396	4.4	57.5	16.5	2.0
Fairy, Average	1 Cake/23g	96	4.6	416	5.1	53.0	20.2	1.5
Fairy, Holly Lane*	1 Cake/26g	118	6.7	460	3.7	52.5	26.1	3.5
Fairy, Iced, Average	1 Cake/23g	91	3.4	394	4.2	60.8	14.8	0.9
Fairy, Lemon Iced, Average	1 Cake/23g	90	3.1	393	4.4	63.2	13.6	1.1
Fairy, Plain, Average	1 Cake/23g	95	4.6	413	5.5	51.1	20.2	1.5
Fairy, Snowman, Christmas, Tesco*	1 Cake/24g	114	6.8	471	4.6	49.8	28.1	2.9
Fairy, Strawberry Iced, Tesco*	1 Cake/24g	94	3.2	392	4.9	62.9	13.4	1.4
Farmhouse, Country, Waitrose*	1 Serving/80g	308	12.1	385	4.7	57.5	15.1	1.4
Farmhouse Loaf, The Handmade Flapjack Company*	1 Cake/75g	274	12.9	365	4.5	48.4	17.2	0.0
Farmhouse Slice, Weight Watchers*	1 Slice/23g	73	0.9	317	5.5	64.9	4.0	1.3

	Measure INFO/WEIGHT	per Measure KCAL	FAT	Nutrition Values per 100g / 100ml KCAL	PROT	CARB	FAT	FIBRE
CAKE								
Flake, Cadbury*	1 Cake/20g	90	4.5	445	6.3	54.5	22.3	0.0
Fondant, Dark Chocolate, Graze*	1 Pack/40g	157	5.8	393	3.5	66.2	14.5	0.0
Fondant Fancies, Lemon, Waitrose*	1 Cake/40g	176	7.1	441	2.5	67.9	17.7	0.6
Fondant Fancies, Sainsbury's*	1 Cake/27g	95	2.4	353	2.4	65.7	9.0	0.4
Fondants, with Chocolate, Mini, Delhaize*	1 Cake/20g	88	6.2	440	4.6	36.3	30.8	3.8
French Fancies, Average	1 Cake/27g	100	2.5	371	2.7	69.6	9.1	0.8
French Fancies, Big, Mr Kipling*	1/8th Cake/236g	463	13.1	196	1.5	35.1	5.5	0.4
French Fancies, Lemon, Average	1 Cake/28g	106	2.7	378	2.5	69.9	9.8	0.5
French Fancies, Lemon, Mr Kipling*	1 Cake/28g	106	2.7	378	2.5	69.9	9.8	0.5
French Fancies, M & S*	1 Cake/25g	91	2.0	365	2.7	70.6	8.1	1.3
French Fancies, Mr Kipling*	1 Cake/28g	106	2.8	378	2.6	69.7	9.9	0.6
French Fancies, Strawberry, Mr Kipling*	1 Cake/28g	106	2.7	379	2.5	70.6	9.6	0.4
Fruit, Iced, Smart Price, Asda*	1 Serving/100g	371	8.2	371	4.0	70.2	8.2	3.0
Fruit, Luxury, Fully Iced Slice, The Best, Morrisons*	1 Serving/50g	178	3.8	356	3.7	66.6	7.6	3.1
Fruit, Parisienne, Rich, Finest, Tesco*	1 Serving/69g	262	9.7	380	4.7	55.2	14.1	1.9
Fruit, Plain, Average	1 Slice/90g	319	11.6	354	5.1	57.9	12.9	0.0
Fruit, Rich, Average	1 Slice/70g	225	8.8	322	4.9	50.7	12.5	1.7
Fruit, Rich, Iced	1 Slice/70g	249	8.0	356	4.1	62.7	11.4	1.7
Fruit, Slices, Gluten & Wheat Free, Lovemore*	1 Slice/40g	122	3.8	304	2.3	51.1	9.4	1.5
Fruit, Slices, Rich, Iced, Finest, Tesco*	1 Slice/41g	152	3.4	370	3.2	69.4	8.3	2.1
Fruit, Slices, Value, Tesco*	1 Slice/23g	84	4.0	372	4.0	48.7	17.7	1.3
Fruit & Nut Cluster, Finest, Tesco*	1 Slice/77g	262	10.3	338	4.5	50.1	13.3	2.7
Fruit & Nut Cluster, TTD, Sainsbury's*	1 Slice/62g	239	9.2	383	5.7	56.8	14.8	4.2
Fudge Brownie, The Handmade Flapjack Company*	1 Cake/75g	286	9.2	381	4.9	62.8	12.3	0.0
Genoa, Tesco*	1 Serving/44g	150	3.9	340	3.7	59.1	8.8	3.1
Ginger Drizzle, Iced, Co-Op*	1/6 Cake/65g	226	7.7	350	3.0	58.0	12.0	1.0
Ginger Orange, The Handmade Flapjack Company*	1 Cake/75g	289	15.2	385	4.3	46.3	20.3	0.0
Happy Birthday, Sainsbury's*	1 Slice/50g	207	8.0	414	2.8	64.5	16.1	0.6
Holly Hedgehog, Tesco*	1 Serving/55g	227	7.9	413	2.0	69.0	14.3	0.8
Jamaica Ginger, McVitie's*	1 Cake/291g	1056	30.6	363	3.7	63.4	10.5	1.6
Jamaica Ginger, with Lemon Filling, McVitie's*	1 Cake/33g	143	8.2	434	4.0	48.3	25.0	0.8
La Madeleine, Bonne Maman*	1 Cake/113g	512	30.3	453	6.3	46.2	26.8	0.8
Lardy, Warings The Bakers*	1 Slice/120g	379	14.8	316	0.0	48.0	12.3	0.0
Lemon, Average	1 Slice/81g	320	14.5	396	4.1	54.8	18.0	0.6
Lemon, Half Moon, Bobby's*	1/6 Cake/60g	244	11.0	406	4.1	55.7	18.4	0.0
Lemon, Home Bake, McVitie's*	1oz/28g	108	5.1	384	4.6	53.9	18.2	1.0
Lemon, Loaf, M & S*	1 Slice/47g	190	8.8	400	2.1	55.8	18.6	0.6
Lemon, Mini, Weight Watchers*	1 Cake/27g	90	3.0	333	3.7	66.7	11.1	11.1
Lemon, The Handmade Flapjack Company*	1 Cake/75g	312	16.4	416	4.5	50.5	21.8	0.0
Lemon & Orange, Finest, Tesco*	1 Serving/53g	216	10.7	410	4.5	52.4	20.3	1.1
Lemon Bakewell, Mr Kipling*	1 Cake/48g	195	7.3	407	2.6	65.0	15.2	0.7
Lemon Buttercream & Lemon Curd, The Cake Shop*	1 Cake/28g	124	7.8	444	3.5	43.4	27.8	0.6
Lemon Crunchy, Devondale*	1 Cake/80g	346	17.6	432	3.3	57.0	22.0	2.4
Lemon Drizzle, Asda*	1 Serving/50g	150	6.0	299	2.8	45.0	12.0	0.4
Lemon Drizzle, M & S*	1/6 Cake/63g	230	8.8	365	4.2	55.8	13.9	1.4
Lemon Madeira, Half Moon, Dan Cake*	1 Slice/50g	215	10.0	430	3.5	59.0	20.0	0.0
Lemon Slices, BGTY, Sainsbury's*	1 Slice/26g	84	0.4	323	3.7	74.0	1.4	1.3
Lemon Slices, Low Fat, Weight Watchers*	1 Slice/26g	79	0.5	303	3.1	68.1	2.0	2.2
Lemon Slices, Mr Kipling*	1 Slice/27g	109	4.5	405	4.1	59.4	16.7	0.7
Lemon Tartlette, Go Ahead, McVitie's*	1 Cake/45g	161	4.3	357	3.7	67.9	9.5	1.1
Leo the Lion, Birthday, Asda*	1 Slice/81g	325	12.9	402	2.6	62.0	16.0	0.5
Madeira	1 Slice/40g	157	6.8	393	5.4	58.4	16.9	0.9
Madeira, All Butter, Sainsbury's*	1 Serving/30g	116	5.9	388	5.2	47.4	19.7	0.8

	Measure INFO/WEIGHT	per Measure KCAL	FAT	Nutrition Values per 100g / 100ml KCAL	PROT	CARB	FAT	FIBRE
CAKE								
Madeira, Cherry, Tesco*	¼ Cake/100g	342	11.2	342	4.3	55.9	11.2	2.6
Madeira, Iced, Tesco*	1/16 Cake/56g	218	6.8	389	2.6	67.2	12.2	0.4
Madeira, Lemon Iced, Tesco*	1 Slice/30g	122	5.2	407	4.5	57.8	17.5	0.9
Madeira, Tesco*	1 Serving/50g	197	7.8	394	5.5	57.9	15.6	1.2
Magic Roundabout, Dougal, Tesco*	1 Serving/50g	214	8.0	428	2.3	68.7	16.0	0.2
Manor House, Mr Kipling*	1 Serving/69g	277	13.8	400	5.3	49.7	20.0	1.4
Marble, Home Bake, McVitie's*	1oz/28g	115	5.3	411	3.7	56.9	18.8	0.9
Marble, Tesco*	1/8 Cake/45g	184	8.4	410	4.4	55.9	18.7	1.5
Marmalade, Orange, M & S*	1 Slice/50g	195	9.2	390	3.6	53.2	18.3	1.8
Mini Rolls, Blackforest, Weight Watchers*	1 Cake/24g	89	3.4	374	5.3	58.9	14.2	4.4
Mini Rolls, Cadbury*	1 Roll/27g	120	6.1	445	4.4	56.4	22.5	1.3
Mini Rolls, Chocolate, Average	1 Cake/27g	122	6.2	453	4.8	56.9	22.9	0.9
Mini Rolls, Chocolate, Milk, Cadbury*	1 Roll/27g	120	6.0	445	4.4	56.5	22.2	0.0
Mini Rolls, Chocolate Orange, Milk, Shapers, Boots*	1 Roll/25g	97	3.0	386	4.6	64.0	12.0	2.4
Mini Rolls, Easter Selection, Cadbury*	1oz/28g	122	5.8	434	5.5	55.6	20.6	0.0
Mini Rolls, Jaffa, Average	1 Cake/29g	111	3.3	382	3.5	67.2	11.2	1.4
Mini Rolls, Jam, Average	1 Cake/29g	115	4.5	395	3.8	59.8	15.6	1.8
Mini Rolls, Jammy Strawberry, Cadbury*	1 Cake/29g	119	4.8	411	4.9	59.8	16.5	0.5
Mini Rolls, Juicy Orange, Cadbury*	1 Cake/28g	110	4.7	390	5.0	55.0	16.8	0.0
Mini Rolls, Lemon, Average	1 Cake/29g	125	5.8	430	4.8	58.6	19.9	0.9
Mini Rolls, Mint, Cadbury*	1 Roll/27g	123	6.2	455	5.0	55.4	23.1	1.4
Mini Rolls, Rolo, Nestle*	1 Cake/29g	111	5.4	388	4.8	49.5	19.0	1.0
Panettone, Average	1 Portion/90g	345	15.3	383	8.0	52.0	17.0	0.0
Panettone, Bauli*	1 Serving/75g	314	15.1	418	5.9	53.5	20.1	0.0
Panettone, Luxury, Christmas, Tesco*	1 Serving/83g	307	11.6	370	7.0	53.5	14.0	2.5
Raisin, Dernys*	1 Cake/45g	175	7.6	388	5.0	54.0	17.0	0.0
Raisin, Sainsbury's*	1 Cake/40g	161	7.6	403	4.7	53.5	18.9	3.0
Rock	1 Sm Cake/40g	158	6.6	396	5.4	60.5	16.4	1.5
Shrek Birthday, Tesco*	1/16 Cake/72g	248	8.8	344	3.3	64.0	12.2	0.5
Simnel, Slices, Mr Kipling*	1 Slice/47g	177	5.9	379	2.9	63.4	12.6	1.2
Snowballs, Sainsbury's*	1 Snowball/18g	80	4.1	445	2.5	55.6	23.0	3.6
Snowballs, Tesco*	1 Snowball/18g	79	4.0	432	2.5	55.8	22.1	5.4
Sponge	1 Slice/53g	243	13.9	459	6.4	52.4	26.3	0.9
Sponge, Chocolate, Less Than 5% Fat, Asda*	1 Sponge/110g	198	4.2	180	4.4	32.0	3.8	1.1
Sponge, Chocolate, Morrisons*	1 Serving/59g	179	7.6	303	4.4	42.5	12.8	0.7
Sponge, Fatless	1 Slice/53g	156	3.2	294	10.1	53.0	6.1	0.9
Sponge, Fresh Cream & Strawberry, Asda*	1/12 Cake/60g	170	6.0	284	4.6	44.0	10.0	1.1
Sponge, Iced, M & S*	1 Serving/100g	400	17.0	400	3.4	58.4	17.0	1.3
Sponge, Jam Filled	1 Slice/65g	196	3.2	302	4.2	64.2	4.9	1.8
Sponge, Victoria, TTD, Sainsbury's*	1 Slice/57g	229	11.0	401	5.0	51.8	19.3	1.4
Sponge, with Butter Icing	1 Slice/65g	318	19.9	490	4.5	52.4	30.6	0.6
Spooky, Birthday, Memory Lane Cakes*	1 Slice/75g	295	14.6	393	3.5	50.8	19.5	0.7
St. Clements, Finest, Tesco*	1 Serving/49g	194	10.5	395	3.1	47.2	21.5	0.4
Stem Ginger, 96% Fat Free, Trimlyne*	¼ Cake/63g	170	2.2	272	4.4	58.1	3.6	1.2
Stem Ginger, Mrs Crimble's*	1 Slice/48g	158	1.1	329	2.7	73.3	2.2	2.7
Stollen, Bites, Finest, Tesco*	1 Piece/22g	81	3.2	370	6.5	52.7	14.4	4.4
Stollen, Kuchenmeister*	1 Serving/80g	357	16.0	446	5.0	61.2	20.0	2.5
Stollen, Slices, Finest, Tesco*	1 Slice/45g	164	5.2	365	6.9	57.3	11.6	4.2
Sultana, Apple & Cranberry, 99% Fat Free, Trimlyne*	1/6 Cake/67g	130	0.6	195	4.6	45.5	0.9	3.3
Sultana, Fair Trade, Co-Op*	1/8 Cake/45g	155	4.0	345	5.0	60.0	9.0	1.0
Sultana & Cherry, Tesco*	1 Cake/37g	124	4.0	334	4.7	54.4	10.8	2.5
Sultana & Cherry Slice, Co-Op*	1oz/28g	87	3.4	310	3.0	48.0	12.0	2.0
Swiss Roll, Average	1oz/28g	77	1.2	276	7.2	55.5	4.4	0.8

	Measure INFO/WEIGHT	per Measure KCAL	per Measure FAT	Nutrition Values per 100g / 100ml KCAL	PROT	CARB	FAT	FIBRE
CAKE								
Swiss Roll, Chocolate, Individual	1 Roll/26g	88	2.9	337	4.3	58.1	11.3	0.0
Swiss Roll, Chocolate, Lyons*	1 Serving/50g	190	9.6	379	4.3	47.0	19.3	0.9
Swiss Roll, Chocolate, M & S*	1 Serving/46g	168	11.1	365	4.6	32.6	24.2	1.2
Swiss Roll, Chocolate, Morrisons*	1/6 Roll/26g	103	4.9	401	4.4	56.4	18.9	3.1
Swiss Roll, Raspberry, Average	1 Slice/35g	107	1.2	305	3.8	64.8	3.5	0.6
Swiss Roll, Raspberry, Lyons*	1 Roll/175g	485	2.4	277	5.2	60.6	1.4	0.0
Swiss Roll, Raspberry & Vanilla, Morrisons*	1 Serving/28g	98	2.7	350	4.2	61.8	9.5	0.0
Swiss Roll, Raspberry Jam, Mr Kipling*	1/6 Cake/52g	184	5.3	355	2.8	63.0	10.2	1.0
Syrup & Ginger, Tesco*	1 Serving/32g	134	7.0	420	4.5	51.4	21.8	0.7
Tiffin, Chocolate, Sainsbury's*	1 Cake/61g	184	11.6	301	2.7	29.8	19.0	1.3
Toffee, & Pecan Slices, M & S*	1 Slice/36g	160	8.5	445	4.7	54.0	23.7	1.3
Toffee, Iced, Tesco*	1 Serving/35g	132	5.2	376	3.3	57.2	14.9	1.6
Toffee, Slices, BGTY, Sainsbury's*	1 Slice/27g	88	0.7	327	4.3	71.7	2.5	1.8
Toffee, Slices, Value, Tesco*	1 Slice/14g	62	3.2	440	4.2	54.9	22.6	0.6
Toffee, The Handmade Flapjack Company*	1 Cake/75g	346	18.8	462	5.1	54.0	25.1	0.0
Toffee, Thorntons*	1/6 Cake/70g	302	16.8	431	4.6	49.2	24.0	0.8
Toffee Apple, McVitie's*	1 Slice/29g	104	3.2	354	3.5	60.2	11.0	1.5
Toffee Bakewell, Tesco*	1 Cake/49g	203	7.9	414	3.9	63.5	16.1	1.4
Toffee Flavour, Slices, Low Fat, Weight Watchers*	1 Slice/27g	80	0.7	297	4.2	63.9	2.6	3.2
Toffee Fudge, Entenmann's*	1 Serving/65g	274	14.1	421	3.4	53.0	21.7	0.5
Toffee Snap, The Handmade Flapjack Company*	1 Cake/75g	365	19.6	487	4.6	62.2	26.1	0.0
Toffee Temptation, Finest, Tesco*	1 Serving/50g	212	11.6	423	4.7	49.0	23.1	0.6
Victoria Sandwich, Average	1 Slice/68g	267	12.9	392	4.4	50.9	19.0	1.0
Victoria Sponge, Fresh Cream, Value, Tesco*	1 Serving/50g	168	8.7	337	4.4	40.7	17.4	0.6
Victoria Sponge, Kate's Cakes Ltd*	1 Serving/100g	410	19.7	410	4.0	52.8	19.7	0.9
Victoria Sponge, Lemon, Co-Op*	1 Slice/42g	151	8.0	360	4.0	44.0	19.0	0.7
Victoria Sponge, Mini, Mr Kipling*	1 Cake/36g	152	6.9	420	3.9	58.5	19.0	0.8
Victoria Sponge, Mini, Weight Watchers*	1 Cake/30g	103	2.5	343	5.7	57.2	8.3	8.4
Viennese, M & S*	1 Cake/51g	250	14.1	495	4.1	58.9	28.0	2.8
Viennese Whirl, Average	1 Cake/28g	131	6.9	467	4.1	56.7	24.8	1.1
Viennese Whirl, Chocolate, Mr Kipling*	1 Whirl/28g	134	7.8	484	4.6	53.1	28.0	2.1
Viennese Whirl, Lemon, Mr Kipling*	1 Cake/28g	115	4.5	409	4.2	62.2	15.9	0.7
Viennese Whirl, Mr Kipling*	1 Cake/28g	141	7.8	504	3.9	59.1	28.0	1.4
Walnut, Sandwich, Sainsbury's*	1/8 Cake/48g	182	8.3	379	5.4	53.8	17.3	1.3
Welsh, Average	1oz/28g	121	5.5	431	5.6	61.8	19.6	1.5
CAKE BAR								
Blueberry, Trimlyne*	1 Cake/50g	142	1.1	283	3.9	64.0	2.2	2.2
Boost, Cadbury*	1 Bar/40g	190	10.8	475	5.3	52.8	26.9	1.1
Bounty, McVitie's*	1 Cake/36g	166	8.8	461	5.1	55.2	24.5	0.0
Caramel, Tesco*	1 Cake/26g	103	4.9	395	5.1	50.8	19.0	8.2
Caramel, Weight Watchers*	1 Bar/23g	89	3.0	381	5.3	56.2	12.8	9.9
Carrot, Gu*	1 Slice/38g	135	6.6	354	1.4	17.2	17.5	0.9
Carrot, Tesco*	1 Bar/68g	239	12.6	351	4.7	41.4	18.5	2.4
Carrot, with Cheese Cream Icing, Kate's Cakes Ltd*	1 Serving/100g	345	15.6	345	3.3	48.3	15.6	1.5
Choc Chip, Go Ahead, McVitie's*	1 Cake/28g	100	3.5	356	6.4	56.9	12.4	1.0
Choc Chip, Mini, Go Ahead, McVitie's*	1 Bar/27g	93	3.3	343	5.7	55.3	12.1	0.9
Chocolate, Average	1 Cake/28g	125	6.2	446	5.6	56.3	22.1	1.9
Chocolate, High Lights, Cadbury*	1 Bar/25g	95	3.5	380	5.5	58.8	14.0	1.1
Chocolate, Snack Cakes, Penguin, McVitie's*	1 Bar/24g	122	7.2	510	4.8	54.6	30.2	1.6
Chocolate & Orange, Go Ahead, McVitie's*	1 Cake/33g	109	2.0	330	4.3	64.9	6.0	1.0
Chocolate Chip, Average	1 Cake/28g	428	21.6	428	6.3	51.9	21.6	1.6
Chocolate Chip, HL, Tesco*	1 Serving/37g	109	1.0	295	4.8	63.6	2.6	0.6
Chocolate Chip, Mr Kipling*	1 Bar/32g	151	8.4	472	5.3	53.5	26.3	1.2

	Measure INFO/WEIGHT	per Measure KCAL	FAT	Nutrition Values per 100g / 100ml KCAL	PROT	CARB	FAT	FIBRE
CAKE BAR								
Chocolate Chip, Sainsbury's*	1 Cake/25g	108	5.6	430	6.1	51.2	22.3	0.6
Crunchie, Cadbury*	1 Cake/32g	147	7.2	460	5.9	58.3	22.6	0.0
Dream, Cadbury*	1 Cake/38g	170	8.5	450	4.5	57.2	22.6	0.0
Flake, Cadbury*	1 Cake/22g	97	5.1	442	6.5	51.8	23.3	0.5
Fudge, Cadbury*	1 Pack/52g	220	9.2	420	5.7	60.3	17.6	0.0
Jaffa, McVitie's*	1 Bar/25g	94	3.5	385	3.2	61.1	14.2	2.4
Jaffa Cakes, Spooky, McVitie's*	1 Bar/25g	96	3.5	390	3.2	62.1	14.2	2.7
Jamaica Ginger, McVitie's*	1 Cake/33g	128	4.9	388	3.5	60.2	14.7	1.2
Milky Way, McVitie's*	1 Cake/26g	124	6.2	476	5.1	58.5	23.6	1.2
Strawberry & Vanilla, HE, Tesco*	1 Serving/42g	124	1.1	295	3.7	64.4	2.6	0.8
CAKE MIX								
Carrot Cake, Betty Crocker*	¼ Pack/125g	504	8.4	403	5.8	78.9	6.7	1.4
Cheesecake, Original, Made Up, Asda*	1/6 Cake/85g	228	10.2	268	4.1	36.0	12.0	1.4
Cheesecake, Strawberry, Real, Green's*	1 Serving/100g	254	12.8	253	3.9	30.6	12.8	0.6
Cheesecake, Tesco*	1 Serving/76g	199	7.9	262	4.1	38.0	10.4	1.6
Chocolate Brownie, Chocolate Chips, Weight Watchers*	1 Pack/190g	568	13.5	299	3.2	55.6	7.1	2.1
Christmas, Mini, Jane Asher*	1oz/28g	104	3.4	372	5.2	65.8	12.0	1.3
Dennis, Green's*	1 Cake/17g	55	1.3	319	4.6	57.8	7.7	0.0
Free From, Sainsbury's*	1 Serving/50g	173	0.2	346	1.3	84.4	0.3	2.2
Sponge, Value, Tesco*	1 Slice/55g	181	4.8	329	4.6	57.9	8.8	1.4
Yellow, Super Moist, Betty Crocker*	1 Cake/128g	517	9.5	404	3.3	81.6	7.4	1.1
CALLALOO								
Leaves, Raw, Unprepared	1 Cup/28g	6	0.1	23	2.5	4.0	0.3	0.0
CANNELLONI								
Beef, & Red Wine, TTD, Sainsbury's*	½ Pack/180g	448	11.5	249	14.8	32.1	6.4	1.8
Beef, & Red Wine, Waitrose*	½ Pack/170g	355	16.0	209	17.5	13.8	9.4	1.0
Beef, Great Value, Asda*	1 Pack/400g	384	10.8	96	6.0	12.0	2.7	1.6
Beef, Italian, Sainsbury's*	1 Pack/400g	498	26.2	124	5.9	10.5	6.6	1.6
Beef, Ready Meal	1 Serving/335g	501	21.8	149	8.4	14.1	6.5	1.4
Beef, Ready Meal, Healthy Range, Average	1 Serving/300g	267	7.0	89	6.0	11.0	2.4	1.6
Chicken, & Pesto, Italian, Sainsbury's*	1 Pack/450g	675	33.8	150	6.1	14.4	7.5	1.1
Mushroom, Italian, Sainsbury's*	1 Pack/450g	598	31.0	133	5.2	12.5	6.9	0.5
Parmesan & Basil, M & S*	1 Pack/360g	504	28.4	140	5.9	11.4	7.9	0.8
Salmon, Smoked, & Spinach, Sainsbury's*	1 Pack/450g	598	27.9	133	5.7	13.5	6.2	0.4
Spinach, & Wild Mushroom, Linda McCartney*	1 Pack/340g	381	13.6	112	4.9	14.1	4.0	1.7
Spinach & Cheese, Finest, Tesco*	1 Pack/350g	532	31.8	152	5.4	12.1	9.1	1.5
Spinach & Ricotta, Charlie Bigham's*	½ Pack/330g	489	30.4	148	5.9	10.5	9.2	0.7
Spinach & Ricotta, Frozen, Sainsbury's*	1 Pack/350g	513	25.8	147	6.1	13.9	7.4	1.1
Spinach & Ricotta, Italian Style, Co-Op*	1 Pack/450g	540	27.0	120	5.0	12.0	6.0	2.0
Spinach & Ricotta, Ready Meal, Average	1 Serving/300g	426	22.0	142	5.6	13.3	7.3	1.4
Spinach & Ricotta, Ross*	1 Pack/299g	296	8.1	99	3.3	15.2	2.7	1.6
Tubes, Dry, Average	***1oz/28g***	***101***	***1.0***	***361***	***12.5***	***69.1***	***3.6***	***1.2***
Vegetable, Mediterranean, Waitrose*	1 Serving/170g	330	15.3	194	9.7	18.7	9.0	1.9
Vegetable, Roasted, Morrisons*	1 Serving/350g	312	8.8	89	3.9	12.5	2.5	2.3
Vegetarian, Linda McCartney*	1 Pack/375g	386	12.4	103	3.4	13.2	3.3	1.0
Vegetarian, Tesco*	1 Pack/400g	552	34.4	138	5.3	9.8	8.6	1.5
CAPERS								
in Vinegar, Average	1 Tsp/5g	2	0.0	34	1.7	3.0	0.6	0.0
CAPRI SUN								
Orange	1 Pouch/200ml	90	0.0	45	0.0	11.0	0.0	0.0
Orange, 100%, Juice	1 Pouch/200ml	75	0.0	38	0.5	9.2	0.0	0.1
CARAMAC								
Nestle*	1 Bar/30g	174	11.0	571	5.9	55.5	36.1	0.0

	Measure INFO/WEIGHT	per Measure KCAL	FAT	Nutrition Values per 100g / 100ml KCAL	PROT	CARB	FAT	FIBRE
CARAMBOLA								
Average	***1oz/28g***	***9***	***0.1***	***32***	***0.5***	***7.3***	***0.3***	***1.3***
CARAWAY								
Seeds, Schwartz*	1 Pack/38g	170	8.1	448	23.3	40.9	21.2	0.0
CARDAMOM								
Black, Ground, Average	***1 Tsp/2g***	***6***	***0.1***	***311***	***10.8***	***68.5***	***6.7***	***28.0***
Ground, Average	***1 Tsp/2g***	***6***	***0.1***	***314***	***10.7***	***53.6***	***7.1***	***28.6***
CAROB POWDER								
Average	***1 Tsp/2g***	***3***	***0.0***	***159***	***4.9***	***37.0***	***0.1***	***0.0***
CARP								
Fillet, Raw, Average	1 Fillet/218g	244	10.2	112	17.5	0.0	4.7	0.0
CARROT & SWEDE								
Diced, for Mashing, Average	***½ Pack/250g***	***58***	***0.7***	***23***	***0.6***	***4.7***	***0.3***	***1.9***
Mash, From Supermarket, Average	1 Serving/150g	138	7.5	92	1.3	10.4	5.0	1.3
Mash, Healthy Range, Average	1 Serving/150g	98	4.2	66	1.3	8.6	2.8	2.1
CARROTS								
& Cauliflower, M & S*	1 Serving/335g	74	1.3	22	0.6	4.4	0.4	2.3
& Peas, Sainsbury's*	1 Serving/200g	100	1.0	50	3.3	8.3	0.5	3.8
Baby, Canned, Average	***1 Can/195g***	***40***	***0.5***	***21***	***0.5***	***4.2***	***0.3***	***2.1***
Baby, Fresh, Average	***1 Serving/80g***	***28***	***0.1***	***35***	***0.6***	***8.2***	***0.1***	***2.9***
Batons, Fresh, Average	***½ Pack/150g***	***41***	***0.4***	***28***	***0.6***	***5.7***	***0.3***	***2.6***
Boiled, Average	***1oz/28g***	***6***	***0.1***	***22***	***0.6***	***4.4***	***0.4***	***2.3***
Canned, Average	***1oz/28g***	***6***	***0.1***	***22***	***0.6***	***4.4***	***0.2***	***2.1***
Chantenay, Frozen, Morrisons*	1 Serving/80g	28	0.3	35	0.4	6.7	0.4	3.2
Crunchies, Shapers, Boots*	1 Bag/80g	28	0.2	35	0.6	7.5	0.3	3.0
Raw, Scrubbed, Average	1 Serving/80g	24	0.4	30	0.7	6.0	0.5	2.4
Roasting, with Honey & Ginger Glaze, Aunt Bessie's*	1 Serving/133g	80	4.1	60	0.7	6.1	3.1	2.5
Sliced, Canned, Average	***1 Serving/180g***	***36***	***0.2***	***20***	***0.7***	***4.1***	***0.1***	***1.5***
Sliced, Canned, Basics, Sainsbury's*	1 Can/160g	30	0.3	19	0.4	3.9	0.2	2.5
Sliced, Fresh, Average	***1 Serving/60g***	***17***	***0.2***	***28***	***0.7***	***5.7***	***0.3***	***2.0***
Whole, Raw, Peeled, Average	***1 Carrot/75g***	***21***	***0.2***	***29***	***0.6***	***6.4***	***0.3***	***2.2***
CASHEW NUTS								
Bbq, Graze*	1 Pack/26g	142	10.8	546	13.9	37.0	41.7	0.0
Ca-shew! Bless You, Graze*	1 Punnet/40g	146	5.8	365	6.1	57.2	14.5	0.0
Cheese Flavour, Graze*	1 Pack/26g	140	10.8	540	15.3	35.7	41.5	0.0
Cracking Black Pepper, Graze*	1 Punnet/36g	216	16.6	600	19.0	26.0	46.0	4.0
Frosted, Graze*	1 Pack/26g	134	8.4	516	10.5	53.0	32.2	0.0
Honey, Graze*	½ Pack/13g	67	4.2	516	10.5	53.0	32.2	0.0
Hot Chilli, Graze*	1 Box/26g	139	10.9	535	14.5	33.6	41.8	0.0
Mexican Chilli, Graze*	1 Pack/26g	140	10.8	539	14.3	34.9	41.6	0.0
Natural, Roasted, Love Life, Waitrose*	1 Serving/25g	160	12.5	640	22.0	23.6	50.1	4.3
Plain, Average	***½ Pack/25g***	***146***	***12.2***	***584***	***15.7***	***18.8***	***48.9***	***3.4***
Raw, Wholesome, Love Life, Waitrose*	1 Pack/150g	866	72.3	577	17.7	18.1	48.2	3.3
Roasted & Salted, Average	***1 Serving/50g***	***306***	***25.6***	***612***	***18.8***	***19.6***	***51.1***	***3.1***
Roasted & Salted, Snacking, Asda*	1/8 Pack/50g	291	24.2	582	20.2	16.1	48.5	1.9
CASSAVA								
Baked, Average	***1oz/28g***	***43***	***0.1***	***155***	***0.7***	***40.1***	***0.2***	***1.7***
Boiled in Unsalted Water, Average	***1oz/28g***	***36***	***0.1***	***130***	***0.5***	***33.5***	***0.2***	***1.4***
Gari, Average	***1oz/28g***	***100***	***0.1***	***358***	***1.3***	***92.9***	***0.5***	***0.0***
Raw, Average	***1oz/28g***	***40***	***0.1***	***142***	***0.6***	***36.8***	***0.2***	***1.6***
Steamed, Average	***1oz/28g***	***40***	***0.1***	***142***	***0.6***	***36.8***	***0.2***	***1.6***
CASSEROLE								
Bean, Spicy, BGTY, Sainsbury's*	1 Pack/300g	171	2.7	57	3.0	9.1	0.9	4.2
Bean & Lentil, Morrisons*	1 Can/410g	287	1.6	70	4.1	12.5	0.4	0.0

	Measure INFO/WEIGHT	per Measure KCAL	FAT	Nutrition Values per 100g / 100ml KCAL	PROT	CARB	FAT	FIBRE
CASSEROLE								
Bean Cassoulet, Organic, Free & Easy*	1 Tin/400g	256	1.2	64	3.4	11.9	0.3	2.3
Beef	1 Serving/336g	490	23.0	146	16.3	4.6	6.8	0.6
Beef, & Ale, Average	1 Serving/300g	251	6.8	84	9.4	6.5	2.2	1.3
Beef, & Red Wine, Average	1 Serving/350g	290	7.3	83	7.2	8.2	2.1	1.5
Beef, Diet Chef Ltd*	1 Pack/300g	177	3.0	59	7.8	4.7	1.0	2.4
Beef, Meal for One, Tesco*	1 Pack/450g	425	18.9	94	3.6	10.6	4.2	1.7
Beef, Mini Favourites, M & S*	1 Pack/200g	210	8.4	105	7.1	9.3	4.2	1.4
Beef, with Dumplings, Ready Meal, Average	1 Serving/350g	464	21.1	132	9.5	10.1	6.0	1.5
Beef, with Herb Potatoes, Ready Meal, Average	1 Serving/475g	504	17.1	106	6.8	11.5	3.6	1.6
Beef & Ale, with Dumplings, Sainsbury's*	1 Pack/450g	711	32.8	158	7.7	15.4	7.3	0.6
Beef & Ale, with Mashed Potato, HL, Tesco*	1 Pack/450g	364	11.2	81	5.1	10.9	2.5	0.6
Beef & Dumplings, M Kitchen, Morrisons*	1 Pack/450g	596	28.0	132	7.3	11.0	6.2	1.7
Beef & Kidney, 153, Oakhouse Foods Ltd*	1 Meal/400g	384	16.8	96	6.7	7.2	4.2	0.7
Beef & Onion, Minced, British Classics, Tesco*	1 Pack/340g	367	19.0	108	5.0	9.3	5.6	0.8
Beef & Red Wine, BGTY, Sainsbury's*	1 Pack/300g	192	1.8	64	8.0	6.7	0.6	0.9
Beef & Red Wine, Fuller Longer, M & S*	1 Pack/420g	355	11.7	85	7.2	6.9	2.8	1.7
Beef & Red Wine, Weight Watchers*	1 Pack/330g	254	9.2	77	4.3	8.6	2.8	0.3
Beef & Red Wine, You Count, Love Life, Waitrose*	1 Pack/381g	297	5.2	78	6.5	9.5	1.4	0.9
Chicken, Diet Chef Ltd*	1 Pack/300g	219	2.7	73	9.0	7.2	0.9	2.5
Chicken, Leek & Mushroom, Tesco*	1 Pack/350g	382	22.0	109	4.5	8.6	6.3	1.0
Chicken, Mediterranean, Tesco*	1 Pack/400g	260	9.2	65	6.7	4.5	2.3	0.9
Chicken, Perfectly Balanced, Waitrose*	1 Pack/400g	392	14.4	98	6.6	9.8	3.6	1.2
Chicken, Skinny Chef, All About Weight*	1 Meal/269g	277	0.8	103	11.2	11.9	0.3	3.8
Chicken, with Dumplings, M & S*	½ Pack/227g	261	10.0	115	9.7	9.0	4.4	0.9
Chicken, You Count, Love Life, Waitrose*	1 Pack/400g	297	4.8	74	7.4	7.9	1.2	1.2
Chicken & Dumpling, Weight Watchers*	1 Pack/328g	243	6.9	74	5.3	8.3	2.1	0.3
Chicken & Dumplings, HL, Tesco*	1 Pack/450g	441	12.2	98	7.4	11.1	2.7	0.6
Chicken & Red Wine, Duchy Originals*	½ Pack/175g	187	7.5	107	14.0	5.1	4.3	1.6
Chicken & Tomato, Asda*	¼ Pack/273g	569	41.0	208	16.0	2.2	15.0	0.5
Chicken & Vegetable, Apetito*	1 Pack/330g	286	9.9	87	6.3	9.4	3.0	1.6
Chicken & Vegetable, Long Life, Sainsbury's*	1 Pack/300g	186	4.5	62	4.6	7.4	1.5	0.8
Chicken & White Wine, BGTY, Sainsbury's*	1 Serving/300g	216	6.6	72	7.2	5.9	2.2	1.3
Cowboy, Iceland*	1 Pack/400g	500	26.0	125	5.8	10.9	6.5	1.7
Ham Hock, & Mash, Tesco*	1 Pack/250g	225	8.0	90	6.1	9.0	3.2	0.8
Lamb, Braised, British Classics, Tesco*	1 Pack/350g	332	18.2	95	7.5	4.6	5.2	1.2
Lamb, Ready Meal, Healthy Range, Average	1 Serving/220g	200	7.3	91	10.5	4.9	3.3	1.0
Lamb, with Mint Dumplings, Minced, Sainsbury's*	1 Pack/450g	558	30.6	124	5.4	10.4	6.8	1.1
Lamb & Rosemary, Eat Well, M & S*	1 Pack/380g	325	11.0	86	7.6	7.0	2.9	2.2
Mushroom, & Onion, Iceland*	1 Pack/400g	272	12.4	68	1.3	8.8	3.1	1.9
Pork, Normandy Style, Finest, Tesco*	1 Pack/450g	405	21.6	90	7.6	4.1	4.8	2.3
Rabbit, Average	1oz/28g	29	1.4	102	11.6	2.6	5.1	0.4
Sausage, 154, Oakhouse Foods Ltd*	1 Meal/400g	484	28.0	121	4.8	10.0	7.0	0.7
Sausage, 328, Wiltshire Farm Foods*	1 Pack/420g	394	20.4	94	3.0	9.7	4.9	1.4
Sausage, Chosen By You, Asda*	1 Pot/400g	240	15.2	60	3.6	1.9	3.8	2.1
Sausage, Pork, Diet Chef Ltd*	1 Pack/300g	303	18.3	101	6.6	4.9	6.1	1.4
Sausage & Potato, M & S*	1 Serving/200g	190	11.8	95	3.3	7.5	5.9	0.9
Seafood, Mediterranean, HL, Tesco*	1 Pack/344g	292	6.9	85	5.8	10.5	2.0	3.2
Steak & Ale, Average	1 Serving/275g	324	14.4	118	9.0	8.8	5.2	1.0
Steak & Ale, British Classics, Tesco*	1 Serving/100g	93	3.4	93	11.2	4.5	3.4	1.1
Steak & Ale, Sainsbury's*	1 Pack/300g	288	10.5	96	10.6	5.6	3.5	0.4
Steak & Kidney, Mini, Favourites, M & S*	1 Pack/200g	240	10.8	120	7.9	9.5	5.4	1.5
Steak & Mushroom, 214, Wiltshire Farm Foods*	1 Pack/360g	322	16.2	89	5.0	7.2	4.5	1.3
Steak & Mushroom, Average	1 Serving/275g	274	15.5	100	6.2	6.0	5.6	1.0

	Measure INFO/WEIGHT	per Measure KCAL	FAT	Nutrition Values per 100g / 100ml KCAL	PROT	CARB	FAT	FIBRE
CASSEROLE								
Steak & Mushroom with Mustard Mash, Finest, Tesco*	1 Pack/550g	522	21.4	95	5.9	9.0	3.9	1.1
Vegetable, & Lentil, Canned, Granose*	1 Can/400g	272	8.0	68	3.5	9.0	2.0	3.0
Vegetable, Average	1 Serving/275g	77	0.8	28	0.8	5.5	0.3	1.5
Vegetable, with Dumplings, Ready Meal, Average	1 Serving/400g	376	13.8	94	2.1	13.0	3.5	2.7
Venison, Wild, Scottish, & Beaujolais, Tesco*	1 Pack/425g	366	8.9	86	11.9	4.9	2.1	0.6
CASSEROLE MIX								
Beef, Colman's*	1 Pack/40g	123	0.6	308	7.5	66.0	1.5	2.5
Beef, Recipe, Colman's*	1 Pack/42g	142	0.5	338	9.1	13.1	1.1	4.0
Beef, Recipe, Schwartz*	1 Pack/43g	123	0.9	287	7.0	56.6	2.1	6.6
Beef & Ale, Colman's*	1 Pack/45g	144	0.9	320	9.2	66.3	2.0	2.3
Chicken, Authentic, Schwartz*	1 Pack/36g	131	1.5	363	10.4	70.7	4.3	2.0
Chicken, Traditional, Colman's*	1 Pack/40g	124	0.5	311	5.7	69.4	1.3	1.5
Chicken Chasseur, Asda*	1 Pack/80g	273	0.8	341	9.0	74.0	1.0	1.4
Farmhouse Sausage, Schwartz*	1 Pack/39g	124	1.1	317	8.1	64.6	2.9	0.5
Honey Chicken, Colman's*	1 Pack/50g	128	0.6	257	3.4	58.3	1.1	1.8
Lamb, Authentic, Schwartz*	1 Pack/35g	116	1.2	332	7.7	68.0	3.3	1.3
Liver & Bacon, Colman's*	1 Pack/40g	121	0.7	303	10.3	61.6	1.7	4.7
Moroccan Lamb, As Sold, Schwartz*	1 Pack/35g	114	0.9	327	5.5	67.4	2.6	5.8
Peppered Beef, Schwartz*	1 Pack/40g	129	2.0	323	7.0	62.9	4.9	7.3
Pork, Colman's*	1 Pack/40g	131	0.6	328	6.7	72.0	1.4	2.8
Pork, Morrisons*	1 Pack/36g	118	0.5	327	8.1	70.6	1.4	0.0
Sausage, Asda*	¼ Pack/25g	80	1.0	321	6.0	65.0	4.1	3.0
Sausage, Classic, Schwartz*	1 Pack/35g	96	0.9	275	12.4	50.1	2.7	14.9
Sausage, Colman's*	1 Pack/40g	144	0.6	361	8.9	77.7	1.6	1.6
Sausage & Onion, Colman's*	1 Pack/45g	143	1.2	318	9.6	64.2	2.6	2.6
Somerset Pork, Colman's*	1 Pack/45g	144	0.6	321	7.1	70.2	1.3	2.2
Spicy Chicken, Colman's*	1 Pack/45g	151	0.8	336	6.5	73.4	1.8	1.5
Turkey, Colman's*	1 Pack/50g	156	1.0	313	5.9	68.0	1.9	3.5
CATFISH								
Cooked, Steamed, Weighed with Bone, Average	***1 Serving/100g***	***101***	***3.1***	***101***	***18.2***	***0.0***	***3.1***	***0.7***
Raw, Average	***1oz/28g***	***27***	***0.8***	***96***	***17.6***	***0.0***	***2.8***	***0.0***
CAULIFLOWER								
Boiled, Average	***1 Serving/80g***	***22***	***0.7***	***28***	***2.9***	***2.1***	***0.9***	***1.6***
Florets, Peas & Carrots, Frozen, Asda*	1 Serving/100g	37	0.6	37	3.0	5.0	0.6	2.8
Organic, Tesco*	1 Serving/100g	35	0.9	35	3.6	3.0	0.9	1.8
Peas & Carrots, Birds Eye*	1oz/28g	9	0.1	32	2.2	4.8	0.4	2.6
Raw, Average	***1 Serving/80g***	***25***	***0.7***	***31***	***3.2***	***2.7***	***0.8***	***1.6***
Steamed, Average	1 Serving/100g	28	0.9	28	2.9	2.1	0.9	1.6
CAULIFLOWER CHEESE								
& Bacon, Gastropub, M & S*	1 Pack/300g	318	21.0	106	6.3	4.5	7.0	1.0
& Broccoli, Average	1 Serving/200g	127	6.4	64	3.8	4.6	3.2	2.0
Average	1 Meal/400g	362	23.3	90	4.5	4.6	5.8	1.3
Birds Eye*	1 Pack/330g	248	13.9	75	4.0	4.9	4.2	0.9
Florets, in a Cheese Sauce, Sainsbury's*	1 Pack/400g	400	26.4	100	4.8	5.4	6.6	0.9
Frozen, Iceland*	1 Serving/200g	190	12.0	95	4.0	5.5	6.0	1.6
Great Value, Asda*	1 Pack/396g	352	23.8	89	3.9	4.9	6.0	0.8
Grills, Grassington's Food Co*	1 Grill/92g	157	4.6	171	6.1	25.3	5.0	2.6
Grills, Meat Free, Tesco*	1 Grill/91g	160	7.4	175	5.3	20.0	8.1	2.9
Grills, Tesco*	1 Grill/92g	207	10.9	225	6.5	22.2	11.9	4.0
Healthy Range, Average	1 Serving/200g	123	4.9	61	4.4	4.9	2.4	1.3
Made with Semi-Skimmed Milk	1oz/28g	28	1.8	100	6.0	5.2	6.4	1.3
Made with Skimmed Milk	1oz/28g	27	1.7	97	6.0	5.2	6.0	1.3
Made with Whole Milk	1oz/28g	29	1.9	105	6.0	5.2	6.9	1.3

	Measure INFO/WEIGHT	per Measure KCAL	FAT	Nutrition Values per 100g / 100ml KCAL	PROT	CARB	FAT	FIBRE
CAULIFLOWER CHEESE								
Ross*	1 Pack/300g	300	19.8	100	4.9	5.5	6.6	0.1
with Crispy Bacon, Finest, Tesco*	1/3 Pack/166g	211	14.1	127	6.5	6.1	8.5	0.4
with Roasted Potatoes, M & S*	1 Pack/200g	500	23.6	250	10.8	24.8	11.8	3.2
CAVIAR								
Average	***1oz/28g***	***26***	***1.3***	***92***	***12.0***	***0.5***	***4.7***	***0.0***
CELERIAC								
Boiled in Salted Water, Average	***1oz/28g***	***4***	***0.1***	***15***	***0.9***	***1.9***	***0.5***	***3.2***
Raw, Average	***1 Serving/100g***	***42***	***0.3***	***42***	***1.5***	***9.2***	***0.3***	***1.8***
CELERY								
Boiled in Salted Water	***1 Serving/50g***	***4***	***0.2***	***8***	***0.5***	***0.8***	***0.3***	***1.2***
Raw, Trimmed	***1 Stalk/40g***	***3***	***0.1***	***7***	***0.5***	***0.9***	***0.2***	***1.1***
CHAMPAGNE								
Average	***1 Sm Glass/125ml***	***95***	***0.0***	***76***	***0.3***	***1.4***	***0.0***	***0.0***
CHANNA MASALA								
Indian, Sainsbury's*	1 Serving/149g	165	7.3	111	4.2	12.4	4.9	3.3
M & S*	1 Pack/225g	360	23.7	160	5.6	11.2	10.5	8.2
Waitrose*	1 Pack/300g	300	18.3	100	3.7	7.4	6.1	7.9
CHAPATIS								
Brown Wheat Flour, Waitrose*	1 Chapati/42g	128	3.4	305	8.6	49.4	8.0	4.6
Indian Style, Asda*	1 Chapati/43g	95	0.4	221	8.0	45.0	1.0	2.9
Made with Fat	1 Chapati/60g	197	7.7	328	8.1	48.3	12.8	0.0
Made without Fat	1 Chapati/55g	111	0.6	202	7.3	43.7	1.0	0.0
Morrisons*	1 Chapati/40g	108	2.8	269	8.6	49.8	6.9	0.0
Plain, Wraps, Original, Patak's*	1 Chapati/42g	115	3.2	273	9.4	48.8	7.5	0.0
Wholemeal, Patak's*	1 Chapati/42g	130	4.0	310	11.2	44.9	9.5	9.0
CHAR								
Arctic, Whole, Raw	1 Serving/100g	137	6.0	137	20.8	0.0	6.0	0.0
CHARD								
Average	1 Serving/80g	15	0.2	19	1.4	3.3	0.2	0.8
Swiss, Boiled in Unsalted Water	***1oz/28g***	***6***	***0.0***	***20***	***1.9***	***4.1***	***0.1***	***2.1***
Swiss, Raw	***1oz/28g***	***5***	***0.1***	***19***	***1.8***	***3.7***	***0.2***	***1.6***
CHEDDARS								
Baked, Mini, Cheese & Ham Flavour, McVitie's*	1 Bag/30g	160	8.9	534	11.0	55.5	29.8	2.0
Baked, Mini, Original, Cheddar Cheese, Jacob's*	1 Bag/25g	129	7.4	516	10.7	50.3	29.5	2.5
Baked, Mini, Peperami, McVitie's*	1 Bag/30g	160	9.1	532	9.7	55.2	30.2	2.0
Baked, Mini, Tangy Salsa, McVitie's*	1 Bag/50g	266	15.0	532	11.0	54.7	29.9	2.1
Branston Pickle, McVitie's*	1 Bag/30g	155	8.9	517	9.1	53.1	29.8	2.7
CHEESE								
Ail & Fines Herbes, Boursin*	1oz/28g	116	11.8	414	7.0	2.0	42.0	0.0
Appenzellar, Sainsbury's*	1 Serving/25g	96	7.9	386	25.4	0.0	31.6	0.0
Asiago, M & S*	1oz/28g	105	7.6	375	33.0	0.1	27.0	0.0
Babybel, Cheddar Variety, Mini, Fromageries Bel*	1 Cheese/20g	75	6.2	375	24.0	0.0	31.0	0.0
Babybel, Emmental, Fromageries Bel*	1 Cheese/20g	63	4.9	316	23.0	1.0	24.5	0.0
Babybel, Goat's Variety, Mini, Fromageries Bel*	1 Cheese/20g	65	5.4	327	21.0	0.0	27.0	0.0
Babybel, Gouda Variety, Mini, Fromageries Bel*	1 Cheese/20g	68	5.6	340	22.0	0.0	28.0	0.0
Babybel, Light, Mini, Fromageries Bel*	1 Cheese/20g	40	2.3	208	25.0	0.0	12.0	0.0
Babybel, Original, Mini, Fromageries Bel*	1 Cheese/20g	61	4.8	304	22.0	0.1	24.0	0.0
Bavarian, Smoked, Slices, Asda*	1 Slice/18g	50	4.1	277	17.0	0.4	23.0	0.0
Bavarian, Smoked, with Ham, Sainsbury's*	1 Serving/30g	89	7.2	298	19.4	0.8	24.1	0.0
Bleu d'Auvergne, TTD, Sainsbury's*	1 Serving/100g	322	26.0	322	22.0	0.0	26.0	0.0
Blue, Basics, Sainsbury's*	1 Serving/100g	410	35.0	410	23.7	0.1	35.0	0.0
Blue, Castello, Soft, Castello*	¼ Pack/38g	162	15.6	432	14.0	0.5	41.5	0.0
Blue, French, Chosen By You, Asda*	1 Serving/30g	90	7.4	301	20.0	0.0	24.5	0.0

C

	Measure INFO/WEIGHT	per Measure KCAL	FAT	Nutrition Values per 100g / 100ml KCAL	PROT	CARB	FAT	FIBRE
CHEESE								
Blue, Saint Agur*	1 Serving/30g	109	9.9	363	16.0	0.2	33.0	0.0
Brie, Average	***1 Serving/25g***	***74***	***6.0***	***296***	***19.7***	***0.3***	***24.0***	***0.0***
Brie, Reduced Fat, Average	***1 Serving/50g***	***99***	***5.7***	***198***	***23.0***	***0.8***	***11.4***	***0.0***
Caerphilly, Average	***1 Serving/50g***	***187***	***15.6***	***374***	***23.0***	***0.1***	***31.3***	***0.0***
Cambazola, Tesco*	1 Serving/30g	128	12.3	425	13.5	0.5	41.0	0.0
Camembert, Average	***1 Serving/50g***	***141***	***11.1***	***283***	***20.5***	***0.1***	***22.2***	***0.0***
Camembert, Breaded, Average	1 Serving/90g	307	20.9	342	16.6	14.2	23.2	0.4
Cantal, French, Sainsbury's*	1 Serving/30g	106	8.7	353	23.0	0.1	29.0	0.0
Cantenaar, M & S*	1 Serving/28g	84	5.4	300	32.2	0.1	19.2	0.0
Cheddar, Average	1 Serving/30g	123	10.3	410	25.0	0.1	34.4	0.0
Cheddar, Extra Mature, Average	***1 Serving/30g***	***123***	***10.3***	***410***	***25.1***	***0.1***	***34.4***	***0.0***
Cheddar, Grated, Average	***1 Serving/50g***	***206***	***17.2***	***413***	***24.4***	***1.5***	***34.3***	***0.0***
Cheddar, Mature, Average	***1 Serving/30g***	***123***	***10.3***	***410***	***25.0***	***0.1***	***34.4***	***0.0***
Cheddar, Mature, Grated, Average	***1 Serving/28g***	***113***	***9.3***	***404***	***24.7***	***1.6***	***33.2***	***0.0***
Cheddar, Mature, Lighter, 30% Less Fat, Mu, Adams*	1 Serving/30g	91	6.6	302	26.0	0.1	22.0	0.0
Cheddar, Mature, Lighter, Less Fat, Pilgrims Choice*	1 Serving/30g	91	6.6	302	26.0	0.1	22.0	0.0
Cheddar, Mature, Reduced Fat, Average	***1 Serving/25g***	***68***	***4.2***	***271***	***30.0***	***0.1***	***16.7***	***0.0***
Cheddar, Medium, Average	***1 Serving/30g***	***123***	***10.4***	***411***	***24.9***	***0.2***	***34.5***	***0.0***
Cheddar, Mild, Average	***1 Serving/30g***	***123***	***10.3***	***409***	***25.0***	***0.1***	***34.3***	***0.0***
Cheddar, Original, Cheestrings*	1 Stick/21g	69	5.0	328	28.0	0.0	24.0	0.0
Cheddar, Reduced Fat, Average	***1 Serving/30g***	***76***	***4.2***	***255***	***32.2***	***0.1***	***14.0***	***0.0***
Cheddar, Sharp, Shredded, Sargento*	1 Serving/30g	118	9.6	393	25.0	3.6	32.1	0.0
Cheddar, Smoked, Average	***1 Serving/30g***	***123***	***10.3***	***411***	***25.2***	***0.1***	***34.4***	***0.0***
Cheddar, West Country Farmhouse, Average	***1 Serving/28g***	***115***	***9.6***	***410***	***25.0***	***0.1***	***34.4***	***0.0***
Cheddar, Wexford, Average	***1 Serving/20g***	***82***	***6.9***	***410***	***25.0***	***0.1***	***34.4***	***0.0***
Cheddar, with Caramelised Onion, Sainsbury's*	1 Serving/28g	109	8.7	391	22.8	5.1	31.0	0.0
Cheddar, with Onion & Chives, Davidson*	1 Serving/25g	100	8.3	400	24.3	0.6	33.3	0.0
Cheddar, with Pickled Onion Relish, Christmas, Tesco*	¼ Cheese/50g	191	15.5	382	23.0	2.7	31.0	0.1
Cheddar, with Winter Berries, Christmas, Tesco*	1oz/28g	106	8.5	378	22.9	3.4	30.3	0.2
Chedds, Bricks, Cathedral City, Dairy Crest Ltd*	1 Brick/18g	75	6.3	416	25.4	0.1	34.9	0.0
Chedds, Nibbles, Cathedral City, Dairy Crest Ltd*	1 Mini Bag/18g	75	6.3	416	25.4	0.1	34.9	0.0
Cheshire	***1oz/28g***	***106***	***8.8***	***379***	***24.0***	***0.1***	***31.4***	***0.0***
Chevre Pave D'affinois, Finest, Tesco*	1 Pack/150g	404	32.6	269	18.5	0.0	21.7	0.0
Cottage, Arla*	1 Serving/25g	22	1.0	90	12.0	2.0	4.0	0.0
Cottage, Crunchy Vegetable, GFY, Asda*	1 Serving/50g	37	0.6	74	11.0	4.5	1.3	0.6
Cottage, Danone*	1 Serving/100g	89	3.9	89	11.2	2.3	3.9	0.0
Cottage, Fat Free, Longley Farm*	½ Pot/125g	79	0.4	63	10.8	3.9	0.3	0.0
Cottage, Garlic & Herb, Diet, Yoplait*	1 Pot/225g	180	4.3	80	12.0	3.9	1.9	0.0
Cottage, Jocca, Kraft*	1 Serving/50g	54	2.8	109	9.3	5.0	5.5	0.0
Cottage, Less Than 5% Fat, Sainsbury's*	½ Pot/125g	131	5.2	105	12.3	4.4	4.2	0.0
Cottage, Low Fat, 2% Fat, Natural, Average	1 Serving/75g	68	1.4	90	13.7	3.6	1.9	0.0
Cottage, Natural, 1.5% Fat, Waitrose*	1 Serving/60g	44	0.9	73	10.7	4.3	1.5	0.0
Cottage, Natural, Longley Farm*	1 Pot/250g	260	15.0	104	10.3	2.2	6.0	0.0
Cottage, Natural, Loseley*	½ Tub/100g	115	7.1	115	9.4	2.9	7.1	0.0
Cottage, Natural, Plain, Average	***1oz/28g***	***27***	***1.1***	***98***	***11.8***	***3.9***	***3.8***	***0.1***
Cottage, Natural, with Creme Fraiche, Tesco*	½ Pack/125g	131	6.0	105	12.1	2.7	4.8	0.6
Cottage, Onion & Chive, 1.4% Fat, Waitrose*	1 Serving/60g	42	0.8	70	9.5	4.6	1.4	0.5
Cottage, Onion & Chive, Waitrose*	1 Serving/20g	18	0.6	91	10.8	4.9	3.1	0.3
Cottage, Onion & Chives, LC, Tesco*	1 Serving/60g	51	0.9	85	11.4	4.8	1.5	0.1
Cottage, Pineapple, LC, Tesco*	1 Serving/60g	54	0.8	90	9.8	8.5	1.3	0.4
Cottage, Pineapple, Perfectly Balanced, Waitrose*	½ Pot/125g	106	1.8	85	8.4	9.7	1.4	0.5
Cottage, Plain, Average	***1 Tbsp/20g***	***19***	***0.7***	***93***	***12.0***	***3.3***	***3.5***	***0.1***
Cottage, Plain, Reduced Fat, Average	***1oz/28g***	***24***	***0.5***	***85***	***12.3***	***4.4***	***1.9***	***0.1***

	Measure INFO/WEIGHT	per Measure KCAL	FAT	Nutrition Values per 100g / 100ml KCAL	PROT	CARB	FAT	FIBRE
CHEESE								
Cottage, Red Pepper, GFY, Asda*	¼ Pot/75g	66	1.9	88	11.1	4.3	2.5	0.1
Cottage, Slimline*	1 Serving/70g	43	0.1	62	12.0	3.0	0.2	0.0
Cottage, Stilton & Celery, BGTY, Sainsbury's*	½ Pot/125g	99	2.8	79	10.8	4.0	2.2	1.5
Cottage, Tropical, Westacre*	1 Serving/100g	89	1.2	89	13.1	6.4	1.2	1.4
Cottage, Tuna & Sweetcorn, GFY, Asda*	½ Pot/113g	104	2.7	92	12.4	5.3	2.4	0.3
Cottage, Value, Tesco*	½ Tub/150g	98	0.8	65	9.5	5.0	0.5	0.0
Cottage, Virtually Fat Free, Average	1 Tbsp/20g	16	0.2	79	13.0	4.5	1.0	0.0
Cottage, Virtually Fat Free, Eden Vale*	1oz/28g	22	0.1	80	12.9	6.5	0.3	0.0
Cottage, Virtually Fat Free, Longley Farm*	½ Pot/125g	84	0.1	67	13.4	3.0	0.1	0.0
Cottage, West Country, Low Fat, Eat Well, M & S*	1 Serving/80g	64	1.2	80	12.2	4.5	1.5	0.0
Cottage, West Country, Low Fat 1.5%, Waitrose*	1 Serving/100g	77	1.5	77	11.8	4.4	1.5	0.0
Cottage, West Country, Waitrose*	1 Serving/100g	113	6.1	113	6.1	3.3	6.1	0.0
Cottage, Whole Milk, Natural, Average	1 Serving/75g	77	3.4	103	12.5	2.7	4.5	0.0
Cottage, with Black Pepper, HE, Tesco*	1 Pot/125g	101	2.2	81	12.1	4.0	1.8	0.0
Cottage, with Chives, Low Fat, Westacre*	1 Pot/100g	81	1.4	81	13.7	3.5	1.4	1.2
Cottage, with Chives, M & S*	1oz/28g	28	1.1	100	11.9	3.5	3.9	0.0
Cottage, with Chives, Virtually Fat free, Longley Farm*	½ Pot/125g	88	0.1	70	14.3	2.9	0.1	0.0
Cottage, with Coronation Chicken, BGTY, Sainsbury's*	1oz/28g	25	0.3	91	11.3	8.7	1.2	0.1
Cottage, with Cucumber & Mint, COU, M & S*	1 Pot/113g	85	1.7	75	11.6	3.1	1.5	0.2
Cottage, with Mango & Peach, HE, Tesco*	1 Pot/250g	188	4.0	75	10.4	4.8	1.6	0.1
Cottage, with Mango & Pineapple, BGTY, Sainsbury's*	½ Pot/125g	112	0.9	90	10.7	10.4	0.7	0.2
Cottage, with Onion & Chive, GFY, Asda*	¼ Tub/75g	50	1.0	66	9.3	3.8	1.4	0.5
Cottage, with Onion & Chive, HL, Tesco*	1 Serving/60g	45	1.0	75	10.0	5.0	1.6	0.5
Cottage, with Onion & Chive, Iceland*	½ Pot/100g	81	1.3	81	8.5	8.9	1.3	0.3
Cottage, with Onion & Chive, M & S*	¼ Pot/65g	88	5.5	135	10.4	4.0	8.5	0.1
Cottage, with Onion & Chive, Nisa Heritage*	1 Pot/227g	168	3.6	74	11.1	3.8	1.6	0.3
Cottage, with Peach & Mango, COU, M & S*	1 Pot/113g	96	1.1	85	9.1	9.7	1.0	0.4
Cottage, with Pineapple, BGTY, Sainsbury's*	1 Serving/125g	105	0.9	84	10.5	8.9	0.7	0.1
Cottage, with Pineapple, Iceland*	½ Pot/100g	81	1.3	81	8.5	8.9	1.3	0.3
Cottage, with Pineapple, NUME, Morrisons*	½ Tub/125g	100	1.6	80	8.7	8.1	1.3	0.5
Cottage, with Pineapple, Shape, Danone*	1oz/28g	20	0.1	73	9.8	8.0	0.2	0.1
Cottage, with Prawn, GFY, Asda*	1oz/28g	22	0.5	79	10.0	6.0	1.7	0.3
Cottage, with Prawn Cocktail, BGTY, Sainsbury's*	1oz/28g	25	0.3	91	12.3	8.3	0.9	0.1
Cottage, with Salmon & Dill, HE, Tesco*	1oz/28g	25	0.7	89	12.0	4.7	2.5	0.5
Cottage, with Smoked Cheese & Onion, GFY, Asda*	1 Serving/50g	39	0.8	78	12.0	3.9	1.6	0.4
Cottage, with Sweet Chilli Chicken, M & S*	1 Serving/200g	190	4.2	95	13.8	4.7	2.1	0.5
Cottage, with Tomato & Cracked Black Pepper, Asda*	½ Pot/113g	86	2.4	76	10.0	3.1	2.1	1.3
Cottage, with Tuna & Pesto, Asda*	1 Serving/170g	184	10.2	108	10.0	3.5	6.0	0.7
Cottage, with Tuna & Sweetcorn, HL, Tesco*	1 Serving/150g	136	3.2	91	12.8	4.8	2.1	0.4
Cream, Average	***1 Portion/30g***	***132***	***14.2***	***439***	***3.1***	***0.0***	***47.4***	***0.0***
Cream, Garlic & Herbs, Light, Boursin*	1 Portion/20g	28	1.8	140	12.0	2.5	9.0	0.0
Cream, Reduced Fat, Average	***1 Serving/20g***	***23***	***1.1***	***117***	***13.0***	***4.0***	***5.3***	***0.1***
Cream, with Onion & Chives, Morrisons*	1 Serving/20g	38	3.0	190	11.0	3.0	15.0	0.0
Cream, with Pineapple, Asda*	1 Serving/40g	77	5.2	193	8.0	11.0	13.0	0.0
Cream, with Red Peppers & Onion, GFY, Asda*	1 Serving/32g	42	1.9	130	13.0	6.0	6.0	0.0
Creme de Saint Agur, Saint Agur*	1 Serving/10g	28	2.5	285	13.5	2.3	24.7	0.0
Dairylea, Light, Slices, Kraft*	1 Slice/25g	51	2.6	205	17.0	8.6	10.5	0.0
Dairylea, Rippers, Straight, Kraft*	1 Ripper/21g	60	3.9	285	28.0	1.0	18.5	0.0
Dairylea, Slices, Kraft*	1 Slice/25g	69	5.1	275	13.0	8.6	20.5	0.0
Danish Blue, Average	***1 Serving/30g***	***106***	***8.7***	***352***	***20.8***	***0.0***	***29.1***	***0.0***
Demi Pont L'eveque, Finest, Tesco*	1 Serving/46g	138	10.6	301	21.1	0.4	23.0	0.0
Dolcelatte, Average	***1 Serving/30g***	***110***	***9.7***	***366***	***17.8***	***0.4***	***32.3***	***0.4***
Double Cheese Flavour, Cheestrings*	1 Stick/21g	69	5.0	328	28.0	0.0	24.0	0.0

C

	Measure INFO/WEIGHT	per Measure KCAL	FAT	Nutrition Values per 100g / 100ml KCAL	PROT	CARB	FAT	FIBRE
CHEESE								
Double Gloucester, Average	***1 Serving/30g***	***121***	***10.2***	***404***	***24.5***	***0.1***	***34.0***	***0.0***
Double Gloucester, Belton Farm, TTD, Sainsbury's*	1 Serving/30g	121	10.2	404	24.4	0.1	34.0	0.0
Double Gloucester with Onion & Chives, Sainsbury's*	1 Serving/30g	110	8.5	365	22.2	5.5	28.2	0.0
Doux De Montagne, Average	***1 Serving/25g***	***88***	***7.1***	***352***	***22.9***	***1.5***	***28.3***	***0.0***
Edam, Average	***1 Serving/10g***	***33***	***2.5***	***326***	***25.3***	***0.0***	***24.9***	***0.0***
Edam, Dutch, Garlic & Herb Wedge, Asda*	1 Serving/60g	197	15.0	329	26.0	0.0	25.0	0.0
Edam, Reduced Fat, Average	***1 Serving/30g***	***69***	***3.3***	***230***	***32.4***	***0.1***	***11.1***	***0.0***
Edam, Slices, Average	***1 Slice/30g***	***96***	***7.2***	***320***	***25.0***	***0.4***	***24.1***	***0.0***
Emmental, Average	***1 Serving/10g***	***37***	***2.8***	***368***	***28.4***	***0.0***	***28.4***	***0.0***
Emmental, Grated, President*	1 Pack/200g	728	56.0	364	28.0	0.0	28.0	0.0
Emmental, Light, Slices, President*	1 Slice/20g	60	3.6	298	34.0	0.0	18.0	0.0
Farmhouse, Reduced Fat, Healthy Range, Average	***1 Serving/30g***	***78***	***4.6***	***260***	***30.4***	***0.0***	***15.4***	***0.0***
Feta, Apetina, Light, 10 % Fat, Arla*	1 Serving/30g	52	3.0	173	18.4	0.6	10.1	0.0
Feta, Average	***1 Serving/30g***	***79***	***6.4***	***262***	***16.3***	***1.0***	***21.5***	***0.0***
Feta, Lemon, Asda*	1 Serving/25g	76	6.8	302	13.2	1.0	27.2	0.6
Feta, Light, Greek, Salad, 40% Reduced Fat, Attis*	1 Portion/30g	51	3.6	170	20.0	0.6	12.0	0.0
Fondue, Original, Fromalp*	1 Pack/400g	888	68.0	222	15.0	2.5	17.0	0.0
Fondue, Swiss, Easy Cook, Tesco*	¼ Pack/100g	235	17.0	235	15.5	4.0	17.0	0.0
Fondue, Traditionnelle, Co-Op*	1 Serving/100g	409	34.0	409	26.0	0.9	34.0	0.0
Fontina, Average	***1 Serving/28g***	***109***	***9.0***	***389***	***25.0***	***0.0***	***32.1***	***0.0***
for Pizza, Grated	***1 Serving/50g***	***163***	***12.2***	***326***	***25.0***	***1.6***	***24.4***	***0.0***
Goats, Breaded, Bites, Sainsbury's*	1 Bite/25g	84	6.2	337	13.0	15.1	25.0	0.8
Goats, French, Mild, Average	***1 Serving/30g***	***49***	***3.5***	***163***	***11.2***	***3.0***	***11.8***	***0.0***
Goats, Honey, Delamere Dairy Ltd*	1 Serving/20g	52	4.4	262	14.0	10.0	22.0	0.0
Goats, Mature, TTD, Sainsbury's*	1 Serving/30g	118	9.6	394	25.2	1.3	32.0	3.8
Goats, Premium, Average	***1 Serving/30g***	***98***	***7.8***	***327***	***20.5***	***0.6***	***26.1***	***0.0***
Goats, Soft, Average	1 Serving/30g	79	6.3	262	16.7	1.8	20.8	0.5
Goats, Somerset, Mild Cream Soft Cheese, Capricorn*	1 Serving/30g	99	8.6	329	17.8	0.0	28.6	0.0
Goats, Welsh with Garlic & Chives, Tesco*	1 Serving/32g	93	7.7	290	15.1	3.3	24.1	0.1
Goats, Welsh with Herbs, Sainsbury's*	1 Serving/30g	90	7.4	299	15.3	3.6	24.8	0.1
Gorgonzola, Average	***1 Serving/30g***	***100***	***8.1***	***334***	***20.0***	***0.0***	***27.0***	***0.0***
Gouda, Average	***1 Serving/30g***	***113***	***9.4***	***376***	***24.0***	***0.0***	***31.5***	***0.0***
Grana Padano, Italian Cheese, Waitrose*	1 Serving/14g	54	4.0	388	33.0	0.0	28.4	0.0
Gruyere	***1oz/28g***	***115***	***9.3***	***409***	***27.2***	***0.0***	***33.3***	***0.0***
Halloumi, Average	***1 Serving/80g***	***253***	***19.7***	***316***	***20.8***	***1.6***	***24.7***	***0.0***
Halloumi, Light, Pittas*	1 Pack/225g	590	36.0	262	27.0	2.5	16.0	0.0
Halloumi, Light Average	1 Serving/100g	245	15.3	245	24.7	1.7	15.3	0.0
Havarti, Slices, Tesco*	1 Slice/25g	85	6.5	340	24.0	1.4	26.0	0.0
Healthy Range, Slices, Average	1 Slice/25g	45	2.2	180	19.5	5.4	9.0	0.0
Italian, Grated, Average	***1 Serving/30g***	***144***	***10.0***	***481***	***44.0***	***1.1***	***33.4***	***0.0***
Italian Hard, Basics, Sainsbury's*	1 Portion/30g	122	9.6	408	28.1	1.8	32.0	0.1
Jarlsberg, Slices, Average	***1 Slice/15g***	***54***	***4.0***	***360***	***27.0***	***0.0***	***27.0***	***0.0***
Lactose Free, Arla*	1 Serving/30g	103	8.1	344	25.3	1.0	27.0	0.0
Lactose Free, Semi Hard, Lactofree, Arla*	1 Portion/30g	103	8.1	344	25.3	1.0	27.0	0.0
Lancashire	***1oz/28g***	***104***	***8.7***	***373***	***23.3***	***0.1***	***31.0***	***0.0***
Light, Slices, The Laughing Cow, Fromageries Bel*	1 Slice/20g	41	2.1	203	21.0	6.0	10.5	0.0
Manchego	***1 Serving/70g***	***340***	***30.8***	***485***	***22.2***	***0.1***	***44.0***	***0.0***
Mascarpone, 25% Less Fat, Sainsbury's*	1 Portion/30g	95	9.0	316	6.7	4.8	30.0	0.0
Mascarpone, Average	***1 Serving/30g***	***131***	***13.1***	***437***	***5.6***	***4.1***	***43.6***	***0.0***
Mild, Reduced Fat, Grated, Average	***1 Serving/30g***	***70***	***3.3***	***235***	***31.5***	***2.2***	***11.1***	***0.0***
Monterey Jack, Iga*	1 Serving/28g	110	9.0	393	25.0	0.0	32.1	0.0
Monterey Jack, Shredded, Kraft*	¼ Cup/28g	101	8.1	360	22.0	3.6	28.8	0.0
Morbier, Sainsbury's*	1 Serving/10g	33	2.4	330	28.0	0.1	24.2	0.0

	Measure INFO/WEIGHT	per Measure KCAL	FAT	Nutrition Values per 100g / 100ml KCAL	PROT	CARB	FAT	FIBRE
CHEESE								
Mozarella, Italian, Lighter, Chosen By You, Asda*	1 Pack/125g	233	15.0	187	20.0	0.0	12.0	0.0
Mozza-Cheddar, Light, Shredded, Kraft*	1/3 of a Cup/30g	80	6.0	267	26.7	3.3	20.0	0.0
Mozzarella, Average	***½ Ball/63g***	***172***	***12.9***	***275***	***21.2***	***1.2***	***20.6***	***0.0***
Mozzarella, Reduced Fat, Average	***½ Ball/63g***	***115***	***6.4***	***184***	***21.2***	***1.0***	***10.2***	***0.0***
Neufchâtel, Soft, Average	1 Serving/30g	76	6.9	253	9.0	3.6	23.0	0.0
Norvegia, Sliced Light, Tine*	1 Slice/10g	27	1.6	272	32.0	0.0	16.0	0.0
Ossau-Iraty, Average	***1 Serving/30g***	***120***	***10.2***	***400***	***22.3***	***0.2***	***34.0***	***0.0***
Parmesan, Average	***1 Tbsp/10g***	***40***	***2.9***	***401***	***35.2***	***0.0***	***29.4***	***0.0***
Parmigianino Reggiano, TTD, Sainsbury's*	1 Serving/30g	116	8.5	388	33.0	0.0	28.4	0.0
Pastrami Flavour, Sandwich, Swiss Processed, Gerber*	1 Slice/13g	44	3.5	348	24.0	0.0	28.0	0.0
Pecorino, Italian, Tesco*	1 Serving/30g	119	9.9	397	22.0	0.0	33.0	0.0
Philadelphia for Salad, Kraft*	1 Pot/50g	158	15.2	315	6.6	2.6	30.5	0.5
Piccante Gorgonzola, TTD, Sainsbury's*	1 Serving/30g	108	9.0	359	22.1	0.5	29.8	0.1
Poivre, Boursin*	1oz/28g	116	11.8	414	7.0	2.0	42.0	0.0
Port Salut, M & S*	1oz/28g	90	7.3	322	21.0	1.0	26.0	0.0
Provolone Piccante, Sainsbury's*	1 Serving/30g	119	9.9	398	25.0	0.2	33.0	0.0
P'tit Louis, St Moret*	1 Serving/20g	49	4.6	247	5.0	5.0	23.0	0.0
Quark, Average	***1 Serving/20g***	***13***	***0.0***	***66***	***11.9***	***4.0***	***0.2***	***0.0***
Raclette, Richsmonts*	1 Slice/28g	100	8.0	357	25.0	0.0	28.6	0.0
Reblochon	***1 Serving/30g***	***95***	***8.0***	***318***	***19.7***	***0.0***	***26.6***	***0.0***
Red Leicester, Average	***1 Serving/30g***	***120***	***10.1***	***400***	***23.8***	***0.1***	***33.7***	***0.0***
Red Leicester, Reduced Fat, Average	***1 Serving/30g***	***78***	***4.6***	***261***	***30.2***	***0.1***	***15.4***	***0.0***
Ricotta, Average	***1 Serving/50g***	***67***	***4.8***	***134***	***9.3***	***2.9***	***9.5***	***0.0***
Roquefort, Average	***1oz/28g***	***105***	***9.2***	***375***	***19.7***	***0.0***	***32.9***	***0.0***
Roule, French, Sainsbury's*	1 Serving/30g	96	9.2	321	8.5	3.0	30.5	0.0
Roule, Garlic & Parsley, Light, BGTY, Sainsbury's*	1 Serving/30g	51	3.2	171	16.4	2.6	10.6	0.0
Sage Derby	***1oz/28g***	***113***	***9.5***	***402***	***24.2***	***0.1***	***33.9***	***0.0***
Shropshire, Blue, Average	***1 Serving/50g***	***196***	***17.1***	***391***	***21.0***	***0.0***	***34.2***	***0.0***
Slices, Average	1 Slice/23g	82	6.6	358	24.0	0.8	28.6	0.0
Slices, GFY, Asda*	1 Slice/20g	37	2.0	185	20.0	4.0	10.0	0.0
Slices, Leerdammer*	1 Slice/20g	71	5.5	356	27.0	0.1	27.5	0.0
Slices, Smoked, with Ham, Aldi*	1 Slice/21g	66	5.2	313	21.0	1.0	25.0	0.1
Soft, & Creamy with Onions & Garlic, GFY, Asda*	1 Serving/25g	32	1.5	126	13.0	5.0	6.0	0.0
Soft, Blue, Philadelphia, Kraft*	1 Serving/28g	76	7.1	270	6.8	3.4	25.5	0.2
Soft, Cracked Pepper, Less Than 5% Fat, M & S*	1 Serving/30g	30	1.4	100	11.0	4.2	4.5	0.3
Soft, Extra Light, Average	***1 Serving/20g***	***25***	***1.2***	***125***	***14.3***	***3.6***	***5.9***	***0.1***
Soft, Fruit & Rum Halo, Discover*	1 Serving/25g	104	8.5	414	8.6	11.7	34.1	0.0
Soft, Full Fat, Average	***1 Serving/50g***	***156***	***15.2***	***312***	***8.2***	***1.7***	***30.3***	***0.0***
Soft, Full Fat, Original, Lactose Free, Kraft*	1 Serving/30g	84	8.2	280	4.5	2.7	27.5	0.3
Soft, Garlic & Herb, Extra Light, LC, Tesco*	1 Serving/38g	49	2.4	130	12.3	5.1	6.3	0.3
Soft, Garlic & Herb, Roulade, M & S*	1 Portion/100g	295	27.3	295	7.8	4.1	27.3	1.3
Soft, Garlic & Herb, Soft & Creamy, Extra Light, Asda*	¼ Pack/50g	65	3.0	130	13.0	6.0	6.0	0.0
Soft, Light, Average	***1 Tbsp/30g***	***54***	***3.9***	***179***	***12.1***	***3.2***	***13.1***	***0.0***
Soft, Light, Philadelphia, Kraft*	1 Serving/30g	47	3.5	157	8.7	4.0	11.7	0.3
Soft, Light, with Garlic & Herbs, Sainsbury's*	2 Servings/100g	157	11.4	157	10.6	3.1	11.4	0.0
Soft, Light, with Grilled Peppers, Philadelphia*	1 Portion/30g	44	3.2	147	7.0	5.4	10.5	0.7
Soft, Lighter, Asda*	1 Serving/33g	36	1.3	109	14.0	3.7	4.0	0.0
Soft, Low Fat, Linessa, Lidl*	1 Serving/50g	30	0.1	61	11.0	3.9	0.2	1.4
Soft, Medium Fat, Average	***1 Serving/30g***	***62***	***5.4***	***207***	***8.4***	***3.0***	***17.9***	***0.0***
Soft, Onion & Chives, Extra Light, LC, Tesco*	1 Serving/30g	38	1.8	125	11.7	5.6	6.0	0.2
Soft, Onion & Chives, Less Than 5% Fat, M & S*	1 Serving/30g	30	1.4	100	10.7	4.4	4.7	1.2
Soft, Philadelphia, Cadbury Chocolate, Mini Tubs, Kraft*	1 Mini Tub/30g	86	4.0	287	6.5	34.0	13.3	1.7
Soft, Philadelphia, Cucumber, Light, Kraft*	1 Serving/30g	44	3.2	145	7.5	4.9	10.6	0.3

	Measure INFO/WEIGHT	per Measure KCAL	FAT	Nutrition Values per 100g / 100ml KCAL	PROT	CARB	FAT	FIBRE
CHEESE								
Soft, Philadelphia, Extra Light, Kraft*	1 Serving/30g	33	1.4	110	11.7	5.0	4.7	0.3
Soft, Philadelphia, Garlic & Herb, Light, Kraft*	1 Serving/30g	46	3.3	154	7.8	5.4	11.0	0.3
Soft, Philadelphia, Light, Basil, Philadelphia, Kraft*	1 Serving/35g	51	3.7	146	8.0	4.0	10.5	0.5
Soft, Philadelphia, Mini Tubs, Cracked Pepper, Kraft*	1 Tub/35g	56	4.6	161	7.7	2.5	13.0	0.4
Soft, Philadelphia, Mini Tubs, Extra Light, Kraft*	1 Tub/35g	38	1.8	108	11.0	4.2	5.0	0.6
Soft, Philadelphia, Mini Tubs, Light, Kraft*	1 Tub/35g	55	4.0	158	8.7	4.0	11.5	0.4
Soft, Philadelphia, with Chives, Light, Kraft*	1 Serving/30g	48	3.6	160	8.3	4.3	12.0	0.7
Soft, Pineapple Halo, Discover*	1 Serving/25g	101	8.2	404	7.2	16.6	32.6	1.2
Soft, White, Lactofree, Arla*	1 Serving/30g	59	5.0	197	8.6	3.0	16.5	0.0
Soft, with Black Pepper, Light, Sainsbury's*	½ Pack/100g	205	16.5	205	11.0	3.0	16.5	0.0
Soft, with Garlic & Herbs, Full Fat, Deli, Boursin*	1 Serving/28g	84	8.3	299	3.5	5.0	29.5	0.0
Soft, with Garlic & Herbs, Lighter, Asda*	½ Pack/100g	106	4.4	106	11.8	4.3	4.4	0.1
Soft, with Garlic & Herbs, Medium Fat, Westacre*	1 Serving/30g	56	4.8	188	8.0	3.0	16.0	0.1
Soft, with Garlic & Herbs, Sainsbury's*	1 Serving/33g	89	8.6	269	6.1	2.7	26.0	0.0
Soft, with Onion & Chives, Lighter, Asda*	1 Serving/30g	32	1.3	105	11.6	4.5	4.3	0.2
Soya	***1oz/28g***	***89***	***7.6***	***319***	***18.3***	***0.0***	***27.3***	***0.0***
Stilton, Average	***1 Serving/30g***	***123***	***10.6***	***410***	***22.4***	***0.1***	***35.5***	***0.0***
Stilton, Blue, Average	***1 Serving/30g***	***124***	***10.7***	***412***	***22.8***	***0.1***	***35.7***	***0.0***
Stilton, White, & Apricot, M & S*	1oz/28g	94	6.5	337	13.8	18.5	23.1	0.0
Stilton, White, Average	***1oz/28g***	***101***	***8.8***	***362***	***19.9***	***0.1***	***31.3***	***0.0***
Stilton, White, with Mango & Ginger, Tesco*	1/3 Pack/65g	228	14.0	350	13.1	25.8	21.6	0.6
Stilton White, & Cranberry, M & S*	1oz/28g	101	7.1	362	18.2	15.5	25.3	0.0
Triangles, Light, Creamy Swiss, The Laughing Cow*	1 Triangle/18g	25	1.2	143	13.7	6.8	6.8	0.0
Triangles, Spread, Eat Smart, Morrisons*	1 Triangle/18g	30	1.4	166	15.0	8.5	8.0	0.0
Wedge, Leerdammer*	1 Serving/30g	107	8.3	357	27.0	0.0	27.7	0.0
Wensleydale, & Ginger, Truckle, Morrisons*	1 Truckle/90g	330	23.7	367	18.0	14.0	26.3	1.1
Wensleydale, Average	***1 Serving/25g***	***92***	***7.8***	***369***	***22.4***	***0.1***	***31.0***	***0.0***
Wensleydale, Cranberry & Mustard, Lozzas	1 Block/50g	179	13.9	359	20.7	6.4	27.8	0.0
Wensleydale, with Blueberries, M & S*	1 Portion/30g	111	7.9	370	18.7	13.4	26.4	0.9
Wensleydale, with Cranberries, Sainsbury's*	1 Serving/50g	180	13.9	359	20.7	6.4	27.8	0.0
CHEESE ALTERNATIVE								
Cheezly, Cream, Garlic & Herb, The Redwood Co*	1 Pack/113g	360	34.5	319	5.8	5.4	30.5	0.0
Cheezly, Cream, Original, The Redwood Co*	1 Pack/113g	357	34.5	316	5.6	4.8	30.5	0.0
Cheezly, Feta Style in Oil, The Redwood Co*	1 Serving/25g	119	11.8	475	2.5	10.6	47.0	0.0
Cheezly, Grated Cheddar Style, The Redwood Co*	1 Pack/150g	242	11.2	161	3.1	21.5	7.5	0.0
Cheezly, Mozzarella Style, The Redwood Co*	1 Portion/25g	69	6.4	274	5.4	5.9	25.4	1.0
Cheezly, Nacho Style, The Redwood Co*	1 Serving/25g	42	2.0	169	3.3	21.1	7.9	0.0
Cheezly, Sour Cream & Chive, The Redwood Co*	1 Serving/25g	80	7.6	318	5.7	5.1	30.5	0.0
Mozzarella, Slices, Dairy Free	1 Slice/19g	80	6.0	420	10.5	10.5	31.5	0.0
Vegetarian, Average	1 Serving/30g	110	8.4	368	28.2	0.0	28.1	0.0
CHEESE DIPPERS								
Original, The Laughing Cow, Fromageries Bel*	1 Pack/35g	101	6.0	288	11.0	25.0	17.0	0.0
CHEESE ON TOAST								
Average	1 Slice/130g	494	34.2	380	13.8	23.8	26.3	0.7
CHEESE PUFFS								
Average	1 Bag/25g	129	7.4	517	7.8	54.8	29.5	1.5
Healthy Range, Average	1 Bag/25g	113	3.8	454	7.6	71.2	15.0	2.2
CHEESE SINGLES								
American, 2% Milk, Kraft*	1 Slice/19g	45	3.0	237	21.0	5.3	15.8	0.0
Healthy Range, Average	1 Slice/20g	39	2.1	197	20.6	5.2	10.4	0.0
Kraft*	1 Single/20g	52	3.7	260	13.5	7.6	18.5	0.0
CHEESE SPREAD								
Average	1 Serving/30g	76	6.4	254	9.4	5.9	21.4	0.1

	Measure INFO/WEIGHT	per Measure KCAL	FAT	Nutrition Values per 100g / 100ml KCAL	PROT	CARB	FAT	FIBRE
CHEESE SPREAD								
Cheese & Garlic, Primula*	1 Serving/20g	49	3.7	247	15.7	4.3	18.6	0.0
Cheese & Ham, Primula*	1 Serving/20g	40	3.0	200	12.3	3.1	15.0	4.9
Cheese & Salmon with Dill, Primula*	1 Serving/30g	78	5.8	261	17.6	3.8	19.5	0.0
Cheez Whiz, Original, Light, 41% Less Fat, Kraft*	1 Tbsp/15g	32	1.7	210	15.7	11.7	11.3	0.0
Dairylea, Light, Tub, Kraft*	1 Serving/30g	44	2.1	147	14.5	6.1	7.0	0.0
Dairylea, Tub, Kraft*	1 Serving/25g	60	4.9	240	11.0	5.3	19.5	0.0
Flavoured	1oz/28g	72	5.7	258	14.2	4.4	20.5	0.0
Garlic & Herbs, Light, Benecol*	1 Serving/20g	35	2.8	174	7.8	4.2	14.0	0.7
Healthy Range, Average	1 Serving/30g	31	1.0	102	14.3	3.8	3.2	0.9
Kerrygold*	1oz/28g	60	4.2	213	11.0	8.5	15.0	0.0
Light, Primula*	1 Serving/20g	30	1.8	149	15.2	3.0	8.9	3.6
Low Fat, Weight Watchers*	1 Serving/50g	56	1.4	112	18.1	3.4	2.9	1.2
Mediterranean, Soft & Creamy, Extra Light, Asda*	1 Serving/32g	42	1.9	130	13.0	6.0	6.0	0.0
Plain, Original, Primula*	1 Serving/25g	49	3.8	196	12.8	4.1	15.2	5.9
Squeeze, Light, Laughing Cow, Fromageries Bel*	1 Portion/30g	42	2.1	139	12.0	7.0	7.0	5.0
Squeeze, Original, Laughing Cow, Fromageries Bel*	1 Portion/30g	71	6.0	236	9.0	5.0	20.0	0.0
with Chives, Primula*	1 Serving/30g	57	4.3	190	12.5	2.9	14.2	4.5
with Prawn, Primula*	1 Squeeze/25g	48	3.6	190	12.5	3.3	14.4	3.6
CHEESE STRAWS								
& Bacon, Party, Tesco*	1 Straw/13g	40	2.6	321	10.5	23.8	20.4	2.1
Cheddar, M & S*	1 Straw/11g	59	3.8	535	14.9	40.1	34.9	2.4
Finest, Tesco*	1 Straw/7g	39	2.6	558	13.3	41.5	37.6	1.5
Fudges*	1 Serving/10g	53	3.5	534	14.9	40.1	34.9	0.0
Homemade or Bakery, Average	1 Straw/41g	173	12.6	422	12.0	24.2	30.7	0.7
Selection, Sainsbury's*	1 Straw/7g	41	2.9	558	16.6	34.5	39.3	2.8
CHEESE TRIANGLES								
Average	1 Triangle/14g	33	2.2	238	10.3	14.2	15.6	0.2
Dairylea, Light, Kraft*	1 Triangle/18g	36	2.2	205	15.5	6.3	12.5	0.0
Extra Light, The Laughing Cow, Fromageries Bel*	1 Triangle/18g	20	0.5	116	15.0	6.5	3.0	0.0
LC, Tesco*	1 Triangle/18g	30	1.2	170	17.5	8.5	7.0	0.0
Original, The Laughing Cow, Fromageries Bel*	1 Triangle/18g	42	3.3	239	11.0	6.0	19.0	0.0
Reduced Fat, Average	1 Triangle/18g	27	1.2	154	15.4	7.0	7.0	0.0
Tri-Bites, Dairylea, Kraft*	1 Triangle/20g	60	4.6	300	20.0	3.2	23.0	0.0
CHEESE TWISTS								
All Butter, M & S*	1 Pack/125g	625	33.4	500	14.2	50.2	26.7	3.2
Gruyere & Poppy Seed, Truly Irresistible, Co-Op*	1 Twist/8g	42	2.4	520	13.2	48.8	30.1	2.5
Pre Packed, Average	1 Twist/8g	41	2.2	515	13.7	47.9	27.7	2.3
CHEESECAKE								
After Noon, Mango & Passionfruit, 3 Pack, Gu*	1 Portion/45g	155	11.3	345	3.4	26.5	25.2	0.4
American Red White & Blueberry, Sainsbury's*	1/6 Cake/83g	264	15.4	318	3.8	35.1	18.5	0.4
Apple & Cinnamon, Baked, M & S*	1 Serving/116g	390	22.0	335	3.7	39.7	18.9	2.1
Apricot, Co-Op*	1 Cake/100g	230	11.0	230	4.0	29.0	11.0	0.9
Apricot, HL, Tesco*	1 Pot/100g	179	2.3	179	4.9	34.7	2.3	1.6
Autumn Berry, Waitrose*	1 Slice/92g	316	20.3	343	4.4	31.5	22.1	2.0
Average	1 Slice/115g	490	40.8	426	3.7	24.6	35.5	0.4
Blackcurrant, Average	1 Serving/90g	237	11.9	263	3.6	32.3	13.2	2.4
Blackcurrant, Healthy Range, Average	1 Serving/90g	182	4.7	203	4.7	33.6	5.3	2.1
Blackcurrant, VLH Kitchens	1 Serving/120g	341	13.7	285	3.4	32.0	16.4	0.9
Blackcurrant, Weight Watchers*	1 Cake/103g	191	2.9	185	4.6	35.4	2.8	3.5
Blackcurrant Devonshire, McVitie's*	1/6 Cake/67g	193	11.5	288	3.8	29.7	17.1	1.7
Blackcurrant Swirl, Heinz*	1/5 Cake/87g	241	13.4	277	4.1	30.3	15.4	3.6
Blueberry & Vanilla, TTD, Sainsbury's*	1 Serving/95g	353	24.8	372	5.4	28.9	26.1	2.1
Caramel Swirl, Cadbury*	1 Slice/91g	373	23.5	410	6.0	40.1	25.8	0.0

	Measure INFO/WEIGHT	per Measure KCAL	FAT	Nutrition Values per 100g / 100ml KCAL	PROT	CARB	FAT	FIBRE
CHEESECAKE								
Cherry, Healthy Range, Average	1 Serving/90g	172	3.0	191	3.7	36.4	3.3	1.1
Chocolate, & Hazelnut, Sara Lee*	1 Serving/65g	224	13.9	345	6.5	31.2	21.4	1.2
Chocolate, & Irish Cream Liqueur, Tesco*	1 Serving/93g	385	28.0	414	5.0	30.7	30.1	0.8
Chocolate, & Vanilla, Gu*	1 Pot/90g	379	27.1	421	4.1	34.6	30.1	1.6
Chocolate, & Vanilla, Reduced Fat, M & S*	1 Serving/114g	319	13.7	280	7.0	37.9	12.0	1.5
Chocolate, & Vanilla, Tesco*	1 Serving/90g	330	19.4	365	5.2	37.1	21.5	1.6
Chocolate, Average	1 Serving/75g	265	15.7	353	5.7	35.6	20.9	1.9
Chocolate, Baked, Ultimate, Entenmann's*	1 Serving/100g	331	19.0	331	5.7	34.2	19.0	2.8
Chocolate, Belgian, M & S*	1 Slice/100g	385	23.9	385	5.3	39.2	23.9	2.5
Chocolate, Kate's Cakes Ltd*	1 Serving/100g	415	27.4	415	5.7	34.7	27.4	2.2
Chocolate, Pure Indulgence, Thorntons*	1 Serving/75g	308	17.6	410	5.6	44.3	23.4	0.6
Chocolate, Weight Watchers*	1 Cake/95g	143	3.8	151	7.5	20.7	4.0	0.7
Chocolate Chip, M & S*	1oz/28g	109	6.6	391	5.1	39.7	23.6	0.2
Chocolate Swirl, Deeply Delicious, Heinz*	1/5 Cake/82g	221	9.4	271	4.6	37.4	11.5	4.7
Chocolate Truffle, HL, Tesco*	1 Slice/96g	250	13.2	260	10.3	23.7	13.8	6.5
Citrus, Good Choice, Mini, Iceland*	1 Cake/111g	198	4.7	178	3.5	31.6	4.2	0.4
Commercially Prepared	1/6 Cake/80g	257	18.0	321	5.5	25.5	22.5	0.4
Fruit, Average	1 Serving/75g	207	10.9	276	5.3	32.3	14.5	1.6
Fudge, Tesco*	1 Serving/102g	384	23.6	376	4.6	37.5	23.1	0.5
Homestyle Chocolate, M & S*	1oz/28g	105	6.2	376	6.0	38.0	22.2	0.7
Irish Cream, McVitie's*	¼ Slice/190g	616	36.9	324	4.4	33.0	19.4	0.4
Lemon, Average	1 Serving/90g	307	19.5	341	4.1	33.0	21.6	1.8
Lemon, Healthy Range, Average	1 Serving/90g	185	4.0	205	5.4	33.6	4.4	1.2
Lemon, Weight Watchers*	1 Serving/100g	211	5.0	211	6.3	30.1	5.0	1.8
Lemon, Zesty, M & S*	1/6 Cake/97g	325	18.9	335	4.0	38.7	19.5	2.6
Lemon Meringue, Tesco*	1 Slice/94g	352	25.0	375	3.8	30.1	26.6	0.3
Lemon Swirl, Individual, Sainsbury's*	1 Pot/125g	380	23.0	304	3.0	31.1	18.4	0.9
Lemon Swirl, Sainsbury's*	1/6 Cake/95g	350	21.0	369	4.8	37.2	22.1	1.0
Mandarin, Co-Op*	1 Slice/99g	297	16.8	300	4.0	32.0	17.0	0.3
Mandarin, GFY, Asda*	1/6 Cake/92g	178	4.0	194	3.6	35.0	4.4	1.2
Mandarin, LC, Tesco*	1/6 Cake/92g	170	3.5	185	4.1	33.1	3.8	1.5
Mandarin, Morrisons*	1 Serving/135g	335	16.9	248	3.8	32.2	12.5	0.8
Mandarin, Weight Watchers*	1 Cake/103g	180	2.9	175	4.6	32.9	2.8	1.5
Praline, Asda*	1/8 Cake/62g	226	14.9	364	7.0	30.0	24.0	3.2
Raspberry, BGTY, Sainsbury's*	1 Pot/95g	154	2.5	163	6.6	28.2	2.6	2.8
Raspberry, Creamy, Tesco*	1 Serving/100g	365	23.4	365	5.9	32.1	23.4	0.9
Raspberry, LC, Tesco*	1 Cake/95g	185	4.1	195	4.3	34.7	4.3	1.3
Raspberry, Low Saturated Fat, Waitrose*	1/6th Cake/108g	187	2.2	174	3.6	35.4	2.0	0.4
Raspberry, M & S*	1 Slice/105g	331	21.5	315	5.0	32.2	20.5	1.0
Raspberry, Perfectly Balanced, Waitrose*	1 Serving/106g	212	3.7	200	4.0	36.2	3.5	1.7
Raspberry, Weight Watchers*	1 Serving/100g	213	4.3	213	5.9	29.7	4.3	1.9
Raspberry & Mascarpone, Best, Morrisons*	1 Cake/84g	257	14.0	306	3.9	34.8	16.7	1.0
Raspberry & Strawberry, M & S*	1 Slice/105g	340	21.1	325	3.9	33.4	20.2	1.2
Strawberries & Cream, Finest, Tesco*	1 Serving/104g	325	22.4	312	4.3	25.3	21.5	0.5
Strawberries & Devonshire Cream, Heinz*	1/6 Cake/66g	184	10.1	279	3.9	31.4	15.3	3.7
Strawberry, Baked New York, Sara Lee*	1 Serving/100g	248	9.9	248	4.7	34.9	9.9	0.7
Strawberry, Creamy, Weight Watchers*	1 Cake/105g	187	2.6	178	4.7	34.2	2.5	2.2
Strawberry, Finest, Tesco*	1 Slice/113g	383	25.1	339	4.8	30.1	22.2	0.9
Strawberry, Fresh, M & S*	¼ Cake/125g	300	19.2	240	2.8	23.1	15.4	1.1
Strawberry, Frozen, Sainsbury's*	1/6 Cake/83.5	277	14.2	332	4.3	40.4	17.0	2.3
Strawberry, Heinz*	1 Pack/245g	588	31.1	240	3.4	28.1	12.7	2.4
Strawberry, Tesco*	1 Serving/100g	254	12.0	254	3.9	32.5	12.0	0.0
Strawberry Shortcake, Sara Lee*	1/6 Slice/68g	230	15.7	337	4.9	27.6	23.0	0.5

	Measure INFO/WEIGHT	per Measure KCAL	FAT	Nutrition Values per 100g / 100ml KCAL	PROT	CARB	FAT	FIBRE
CHEESECAKE								
Strawberry Swirl, Chosen By You, Asda*	1 Serving/100g	329	15.9	329	4.5	41.5	15.9	1.0
Summerfruit, GFY, Asda*	1/6 Cake/92g	175	3.8	191	3.7	34.5	4.2	1.4
Toffee, American Style, Asda*	1 Serving/75g	269	15.8	359	4.5	38.0	21.0	3.8
Toffee, Asda*	1 Cake/87g	295	19.1	339	4.3	31.0	22.0	3.5
Toffee, M & S*	1 Serving/105g	357	22.6	340	5.2	37.2	21.5	0.9
Toffee & Pecan, Wedge, Sainsbury's*	1 Serving/75g	296	21.8	395	5.4	28.1	29.0	3.1
Toffee Swirl, Chosen By You, Asda*	1 Serving/100g	334	16.1	334	5.5	41.4	16.1	0.9
Vanilla	1 Serving/100g	395	26.2	395	5.3	42.8	26.2	1.1
Vanilla Chocolate, Baked, Slice, Sainsbury's*	1 Slice/90g	349	23.0	388	5.7	33.8	25.6	2.7
CHERRIES								
Black, Fresh, Average	***1 Serving/80g***	***41***	***0.1***	***51***	***0.9***	***11.5***	***0.1***	***1.6***
Black, in Syrup, Average	***1 Serving/242g***	***160***	***0.0***	***66***	***0.6***	***16.0***	***0.0***	***0.7***
Dried, Love Life, Waitrose*	1 Portion/10g	35	0.1	348	0.2	84.3	1.1	2.1
Dried, Sainsbury's*	1 Tbsp/14g	45	0.2	319	3.8	72.4	1.5	6.2
Dried, Wholefoods, Tesco*	1 Serving/25g	86	0.2	345	1.9	81.6	0.8	4.6
Glace, Average	***1oz/28g***	***79***	***0.0***	***280***	***0.4***	***71.2***	***0.2***	***1.1***
Morello, Dried, Graze*	1 Pack/30g	100	0.4	335	4.5	82.0	1.5	0.0
Picota, Average	1 Serving/80g	42	0.1	52	0.9	11.4	0.1	1.2
Raw, Average	***1oz/28g***	***14***	***0.0***	***49***	***0.9***	***11.2***	***0.1***	***1.4***
Stewed with Sugar, Average	***1oz/28g***	***23***	***0.0***	***82***	***0.7***	***21.0***	***0.1***	***0.7***
Stewed without Sugar, Average	***1oz/28g***	***12***	***0.0***	***42***	***0.8***	***10.1***	***0.1***	***0.8***
CHESTNUTS								
Roasted, Peeled, Average	***1 Nut/10g***	***17***	***0.3***	***170***	***2.0***	***36.6***	***2.7***	***4.1***
CHEWING GUM								
Airwaves, Sugar Free, Wrigleys*	1 Pack/15g	23	0.0	155	0.0	62.0	0.0	0.0
Extra, Cool Breeze, Wrigleys*	1 Piece/2g	3	0.0	153	0.0	64.0	0.0	0.0
Extra, Peppermint, Sugar Free, Wrigleys*	1 Piece/2g	3	0.0	155	0.0	39.0	0.0	0.0
Peppermint, Soft, Sugar Free, Trident*	1 Stick/3g	4	0.0	155	0.4	62.3	0.4	0.0
Peppermint, Sugar Free, Active, Aldi*	2 Pieces/3g	4	0.0	146	0.0	61.0	0.0	0.0
Spearmint, Extra, Wrigleys*	1 Piece/1g	1	0.0	143	0.0	64.3	0.0	0.0
Spearmint, Wrigleys*	1 Piece/3g	9	0.0	295	0.0	73.0	0.0	0.0
Splash, Raspberry & Peach, Trident*	1 Piece/2g	4	0.0	180	1.6	68.5	0.5	0.0
Sugar Free, Pulse, Crisp Tropical Flavour, Wrigleys*	1 Stick/1g	2	0.0	161	0.0	65.0	0.0	0.0
CHICK PEAS								
Canned, Drained, Average	1 Can/240g	276	6.0	115	7.4	15.2	2.5	4.6
Canned, Kikkererwten, Albert Heijn*	1 Serving/200g	260	6.0	130	7.5	15.0	3.0	6.5
Dried, Average	***1 Serving/100g***	***319***	***5.4***	***319***	***21.7***	***47.4***	***5.4***	***8.0***
Dried, Boiled, Average	***1 Serving/75g***	***85***	***1.7***	***114***	***7.3***	***16.4***	***2.2***	***2.6***
in Salted Water, Canned, Average	***1 Can/179g***	***204***	***5.2***	***114***	***7.2***	***14.9***	***2.9***	***4.1***
in Water, Canned, Average	***1 Can/250g***	***282***	***6.6***	***113***	***7.2***	***15.3***	***2.6***	***4.8***
CHICKEN								
Bites, Battered, Tesco*	1 Pack/200g	440	28.6	220	15.2	7.6	14.3	2.0
Bites, Hot & Spicy, Tesco*	1 Pack/110g	143	1.8	130	18.9	9.6	1.6	2.5
Bites, Southern Fried, Tesco*	1 Pack/300g	720	33.3	240	18.1	16.9	11.1	2.1
Bites, Tikka, Average	1 Serving/50g	96	5.3	193	20.7	3.8	10.5	1.9
Breast, Chargrilled, Premium, Average	1 Piece/10g	20	1.1	197	21.6	1.5	11.2	0.3
Breast, Chargrilled, Sliced, Average	1 Slice/19g	24	0.5	124	24.4	0.5	2.7	0.4
Breast, Chargrilled, Sliced, M & S*	1 Pack/130g	182	3.8	140	27.6	0.4	2.9	0.1
Breast, Chilli & Ginger, COU, M & S*	1 Breast/120g	156	2.4	130	19.5	8.6	2.0	1.7
Breast, Chinese Style, Cooked, Sliced, Sainsbury's*	½ Pack/65g	96	1.2	148	28.3	4.7	1.8	0.1
Breast, Diced, Average	***1 Serving/188g***	***242***	***4.4***	***129***	***26.9***	***0.1***	***2.4***	***0.1***
Breast, Eastern Spices, Birds Eye*	1 Portion/175g	308	20.8	176	13.5	3.8	11.9	1.5
Breast, Escalope, Pesto Chargrilled, M & S*	1 Serving/100g	135	6.2	135	19.6	0.7	6.2	0.6

C

	Measure INFO/WEIGHT	per Measure KCAL	FAT	Nutrition Values per 100g / 100ml KCAL	PROT	CARB	FAT	FIBRE
CHICKEN								
Breast, Escalope, Plain, Average	***1 Serving/100g***	***110***	***2.2***	***110***	***22.3***	***0.7***	***2.2***	***0.5***
Breast, Fillet, Mesquite, KP Snacks*	1 Serving/85g	130	7.0	153	20.0	1.2	8.2	0.0
Breast, Fillets, Breaded, Average	1 Fillet/112g	246	11.6	220	17.6	14.0	10.4	1.3
Breast, Fillets, Breaded, Lemon & Pepper, Average	1 Fillet/89g	133	2.0	150	22.0	10.1	2.3	1.3
Breast, Fillets, Cajun, Average	1 Fillet/93g	124	2.6	134	23.6	3.5	2.8	0.3
Breast, Fillets, Chargrilled, Average	1 Serving/100g	120	1.1	120	27.3	0.3	1.1	0.3
Breast, Fillets, Frozen, Value, Tesco*	1 Breast/125g	125	2.1	100	20.4	0.7	1.7	0.0
Breast, Fillets, Garlic & Herb, Marinated, Mini, Morrisons*	1 Pack/300g	336	3.0	112	20.2	4.9	1.0	0.5
Breast, Fillets, Garlic & Herb, Tesco*	1 Fillet/135g	290	12.2	215	18.9	14.4	9.0	1.3
Breast, Fillets, Korma Style, Average	1 Serving/100g	132	2.8	132	27.4	0.8	2.8	0.6
Breast, Fillets, Lemon Parsley, M & S*	½ Pack/145g	232	3.5	160	14.3	20.7	2.4	4.3
Breast, Fillets, Mexican, Ready to Eat, Asda*	½ Pack/100g	147	1.5	147	27.8	5.5	1.5	0.1
Breast, Fillets, Mini, Raw, Average	***1oz/28g***	***34***	***0.4***	***121***	***26.9***	***0.2***	***1.5***	***0.1***
Breast, Fillets, Organic, Average	***1 Serving/150g***	***153***	***1.1***	***102***	***24.0***	***0.0***	***0.8***	***0.0***
Breast, Fillets, Skin On, Free Range, TTD, Sainsbury's*	1 Fillet/162g	235	7.6	145	25.7	0.0	4.7	0.0
Breast, Fillets, Skinless & Boneless, Raw, Average	***1 Breast/100g***	***129***	***2.0***	***129***	***27.8***	***0.0***	***2.0***	***0.0***
Breast, Fillets, Slices, Red Thai, Mini, Tesco*	2 Slices/65g	81	0.6	125	25.8	2.4	0.9	0.5
Breast, Fillets, Smokey Maple, Roast, Waitrose*	1 Fillet/96g	140	1.9	146	27.9	4.2	2.0	0.1
Breast, Fillets, Smoky Chilli, Tesco*	1 Fillet/92g	111	1.2	121	21.2	6.0	1.3	0.1
Breast, Fillets, Tikka, Mini, Ready to Eat, Tesco*	½ Pack/95g	120	1.8	125	22.4	4.2	1.9	0.2
Breast, Garlic & Herb, Premium, Bernard Matthews*	1 Serving/50g	50	1.2	101	17.9	1.6	2.5	1.8
Breast, Garlic & Herb Flavour, Co-Op*	1 Serving/170g	280	15.3	165	19.0	2.0	9.0	0.3
Breast, Grilled, Average	***1 Breast/130g***	***174***	***2.8***	***134***	***29.0***	***0.1***	***2.2***	***0.0***
Breast, Joint, Lemon & Tarragon, Finest, Tesco*	1 Serving/175g	247	11.0	141	18.8	2.3	6.3	0.2
Breast, Latino Style, Asda*	1 Breast/65g	99	2.0	152	27.0	4.1	3.1	0.5
Breast, Lemon & Herb, Chargrilled, Bernard Matthews*	1 Serving/100g	154	4.5	154	23.7	4.7	4.5	0.0
Breast, Lemon & Pepper, Breaded, Asda*	1 Portion/90g	187	7.6	208	15.3	17.7	8.4	1.8
Breast, Lemon Pepper, Cooked, Birds Eye*	1 Piece/101g	261	14.1	260	15.0	19.0	14.0	0.9
Breast, Lime & Coriander, Chargrilled, Asda*	1 Breast/160g	260	11.2	163	25.0	0.1	7.0	1.5
Breast, Meat & Skin, Raw, Average	***1 Serving/145g***	***249***	***13.4***	***172***	***20.8***	***0.0***	***9.2***	***0.0***
Breast, Meat & Skin, Weighed with Bone, Raw, Average	***1oz/28g***	***48***	***2.6***	***172***	***20.8***	***0.0***	***9.2***	***0.0***
Breast, Meat Only, Fried	***1 Serving/50g***	***94***	***2.4***	***187***	***33.4***	***0.5***	***4.7***	***0.0***
Breast, Pieces, Tikka, Average	1 Serving/100g	154	3.4	154	28.2	2.8	3.4	0.4
Breast, Platter, 237, Oakhouse Foods Ltd*	1 Platter/405g	409	8.1	101	8.3	12.6	2.0	1.0
Breast, Roast, Sliced, From Supermarket, Average	***1 Slice/13g***	***17***	***0.4***	***139***	***25.0***	***1.8***	***3.5***	***0.2***
Breast, Roast, without Skin, Average	***1oz/28g***	***42***	***1.3***	***149***	***25.4***	***1.0***	***4.7***	***0.2***
Breast, Roll, Average	***1 Slice/10g***	***17***	***1.0***	***167***	***16.1***	***3.2***	***10.0***	***0.2***
Breast, Smoked, Sliced, Average	***1 Slice/20g***	***22***	***0.5***	***110***	***20.7***	***0.9***	***2.6***	***0.1***
Breast, Southern Fried, Premium, Bernard Matthews*	1 Serving/60g	70	1.7	117	19.6	3.1	2.9	0.6
Breast, Strips, Raw, Average	***1 Serving/280g***	***358***	***5.7***	***128***	***27.1***	***0.4***	***2.0***	***0.3***
Breast, Strips, with Garlic & Rosemary, Sainsbury's*	1 Serving/58g	87	2.9	150	25.9	0.3	5.0	0.0
Breast, Tandoori Style, Average	1 Serving/180g	237	6.8	132	22.3	2.3	3.8	1.0
Breast, Tikka, Sliced, Average	1oz/28g	34	0.5	120	24.9	2.0	1.7	0.6
Dippers, Crispy, Average	5 Dippers/93g	231	14.3	249	13.2	14.4	15.4	0.6
Drumsticks, & Thighs, Garlic & Herb, Sainsbury's*	1 Serving/120g	184	10.7	153	16.6	1.5	8.9	0.1
Drumsticks, BBQ Flavour, Average	1 Serving/200g	348	16.0	174	22.6	3.1	8.0	0.4
Drumsticks, Breaded, Fried, Average	1oz/28g	70	4.1	248	19.6	9.9	14.6	0.6
Drumsticks, Chinese Style, Average	1 Drumstick/100g	178	8.1	178	22.6	3.6	8.1	0.7
Drumsticks, Free Range, TTD, Sainsbury's*	1 Piece/67g	126	6.7	188	24.4	0.0	10.0	0.0
Drumsticks, Meat & Skin, with Bone, Raw, Average	1 Drumstick/133g	281	16.4	211	23.4	0.2	12.4	0.0
Drumsticks, Meat Only, with Bone, Raw, Average	1 Drumstick/122g	237	13.8	194	21.5	0.1	11.3	0.0
Drumsticks, with Skin, Average	***1 Piece/125g***	***268***	***16.6***	***215***	***22.1***	***1.8***	***13.3***	***0.3***

	Measure INFO/WEIGHT	per Measure KCAL	FAT	Nutrition Values per 100g / 100ml KCAL	PROT	CARB	FAT	FIBRE
CHICKEN								
Escalope, Cheese Topped, Asda*	1 Escalope/173g	411	22.5	237	12.0	18.0	13.0	1.9
Escalope, Lemon & Pepper, Sainsbury's*	1 Escalope/143g	428	27.6	299	12.8	18.7	19.3	1.9
Fillets, Battered, Average	1 Fillet/90g	199	10.4	221	16.1	13.3	11.5	0.5
Fillets, BBQ, Hickory Style, Tesco*	1 Fillet/80g	112	1.8	140	28.4	1.5	2.2	0.5
Fillets, Breaded, Average	1 Piece/98g	214	10.5	219	14.2	15.9	10.7	1.9
Fillets, Chinese Style, Average	1oz/28g	37	0.5	132	24.4	4.6	1.8	0.5
Fillets, Coronation, BGTY, Sainsbury's*	1 Fillet/100g	136	2.6	136	27.1	2.4	2.6	1.0
Fillets, Green Thai, Marinated, Mini, Love Life, Waitrose*	½ Pack/138g	153	3.3	111	21.2	1.2	2.4	0.6
Fillets, Hickory Barbecue & Chilli, BGTY, Sainsbury's*	1 Fillet/100g	133	1.2	133	26.9	3.6	1.2	0.9
Fillets, Honey & Maple, Roast, Mini, Waitrose*	½ Pack/100g	131	0.5	131	23.0	8.6	0.5	1.5
Fillets, Honey & Mustard, Average	1 Serving/100g	138	3.7	138	18.4	7.5	3.7	0.8
Fillets, Hot & Spicy, Average	1oz/28g	58	3.1	206	16.4	10.5	11.0	1.1
Fillets, Lime & Coriander, Mini, Average	1 Fillet/42g	49	0.5	118	24.3	2.6	1.3	0.6
Fillets, Red Thai, Mini, Average	1oz/28g	36	0.6	128	21.7	5.4	2.0	0.6
Fillets, Southern Fried, Meat Only, Average	1 Piece/100g	222	12.0	222	16.4	12.2	12.0	1.1
Fillets, Tandoori Style, Mini, Average	1 Serving/100g	128	2.0	128	24.7	2.6	2.0	0.4
Fillets, Tikka, Average	1 Serving/100g	141	5.0	141	22.4	1.7	5.0	1.1
Fillets, Tikka, Mini, Average	1oz/28g	35	0.6	124	25.1	1.3	2.2	1.2
Fillets, Tomato & Basil, Mini, Average	1oz/28g	34	0.6	123	23.4	2.5	2.1	0.4
Fingers, Average	1 Serving/75g	188	9.9	250	13.7	18.8	13.2	1.2
Fricassee, Diet Chef Ltd*	1 Packet/300g	345	18.3	115	8.3	6.6	6.1	0.9
Goujons, Breaded, Average	1 Serving/114g	293	17.1	258	15.8	15.2	15.0	1.0
Goujons, Breast, Fresh, Average	1oz/28g	36	0.5	127	28.0	0.0	1.6	0.0
Honey Roast, Sliced, Average	1 Slice/13g	15	0.3	117	21.6	2.2	2.4	0.1
Hunter's, Asda*	½ Pack/190g	348	14.1	183	19.1	10.1	7.4	0.0
Hunters, Restaurant Favourites, Birds Eye*	1 Portion/178g	215	5.9	121	13.5	9.1	3.3	0.6
Leg, Meat Only, Raw, Average	***1oz/28g***	***34***	***1.1***	***120***	***20.1***	***0.0***	***3.8***	***0.0***
Leg, Meat Only, Raw, Weighed Skin & Bone, Average	***1oz/28g***	***38***	***1.2***	***134***	***22.5***	***0.0***	***4.3***	***0.0***
Leg, Meat Only, Stewed with Bone & Skin, Average	***1oz/28g***	***52***	***2.3***	***185***	***26.3***	***0.0***	***8.1***	***0.0***
Leg, with Skin, Raw, Average	***1oz/28g***	***48***	***2.9***	***172***	***19.1***	***0.0***	***10.4***	***0.0***
Leg, with Skin, Roasted, Weighed with Bone, Average	***1oz/28g***	***66***	***4.6***	***234***	***21.5***	***0.1***	***16.4***	***0.0***
Leg or Thigh, Hot & Spicy, Average	1oz/28g	50	3.0	179	19.4	1.0	10.8	0.4
Leg Portion, Roast, weighed with Bone, without Skin	1 Portion/114g	246	15.5	216	43.5	0.0	13.6	0.0
Light Meat, Raw	***1oz/28g***	***30***	***0.3***	***106***	***24.0***	***0.0***	***1.1***	***0.0***
Light Meat, Roasted	***1oz/28g***	***43***	***1.0***	***153***	***30.2***	***0.0***	***3.6***	***0.0***
Meat, Roasted, Average	***1oz/28g***	***50***	***2.1***	***177***	***27.3***	***0.0***	***7.5***	***0.0***
Meat & Skin, Raw, Average	***1oz/28g***	***64***	***5.0***	***230***	***17.6***	***0.0***	***17.7***	***0.0***
Meat & Skin, Roasted, Average	***1oz/28g***	***60***	***3.9***	***216***	***22.6***	***0.0***	***14.0***	***0.0***
Meat & Skin Portions, Deep Fried, Average	1oz/28g	73	4.7	259	26.9	0.0	16.8	0.0
Mince, Average	***1oz/28g***	***39***	***1.7***	***140***	***20.9***	***0.1***	***6.0***	***0.2***
Nuggets, Battered, Average	1 Nugget/20g	50	2.9	251	13.5	16.9	14.4	0.9
Nuggets, Breaded, Average	1 Nugget/14g	37	2.0	263	14.8	19.8	13.8	1.9
Nuggets, Free From Gluten & Wheat, Sainsbury's*	1 Nugget/19g	47	2.5	251	13.4	19.7	13.2	0.8
Nuggets, Southern Style, Tyson*	5 Nuggets/90g	290	22.0	322	12.2	13.3	24.4	1.1
Pieces, Boneless, Breaded, Fried, From Restaurant	1 Piece/17g	51	3.3	301	17.0	14.4	19.4	0.0
Pieces, Garlic, Crunchy, Birds Eye*	1 Piece/99g	259	15.0	262	14.4	16.9	15.2	0.9
Pops, Southern Fried, Frozen, Tesco*	1 Pack/225g	518	25.9	230	13.1	18.1	11.5	1.9
Shashlik, Patak's*	1 Serving/250g	203	3.6	81	12.4	4.4	1.4	0.0
Skewers, BBQ, George Foreman's Lean Mean Grillers*	1 Skewer/60g	68	0.8	114	20.0	5.5	1.4	0.4
Skewers, Marinated, Asda*	1 Skewer/35g	50	0.4	142	24.9	8.0	1.2	0.9
Sliced, Cooked, Average	***1 Slice/15g***	***18***	***0.4***	***118***	***22.4***	***1.6***	***2.4***	***0.1***
Spatchcock, Poussin, Sainsbury's*	1 Serving/122g	168	6.6	138	21.1	0.1	5.4	0.2
Spatchcock, Salt & Cracked Pepper, Sainsbury's*	1 Serving/122g	168	6.6	138	21.1	0.1	5.4	0.2

	Measure INFO/WEIGHT	per Measure KCAL	FAT	Nutrition Values per 100g / 100ml KCAL	PROT	CARB	FAT	FIBRE
CHICKEN								
Steaks, Average	***1 Serving/100g***	***205***	***9.4***	***205***	***21.1***	***9.0***	***9.4***	***0.7***
Strips or Tenders, Chinese Style, Average	1oz/28g	41	1.1	145	19.6	8.0	4.1	1.0
Thigh, Fillets, Tesco*	1 Serving/100g	165	9.8	165	18.3	0.0	9.8	0.0
Thigh, Meat & Skin, Casseroled, Average	***1oz/28g***	***65***	***4.6***	***233***	***21.5***	***0.0***	***16.3***	***0.0***
Thigh, Meat & Skin, Raw, Average	***1 Serving/100g***	***218***	***14.7***	***218***	***21.4***	***0.0***	***14.7***	***0.0***
Thigh, Meat & Skin, Weighed with Bone, Raw, Average	1 Serving/100g	219	16.6	219	16.2	0.2	16.6	0.0
Thigh, Meat Only, Diced, Casseroled	***1oz/28g***	***50***	***2.4***	***180***	***25.6***	***0.0***	***8.6***	***0.0***
Thigh, Meat Only, Raw, Average	***1 Thigh/90g***	***113***	***4.9***	***126***	***19.4***	***0.0***	***5.4***	***0.0***
Thigh, Roast, Average	***1 Serving/100g***	***238***	***15.6***	***238***	***23.8***	***0.4***	***15.6***	***0.0***
Tikka, Steaks, Cooked, Butchers Selection, Asda*	1 Serving/100g	160	3.7	160	29.7	1.8	3.7	0.1
Wafer Thin, Average	1 Slice/10g	12	0.4	120	19.0	2.8	3.6	0.2
Wafer Thin, Coronation, Sainsbury's*	½ Pack/50g	68	2.2	135	19.1	4.5	4.5	0.1
Whole, Roast, Average	***1oz/28g***	***59***	***3.7***	***211***	***21.2***	***1.5***	***13.4***	***0.2***
Wing, Breaded, Fried, Average	1oz/28g	82	5.2	294	18.4	14.0	18.5	0.4
Wing, Meat & Skin, Cooked, Average	***1oz/28g***	***67***	***4.4***	***241***	***23.3***	***1.9***	***15.6***	***0.3***
Wing Quarter, Meat Only, Casseroled	***1oz/28g***	***46***	***1.8***	***164***	***26.9***	***0.0***	***6.3***	***0.0***
Wings, BBQ Flavour, Average	1oz/28g	61	3.5	220	20.3	6.6	12.4	0.6
Wings, Chinese Style, Average	1oz/28g	72	4.3	256	24.2	5.1	15.5	0.6
Wings, Hot & Spicy, Average	1oz/28g	65	3.8	231	21.8	5.2	13.6	0.8
Wings, Meat & Skin, Raw, Average	***1oz/28g***	***52***	***3.3***	***184***	***19.0***	***0.5***	***11.8***	***0.2***
CHICKEN &								
Apricot Rice, COU, M & S*	1 Pack/400g	360	3.6	90	9.4	10.6	0.9	0.7
Asparagus, in a Champagne Sauce, Finest, Tesco*	1 Pack/500g	615	33.5	123	8.8	7.0	6.7	0.9
Asparagus, with Rice, Frozen, Low Fat, Waitrose*	1 Pack/380g	403	7.6	106	8.5	13.6	2.0	0.6
Bacon, Easy Steam, Tesco*	1 Pack/400g	728	36.4	182	11.7	13.6	9.1	0.8
Black Bean, Chinese, Tesco*	1 Pack/350g	382	17.2	109	8.9	7.4	4.9	0.7
Black Bean, Special Fried Rice, HL, Tesco*	1 Pack/450g	360	6.3	80	6.8	9.5	1.4	0.9
Black Bean, with Chinese Rice, COU, M & S*	1 Pack/400g	320	9.6	80	7.4	7.6	2.4	1.1
Black Bean, with Noodles, Tesco*	1 Pack/475g	470	7.6	99	7.6	13.6	1.6	0.2
Black Bean, with Rice, Chinese, Tesco*	1 Serving/450g	459	9.5	102	5.3	15.4	2.1	0.5
Black Bean, with Rice, HL, Tesco*	1 Pack/450g	464	7.2	103	6.9	19.6	1.6	0.6
Broccoli, with Herb Potatoes, Tesco*	1 Pack/475g	499	10.9	105	7.8	12.5	2.3	1.5
Butternut Squash, Curry Pot, Weight Watchers*	1 Pot/250g	232	3.5	93	6.6	12.5	1.4	1.6
Cashew Nuts, Chinese, Cantonese, Sainsbury's*	½ Pack/175g	172	8.8	98	8.4	4.9	5.0	1.3
Cashew Nuts, Chinese, Ready Meal, Average	1 Serving/400g	497	24.0	124	9.2	7.5	6.0	1.2
Cashew Nuts, Oriental, HL, Tesco*	1 Pack/450g	436	4.5	97	7.0	15.1	1.0	0.7
Chips, BBQ, BGTY, Sainsbury's*	1 Pack/381g	423	6.9	111	7.9	15.9	1.8	2.5
Chorizo Paella, Go Cook, Asda*	½ Pack/475g	591	10.5	124	10.2	15.9	2.2	2.6
Cous Cous, HE, Tesco*	1 Pack/351g	263	1.8	75	10.3	7.3	0.5	1.4
Cranberry, Perfectly Balanced, Waitrose*	1 Pack/240g	161	1.0	67	11.8	4.1	0.4	1.1
Fries, Southern Fried, Sainsbury's*	½ Pack/250g	562	21.8	225	10.5	26.2	8.7	0.8
Gravy, COU, M & S*	1 Pack/300g	216	3.9	72	7.2	7.8	1.3	1.6
Mushroom, Al Forno, Charlie Bigham's*	½ Pack/324g	509	29.2	157	7.2	11.2	9.0	0.6
Mushroom, Chinese, Iceland*	1 Pack/400g	276	9.2	69	8.2	3.8	2.3	0.4
Mushroom, Chinese, Sainsbury's*	½ Pack/175g	116	3.5	66	7.6	4.4	2.0	0.9
Mushroom, Skinny Chef, All About Weight*	1 Meal/268g	204	2.7	76	12.1	3.0	1.0	3.1
Mushroom, with Puff Pastry, 134, Oakhouse Foods Ltd*	1 Meal/400g	516	23.2	129	7.9	11.1	5.8	1.3
Mushroom, with Rice, Egg Fried, Average	1 Serving/400g	421	10.1	105	6.3	14.4	2.5	0.8
Mushroom, with Vegetable Rice, BGTY, Sainsbury's*	1 Pack/400g	376	7.2	94	6.4	13.0	1.8	0.9
Noodles, Chinese Style, HE, Tesco*	1 Pack/370g	422	6.3	114	8.5	15.9	1.7	1.5
Peppers, M & S*	1 Serving/240g	264	10.8	110	14.7	2.3	4.5	0.6
Pineapple, Chilled, Tesco*	1 Pack/350g	364	8.4	104	9.6	11.1	2.4	5.5
Pineapple, with Egg Fried Rice, HL, Tesco*	1 Pack/450g	414	3.2	92	6.0	15.4	0.7	0.6

	Measure INFO/WEIGHT	per Measure KCAL	FAT	Nutrition Values per 100g / 100ml KCAL	PROT	CARB	FAT	FIBRE
CHICKEN &								
Pineapple, with Egg Fried Rice, Tesco*	1 Pack/450g	450	10.8	100	7.6	12.1	2.4	1.2
Pineapple, with Vegetable Rice, M & S*	1 Pack/400g	400	7.6	100	7.2	13.0	1.9	1.6
Rice, Mexican Mojito, Cooked, Sainsbury's*	1 Pack/441g	560	11.9	127	5.6	18.8	2.7	2.8
Stuffing, Roast, HL, Tesco*	1 Serving/17g	19	0.2	111	23.3	1.3	1.4	0.2
Tomato & Basil, COU, M & S*	½ Pack/200g	180	4.6	90	14.3	3.4	2.3	0.8
Tomato Saag, with Pilau Rice, BGTY, Sainsbury's*	1 Pack/400g	404	4.0	101	7.3	15.6	1.0	1.0
Vegetable Medley, Chargrilled, HE, Tesco*	1 Pack/450g	270	5.4	60	6.5	5.8	1.2	0.9
Vegetables, in Gravy, Chosen By You, Asda*	1 Pack/420g	441	10.9	105	13.9	6.0	2.6	0.8
White Wine, with Rice, HE, Tesco*	1 Pack/450g	450	6.3	100	7.1	14.8	1.4	1.0
CHICKEN ALFREDO								
Average	1 Pack/400g	416	10.0	104	12.2	8.2	2.5	0.8
BGTY, Sainsbury's*	1 Serving/200g	208	5.4	104	18.0	1.9	2.7	0.5
CHICKEN ARRABBIATA								
Al Forno, Sainsbury's*	1 Pack/900g	1026	22.5	114	6.5	16.4	2.5	1.4
Bistro, Waitrose*	½ Pack/175g	156	5.2	89	12.9	2.5	3.0	0.5
Easy Steam, HL, Tesco*	1 Pack/400g	284	3.2	71	8.4	7.6	0.8	1.2
GFY, Asda*	1 Pack/448g	394	3.1	88	5.2	15.1	0.7	1.1
Weight Watchers, Heinz*	1 Serving/300g	222	1.8	74	5.4	11.5	0.6	0.8
CHICKEN BANG BANG								
Oriental Express*	½ Pack/200g	170	3.4	85	6.4	11.0	1.7	3.2
Waitrose*	1 Pack/350g	368	17.2	105	9.4	5.9	4.9	1.2
CHICKEN BUTTER								
with Rice, Average	1 Serving/400g	561	27.6	140	10.6	8.9	6.9	1.4
CHICKEN CAJUN								
& Potato Hash, HL, Tesco*	1 Pack/450g	428	6.3	95	6.5	14.1	1.4	1.5
HE, Tesco*	1 Pack/365g	412	4.7	113	7.9	17.3	1.3	0.7
CHICKEN CANTONESE								
& Rice, Sizzler, Tesco*	1 Serving/450g	639	25.6	142	7.7	14.9	5.7	0.9
Breast, Fillets, Sainsbury's*	1 Serving/154g	168	2.3	109	20.3	3.6	1.5	0.6
Chinese, Tesco*	½ Pack/175g	196	6.5	112	10.3	9.4	3.7	0.4
Honey, Sesame, Sainsbury's*	1/3 Pack/135g	116	3.6	86	9.8	5.5	2.7	0.8
CHICKEN CARIBBEAN								
Fruity, with Rice & Peas, New, BGTY, Sainsbury's*	1 Pack/400g	352	3.6	88	6.9	13.1	0.9	2.2
Style, Breasts, COU, M & S*	1 Serving/205g	205	3.1	100	14.6	7.3	1.5	1.3
CHICKEN CHASSEUR								
Average	1 Serving/400g	363	9.2	91	12.2	4.9	2.3	0.9
BGTY, Sainsbury's*	1 Pack/320g	243	3.5	76	6.8	9.5	1.1	1.0
CHICKEN CHILLI								
Sweet, & Egg Fried Rice, HL, Tesco*	1 Serving/450g	446	8.1	99	5.7	15.0	1.8	0.4
Sweet, Chosen By You, Asda*	½ Pack/170g	253	6.8	149	19.1	8.9	4.0	0.7
Sweet, Findus*	1 Pack/350g	420	12.2	120	6.0	15.0	3.5	1.5
Sweet, Just Cook, Sainsbury's*	½ Pack/191g	200	1.3	105	15.2	9.4	0.7	0.5
Sweet, Pieces, Morrisons*	1 Pack/200g	282	5.0	141	25.5	4.1	2.5	0.5
Sweet, with Noodles, Ready Meal, Average	1 Serving/400g	404	5.8	101	6.5	15.5	1.4	1.4
CHICKEN CHINESE								
& Prawns, Sizzler, House Special, Tesco*	1 Serving/450g	684	23.4	152	7.5	18.8	5.2	1.2
Balls, M & S*	1 Ball/16g	45	2.2	280	10.8	29.2	13.6	2.1
Battered, with Plum Sauce, Tesco*	1 Pack/350g	648	20.3	185	6.7	26.5	5.8	0.8
Crispy Aromatic, Half, Tesco*	1 Serving/233g	524	24.2	225	16.3	16.7	10.4	1.2
Fillets, with Sweet Chilli Sauce, Tesco*	1 Serving/350g	592	22.0	169	8.8	19.2	6.3	0.7
Stir Fry, Morrisons*	1 Serving/319g	341	5.4	107	5.7	17.0	1.7	1.5
with Ginger & Spring Onion, Tesco*	1 Serving/350g	299	10.1	85	7.6	7.3	2.9	0.6

	Measure INFO/WEIGHT	per Measure KCAL	FAT	Nutrition Values per 100g / 100ml KCAL	PROT	CARB	FAT	FIBRE
CHICKEN CORDON BLEU								
Breast, Fillets, Sainsbury's*	1 Serving/150g	304	14.3	203	17.5	11.5	9.5	1.6
Waitrose*	1 Serving/160g	325	15.4	203	20.1	9.1	9.6	2.4
CHICKEN CORONATION								
COU, M & S*	1oz/28g	34	0.6	120	16.3	8.6	2.2	0.7
M & S*	1 Serving/200g	420	26.4	210	12.6	10.6	13.2	1.3
CHICKEN CURRIED								
with Vegetables, Plumrose*	1 Serving/196g	253	16.1	129	5.8	8.0	8.2	0.0
CHICKEN DINNER								
Breast, with Pork, Sage & Onion Stuffing, Tesco*	1 Serving/180g	277	14.8	154	19.4	0.7	8.2	0.5
Kershaws*	1 Pack/350g	210	3.5	60	4.3	8.4	1.0	1.2
Roast, 104, Oakhouse Foods Ltd*	1 Dinner/400g	608	16.0	152	6.6	10.2	4.0	1.3
Tesco*	1 Serving/400g	388	7.2	97	9.2	10.9	1.8	1.2
with Gravy, The Crafty Cook*	1 Serving/320g	330	6.7	103	5.6	15.3	2.1	1.9
CHICKEN EN CROUTE								
Breast, Tesco*	1 Serving/215g	555	33.1	258	9.4	20.4	15.4	0.6
Charlie Bigham's*	½ Pack/230g	568	36.8	247	11.1	14.1	16.0	0.6
Just Cook, Sainsbury's*	1 Serving/180g	481	27.2	267	16.8	15.9	15.1	0.4
CHICKEN ESCALOPE								
Cheese & Chive, Asda*	1 Escalope/159g	377	21.1	237	11.5	15.9	13.3	0.7
Creamy Peppercorn, Sainsbury's*	1 Serving/150g	367	24.5	245	13.3	11.2	16.3	1.1
Lemon & Herb, Waitrose*	1 Serving/200g	242	6.4	121	22.0	1.0	3.2	0.6
Sour Cream & Chive, Tesco*	1 Escalope/143g	390	24.8	274	13.3	16.1	17.4	2.0
Spinach & Ricotta, Sainsbury's*	1 Escalope/150g	354	22.9	236	13.1	11.5	15.3	0.9
Topped with Cheese, Ham & Mushrooms, Asda*	½ Pack/149g	217	9.0	145	22.0	0.8	6.0	0.4
CHICKEN FLORENTINE								
Asda*	1 Serving/200g	322	18.0	161	18.0	2.1	9.0	0.9
Finest, Tesco*	½ Pack/225g	358	19.1	159	11.0	9.7	8.5	1.3
HL, Tesco*	1 Pack/400g	340	10.8	85	12.1	3.0	2.7	0.9
CHICKEN FORRESTIERE								
COU, M & S*	1 Serving/220g	187	3.7	85	14.5	2.2	1.7	0.6
CHICKEN FU YUNG								
Chinese Takeaway, Tesco*	1 Pack/350g	315	3.5	90	5.6	14.5	1.0	0.8
CHICKEN GINGER								
& Plum, with Rice, Perfectly Balanced, Waitrose*	1 Pack/400g	492	2.0	123	6.3	23.5	0.5	1.0
& Spring Onion with Rice, Sharwood's*	1 Pack/375g	347	6.4	93	5.1	14.2	1.7	1.7
CHICKEN GLAZED								
Balsamic, HL, Tesco*	1 Pack/400g	288	3.6	72	5.1	10.8	0.9	0.9
CHICKEN HARISSA								
BGTY, Sainsbury's*	1 Serving/250g	211	3.0	84	10.4	8.0	1.2	1.5
with Cous Cous, Perfectly Balanced, Waitrose*	1 Pack/400g	348	8.0	87	7.6	9.5	2.0	1.7
CHICKEN HAWAIIAN								
with Rice, Birds Eye*	1 Pack/350g	406	5.2	116	5.5	20.2	1.5	0.6
CHICKEN HERB								
Steam Cuisine, M & S*	1 Pack/400g	280	6.4	70	8.2	6.0	1.6	0.9
CHICKEN IN								
Bacon, Mushroom & Red Wine Sauce, Asda*	1 Serving/151g	145	3.9	96	16.0	2.2	2.6	0.5
Barbecue Sauce, COU, M & S*	1 Pack/352g	370	5.6	105	8.6	13.8	1.6	1.2
Barbeque Sauce, Breasts, COU, M & S*	1 Pack/350g	420	6.7	120	8.5	20.6	1.9	0.6
Barbeque Sauce, HE, Tesco*	1 Breast/170g	177	2.4	104	18.3	4.5	1.4	0.9
BBQ Sauce, Breast, Sainsbury's*	1 Serving/170g	199	1.2	117	14.5	13.1	0.7	1.3
BBQ Sauce, Chargrilled, Breast, GFY, Asda*	1 Serving/166g	214	6.1	129	19.0	5.0	3.7	1.0
BBQ Sauce, GFY, Asda*	1 Pack/380g	494	2.7	130	18.0	13.0	0.7	0.2
BBQ Sauce, Weight Watchers*	1 Pack/339g	332	11.9	98	5.8	10.8	3.5	0.9

	Measure INFO/WEIGHT	per Measure KCAL	FAT	Nutrition Values per 100g / 100ml KCAL	PROT	CARB	FAT	FIBRE
CHICKEN IN								
Black Bean Sauce, & Rice, Morrisons*	1 Pack/400g	408	9.2	102	3.9	16.4	2.3	1.2
Black Bean Sauce, Asia, Aldi*	1 Pack/375g	364	10.9	97	10.9	6.1	2.9	1.3
Black Bean Sauce, Budgens*	1 Pack/350g	332	14.0	95	9.9	4.9	4.0	0.9
Black Bean Sauce, Canned, BGTY, Sainsbury's*	1 Can/400g	308	3.6	77	9.3	7.9	0.9	0.7
Black Bean Sauce, Chinese Takeaway, Iceland*	1 Pack/400g	348	12.8	87	9.3	5.3	3.2	0.7
Black Bean Sauce, Frozen, BGTY, Sainsbury's*	1 Pack/400g	380	4.4	95	4.5	16.6	1.1	0.5
Black Bean Sauce, M & S*	1 Pack/350g	298	7.0	85	8.7	8.0	2.0	1.1
Black Bean Sauce, Sainsbury's*	1 Pack/465g	484	7.9	104	5.0	17.3	1.7	0.3
Black Bean Sauce, Tinned, Tesco*	1 Serving/200g	164	2.6	82	10.0	7.7	1.3	1.1
Black Bean Sauce, Waitrose*	1 Pack/300g	243	3.6	81	10.9	6.6	1.2	0.8
Black Bean Sauce, with Noodles, Pro Cuisine*	1 Pack/600g	366	3.6	61	5.6	8.5	0.6	0.0
Black Bean Sauce, with Rice, Asda*	1 Pack/400g	500	7.6	125	7.0	20.0	1.9	0.6
Black Bean Sauce, with Rice, Iceland*	1 Pack/400g	388	6.0	97	5.1	15.8	1.5	0.8
Breadcrumbs, Breast, Grills, Birds Eye*	1 Fillet/93g	246	11.8	264	15.1	21.8	12.7	0.9
Breadcrumbs, Southern, Breast, Cooked, Birds Eye*	1 Breast/88g	240	12.0	273	15.9	20.4	13.6	1.2
Cheese & Bacon, Wrapped, Breast, Tesco*	1 Serving/300g	474	23.4	158	20.7	1.2	7.8	0.5
Chilli & Lemon Grass, with Rice, Sainsbury's*	1 Pack/450g	526	11.2	117	6.2	17.4	2.5	0.7
Coconut, Sizzler, HL, Tesco*	1 Pack/350g	280	7.7	80	9.8	4.5	2.2	2.1
Garlic & Cream Sauce, Breast Fillet, Morrisons*	1 Serving/180g	262	15.8	146	14.9	1.8	8.8	0.6
Garlic & Herbs, Breast, Sainsbury's*	1 Serving/200g	316	5.2	158	28.3	5.4	2.6	0.1
Ginger & Chilli, with Veg Noodles, COU, M & S*	1 Pack/400g	300	2.4	75	6.4	10.7	0.6	1.1
Gravy, Breast, Sainsbury's*	1 Pack/200g	124	1.0	62	11.8	2.9	0.5	0.2
Gravy, Chunky, M & S*	1 Can/489g	465	19.1	95	13.6	1.4	3.9	0.8
Honey Mustard & Parsnip Mash, LC, Tesco*	1 Pack/400g	340	6.8	85	8.0	9.0	1.7	2.0
Hot Ginger Sauce, with Thai Sticky Rice, Sainsbury's*	1 Pack/450g	603	20.7	134	6.8	16.3	4.6	0.5
Hunter's BBQ Sauce, Asda*	½ Pack/190g	348	14.1	183	19.1	10.3	7.4	0.0
Leek & Bacon Sauce, Chilled, Co-Op*	1 Pack/400g	460	20.0	115	15.0	2.0	5.0	0.2
Leek & Bacon Sauce, with Mash, HL, Tesco*	1 Pack/450g	338	8.1	75	6.7	8.0	1.8	1.6
Lemon & Garlic Marinade, Thighs, Go Cook, Asda*	½ Pack/265g	493	30.2	186	19.7	1.2	11.4	0.8
Lemon Sauce, Breast, HE, Tesco*	1 Pack/385g	385	7.3	100	15.9	4.7	1.9	0.5
Lemon Sauce with Rice, Sainsbury's*	1 Pack/450g	513	6.8	114	8.1	17.0	1.5	0.7
Light Batter, Bites, Captain Birds Eye, Birds Eye*	1 Piece/15g	32	1.9	210	18.6	5.8	12.5	0.2
Lime & Coriander Marinade, Chargrilled, Asda*	½ Pack/163g	286	14.7	175	23.0	0.5	9.0	0.0
Madeira Sauce, with Mushrooms, Finest, Tesco*	½ Pack/200g	210	8.3	105	13.8	3.0	4.2	1.0
Masala, with Spiced Indian Lentils, M & S*	1 Pack/330g	297	8.2	90	10.3	6.1	2.5	5.9
Mediterranean Sauce, Iceland*	1 Pack/500g	640	6.0	128	7.4	21.8	1.2	0.5
Mexican Salsa, Tesco*	1 Pack/320g	368	8.6	115	19.5	3.1	2.7	0.6
Mexican Style Sauce, Tesco*	1 Serving/180g	128	1.4	71	13.3	2.6	0.8	0.7
Mushroom & Red Wine Sauce, Breast Fillets, Morrisons*	1 Serving/177g	184	4.4	104	15.7	4.6	2.5	0.7
Mushroom Sauce, 124, Oakhouse Foods Ltd*	1 Meal/380g	334	8.0	88	8.5	9.7	2.1	1.7
Mushroom Sauce, Diet Chef Ltd*	1 Pack/300g	225	6.9	75	7.9	5.7	2.3	0.1
Oyster Sauce, & Mushrooms, Tesco*	1 Pack/350g	252	5.6	72	8.0	6.3	1.6	0.7
Oyster Sauce, with Mushrooms, Tesco*	1 Pack/350g	189	3.2	54	8.0	3.5	0.9	0.8
Peanut Sauce, Cafe Classics, Lean Cuisine	1 Pack/255g	300	9.0	118	7.8	13.7	3.5	1.2
Peppercorn Sauce, GFY, Asda*	1 Serving/399g	431	7.2	108	6.0	17.0	1.8	0.5
Peppers, Fillets, Sainsbury's*	1 Pack/360g	378	13.3	105	13.7	4.2	3.7	1.1
Pesto Style Dressing, Asda*	1 Serving/150g	210	10.0	140	18.7	1.3	6.7	0.0
Prosciutto, Wrapped, Charlie Bigham's*	½ Pack/185g	263	12.8	142	17.0	2.9	6.9	0.4
Red Pepper Dressing, Tesco*	1 Serving/140g	228	13.3	163	19.2	0.1	9.5	0.5
Red Thai Marinade, Breasts, Mini, HE, Tesco*	1 Serving/200g	276	5.0	138	26.8	2.0	2.5	0.5
Red Wine, with Mash, Morrisons*	1 Serving/400g	288	5.2	72	9.1	6.1	1.3	1.4
Red Wine Sauce, Breasts, Fresh Tastes, Asda*	½ Pack/190g	245	8.0	129	20.5	2.4	4.2	0.5
Reggae Reggae Sauce, Drumsticks, Levi Roots*	1 Serving/100g	165	7.3	165	21.5	3.4	7.3	0.0

	Measure INFO/WEIGHT	per Measure KCAL	FAT	Nutrition Values per 100g / 100ml KCAL	PROT	CARB	FAT	FIBRE
CHICKEN IN								
Smoky Barbecue Sauce, Breast, Fresh Tastes, Asda*	1 Breast/160g	258	6.2	161	21.9	9.6	3.9	0.9
Smoky Barbeque Sauce, Tesco*	1 Serving/185g	229	3.9	124	16.3	9.9	2.1	1.0
Spicy Chilli Sauce, Topped with Cheese, Breast, Asda*	½ Pack/190g	241	7.0	127	20.0	3.4	3.7	0.0
Sticky Balsamic Glaze, Chargrilled, COU, M & S*	1 Pack/370g	296	2.2	80	7.0	11.2	0.6	1.3
Sun Dried Tomato & Basil, Breast, Fillets, M & S*	½ Pack/110g	165	4.5	150	22.5	4.7	4.1	1.1
Sun Dried Tomato & Basil Sauce, Breast, Iceland*	1 Serving/156g	134	2.5	86	14.6	3.3	1.6	1.0
Sweet Chilli Sauce, Breast, Fresh Tastes, Asda*	½ Pack/180g	288	9.0	160	18.4	10.3	5.0	0.5
Tarragon Sauce, Lean Cuisine*	1 Pack/338g	270	6.8	80	4.0	11.0	2.0	1.5
Tomato & Basil Sauce, Breast, Fresh Tastes, Asda*	½ Pack/130g	136	2.7	105	19.3	2.3	2.1	0.7
Tomato & Basil Sauce, Breast, GFY, Asda*	1 Pack/392g	447	13.3	114	12.0	9.0	3.4	1.5
Tomato & Basil Sauce, Breast Fillets, Morrisons*	½ Pack/171g	231	7.5	135	21.3	2.5	4.4	1.4
Tomato & Basil Sauce, Eat Smart, Morrisons*	1 Pack/375g	300	6.4	80	8.3	7.8	1.7	2.4
Tomato & Basil Sauce, GFY, Asda*	½ Pack/189g	231	6.1	122	22.0	1.2	3.2	2.0
Tomato & Basil Sauce, Good Choice, Iceland*	½ Pack/170g	153	4.4	90	13.3	3.3	2.6	0.6
White Sauce, BGTY, Sainsbury's*	1 Can/200g	162	4.2	81	1.2	2.4	2.1	1.1
White Sauce, Canned, Asda*	½ Can/400g	644	44.0	161	12.0	3.5	11.0	0.0
White Sauce, Canned, HL, Tesco*	½ Can/200g	180	5.8	90	14.3	1.3	2.9	5.4
White Wine, with Pasta, Perfectly Balanced, Waitrose*	1 Pack/400g	400	10.0	100	8.2	12.1	2.5	2.5
White Wine, with Rice, HE, Tesco*	1 Serving/450g	513	12.2	114	7.1	15.3	2.7	0.7
White Wine & Asparagus Panzerotti, Asda*	½ Pack/150g	238	2.6	159	8.0	28.0	1.7	0.0
White Wine & Tarragon Sauce, Breasts, Finest, Tesco*	½ Pack/200g	326	20.2	163	16.8	1.3	10.1	0.0
White Wine & Tarragon Sauce, Waitrose*	½ Pack/225g	281	17.3	125	10.7	3.1	7.7	0.3
White Wine Sauce, Breasts, Tesco*	1 Serving/370g	388	14.1	105	16.9	0.8	3.8	0.6
White Wine Sauce, Wild Rice, Pub Specials, Birds Eye*	1 Pack/450g	335	5.9	74	7.1	8.4	1.3	2.1
White Wine Sauce, with Pasta, LowLow*	1 Pack/320g	330	6.7	103	5.8	14.4	2.1	1.7
Wild Mushroom Sauce, Breasts, HL, Tesco*	1 Serving/212g	191	5.1	90	15.1	2.1	2.4	1.5
Wild Mushroom Sauce, Extra Special, Asda*	1 Serving/225g	319	19.0	142	14.2	2.2	8.4	0.3
CHICKEN ITALIAN								
Good Choice, Iceland*	1 Pack/400g	388	2.0	97	4.7	18.3	0.5	0.6
Style, BGTY, Sainsbury's*	1 Pack/400g	364	4.4	91	6.0	14.5	1.1	0.9
Style, Dinner, Asda*	1 Pack/400g	244	4.0	61	6.0	7.0	1.0	1.1
Style, Meal, Asda*	1 Pack/408g	241	3.3	59	6.0	7.0	0.8	0.8
Style, Sainsbury's*	½ Pack/190g	222	7.6	117	16.3	3.9	4.0	0.1
with a Spicy Tomato, Chilli & Herb Sauce, Slim Fast*	1 Pack/371g	390	4.1	105	7.1	16.6	1.1	0.4
CHICKEN JEERA								
Sainsbury's*	½ Pack/201g	247	14.1	123	10.5	4.6	7.0	1.8
CHICKEN KUNG PO								
Sainsbury's*	½ Pack/175g	131	4.4	75	9.2	4.0	2.5	1.0
Waitrose*	1 Pack/350g	318	3.9	91	8.2	12.1	1.1	1.2
with Egg Fried Rice, Asda*	1 Pack/450g	688	22.5	153	6.0	21.0	5.0	1.0
CHICKEN LEMON								
Balls, Asda*	1 Ball/15g	42	2.6	279	14.0	19.0	17.0	1.6
Battered, Cantonese, Sainsbury's*	1 Pack/350g	560	19.6	160	10.7	16.6	5.6	0.9
Battered, Chinese Meal for Two, Tesco*	½ Serving/175g	294	13.0	168	6.6	18.8	7.4	2.0
Battered, HE, Tesco*	1 Pack/350g	399	9.1	114	8.8	13.9	2.6	0.4
Breast, Fillets, BGTY, Sainsbury's*	1 Fillet/113g	195	2.4	173	18.4	19.9	2.1	1.9
Cantonese, Sainsbury's*	½ Pack/140g	218	8.8	156	11.0	13.9	6.3	0.6
Cantonese Style with Egg Fried Rice, Farmfoods*	1 Pack/324g	486	15.6	150	4.9	21.8	4.8	0.1
Chinese, Tesco*	1 Serving/350g	564	11.2	161	7.0	26.0	3.2	0.3
COU, M & S*	1 Pack/150g	150	1.4	100	17.9	5.6	0.9	0.8
Tesco*	½ Pack/175g	214	7.4	122	11.0	10.1	4.2	0.6
with Vegetable Rice, BGTY, Sainsbury's*	1 Pack/400g	428	6.4	107	6.5	16.8	1.6	0.8

	Measure INFO/WEIGHT	per Measure KCAL	per Measure FAT	Nutrition Values per 100g / 100ml KCAL	PROT	CARB	FAT	FIBRE
CHICKEN MEAL								
American, Fillets, Asda*	1 Pack/345g	838	38.0	243	9.0	27.0	11.0	2.3
Breast Fillets, Meal For One, Eat Well, M & S*	1 Pack/400g	340	10.4	85	7.0	7.9	2.6	1.5
Roast, M & S*	1 Pack/280g	294	9.2	105	6.6	11.6	3.3	1.9
CHICKEN MEXICAN								
Style, BGTY, Sainsbury's*	1 Serving/260g	255	6.5	98	6.9	12.1	2.5	2.2
Style, Combo, Asda*	1 Pack/380g	562	16.7	148	21.0	6.0	4.4	2.0
Style, GFY, Asda*	½ Pack/200g	256	10.0	128	17.0	3.7	5.0	0.3
Style, with Rice, Morrisons*	1 Pack/400g	360	5.2	90	5.1	14.1	1.3	0.8
Style Sauce, Breast, Tesco*	1 Serving/180g	128	1.4	71	13.3	2.6	0.8	0.7
CHICKEN MOROCCAN								
Style, Sainsbury's*	½ Pack/269g	334	7.0	124	14.7	10.4	2.6	3.1
Style, with Spicy Cous Cous, BGTY, Sainsbury's*	1 Serving/225g	304	3.8	135	9.2	20.6	1.7	0.0
with Cous Cous, & Fruity Sauce, BGTY, Sainsbury's*	1 Pack/400g	440	8.0	110	10.0	13.1	2.0	2.6
with Cous Cous, GFY, Asda*	1 Serving/450g	414	5.8	92	8.0	12.0	1.3	0.8
CHICKEN MUSTARD								
with Gratin Potatoes, HL, Tesco*	1 Pack/450g	464	12.2	103	9.0	10.7	2.7	2.5
CHICKEN ORIENTAL								
& Pineapple, HL, Tesco*	1 Serving/450g	414	3.2	92	6.0	15.4	0.7	0.6
with Noodles, SteamFresh, Birds Eye*	1 Pack/400g	336	8.8	84	7.1	9.0	2.2	0.3
CHICKEN PAPRIKA								
COU, M & S*	1 Pack/400g	380	6.4	95	9.0	11.7	1.6	2.0
with Savoury Rice, & Vegetables, BGTY, Sainsbury's*	1 Pack/400g	383	2.4	96	7.2	15.5	0.6	1.1
CHICKEN PARMESAN								
& Sun Dried Tomato, Fillets, Mini, Sainsbury's*	1 Pack/200g	278	5.8	139	22.1	6.0	2.9	0.5
Sun Dried Tomato, Fillets, BGTY, Sainsbury's*	½ Pack/100g	138	2.9	138	22.1	6.0	2.9	0.5
CHICKEN PENANG								
Waitrose*	1 Pack/400g	364	10.8	91	10.1	6.6	2.7	0.8
CHICKEN PEPPERCORN								
BGTY, Sainsbury's*	1 Pack/252g	214	6.5	85	11.0	4.5	2.6	0.9
CHICKEN PICCATA								
HE, Tesco*	1 Pack/405g	518	15.4	128	15.7	7.7	3.8	0.5
CHICKEN PIRI PIRI								
& Rice, HE, Tesco*	1 Pack/395g	395	7.9	100	8.2	12.0	2.0	1.7
Breast, Fillets, Mini, Tesco*	½ Pack/100g	135	1.1	135	22.7	7.6	1.1	0.0
GFY, Asda*	1 Pack/400g	406	2.8	102	5.8	18.0	0.7	1.4
M & S*	1 Pack/300g	420	23.1	140	10.0	7.3	7.7	1.3
Sainsbury's*	½ Pack/200g	248	10.8	124	14.0	4.8	5.4	0.5
with Paprika Potatoes, TTD, Sainsbury's*	1 Pack/400g	408	12.0	102	8.9	7.5	3.0	4.4
with Rice, BGTY, Sainsbury's*	1 Serving/399g	395	4.4	99	10.3	11.9	1.1	1.6
CHICKEN ROAST								
in a Pot, Sainsbury's*	1 Pack/450g	477	13.0	106	9.6	10.3	2.9	0.7
CHICKEN SIZZLER								
GFY, Asda*	1 Pack/350g	289	5.0	83	12.9	4.6	1.4	1.4
HL, Tesco*	1 Serving/350g	273	7.0	78	11.1	3.8	2.0	4.3
CHICKEN SPANISH								
Style, Asda*	½ Pack/275g	322	13.5	117	14.0	4.1	4.9	0.7
CHICKEN STUFFED								
Asparagus & Ricotta, with Herb Rice, BGTY, Sainsbury's*	1 Pack/400g	444	10.4	111	8.1	13.8	2.6	0.3
Breast with Mushrooms, HE, Tesco*	1 Serving/175g	152	3.2	87	16.3	1.5	1.8	0.2
with Moroccan Style Cous Cous, GFY, Asda*	½ Pack/180g	259	4.9	144	20.0	10.0	2.7	0.0
with Mushrooms, Finest, Tesco*	1 Serving/150g	177	7.6	118	15.9	2.0	5.1	0.6
CHICKEN SUPREME								
BGTY, Sainsbury's*	1 Pack/350g	416	4.9	119	9.4	17.2	1.4	0.5

	Measure INFO/WEIGHT	per Measure KCAL	FAT	Nutrition Values per 100g / 100ml KCAL	PROT	CARB	FAT	FIBRE
CHICKEN SUPREME								
Breast, Sainsbury's*	1 Serving/187g	421	29.5	225	20.6	0.3	15.8	0.6
with Rice, Asda*	1 Pack/450g	616	31.5	137	15.0	3.4	7.0	1.1
with Rice, Birds Eye*	1 Pack/376g	470	9.8	125	6.6	18.8	2.6	0.5
with Rice, HE, Tesco*	1 Pack/400g	384	6.4	96	4.9	15.6	1.6	1.5
with Rice, Oakhouse Foods Ltd*	1 Meal/400g	520	16.8	130	6.7	16.5	4.2	0.5
with Rice, Weight Watchers*	1 Pack/300g	255	4.8	85	5.6	11.9	1.6	0.5
CHICKEN SZECHUAN								
Chilli & Peppercorn, Sainsbury's*	1 Pack/400g	352	16.0	88	9.9	3.2	4.0	0.5
Tesco*	1 Pack/350g	385	10.5	110	7.2	13.6	3.0	0.3
with Noodles, Sainsbury's*	1 Pack/450g	423	14.0	94	6.0	10.4	3.1	0.9
CHICKEN TAGINE								
with Cous Cous, BGTY, Sainsbury's*	1 Pack/450g	626	17.6	139	10.1	15.9	3.9	1.5
CHICKEN TANDOORI								
Fresh Tastes, Asda*	1 Pack/400g	356	5.6	89	6.4	12.7	1.4	2.1
GFY, Asda*	1 Pack/400g	324	9.6	81	7.5	7.3	2.4	1.7
Masala, Asda*	1 Pack/400g	580	20.0	145	7.0	18.0	5.0	1.3
Masala, Indian, Tesco*	1 Serving/350g	430	25.9	123	10.2	4.0	7.4	1.8
Masala, Sainsbury's*	1 Pack/400g	536	27.2	134	13.2	5.0	6.8	0.5
Masala & Rice, HL, Tesco*	1 Serving/450g	410	7.6	91	6.6	12.9	1.7	0.6
Sizzler, HL, Tesco*	1 Pack/350g	275	7.0	79	11.1	3.8	2.0	4.3
Sizzler, Sainsbury's*	1 Pack/400g	536	29.2	134	12.8	4.3	7.3	1.7
Sizzler, Tesco*	1 Serving/175g	243	11.6	139	10.0	10.0	6.6	1.0
Skewers, Six, M Kitchen, Morrisons*	½ Pack/90g	158	5.0	175	28.9	2.0	5.6	0.5
Tesco*	1 Serving/175g	198	8.6	113	10.6	6.7	4.9	1.0
with Rice, Easy Steam, Tesco*	1 Pack/400g	484	12.0	121	8.7	14.7	3.0	0.7
with Spicy Potatoes, & Dip, HE, Tesco*	1 Pack/370g	322	3.0	87	9.7	10.3	0.8	1.3
with Vegetable Pilau Rice, HL, Tesco*	1 Pack/348g	400	9.0	115	8.4	14.1	2.6	1.9
CHICKEN TERIYAKI								
& Noodles, Asda*	½ Pack/340g	445	8.8	131	9.0	18.0	2.6	0.9
Asda*	1 Pack/360g	299	5.0	83	9.1	8.6	1.4	0.8
Japanese with Ramen Noodles, Sainsbury's*	1 Pack/450g	482	9.4	107	6.5	15.5	2.1	0.8
CHICKEN THAI								
& Siu Mai Dumplings, M & S*	1 Dumpling/21g	35	1.6	170	16.0	9.4	7.6	0.8
& Vegetables, Eat Positive, Birds Eye*	1 Packet/400g	412	12.0	103	5.9	13.0	3.0	1.0
Chiang Mai, & Noodles, BGTY, Sainsbury's*	1 Pack/448g	484	17.9	108	6.9	11.0	4.0	1.7
Green, Fillets, Mini, Sainsbury's*	½ Pack/100g	130	1.6	130	27.9	0.9	1.6	0.8
Style, with Noodles, Tesco*	1 Pack/400g	332	6.8	83	7.5	9.5	1.7	1.0
Style Marinade, Breast, Chargrilled, GFY, Asda*	½ Pack/178g	178	5.3	100	17.0	1.3	3.0	0.5
with Rice, SteamFresh, Birds Eye*	1 Serving/400g	380	7.6	95	6.8	12.8	1.9	0.9
CHICKEN TIKKA								
& Coriander Rice, Weight Watchers*	1 Pack/400g	348	2.4	87	6.2	14.3	0.6	1.6
& Cous Cous, Boots*	1 Pack/160g	307	17.6	192	6.2	17.0	11.0	1.3
& Lemon Rice, Deli Meal, M & S*	1 Pack/360g	342	7.2	95	9.8	10.2	2.0	0.7
& Rice, Everyday, Value, Tesco*	1 Pack/396g	535	21.4	135	7.3	12.8	5.4	2.5
BGTY, Sainsbury's*	1 Serving/188g	265	3.0	141	10.5	21.2	1.6	0.0
Creamy, Breast, Tesco*	1 Breast/190g	215	10.4	113	15.1	0.7	5.5	0.8
Satay, Mini, Asda*	1 Pack/80g	178	12.4	222	15.5	5.2	15.5	2.4
with Basmati Rice, GFY, Asda*	1 Pack/400g	592	7.2	148	9.0	24.0	1.8	1.6
with Pilau Rice, GFY, Asda*	1 Pack/450g	382	2.7	85	7.0	13.0	0.6	1.8
CHICKEN VINDALOO								
Average	1 Serving/410g	787	51.2	192	18.5	2.6	12.5	0.3
Waitrose*	1 Pack/340g	398	18.4	117	10.6	6.4	5.4	1.6

C

	Measure INFO/WEIGHT	per Measure KCAL	FAT	Nutrition Values per 100g / 100ml KCAL	PROT	CARB	FAT	FIBRE
CHICKEN WITH								
Apricots & Almonds, HE, Tesco*	1 Pack/500g	465	9.5	93	11.8	7.3	1.9	0.5
Asparagus & Rice, BGTY, Sainsbury's*	1 Pack/400g	428	5.6	107	9.1	14.5	1.4	0.9
Bacon & Leeks, GFY, Asda*	1 Pack/400g	328	8.0	82	13.0	3.0	2.0	0.6
Basil, Puy Lentils & Spelt, Roasted, The Food Doctor*	1 Pack/350g	210	7.4	60	9.6	0.7	2.1	10.2
Basil Pesto & Parmesan Crust, Breast, COOK!, M & S*	½ Pack/150g	240	11.0	160	20.9	1.8	7.3	0.8
BBQ Dip, Chargrilled, Fillets, Mini, Eat Well, M & S*	1 Pack/120g	144	0.7	120	23.3	5.8	0.6	0.0
Black Bean Sauce, Green Peppers & Rice, Farmfoods*	1 Meal/324g	408	12.6	126	5.5	17.1	3.9	0.4
Broccoli & Pesto Pasta, BGTY, Sainsbury's*	1 Pack/301g	328	5.1	109	10.3	13.2	1.7	2.5
Butternut Squash Rice, Reggae Reggae, Levi Roots*	1 Pack/450g	495	13.5	110	5.8	14.0	3.0	1.1
Caesar Melt, & Prosciutto, Breast, M & S*	1 Pack/375g	488	18.8	130	19.6	1.3	5.0	1.0
Caramelised Peppers, Chargrilled, M & S*	½ Pack/237g	225	9.0	95	12.9	2.1	3.8	1.3
Cheese, Leek & Ham, Breast, Fresh Tastes, Asda*	1 Pack/430g	658	30.5	153	18.9	3.4	7.1	0.7
Cheese & Chive Sauce, Carb Control, Tesco*	1 Serving/400g	400	25.6	100	8.4	2.0	6.4	1.6
Cheese Croutons & Onion, Asda*	1 Serving/200g	200	6.4	100	16.0	2.0	3.2	0.9
Cherrywood Barbecue Sauce, Simply Cook, Tesco*	1 Serving/147g	165	2.5	112	16.6	7.6	1.7	0.4
Chorizo, Skewers, Charlie Bigham's*	1 Skewer/95g	129	6.5	136	17.1	1.5	6.9	0.5
Chorizo & Patatas Bravas, COU, M & S*	1 Pack/400g	380	9.2	95	7.8	10.8	2.3	1.7
Chorizo & Tomato Sauce, Catalan, Charlie Bigham's*	1 Pack/479g	407	15.8	85	10.9	2.8	3.3	0.7
Coriander & Lime, Asda*	1 Serving/105g	122	0.9	116	24.0	2.9	0.9	0.2
Cous Cous, Lemon & Herb, Finest, Tesco*	1 Pack/370g	492	18.5	133	10.5	11.5	5.0	0.9
Couscous, Spiced, Love Life, Waitrose*	1 Pack/365g	391	3.3	107	7.9	15.3	0.9	2.8
Cranberry & Orange Stuffing, Sainsbury's*	1 Serving/100g	201	10.3	201	23.0	4.1	10.3	0.8
Cranberry Stuffing, Breast, Finest, Tesco*	½ Pack/200g	252	4.8	126	16.2	9.9	2.4	0.9
Fresh Mango, Chilli & Coriander, British, COU, M & S*	1 Pack/169g	270	3.9	160	12.1	22.8	2.3	1.9
Fusilli & Courgette, Sainsbury's*	1 Pack/450g	675	28.8	150	8.6	14.6	6.4	0.5
Garlic & Herbs, Asda*	1 Slice/25g	28	0.4	114	23.9	1.1	1.5	0.0
Garlic Mushrooms, Asda*	1 Serving/320g	342	16.0	107	13.8	1.8	5.0	2.2
Garlic Mushrooms, Breast, Simply Cook, Tesco*	½ Pack/125g	170	6.6	136	22.0	0.1	5.3	0.1
Grapes & Asparagus, Sainsbury's*	½ Pack/200g	240	13.2	120	13.3	1.8	6.6	1.0
Gravy & Stuffing, Breasts, Tesco*	½ Pack/173g	257	11.1	149	14.4	8.3	6.4	2.2
Gruyere Cheese & Parma Ham, Breast, COOK!, M & S*	1 Breast/194g	349	21.3	180	18.0	2.5	11.0	0.9
Hoi Sin Sauce, Ooodles of Noodles, Oriental Express*	1 Pack/425g	400	9.4	94	5.3	13.2	2.2	1.7
Honey & Ginger Sauce, 125, Oakhouse Foods Ltd*	1 Dinner/365g	339	8.0	93	8.7	9.8	2.2	1.2
Honey & Mustard Sauce, Breasts, Simply Cook, Tesco*	½ Pack/219g	230	1.3	105	16.3	8.0	0.6	0.3
Honey & Sesame, with Rice, LC, Tesco*	1 Pack/400g	432	12.0	108	5.3	14.9	3.0	2.2
Leek & Bacon, 119, Oakhouse Foods Ltd*	1 Meal/400g	340	13.6	85	7.0	6.6	3.4	1.2
Lemon Grass, Thai Greens & Baby Corn, Sainsbury's*	1 Serving/200g	196	6.8	98	10.0	6.9	3.4	1.4
Lime & Coriander, Chargrilled, Asda*	1 Serving/190g	352	17.1	185	24.0	2.0	9.0	1.1
Lime & Coriander, Easy, Waitrose*	½ Pack/168g	203	7.9	121	18.9	0.7	4.7	0.5
Lime & Tequila, Asda*	1 Serving/150g	194	2.7	129	24.0	4.3	1.8	0.5
Lyonnaise Potatoes, M & S*	½ Pack/260g	286	8.1	110	12.6	8.0	3.1	0.9
Mango, Lime & Coriander, Asda*	1 Pack/400g	416	6.0	104	6.6	15.9	1.5	1.4
Mango Salsa & Potato Wedges, BGTY, Sainsbury's*	1 Pack/400g	336	6.4	84	7.0	10.4	1.6	1.5
Mascarpone, Bacon & Roasted Onions, Finest, Tesco*	1 Serving/200g	312	17.6	156	14.5	4.7	8.8	0.5
Mozzarella & Pancetta, Breast, Finest, Tesco*	½ Pack/225g	326	14.0	145	14.4	7.9	6.2	1.1
Mozzarella & Pesto Melt, Breasts, COOK!, M & S*	½ Pack/165g	206	10.2	125	16.4	1.3	6.2	0.7
Mushroom & Bacon, Fillets, M & S*	½ Pack/188g	225	11.2	120	15.5	0.5	6.0	1.7
Mushroom & Garlic Butter, Breasts, Sainsbury's*	½ Pack/195g	388	20.1	199	20.0	4.6	10.3	0.1
Mushroom & Tomato Sauce, GFY, Asda*	1 Serving/175g	180	3.7	103	19.0	2.0	2.1	2.7
Mushroom Pilaff, BGTY, Sainsbury's*	1 Serving/400g	320	2.0	80	8.0	10.5	0.5	1.4
Mushroom Risotto, M & S*	1 Pack/400g	480	11.6	120	6.9	16.7	2.9	0.8
Mushroom Sauce & Herby Rice, Fillets, M & S*	1 Pack/380g	475	19.4	125	7.7	12.0	5.1	1.3
Pancakes & Plum Sauce, COU, M & S*	1 Pack/245g	257	5.6	105	7.9	12.7	2.3	0.3

	Measure INFO/WEIGHT	per Measure KCAL	FAT	Nutrition Values per 100g / 100ml KCAL	PROT	CARB	FAT	FIBRE
CHICKEN WITH								
Pasta, Chianti & Balsamic, BGTY, Sainsbury's*	1 Pack/400g	372	7.6	93	9.4	9.5	1.9	1.9
Pesto & Linguine Pasta, Meal, SteamFresh, Birds Eye*	1 Pack/400g	440	16.0	110	8.5	10.0	4.0	1.3
Plum Sauce, Battered, Tesco*	1 Serving/175g	324	10.2	185	6.7	26.5	5.8	0.8
Plum Tomatoes & Basil, Breast, Birds Eye*	1 Serving/172g	200	8.1	116	13.3	5.0	4.7	0.6
Pork, Parsnip Herb Stuffing, Sainsbury's*	1 Serving/100g	181	9.0	181	22.9	2.1	9.0	0.7
Pork Stuffing, Breast, Roast, M & S*	1 Serving/100g	165	6.5	165	24.1	3.0	6.5	0.0
Pork Stuffing & Chipolatas, Breast Joint, Tesco*	½ Pack/340g	524	27.9	154	16.7	3.4	8.2	0.5
Potato & Smoked Bacon Topping, M & S*	1 Serving/175g	228	8.4	130	17.8	3.2	4.8	1.2
Potato Wedges, Tomato & Basil, Weight Watchers*	1 Pack/330g	254	6.6	77	4.7	9.2	2.0	1.6
Prosciutio, Dolcelatte & 3 Cheese Sauce, Asda*	½ Pack/195g	355	11.7	182	30.0	1.9	6.0	1.2
Rice, Breast, Chargrilled, Spicy, Asda*	1 Pack/400g	372	2.4	93	6.0	16.0	0.6	1.0
Rice, Fiesta, Weight Watchers*	1 Pack/330g	307	6.6	93	6.1	12.8	2.0	0.4
Rice, Jamaican Jerk, Healthier Choice, Co-Op*	1 Pack/406g	365	9.3	90	7.8	9.8	2.3	3.4
Rice 'n' Peas, Sainsbury's*	1 Pack/300g	489	18.3	163	12.5	14.4	6.1	2.1
Sage & Onion Stuffing, Breast, Roast, Sliced, M & S*	1 Slice/17g	27	1.1	165	24.1	3.0	6.5	0.0
Sea Salt & Black Pepper Crust, Breasts, Asda*	1 Serving/154g	186	4.3	121	19.0	5.0	2.8	0.0
Soured Cream, Cajun Spiced, Breast, COOK!, M & S*	½ Pack/200g	230	10.2	115	14.7	2.1	5.1	1.1
Soy & Ginger Noodles, Love Life, Waitrose*	1 Pot/360g	212	4.7	59	5.0	6.7	1.3	2.3
Spiced Butter, Jerk, Spicy, Half, Waitrose*	1 Pack/679g	1331	75.4	196	22.8	0.9	11.1	0.8
Spinach, Honey Mustard, American Style, Asda*	1 Serving/240g	394	24.0	164	14.0	4.4	10.0	0.3
Spirelli, Steam Meal, Tesco*	1 Serving/400g	400	10.8	100	6.6	12.0	2.7	1.2
Spring Vegetables, Chargrilled, COU, M & S*	1 Pack/414g	290	3.7	70	8.8	7.3	0.9	1.8
Sticky Honey & Chilli Sauce, Breast, Asda*	1 Serving/175g	247	5.6	141	20.0	8.0	3.2	0.0
Stilton & Port Sauce, Breasts, Finest, Tesco*	1 Serving/400g	668	34.4	167	18.5	3.9	8.6	0.7
Stuffing, TTD, Sainsbury's*	1 Slice/34g	50	2.0	148	22.7	1.3	5.8	0.9
Sun Dried Tomato & Basil Butter, Sainsbury's*	1 Breast/185g	363	17.6	196	25.0	2.5	9.5	0.2
Sun Dried Tomato & Basil Sauce, Bistro, Waitrose*	½ Pack/175g	254	14.2	145	14.2	3.7	8.1	0.3
Sweet Chilli & Garlic, Chinese, Asda*	1 Serving/400g	436	2.4	109	8.0	18.0	0.6	2.1
Sweet Chilli Sauce & Egg Fried Rice, Tesco*	1 Pack/380g	494	10.3	130	7.5	18.2	2.7	1.3
Sweet Potato Mash, Jerk, Super Naturals, Sainsbury's*	1 Pack/400g	284	4.4	71	6.1	9.2	1.1	2.2
Tagine, Cous Cous, Perfectly Balanced, Waitrose*	1 Pack/400g	516	14.0	129	8.2	16.2	3.5	1.0
Tangy Lemon Sauce, Breasts, Just Cook, Sainsbury's*	1 Serving/164g	244	3.0	149	16.2	16.9	1.8	0.1
Tomato & Basil, HE, Tesco*	1 Serving/225g	189	3.8	84	11.2	6.1	1.7	1.2
Tomato & Basil, Steam Cuisine, M & S*	1 Pack/400g	460	13.6	115	9.6	11.6	3.4	2.0
Tomato & Basil Sauce, HL, Tesco*	1 Breast/200g	154	2.4	77	12.0	3.9	1.2	1.2
CHICORY								
Fresh, Raw, Average	***1 Head/150g***	***30***	***0.9***	***20***	***0.6***	***2.8***	***0.6***	***0.9***
CHILLI								
& Potato Wedges, Good Choice, Iceland*	1 Pack/400g	368	13.6	92	5.5	9.8	3.4	1.2
& Potato Wedges, Sainsbury's*	1 Pack/371g	393	15.2	106	7.2	10.1	4.1	2.2
& Rice, Birds Eye*	1 Serving/285g	305	7.7	107	3.4	17.2	2.7	1.0
& Rice, Frozen, Sainsbury's*	1 Pack/400g	436	7.6	109	4.8	18.4	1.9	0.6
& Rice, GFY, Asda*	1 Pack/400g	352	1.6	88	5.0	16.0	0.4	1.8
& Rice, Morrisons*	1 Serving/500g	630	15.5	126	5.7	18.9	3.1	1.1
& Wedges, BBQ, HL, Tesco*	1 Pack/420g	391	10.9	93	5.4	12.2	2.6	1.9
& Wedges, GFY, Asda*	1 Pack/400g	364	10.0	91	7.0	10.1	2.5	2.5
Beef, & Mushrooms, GFY, Asda*	1 Pack/400g	364	6.0	91	9.1	10.2	1.5	1.2
Beef, & Potato Crush, Weight Watchers*	1 Pack/400g	232	6.0	58	5.0	5.9	1.5	3.4
Beef, Asda*	½ Pack/200g	190	7.8	95	7.0	8.0	3.9	1.2
Beef, with Potato Wedges, Naturally Good Food, Tesco*	1 Pack/440g	352	12.3	80	7.2	6.2	2.8	1.8
Beef, with Rice, GFY, Asda*	1 Serving/402g	354	6.0	88	4.7	14.0	1.5	0.9
Beef, with Rice, Sainsbury's*	1 Serving/300g	360	5.1	120	5.6	20.6	1.7	1.1
Bowl, American Style, Sainsbury's*	½ Pack/300g	255	10.5	85	8.8	4.6	3.5	2.0

	Measure INFO/WEIGHT	per Measure KCAL	FAT	Nutrition Values per 100g / 100ml KCAL	PROT	CARB	FAT	FIBRE
CHILLI								
Chicken Grande, Stagg*	1 Serving/205g	168	1.2	82	9.7	9.4	0.6	1.6
Con Carne, & Sweetcorn Mash, Fuller Longer, M & S*	1 Pack/400g	380	13.2	95	8.5	7.4	3.3	3.9
Con Carne, 2 Minute Meals, Sainsbury's*	1 Pouch/200g	146	3.2	73	6.0	8.6	1.6	2.7
Con Carne, Asda*	1 Can/392g	376	13.7	96	7.0	9.0	3.5	0.0
Con Carne, Baked Bean, Heinz*	1 Can/390g	324	5.8	83	7.0	10.3	1.5	2.8
Con Carne, Canned, La Caldera, Lidl*	¼ Can/200g	240	12.8	120	6.9	8.6	6.4	0.0
Con Carne, Canned, Sainsbury's*	½ Can/200g	162	4.2	81	6.6	8.9	2.1	2.5
Con Carne, Cooked, BGTY, Sainsbury's*	1 Pack/400g	356	6.8	94	4.9	13.4	1.8	2.2
Con Carne, Diet Chef Ltd*	1 Pack/300g	333	13.5	111	7.3	10.4	4.5	2.1
Con Carne, Dynamite Hot, Stagg*	1 Serving/250g	310	15.5	124	7.6	9.6	6.2	2.5
Con Carne, From Restaurant, Average	1 Serving/253g	256	8.3	101	9.7	8.7	3.3	0.0
Con Carne, Frozen, Co-Op*	1 Pack/340g	306	3.4	90	6.0	15.0	1.0	1.0
Con Carne, Good Choice, Iceland*	1 Pack/400g	476	4.0	119	5.5	21.9	1.0	1.0
Con Carne, Homepride*	1 Can/390g	234	2.3	60	2.5	11.2	0.6	0.0
Con Carne, M & S*	1 Pack/285g	285	10.5	100	8.7	7.4	3.7	2.0
Con Carne, Recipe Mix, Colman's*	1 Pack/50g	158	1.2	316	10.4	62.9	2.5	6.8
Con Carne, Restaurant, Sainsbury's*	1 Serving/100g	80	2.7	80	6.9	7.0	2.7	1.5
Con Carne, Slim Fast*	1 Pack/375g	394	7.1	105	5.5	16.2	1.9	1.5
Con Carne, with Long Grain Rice, COU, M & S*	1 Pack/400g	380	7.6	95	5.0	13.9	1.9	1.9
Con Carne, with Rice, Birds Eye*	1 Pack/285g	291	7.1	102	3.3	16.6	2.5	0.8
Con Carne, with Rice, GFY, Asda*	1 Serving/400g	456	6.4	114	6.0	19.0	1.6	0.9
Con Carne, with Rice, Healthy Choice, Asda*	1 Pack/400g	412	8.4	103	6.0	15.0	2.1	0.9
Con Carne, with Rice, Morrisons*	1 Pack/400g	328	5.2	82	5.3	12.2	1.3	1.4
Con Carne, with Rice, Organic, Sainsbury's*	1 Pack/400g	472	10.8	118	5.0	18.5	2.7	1.8
Con Carne, with Rice, Perfectly Balanced, Waitrose*	1 Pack/400g	404	7.2	101	5.8	15.3	1.8	1.7
Con Carne, with Rice, Weight Watchers*	1 Serving/301g	262	3.3	87	4.6	14.7	1.1	0.4
Mexican, with Long Grain Rice, Rice Time, Uncle Ben's*	1 Pot/300g	339	3.0	113	2.5	22.8	1.0	1.3
Mixed Vegetable, Tesco*	1 Pack/400g	352	11.6	88	3.9	11.0	2.9	3.2
Non Carne, with Rice, Linda McCartney*	1 Pack/400g	364	9.2	91	4.2	14.9	2.3	3.1
Peruvian, Hot in Sunflower Oil, Barts*	1 Serving/100g	62	1.5	62	1.5	10.7	1.5	0.0
Three Bean, Diet Chef Ltd*	1 Pack/300g	195	2.7	65	4.0	10.3	0.9	3.6
Uncle Ben's*	1oz/28g	17	0.2	59	1.8	11.1	0.8	0.0
Vegetable	1oz/28g	16	0.2	57	3.0	10.8	0.6	2.6
Vegetable, & Rice, BGTY, Sainsbury's*	1 Pack/450g	410	5.0	91	3.5	16.7	1.1	3.5
Vegetable, & Rice, HE, Tesco*	1 Pack/450g	392	5.4	87	2.8	16.1	1.2	1.5
Vegetable, Canned, Heated, Asda*	½ Can/200g	158	1.0	79	3.2	14.1	0.5	2.5
Vegetable, Canned, Sainsbury's*	1 Can/400g	230	1.6	58	3.1	10.4	0.4	3.2
Vegetable, Diet Chef Ltd*	1 Pack/300g	258	4.8	86	3.4	14.5	1.6	4.4
Vegetable, Retail	1oz/28g	20	0.6	70	4.0	9.4	2.1	0.0
Vegetable Garden, Stagg*	1 Can/410g	254	2.0	62	3.6	10.8	0.5	2.3
Vegetarian, with Rice, Ready Meal, Average	1 Serving/400g	434	6.0	108	3.8	20.0	1.5	1.3
Vegetarian, with Rice, Tesco*	1 Pack/500g	575	13.0	115	4.0	19.0	2.6	1.8
CHINESE LEAF								
Fresh, Raw, Average	***1oz/28g***	***4***	***0.1***	***14***	***1.5***	***1.5***	***0.2***	***1.7***
CHIPS								
& Curry Sauce, Tesco*	1 Serving/400g	440	20.0	110	2.1	14.1	5.0	1.0
11mm Fresh, Deep Fried, McCain*	1oz/28g	66	3.0	235	3.2	31.8	10.6	0.0
14mm Fresh, Deep Fried, McCain*	1oz/28g	59	1.9	209	2.7	34.2	6.8	0.0
14mm Friers Choice, Deep Fried, McCain*	1oz/28g	56	2.2	199	3.5	29.3	8.0	0.0
9/16" Straight Cut Caterpack, Deep Fried, McCain*	1oz/28g	63	2.6	225	3.1	32.1	9.4	0.0
American Style, Oven, Sainsbury's*	1 Serving/165g	314	13.7	190	5.4	23.6	8.3	1.3
American Style, Thin, Oven, Tesco*	1 Serving/125g	210	8.1	168	2.7	24.6	6.5	2.1
Beefeater, Deep Fried, McCain*	1oz/28g	71	2.8	253	3.3	37.7	9.9	0.0

	Measure INFO/WEIGHT	per Measure KCAL	FAT	Nutrition Values per 100g / 100ml KCAL	PROT	CARB	FAT	FIBRE
CHIPS								
Beefeater, Oven Baked, McCain*	1oz/28g	55	1.6	195	4.0	32.2	5.6	0.0
British Classics, HL, Tesco*	½ Pack/200g	250	1.6	125	2.6	26.9	0.8	1.3
Chippy, Microwave, McCain*	1oz/28g	49	2.0	176	2.6	25.2	7.2	1.7
Chunky, Baked, Organic, M & S*	1 Serving/100g	150	3.7	150	1.7	27.1	3.7	2.2
Chunky, British, Oven, Frozen, Cooked, Finest, Tesco*	1 Serving/125g	240	5.1	192	2.3	35.1	4.1	2.7
Chunky, COU, M & S*	1 Serving/150g	158	2.4	105	2.1	20.5	1.6	2.3
Chunky, Crisp & Golden, Waitrose*	½ Pack/225g	259	7.0	115	2.1	17.7	3.1	3.9
Chunky, Fresh, Chilled, Finest, Tesco*	1 Pack/450g	608	18.0	135	2.1	22.3	4.0	2.7
Chunky, Gastropub, M & S*	1 Pack/400g	520	12.4	130	2.6	22.4	3.1	2.3
Chunky, Ready to Bake, M & S*	1 Serving/200g	310	8.4	155	2.2	26.8	4.2	2.0
Crinkle Cut, Frozen, Aunt Bessie's*	1 Serving/100g	163	7.3	163	3.1	21.3	7.3	2.2
Crinkle Cut, Frozen, Fried in Corn Oil	1oz/28g	81	4.7	290	3.6	33.4	16.7	2.2
Crinkle Cut, M & S*	1 Serving/150g	270	8.1	180	3.3	29.5	5.4	2.4
Fine Cut, Frozen, Fried in Blended Oil	1oz/28g	102	6.0	364	4.5	41.2	21.3	2.4
Fine Cut, Frozen, Fried in Corn Oil	1oz/28g	102	6.0	364	4.5	41.2	21.3	2.7
Fried, Average	1 Serving/130g	266	10.9	204	3.2	29.6	8.4	1.2
Fried, Chip Shop, Average	1 Serving/100g	239	12.4	239	3.2	30.5	12.4	2.2
Frying, Crinkle Cut, Tesco*	1 Serving/125g	161	4.1	129	2.6	22.2	3.3	1.9
Homefries, Chunky, Weighed Baked, McCain*	1 Serving/100g	153	3.1	153	3.2	28.0	3.1	2.3
Homefries, Chunky, Weighed Frozen, McCain*	1 Serving/100g	123	2.5	123	2.5	22.6	2.5	1.6
Homefries, Crinkle Cut, Weighed Baked, McCain*	1 Serving/100g	176	5.0	176	2.6	30.1	5.0	2.3
Homefries, Crinkle Cut, Weighed Frozen, McCain*	1 Serving/100g	142	5.1	142	1.9	22.2	5.1	1.3
Homefries, Jacket Oven, McCain*	1 Serving/100g	220	7.4	220	3.9	37.9	7.4	0.0
Homefries, Straight Cut, Weighed Baked, McCain*	1 Serving/100g	181	6.2	181	3.1	28.1	6.2	2.4
Homefries, Straight Cut, Weighed Frozen, McCain*	1 Serving/100g	134	4.6	134	2.2	21.0	4.6	1.7
Homefries, Thin & Crispy, Weighed Frozen, McCain*	1 Serving/100g	143	4.1	143	2.6	24.0	4.1	1.5
Homemade, Actify, 1000g Potatoes, 3ml Oil, Actifry*	1 Portion/250g	197	1.2	79	1.9	16.9	0.5	1.2
Homemade, Fried in Blended Oil, Average	1oz/28g	53	1.9	189	3.9	30.1	6.7	2.2
Homemade, Fried in Corn Oil, Average	1oz/28g	53	1.9	189	3.9	30.1	6.7	2.2
Homemade, Fried in Dripping, Average	1oz/28g	53	1.9	189	3.9	30.1	6.7	2.2
Homestyle, Frozen, Aunt Bessie's*	1 Serving/200g	260	11.2	130	2.2	17.6	5.6	2.7
Homestyle, Oven Cooked, Aunt Bessie's*	1 Serving/100g	191	7.8	191	3.1	27.0	7.8	2.9
Homestyle Oven, Sainsbury's*	1 Serving/125g	206	5.4	165	2.4	29.2	4.3	2.1
Micro, Asda*	1 Serving/112g	221	7.8	197	3.5	30.0	7.0	4.0
Micro, Crinkle Cut, Tesco*	1 Serving/100g	203	8.0	203	3.3	29.5	8.0	1.8
Micro Chips, Crinkle Cut, Cooked, McCain*	1 Pack/100g	166	4.2	166	2.9	28.9	4.2	2.4
Micro Chips, Straight Cut, Cooked, McCain*	1 Pack/100g	163	4.8	163	2.3	27.7	4.8	2.0
Microwave, Cooked	1oz/28g	62	2.7	221	3.6	32.1	9.6	2.9
Oven, 5% Fat, Frozen, McCain*	1 Serving/200g	238	6.0	119	1.9	21.0	3.0	1.6
Oven, American Style, Champion*	1 Serving/200g	372	14.4	186	2.2	28.2	7.2	2.0
Oven, Best in the World, Iceland*	1 Serving/175g	332	11.7	190	3.4	28.9	6.7	3.5
Oven, Champion*	1 Pack/133g	210	6.0	158	2.5	27.0	4.5	0.0
Oven, Chunky, Extra Special, Asda*	1 Serving/125g	238	7.0	190	3.4	31.5	5.6	3.2
Oven, Chunky, Harry Ramsden's*	1 Serving/150g	184	5.4	123	2.8	19.9	3.6	1.6
Oven, Chunky, Ross*	1 Serving/100g	177	6.5	177	3.1	26.6	6.5	3.9
Oven, Chunky, TTD, Sainsbury's*	1 Serving/166g	250	5.3	151	2.0	28.6	3.2	2.3
Oven, Cooked, Value, Tesco*	1 Serving/125g	308	9.8	246	4.5	39.5	7.8	2.9
Oven, Cooked, Weight Watchers*	1 Serving/100g	150	3.0	150	2.8	33.7	3.0	5.9
Oven, Crinkle Cut, 5% Fat, Weighed Baked, McCain*	1 Serving/100g	163	4.3	163	3.1	27.9	4.3	3.0
Oven, Crinkle Cut, 5% Fat, Weighed Frozen, McCain*	1 Serving/100g	134	3.6	134	2.4	23.2	3.6	2.4
Oven, Crinkle Cut, Frozen, Essential, Waitrose*	1 Serving/165g	225	6.4	136	2.7	22.6	3.9	1.7
Oven, Crinkle Cut, Sainsbury's*	1 Serving/165g	297	9.1	180	3.3	29.5	5.5	2.4
Oven, Frozen, Baked	1 Portion/80g	130	3.4	162	3.2	29.8	4.2	2.0

	Measure INFO/WEIGHT	per Measure KCAL	FAT	Nutrition Values per 100g / 100ml KCAL	PROT	CARB	FAT	FIBRE
CHIPS								
Oven, Homefries, McCain*	1 Serving/100g	134	4.6	134	2.2	21.0	4.6	1.7
Oven, Organic, Waitrose*	1 Serving/165g	233	6.3	141	1.5	25.1	3.8	1.6
Oven, Original, McCain*	1 Serving/100g	158	3.8	158	2.5	28.5	3.8	2.3
Oven, Original, Straight Cut, 5% Fat, Cooked, McCain*	1 Serving/100g	158	3.8	158	3.8	28.5	3.8	2.3
Oven, Original, Straight Cut, 5% Fat, Frozen, McCain*	1 Serving/100g	138	4.0	138	2.5	26.2	4.0	1.9
Oven, Rooster, Albert Bartlett & Sons Ltd*	1 Serving/125g	156	2.4	125	2.9	27.7	1.9	3.7
Oven, Steak Cut, Asda*	1 Serving/100g	153	4.1	153	2.0	27.0	4.1	2.5
Oven, Steak Cut, Waitrose*	1 Serving/165g	218	5.6	132	2.7	22.7	3.4	1.7
Oven, Straight Cut, 5% Fat, Sainsbury's*	1 Serving/165g	280	8.1	170	3.4	28.0	4.9	2.5
Oven, Straight Cut, Asda*	1 Serving/100g	199	5.0	199	3.5	35.0	5.0	3.0
Oven, Straight Cut, Cooked, LC, Tesco*	1 Serving/125g	150	2.1	120	2.4	22.1	1.7	2.6
Oven, Straight Cut, Frozen Weight, HL, Tesco*	1 Serving/125g	132	2.4	106	2.1	20.0	1.9	2.3
Oven, Straight Cut, Reduced Fat, Tesco*	1 Serving/100g	127	3.0	127	2.3	22.7	3.0	2.1
Oven, Sweet Potato, Cooked, Tesco*	¼ Pack/125g	180	7.1	145	2.5	18.2	5.7	3.7
Oven, Thin & Crispy, Tesco*	1 Portion/100g	205	4.9	205	2.7	37.6	4.9	5.8
Oven, Thin Cut, American Style, Asda*	1 Serving/100g	240	10.0	240	3.4	34.0	10.0	3.0
Oven, Thin Fries, Morrisons*	1 Serving/100g	161	6.1	161	2.9	23.6	6.1	1.2
Potato, Lights, Reduced Fat, Lay's*	1 Serving/25g	118	5.5	470	7.5	60.0	22.0	5.0
Steak Cut, Frying, Asda*	1 Serving/97g	181	6.8	187	2.9	28.0	7.0	2.8
Steak Cut, Oven, Tesco*	1 Serving/165g	233	6.4	141	2.0	24.4	3.9	2.0
Straight Cut, Frozen, Fried in Blended Oil	1oz/28g	76	3.8	273	4.1	36.0	13.5	2.4
Straight Cut, Frozen, Fried in Corn Oil	1oz/28g	76	3.8	273	4.1	36.0	13.5	2.4
Straight Cut, Low Fat, Tesco*	1 Serving/125g	159	3.8	127	2.3	22.7	3.0	2.1
Straight Cut, Microwave Baked, McCain*	1oz/28g	70	3.0	251	3.5	35.0	10.7	0.0
Straight Cut, Oven, BGTY, Sainsbury's*	1 Portion/165g	226	3.5	137	2.7	26.8	2.1	4.1
The Big Chip, Frozen, Tesco*	1 Serving/200g	220	4.8	110	1.8	20.3	2.4	2.1
Thick Cut, Caterpack, Deep Fried, McCain*	1oz/28g	60	2.7	215	3.1	28.8	9.7	0.0
Thick Cut, Frozen, Fried in Corn Oil, Average	1oz/28g	66	2.9	234	3.6	34.0	10.2	2.4
CHIVES								
Fresh, Average	***1 Tsp/2g***	***0***	***0.0***	***23***	***2.8***	***1.7***	***0.6***	***1.9***
CHOC ICES								
Chocolate, Dark, Seriously Creamy, Waitrose*	1 Ice/82g	195	12.9	238	2.6	21.6	15.7	1.7
Chocolate, Real Milk, Sainsbury's*	1 Ice/48g	151	9.5	312	3.5	30.3	19.7	0.8
Chocolate, White, Sainsbury's*	1 Ice/48g	140	8.9	292	3.8	27.3	18.6	0.1
Chunky, Wall's Ice Cream*	1 Ice/81g	162	10.6	200	2.6	18.9	13.1	0.0
Dark, Sainsbury's*	1 Ice/43g	136	9.5	315	3.8	25.5	22.0	0.4
Dark, Tesco*	1 Ice/43g	141	9.1	325	2.8	30.2	21.0	0.1
Everyday, Value, Tesco*	1 Ice/31g	95	6.3	300	2.3	26.7	19.9	1.0
Mini Mix, Eis Stern*	1 Ice/39g	129	8.9	334	4.2	29.0	23.0	0.0
Neapolitan Chocolate, Co-Op*	1 Ice/62g	120	8.2	194	2.0	16.9	13.2	0.4
CHOCOLATE								
Advent Calendar, Dairy Milk, Cadbury*	1 Chocolate/4g	22	1.3	525	7.5	56.6	30.1	0.7
Advent Calendar, Magic of Christmas, Cadbury*	1 Chocolate/10g	48	2.7	510	7.0	57.7	28.0	0.7
Advent Calendar, Maltesers, Mars*	1 Chocolate/4g	21	1.2	537	6.8	57.9	30.9	0.0
Advent Calendar, Pirates of the Caribbean, Kinnerton*	1 Chocolate/4g	19	1.0	525	5.4	61.2	28.6	1.6
Advent Calendar, Sainsbury's*	1 Chocolate/4g	20	1.2	557	7.2	52.7	34.3	2.1
Advent Calendar, The Simpsons, Kinnerton*	1 Chocolate/4g	20	1.1	526	5.3	63.2	29.0	1.6
Advent Calendar, The Snowman, M & S*	1 Chocolate/4g	21	1.2	550	6.6	60.4	31.0	0.0
Almond & Honey, Dairy Milk, Cadbury*	1 Sm Bar/54g	281	15.6	520	8.0	57.1	28.9	1.0
Baking, Continental, for Home Baking, Luxury, Tesco*	1 Pack/150g	822	67.6	548	2.7	27.7	45.1	0.9
Baking, Milk, for Home Baking, Luxury, Tesco*	1 Pack/150g	838	54.3	559	7.0	51.4	36.2	1.7
Bar, Alpini, Continental, Thorntons*	1 Bar/36g	192	11.4	538	6.9	55.3	32.0	2.7
Bar, Animal, Nestle*	1 Bar/19g	97	5.0	513	5.8	63.6	26.1	0.0

C

	Measure INFO/WEIGHT	per Measure KCAL	FAT	Nutrition Values per 100g / 100ml KCAL	PROT	CARB	FAT	FIBRE
CHOCOLATE								
Bar, Apricot & Raisin, Thorntons*	1 Bar/40g	185	10.9	462	8.0	46.0	27.3	3.5
Bar, Baby Ruth, Candy, Nestlé*	1 Bar/60g	296	14.1	494	6.7	63.9	23.5	1.7
Bar, Bliss, Hazelnut Truffle, Cadbury*	1 Serving/100g	565	37.9	565	7.2	47.7	37.9	2.6
Bar, Bliss Truffle, Cadbury*	1 Bar/40g	226	14.9	565	6.6	48.8	37.3	2.8
Bar, Bubbles, Galaxy, Mars*	1 Bar/31g	172	10.6	555	6.5	54.7	34.2	1.5
Bar, Candy, Reese's, Fast Break, Hershey*	1 Bar/56g	260	12.0	464	8.9	62.5	21.4	3.6
Bar, Cappuccino, Thorntons*	1 Bar/38g	201	13.2	529	5.2	49.7	34.7	0.5
Bar, Cherry, Lindt*	1 Bar/100g	470	22.8	470	4.5	61.7	22.8	0.0
Bar, Chocolate Cream, Fry's*	1 Piece/10g	42	1.3	415	2.8	70.8	13.2	1.2
Bar, Cookies & Cream, Hello, Lindt*	1 Square/10g	56	3.7	565	7.0	52.0	37.0	0.0
Bar, Dark, 60% Cocoa with Macadamia, Thorntons*	1 Bar/70g	183	12.8	523	6.5	42.3	36.5	12.6
Bar, Dark, Diabetic, Thorntons*	1 Bar/75g	345	26.8	460	5.4	28.5	35.8	8.1
Bar, Dark, Thorntons*	1 Sm Bar/48g	250	17.7	521	7.3	39.9	36.9	10.9
Bar, Extra Dark, 60% Cocoa, Lindor, Lindt*	1 Bar/150g	900	73.5	600	5.0	35.0	49.0	2.0
Bar, Flake Allure, Cadbury*	1 Bar/30g	170	10.9	567	6.7	51.0	36.3	0.7
Bar, Hazel Nut & Cashew, Dairy Milk, Cadbury*	3 Chunks/18g	96	6.0	540	8.8	50.6	33.5	1.8
Bar, Jazz Orange, Thorntons*	1 Bar/56g	304	18.1	543	6.8	55.7	32.3	1.2
Bar, Milk, Galaxy, Mars*	1 Bar/46g	250	15.0	544	6.6	56.3	32.5	1.5
Bar, Milk, Gold, Lindt*	1 Bar/300g	1605	92.9	535	6.6	58.7	31.0	0.0
Bar, Milk, Hazelnut, Gold, Lindt*	1 Bar/300g	1665	108.2	555	7.9	50.7	36.1	0.0
Bar, Milk, Hazelnut, Lindt*	1 Bar/100g	570	38.8	570	8.5	47.0	38.8	0.0
Bar, Milk, Lindt*	1 Bar/100g	535	31.0	535	6.6	57.6	31.0	0.0
Bar, Milk, Raisin & Hazelnut, Gold, Lindt*	1 Bar/300g	1590	94.8	530	6.8	54.7	31.6	0.0
Bar, Milk, Raisin & Hazelnut, Lindt*	1 Bar/100g	530	31.6	530	3.1	54.7	31.6	0.0
Bar, Milk, Thorntons*	1 Sm Bar/50g	269	16.0	538	7.5	54.8	32.0	1.0
Bar, Milk, with Marmite Flavour, Very Peculiar, Marmite*	4 Squares/13g	70	4.2	540	6.9	54.9	32.1	2.0
Bar, Pistacho, Lindt*	1 Bar/100g	585	40.6	585	7.1	48.2	40.6	0.0
Bar, Snack, Kinder*	1 Bar/21g	116	7.1	554	10.0	52.0	34.0	0.0
Bar, Strawberry, Lindt*	1 Bar/100g	470	22.8	470	4.5	61.6	22.8	0.0
Bar, Taz, Cadbury*	1 Bar/25g	121	6.0	485	4.8	62.0	24.0	0.0
Bar, Truffle, M & S*	1 Bar/35g	168	11.4	480	5.9	41.7	32.5	8.3
Bar, Truffle, Orange, M & S*	1 Bar/33g	177	10.5	535	6.6	55.6	31.9	1.4
Bar, Turkish Delight, Large, Dairy Milk, Cadbury*	1 Square/8g	35	1.6	470	5.6	63.2	21.4	0.5
Bar, Twisted, Creme Egg, Cadbury*	1 Bar/45g	210	9.4	465	5.2	64.6	20.8	0.5
Bar, Viennese, Continental, Thorntons*	1 Bar/38g	206	13.0	542	4.2	54.0	34.2	0.8
Bar, White, Swiss, M & S*	1oz/28g	152	8.7	543	8.0	58.3	30.9	0.0
Bar, White, Thorntons*	1 Bar/50g	274	15.6	547	6.5	59.5	31.3	0.0
Bar, Wildlife, Cadbury*	1 Bar/21g	109	6.2	520	7.8	56.8	29.3	0.0
Beans, Coffee, Dark, Solid, M & S*	1 Serving/10g	53	3.8	532	4.7	42.4	37.6	11.6
Beans, Non Dairy, Graze*	1 Pack/40g	196	8.8	491	3.3	70.0	22.0	0.0
Beans, Plain, Carl Brandt*	4 Beans/5g	25	1.4	501	5.7	54.6	28.9	0.0
Bear, Lindt*	1 Bear/11g	60	3.6	572	7.5	57.7	34.6	0.0
Bubbly, Dairy Milk, Cadbury*	1 Bar/35g	185	10.5	525	7.7	56.9	29.7	0.7
Bubbly Santa, M & S*	1 Santa/23g	124	7.3	540	7.0	55.8	31.7	2.7
Bunny, Easter, Mars*	1 Bunny/29g	155	9.2	535	6.2	56.2	31.7	0.0
Bunny, Lindt*	1 Bunny/11g	60	3.6	572	7.5	57.5	34.6	0.0
Cappuccino, Nestle*	1 Serving/20g	109	6.6	545	6.1	56.0	32.9	0.0
Caramel, Dairy Milk, Cadbury*	1 Bar/45g	215	10.4	480	4.9	62.8	23.2	0.4
Chocolat Noir, Lindt*	1/6 Bar/17g	87	5.4	510	6.0	50.0	32.0	0.0
Chocolate Favourites, Tesco*	½ Box/227g	1015	43.6	447	4.2	64.3	19.2	0.3
Chomp, Cadbury*	1 Bar/24g	112	4.8	465	3.3	67.9	20.0	0.2
Christmas Decorations, Dairy Milk, Caramel, Cadbury*	1 Chocolate/11g	53	2.8	485	5.6	59.7	25.1	0.0
Christmas Tree Decoration, Average	1 Chocolate/12g	63	3.6	522	7.6	56.4	29.9	0.4

	Measure INFO/WEIGHT	per Measure KCAL	FAT	Nutrition Values per 100g / 100ml KCAL	PROT	CARB	FAT	FIBRE
CHOCOLATE								
Christmas Tree Decoration, Cadbury*	1 Picco/12g	60	3.4	525	7.6	56.2	29.9	0.0
Coconut, White, Excellence, Lindt*	1 Square/10g	61	4.4	610	6.0	48.0	44.0	0.0
Coins, Milk, Sainsbury's*	1 Coin/5g	26	1.4	502	5.5	58.8	27.1	2.5
Counters, Galaxy, Mars*	4 Counters/10g	53	2.9	529	6.8	59.4	29.1	1.4
Creme Egg Splats, Cadbury*	¼ Pack/40g	192	9.0	480	5.7	64.5	22.5	0.5
Crispy, Sainsbury's*	4 Squares/19g	99	5.4	521	9.1	56.9	28.5	2.1
Dairy Milk, Cadbury*	1 Bar/45g	240	13.8	530	7.5	56.5	30.5	0.7
Dairy Milk, Chunk Bar, Cadbury*	1 Chunk/7g	35	2.0	525	7.5	57.0	29.8	0.1
Dairy Milk, Cool & Delicious, Cadbury*	1 Bar/21g	110	6.3	525	7.6	56.1	30.1	0.0
Dairy Milk, Crispies, Cadbury*	1 Bar/49g	250	13.4	510	7.6	58.6	27.4	0.0
Dairy Milk, King Size, Cadbury*	1 Serving/85g	446	25.2	525	7.6	56.4	29.7	0.0
Dairy Milk, Toffee Popcorn, Dairy Milk, Cadbury*	1 Bar/150g	765	39.8	510	7.0	59.5	26.5	1.7
Dairy Milk, Treatsize, Cadbury*	1 Bar/14g	73	4.2	525	7.5	57.0	29.8	0.7
Dairy Milk, with Oreo, Cadbury*	3 Chunks/15g	85	5.4	560	6.1	53.5	35.5	0.7
Dark, 70% Cocoa Solids, Extra Fine, Lindt*	1 Square/10g	54	4.1	537	8.0	33.0	41.0	0.0
Dark, 70% Cocoa Solids, Organic, Green & Black's*	1 Sm Bar/35g	193	14.4	551	9.3	36.0	41.1	11.5
Dark, 70% Cocoa Solids, Organic, Morrisons*	½ Bar/50g	266	20.6	531	7.9	31.6	41.1	11.0
Dark, 75% Cacao, Rausch*	1 Row/31g	163	12.9	522	8.8	28.5	41.1	15.0
Dark, 85% Cocoa, Excellence, Lindt*	1 Serving/40g	212	18.4	530	11.0	19.0	46.0	0.0
Dark, 85% Cocoa, Finest, Moser Roth, Aldi*	1 Bar/25g	147	12.3	589	9.3	21.0	49.3	11.9
Dark, 85% Cocoa, TTD, Sainsbury's*	1 Serving/25g	142	12.8	569	9.7	17.0	51.4	14.1
Dark, 99% Cocoa, Excellence, Lindt*	1 Serving/25g	132	12.5	530	13.0	8.0	50.0	8.0
Dark, Belgian, Continental, Luxury, Sainsbury's*	1 Bar/100g	490	38.7	490	11.1	24.2	38.7	7.4
Dark, Belgian, Extra Special, Asda*	2 Squares/20g	102	8.0	508	11.0	26.0	40.0	16.0
Dark, Bittersweet, Cherries, Organic, Green & Black's*	1 Bar/100g	477	28.2	477	7.9	48.0	28.2	8.7
Dark, Chilli, Excellence, Lindt*	1 Serving/40g	202	12.8	506	5.4	49.0	32.0	0.0
Dark, Classic, Bourneville, Cadbury*	4 Squares/25g	125	6.8	505	4.7	58.8	27.3	2.0
Dark, Continental, Luxury, Tesco*	1 Bar/100g	571	37.8	571	11.3	46.5	37.8	0.1
Dark, Espresso, Arabica, 70% Cocoa, Green & Black's*	½ Bar/50g	290	20.8	580	9.0	37.2	41.7	11.0
Dark, Espresso with Coffee, Organic, Green & Black's*	1 Bar/150g	824	62.4	549	9.8	33.8	41.6	11.7
Dark, Fair Trade, Co-Op*	1 Bar/45g	214	13.0	475	4.0	49.0	29.0	6.0
Dark, Feuilles with Orange, Nestle*	1 Piece/8g	42	2.6	524	4.6	54.4	32.0	0.0
Dark, Luxury Continental, Sainsbury's*	½ Bar/50g	252	20.0	504	10.7	25.5	40.0	16.1
Dark, Mint, Intense, Lindt*	1 Square/10g	51	3.2	510	5.0	50.0	32.0	0.0
Dark, Orange & Spices, Maya Gold, Green & Black's*	1 Sm Bar/35g	184	11.8	526	7.3	48.2	33.8	8.2
Dark, Plain, Average	***1oz/28g***	***143***	***7.8***	***510***	***5.0***	***63.5***	***28.0***	***2.5***
Dark, Raspberry, Ruffles, Jameson's*	1oz/28g	123	5.3	441	1.9	65.9	18.9	4.4
Dark, Raw Organic, Loving Earth*	1 Serving/20g	99	7.9	495	9.3	46.4	39.5	0.0
Dark, Smooth, Bar, Galaxy, Mars*	1 Bar/125g	651	42.0	521	6.2	48.0	33.6	9.3
Dark, Special, Hershey*	1 Pack/41g	180	12.0	439	4.9	61.0	29.3	7.3
Dark, Whole Nut, Tesco*	1 Serving/13g	67	4.5	539	6.1	48.3	35.7	6.5
Dark, with a Soft Mint Centre, Organic, Green & Black's*	1 Bar/100g	478	27.3	478	7.4	50.5	27.3	8.6
Dark, with Chilli, Thorntons*	4 Squares/20g	107	7.9	533	7.2	36.3	39.5	10.4
Diet, Ritter Sport*	1 Square/6g	25	1.8	412	6.0	44.0	30.0	0.0
Double, Nestle*	1 Serving/25g	133	8.3	532	9.1	49.4	33.1	0.0
Double Blend, Nestle*	1 Rectangle/11g	61	3.6	553	7.3	55.9	33.0	0.0
Dream, with Real Strawberries, Cadbury*	1 Bar/45g	250	14.9	555	4.5	59.6	33.1	0.0
Drops, Plain, Sainsbury's*	1 Serving/125g	638	34.5	510	5.3	60.1	27.6	4.0
Egg, Double Cream, Nestle*	1 Egg/28g	163	11.1	582	6.9	49.2	39.7	0.4
Egg, Mars*	1 Egg/33g	166	9.3	503	4.6	57.3	28.2	0.0
Elves, Magical, with Popping Candy, Cadbury*	1 Elf/15g	77	4.2	515	6.9	60.0	27.7	0.0
Ferrero Rocher, Ferrero*	1 Chocolate/13g	74	5.1	593	7.0	49.0	41.0	0.0
Freddo, Caramel, Dairy Milk, Cadbury*	1 Freddo/19g	93	4.7	490	5.5	60.5	24.8	0.5

	Measure INFO/WEIGHT	per Measure KCAL	FAT	Nutrition Values per 100g / 100ml KCAL	PROT	CARB	FAT	FIBRE
CHOCOLATE								
Freddo, Dairy Milk, Cadbury*	1 Freddo/18g	95	5.4	530	7.5	57.0	29.8	0.7
Fruit & Nut, Belgian, Waitrose*	1 Serving/50g	254	14.6	508	8.6	54.6	29.2	3.4
Fruit & Nut, Dark, Tesco*	4 Squares/25g	124	7.0	494	5.8	54.8	27.9	6.5
Fudge, Keto Bar*	1 Serving/65g	250	7.0	385	36.9	36.9	10.8	32.3
Ginger, Traidcraft*	1 Bar/50g	212	7.4	424	3.9	68.2	14.8	0.0
Golf Balls, Milk Chocolate, Lindt*	1 Packet/110g	619	39.5	563	6.5	53.6	35.9	0.0
Kinder, Bueno, Bar, White, Ferrero*	1 Piece/20g	111	7.0	571	8.8	52.6	35.9	1.0
Kinder, Bueno Bar, Milk, Ferrero*	1 Bar/22g	123	8.0	575	9.2	49.5	37.3	2.0
Kinder, Riegel, Ferrero*	1 Bar/21g	117	7.1	558	10.0	53.0	34.0	0.0
Kinder Maxi, Ferrero*	1 Bar/21g	116	7.1	550	10.0	51.0	34.0	0.0
Kinder Surprise, Ferrero*	1 Egg/20g	113	7.1	564	9.0	52.5	35.3	1.0
Kitten, Milk Chocolate, Lindt*	1 Kitten/11g	60	3.6	572	7.5	57.7	34.6	0.0
Light & Whippy, Bite Sized, Sainsbury's*	1 Bar/15g	66	2.4	439	3.3	69.7	16.3	0.1
Macadamia Nut, Excellence, Lindt*	1 Bar/100g	560	37.0	560	7.0	51.0	37.0	0.0
Matchmakers, Mint, Nestle*	1 Stick/4g	20	0.8	477	4.3	69.7	20.1	0.9
Milk, a Darker Shade of Milk Choc, Green & Black's*	1 Sm Bar/35g	183	10.4	523	9.9	54.0	29.7	3.7
Milk, Average	***1oz/28g***	***146***	***8.6***	***520***	***7.7***	***56.9***	***30.7***	***0.8***
Milk, Belgian, Mini Eggs, M & S*	1 Egg/8g	43	2.5	535	7.0	55.8	31.7	2.7
Milk, Belgian, TTD, Sainsbury's*	1 Piece/10g	55	3.5	549	9.6	48.3	35.3	2.0
Milk, Biscuit Sticks, Mikado, Kraft*	1 Stick/2g	11	0.5	475	7.8	67.0	19.8	3.1
Milk, Bubbly, Swiss, M & S*	1 Serving/40g	218	13.7	545	8.0	52.0	34.3	2.5
Milk, Creamy, Organic, Green & Black's*	6 Pieces/20g	110	7.0	560	9.1	50.3	35.5	1.6
Milk, Extra Au Lait, Milch Extra, Lindt*	½ Bar/50g	268	15.5	535	6.5	57.0	31.0	0.0
Milk, Extra Creamy, Excellence, Lindt*	1 Bar/100g	560	37.1	560	6.0	51.1	37.1	0.0
Milk, Extra Fine, Swiss, M & S*	1 Serving/25g	141	9.2	565	7.2	50.9	36.7	2.3
Milk, Figures, Hollow, Dairyfine, Aldi*	1 Serving/11g	58	3.2	523	5.5	59.9	29.0	3.1
Milk, Fimbles Bar, Kinnerton*	1 Bar/12g	65	3.8	539	5.8	57.0	31.8	1.9
Milk, for Baking, Value, Tesco*	½ Bar/50g	265	14.5	530	6.7	60.0	29.0	2.2
Milk, Honey, Traidcraft*	1 Bar/50g	272	16.5	545	6.0	54.0	33.0	0.0
Milk, Italian, Low Sugar, Groder*	1 Serving/40g	199	14.6	498	6.9	51.2	36.5	1.9
Milk, Less Than 99 Calories, M & S*	1 Bar/16g	85	4.6	531	7.5	61.2	28.8	0.6
Milk, Lindor, Lindt*	1 Square/11g	68	5.2	615	4.7	43.0	47.0	0.0
Milk, Ryelands*	4 Squares/29g	155	8.2	520	7.3	60.7	27.6	1.7
Milk, Santas, Tesco*	1 Bag/90g	433	21.8	481	4.5	61.4	24.2	1.4
Milk, Shapes, Easter Friends, Tesco*	1 Chocolate/13g	68	4.3	540	8.0	52.3	34.2	2.3
Milk, Soft Caramel Centre, Organic, Green & Black's*	1 Bar/100g	495	26.4	495	8.3	56.2	26.4	2.8
Milk, Super Naturals, Sainsbury's*	4 Pieces/40g	85	4.9	212	2.4	23.0	12.2	0.9
Milk, Swiss, Diabetic with Fruit & Nuts, Boots*	½ Bar/21g	97	6.7	462	7.0	55.0	32.0	2.7
Milk, Swiss Made, Organic, Traidcraft*	4 Squares/17g	91	5.6	550	7.0	50.0	34.0	0.0
Milk, Whole Nut, Tesco*	1 Serving/25g	129	8.4	517	8.7	53.4	33.8	9.0
Milk, Winnie the Pooh, Solid Shapes, M & S*	1 Chocolate/6g	32	1.9	540	8.1	54.1	32.4	1.3
Milk, with Biscuit Pieces, Asda*	2 Squares/14g	73	4.1	521	8.0	57.0	29.0	1.9
Milk, with Butterscotch, Organic, Green & Black's*	1 Bar/100g	555	34.5	555	8.8	50.5	34.5	2.7
Milk, with Crisped Rice, Dubble*	1 Bar/40g	211	11.8	528	6.4	59.6	29.4	0.0
Milk, with Honey & Almond Nougat, Swiss, Toblerone*	1 Piece/8g	42	2.4	525	5.4	59.0	29.5	2.2
Milk, with Peanut Butter Filling, Ghirardelli*	1 Serving/45g	250	17.0	556	8.9	48.9	37.8	2.2
Milk, with Raisins & Hazelnuts, Green & Black's*	1 Bar/100g	556	36.9	556	9.2	46.8	36.9	3.2
Milk, with Whole Almonds, Organic, Green & Black's*	1 Bar/100g	578	42.2	578	11.8	37.7	42.2	5.2
Mini, Toblerone*	1 Serving/6g	32	1.8	525	5.6	57.5	30.0	3.5
Mini Bites, Chunky, Moments, Fox's*	1 Roll/20g	90	4.9	450	5.7	52.4	24.6	2.2
Mini Eggs, Cadbury*	1 Egg/3g	16	0.7	490	4.6	67.8	21.9	1.3
Mini Eggs, Caramel, Cadbury*	1 Mini Egg/11g	55	2.9	485	5.7	59.0	25.7	0.4
Mini Eggs, Lindor, Lindt*	3 Eggs/15g	92	6.8	611	5.4	45.0	45.0	0.0

	Measure INFO/WEIGHT	per Measure KCAL	FAT	Nutrition Values per 100g / 100ml KCAL	PROT	CARB	FAT	FIBRE
CHOCOLATE								
Mint, Lamb, Aero, Nestle*	1 Lamb/27g	147	8.3	543	5.3	60.2	30.7	0.0
Mint Chips, Chunk, Dairy Milk, Cadbury*	1 Chunk/32g	162	8.4	505	6.5	61.2	26.1	0.0
Mint Chips, Dairy Milk, Cadbury*	1 Bar/49g	247	12.8	505	6.6	61.6	26.1	0.6
Mint Creme, Sainsbury's*	1 Serving/20g	93	4.9	467	2.8	62.7	24.5	2.1
Mint Crisp, Sainsbury's*	4 Squares/19g	95	4.8	501	5.0	63.7	25.0	3.6
Mistletoe Kisses, Mars*	1 Packet/42g	209	11.5	498	5.3	57.0	27.3	0.0
Natural Orange, Excellence, Lindt*	1 Bar/100g	560	37.0	560	7.0	50.0	37.0	0.0
Natural Vanilla, Excellence, Lindt*	1 Bar/100g	590	40.0	590	6.0	51.0	40.0	0.0
Neapolitans, Terry's*	1oz/28g	146	8.3	522	6.0	57.3	29.7	4.1
Nibs, Raw, Cacao, Organic, Navitas Naturals*	1 Serving/28g	130	12.0	464	14.3	35.7	42.9	32.1
Noir, Special, Frey*	1 Bar/35g	197	15.8	562	8.0	30.0	45.0	0.0
NutRageous, Reese's, Hershey*	1 Bar/51g	260	16.0	510	11.8	54.9	31.4	3.9
Nuts About Caramel, Cadbury*	1 Bar/55g	272	15.1	495	5.8	56.6	27.4	0.0
Nutty Caramel, Dairy Milk, Cadbury*	4 Squares/28g	155	9.9	550	6.9	51.0	35.0	1.2
Nutty Nougat, Bite Sized, Sainsbury's*	1 Bar/23g	111	5.5	481	7.6	59.0	23.8	0.6
Old Jamaica, Bournville, Cadbury*	4 Chunks/23g	107	5.4	465	4.2	59.6	23.4	2.0
Orange, Fair Trade, Divine Foods*	4 Squares/17g	92	5.4	541	6.5	57.7	31.5	0.0
Orange, Sainsbury's*	4 Squares/19g	100	5.8	531	9.2	54.3	30.7	2.2
Orange Cream, Cadbury*	1 Bar/51g	217	7.9	425	2.6	68.6	15.4	0.0
Orange Cream, Fry's*	1 Bar/50g	210	6.8	420	2.8	72.3	13.7	0.0
Panna Cotta & Raspberry, M & S*	1 Bar/36g	190	12.1	528	4.7	51.4	33.6	0.3
Peanut Butter Cup, Big Cup, Reese's, Hershey*	1 Cup/39g	210	12.0	538	10.3	53.8	30.8	2.6
Peanut Butter Cup, Miniature, Reese's, Hershey*	1 Cup/9g	44	2.6	500	9.1	59.1	29.6	2.3
Peanut Butter Cup, Reese's, Hershey*	1 Cup/21g	105	6.5	500	11.9	57.1	31.0	5.9
Peanut Butter Cup, White, Mini, Reese's, Hershey*	5 Cups/39g	210	12.0	538	12.8	53.8	30.8	2.6
Peppermint, Ritter Sport*	1 Bar/100g	483	26.0	483	3.0	60.0	26.0	0.0
Peppermint Cream, Fry's*	1 Bar/51g	217	7.9	425	2.6	68.8	15.4	0.0
Peppermint Patty, Hershey*	3 Patties/41g	160	3.0	390	2.4	80.5	7.3	0.0
Plain, 50% Cocoa Solids Minimum, Tesco*	4 Squares/22g	115	6.2	523	7.4	60.0	28.1	1.8
Plain, 72% Cocoa Solids, Finest, Tesco*	1 Square/10g	60	4.4	603	7.7	44.0	44.0	3.7
Plain, Belgian, Organic, Waitrose*	1 Bar/100g	505	37.6	505	9.6	32.0	37.6	5.6
Plain, Belgian, TTD, Sainsbury's*	1 Piece/10g	57	4.7	570	7.0	29.3	47.2	10.2
Plain, Continental, Waitrose*	1 Square/4g	23	1.8	558	7.7	32.9	44.0	5.9
Plain, Dark, Fruit & Nut, Rich, Sainsbury's*	4 Squares/25g	122	7.0	489	5.2	53.9	27.9	5.7
Plain, Fair Trade, Tesco*	1 Bar/40g	200	11.8	501	4.8	53.8	29.6	6.6
Plain, Whole Nut, Belgian, Waitrose*	4 Squares/25g	135	9.5	540	6.3	45.4	38.0	7.8
Plain, Wholenut, Sainsbury's*	1 Serving/25g	142	9.0	567	5.7	54.6	36.2	2.5
Plain, with Ginger, Swiss, Waitrose*	4 Squares/17g	88	5.0	519	5.3	58.3	29.4	2.0
Plain, with Hazelnuts, Tesco*	4 Squares/25g	135	8.9	539	6.1	48.3	35.7	6.5
Planets, Mars*	1 Pack/37g	178	8.3	481	4.9	65.4	22.4	0.0
Praline, M & S*	1 Bar/34g	185	12.0	545	7.3	49.6	35.2	3.1
Probiotic, Bar, Ohso*	1 Bar/14g	72	5.0	514	5.0	47.0	36.0	15.5
Rafaello, Roche, Ferrero*	1 Sweet/10g	60	4.7	600	9.7	35.4	46.6	0.0
Reese's Pieces, Bite Size, Minis, Hershey*	11 Pieces/39g	200	12.0	513	7.7	59.0	30.8	2.6
Rocky Road, Clusters, Tesco*	1 Serving/32g	160	9.5	500	7.1	51.0	29.7	6.7
Shots, Cadbury*	1 Pack/160g	752	37.1	470	5.9	59.7	23.2	0.0
Snaps, Hazelnut, Cadbury*	1 Curl/4g	20	1.1	520	6.8	57.8	28.8	0.0
Snaps, Milk, Cadbury*	1 Snap/3g	15	0.8	505	6.3	60.5	27.0	1.0
Snaps, Orange, Cadbury*	1 Snap/3g	15	0.8	505	6.3	60.4	27.0	1.0
Snickers, More Nuts, Snickers*	1 Bar/58g	299	17.3	515	10.1	52.8	29.8	0.0
Snowman, Mousse, Dairy Milk, Cadbury*	1 Snowman/29g	162	10.2	560	6.7	54.5	35.0	0.4
Speckled Eggs, M & S*	1 Egg/6g	25	1.0	440	6.6	63.1	18.2	1.5
Tasters, Dairy Milk, Cadbury*	1 Bag/45g	238	13.7	530	7.6	56.4	30.5	0.0

	Measure INFO/WEIGHT	per Measure KCAL	FAT	Nutrition Values per 100g / 100ml KCAL	PROT	CARB	FAT	FIBRE
CHOCOLATE								
Teddy Bear, Milk Chocolate, Thorntons*	1 Teddy/250g	1358	83.8	543	7.6	52.6	33.5	1.0
Toffifee, Storck*	1 Sweet/6g	32	1.9	535	6.0	58.0	31.0	0.0
Twirl, Bites, Cadbury*	1 Bite/2g	11	0.6	530	7.7	56.5	30.3	0.8
Wafer, Dairy Milk, Cadbury*	1 Bar/46g	235	12.9	510	7.7	57.0	28.0	0.0
White, Average	***1oz/28g***	***148***	***8.7***	***529***	***8.0***	***58.3***	***30.9***	***0.0***
White, Belgian, No Added Sugar, Boots*	1 Serving/30g	146	10.8	488	6.0	47.8	36.0	7.0
White, Belgian, Sugar Less, Sweet' N Low*	1 Piece/25g	128	9.6	512	5.8	63.1	38.3	0.0
White, Creamy Vanilla, Green & Black's*	1 Sm Bar/35g	201	12.8	573	7.4	53.5	36.6	0.1
White, Crispy, Fair Trade, Co-Op*	½ Bar/50g	278	17.5	555	9.0	51.0	35.0	0.1
White, Double Berry, Nestle*	¼ Bar/30g	167	10.4	556	6.6	54.9	34.5	0.0
White, Nestle*	4 Pieces/40g	220	13.0	550	7.5	55.0	32.5	0.0
White, Organic, Waitrose*	1oz/28g	160	10.3	572	6.1	53.9	36.8	0.0
White, with Honey & Almond Nougat, Toblerone*	1 Serving/25g	132	7.2	530	6.2	60.5	29.0	0.2
White, with Strawberries, Divine*	1 Piece/3g	16	0.9	534	7.6	59.9	29.3	0.1
White, with Strawberry Pieces, Under 99 Cals, M & S*	1 Bar/16g	86	4.9	540	6.6	60.4	30.4	0.3
Whole Nut, Dairy Milk, Cadbury*	1 Bar/49g	270	17.4	550	8.9	49.5	35.4	1.7
Whole Nut, Sainsbury's*	4 Chunks/25g	142	9.4	566	8.5	48.5	37.6	2.6
Wispa, Bitsa Wispa, Cadbury*	¼ Bag/43g	238	14.7	550	7.3	53.0	34.0	0.9
CHOCOLATE DROPS								
Plain, Asda*	1 Serving/100g	489	29.0	489	7.0	50.0	29.0	10.0
White for Cooking & Decorating, Sainsbury's*	1oz/28g	152	8.6	544	6.5	60.3	30.8	0.0
CHOCOLATE ORANGE								
Bar, Montana*	1 Serving/25g	131	6.8	523	7.0	62.2	27.4	0.0
Crunchball, Terry's*	1 Segment/9g	45	2.4	520	6.9	59.8	28.1	2.0
Dark, Terry's*	1 Segment/9g	45	2.6	511	4.3	57.0	29.3	6.2
Egg & Spoon, Terry's*	1 Egg/34g	195	12.9	575	5.5	51.6	38.0	1.7
Goes Minty, Terry's*	3 Slices/26g	133	7.7	510	4.3	57.0	29.5	6.2
Milk, Mini Segments, Minis, Terry's*	1 Segment/4g	21	1.1	525	5.4	60.5	28.5	2.1
Milk, Terry's*	1 Orange/175g	931	51.6	532	7.4	57.8	29.5	2.1
Plain, Terry's*	1 Orange/175g	889	51.4	508	3.8	56.8	29.4	6.2
Segsations, Terry's*	1 Segsation/8g	43	2.3	520	6.9	58.5	28.5	2.8
White, Terry's*	1 Segment/11g	61	3.4	535	6.3	60.9	29.4	0.0
CHOCOLATE RAISINS								
Assorted, Thorntons*	1 Bag/140g	601	27.6	429	4.2	58.8	19.7	2.9
Californian, Tesco*	½ Bag/57g	268	11.7	472	5.2	66.2	20.7	1.3
Californian, White, Belgian, M & S*	1 Pack/100g	450	20.9	450	4.3	60.6	20.9	0.8
Coated, Californian, M & S*	1 Bag/130g	520	19.1	400	4.3	63.2	14.7	1.9
Jameson's*	1 Serving/23g	96	3.8	418	4.7	62.7	16.5	1.4
Milk Chocolate Coated, Average	1 Serving/50g	207	7.7	415	4.4	64.6	15.4	2.0
CHOCOLATE SPREAD								
& Caramel, Chosen By You, Asda*	1 Serving/100g	564	34.7	564	2.5	60.1	34.7	0.8
Average	***1 Tsp/12g***	***68***	***4.5***	***569***	***4.1***	***57.1***	***37.6***	***0.0***
Chilli, Atkins & Potts*	1 Tbsp/25g	112	6.9	447	3.5	43.4	27.7	4.8
Hazelnut, Nutella, Ferrero*	1oz/28g	149	8.7	533	6.6	56.4	31.0	3.5
Hazelnut, Weight Watchers*	1 Serving/15g	50	1.8	333	4.7	45.3	12.0	12.0
Snickers, Mars*	1 Serving/7g	38	2.6	548	8.7	43.3	37.8	0.0
with Nuts	***1 Tsp/12g***	***66***	***4.0***	***549***	***6.2***	***60.5***	***33.0***	***0.8***
CHOCOLATES								
All Gold, Dark, Terry's*	1 Serving/30g	152	8.7	505	4.0	57.5	29.0	4.3
All Gold, Milk, Terry's*	1 Serving/30g	158	9.2	525	4.8	58.0	30.5	1.5
Almond Marzipan, Milk Chocolate, Thorntons*	1 Chocolate/13g	60	2.9	464	6.6	59.4	22.6	5.6
Almond Mocca Mousse, Thorntons*	1 Chocolate/14g	76	5.3	543	8.5	40.7	37.9	2.9
Alpini, Thorntons*	1 Chocolate/13g	70	4.2	538	7.0	54.6	32.3	2.3

	Measure INFO/WEIGHT	per Measure KCAL	FAT	Nutrition Values per 100g / 100ml KCAL	PROT	CARB	FAT	FIBRE
CHOCOLATES								
Assortment, Belgian, Waitrose*	1oz/28g	127	7.6	453	6.3	45.5	27.3	3.8
Assortment, Occasions, Tesco*	1 Chocolate/15g	70	3.1	470	4.6	65.8	20.9	0.5
Bites, Galaxy, Mars*	1 Pack/40g	197	9.7	492	5.0	63.0	24.2	0.8
Bittermint, Bendicks*	1 Mint/18g	80	3.0	440	4.3	68.9	16.3	2.4
Brandy Liqueurs, Asda*	1 Chocolate/8g	34	1.4	409	4.0	60.0	17.0	0.8
Brazil Nut Assortment, M & S*	1oz/28g	163	12.7	581	9.6	37.5	45.3	1.5
Cafe Au Lait, from Continental Selection, Thorntons*	1 Chocolate/16g	77	4.0	481	5.3	58.1	25.0	0.6
Cappuccino, from Continental Selection, Thorntons*	1 Chocolate/13g	70	4.7	538	5.9	48.5	36.2	0.8
Caramels, Sainsbury's*	1 Sweet/12g	57	2.6	490	3.5	69.0	22.2	0.2
Celebrations, Mars*	1 Sweet/8g	41	2.2	512	5.7	61.5	27.0	1.7
Cherry Liqueur, M & S*	1 Chocolate/13g	55	2.6	435	3.2	50.6	20.2	4.1
Chocolate Mousse, Thorntons*	1 Chocolate/13g	67	4.7	515	7.5	40.0	36.2	3.1
Classic Collection, Thorntons*	1 Chocolate/12g	58	2.8	472	4.3	62.7	22.8	2.4
Coconut, Lindor, Lindt*	1 Ball/13g	79	6.0	632	5.4	42.0	48.0	0.0
Coffee Cream, Average	1 Chocolate/12g	54	2.0	446	3.3	70.4	17.0	2.4
Coffee Creme, Dark, Thorntons*	1 Chocolate/13g	52	1.4	400	3.0	71.5	10.8	0.8
Coffee Creme, Milk, Thorntons*	1 Chocolate/13g	52	1.3	400	2.8	74.6	10.0	0.8
Continental, Belgian, Thorntons*	1 Chocolate/13g	67	3.9	514	5.8	53.5	30.3	2.9
Continental, Thorntons*	1 Chocolate/15g	76	4.4	506	5.6	54.5	29.3	2.7
Country Caramel, Milk, Thorntons*	1 Chocolate/9g	45	2.4	500	4.6	62.2	26.7	0.0
Dairy Box, Milk, Nestle*	1 Piece/11g	50	2.1	456	4.4	65.9	19.4	0.7
Dark, Elegant, Elizabeth Shaw*	1 Chocolate/8g	38	1.8	469	2.9	62.5	23.1	0.0
Dark, Rose & Violet Creams	1 Chocolate/13g	55	1.6	422	2.2	76.1	12.5	1.7
Dark, Swiss Thins, Lindt*	1 Pack/125g	681	46.2	545	4.8	49.2	37.0	0.0
Eclipse, Truffle, Plain, Dark, Montezuma*	1 Truffle/16g	93	8.5	581	0.6	21.9	53.1	0.0
Filled, Average	1 Chocolate/13g	58	2.8	447	4.9	62.9	21.3	1.3
Fondant, Chocolate Coated, Usda Average*	1 Chocolate/11g	40	1.0	366	2.2	80.4	9.3	2.1
Gorgeous, Bendicks*	3 Sweets/15g	82	5.0	550	6.6	55.3	33.3	1.1
Heroes, Cadbury*	1 Sweet/8g	38	1.8	480	4.8	65.1	22.4	0.4
Italian Collection, Amaretto, M & S*	1 Chocolate/13g	60	3.1	480	4.4	59.7	25.1	2.3
Italian Collection, Cappuccino, M & S*	1 Bag/100g	545	37.0	545	6.3	46.7	37.0	1.8
Italian Collection, Favourites, M & S*	1 Chocolate/14g	74	4.7	530	5.7	50.4	33.7	1.6
Italian Collection, Panna Cotta, M & S*	1 Chocolate/13g	70	4.7	545	5.3	49.4	36.4	0.1
Liqueur, Barrels, Cointreau	1 Chocolate/10g	44	1.8	435	3.5	57.0	18.0	0.0
Liqueur, Cognac Truffle, Thorntons*	1 Chocolate/14g	65	3.8	464	7.3	40.0	27.1	2.9
Milk, Mini Eggs, Green & Black's*	1 Mini Egg/8g	42	2.7	562	8.6	48.3	35.5	3.8
Milk, Swiss Thins, Lindt*	1 Pack/125g	688	43.3	550	5.8	53.6	34.6	0.0
Milk Tray, Cadbury*	1 Chocolate/9g	47	2.4	495	4.7	61.5	25.8	0.7
Mingles, Bendicks*	1 Chocolate/5g	27	1.6	540	6.5	58.6	31.3	0.1
Mint Creams, Dark, Smooth & Fragrant, Waitrose*	1 Sweet/10g	42	0.9	410	3.0	77.9	9.1	2.4
Mint Crisp, Bendicks*	1 Mint/8g	38	2.3	494	5.2	55.0	29.9	0.0
Mint Crisp, Dark, Elizabeth Shaw*	1 Chocolate/6g	27	1.2	458	1.9	68.0	20.7	0.0
Mint Crisp, Milk, Elizabeth Shaw*	1 Chocolate/6g	30	1.3	493	4.0	70.9	21.4	0.0
Mint Crisp, Thorntons*	1 Chocolate/7g	34	2.2	486	7.7	40.0	31.4	4.3
Mints, After Eight, Dark, Nestle*	1 Sweet/7g	32	0.9	461	5.0	63.0	12.9	2.0
Mints, After Eight, Orange, Nestle*	1 Sweet/7g	29	0.9	417	2.5	72.6	12.9	1.1
Mints, After Eight, Straws, Nestle*	1 Sweet/5g	24	1.4	526	5.1	56.6	31.0	4.0
Misshapes, Assorted, Cadbury*	1 Chocolate/8g	41	2.3	515	5.2	57.5	29.1	0.0
Moments, Thorntons*	1 Chocolate/7g	37	2.0	511	5.4	59.9	27.8	1.9
Orange Cream, Average	1 Chocolate/12g	53	2.0	440	3.2	69.3	16.7	0.0
Orange Crisp, Elizabeth Shaw*	1 Chocolate/6g	29	1.3	478	2.9	68.2	21.5	0.0
Peppermint Cream, Average	1 Chocolate/12g	50	1.4	418	1.9	76.4	11.4	1.6
Praline, Coffee, Thorntons*	1 Chocolate/7g	37	2.4	529	7.0	47.1	34.3	2.9

	Measure INFO/WEIGHT	per Measure KCAL	FAT	Nutrition Values per 100g / 100ml KCAL	PROT	CARB	FAT	FIBRE
CHOCOLATES								
Praline, Hazelnut, Thorntons*	1 Chocolate/5g	27	1.8	540	7.0	48.0	36.0	4.0
Praline, Marzipan, Thorntons*	1 Chocolate/14g	63	3.0	450	5.9	58.6	21.4	2.1
Praline, Roast Hazelnut, Thorntons*	1 Chocolate/13g	70	4.4	538	6.0	51.5	33.8	3.1
Quality Street, Nestle*	1 Sweet/9g	44	1.9	470	3.5	67.3	20.5	1.5
Rocher, Continental, Thorntons*	1 Chocolate/15g	76	5.0	507	6.8	45.3	33.3	2.0
Roses, Cadbury*	1 Chocolate/9g	42	2.2	495	4.8	62.6	25.3	0.7
Sea Shells, Belgian, Guylian*	1 Shell/11g	62	3.8	550	7.6	52.0	34.0	0.0
Seashells, Milk & White, Belgian, Waitrose*	1 Serving/15g	77	4.6	511	5.0	53.1	31.0	2.8
Stars, Mini Wishes, Truffle Centre, Cadbury*	1 Star/13g	70	4.1	540	6.9	55.6	31.8	1.3
Strawberries & Cream, Thorntons*	1 Chocolate/12g	64	3.9	533	5.1	54.2	32.5	0.8
Swiss Tradition, De Luxe, Lindt*	1 Packet/250g	1388	90.7	555	6.3	51.9	36.3	0.0
Swiss Tradition, Mixed, Lindt*	1 Packet/392g	2215	149.4	565	6.1	49.8	38.1	0.0
Tartufo, Thorntons*	1 Chocolate/15g	77	5.4	513	7.4	40.0	36.0	3.3
Truffle, Amaretto, Thorntons*	1 Chocolate/14g	66	3.6	471	5.5	55.0	25.7	2.9
Truffle, Belgian, Flaked, Tesco*	1 Truffle/14g	80	5.4	575	4.4	52.7	38.5	2.3
Truffle, Brandy, Thorntons*	1 Chocolate/14g	68	3.8	486	6.1	52.1	27.1	0.7
Truffle, Caramel, Thorntons*	1 Chocolate/14g	67	3.6	479	4.2	57.9	25.7	2.1
Truffle, Champagne, Petit, Thorntons*	1 Chocolate/6g	31	1.9	517	7.5	48.3	31.7	3.3
Truffle, Champagne, Premier, Thorntons*	1 Chocolate/17g	88	5.6	518	6.9	45.3	32.9	2.4
Truffle, Cherry, Thorntons*	1 Chocolate/14g	58	3.0	414	4.2	50.7	21.4	1.4
Truffle, Continental Champagne, Thorntons*	1 Chocolate/16g	78	4.5	488	6.1	51.3	28.0	0.6
Truffle, Dark, Balls, Lindor, Lindt*	1 Ball/12g	76	6.2	630	3.4	38.5	51.4	0.0
Truffle, French Cocoa Dusted, Sainsbury's*	1 Truffle/10g	57	4.5	570	4.0	37.0	45.0	0.0
Truffle, Grand Marnier, Thorntons*	1 Chocolate/15g	77	5.1	513	7.2	40.7	34.0	4.0
Truffle, Hazelnut, Balls, Lindor, Lindt*	1 Ball/12g	76	6.1	632	5.0	39.1	50.6	0.0
Truffle, Irish Milk Chocolate Cream, Elizabeth Shaw*	1 Chocolate/12g	57	2.7	477	3.9	63.4	22.8	0.0
Truffle, Lemon, White, Thorntons*	1 Chocolate/14g	63	3.5	450	4.6	64.3	25.0	0.7
Truffle, Milk Chocolate, Balls, Lindor, Lindt*	1 Ball/12g	73	6.0	611	5.6	41.7	50.0	2.8
Truffle, Rum, Thorntons*	1 Chocolate/13g	63	3.2	485	4.8	58.5	24.6	4.8
Truffle, Selection, Tesco*	1 Chocolate/14g	75	4.2	539	5.1	62.0	29.8	0.5
Truffle, Seville, Thorntons*	1 Chocolate/14g	76	4.7	543	7.1	53.6	33.6	1.4
Truffle, Thorntons*	1 Chocolate/7g	33	1.9	471	6.0	48.6	27.1	1.4
Truffle, Vanilla, Thorntons*	1 Chocolate/13g	64	3.5	492	4.8	57.7	26.9	1.5
Truffle, Viennese, Dark, Thorntons*	1 Chocolate/10g	53	3.6	530	5.9	47.0	36.0	3.0
Truffle, Viennese, Milk, Thorntons*	1 Chocolate/10g	56	3.6	560	4.9	54.0	36.0	0.0
Truffle, White Chocolate, Balls, Lindor, Lindt*	1 Ball/12g	78	6.2	649	5.2	40.2	51.9	0.0
Truffle Filled, Swiss, Balls, Finest, Tesco*	3 Balls/37g	240	19.0	640	5.0	40.7	50.8	1.5
Truffle Hearts, Baileys*	1 Chocolate/15g	76	4.3	506	5.2	52.6	28.9	1.3
Twilight, Dark with Mint, Terry's*	1 Chocolate/6g	33	1.9	530	3.1	59.5	30.5	4.2
Valentine, Thorntons*	1 Chocolate/11g	60	3.8	542	5.7	52.0	34.5	2.1
Winter Selection, Thorntons*	1 Chocolate/10g	51	3.1	506	6.2	51.3	30.6	3.8
CHOP SUEY								
Chicken, with Noodles, Sainsbury's*	1 Pack/300g	300	7.5	100	5.7	13.6	2.5	1.2
Vegetable, M & S*	½ Pack/150g	90	6.2	60	2.0	3.1	4.1	2.9
CHOW MEIN								
Beef, Ready Meal, Average	1 Serving/400g	422	12.2	106	6.0	13.4	3.0	1.0
Char Sui, Cantonese, Sainsbury's*	½ Pack/225g	205	7.0	91	5.7	10.0	3.1	1.1
Chicken, Ainsley Harriott*	1 Serving/250g	447	11.8	179	14.0	21.2	4.7	2.0
Chicken, Chinese, Asda*	1 Pack/400g	479	20.4	120	6.7	11.0	5.1	1.5
Chicken, Chinese Takeaway, Sainsbury's*	1 Pack/316g	338	8.5	107	9.1	11.6	2.7	0.7
Chicken, Chosen By You, Asda*	1 Pack/400g	312	2.8	78	8.3	9.2	0.7	0.9
Chicken, COOK!, M & S*	1 Pack/375g	356	7.9	95	7.9	10.5	2.1	1.7
Chicken, COU, M & S*	1 Pack/200g	170	5.4	85	5.9	9.5	2.7	1.4

	Measure INFO/WEIGHT	per Measure KCAL	FAT	Nutrition Values per 100g / 100ml KCAL	PROT	CARB	FAT	FIBRE
CHOW MEIN								
Chicken, Frozen, Sainsbury's*	1 Pack/404g	424	12.1	105	6.1	13.4	3.0	0.9
Chicken, Ready Meal, Average	1 Serving/400g	375	9.4	94	6.5	11.5	2.4	1.2
Chicken, Ready Meal, Healthy Range, Average	1 Serving/400g	329	8.5	82	5.9	9.9	2.1	1.3
Chicken, with Vegetable Spring Roll, Oriental Express*	1 Pack/300g	213	1.8	71	5.5	12.4	0.6	1.9
Chinese, Special, Farmfoods*	1 Pack/400g	276	11.2	69	4.3	6.7	2.8	0.8
Pork, Perfectly Balanced, Waitrose*	½ Pack/310g	332	2.8	107	7.6	17.2	0.9	1.6
Special, COU, M & S*	1 Pack/400g	400	15.2	100	6.6	10.3	3.8	1.4
Special, Perfectly Balanced, Waitrose*	1 Pack/400g	316	4.4	79	7.4	10.0	1.1	0.9
Special, Ready Meal, Average	1 Serving/400g	383	9.7	96	6.5	12.1	2.4	1.0
Stir Fry, Asda*	1 Pack/350g	270	17.5	77	2.1	6.0	5.0	0.0
Stir Fry, Tesco*	½ Pack/240g	180	3.4	75	2.8	12.0	1.4	1.6
Stir Fry, Vegetable, Cantonese, Sainsbury's*	¼ Pack/100g	85	3.8	85	2.2	10.6	3.8	1.2
Vegetable, Ready Meal, Average	1 Serving/400g	337	6.7	84	4.2	12.8	1.7	2.0
Vesta*	1 Pack/433g	594	17.3	137	4.8	20.4	4.0	3.3
CHRISTMAS PUDDING								
Average	1oz/28g	81	2.7	291	4.6	49.5	9.7	1.3
BGTY, Sainsbury's*	1 Serving/114g	302	2.8	266	2.8	58.2	2.5	4.6
Cooked, Fox's*	¼ Pudding/114g	384	11.1	338	3.6	56.0	9.8	5.7
Luxury	1 Serving/114g	416	18.8	365	2.5	48.6	16.4	1.0
Nut Free & Alcohol Free, HE, Tesco*	1 Serving/100g	258	2.7	258	2.8	55.6	2.7	4.3
Retail	1oz/28g	92	3.3	329	3.0	56.3	11.8	1.7
Sticky Toffee, Tesco*	¼ Pudding/114g	372	7.3	326	2.5	64.5	6.4	0.8
Toffee Sauce Coated, Morrisons*	1 Pudding/100g	324	6.4	324	2.5	64.5	6.4	0.0
VLH Kitchens	1 Serving/114g	310	2.2	272	3.1	59.3	2.5	4.6
Wheat Free, GF, Tesco*	1oz/28g	84	2.0	295	1.9	60.4	7.1	4.5
with Cider, Value, Tesco*	1 Serving/100g	312	7.0	312	2.7	59.6	7.0	3.3
with Cider & Sherry, Waitrose*	¼ Pudding/113g	344	7.2	303	2.5	59.0	6.3	3.2
CHUTNEY								
Albert's Victorian, Baxters*	1 Serving/25g	40	0.1	159	1.1	37.9	0.3	1.5
Apple, Tomato & Sultana, Tesco*	1 Serving/50g	88	0.1	176	1.1	42.4	0.2	1.3
Apple & Pear, TTD, Sainsbury's*	1 Serving/20g	38	0.2	190	0.6	45.2	0.8	1.7
Apple & Walnut, Waitrose*	1 Serving/20g	49	0.5	243	12.0	53.8	2.6	3.8
Apricot, Sharwood's*	1 Tsp/16g	21	0.0	131	0.6	32.0	0.1	2.3
Caramelised Onion, Sainsbury's*	1 Serving/25g	28	0.4	111	1.1	23.5	1.4	1.1
Caramelised Onion, TTD, Sainsbury's*	1 Serving/20g	31	0.1	157	0.8	37.3	0.5	2.1
Caramelised Red Onion, Loyd Grossman*	1 Serving/10g	11	0.0	111	0.5	27.2	0.0	0.5
Cheese Board, Cottage Delight Ltd*	1 Tbsp/15g	42	0.5	277	1.0	46.6	3.1	0.0
Cranberry & Caramelised Red Onion, Baxters*	1 Serving/20g	31	0.0	154	0.3	38.0	0.1	0.3
Fruit, Spiced, Baxters*	1 Tsp/16g	23	0.0	143	6.0	34.8	0.1	0.0
Indian Appetisers, Pot, Waitrose*	1 Pot/158g	330	2.2	209	1.8	47.3	1.4	1.8
Lime & Chilli, Geeta's*	1 Serving/25g	69	0.4	277	2.0	64.0	1.4	1.9
Mango, Bengal, Spice, Sharwood's*	1 Tsp/5g	12	0.0	236	0.5	58.0	0.2	1.2
Mango, Budgens*	1oz/28g	66	0.0	235	0.3	58.2	0.1	0.0
Mango, Green Label, Sharwood's*	1 Tsp/10g	24	0.0	241	0.3	59.7	0.1	0.9
Mango, Hot, Patak's*	1 Jar/340g	877	0.7	258	0.4	67.1	0.2	0.7
Mango, Hot & Spicy, Waitrose*	1 Serving/20g	46	0.1	230	0.6	51.6	0.3	1.8
Mango, Indian Takeaway, Asda*	1 Pack/70g	145	0.1	207	0.3	50.9	0.2	1.0
Mango, Major Grey, Patak's*	1 Tbsp/15g	38	0.0	255	0.4	66.0	0.2	0.7
Mango, Premium, Geeta's*	1 Serving/50g	126	0.1	253	0.8	62.0	0.2	0.8
Mango, Sensations, Walkers*	¼ Jar/57g	122	0.1	214	0.3	53.0	0.1	0.6
Mango, Spiced, M & S*	1 Serving/15g	26	0.1	175	1.2	42.3	0.4	3.2
Mango, Spicy, Sainsbury's*	1 Tbsp/15g	24	0.1	160	0.7	37.0	0.7	1.3
Mango, Sweet	***1 Heap Tsp/16g***	***30***	***0.0***	***189***	***0.7***	***48.3***	***0.1***	***0.0***

	Measure INFO/WEIGHT	per Measure KCAL	FAT	KCAL	PROT	CARB	FAT	FIBRE
				Nutrition Values per 100g / 100ml				
CHUTNEY								
Mango, with Hint of Chilli & Ginger, Waitrose*	1 Serving/20g	52	0.0	259	0.5	64.2	0.0	0.7
Mango & Apple, Sharwood's*	1oz/28g	65	0.0	233	0.4	57.6	0.1	1.1
Mango & Chilli, Geeta's*	1 Serving/30g	74	0.0	246	0.5	60.7	0.1	0.2
Mango & Ginger, Baxters*	1 Jar/320g	598	0.6	187	5.0	45.7	0.2	0.9
Mango & Lime, Sharwood's*	1oz/28g	58	0.1	206	0.4	50.5	0.3	0.8
Mango & Mint, Cofresh*	1 Tbsp/20g	31	0.1	155	1.7	36.4	0.3	2.0
Mixed Fruit	***1 Heap Tsp/16g***	***25***	***0.0***	***155***	***0.6***	***39.7***	***0.0***	***0.0***
Onion, Spicy, Organic, The English Provender Co.*	1 Serving/10g	24	0.0	245	1.2	59.0	0.5	3.5
Peach, Spicy, Waitrose*	1 Serving/20g	43	0.3	215	1.0	49.0	1.5	1.5
Plum, Ploughman's, The English Provender Co.*	1 Tsp/10g	16	0.0	160	1.3	38.1	0.2	1.6
Red Onion & Sherry Vinegar, Sainsbury's*	1 Serving/10g	24	0.1	236	0.5	57.1	0.6	1.4
Spicy Fruit, Baxters*	1 Serving/15g	22	0.0	146	0.6	35.4	0.2	0.0
Tomato	***1 Heap Tsp/16g***	***20***	***0.0***	***128***	***1.2***	***31.0***	***0.2***	***1.3***
Tomato, Waitrose*	1 Pot/100g	195	0.3	195	1.3	46.8	0.3	0.0
Tomato & Chilli, Sweet, The English Provender Co.*	1 Tsp/10g	19	0.0	189	0.9	46.0	0.2	1.7
Tomato & Red Pepper, Baxters*	1 Jar/312g	512	1.2	164	2.0	38.0	0.4	1.5
CIDER								
Basics, Sainsbury's*	1 Glass/250ml	200	0.0	80	0.0	0.0	0.0	0.0
Berry, Irish, Magner's*	1 Bottle/500ml	215	0.0	43	0.0	4.3	0.0	0.0
Cyder, Organic, Aspall*	1 Serving/200ml	120	0.2	60	0.1	3.1	0.1	0.0
Cyder, Perronelle's Blush, Aspall*	1 Serving/200ml	122	0.2	61	0.1	5.4	0.1	0.5
Cyder, Premier Cru, Aspall*	1 Serving/200ml	120	0.0	60	0.0	3.1	0.0	0.0
Cyder, Suffolk, Medium, Aspall*	1 Serving/200ml	134	0.0	67	0.1	4.4	0.0	0.0
Diamond White*	1 fl oz/30ml	11	0.0	36	0.0	2.6	0.0	0.0
Dry, Average	***1 Pint/568ml***	***205***	***0.0***	***36***	***0.0***	***2.6***	***0.0***	***0.0***
Dry, Strongbow*	1 Bottle/375ml	161	0.0	43	0.0	3.4	0.0	0.0
Gold, Thatchers*	1 Bottle/500ml	230	0.0	46	0.0	4.5	0.0	0.0
Light, Bulmers*	1 Can/500ml	140	0.0	28	0.0	0.8	0.0	0.0
Low Alcohol	***1 Pint/568ml***	***97***	***0.0***	***17***	***0.0***	***3.6***	***0.0***	***0.0***
Low Carb, Stowford*	1 Bottle/500ml	140	0.0	28	0.0	0.2	0.0	0.0
Magner's*	½ Pint/284ml	105	0.0	37	0.0	2.0	0.0	0.0
Organic, Westons*	1 Serving/200ml	96	0.0	48	0.0	3.1	0.0	0.0
Original, Bulmers*	1 Serving/250ml	105	0.0	42	0.0	4.0	0.0	0.0
Original, Gaymers*	1 Bottle/330ml	148	0.0	45	0.0	4.7	0.0	0.0
Pear, Average	***1 Serving/200ml***	***86***	***0.0***	***43***	***0.0***	***3.6***	***0.0***	***0.0***
Pear, Bulmers*	1 Serving/200ml	86	0.0	43	0.0	3.6	0.0	0.0
Pear, Gaymers*	1 Bottle/330ml	168	0.0	51	0.0	6.2	0.0	0.0
Pear, Magner's*	1 Bottle/568ml	179	0.0	32	0.0	0.0	0.0	0.0
Pear, Non Alcoholic, Kopparberg*	1 Bottle/500ml	170	0.5	34	0.0	8.4	0.1	0.0
Pear, Organic, Westons*	1 Serving/200ml	106	0.0	53	0.0	5.1	0.0	0.0
Ritz, Perry, Bulmers*	1 Bottle/330ml	142	0.0	43	0.0	4.0	0.0	0.0
Scrumpy, Average	***1 Serving/200ml***	***93***	***0.0***	***46***	***0.0***	***2.3***	***0.0***	***0.0***
Scrumpy, Westons*	1 Serving/200ml	94	0.0	47	0.0	1.8	0.0	0.0
Sweet, Average	***1 Pint/568ml***	***239***	***0.0***	***42***	***0.0***	***4.3***	***0.0***	***0.0***
Vintage	***1 Pint/568ml***	***574***	***0.0***	***101***	***0.0***	***7.3***	***0.0***	***0.0***
CINNAMON								
Ground, Average	***1 Tsp/3g***	***8***	***0.1***	***261***	***3.9***	***55.5***	***3.2***	***0.0***
Stick, Schwartz*	1 Stick/2g	7	0.0	339	4.7	79.3	0.3	0.0
CLAMS								
in Brine, Average	***1oz/28g***	***22***	***0.2***	***79***	***16.0***	***2.4***	***0.6***	***0.0***
Raw, Average	***20 Sm/180g***	***133***	***1.7***	***74***	***12.8***	***2.6***	***1.0***	***0.0***
CLEMENTINES								
Raw, Weighed with Peel, Average	***1 Med/61g***	***29***	***0.1***	***47***	***0.8***	***12.0***	***0.2***	***1.7***

	Measure INFO/WEIGHT	per Measure KCAL	FAT	Nutrition Values per 100g / 100ml KCAL	PROT	CARB	FAT	FIBRE
CLEMENTINES								
Raw, Weighed without Peel, Average	***1 Med/46g***	***22***	***0.1***	***47***	***0.8***	***12.0***	***0.2***	***1.7***
COCKLES								
Boiled	***1 Cockle/4g***	***2***	***0.0***	***53***	***12.0***	***0.0***	***0.6***	***0.0***
Bottled in Vinegar, Drained	***1oz/28g***	***17***	***0.2***	***60***	***13.3***	***0.0***	***0.7***	***0.0***
COCKTAIL								
Alcoholic, Juice Based, Average	1 Glass/200ml	464	29.2	232	6.4	18.7	14.6	1.4
Bucks Fizz, Premixed, M & S*	1 Glass/250ml	152	0.0	61	0.0	9.0	0.0	0.0
Cosmopolitan, Canned, M & S*	1 Serving/200ml	456	0.0	228	0.0	22.0	0.0	0.0
Grenadine, Orange Juice, Pineapple Juice	1 Serving/200ml	158	0.3	79	0.5	19.2	0.1	0.2
Mai Tai, Average	1 Serving/200ml	209	0.1	105	0.2	13.9	0.1	0.1
Pina Colada	1 Glass/250ml	592	20.0	237	1.0	28.0	8.0	0.0
COCOA								
Nibs, Naturya*	1 Serving/10g	58	5.0	578	13.0	18.2	50.3	13.4
COCOA BUTTER								
Average	***1oz/28g***	***251***	***27.9***	***896***	***0.0***	***0.0***	***99.5***	***0.0***
COCOA POWDER								
Cadbury*	1 Tbsp/16g	52	3.3	322	23.1	10.5	20.8	0.0
Dry, Unsweetened, Average	1 Tbsp/5g	11	0.7	229	19.6	54.3	13.7	33.2
Organic, Green & Black's*	1 Tbsp/7g	25	1.7	345	22.5	12.5	22.6	30.5
COCONUT								
Chips, Organic, Infinity Foods*	1 Serving/100g	604	62.0	604	5.6	6.4	62.0	13.7
Creamed, Average	***1oz/28g***	***186***	***19.2***	***666***	***6.0***	***6.7***	***68.4***	***7.0***
Desiccated, Average	***1oz/28g***	***169***	***17.4***	***604***	***5.6***	***6.4***	***62.0***	***13.7***
Desiccated, Whitworths*	1oz/28g	170	17.4	606	5.6	6.4	62.0	13.7
Fresh, Flesh Only, Average	***1oz/28g***	***98***	***10.1***	***351***	***3.2***	***3.7***	***36.0***	***7.3***
Ice, Average	***1oz/28g***	***104***	***3.6***	***371***	***1.7***	***66.7***	***12.7***	***2.6***
Milk, Average	***1 Can/400ml***	***698***	***69.7***	***174***	***1.4***	***2.9***	***17.4***	***2.9***
Milk, KTC*	1 Can/400g	776	73.2	194	0.9	1.2	18.3	0.0
Milk, Organic, Tesco*	1/8 Can/49g	85	8.3	175	1.8	2.7	17.0	1.3
Milk, Reduced Fat, Amoy*	1 Tin/400ml	440	44.0	110	1.0	2.0	11.0	1.0
Milk, Reduced Fat, Average	***1 Serving/100g***	***104***	***10.0***	***104***	***1.0***	***2.4***	***10.0***	***0.4***
Sliced, Dried, Forest Feast*	1oz/28g	166	17.4	593	5.6	6.4	62.0	13.7
Water, with Pineapple, Vita Coco*	1 Carton/330ml	82	0.0	25	0.0	6.0	0.0	0.0
COD								
Baked, Average	***1oz/28g***	***27***	***0.3***	***96***	***21.4***	***0.0***	***1.2***	***0.0***
Dried, Salted, Average	***1oz/28g***	***82***	***0.7***	***290***	***62.8***	***0.0***	***2.4***	***0.0***
Dried, Salted, Boiled, Average	***1oz/28g***	***39***	***0.3***	***138***	***32.5***	***0.0***	***0.9***	***0.0***
Fillets, Battered, Average	1 Fillet/125g	219	10.2	176	12.6	13.0	8.2	1.0
Fillets, Battered, Harry Ramsdens, Birds Eye*	1 Fillet/122g	310	18.8	254	11.4	17.2	15.4	0.6
Fillets, Breaded, Average	1 Fillet/125g	258	12.2	206	13.0	16.7	9.8	1.0
Fillets, Breaded, Chunky, Average	1 Piece/135g	204	8.0	151	13.7	10.9	5.9	1.4
Fillets, Breaded, Light, Healthy Range, Average	1 Fillet/135g	209	6.9	154	13.6	13.3	5.1	1.2
Fillets, Chunky, Average	***1 Fillet/198g***	***267***	***7.3***	***135***	***17.1***	***8.2***	***3.7***	***0.8***
Fillets, Portions, Large, Battered, Morrisons*	1 Fillet/118g	219	11.9	186	9.6	14.1	10.1	1.3
Fillets, Skinless & Boneless, Raw, Average	***1 Fillet/140g***	***137***	***2.4***	***98***	***17.8***	***2.7***	***1.8***	***0.4***
Fillets, Smoked, Average	***1 Serving/150g***	***152***	***2.4***	***101***	***21.6***	***0.0***	***1.6***	***0.0***
Loins, Average	***1 Serving/145g***	***116***	***1.2***	***80***	***17.9***	***0.1***	***0.8***	***0.2***
Loins, Beer Battered, TTD, Sainsbury's*	1 Fillet/93g	182	10.8	196	14.4	8.5	11.6	2.7
Loins, Skinless, TTD, Sainsbury's*	1 Serving/100g	83	0.9	83	18.6	0.0	0.9	0.0
Loins, Steaks, Skinless & Boneless, TTD, Sainsbury's*	1 Steak/100g	105	0.4	105	25.2	0.1	0.4	0.1
Poached, Average	***1oz/28g***	***26***	***0.3***	***94***	***20.9***	***0.0***	***1.1***	***0.0***
Smoked, Raw, Average	***1oz/28g***	***22***	***0.2***	***79***	***18.3***	***0.0***	***0.6***	***0.0***
Steaks, Battered, Chip Shop Style, Average	1 Serving/150g	321	18.0	214	12.5	14.3	12.0	1.1

	Measure INFO/WEIGHT	per Measure KCAL	FAT	Nutrition Values per 100g / 100ml KCAL	PROT	CARB	FAT	FIBRE
COD								
Steamed, Average	***1oz/28g***	***23***	***0.3***	***83***	***18.6***	***0.0***	***0.9***	***0.0***
COD &								
Cauliflower Bake, Asda*	1 Pack/400g	492	28.0	123	9.5	5.5	7.0	1.0
Cauliflower Cheese, Fillets, Iceland*	½ Pack/176g	234	13.5	133	12.7	3.3	7.7	1.7
Salmon, Steam Cuisine, COU, M & S*	1 Pack/400g	340	7.2	85	6.8	8.9	1.8	1.2
COD IN								
Beer Batter, Crispy, Finest, Tesco*	1 Portion/250g	575	35.0	230	12.0	13.4	14.0	1.3
Butter Sauce, Rich, Steaks, Ocean Trader*	1 Pouch/150g	136	6.2	91	10.3	3.3	4.1	0.1
Butter Sauce, Ross*	1 Serving/150g	126	5.8	84	9.1	3.2	3.9	0.1
Butter Sauce, Sainsbury's*	1 Serving/170g	224	15.3	132	10.6	2.0	9.0	0.1
Butter Sauce, Steaks, Birds Eye*	1 Pack/170g	185	9.4	109	9.8	5.0	5.5	0.1
Butter Sauce, Steaks, Frozen, Asda*	1 Pouch/152g	163	4.0	107	16.0	5.0	2.6	0.8
Butter Sauce, Steaks, Youngs*	1 Pack/139g	107	3.2	77	9.7	4.1	2.3	0.4
Cheese Sauce, BGTY, Sainsbury's*	1 Serving/170g	144	4.1	85	12.8	3.1	2.4	0.0
Cheese Sauce, Pre Packed, Average	1 Serving/150g	136	4.4	90	11.8	4.2	3.0	0.0
Cheese Sauce, Steaks, Birds Eye*	1 Pack/182g	175	6.4	96	10.9	5.2	3.5	0.1
Mushroom Sauce, BGTY, Sainsbury's*	1 Serving/170g	112	2.9	66	9.9	2.8	1.7	0.1
Parsley Sauce, COU, M & S*	1 Pack/185g	130	4.6	70	10.6	1.4	2.5	0.6
Parsley Sauce, Frozen, M & S*	1 Pack/184g	156	7.2	85	11.1	1.9	3.9	1.0
Parsley Sauce, Portions, Ocean Trader*	1 Serving/120g	112	4.7	93	9.4	4.0	3.9	0.1
Parsley Sauce, Pre Packed, Average	1 Serving/150g	123	4.7	82	10.1	3.3	3.1	0.5
Parsley Sauce, Steaks, Birds Eye*	1 Steak/172g	155	4.8	90	10.5	5.6	2.8	0.1
Red Pepper Sauce, SteamFresh, Birds Eye*	1 Serving/125g	115	2.4	92	14.4	4.7	1.9	0.3
COD WITH								
Chips & Peas, 240, Oakhouse Foods Ltd*	1 Meal/300g	510	18.6	170	6.4	22.3	6.2	2.2
Chunky Chips, M & S*	1 Serving/340g	510	20.4	150	6.5	17.5	6.0	1.5
Fish Pesto, Fillets, COOK!, M & S*	½ Pack/165g	210	5.1	127	16.4	8.4	3.1	4.2
Mediterranean Butter, Sainsbury's*	1 Pack/170g	196	8.9	115	17.0	0.1	5.2	0.1
Parma Ham & Sardinian Chick Peas, M & S*	½ Pack/255g	268	12.5	105	9.8	5.3	4.9	0.5
Roasted Vegetables, M & S*	1 Serving/280g	238	10.6	85	8.0	4.9	3.8	1.7
Salsa & Rosemary Potatoes, BGTY, Sainsbury's*	1 Pack/450g	356	4.0	79	4.7	13.1	0.9	1.6
Sunblush Tomato Sauce, GFY, Asda*	½ Pack/177g	117	2.7	66	13.0	0.1	1.5	1.0
Sweet Chilli, COU, M & S*	1 Pack/400g	360	2.0	90	7.7	13.1	0.5	1.6
Tomato Sauce, Fillets, Asda*	1 Serving/181g	210	10.9	116	13.0	2.6	6.0	2.3
Vegetables, Haches, Steaks, Peche Ocean*	1 Serving/200g	184	7.8	92	12.0	2.1	3.9	0.0
COFFEE								
Azera, Barista Style Instant, Nescafe*	1 Serving/200ml	2	0.0	1	0.1	0.0	0.0	0.0
Black, Average	1 Mug/270ml	5	0.0	2	0.2	0.3	0.0	0.0
Cafe Caramel, Cafe Range, Nescafe*	1 Sachet/17g	72	2.4	423	9.2	64.6	14.1	1.3
Cafe Hazelnut, Nescafe*	1 Sachet/17g	73	2.4	428	9.3	66.0	14.1	0.0
Cafe Irish Cream, Cafe Range, Nescafe*	1 Sachet/23g	98	3.2	425	8.2	65.2	14.1	1.2
Cafe Latte, Dry, Douwe Egberts*	1 Serving/12g	58	2.6	480	10.0	60.0	22.0	0.0
Cafe Latte, Instant, Maxwell House*	1 Serving/16g	67	3.0	420	17.0	45.5	18.9	0.1
Cafe Mocha, Cafe Range, Nescafe*	1 Sachet/22g	92	2.9	418	8.5	66.6	13.1	0.0
Cafe Vanilla, Latte, Cafe Range, Nescafe*	1 Sachet/19g	73	1.6	395	9.2	68.3	8.5	4.1
Cappuccino, Cafe Mocha, Dry, Maxwell House*	1 Serving/23g	100	2.5	434	4.3	78.2	10.8	0.0
Cappuccino, Cafe Specials, Dry, M & S*	1 Serving/14g	55	1.6	395	14.0	59.0	11.5	0.7
Cappuccino, Cappio, Iced, Kenco*	1 Can/200ml	138	6.0	69	3.0	7.0	3.0	0.0
Cappuccino, Cappio, Kenco*	1 Sachet/18g	79	1.9	439	11.7	73.9	10.6	0.6
Cappuccino, Chocolate, Organic, Traidcraft*	1 Serving/25g	139	9.5	555	7.0	43.0	38.0	0.0
Cappuccino, Chocolate, Swiss, Nescafe*	1 Sachet/20g	81	2.3	404	10.5	65.3	11.5	2.9
Cappuccino, Co-Op*	1 Serving/13g	55	2.0	440	16.0	64.0	16.0	8.0
Cappuccino, Decaff, Instant, Made Up, Nescafe*	1 Mug/200ml	68	2.3	34	1.0	5.0	1.2	0.0

	Measure INFO/WEIGHT	per Measure KCAL	FAT	Nutrition Values per 100g / 100ml KCAL	PROT	CARB	FAT	FIBRE
COFFEE								
Cappuccino, Decaff, Nescafe*	1 Sachet/16g	68	2.3	428	11.6	62.6	14.6	0.0
Cappuccino, Decaff, Unsweetened, Nescafe*	1 Sachet/16g	70	3.1	437	14.5	51.2	19.4	4.3
Cappuccino, Dreamy, Cafe, Options*	1 Serving/30g	77	5.1	256	12.9	58.1	16.9	0.0
Cappuccino, Dry, Maxwell House*	1 Mug/15g	52	1.4	350	12.0	64.0	9.6	0.4
Cappuccino, Dry, Waitrose*	1 Sachet/13g	58	2.3	439	15.1	56.0	17.2	4.4
Cappuccino, for Filter Systems, Kenco*	1 Sachet/6g	22	0.8	375	19.0	44.0	13.5	0.0
Cappuccino, Instant, Aldi*	1 Sachet/13g	49	1.7	393	12.5	55.1	13.6	0.0
Cappuccino, Instant, Asda*	1 Sachet/15g	60	2.3	399	13.0	53.0	15.2	0.9
Cappuccino, Instant, Kenco*	1 Sachet/20g	80	2.8	401	13.5	55.7	13.8	0.0
Cappuccino, Instant, Made Up, Maxwell House*	1 Serving/280g	123	5.3	44	0.6	5.8	1.9	0.0
Cappuccino, Instant, Unsweetened, Douwe Egberts*	1 Serving/12g	48	1.9	400	11.0	53.0	16.0	0.0
Cappuccino, Italian, Nescafe*	1 Cup/150ml	60	2.9	40	1.2	4.4	1.9	0.0
Cappuccino, Made Up, Dolce Gusto, Nescafe*	1 Serving/240ml	84	3.7	35	1.6	4.0	1.5	0.3
Cappuccino, Original, Sachets, Nescafe*	1 Sachet/18g	80	3.1	444	11.7	60.3	17.4	0.0
Cappuccino, Sainsbury's*	1 Serving/12g	49	1.9	411	14.9	52.9	15.5	0.4
Cappuccino, Semi Skimmed Milk, Average	1 Serving/200ml	63	2.3	31	2.2	3.2	1.2	0.0
Cappuccino, to Go, Original, Nescafe*	1 Serving/19g	84	3.3	444	11.7	60.3	17.4	0.0
Cappuccino, to Go, Unsweetened, Nescafe*	1 Serving/17g	79	4.0	464	15.0	47.3	23.8	0.0
Cappuccino, Unsweetened, Cappio, Kenco*	1 Serving/18g	73	1.8	406	12.2	66.7	10.0	0.6
Cappuccino, Unsweetened, Nescafe*	1 Sachet/16g	74	3.8	464	15.0	47.3	23.8	0.0
Cappuccino, Unsweetened Taste, Maxwell House*	1 Serving/15g	65	2.9	434	17.4	47.6	19.3	0.3
Cappuccino Ice, Made Up, Dolce Gusto, Nescafe*	1 Serving/240ml	111	2.8	46	1.8	7.2	1.2	0.2
Chococino, Made up, Dolce Gusto, Nescafe*	1 Serving/210g	147	5.4	70	2.3	9.4	2.6	0.7
Columbian, Nescafe*	1 Serving/2g	2	0.0	111	16.7	11.1	0.0	5.6
Compliment*	1 Serving/14ml	20	1.8	143	1.4	6.4	12.9	0.0
Dandelion, Symingtons*	1 Round Tsp/6g	19	0.0	320	2.8	79.3	0.0	0.0
Espresso, Instant, Nescafe*	1 Tsp/2g	2	0.0	118	7.8	3.1	0.2	34.1
Espresso, Made Up, Dolce Gusto, Nescafe*	1 Serving/60ml	1	0.1	2	0.1	0.0	0.2	0.3
Frappe, Iced, Nestle*	1 Sachet/24g	92	1.0	384	15.0	72.0	4.0	0.5
Gold Blend, Decafefinated, Nescafe*	1 Tsp/5g	3	0.0	63	7.0	9.0	0.2	27.0
Gold Blend, Nescafe*	1 Cup 200ml/5g	3	0.0	63	7.0	9.0	0.2	27.0
Infusion, Average with Semi-Skimmed Milk	1 Cup/220ml	15	0.4	7	0.6	0.7	0.2	0.0
Infusion, Average with Single Cream	1 Cup/220ml	31	2.6	14	0.4	0.3	1.2	0.0
Infusion, Average with Whole Milk	1 Cup/220ml	15	0.9	7	0.5	0.5	0.4	0.0
Instant, Alta Rica, Nescafe*	1 Tsp/2g	2	0.0	98	13.8	10.0	0.3	21.0
Instant, Decaffeinated, Nescafe*	1 Tsp/2g	2	0.0	101	14.9	10.0	0.2	8.4
Instant, Fine Blend, Nescafe*	1 Tsp/2g	1	0.0	63	7.0	9.0	0.2	27.0
Instant, Made with Skimmed Milk	1 Serving/270ml	15	0.0	6	0.6	0.8	0.0	0.0
Instant, Made with Water & Semi-Skimmed Milk	1 Serving/350ml	24	1.4	7	0.4	0.5	0.4	0.0
Instant, Original, Nescafe*	1 Tsp/2g	1	0.0	63	7.0	9.0	0.2	27.0
Instant, with Skimmed Milk, Costa Rican, Kenco*	1 Mug/300ml	17	0.1	6	0.6	0.8	0.0	0.0
Latte, Cafe, M & S*	1 Serving/190g	142	5.3	75	4.3	8.3	2.8	0.0
Latte, Instant, Skinny, Douwe Egberts*	1 Serving/12g	35	1.3	290	11.0	38.0	11.0	29.0
Latte, Luscious, Options*	1 Serving/14g	62	2.4	443	14.3	57.9	17.1	3.6
Latte, Macchiato, Tassimo*	1 Cup/275ml	135	7.7	49	2.3	3.6	2.8	0.0
Latte, Nescafe*	1 Sachet/22g	110	6.3	498	14.5	45.7	28.5	0.0
Latte, No Sugar, in Cup, from Machine, Kenco*	1 Cup/4g	17	0.9	400	7.6	44.0	22.0	0.0
Latte, Skinny, Nescafe*	1 Sachet/20g	72	1.1	359	24.1	54.3	5.3	1.1
Latte Macchiato, Made Up, Dolce Gusto, Nescafe*	1 Serving/220ml	89	4.2	40	2.0	4.1	1.9	0.3
Mocha, Instant, Skinny, Douwe Egberts*	1 Serving/12g	37	1.3	308	10.8	40.8	10.8	5.0
Mocha, Made Up, Dolce Gusto, Nescafe*	1 Serving/210g	117	5.1	56	2.4	6.1	2.4	0.6
Mocha, Sainsbury's*	1 Serving/22g	84	3.0	383	14.0	51.0	13.7	1.3
Regular, Ground or Instant	1 Cup/177g	6	0.0	4	0.2	0.7	0.0	0.0

	Measure INFO/WEIGHT	per Measure KCAL	FAT	Nutrition Values per 100g / 100ml KCAL	PROT	CARB	FAT	FIBRE
COFFEE								
Skinny Cappuccino, Made Up, Dolce Gusto, Nescafe*	1 Mug/15g	49	0.1	337	33.3	48.8	0.9	2.3
COFFEE MATE								
Creamer, Hazelnut, Fat Free, Nestle*	1 Tbsp/15ml	25	0.0	167	0.0	33.3	0.0	0.0
Original, Nestle*	1 Tsp/4g	19	1.2	547	2.4	56.7	34.4	0.0
Virtually Fat Free, Nestle*	1 Tsp/5g	10	0.2	200	1.0	42.0	3.0	0.0
COFFEE SUBSTITUTE								
Bambu, Vogel*	1 Tsp/3g	10	0.0	320	3.5	75.3	0.5	0.0
COFFEE WHITENER								
Half Fat, Co-Op*	1 Tsp/5g	22	0.6	430	0.9	78.0	13.0	0.0
Light, Asda*	1 Serving/3g	13	0.4	433	0.9	78.0	13.0	0.0
Light, HE, Tesco*	1 Tsp/6g	27	1.0	449	3.5	71.0	16.8	0.0
Light, Tesco*	1 Tsp/3g	13	0.4	429	0.9	77.7	12.7	0.0
Morrisons*	1 Serving/10g	54	3.3	535	2.6	57.5	32.8	0.0
Tesco*	1 Tsp/3g	16	0.9	533	1.2	61.3	31.4	0.0
COGNAC								
40% Volume	***1 Shot/35ml***	***78***	***0.0***	***222***	***0.0***	***0.0***	***0.0***	***0.0***
French, All Flavours, Alize*	1 fl oz/30ml	69	0.0	230	0.0	6.7	0.0	0.0
COLA								
Average	1 Can/330ml	135	0.0	41	0.0	10.9	0.0	0.0
Coca Cola, Abokado*	1 Serving/330ml	135	0.0	41	0.0	10.9	0.0	0.0
Coca Cola, Diet, Abokado*	1 Serving/330ml	3	0.0	1	0.0	0.0	0.0	0.0
Coke, Cherry, Coca-Cola*	1 Bottle/500ml	225	0.0	45	0.0	11.2	0.0	0.0
Coke, Coca-Cola*	1 Can/330ml	142	0.0	43	0.0	10.7	0.0	0.0
Coke, Diet, Caffeine Free, Coca-Cola*	1 Can/330ml	1	0.0	0	0.0	0.1	0.0	0.0
Coke, Diet, Coca-Cola*	1 Can/330ml	1	0.0	0	0.0	0.0	0.0	0.0
Coke, Diet with Cherry, Coca-Cola*	1 Bottle/500ml	5	0.0	1	0.0	0.0	0.0	0.0
Coke, Vanilla, Coca-Cola*	1 Bottle/500ml	215	0.0	43	0.0	10.7	0.0	0.0
Coke, with Lemon, Diet, Coca-Cola*	1 Can/330ml	5	0.0	1	0.0	0.0	0.0	0.0
Coke, with Vanilla, Diet, Coca-Cola*	1 Glass/200ml	1	0.0	0	0.0	0.1	0.0	0.0
Curiosity, Fentiman's*	1 Bottle/275ml	129	0.0	47	0.1	11.6	0.0	0.0
Diet, Average	1 Serving/200ml	1	0.0	1	0.0	0.0	0.0	0.0
Diet, Pepsi*	1 Can/330ml	1	0.0	0	0.0	0.0	0.0	0.0
Diet, Virgin Trains*	1 Glass/250ml	1	0.2	0	0.1	0.1	0.1	0.0
Max, Pepsi*	1 Can/330ml	2	0.0	1	0.1	0.1	0.0	0.0
Pepsi*	1 Can/330ml	145	0.0	44	0.0	11.1	0.0	0.0
Royal Crown*	1 Serving/200ml	1	0.0	0	0.1	0.1	0.0	0.0
Twist, Light, Pepsi*	1 Bottle/500ml	4	0.0	1	0.0	0.1	0.0	0.0
Twist, Pepsi*	1 Bottle/500ml	235	0.0	47	0.0	11.7	0.0	0.0
Zero, Caffeine Free, Coca-Cola*	1 Glass/200ml	0	0.0	0	0.0	0.0	0.0	0.0
Zero, Coca-Cola*	1 Can/330ml	2	0.0	0	0.0	0.0	0.0	0.0
COLESLAW								
20% Less Fat, Asda*	1 Serving/100g	88	6.0	88	1.5	7.0	6.0	1.7
50% Less Fat, Asda*	1oz/28g	17	0.8	61	2.1	6.8	2.8	0.9
99% Fat Free, Kraft*	1 Serving/40ml	50	0.4	126	1.0	28.9	1.0	0.0
Aldi*	1 Serving/100g	206	18.7	206	0.8	8.6	18.7	0.0
Apple, Raisin & Walnut, TTD, Sainsbury's*	2 Heap Tbsp/75g	212	19.6	283	2.3	8.0	26.2	2.8
Asda*	1 Serving/100g	190	18.0	190	1.0	6.0	18.0	1.4
Bryn Wharf Food Co*	1 Serving/90g	109	9.4	121	1.4	5.7	10.4	1.8
Cheese, Asda*	1 Serving/100g	242	22.0	242	4.8	6.3	22.0	1.6
Cheese, Supreme, Waitrose*	¼ Pack/88g	197	18.2	225	4.5	5.0	20.8	1.2
Cheese, TTD, Sainsbury's*	¼ Pot/75g	213	20.4	284	5.0	4.7	27.2	2.7
Coronation, Sainsbury's*	¼ Pot/75g	145	11.6	193	1.0	11.4	15.5	1.9
COU, M & S*	½ Pack/125g	75	3.4	60	1.3	7.4	2.7	1.7

	Measure INFO/WEIGHT	per Measure KCAL	FAT	Nutrition Values per 100g / 100ml KCAL	PROT	CARB	FAT	FIBRE
COLESLAW								
Creamy, Asda*	1 Serving/25g	62	6.0	248	0.9	7.0	24.0	1.8
Creamy, GFY, Asda*	1 Serving/100g	163	14.9	163	0.7	6.5	14.9	0.8
Creamy, LC, Tesco*	1/3 Pot/100g	105	8.8	105	1.2	4.9	8.8	1.6
Crunchy, Premium, Millcroft*	1 Pack/400g	756	69.6	189	0.9	7.3	17.4	1.5
Deli Style, BGTY, Sainsbury's*	1 Serving/75g	75	5.6	100	1.1	6.2	7.5	1.7
Deli Style, M & S*	1 Serving/50g	110	10.6	220	1.0	4.8	21.2	1.9
Fruity, Asda*	½ Pot/125g	101	6.1	81	1.3	8.0	4.9	1.7
Fruity, M & S*	1 Serving/63g	151	14.3	240	1.1	8.3	22.7	3.1
Garlic & Herb, Asda*	1 Tbsp/15g	22	2.0	147	0.9	5.8	13.3	1.7
GFY, Asda*	1 Serving/50g	28	1.4	55	1.3	6.0	2.9	2.3
Iceland*	1 Serving/110g	112	8.2	102	0.7	7.8	7.5	1.6
Jalapeno, Sainsbury's*	1 Serving/75g	142	13.4	190	0.9	5.6	17.9	1.6
Luxury, Asda*	1 Serving/50g	108	10.5	217	0.9	6.0	21.0	0.0
Luxury, Lidl*	1 Serving/50g	102	9.7	203	0.9	5.9	19.4	0.0
Luxury, M & S*	1oz/28g	43	3.9	152	1.0	6.0	13.8	1.0
Luxury, Morrisons*	1 Serving/50g	136	13.5	273	1.2	6.4	27.0	0.0
Mango & Chilli, Sainsbury's*	1 Serving/75g	97	7.7	129	0.9	7.2	10.3	1.8
Organic, M & S*	1oz/28g	41	3.5	145	1.1	7.3	12.4	1.0
Piri Piri, Sainsbury's*	½ Tub/70g	113	9.9	162	1.1	6.6	14.2	1.8
Prawn, Chosen By You, Asda*	1 Pot/280g	490	43.1	175	2.2	6.8	15.4	1.8
Premium, Co-Op*	1 Serving/50g	160	17.0	320	1.0	3.0	34.0	2.0
Reduced Calorie, Iceland*	1 Serving/50g	51	3.8	102	0.7	7.8	7.5	1.6
Reduced Fat, Average	1 Tbsp/20g	23	1.9	113	1.0	6.4	9.3	2.0
Smart Price, Asda*	1oz/28g	30	2.2	107	0.8	8.0	8.0	2.0
Supreme, Waitrose*	1oz/28g	53	5.1	190	1.8	4.9	18.1	1.7
Tesco*	1 Serving/50g	79	7.2	158	2.2	5.2	14.3	1.6
Three Cheese, Asda*	1 Serving/78g	203	18.7	260	5.0	6.0	24.0	1.7
Three Cheese, Finest, Tesco*	1/3 Pack/100g	255	22.7	255	6.4	5.8	22.7	1.1
with Reduced Calorie Dressing, Retail	1 Serving/40g	27	1.8	67	0.9	6.1	4.5	1.4
COLEY								
Portions, Raw, Average	***1 Serving/92g***	***75***	***0.7***	***82***	***18.4***	***0.0***	***0.7***	***0.0***
Steamed, Average	***1oz/28g***	***29***	***0.4***	***105***	***23.3***	***0.0***	***1.3***	***0.0***
CONCHIGLIE								
Cooked, Average	***1 Serving/185g***	***247***	***1.6***	***134***	***4.8***	***26.6***	***0.8***	***0.6***
Dry Weight, Average	***1 Serving/100g***	***352***	***1.7***	***352***	***12.5***	***71.6***	***1.7***	***2.6***
Whole Wheat, Dry Weight, Average	***1 Serving/75g***	***237***	***1.5***	***316***	***12.6***	***62.0***	***2.0***	***10.7***
CONSERVE								
Apricot, Average	***1 Tbsp/15g***	***37***	***0.0***	***244***	***0.5***	***59.3***	***0.2***	***1.5***
Apricot, Reduced Sugar, Streamline*	1 Tbsp/20g	37	0.0	184	0.5	45.0	0.2	0.0
Black Cherry with Amaretto, Finest, Tesco*	1 Serving/10g	26	0.0	261	0.5	64.4	0.1	0.8
Blackcurrant, Average	***1 Tbsp/15g***	***37***	***0.0***	***245***	***0.6***	***60.0***	***0.1***	***1.9***
Blueberry, M & S*	1 Tsp/8g	15	0.0	206	0.3	51.1	0.1	1.3
Hedgerow, TTD, Sainsbury's*	1 Tbsp/15g	41	0.0	276	0.5	68.2	0.1	0.5
Morello Cherry, Waitrose*	1 Tbsp/15g	39	0.0	258	0.4	64.2	0.0	1.4
Plum, TTD, Sainsbury's*	1 Tbsp/15g	44	0.0	295	0.3	73.1	0.1	0.5
Raspberry, Average	***1 Tbsp/15g***	***37***	***0.1***	***249***	***0.6***	***61.0***	***0.3***	***1.3***
Red Cherry, TTD, Sainsbury's*	1 Tbsp/15g	43	0.0	283	0.4	70.2	0.1	0.5
Rhubarb & Ginger, M & S*	1 Tbsp/15g	29	0.0	194	0.3	47.9	0.1	1.0
Strawberry, 60% Fruit, Reduced Sugar, M & S*	1 Tsp/7g	9	0.0	135	0.4	30.1	0.2	1.9
Strawberry, Average	***1 Tbsp/15g***	***37***	***0.0***	***250***	***0.4***	***61.6***	***0.1***	***0.5***
CONSOMME								
Average	***1oz/28g***	***3***	***0.0***	***12***	***2.9***	***0.1***	***0.0***	***0.0***
Beef, Luxury, with Sherry, Baxters*	1 Can/415g	62	0.0	15	2.7	1.0	0.0	0.0

C

C

	Measure INFO/WEIGHT	per Measure KCAL	FAT	Nutrition Values per 100g / 100ml KCAL	PROT	CARB	FAT	FIBRE
COOKIES								
All Butter, Almond, Italian Style, M & S*	1 Cookie/23g	120	6.4	515	6.7	59.4	27.6	3.6
All Butter, Ginger Bread, M & S*	1 Cookie/23g	102	5.0	445	4.3	57.5	21.8	2.4
All Butter, Italian Style Sorrento Lemon, M & S*	1 Cookie/24g	120	6.4	500	4.9	60.4	26.7	2.1
All Butter, Melting Moment, M & S*	1 Cookie/23g	110	6.4	470	4.5	51.5	27.5	3.4
All Butter, Sultana, TTD, Sainsbury's*	1 Biscuit/17g	79	3.8	476	5.4	62.7	22.6	2.0
Almond, Ose*	1 Cookie/10g	46	1.4	456	8.4	74.0	14.0	0.0
Apple & Raisin, Go Ahead, McVitie's*	1 Cookie/15g	66	1.9	443	5.3	76.8	12.7	3.4
Apple Crumble, M & S*	1 Cookie/26g	90	0.5	345	4.6	76.8	2.0	2.9
Apple Pie, The Biscuit Collection*	1 Cookie/19g	90	4.2	474	3.9	65.0	22.1	0.0
Bites, Weight Watchers*	1 Pack/21g	97	4.0	464	5.8	67.0	19.2	4.3
Blueberry & Oatmeal, M & S*	1 Cookie/100g	90	3.5	90	1.1	13.4	3.5	0.5
Brazil Nut, Organic, Traidcraft*	1 Cookie/17g	91	5.4	547	5.8	57.7	32.6	2.1
Brazil Nut, Prewett's*	1 Cookie/50g	122	7.4	244	2.6	25.2	14.8	1.0
Butter & Sultana, Sainsbury's*	1 Cookie/13g	61	2.6	473	4.5	68.4	20.1	1.6
Cherry Bakewell, COU, M & S*	1 Cookie/25g	90	0.6	355	6.0	77.2	2.5	3.4
Choc, Double, Cadbury*	1 Biscuit/11g	55	2.5	485	7.3	64.3	22.2	0.0
Choc, Double, Maryland*	1 Cookie/10g	51	2.6	510	5.2	64.4	25.7	0.0
Choc Chip, Cadbury*	1 Cookie/11g	55	2.8	503	5.9	62.2	25.6	0.0
Choc Chip, Double, Giant, Paterson's*	1 Cookie/60g	293	15.2	489	0.3	61.3	25.3	3.7
Choc Chip, Double, Mini, M & S*	1 Cookie/22g	108	5.2	490	5.3	63.6	23.7	1.8
Choc Chip, Double, Tesco*	1 Cookie/11g	55	2.7	500	4.2	65.3	24.7	3.0
Choc Chip, Double, Weight Watchers*	1 Biscuit/11g	49	1.9	443	7.6	65.4	17.2	4.6
Choc Chip, Giant, Paterson's*	1 Cookie/60g	296	15.2	493	0.1	61.3	25.3	3.2
Choc Chip, Lyons*	1 Cookie/11g	57	2.7	499	5.2	68.3	23.4	1.7
Choc Chip, Maryland*	1 Cookie/11g	56	2.6	511	6.2	68.0	23.9	1.3
Choc Chip, Parkside*	1 Cookie/11g	56	2.7	495	5.3	64.5	23.7	0.0
Choc Chip, Reduced Fat, Maryland*	1 Cookie/11g	51	1.9	478	5.9	73.0	18.0	0.0
Choc Chip & Coconut, Maryland*	1 Cookie/10g	55	2.5	512	5.1	62.9	23.7	0.0
Choc Chip & Hazelnut, Maryland*	1 Cookie/11g	55	2.7	513	6.3	65.3	25.0	0.0
Choc Chip 'n' Chunk, McVitie's*	1 Cookie/11g	55	2.9	498	5.8	59.2	26.4	3.5
Choc Chunk, & Hazelnut, Luxury, Cadbury*	1oz/28g	146	8.0	521	6.3	60.0	28.7	0.0
Choc Chunk, Fabulous Bakin' Boys*	1 Cookie/60g	270	12.6	450	5.0	59.0	21.0	3.0
Choc Chunk, Finest, Tesco*	1 Cookie/80g	355	14.1	445	5.7	65.3	17.7	1.8
Chocolate, Almond & Toffee, Kate's Cakes Ltd*	1 Serving/100g	406	14.9	406	5.5	62.5	14.9	2.4
Chocolate, Belgian, Extra Special, Asda*	1 Cookie/26g	138	8.0	535	6.0	58.0	31.0	2.0
Chocolate, Double, & Walnut, Soft, Tesco*	1 Cookie/25g	116	6.4	463	5.8	52.1	25.7	4.7
Chocolate, Double, Premium, Co-Op*	1 Cookie/17g	86	4.6	505	5.0	62.0	27.0	2.0
Chocolate, Milk, Classic, Millie's Cookies*	1 Cookie/45g	190	10.2	422	5.1	49.3	22.7	1.3
Chocolate, Milk, Free From, Tesco*	1 Cookie/20g	100	6.1	500	5.6	50.4	30.7	4.1
Chocolate, Quadruple, Sainsbury's*	1 Cookie/20g	117	6.6	585	6.0	66.5	33.0	1.5
Chocolate, Soft, American Style, Budgens*	1 Cookie/50g	216	9.3	431	5.1	60.8	18.6	2.2
Chocolate, Triple, Greggs*	1 Serving/100g	489	24.5	489	5.8	61.4	24.5	4.2
Chocolate, White, & Cranberry, Devondale*	1 Cookie/65g	300	15.3	462	4.7	60.7	23.5	2.1
Chocolate, White, & Cranberry, Kate's Cakes Ltd*	1 Serving/100g	389	13.4	389	4.7	62.3	13.4	2.0
Chocolate, White, & Raspberry, Finest, Tesco*	1 Cookie/76g	304	9.6	400	5.2	66.3	12.6	2.4
Chocolate, White, & Raspberry, McVitie's*	1 Cookie/17g	87	4.4	512	4.7	64.1	25.9	1.8
Chocolate, White, Asda*	1 Cookie/54g	256	11.9	474	5.0	64.0	22.0	2.1
Chocolate, White, Maryland*	1 Cookie/10g	51	2.5	512	5.7	64.0	25.0	0.0
Chocolate & Nut, Organic, Evernat*	1 Cookie/69g	337	15.6	489	7.2	64.1	22.6	0.0
Chocolate & Orange, COU, M & S*	1 Cookie/26g	90	0.7	350	5.7	77.2	2.6	3.2
Chocolate Chip, Average	1 Cookie/10g	49	2.5	489	5.5	64.1	24.7	2.9
Chocolate Chip, BGTY, Sainsbury's*	1 Cookie/17g	72	2.0	428	4.5	75.6	11.9	2.5
Chocolate Chip, Carb Check, Heinz*	1 Cookie/20g	91	5.0	457	7.2	43.1	24.9	7.2

	Measure INFO/WEIGHT	per Measure KCAL	FAT	Nutrition Values per 100g / 100ml KCAL	PROT	CARB	FAT	FIBRE
COOKIES								
Chocolate Chip, Chips Ahoy*	1 Cookie/11g	55	2.8	500	6.0	65.0	25.0	3.0
Chocolate Chip, Double, Co-Op*	1 Cookie/17g	87	4.6	510	5.0	63.0	27.0	2.0
Chocolate Chip, Double, Organic, Waitrose*	1 Cookie/18g	96	5.6	535	5.1	58.6	31.0	1.9
Chocolate Chip, GF, Organic, Dove's Farm*	1 Cookie/17g	77	3.1	451	4.3	66.9	18.5	0.0
Chocolate Chip, GFY, Asda*	1 Cookie/10g	48	2.0	463	5.0	68.0	19.0	3.5
Chocolate Chip, Gluten & Wheat Free, Lovemore*	1 Cookie/17g	81	4.5	483	3.8	57.8	26.8	3.5
Chocolate Chip, Handbaked, Border*	1 Cookie/15g	72	3.4	480	5.9	67.4	22.6	0.0
Chocolate Chip, Lyons*	1 Cookie/12g	56	2.5	483	5.6	66.5	21.6	1.7
Chocolate Chip, McVitie's*	1 Cookie/11g	54	2.8	496	5.8	60.2	25.8	3.0
Chocolate Chip, Mini, McVitie's*	1 Bag/40g	196	9.2	491	5.5	65.1	23.1	2.8
Chocolate Chip, Organic, Sainsbury's*	1 Cookie/17g	89	4.9	530	5.0	61.8	29.2	0.3
Chocolate Chip, Weight Watchers*	1 Cookie/11g	49	1.9	443	7.6	65.4	17.2	4.6
Chocolate Chip & Hazelnut, Extra Special, Asda*	1 Cookie/25g	130	8.1	516	6.0	51.0	32.0	2.5
Chocolate Chunk, Cadbury*	1 Cookie/22g	119	6.9	540	6.5	58.0	31.2	0.0
Chocolate Chunk, Devondale*	1 Cookie/65g	308	16.3	474	4.6	59.2	25.1	2.8
Chocolate Chunk, Milk, Average	1 Cookie/25g	129	6.9	515	6.6	60.0	27.6	1.6
Chocolate Chunk, Triple, Bakery, Finest, Tesco*	1 Cookie/80g	360	15.9	450	7.4	59.2	19.9	2.1
Chocolate Chunk, White, Average	1 Cookie/25g	124	6.2	498	5.5	62.8	24.8	1.0
Coconut, Gluten-Free, Sainsbury's*	1 Cookie/20g	103	6.1	516	5.6	54.4	30.7	4.1
Coconut & Raspberry, GF, Sainsbury's*	1 Cookie/20g	102	5.9	511	5.9	56.0	29.3	6.7
Cranberry & Orange, Finest, Tesco*	1 Cookie/26g	125	5.8	490	4.1	67.4	22.6	3.2
Cranberry & Orange, Go Ahead, McVitie's*	1 Cookie/17g	77	2.2	452	5.3	78.0	13.2	2.4
Crunchy Muesli, Mini, Shapers, Boots*	1 Pack/30g	134	4.5	448	6.7	71.0	15.0	1.8
Danish Butter, Tesco*	1 Cookie/26g	133	6.6	516	4.7	66.7	25.6	1.3
Fortune, Average	1 Cookie/8g	30	0.2	378	4.2	84.0	2.7	1.6
Fruit, Giant, Cookie Coach*	1 Cookie/60g	280	13.2	466	4.9	62.0	22.0	0.0
Fudge Brownie, Maryland*	1 Cookie/11g	56	2.8	510	5.8	63.0	25.0	0.0
Fudge Brownie American Cream, Sainsbury's*	1 Cookie/12g	60	2.8	499	4.8	67.9	23.2	2.2
Ginger, GF, Barkat*	1 Cookie/17g	85	4.4	501	3.2	63.8	25.9	0.0
Ginger, Low Fat, M & S*	1 Cookie/23g	82	1.0	358	5.1	74.9	4.3	2.4
Glace Cherry, Border*	1 Cookie/15g	74	3.8	493	5.4	64.3	25.6	0.0
Hazelnut, GF, Organic, Dove's Farm*	1 Cookie/17g	79	3.7	463	4.8	61.5	21.9	1.8
Lemon & Currant, Weight Watchers*	2 Cookies/19g	86	3.4	451	5.1	63.6	17.7	8.4
Lemon Meringue, COU, M & S*	1 Cookie/25g	89	0.6	355	5.6	77.6	2.6	3.0
Lemon Zest, GF, Organic, Dove's Farm*	1 Cookie/17g	80	3.1	473	3.3	73.7	18.3	0.0
Oat, Giant Jumbo, Paterson's*	1 Cookie/60g	299	16.2	499	0.4	58.4	27.0	3.2
Oat & Cranberry, BGTY, Sainsbury's*	1 Cookie/28g	126	5.0	449	6.8	65.0	18.0	5.1
Oat & Fruit, Kate's Cakes Ltd*	1 Serving/100g	418	18.2	418	4.2	59.5	18.2	3.0
Oat & Raisin, Health Matters*	1 Cookie/8g	33	0.7	414	7.0	76.6	8.8	3.3
Oatflake & Raisin, Waitrose*	1 Cookie/17g	80	3.8	469	5.8	61.7	22.1	4.7
Oatmeal, Chocolate Chip, Chewy, Dad's*	1 Cookie/15g	70	3.0	467	6.7	66.7	20.0	3.3
Oreo, Mini, Oreo*	1 Pack/25g	120	4.8	480	4.8	70.0	19.2	2.4
Oreo*	1 Cookie/11g	52	2.3	471	5.9	70.6	20.6	2.9
Pecan & Maple, Mini, Bronte*	1 Pack/100g	509	27.3	509	5.4	60.3	27.3	1.6
Praline Nougatine, Belle France*	1 Cookie/17g	84	4.2	506	8.0	63.0	25.0	0.0
Raisin & Cinnamon, Low Fat, M & S*	1 Cookie/22g	78	0.9	355	6.2	73.0	4.1	3.2
Raspberry Spritz, Heaven Scent*	1 Cookie/19g	90	6.0	474	5.3	52.6	31.6	0.0
Rolo, Nestle*	1 Cookie/39g	178	7.4	456	5.4	64.8	19.0	2.2
Stem Ginger, Aldi*	1 Cookie/13g	58	2.4	463	3.6	68.5	19.4	0.0
Stem Ginger, BGTY, Sainsbury's*	1 Cookie/17g	73	2.0	431	4.5	76.5	11.9	1.7
Stem Ginger, Free From, Sainsbury's*	1 Cookie/17g	84	4.8	489	6.5	58.0	28.0	6.8
Stem Ginger, Reduced Fat, Waitrose*	1 Cookie/17g	75	2.7	448	4.5	71.0	16.2	1.6
Stem Ginger, Tesco*	1 Cookie/20g	98	4.8	489	4.2	64.0	24.0	2.0

	Measure INFO/WEIGHT	per Measure KCAL	FAT	Nutrition Values per 100g / 100ml KCAL	PROT	CARB	FAT	FIBRE
COOKIES								
Stem Ginger, TTD, Sainsbury's*	1 Cookie/17g	79	3.7	476	5.2	64.3	22.0	2.3
Sultana, All Butter, Reduced Fat, M & S*	1 Cookie/17g	70	2.4	420	4.9	68.6	14.2	2.6
Sultana, Soft & Chewy, Sainsbury's*	1 Cookie/25g	104	3.5	414	4.4	67.8	13.9	2.5
Sultana & Cinnamon, Weight Watchers*	1 Cookie/12g	46	1.4	398	5.0	67.1	12.1	1.8
Tennessee American Style, Stiftung & Co*	1 Cookie/19g	96	4.6	504	6.0	66.0	24.0	0.0
Toffee, Weight Watchers*	1 Cookie/12g	52	1.9	456	5.2	71.1	16.8	2.9
COQ AU VIN								
Diet Chef Ltd*	1 Pack/300g	285	13.2	95	7.7	6.1	4.4	2.2
Finest, Tesco*	1 Serving/273g	251	9.8	92	14.3	0.7	3.6	1.8
HL, Tesco*	½ Pack/200g	172	3.8	86	15.2	2.1	1.9	0.4
M & S*	1 Serving/295g	398	22.7	135	14.2	1.5	7.7	1.0
Perfectly Balanced, Waitrose*	1 Pack/500g	445	15.5	89	12.6	2.7	3.1	0.6
Sainsbury's*	1 Pack/400g	484	17.6	121	16.8	3.5	4.4	0.2
with Potatoes, Diet Chef Ltd*	1 Pack/300g	285	13.2	95	7.7	6.1	4.4	2.2
CORDIAL								
Blackcurrant, New Zealand Honey Co*	1 Serving/30ml	109	0.3	363	1.0	88.0	1.0	0.0
Elderflower, Made Up, Bottle Green*	1 Glass/200ml	46	0.0	23	0.0	5.6	0.0	0.0
Elderflower, Undiluted, Waitrose*	1 Serving/20ml	22	0.0	110	0.0	27.5	0.0	0.0
Honey & Lemonbalm with Chamomile, Bottle Green*	1 fl oz/30ml	8	0.0	27	0.0	6.8	0.0	0.0
Lemon & Lime, High Juice, M & S*	1 Glass/250ml	75	0.0	30	0.0	7.0	0.0	0.0
Lime, Juice, Diluted, Rose's*	1 Serving/50ml	12	0.0	24	0.0	5.7	0.0	0.0
Lime, with Aromatic Bitters & Ginger, Sainsbury's*	1 Serving/40ml	12	0.1	29	0.0	6.9	0.3	0.3
Lime Juice, Concentrated	1 Serving/20ml	22	0.0	112	0.1	29.8	0.0	0.0
Lime Juice, Diluted	1 Glass/250ml	55	0.0	22	0.0	6.0	0.0	0.0
Pomegranate & Elderflower, Bottle Green*	1 fl oz/30ml	7	0.0	22	0.0	5.6	0.0	0.0
Pomegreat, Original, Pomegreat*	1 Serving/50ml	16	0.0	32	0.0	7.6	0.0	0.0
CORIANDER								
Leaves, Dried, Average	***1oz/28g***	***78***	***1.3***	***279***	***21.8***	***41.7***	***4.8***	***0.0***
Leaves, Fresh, Average	***1 Bunch/20g***	***5***	***0.1***	***23***	***2.1***	***3.7***	***0.5***	***2.8***
Seeds, Ground, Schwartz*	1 Tsp/5g	22	0.9	446	14.2	54.9	18.8	0.0
CORN								
Baby, & Mange Tout, Eat Fresh, Tesco*	1 Serving/100g	31	0.2	31	2.9	3.3	0.2	2.1
Baby, Average	***1 Serving/80g***	***21***	***0.3***	***26***	***2.5***	***3.1***	***0.4***	***1.7***
Baby & Asparagus Tips, Tesco*	1 Pack/150g	38	0.8	25	2.6	2.5	0.5	1.9
Cobs, Boiled, Weighed with Cob, Average	***1 Ear/200g***	***132***	***2.8***	***66***	***2.5***	***11.6***	***1.4***	***1.3***
Creamed Style, Green Giant*	1 Can/418g	238	2.1	57	1.2	11.9	0.5	3.0
CORN CAKES								
M & S*	½ Pack/85g	238	17.0	280	6.4	19.8	20.0	3.4
Organic, Kallo*	1 Cake/5g	16	0.2	340	12.7	74.3	4.1	11.2
Slightly Salted, Mrs Crimble's*	1 Pack/28g	104	0.9	380	7.9	80.0	3.4	5.4
Thick Slices, Orgran*	1 Cake/11g	42	0.4	385	13.2	79.0	3.7	14.2
CORN MEAL								
Yellow, Enriched & Degerminated, Dry, Quaker Oats*	1 Tbsp/9g	30	0.2	333	7.4	77.8	1.8	7.4
CORNED BEEF								
Average	***1 Slice/35g***	***75***	***4.3***	***214***	***25.9***	***0.7***	***12.2***	***0.0***
Lean, Healthy Range, Average	***1 Slice/30g***	***57***	***2.6***	***191***	***27.0***	***1.0***	***8.7***	***0.0***
Sliced, Premium, Average	***1 Slice/31g***	***69***	***3.9***	***222***	***26.6***	***0.5***	***12.6***	***0.0***
Slices, Value, Tesco*	1 Slice/31g	66	3.7	213	26.0	0.8	11.8	0.0
CORNFLOUR								
Average	***1 Tsp/5g***	***18***	***0.1***	***355***	***0.6***	***86.9***	***1.2***	***0.1***
COURGETTE								
Fried, Average	***1oz/28g***	***18***	***1.3***	***63***	***2.6***	***2.6***	***4.8***	***1.2***
Raw, Average	***1 Courgette/224g***	***40***	***0.9***	***18***	***1.8***	***1.8***	***0.4***	***0.9***

	Measure INFO/WEIGHT	per Measure KCAL	FAT	Nutrition Values per 100g / 100ml KCAL	PROT	CARB	FAT	FIBRE
COURGETTE								
Stuffed, Round, Lovely Vegetables, M & S*	½ Pack/200g	110	2.6	55	1.8	7.7	1.3	1.8
COUS COUS								
& Chargrilled Vegetables, M & S*	1 Serving/200g	200	3.0	100	3.9	17.3	1.5	1.6
& Chickpeas, TTD, Sainsbury's*	¼ Pot/72g	121	6.8	167	4.7	15.8	9.4	1.4
& Wok Oriental, Findus*	½ Pack/300g	510	25.5	170	4.5	19.0	8.5	0.0
Citrus Kick, Dry, Ainsley Harriott*	½ Sachet/50g	184	1.2	368	11.6	77.0	2.4	9.2
Cooked, Average	***1 Tbsp/15g***	***24***	***0.3***	***158***	***4.3***	***31.4***	***1.9***	***1.3***
Dry, Average	***1 Serving/50g***	***178***	***0.7***	***356***	***13.7***	***72.8***	***1.5***	***2.6***
Garlic & Coriander, Dry, Waitrose*	1 Serving/70g	235	2.5	336	11.7	64.2	3.6	6.2
Giant, Tesco*	1 Pack/220g	350	14.4	160	4.1	20.7	6.6	1.2
Indian Style, Sainsbury's*	½ Pack/143g	204	3.9	143	4.5	25.1	2.7	1.0
Lemon & Coriander, Dry, Tesco*	1 Pack/110g	375	3.0	341	11.0	68.2	2.7	6.1
Mediterranean Style, Dry, Tesco*	1 Pack/110g	368	3.3	335	11.9	65.1	3.0	5.6
Moroccan Medley, Ainsley Harriott*	½ Sachet/130g	178	2.0	137	5.4	25.4	1.5	2.2
Moroccan Style, Break, GFY, Asda*	1 Pack/150g	215	2.7	143	5.6	26.1	1.8	1.8
Moroccan Style, Cooked, Sainsbury's*	½ Pack/140g	200	1.1	143	6.2	26.4	0.8	2.5
Moroccan Style, Finest, Tesco*	1 Tub/225g	292	5.6	130	4.3	22.6	2.5	3.7
Moroccan Style, Fruity, M & S*	1 Serving/200g	370	5.4	185	3.4	36.7	2.7	3.4
Moroccan Style, TTD, Sainsbury's*	1 Pot/200g	364	7.2	182	4.4	30.3	3.6	5.5
Moroccan Sultana & Pine Nuts, Dry, Sammy's*	1 Serving/50g	172	1.5	343	12.0	72.0	3.0	6.0
Mushroom & Garlic, Cooked, Morrisons*	1 Serving/100g	164	3.0	164	5.7	28.7	3.0	1.7
Mushrooms, Onion, Garlic & Herbs, Dry, Tesco*	½ Pack/50g	166	1.3	333	11.3	66.2	2.6	4.9
Red & Yellow Pepper, Chargrilled, Tesco*	1 Pack/200g	212	3.6	106	4.6	17.8	1.8	0.5
Red Pepper & Chilli, Waitrose*	1 Pack/200g	344	13.8	172	4.5	23.0	6.9	1.3
Spice Fusion, Lyttos*	1 Serving/100g	134	1.5	134	4.3	23.9	1.5	3.4
Spice Sensation, Dry, Ainsley Harriott*	½ Sachet/50g	166	1.2	332	11.6	66.2	2.4	9.2
Tomato, Mediterranean, GFY, Asda*	½ Pack/141g	192	1.3	136	5.0	27.0	0.9	1.7
Tomato, Tangy, Dry, Ainsley Harriott*	½ Sachet/50g	166	0.8	332	12.2	67.2	1.6	8.8
Tomato & Basil, Made Up, Tesco*	1 Serving/200g	348	16.6	174	3.9	21.0	8.3	3.4
Tomato & Onion, Dry Weight, Waitrose*	1 Pack/110g	376	4.0	342	12.6	64.9	3.6	5.1
Vegetable, Chargrilled, Morrisons*	1 Serving/225g	227	5.4	101	3.3	16.5	2.4	1.3
Vegetable, Roast, Veg Pot, Summer, Innocent*	1 Pot/400g	460	9.2	115	3.6	17.5	2.3	4.3
Vegetable, Roasted, Dry, Ainsley Harriott*	½ Sachet/50g	180	2.0	360	14.6	66.4	4.0	6.8
Vegetable, Roasted, Waitrose*	1 Serving/200g	328	13.2	164	3.9	22.0	6.6	0.9
Vegetable, Spicy, GFY, Asda*	½ Pack/55g	71	0.6	129	4.7	25.0	1.1	2.0
Vegetable, Spicy, Morrisons*	1 Pack/110g	187	5.5	170	5.1	26.2	5.0	2.9
Wholewheat, Tesco*	1 Serving/50g	178	1.0	355	12.0	72.0	2.0	5.0
CRAB								
Blue, Soft Shelled, Raw, Average	1 Crab/84g	73	0.9	87	18.1	0.0	1.1	0.0
Boiled, Meat Only, Average	***1 Tbsp/40g***	***51***	***2.2***	***128***	***19.5***	***0.0***	***5.5***	***0.0***
Brown, Cornish, Seafood & Eat It*	1 Pack/100g	171	10.7	171	17.9	1.9	10.7	0.0
Claws, Asda*	1oz/28g	25	0.3	89	11.0	9.0	1.0	0.2
Cocktail, Waitrose*	1 Serving/100g	217	17.6	217	10.8	3.8	17.6	0.4
Cornish 50/50, Seafood & Eat It*	1 Pot/100g	144	5.8	144	21.6	1.2	5.8	0.5
Cornish Potted, Seafood & Eat It*	1 Pack/100g	235	17.5	235	15.0	5.1	17.5	0.8
Dressed, Average	***1 Can/43g***	***66***	***3.4***	***154***	***16.8***	***4.1***	***7.9***	***0.2***
Meat, Raw, Average	***1oz/28g***	***28***	***0.2***	***100***	***20.8***	***2.8***	***0.6***	***0.0***
Meat in Brine, Average	***½ Can/60g***	***46***	***0.3***	***76***	***17.2***	***0.9***	***0.4***	***0.1***
White Cornish, Seafood & Eat It*	1 Pack/100g	81	0.5	81	19.0	0.1	0.5	0.0
White Meat, See Food & Eat It*	1 Pack/100g	81	0.5	81	19.0	0.1	0.5	0.0
CRAB CAKES								
Goan, M & S*	1 Pack/190g	228	7.6	120	8.0	12.9	4.0	1.8
Iceland*	1 Serving/18g	52	3.2	288	7.2	25.6	18.0	1.3

	Measure INFO/WEIGHT	per Measure KCAL	FAT	Nutrition Values per 100g / 100ml KCAL	PROT	CARB	FAT	FIBRE
CRAB CAKES								
Shetland Isles, Dressed, TTD, Sainsbury's*	1 Crab/75g	130	8.3	174	12.4	6.0	11.1	0.5
Tesco*	1 Serving/130g	281	16.0	216	11.0	15.4	12.3	1.1
Thai, TTD, Sainsbury's*	½ Pack/106g	201	9.5	189	9.5	17.8	8.9	1.4
CRAB STICKS								
Average	1 Stick/15g	14	0.0	94	9.1	13.9	0.3	0.0
CRACKERBREAD								
Original, Ryvita*	1 Slice/5g	19	0.1	378	10.8	75.0	2.8	4.8
Wholegrain, Ryvita*	1 Slice/6g	20	0.2	360	12.4	68.7	3.9	9.8
CRACKERS								
Bath Oliver, Jacob's*	1 Cracker/12g	52	1.6	432	9.6	67.6	13.7	2.6
Black Olive, M & S*	1 Cracker/4g	20	1.0	485	8.3	59.4	23.5	4.3
Black Pepper, for Cheese, Ryvita*	1 Cracker/7g	27	0.2	384	13.2	72.9	2.9	6.8
Bran, Jacob's*	1 Cracker/7g	32	1.3	454	9.7	62.8	18.2	3.2
Butter Puff, Sainsbury's*	1 Cracker/10g	54	2.7	523	10.4	60.7	26.5	2.5
Chapati Chips, Tikka, Medium Spicy, Patak's*	1 Serving/25g	127	7.0	508	8.0	56.0	28.0	4.0
Cheese, Cheddar, Crispies, TTD, Sainsbury's*	1 Thin/4g	21	1.5	576	14.2	39.0	40.4	2.2
Cheese, Mini, Heinz*	1 Pack/25g	108	3.6	433	9.4	68.6	14.6	0.6
Cheese, Mini, Shapers, Boots*	1 Serving/23g	97	3.2	421	9.4	65.0	14.0	4.6
Cheese, Ritz*	1 Cracker/4g	17	0.9	486	10.1	55.9	24.7	2.2
Cheese, Trufree*	1 Cracker/8g	42	2.6	524	9.0	50.0	32.0	0.5
Cheese Thins, Asda*	1 Cracker/4g	21	1.3	532	12.0	49.0	32.0	0.0
Cheese Thins, Cheddar, The Planet Snack Co*	1 Serving/30g	153	8.8	509	11.5	50.1	29.2	2.1
Cheese Thins, Co-Op*	1 Cracker/4g	21	1.3	530	12.0	49.0	32.0	3.0
Cheese Thins, Mini, Snack Rite*	1 Bag/30g	144	6.8	480	12.9	55.9	22.7	2.5
Cheese Thins, Waitrose*	1 Cracker/4g	21	1.2	545	11.9	52.6	31.9	2.5
Chinese, Pop Pan*	1 Cracker/8g	40	2.5	533	13.3	53.3	33.3	0.0
Chives, Jacob's*	1 Cracker/6g	28	1.0	457	9.5	67.5	16.5	2.7
Corn Thins, 97% Fat Free, Real Foods*	1 Cracker/6g	23	0.2	378	10.2	81.7	3.0	8.6
Corn Thins, Real Foods*	1 Serving/6g	22	0.2	378	10.2	81.7	3.0	8.6
Cream, 45% Less Fat, Morrisons*	1 Cracker/8g	32	0.6	403	10.5	74.2	7.1	3.3
Cream, Average	1 Cracker/7g	31	1.1	440	9.5	68.3	16.3	2.2
Cream, BFY, Morrisons*	1 Cracker/8g	32	0.6	406	10.9	74.4	7.2	2.8
Cream, Choice Grain, Jacob's*	1 Cracker/7g	30	0.9	400	9.0	64.5	11.8	7.0
Cream, Excelsior*	5 Crackers/30g	120	0.0	400	0.0	80.0	0.0	3.3
Cream, Jacob's*	1 Cracker/8g	34	1.1	431	10.0	67.5	13.5	3.8
Cream, Light, Jacob's*	1 Cracker/8g	31	0.5	388	10.6	72.2	6.3	4.1
Cream, Reduced Fat, Tesco*	1 Cracker/8g	31	0.5	406	10.9	74.4	7.2	2.8
Cream, Roasted Onion, Jacob's*	1 Cracker/8g	35	1.2	441	10.2	66.8	14.8	2.9
Cream, Sun Dried Tomato Flavour, Jacob's*	1 Cracker/8g	35	1.1	434	10.2	66.7	14.0	3.0
Crispy Cheese, M & S*	1 Cracker/4g	20	1.0	470	9.4	58.1	22.1	3.0
Cruskits, Arnotts*	2 Cruskits/12g	40	0.2	331	9.0	63.7	1.5	0.0
Extra Wheatgerm, Hovis*	1 Serving/6g	27	1.1	447	10.2	60.0	18.5	4.4
Firecracker, The, Graze*	1 Punnet/24g	120	6.8	520	10.5	52.6	29.5	2.0
Garden Herbs, Jacob's*	1 Cracker/6g	28	1.0	457	9.5	67.5	16.5	2.7
Garlic, Chosen By You, Asda*	2 Biscuits/12g	58	2.6	483	7.0	63.3	21.5	4.2
Garlic & Herb, Jacob's*	1 Cracker/100g	450	16.7	450	10.0	68.3	16.7	3.3
Glutafin*	1 Serving/11g	52	2.2	470	2.4	70.0	20.0	0.7
Golden Rye, for Cheese, Ryvita*	1 Cracker/7g	27	0.2	384	13.2	72.9	2.9	6.5
Herb & Onion, 99% Fat Free, Rakusen's*	1 Cracker/5g	18	0.0	360	9.1	82.6	1.0	3.9
Herb & Onion, Trufree*	1 Cracker/6g	25	0.7	418	2.5	75.0	12.0	10.0
Herb & Spice, Jacob's*	1 Cracker/6g	27	1.0	457	9.5	67.5	16.5	2.7
Herbs & Spice Selection, Jacob's*	1 Cracker/6g	27	0.9	451	9.5	68.0	15.7	2.7
Krackawheat, McVitie's*	1 Cracker/7g	33	1.4	446	9.7	60.0	18.6	5.8

	Measure INFO/WEIGHT	per Measure KCAL	FAT	Nutrition Values per 100g / 100ml KCAL	PROT	CARB	FAT	FIBRE
CRACKERS								
Light & Crispy, Sainsbury's*	1 Cracker/11g	42	1.2	384	11.3	61.0	10.5	13.0
Lightly Salted, Crispy, Sainsbury's*	1 Cracker/5g	25	1.3	533	7.8	62.6	27.9	2.1
Lightly Salted, Italian, Jacob's*	1 Cracker/6g	26	0.8	429	10.3	67.6	13.0	2.9
Mediterranean, Jacob's*	1 Cracker/6g	27	1.0	450	9.7	66.5	16.1	2.7
Multigrain, Corn Thins, Real Foods*	1 Cracker/6g	23	0.2	388	10.9	71.0	3.7	10.3
Multigrain, Morrisons*	10 Crackers/20g	76	2.2	379	8.8	61.3	11.0	5.1
Multigrain, Savour Bakes, Aldi*	1 Cracker/5g	20	0.8	404	8.3	55.0	16.8	5.1
Multigrain, Snack Crackers, Special K, Kellogg's*	1 Pack/30g	120	3.0	400	10.0	73.3	10.0	6.7
Multigrain, Tesco*	1 Cracker/6g	27	1.1	458	8.5	64.5	18.4	4.1
Peanut, Wasabi, Graze*	1 Pack/26g	125	5.6	479	15.2	53.8	21.4	5.4
Peking Dynasty, Graze*	1 Punnet/26g	130	7.3	498	19.8	43.1	27.9	4.6
Pesto, Jacob's*	1 Cracker/6g	27	1.0	450	9.7	66.5	16.1	2.7
Poppy & Sesame Seed, Sainsbury's*	1 Cracker/4g	21	1.1	530	9.6	58.9	28.4	3.4
Ritz, Mini, Kraft*	1 Bag/25g	126	6.0	504	7.9	63.0	24.0	2.0
Ritz, Original, Jacob's*	1 Cracker/3g	17	1.0	509	6.9	55.6	28.8	2.0
Rye, Organic, Dove's Farm*	1 Cracker/7g	28	1.0	393	7.0	58.4	14.6	8.7
Salt & Black Pepper, Eat Well, M & S*	1 Pack/25g	106	3.7	422	9.6	62.9	14.7	5.1
Salt & Black Pepper, Jacob's*	1 Cracker/6g	27	1.0	457	9.5	67.5	16.5	2.7
Salt & Pepper, Sainsbury's*	1 Cracker/6g	27	1.2	485	7.3	64.5	21.3	3.0
Salted, Ritz, Nabisco*	1 Cracker/3g	17	0.9	493	7.0	57.5	26.1	2.9
Selection, Finest, Tesco*	1 Serving/30g	136	4.3	452	9.6	71.0	14.4	0.0
Sesame & Poppy Thins, Tesco*	1 Cracker/4g	20	1.0	485	9.9	57.6	23.5	4.4
Sweet Chilli, Thins, Savours, Jacob's*	1 Cracker/4g	21	0.9	472	8.0	62.3	21.2	3.6
Tarallini, with Fennel Seeds, Crosta & Mollica*	1 Cracker/4g	21	0.9	529	8.2	67.5	22.0	4.2
Thai Spiced, Blue Dragon*	10 Crackers/10g	54	3.1	536	1.5	61.0	31.2	2.1
The British Barbecue, Graze*	1 Punnet/23g	117	7.4	508	17.4	36.8	32.2	7.4
Tom Yum Yum, Graze*	1 Pack/23g	90	0.6	390	7.2	84.8	2.4	1.4
Tuc, Cheese Sandwich, Jacob's*	1 Cracker/14g	72	4.3	531	8.4	53.8	31.4	0.0
Tuc, Jacob's*	1 Cracker/5g	25	1.4	517	7.7	56.4	28.6	2.1
Unsalted, Tops, Premium Plus, Impress*	1 Cracker/3g	13	0.3	448	10.3	75.9	10.3	0.0
Vegetable, Thai Spicy, Sainsbury's*	1 Pack/50g	231	10.4	462	7.2	61.5	20.8	2.6
Veggie, Heinz, Heinz*	1 Pack/25g	110	3.0	440	7.0	76.0	12.0	3.6
Wasapeas, Graze*	1 Pack/32g	128	2.5	406	14.8	65.2	7.8	7.1
Waterthins, Wafers, Philemon*	1 Crackers/2g	7	0.1	392	10.6	77.9	3.6	5.0
Wheaten, M & S*	1 Cracker/4g	20	0.9	450	10.2	57.0	20.2	5.0
Wholemeal, Tesco*	1 Cracker/7g	29	1.0	414	9.4	60.6	14.9	10.4
Wholewheat, Saiwa*	1 Pack/31g	128	3.9	414	12.5	62.9	12.5	7.9
Wholmeal, Organic, Nairn's*	1 Cracker/14g	58	2.0	413	9.0	61.4	14.6	8.7
CRANBERRIES								
& Blueberries, Delicious, Boots*	1 Pack/75g	220	1.0	293	0.7	70.0	1.3	9.1
& Raisins, Dried, Sweetened, Ocean Spray*	1 Serving/50g	163	0.2	326	0.1	80.3	0.5	4.6
Dried, Fruit bag, The Foodie Market, Aldi*	1 Serving/50g	172	0.7	343	0.3	80.1	1.3	4.7
Dried, Sweetened, Average	***1 Serving/10g***	***34***	***0.1***	***335***	***0.3***	***81.1***	***0.8***	***4.4***
Dried, Wholesome, Love Life, Waitrose*	¼ Pack/25g	92	0.2	370	0.3	86.8	0.8	4.6
Fresh, Raw, Average	***1oz/28g***	***4***	***0.0***	***15***	***0.4***	***3.4***	***0.1***	***3.0***
Organic, Infinity Foods*	1 Serving/100g	334	0.6	334	0.9	80.3	0.6	7.2
CRAYFISH								
Raw	***1oz/28g***	***19***	***0.2***	***67***	***14.9***	***0.0***	***0.8***	***0.0***
Tails, Chilli & Garlic, Asda*	1 Serving/140g	133	4.3	95	16.0	1.1	3.1	0.8
Tails in Brine, Luxury, The Big Prawn Co*	½ Tub/90g	46	0.6	51	10.1	1.0	0.7	0.0
CREAM								
Aerosol, Average	***1oz/28g***	***87***	***8.7***	***309***	***1.8***	***6.2***	***30.9***	***0.0***
Aerosol, Reduced Fat, Average	***1 Serving/55ml***	***33***	***3.0***	***60***	***0.6***	***2.0***	***5.4***	***0.0***

C

	Measure INFO/WEIGHT	per Measure KCAL	FAT	Nutrition Values per 100g / 100ml KCAL	PROT	CARB	FAT	FIBRE
CREAM								
Brandy, Pourable with Remy Martin*, Finest, Tesco*	½ Pot/125ml	460	35.5	368	2.7	19.8	28.4	0.0
Brandy, Really Thick, Tesco*	1 Pot/250ml	1162	98.2	465	1.4	21.3	39.3	0.0
Chantilly, TTD, Sainsbury's*	2 Tbsp/30g	136	14.0	455	1.4	6.9	46.8	0.0
Clotted, Fresh, Average	***1 Serving/28g***	***162***	***17.5***	***579***	***1.6***	***2.3***	***62.7***	***0.0***
Double, Average	***1 Tbsp/15ml***	***68***	***7.3***	***452***	***1.6***	***2.4***	***48.4***	***0.0***
Double, Reduced Fat, Average	***1 Serving/30g***	***73***	***7.0***	***243***	***2.7***	***5.6***	***23.3***	***0.1***
Extra Thick, 99% Real Dairy Cream, Anchor*	1 Serving/13g	51	5.4	409	1.7	3.9	43.0	0.0
Extra Thick, Reduced Fat, Weight Watchers*	1 Serving/30g	42	3.4	140	2.5	6.7	11.5	0.8
Extra Thick, with Baileys, Baileys*	1 fl oz/30ml	129	11.6	431	1.5	13.4	38.6	0.0
Oat Alternative, Dairy Free, Oatly*	1 Carton/250ml	375	32.5	150	1.0	6.0	13.0	0.8
Single, Average	***1 Tbsp/15ml***	***28***	***2.7***	***188***	***2.6***	***3.9***	***18.0***	***0.1***
Single, Extra Thick, Average	***1 Serving/38ml***	***72***	***6.9***	***192***	***2.7***	***4.1***	***18.4***	***0.0***
Sour, Avonmore*	1 Tub/200ml	440	50.0	220	2.4	4.0	25.0	0.5
Soured, Fresh, Average	***1 Tsp/5ml***	***10***	***0.9***	***191***	***2.7***	***3.9***	***18.4***	***0.0***
Soured, Reduced Fat, Average	***1 Tsp/5g***	***6***	***0.4***	***119***	***5.2***	***6.7***	***8.6***	***0.4***
Strawberry, Light, Real Dairy, Uht, Anchor*	1 Serving/13g	25	2.1	198	2.6	8.7	17.0	0.0
Thick, Sterilised, Average	***1 Tbsp/15ml***	***35***	***3.5***	***233***	***2.6***	***3.6***	***23.1***	***0.0***
Uht, Double, Average	***1 Tbsp/15g***	***41***	***3.9***	***274***	***2.2***	***7.4***	***26.3***	***0.0***
Uht, Reduced Fat, Average	***1 Serving/25ml***	***16***	***1.4***	***62***	***0.6***	***2.2***	***5.6***	***0.0***
Uht, Single, Average	***1 Tbsp/15ml***	***29***	***2.8***	***194***	***2.6***	***4.0***	***18.8***	***0.0***
Whipping, Average	***1 Tbsp/15ml***	***52***	***5.5***	***348***	***2.1***	***3.2***	***36.4***	***0.0***
CREAM HORN								
Fresh, Tesco*	1 Horn/57g	244	15.8	428	4.1	40.3	27.8	0.3
CREAM SODA								
American with Vanilla, Tesco*	1 Glass/313ml	75	0.0	24	0.0	5.9	0.0	0.0
Diet, Sainsbury's*	1 Serving/250ml	2	0.0	1	0.0	0.0	0.0	0.0
No Added Sugar, Sainsbury's*	1 Can/330ml	2	0.3	0	0.1	0.1	0.1	0.1
Shapers, Boots*	1 Bottle/300ml	3	0.0	1	0.0	0.0	0.0	0.0
Traditional Style, Tesco*	1 Can/330ml	139	0.0	42	0.0	10.4	0.0	0.0
CREME BRULEE								
Average	1 Serving/100g	313	26.0	313	3.8	15.7	26.0	0.2
Gastropub, M & S*	1 Brulee/84g	285	24.6	340	3.1	15.7	29.3	0.7
CREME CARAMEL								
Average	1 Serving/128g	140	2.8	109	3.0	20.6	2.2	0.0
Carmelle, Green's*	1 Pack/70g	82	2.8	117	3.0	17.0	4.0	0.0
Chosen By You, Asda*	1 Pot/100g	101	1.0	101	2.0	20.8	1.0	0.0
La Laitiere*	1 Pot/100g	135	4.0	135	5.0	20.0	4.0	0.0
CREME EGG								
Cadbury*	1 Egg/39g	180	6.3	462	4.1	73.0	16.1	0.5
Minis, Cadbury*	1 Egg/11g	50	1.8	445	4.1	67.5	16.4	0.4
CREME FRAICHE								
Average	***1 Pot/295g***	***1067***	***112.2***	***362***	***2.2***	***2.6***	***38.0***	***0.0***
Cucumber & Mint, Triangles, Sainsbury's*	1 Serving/25g	105	2.4	421	11.0	72.3	9.7	2.5
Extra Light, President*	1 Tub/200g	182	10.0	91	2.7	8.7	5.0	0.0
Half Fat, Average	***1 Serving/30g***	***54***	***4.9***	***181***	***3.1***	***5.5***	***16.2***	***0.0***
Lemon & Rocket, Sainsbury's*	1 Serving/150g	188	17.2	125	2.2	3.0	11.5	0.5
Low Fat, Average	1 Tbsp/30ml	43	3.6	143	3.3	5.6	12.1	0.1
Low Fat, Weight Watchers*	1 Tbsp/20g	15	0.5	76	5.1	7.7	2.7	0.5
CREPES								
Chocolate Filled, Tesco*	1 Crepe/32g	140	5.8	438	5.9	62.5	18.1	1.6
Lobster, Finest, Tesco*	1 Serving/160g	250	10.2	156	10.7	14.0	6.4	1.2
Mushroom, M & S*	1 Pack/186g	195	4.5	105	5.7	17.1	2.4	2.5

C

	Measure INFO/WEIGHT	per Measure KCAL	FAT	Nutrition Values per 100g / 100ml KCAL	PROT	CARB	FAT	FIBRE
CRISPBAKES								
Beef, Minced, M & S*	1 Bake/113g	226	12.3	200	10.0	15.6	10.9	1.5
Broccoli & Leek, Asda*	1 Bake/132g	263	13.2	199	6.3	21.0	10.0	2.0
Bubble & Squeak, M & S*	1 Bake/47g	79	4.1	170	2.7	19.6	8.8	1.5
Cheese, Spring Onion & Chive, Sainsbury's*	1 Bake/114g	287	16.8	253	7.1	24.5	14.8	1.7
Cheese & Onion, Cooked, Dalepak*	1 Bake/86g	192	8.8	223	4.9	26.9	10.2	1.7
Cheese & Onion, M & S*	1 Bake/114g	285	18.5	250	6.4	19.4	16.2	1.7
Cheese & Onion, Tesco*	1 Bake/109g	275	17.2	252	7.9	19.6	15.8	2.1
Dutch, Asda*	1 Bake/8g	31	0.3	388	14.7	74.9	3.3	4.2
Dutch, HL, Tesco*	1 Bake/8g	30	0.2	385	14.7	74.9	2.7	4.2
Mushroom, Uncooked, Dalepak*	1 Bake/84g	141	7.4	168	3.8	18.5	8.8	2.1
Spinach, Cheese & Sweetcorn, Cauldron Foods*	1 Bake/115g	233	12.2	203	5.6	21.3	10.6	2.1
Vegetable, M & S*	1 Bake/114g	200	10.3	175	2.5	19.2	9.0	2.6
Vegetable, Roast, & Basil, Cauldron Foods*	1 Bake/115g	242	11.0	210	3.5	26.0	9.6	2.9
Vegetable, Sainsbury's*	1 Bake/114g	246	13.0	216	2.0	26.2	11.4	2.0
CRISPBREAD								
3 Seed, Classic, Gourmet, Dr Karg*	1 Bread/25g	108	4.9	430	16.5	46.6	19.7	10.9
3 Seed, Organic, Gourmet	1 Bread/25g	101	4.7	405	15.8	48.8	18.8	14.6
Corn, Orgran*	1 Bread/5g	18	0.1	360	7.5	83.0	1.8	3.0
Corn Thins, Sesame, Real Foods*	1 Thin/6g	23	0.2	384	10.7	69.9	3.4	10.2
Cracked Black Pepper, Ryvita*	1 Slice/11g	38	0.2	344	8.8	66.6	1.6	14.5
Crisp 'n' Light, Wasa*	1 Bread/7g	24	0.1	360	12.0	73.0	2.2	5.3
Dark Rye, Ryvita*	1 Bread/10g	34	0.1	342	8.5	66.5	1.2	15.2
Fruit Crunch, Ryvita*	1 Slice/15g	54	0.8	358	8.3	61.8	5.4	14.9
GF	1 Serving/8g	25	0.1	331	6.4	72.9	1.5	0.0
Hint of Chilli, Ryvita*	1 Slice/12g	42	0.2	349	8.6	66.6	1.9	16.8
Mildly Seasoned, Gourmet, Dr Karg*	1 Bread/25g	101	4.0	405	16.2	48.8	16.1	11.6
Mini, Sesame & Linseed, Dr Karg*	1 Crispbread/3g	13	0.4	424	12.1	57.6	12.1	9.1
Mixed Grain, Jacobs*	1 Cracker/10g	41	1.3	436	9.1	66.7	13.9	4.2
Multigrain, Ryvita*	1 Slice/11g	41	0.8	370	11.2	56.0	7.2	18.3
Original, Ryvita*	1 Bread/10g	35	0.2	350	8.5	66.9	1.7	16.5
Poppyseed, Wasa*	1 Bread/13g	46	1.0	350	13.0	56.0	8.0	14.0
Provita*	1 Bread/6g	26	0.6	416	12.5	68.4	9.9	0.0
Pumpkin Seeds & Oats, Ryvita*	1 Slice/13g	46	0.9	370	11.2	56.0	7.2	18.3
Rice, Original, Sakata*	1 Bread/25g	102	0.6	410	6.9	88.0	2.6	1.3
Rice, Sakata*	1 Bread/25g	26	0.2	102	1.7	22.0	0.7	0.3
Rice & Cracked Pepper, Orgran*	1 Bread/5g	18	0.1	388	8.4	81.9	1.8	2.0
Rounds, Multigrain, Finn Crisp*	1 Bread/13g	41	0.8	330	13.0	56.0	6.0	18.0
Rounds, Wholegrain Wheat, Finn Crisp*	1 Bread/13g	45	0.7	360	11.0	66.0	5.9	10.0
Scan Bran, Slimming World*	1 Slice/10g	31	0.5	310	14.9	29.0	5.3	42.1
Seeded, Spelt, Organic, Dr Karg*	1 Bread/25g	108	4.5	430	17.2	44.4	18.0	11.2
Sesame, Ryvita*	1 Bread/10g	37	0.7	373	10.5	58.3	7.0	17.5
Sesame, Savour Bakes, Aldi*	1 Crispbread/9g	33	0.5	366	12.3	57.2	5.2	20.6
Spelt, Cheese, Sunflower Seeds, Organic, Dr Karg*	1 Bread/25g	103	4.5	411	19.2	42.8	18.1	10.4
Spelt, Muesli, Organic, Dr Karg*	1 Bread/25g	94	2.8	375	14.2	54.4	11.2	10.6
Spelt, Sesame, Sunflower, Amisa*	1 Bread/29g	85	4.3	297	11.7	28.5	15.1	5.0
Sport, Wasa*	1 Bread/15g	46	0.2	310	9.0	64.0	1.5	16.0
Sunflower Seeds & Oats, Ryvita*	1 Bread/12g	46	1.1	384	9.7	58.4	9.0	15.3
Sweet Onion, Ryvita*	1 Crispbread/12g	43	0.2	356	9.0	70.6	1.4	12.6
Trufree*	1 Bread/6g	22	0.1	370	6.0	82.0	2.0	1.0
Wheat, with Poppy Seeds, Morrisons*	1 Serving/12g	45	0.9	390	11.0	68.0	8.0	8.0
Wholegrain, Classic Three Seed, Organic, Dr Karg*	1 Bread/25g	101	4.5	405	15.8	44.8	18.0	14.6
Wholemeal, Light, Allinson*	1 Bread/5g	17	0.1	349	11.7	69.7	2.6	11.0
Wholemeal, Organic, Allinson*	1 Bread/5g	17	0.1	336	14.2	66.0	1.7	12.2

	Measure INFO/WEIGHT	per Measure KCAL	FAT	Nutrition Values per 100g / 100ml KCAL	PROT	CARB	FAT	FIBRE
CRISPBREAD								
Wholemeal, Rye with Milk, Grafschafter*	1 Bread/9g	29	0.1	316	11.4	64.0	1.6	15.0
Wholemeal Rye, Organic, Kallo*	1 Bread/10g	31	0.2	314	9.7	65.0	1.7	15.4
CRISPS								
Apple, Dried, Snapz*	1 Packet/15g	52	0.0	344	2.0	77.0	0.0	14.7
Apple, The Fruit Factory*	1 Packet/10g	33	0.0	334	1.3	81.1	0.5	12.4
Apple, Thyme & Sage, M & S*	1 Bag/55g	253	13.4	460	5.5	55.3	24.3	6.1
Bacon, Shapers, Boots*	1 Bag/23g	99	3.4	431	8.0	66.0	15.0	3.0
Bacon, Webs, Monster Munch*	1 Pack/15g	74	3.4	497	6.5	65.2	23.1	1.6
Bacon & Cheddar, Baked, Walkers*	1 Pack/38g	149	3.2	397	6.5	73.7	8.5	4.7
Bacon Pillows, Light, Shapers, Boots*	1 Pack/12g	44	0.3	367	3.7	83.0	2.3	4.0
Bacon Rashers, Blazin, Tesco*	1 Bag/25g	121	6.6	485	16.5	45.7	26.3	3.8
Bacon Rashers, Iceland*	1 Bag/75g	330	13.2	440	8.3	61.9	17.6	2.9
Bacon Rashers, Tesco*	1 Serving/25g	125	6.4	500	7.1	59.8	25.5	4.0
Bacon Rice Bites, Asda*	1 Bag/30g	136	4.8	452	7.0	70.0	16.0	0.4
Bacon Sizzler, Ridge Cut, McCoys*	1 Bag/32g	165	9.7	516	7.1	53.6	30.3	3.9
Baked, Average	1 Bag/25g	93	1.5	374	6.5	73.5	5.9	5.8
Baked, Ready Salted, Walkers*	1 Packet/38g	146	3.0	390	6.0	74.0	8.0	5.5
Baked, Sour Cream & Chive, Walkers*	1 Packet/38g	148	3.2	395	7.0	73.0	8.5	5.0
Baked Bean Flavour, Walkers*	1 Bag/35g	184	11.6	525	6.5	50.0	33.0	4.0
Barbecue, Handcooked, Tesco*	1 Bag/40g	187	10.0	468	6.6	53.8	25.1	5.2
Barbecue, Savoury Snacks, Weight Watchers*	1 Pack/22g	81	1.9	366	18.6	61.0	8.7	6.1
Barbecue, Snack Rite*	1 Bag/25g	131	8.3	524	5.1	51.3	33.2	0.0
Barbecue, Sunseed Oil, Walkers*	1 Pack/33g	171	10.7	525	6.5	50.0	33.0	4.0
BBQ Rib, Sunseed, Walkers*	1 Bag/25g	131	8.2	525	6.5	50.0	33.0	4.0
Beef, Space Raiders, KP Snacks*	1 Pack/13g	64	2.9	495	6.5	65.3	22.8	1.0
Beef, Squares, Walkers*	1 Bag/25g	105	4.5	420	6.0	59.0	18.0	4.6
Beef & Horseradish, Extra Special, Asda*	1 Serving/100g	516	32.0	516	7.0	50.0	32.0	3.4
Beef & Onion, Tayto*	1 Bag/35g	184	11.9	526	7.6	47.3	34.0	4.5
Beef & Onion, Walkers*	1 Bag/33g	171	10.7	525	6.5	50.0	33.0	4.0
Beef & Onion Flavour, Average	1 Bag/25g	131	8.3	524	6.5	50.0	33.1	4.3
Beefy, Smiths, Walkers*	1 Bag/25g	133	9.2	531	4.3	45.2	37.0	0.0
Beetroot, Seasoned in Salt, Glennans*	1 Bag/27g	130	8.9	480	8.2	36.0	32.8	13.2
Beetroot Chips, Crunchy, Apple Snapz*	1 Bag/20g	52	0.2	260	14.7	76.0	1.0	28.0
Big Snak, Crisp 'n Tasty Potato Chips, Herrs*	1 Pack/43g	212	12.1	494	7.1	56.5	28.2	3.6
Bread, Baked, Sweet Chilli Flavour, Seabrook*	1 Serving/100g	416	10.5	416	12.2	65.2	10.5	6.1
Bread, Baked, Tangy Barbeque Flavour, Seabrook*	1 Serving/100g	405	8.8	405	12.9	65.5	8.8	6.5
Brown Rice Chips, Sesame Soy, Gourmet, Riceworks*	1 Serving/40g	192	8.6	480	7.7	66.0	21.4	4.1
Buffalo Mozzarella, Tomato & Basil, Kettle Chips*	1 Serving/50g	238	12.8	476	6.7	54.4	25.7	4.9
Buffalo Mozzarella & Herbs, Walkers*	1 Serving/35g	172	9.1	490	6.1	57.0	26.0	4.2
Builders Breakfast, Walkers*	1 Sm Bag/25g	131	8.3	524	5.6	50.8	33.2	4.0
Butter & Chive, COU, M & S*	1 Bag/26g	95	0.5	365	7.7	77.3	1.9	4.6
Cajun Squirrel, Walkers*	1 Sm Bag/25g	130	8.2	522	5.8	51.2	32.7	4.2
Cheddar, Mature, & Chive, Kettle Chips*	1 Serving/50g	239	12.7	478	8.1	54.4	25.4	5.0
Cheddar, New York, Kettle Chips*	1 Bag/50g	242	13.4	483	6.7	53.9	26.7	4.5
Cheddar & Onion, Crinkles, Walkers*	1 Packet/28g	150	9.3	538	6.0	51.5	33.3	3.5
Cheddar & Onion, Potato, Hand Cooked, Aldi*	1 Pack/150g	753	41.8	502	7.7	54.9	27.9	4.0
Cheddar & Onion, Ridge Cut, McCoys*	1 Bag/32g	165	9.8	516	7.0	53.2	30.6	3.9
Cheddar & Red Onion Chutney, Sensations, Walkers*	1 Bag/40g	198	11.2	495	6.5	54.0	28.0	4.5
Cheddar & Sour Cream, Extra Crunchy, Walkers*	1 Serving/30g	143	6.8	476	6.6	59.1	22.6	4.7
Cheddar & Spring Onion, 35% Less Fat, Sainsbury's*	1 Pack/20g	93	4.2	463	6.3	62.4	20.9	0.9
Cheese, Space Raiders, KP Snacks*	1 Bag/16g	76	3.5	473	7.1	61.6	22.0	3.1
Cheese & Chive Flavour, GFY, Asda*	1 Bag/25g	119	6.0	476	6.0	59.0	24.0	6.0
Cheese & Chives, Walkers*	1 Bag/33g	172	10.7	530	6.5	50.0	33.0	4.1

	Measure INFO/WEIGHT	per Measure KCAL	FAT	Nutrition Values per 100g / 100ml KCAL	PROT	CARB	FAT	FIBRE
CRISPS								
Cheese & Onion, 30% Less Fat, Sainsbury's*	1 Pack/25g	115	5.4	459	7.5	58.1	21.8	5.4
Cheese & Onion, BGTY, Sainsbury's*	1 Bag/25g	120	6.2	479	7.0	57.0	24.8	5.7
Cheese & Onion, Crinkle, Seabrook*	1 Pack/32g	170	10.5	536	5.9	51.1	33.1	5.2
Cheese & Onion, Crinkle Cut, Low Fat, Waitrose*	1 Bag/25g	122	5.8	490	7.7	62.6	23.2	4.7
Cheese & Onion, Flavour Crinkles, Shapers, Boots*	1 Bag/20g	96	4.8	482	6.6	60.0	24.0	4.0
Cheese & Onion, GFY, Asda*	1 Pack/26g	122	5.7	470	7.0	61.0	22.0	4.2
Cheese & Onion, KP Snacks*	1 Bag/25g	134	8.7	534	6.6	48.7	34.8	4.8
Cheese & Onion, M & S*	1 Bag/25g	134	8.9	535	5.5	48.8	35.5	5.0
Cheese & Onion, Max, Walkers*	1 Pack/50g	262	16.0	525	6.8	52.0	32.0	5.2
Cheese & Onion, Organic, Tesco*	1 Bag/25g	128	8.2	514	5.2	49.9	32.6	7.0
Cheese & Onion, Oven Baked, Tesco*	1 Bag/25g	102	1.6	410	5.3	74.7	6.6	7.7
Cheese & Onion, Pom Bear, Intersnack Ltd*	1 Bag/19g	95	5.3	498	3.8	58.1	27.8	3.2
Cheese & Onion, Potato Heads, Walkers*	1 Pack/23g	108	5.3	470	6.0	60.0	23.0	5.5
Cheese & Onion, Rings, Crunchy, Shapers, Boots*	1 Bag/15g	56	0.4	374	5.9	81.0	2.9	2.0
Cheese & Onion, Sainsbury's*	1 Bag/25g	132	8.7	527	4.6	48.8	34.8	3.9
Cheese & Onion, Snack Rite*	1 Pack/25g	132	8.4	527	5.3	51.3	33.4	0.0
Cheese & Onion, Sprinters*	1 Bag/25g	137	9.2	549	5.4	49.4	36.6	0.0
Cheese & Onion, Squares, Walkers*	1 Bag/25g	108	4.5	430	6.5	61.0	18.0	5.5
Cheese & Onion, Sunseed Oil, Walkers*	1 Bag/33g	171	10.7	525	7.0	50.0	33.0	4.0
Cheese & Onion, Tayto*	1 Bag/25g	132	8.5	526	7.6	47.3	34.0	4.5
Cheese & Onion, Tesco*	1 Pack/25g	135	8.0	535	5.4	54.8	31.8	3.2
Cheese Bites, Weight Watchers*	1 Pack/18g	73	1.0	406	13.9	71.1	5.6	2.2
Cheese Curls, Red Mill*	½ Bag/50g	276	18.0	553	6.6	50.6	36.0	2.0
Cheese Curls, Shapers, Boots*	1 Pack/14g	68	3.8	489	4.5	57.0	27.0	2.7
Cheese Curls, Sprinters*	1 Bag/14g	68	3.8	483	4.1	56.4	26.8	0.0
Cheese Curls, Weight Watchers*	1 Pack/20g	78	1.7	392	5.0	73.8	8.6	3.4
Cheese Moments, Smiths*	1 Pack/28g	148	9.2	530	8.0	50.0	33.0	2.0
Cheese Puffs, Weight Watchers*	1 Pack/18g	80	1.9	444	7.8	77.2	10.6	3.3
Cheese Twirls, Boulevard, Simply Delicious*	1 Pack/25g	138	8.8	550	12.1	46.7	35.0	0.0
Cheese XL, Golden Wonder*	1 Bag/30g	155	9.6	516	6.2	50.6	32.1	4.2
Cheesy & Oniony, Potato, Tasty Little Numbers*	1 Pack/19g	100	6.1	527	7.9	51.6	32.1	2.6
Cheesy Curls, Bobby's*	1 Bag/40g	225	14.8	563	7.6	50.1	36.9	0.0
Cheesy Puffs, Co-Op*	1 Bag/60g	321	20.4	535	3.0	54.0	34.0	2.0
Chicken, Chargrilled, Ridge Cut, McCoys*	1 Pack/32g	167	10.0	521	7.0	52.9	31.3	4.0
Chicken, Firecracker, McCoys*	1 Bag/35g	177	10.3	506	6.2	54.0	29.5	4.0
Chicken, Oven Roasted, with Lemon & Thyme, Walkers*	1 Bag/40g	200	11.2	500	6.5	55.0	28.0	4.5
Chicken, Potato Heads, Walkers*	1 Pack/23g	106	4.8	460	8.5	58.0	21.0	6.0
Chicken & Thyme, Oven Roasted, Tesco*	1 Pack/150g	728	40.5	485	6.5	54.0	27.0	4.5
Chilli, Mexican, & Cheese, Golden Wonder*	1 Pack/45g	230	14.1	511	6.6	50.7	31.3	0.0
Chilli, Mexican, Ridge Cut, McCoys*	1 Bag/32g	164	9.8	514	6.9	53.0	30.5	4.5
Chilli & Chocolate, Walkers*	1 Pack/25g	131	8.3	523	6.1	50.1	33.1	4.2
Chilli & Lemon, Walkers*	1 Pack/25g	131	8.2	525	6.3	51.0	33.0	3.8
Cider Vinegar & Sea Salt, Tyrrells*	1 Pack/40g	192	9.8	481	7.2	60.1	24.6	2.4
Corn Chips, Fritos*	1 Pack/43g	240	15.0	565	4.7	56.5	35.3	0.0
Cream Cheese & Chive, Waffles, Spar*	1 Pack/27g	132	6.8	488	4.2	60.7	25.3	1.3
Crinkle Cut, Lower Fat, No Added Salt, Waitrose*	1 Bag/40g	193	10.0	483	6.5	58.0	25.0	3.9
Crushed Natural Sea Salt, Darling Spuds*	1 Bag/40g	195	12.0	488	5.6	53.4	30.0	4.5
Curls, Cheesy, Asda*	1 Pack/17g	87	4.9	511	3.8	59.7	28.6	1.7
D'lites, Cheddar & Red Onion Bites, The Real Crisp Co.*	1 Pack/20g	83	2.0	414	2.1	78.8	10.0	2.7
Feta Cheese Flavour, Mediterranean, Walkers*	1 Pack/25g	128	8.2	510	6.5	49.0	33.0	4.5
Flame Grilled Steak, Argentinean, Walkers*	1 Bag/35g	182	11.3	520	6.5	50.7	32.4	4.2
Flame Grilled Steak, Extra Crunchy, Walkers*	1 Bag/150g	702	31.6	468	6.9	60.0	21.1	5.0
Flame Grilled Steak, Ridge Cut, McCoys*	1 Bag/32g	165	9.8	516	7.0	53.0	30.7	4.0

	Measure INFO/WEIGHT	per Measure KCAL	FAT	Nutrition Values per 100g / 100ml KCAL	PROT	CARB	FAT	FIBRE
CRISPS								
Flamed Grilled Steak, Deep Ridge, Walkers*	1 Pack/28g	144	8.4	515	6.4	52.6	30.1	4.3
Four Cheese & Red Onion, Sensations, Walkers*	1 Bag/40g	194	10.8	485	6.5	54.0	27.0	4.5
French Garlic Baguette, Walkers*	1 Packet/25g	131	8.2	523	5.9	50.8	32.9	4.1
Garlic & Herbs Creme Fraiche, Kettle Chips*	1 Bag/50g	248	14.2	497	6.0	54.7	28.3	4.2
Guinness, Burts*	1 Bag/40g	206	11.5	514	5.1	58.6	28.8	2.5
Ham & Mustard, Salty Dog*	1 Pack/40g	192	10.8	480	7.5	54.5	27.1	4.2
Ham Flavour, Canadian, Seabrook*	1 Pack/30g	159	9.8	531	5.7	50.9	32.7	5.1
Heinz Tomato Ketchup, Sunseed, Walkers*	1 Bag/35g	179	11.0	520	6.5	51.0	32.0	4.0
Honey & BBQ, Wholgrain, Snacks, M & S*	1 Serving/30g	146	7.5	485	7.8	57.6	24.9	5.2
Honey Roast Gammon & English Mustard, Sainsbury's*	1 Serving/50g	236	12.4	472	7.2	55.0	24.8	5.0
Honey Roasted Ham, Sensations, Walkers*	1 Bag/40g	196	10.8	490	6.5	55.0	27.0	4.0
Hoops, Ready Salted, Weight Watchers*	1 Bag/20g	73	0.3	365	3.4	82.7	1.4	4.1
Hot & Spicy Salami, Tesco*	1 Bag/50g	216	18.0	431	26.2	0.7	35.9	0.0
Jalapeno Peppers, Fire Roasted, Darling Spuds*	1 Pack/40g	191	11.4	478	6.3	53.4	28.5	4.5
Kale, Pret a Manger*	1 Pack/25g	105	6.6	420	14.4	30.8	26.4	17.2
Lamb & Mint, Slow Roasted, Sensations, Walkers*	1 Bag/35g	170	9.4	485	6.5	54.0	27.0	4.5
Lamb & Mint, Sunseed Oil, Walkers*	1 Pack/33g	171	10.7	525	6.5	50.0	33.0	4.0
Lant Chips, Ikea*	1 Serving/25g	126	6.9	505	8.3	55.9	27.6	4.5
Lightly Salted, Baked, COU, M & S*	1 Bag/25g	88	0.6	350	8.5	76.4	2.3	5.7
Lightly Salted, Crinkle Cut, Low Fat, Waitrose*	1 Pack/35g	163	8.0	466	5.2	60.1	22.8	5.1
Lightly Salted, Crinkles, Shapers, Boots*	1 Pack/20g	96	4.8	482	6.6	60.0	24.0	4.0
Lightly Salted, Handcooked, Finest, Tesco*	1 Bag/40g	206	11.5	515	5.1	58.6	28.8	2.5
Lightly Salted, Hoops, Mini, Weight Watchers*	1 Pack/20g	71	0.2	355	4.0	82.0	1.0	3.5
Lightly Salted, Kettle Chips*	1 Serving/50g	255	15.2	510	5.9	50.5	30.3	5.6
Lightly Salted, Low Fat, Waitrose*	1 Bag/25g	125	6.2	500	7.5	61.3	25.0	4.8
Lightly Salted, Potato Bakes, Weight Watchers*	1 Pack/20g	78	1.8	392	5.0	72.0	9.0	5.0
Lightly Salted, Potato Thins, LC, Tesco*	1 Pack/20g	72	0.4	360	5.1	79.5	2.0	4.2
Lightly Salted, Reduced Fat, Crinkles, Eat Well, M & S*	1 Pack/30g	140	6.6	460	6.7	59.4	21.8	4.5
Lightly Sea Salted, Jonathan Crisp*	1 Bag/35g	176	10.2	503	6.5	52.0	29.0	5.4
Lightly Sea Salted, Potato Chips, Hand Fried, Burts*	¼ Bag/50g	252	13.8	504	6.4	57.4	27.7	0.0
Lightly Sea Salted, Tyrrells*	1 Pack/40g	204	10.2	510	5.9	49.0	25.4	5.3
Lime, with a Hint of Chilli, Mexican, Kettle Chips*	1 Serving/50g	242	13.8	484	5.0	54.1	27.5	5.4
Lincolnshire Sausage, Tyrrells*	1 Pack/100g	530	28.2	530	8.6	60.8	28.2	3.0
Mango & Chilli, Baked, Walkers*	1 Packet/38g	147	3.0	392	6.4	74.0	8.0	4.8
Mango Chilli, Kettle Chips*	1 Serving/40g	190	9.6	475	6.3	53.9	24.0	6.1
Marmite*	1 Pack/25g	130	7.7	519	6.2	52.6	30.7	3.7
Munchies, Cheese Fix, Snack Mix, Rold Gold*	1 Serving/28g	140	7.0	500	7.1	64.3	25.0	3.6
Naked, Tyrrells*	1 Pack/150g	748	41.2	499	7.7	56.5	27.5	0.0
Olive Oil, Mozzarella & Oregano, Walkers*	1 Serving/30g	152	8.7	505	6.5	54.0	29.0	4.0
Onion Bhaji, Walkers*	1 Pack/25g	130	8.2	522	6.1	50.7	32.7	4.3
Onion Rings, Corn Snacks, Average	1 Bag/25g	122	6.1	486	5.8	60.9	24.2	2.7
Onion Rings, Crunchy, Shapers, Boots*	1 Bag/12g	61	3.4	507	2.5	62.0	28.0	2.6
Onion Rings, M & S*	1 Pack/40g	186	8.6	465	5.2	62.1	21.5	4.3
Onion Rings, Pickled, HE, Tesco*	1 Pack/15g	51	0.3	340	6.2	74.7	1.8	6.5
Onion Rings, Tayto*	1 Pack/17g	82	4.1	484	3.0	63.4	24.0	2.4
Onion Rings, Tesco*	1 Serving/30g	148	7.6	495	8.4	57.8	25.5	2.5
Oriental Ribs, Ridge Cut, McCoys*	1 Pack/50g	256	15.0	511	7.3	52.7	30.1	4.2
Paprika, Handcooked, Shapers, Boots*	1 Bag/20g	99	4.8	493	7.2	62.0	24.0	5.0
Paprika, Max, Walkers*	1 Bag/50g	260	16.0	520	6.5	52.0	31.9	5.1
Paprika, Mini Hoops, Shapers, Boots*	1 Bag/13g	64	3.5	494	8.7	54.0	27.0	2.2
Parsnip, Passions, Snack Rite*	1 Serving/25g	124	9.4	494	4.5	34.5	37.6	18.8
Parsnip & Black Pepper, Sainsbury's*	1 Serving/35g	166	11.1	473	3.2	43.6	31.8	15.2
Pastrami & Cheese, Crinkle, M & S*	1 Bag/25g	120	5.9	485	6.5	61.0	24.0	3.5

	Measure INFO/WEIGHT	per Measure KCAL	FAT	Nutrition Values per 100g / 100ml KCAL	PROT	CARB	FAT	FIBRE
CRISPS								
Peri Peri Chicken, Nando's*	½ Bag/75g	410	20.2	547	5.1	57.4	27.0	3.4
Pickled Onion, Beastie Bites, Asda*	1 Bag/20g	100	5.2	498	6.0	60.0	26.0	0.0
Pickled Onion, Golden Wonder*	1 Bag/25g	131	8.5	524	5.6	49.0	34.0	2.0
Pickled Onion, Monster Bites, Sainsbury's*	1 Bag/20g	107	6.7	535	5.2	53.5	33.3	1.0
Pickled Onion, Space Raiders, KP Snacks*	1 Bag/13g	64	2.9	495	6.5	65.3	22.8	1.0
Pickled Onion, Stompers, Morrisons*	1 Pack/25g	129	7.9	518	6.1	52.2	31.6	1.3
Pickled Onion, Sunseed, Walkers*	1 Bag/33g	171	10.7	525	6.5	50.0	33.0	4.0
Pickled Onion Flavour, Average	1 Bag/25g	132	8.2	527	6.6	52.5	32.6	3.5
Pickled Onion Flavour Rings, BGTY, Sainsbury's*	1 Serving/10g	34	0.2	345	5.0	81.7	1.5	3.7
Pickled Onion Rings, COU, M & S*	1 Bag/20g	69	0.3	345	5.0	81.7	1.5	3.7
Pom Bear, Salt & Vinegar, Intersnack Ltd*	1 Pack/25g	124	6.8	494	3.0	58.8	27.4	2.7
Pom-Bear, Prawn Cocktail, Intersnack Ltd*	1 Bag/19g	97	5.2	508	3.4	61.6	27.2	1.8
Pom-Bear, Smoky Bacon, Intersnack Ltd*	1 Bag/19g	98	5.1	515	3.9	63.8	27.0	0.7
Pom-Bear, Zoo, Really Cheesy, Potato Snack	1 Bag/19g	100	5.8	525	3.6	57.0	30.7	3.1
Potato, Baked, COU, M & S*	1 Bag/25g	88	0.6	350	8.5	76.4	2.3	5.7
Potato, Low Fat	1oz/28g	128	6.0	458	6.6	63.5	21.5	5.9
Potato, Tyrrells*	1 Pack/261g	1362	72.8	522	6.1	56.5	27.9	0.0
Potato Zoo, Crispy Potato Animals, Kids, Tesco*	1 Bag/30g	57	1.9	190	2.5	24.5	6.3	2.1
Prawn, Spirals, Shapers, Boots*	1 Pack/100g	468	22.0	468	3.1	64.0	22.0	2.8
Prawn Cocktail, 30% Less Fat, Sainsbury's*	1 Pack/25g	118	5.9	470	6.3	58.9	23.6	5.7
Prawn Cocktail, BGTY, Sainsbury's*	1 Bag/25g	118	5.9	473	6.3	58.6	23.7	5.7
Prawn Cocktail, Boots*	1 Pack/21g	99	4.6	470	6.8	60.0	22.0	4.3
Prawn Cocktail, Golden Wonder*	1 Bag/25g	130	8.4	521	5.8	49.0	33.5	2.0
Prawn Cocktail, KP Snacks*	1 Bag/25g	133	8.7	531	5.9	48.4	34.9	4.7
Prawn Cocktail, Lites, Advantage, Tayto*	1 Pack/21g	96	4.1	455	5.3	65.1	19.3	3.8
Prawn Cocktail, Lites, Shapers, Boots*	1 Bag/21g	92	3.8	438	5.1	64.0	18.0	4.1
Prawn Cocktail, Snack Rite*	1 Bag/25g	129	8.3	516	5.0	49.2	33.2	0.0
Prawn Cocktail, Spar*	1 Bag/40g	207	11.7	517	3.2	60.1	29.3	1.3
Prawn Cocktail, Sunseed Oil, Walkers*	1 Bag/33g	171	10.7	525	6.5	50.0	33.0	4.0
Prawn Cocktail, Tayto*	1 Bag/35g	185	12.3	526	7.5	46.6	35.0	4.5
Prawn Cocktail Flavour, Seabrook*	1 Bag/30g	163	10.1	544	5.7	49.2	33.7	4.5
Prawn Crackers, Tesco*	1 Bag/60g	316	17.5	527	3.2	62.8	29.2	0.8
Ready Salted, Average	1 Bag/25g	127	7.4	508	6.1	53.4	29.7	4.0
Ready Salted, BGTY, Sainsbury's*	1 Bag/25g	122	6.6	486	6.8	55.7	26.2	6.6
Ready Salted, Deep Ridge, Walkers*	1 Pack/28g	148	9.0	529	6.4	51.1	32.1	4.6
Ready Salted, GFY, Asda*	1 Bag/23g	109	5.3	475	7.0	60.0	23.0	4.3
Ready Salted, Golden Wonder*	1 Bag/25g	135	8.8	539	5.5	49.9	35.3	2.0
Ready Salted, KP Snacks*	1 Bag/24g	131	8.8	545	5.6	47.9	36.8	4.9
Ready Salted, Lower Fat, Asda*	1 Bag/25g	120	6.2	481	6.0	58.0	25.0	4.8
Ready Salted, Lower Fat, Sainsbury's*	1 Bag/25g	111	5.4	444	7.0	55.0	21.8	5.1
Ready Salted, Oven Baked, Asda*	1 Bag/25g	95	1.9	379	4.4	73.1	7.7	2.6
Ready Salted, Oven Baked, Tesco*	1 Bag/25g	95	1.9	380	4.4	73.1	7.7	8.4
Ready Salted, Potato Squares, Sainsbury's*	1 Bag/50g	192	8.0	384	6.5	53.8	15.9	7.8
Ready Salted, Potato Triangles, Sainsbury's*	½ Pack/50g	243	11.7	486	9.4	59.7	23.4	3.4
Ready Salted, Reduced Fat, Tesco*	1 Pack/25g	114	6.2	456	6.3	52.0	24.7	5.9
Ready Salted, Ridge Cut, McCoys*	1 Bag/49g	257	15.6	524	6.6	52.6	31.9	4.1
Ready Salted, Squares, Walkers*	1 Pack/25g	109	4.8	435	6.5	60.0	19.0	6.0
Ready Salted, Sunseed Oil, Walkers*	1 Bag/33g	175	11.1	537	5.9	49.7	34.1	4.2
Red Leicester & Spring Onion, Handcooked, M & S*	1 Pack/40g	194	10.6	485	6.8	55.0	26.4	5.1
Red Pepper & Lime, Roasted, Potato Chips, Red Sky*	1 Serving/40g	187	9.0	467	6.8	59.5	22.4	4.8
Roast Beef, KP Snacks*	1 Bag/25g	134	8.8	534	6.6	47.5	35.3	4.7
Roast Beef & Mustard, Thick Cut, Brannigans*	1 Bag/40g	203	12.0	507	7.6	51.7	30.0	3.7
Roast Chicken, 30% Less Fat, Sainsbury's*	1 Pack/25g	115	5.5	460	7.4	58.3	21.9	5.2

	Measure INFO/WEIGHT	per Measure KCAL	FAT	Nutrition Values per 100g / 100ml KCAL	PROT	CARB	FAT	FIBRE
CRISPS								
Roast Chicken, Golden Wonder*	1 Bag/25g	130	8.4	522	6.2	48.6	33.6	2.0
Roast Chicken, Highlander*	1 Bag/25g	138	9.7	554	5.3	46.0	38.9	5.1
Roast Chicken, Sunseed Oil, Walkers*	1 Bag/33g	171	10.7	525	6.5	50.0	33.0	4.0
Roast Chicken, Tayto*	1 Bag/35g	184	11.9	526	7.6	47.3	34.0	4.5
Roast Chicken & Sage Flavour, M & S*	1 Bag/25g	135	8.6	540	5.9	50.6	34.6	4.6
Roast Chicken Flavour, Average	1 Bag/25g	132	8.6	528	6.1	48.8	34.2	3.9
Roast Chicken Flavour, BGTY, Sainsbury's*	1 Bag/25g	118	5.9	473	6.2	58.9	23.6	5.7
Roast Chicken Flavour, Crinkle, Weight Watchers*	1 Pack/16g	76	3.3	475	5.6	63.1	20.6	6.2
Roasted Lamb, Moroccan Spices, Sensations, Walkers*	1 Bag/40g	198	11.6	495	6.0	53.0	29.0	4.5
Salt & Balsamic Vinegar, Perfectly Balanced, Waitrose*	1 Bag/20g	69	0.5	347	4.2	76.4	2.7	5.2
Salt & Black Pepper, Handcooked, M & S*	1 Bag/40g	180	9.2	450	5.7	55.0	22.9	5.2
Salt & Cracked Black Pepper, Shapers, Boots*	1 Bag/20g	91	4.4	453	7.2	57.0	22.0	5.0
Salt & Malt Vinegar, Deep Ridge, Walkers*	1 Pack/28g	143	8.6	511	6.1	50.7	30.7	4.3
Salt & Malt Vinegar, Extra Crunchy, Walkers*	1 Pack/30g	139	6.2	463	6.6	59.9	20.8	4.8
Salt & Malt Vinegar, Hunky Dorys*	1 Serving/30g	141	8.6	469	6.3	49.3	28.7	0.0
Salt & Malt Vinegar, Ridge Cut, McCoys*	1 Bag/32g	165	9.8	515	6.7	53.3	30.6	3.9
Salt & Malt Vinegar Flavour, Sainsbury's*	1 Bag/25g	134	8.8	538	4.9	50.3	35.2	2.3
Salt & Shake, Walkers*	1 Pack/24g	128	7.8	533	6.2	52.2	32.3	4.4
Salt & Vinegar, 30% Less Fat, Sainsbury's*	1 Bag/25g	114	5.4	458	7.2	58.3	21.8	5.1
Salt & Vinegar, Average	1 Bag/25g	130	8.2	519	5.5	50.3	32.9	3.4
Salt & Vinegar, Baked, Walkers*	1 Packet/38g	150	3.0	400	6.0	73.5	8.1	4.6
Salt & Vinegar, BGTY, Sainsbury's*	1 Bag/25g	120	6.3	482	6.5	57.3	25.2	5.2
Salt & Vinegar, Crinkle, M & S*	1 Pack/25g	120	5.9	485	6.5	61.0	24.0	3.5
Salt & Vinegar, Crinkle Cut, Seabrook*	1 Bag/32g	181	11.7	569	5.4	54.4	36.7	3.9
Salt & Vinegar, Crinkles, Shapers, Boots*	1 Pack/20g	96	4.8	482	6.6	60.0	24.0	4.0
Salt & Vinegar, Crispy Discs, Shapers, Boots*	1 Bag/92g	404	17.5	439	4.8	63.0	19.0	4.9
Salt & Vinegar, Distinctively, Walkers*	1 Pack/33g	169	10.0	519	5.9	52.6	30.8	4.2
Salt & Vinegar, Fish Shapes, Food Explorers, Waitrose*	1 Bag/20g	86	3.2	430	2.4	69.1	16.0	1.3
Salt & Vinegar, GFY, Asda*	1 Bag/26g	120	5.7	466	6.0	61.0	22.0	4.1
Salt & Vinegar, Golden Lights, Golden Wonder*	1 Bag/21g	94	3.9	446	4.2	65.7	18.5	3.7
Salt & Vinegar, Golden Wonder*	1 Bag/25g	130	8.5	522	5.4	48.5	34.0	2.0
Salt & Vinegar, HE, Tesco*	1 Bag/17g	61	0.3	357	3.2	82.4	1.6	3.0
Salt & Vinegar, KP Snacks*	1 Bag/25g	133	8.8	532	5.5	48.7	35.0	4.7
Salt & Vinegar, Lights, Walkers*	1 Bag/28g	133	6.2	475	7.0	62.0	22.0	4.5
Salt & Vinegar, Oven Baked, Asda*	1 Bag/25g	95	2.0	380	5.1	72.0	8.0	2.9
Salt & Vinegar, Potato Bakes, Weight Watchers*	1 Bag/20g	81	1.8	404	5.3	76.0	8.8	2.3
Salt & Vinegar, Red Mill*	1 Bag/40g	174	7.0	436	3.9	65.8	17.5	2.4
Salt & Vinegar, Rough Cuts, Tayto*	1 Bag/30g	152	9.2	506	4.6	56.8	30.8	0.0
Salt & Vinegar, Space Raiders, KP Snacks*	1 Bag/17g	81	3.8	478	6.9	61.7	22.6	2.2
Salt & Vinegar, Squares, Walkers*	1 Bag/28g	121	4.9	441	6.5	61.0	18.0	5.5
Salt & Vinegar, Sunseed Oil, Walkers*	1 Bag/33g	171	10.7	525	6.5	50.0	33.0	4.0
Salt & Vinegar, Tayto*	1 Bag/35g	184	11.9	526	7.6	47.3	34.0	4.5
Salt & Vinegar, Tubes, HL, Tesco*	1 Bag/17g	61	0.3	357	3.2	82.4	1.6	3.0
Salt & Vinegar Flavour, Half Fat, M & S*	1 Bag/40g	168	6.8	420	5.8	61.0	17.0	7.7
Salt & Vinegar Flavour, Sprinters*	1 Bag/25g	133	8.8	532	4.8	49.1	35.2	0.0
Salt & Vinegar in Sunflower Oil, Sainsbury's*	1 Serving/25g	131	8.4	524	5.2	49.7	33.8	3.7
Salt Your Own, Excluding Salt, Aldi*	1 Pack/24g	130	8.1	536	6.0	52.6	33.5	4.5
Salt Your Own, Jacket, 35% Less Fat, Sainsbury's*	1 Bag/20g	98	4.5	490	7.5	64.5	22.5	9.5
Salt Your Own, Sainsbury's*	1 Pack/24g	127	7.9	520	5.0	52.2	32.3	3.7
Salt Your Own, Snackrite, Aldi*	1 Pack/24g	130	8.1	536	6.0	52.6	33.5	4.5
Salted Tubes, Shapers, Boots*	1 Bag/15g	67	3.0	448	5.1	62.0	20.0	3.6
Sausage & Tomato, Sainsbury's*	1 Pack/25g	131	8.4	525	6.0	49.3	33.8	3.8
Sausage & Tomato Flavour, Golden Wonder*	1 Bag/35g	174	10.6	505	6.1	51.3	30.6	4.5

	Measure INFO/WEIGHT	per Measure KCAL	FAT	Nutrition Values per 100g / 100ml KCAL	PROT	CARB	FAT	FIBRE
CRISPS								
Scotch Bonnet Flavour, Mackies*	1 Pack/150g	732	369.0	488	78.0	574.0	246.0	42.0
Sea Salt, Anglesey, Potato Chips, Red Sky*	1 Serving/40g	185	8.7	463	6.8	59.8	21.8	5.0
Sea Salt, Golden Lights, Golden Wonder*	1 Bag/21g	94	3.9	448	3.9	66.4	18.5	4.4
Sea Salt, Gourmet, TTD, Sainsbury's*	1/3 Pack/50g	249	15.0	498	5.7	51.4	30.0	6.4
Sea Salt, Handcooked, Extra Special, Asda*	1 Pack/31g	149	7.8	477	7.0	56.0	25.0	4.1
Sea Salt, Original, Crinkle Cut, Seabrook*	1 Bag/30g	155	9.3	517	5.7	53.7	31.1	4.2
Sea Salt & Balsamic Vinegar, Kettle Chips*	1 Bag/40g	201	11.4	502	5.4	53.0	28.4	6.1
Sea Salt & Balsamic Vinegar, Low Fat, Peak*	1 Serving/25g	87	0.4	348	7.4	76.6	1.4	6.7
Sea Salt & Black Pepper, GFY, Asda*	1 Bag/100g	476	24.0	476	6.0	59.0	24.0	6.0
Sea Salt & Black Pepper, Highlander*	1 Serving/25g	141	9.6	564	5.6	44.0	38.4	4.8
Sea Salt & Black Pepper, Shapers, Boots*	1 Bag/20g	96	4.8	482	6.6	60.0	24.0	4.0
Sea Salt & Black Pepper, Tyrrells*	¼ Pack/38g	182	9.3	480	7.3	59.9	24.5	2.4
Sea Salt & Cider Vinegar, TTD, Sainsbury's*	1/3 Pack/50g	245	14.3	489	5.5	52.7	28.5	6.1
Sea Salt & Cracked Black Pepper, Lights, Walkers*	1 Bag/24g	115	5.3	480	7.0	63.0	22.0	5.0
Sea Salt & Cracked Black Pepper, Sensations, Walkers*	1 Bag/40g	196	10.8	490	6.5	55.0	27.0	4.0
Sea Salt & Indian Black Pepper, Pipers Crisps*	1 Pack/40g	195	11.6	487	6.6	49.9	29.0	0.0
Sea Salt & Malt Vinegar, Sensations, Walkers*	1 Bag/40g	194	10.8	485	6.5	54.0	27.0	4.5
Sea Salt & Modena Balsamic Vivegar, Darling Spuds*	1 Bag/40g	190	11.4	475	5.4	54.3	28.5	4.2
Shells, Prawn Cocktail, Asda*	1 Bag/18g	90	5.3	501	4.6	54.9	29.2	6.2
Simply Salted, Extra Crunchy, Walkers*	1 Bag/30g	142	6.5	473	6.8	59.8	21.8	5.0
Simply Salted, Lights, Walkers*	1 Bag/24g	113	5.3	470	7.0	61.0	22.0	5.0
Smoked Ham & Pickle, Thick Cut, Brannigans*	1 Bag/40g	203	11.9	507	7.0	52.8	29.8	3.8
Smokey Bacon, Budgens*	1 Bag/25g	130	8.2	519	6.2	49.3	33.0	4.8
Smokey Bacon, Crinkle, Shapers, Boots*	1 Pack/20g	96	4.8	482	6.6	60.0	24.0	4.0
Smokey Bacon, Seabrook*	1 Bag/32g	181	11.7	569	5.4	54.4	36.7	3.9
Smokey Bacon, Select, Tesco*	1 Bag/25g	134	8.7	536	6.4	49.0	34.9	4.3
Smokey Bacon Potato Hoops, COU, M & S*	1 Pack/16g	58	0.4	360	5.6	78.7	2.7	4.5
Smoky Bacon, 30% Lower Fat, Sainsbury's*	1 Bag/25g	118	5.9	471	6.5	58.4	23.6	5.7
Smoky Bacon, BGTY, Sainsbury's*	1 Bag/25g	118	5.9	472	6.5	58.5	23.6	5.7
Smoky Bacon, Golden Wonder*	1 Bag/25g	131	8.4	523	5.9	49.1	33.7	2.0
Smoky Bacon, Sainsbury's*	1 Bag/25g	130	7.7	519	5.8	53.1	30.7	3.6
Smoky Bacon, Snack Rite*	1 Bag/25g	131	8.3	525	5.5	51.2	33.1	0.0
Smoky Bacon, Sunseed Oil, Walkers*	1 Bag/35g	183	11.4	530	6.5	51.0	33.0	4.0
Smoky Bacon, Tayto*	1 Bag/35g	184	11.9	526	7.6	47.3	34.0	4.5
Smoky Bacon Flavour, Average	1 Bag/25g	132	8.4	527	6.2	49.7	33.7	3.2
Snaps, Spicy Tomato Flavour, Walkers*	1 Bag/18g	91	4.8	508	1.5	65.5	26.8	0.0
Snax, Tayto*	1 Pack/17g	82	3.7	483	2.4	70.0	21.5	1.6
Sour Cream & Chilli Lentil Curls, M & S*	1 Pack/60g	243	5.2	405	13.6	65.3	8.7	4.3
Sour Cream & Chive, Crinkle, Reduced Fat, M & S*	1 Bag/40g	178	8.2	445	5.6	58.8	20.6	5.6
Sour Cream & Chive, HE, Tesco*	1 Bag/20g	72	0.8	362	6.7	81.1	3.8	3.4
Sour Cream & Chive, Lights, Walkers*	1 Bag/24g	114	5.3	475	7.5	62.0	22.0	5.0
Sour Cream & Chive, Perfectly Balanced, Waitrose*	1 Pack/20g	69	0.5	347	4.4	76.3	2.7	5.2
Sour Cream & Chive, Potato Bakes, Weight Watchers*	1 Bag/20g	83	1.8	417	3.8	80.7	8.8	3.6
Sour Cream & Chive, Potato Bites, BGTY, Sainsbury's*	1 Pack/20g	73	0.6	365	7.2	77.8	2.8	3.9
Sour Cream & Chive Baked Potato, COU, M & S*	1 Pack/24g	84	0.7	350	7.5	73.2	2.8	7.9
Sour Cream & Chive Crispy Discs, Shapers, Boots*	1 Bag/21g	94	4.0	448	5.7	61.9	19.0	4.3
Sour Cream & Chive Flavour, Average	1 Bag/25g	127	7.7	508	6.8	50.7	30.9	4.6
Sour Cream & Chives, Jordans*	1 Bag/30g	125	3.6	417	7.3	69.9	12.0	2.7
Sour Cream & Green Herbs, Potato Chips, Red Sky*	1 Pack/40g	188	9.4	471	6.8	58.4	23.4	4.8
Sour Cream & Onion, Golden Lights, Golden Wonder*	1 Bag/21g	93	3.8	442	4.1	66.0	17.9	4.4
Spare Rib Flavour, Chinese, Walkers*	1 Bag/35g	181	11.4	525	6.5	50.0	33.0	4.0
Spiced Chilli, McCoys*	1 Bag/35g	175	10.1	500	6.1	54.2	28.8	4.2
Spicy Chilli, Sunseed, Walkers*	1 Pack/35g	183	11.4	530	6.5	51.0	33.0	4.0

	Measure INFO/WEIGHT	per Measure KCAL	FAT	Nutrition Values per 100g / 100ml KCAL	PROT	CARB	FAT	FIBRE
CRISPS								
Spring Onion, Seabrook*	1 Bag/32g	182	11.7	569	5.4	54.4	36.7	3.9
Spring Onion Flavour, M & S*	1 Bag/40g	210	13.7	525	5.9	48.7	34.3	5.1
Spring Onion Flavour, Tayto*	1 Bag/35g	184	11.9	526	7.6	47.3	34.0	4.5
Steak & Onion, Walkers*	1 Pack/33g	169	10.7	520	6.5	49.0	33.0	4.0
Sun Dried Tomato & Basil, Jonathan Crisp*	1 Pack/35g	176	10.2	503	5.6	52.0	29.0	5.4
Sun Dried Tomato & Chilli, Asda*	1 Pack/150g	700	34.5	467	7.0	58.0	23.0	4.1
Sweet Chill, Mexican, Phileas Fogg*	1 Bag/38g	193	11.0	507	6.7	54.8	29.0	4.2
Sweet Chilli, Baked Potato, COU, M & S*	1 Bag/26g	91	0.7	350	7.6	73.9	2.8	8.5
Sweet Chilli, Cracker, Special K, Kellogg's*	21 Crisps/23g	94	2.1	409	5.0	73.0	9.0	8.0
Sweet Chilli, Crinkle Cut, Weight Watchers*	1 Bag/20g	94	4.1	470	5.6	62.9	20.6	5.8
Sweet Chilli, Hand Cooked, Asda*	1 Pack/25g	120	7.1	479	5.7	54.5	28.3	4.5
Sweet Chilli & Red Peppers, Fusion, Tayto*	1 Bag/28g	140	8.3	500	4.9	52.2	29.8	4.6
Sweet Chilli Chicken, Extra Crunchy, Walkers*	1 Bag/30g	143	6.8	477	6.5	59.9	22.5	4.8
Sweet Chilli Flavour, Average	1 Bag/25g	115	5.6	461	5.1	59.9	22.6	4.6
T Bone Steak, Roysters*	1 Pack/28g	148	9.0	530	5.2	55.3	32.0	3.0
Tangy Malaysian Chutney, Sensations, Walkers*	1 Bag/24g	116	6.2	485	0.9	62.0	26.0	0.0
Tangy Toms, Red Mill*	1 Bag/15g	76	4.1	507	6.0	60.0	27.3	0.7
Thai Curry & Coriander, Tyrrells*	1 Pack/50g	261	14.0	522	6.1	56.5	27.9	5.4
Thai Sweet Chicken, Ridge Cut, McCoys*	1 Bag/50g	257	15.0	514	7.0	54.0	30.0	4.1
Thai Sweet Chilli, Sensations, Walkers*	1 Bag/40g	194	10.4	485	6.0	57.0	26.0	4.2
Thai Sweet Chilli Flavour, Velvet Crunch, King*	1 Pack/20g	81	1.9	404	1.6	77.5	9.7	2.0
Tomato & Basil, Mediterranean, Walkers*	1 Pack/25g	128	8.2	510	6.5	49.0	33.0	4.5
Tomato & Herb, Shapers, Boots*	1 Bag/20g	94	4.2	468	3.7	66.0	21.0	3.9
Tomato Ketchup Flavour, Golden Wonder*	1 Bag/25g	135	8.0	521	5.1	54.0	30.8	3.6
Tortillas, Nacho Cheese Flavour, Weight Watchers*	1 Pack/18g	78	2.9	433	6.1	66.7	16.1	3.9
Traditional, Hand Cooked, Finest, Tesco*	1 Bag/150g	708	39.2	472	6.4	52.9	26.1	5.1
Turkey & Paxo, Walkers*	1 Bag/35g	181	11.4	525	6.4	50.1	33.0	4.1
Unsalted, Potato Heads, Walkers*	1 Serving/23g	106	5.1	460	5.0	61.0	22.0	5.0
Unsalted, Seabrook*	1 Bag/30g	163	10.7	544	5.7	47.9	35.8	4.1
Vegetable, Average	1 Bag/25g	118	7.4	470	4.1	46.5	29.6	12.1
Vegetable, Crunchy, Asda*	½ Bag/50g	251	12.0	502	1.4	70.0	24.0	6.0
Vegetable, Finest, Tesco*	1 Serving/50g	203	12.8	406	5.0	39.0	25.5	14.6
Vegetable, TTD, Sainsbury's*	½ Pack/52g	254	17.9	490	4.8	39.9	34.5	12.8
Vegetable, Waitrose*	1 Pack/100g	490	35.2	490	4.7	38.5	35.2	13.0
Waffles, Bacon Flavour, BGTY, Sainsbury's*	1 Serving/12g	41	0.2	345	6.4	79.7	1.4	2.9
Wild Chilli, McCoys*	1 Bag/50g	255	15.2	510	6.0	53.2	30.3	4.8
Wild Paprika Flavour, Croky*	1 Pack/45g	234	13.0	521	6.0	58.0	29.0	0.0
Worcester Sauce, Sunseed Oil, Walkers*	1 Bag/35g	183	11.4	530	6.5	52.0	33.0	4.0
Worcester Sauce Flavour, Hunky Dorys*	1 Bag/45g	211	12.9	469	6.3	49.3	28.7	0.0
Yoghurt & Green Onion, Kettle Chips*	1 Serving/50g	236	13.0	473	6.6	54.1	26.1	5.4
CRISPY PANCAKE								
Beef, Minced, Findus*	1 Pancake/63g	100	2.5	160	6.5	25.0	4.0	1.0
Chicken, Bacon & Sweetcorn, Findus*	1 Pancake/63g	101	2.5	160	5.5	26.0	4.0	1.1
Three Cheeses, Findus*	1 Pancake/62g	118	4.0	190	7.0	25.0	6.5	0.9
CROISSANT								
All Butter, BGTY, Sainsbury's*	1 Croissant/44g	151	6.5	343	9.3	42.7	14.8	1.8
All Butter, M & S*	1 Croissant/54g	222	12.8	415	7.4	45.2	23.8	1.6
All Butter, Mini, Sainsbury's*	1 Croissant/35g	150	8.6	428	9.2	42.6	24.5	1.2
All Butter, Reduced Fat, Tesco*	1 Croissant/52g	164	5.5	315	7.5	47.4	10.6	1.8
All Butter, Sainsbury's*	1 Croissant/44g	188	10.8	428	9.2	42.6	24.5	1.2
Average	1 Croissant/50g	180	10.2	360	8.3	38.3	20.3	1.6
Cheese & Ham, Delice de France*	1 Serving/91g	225	12.3	247	7.0	24.4	13.5	2.5
Cheese & Ham, Mini, Waitrose*	1 Croissant/17g	64	4.1	383	13.2	28.1	24.6	3.0

	Measure INFO/WEIGHT	per Measure KCAL	FAT	Nutrition Values per 100g / 100ml KCAL	PROT	CARB	FAT	FIBRE
CROISSANT								
Continental, Mini, Chosen By You, Asda*	1 Croissant/35g	150	8.9	427	9.2	40.6	25.3	1.6
Creme Patissiere & Raisins, Mini Chinois, Aldi*	1 Chinois/50g	133	3.4	266	0.0	20.2	6.8	0.0
Flaky Pastry, with a Plain Chocolate Filling, Tesco*	1 Croissant/78g	318	19.0	408	6.5	41.0	24.3	2.0
French Butter, Bon Appetit, Aldi*	1 Croissant/40g	171	9.2	428	7.0	47.2	23.0	2.2
French Butter, You Count, Love Life, Waitrose*	1 Croissant/44g	168	7.4	382	9.8	46.4	16.8	3.1
Heart Shaped, Breakfast in Bed, M & S*	1 Croissant/54g	230	13.6	430	8.2	43.7	25.5	1.2
Homebake, Long Life, Stay Fresh Range, Harvestime*	1 Croissant/44g	159	6.0	362	7.6	51.9	13.7	1.9
Low Fat, M & S*	1 Croissant/45g	180	9.1	400	8.2	46.0	20.2	1.8
Mini, Lidl*	1 Croissant/30g	112	5.0	373	7.8	48.0	16.6	0.0
Organic, Tesco*	1 Croissant/45g	195	11.6	433	8.2	42.0	25.8	2.2
Reduced Fat, Asda*	1 Croissant/44g	159	6.5	361	9.7	47.2	14.8	2.0
Reduced Fat, Sainsbury's*	1 Croissant/44g	173	7.7	393	9.8	49.2	17.5	2.2
CROQUETTES								
Morrisons*	1 Serving/150g	231	8.1	154	3.3	23.1	5.4	1.1
Potato, Asda*	3 Croquettes/81g	144	5.7	177	2.0	26.5	7.0	2.2
Potato, Birds Eye*	1 Croquette/29g	44	1.7	152	2.6	22.6	5.7	1.2
Potato, Cheese & Onion, Mash Direct*	2 Croquettes/100g	214	10.0	214	3.7	26.1	10.0	2.3
Potato, Chunky, Aunt Bessie's*	1 Serving/41g	62	2.5	152	2.3	23.9	6.1	1.8
Potato, Crispy, Chilled, Sainsbury's*	3 Croquettes/125g	245	11.5	196	2.5	25.7	9.2	1.9
Potato, Fried in Blended Oil, Average	1 Croquette/80g	171	10.5	214	3.7	21.6	13.1	1.3
Potato, M & S*	1 Croquette/41g	68	3.6	165	2.4	19.3	8.8	2.2
Potato, Sainsbury's*	½ Pack/110g	227	10.9	223	3.3	27.1	10.7	2.8
Potato, Waitrose*	1 Croquette/30g	47	2.4	157	3.0	17.9	8.1	1.5
Potato & Parsnip, Finest, Tesco*	2 Croquettes/74g	155	7.3	210	6.0	23.2	9.9	3.9
Vegetable, Sainsbury's*	1 Serving/175g	392	20.8	224	5.8	23.3	11.9	2.2
CROUTONS								
Fresh, M & S*	1 Serving/10g	53	3.3	530	11.4	50.0	32.8	3.2
Garlic, Waitrose*	1 Serving/40g	209	12.0	522	10.8	52.1	30.0	2.7
Herb, Sainsbury's*	1 Serving/15g	64	1.7	429	13.4	68.2	11.4	2.8
Herb & Garlic, La Rochelle*	¼ Pack/18g	106	7.2	587	6.9	49.8	40.0	2.1
Italian Salad, Sainsbury's*	1 Pack/40g	204	10.0	510	8.5	62.7	25.0	2.5
La Rochelle*	1 Bag/70g	400	28.0	572	7.0	49.0	40.0	0.0
Lightly Sea Salted, Asda*	1 Serving/20g	83	1.9	414	12.9	69.7	9.3	4.3
Migros*	1 Serving/15g	56	0.4	375	14.0	72.0	3.0	3.5
Prepacked, Average	1 Serving/15g	74	3.6	495	10.8	58.7	24.0	2.6
Sun Dried Tomato, Sainsbury's*	¼ Pack/15g	75	3.8	497	11.7	55.2	25.5	2.5
CRUMBLE								
Almond & Apricot, Devondale*	1 Cake/80g	314	13.2	392	3.6	57.0	16.5	9.8
Apple, Average	1 Serving/240g	497	12.0	207	0.9	40.5	5.0	1.1
Apple, Basics, Sainsbury's*	¼ Crumble/125g	235	4.9	188	1.7	36.5	3.9	1.2
Apple, Fresh, Chilled, Tesco*	¼ Pack/150g	368	13.4	245	2.8	38.0	8.9	1.4
Apple, Frozen, Iceland*	1 Serving/97g	240	9.8	247	2.1	36.9	10.1	1.8
Apple, Sara Lee*	1 Serving/200g	606	18.0	303	2.3	53.3	9.0	1.2
Apple, with Custard, Green's*	1 Serving/79g	171	5.3	216	1.9	37.0	6.7	1.2
Apple, with Custard, Individual, Sainsbury's*	1 Pudding/120g	286	13.9	238	2.0	31.4	11.6	2.4
Apple, with Sultanas, Weight Watchers*	1 Dessert/110g	196	4.3	178	1.4	34.2	3.9	1.3
Apple & Blackberry, Asda*	1 Serving/175g	427	15.8	244	2.7	38.0	9.0	1.2
Apple & Blackberry, M & S*	1 Serving/135g	398	15.1	295	3.5	44.9	11.2	1.6
Apple & Blackberry, Sainsbury's*	1 Serving/110g	232	6.2	211	3.0	37.1	5.6	2.1
Apple & Custard, Asda*	1 Serving/125g	250	8.8	200	2.3	32.0	7.0	0.0
Apple & Toffee, Weight Watchers*	1 Pot/98g	190	4.5	194	1.6	36.6	4.6	0.0
Blackcurrant & Apple, Devondale*	1 Cake/80g	314	13.2	393	3.6	57.0	16.5	9.8
Cauliflower & Camembert, Sainsbury's*	1 Pack/400g	588	43.2	147	5.5	6.9	10.8	0.7

	Measure INFO/WEIGHT	per Measure KCAL	FAT	Nutrition Values per 100g / 100ml KCAL	PROT	CARB	FAT	FIBRE
CRUMBLE								
Christmas, Devondale*	1 Cake/100g	359	12.4	359	3.3	58.7	12.4	2.4
Fish & Prawn, Youngs*	1 Pie/375g	476	27.0	127	5.8	9.7	7.2	1.3
Fruit	1 Portion/170g	337	11.7	198	2.0	34.0	6.9	1.7
Fruit, Wholemeal	1oz/28g	54	2.0	193	2.6	31.7	7.1	2.7
Fruit, with Custard	1 Serving/270g	463	17.6	171	2.4	27.0	6.5	1.3
Gooseberry, M & S*	1 Serving/133g	379	14.2	285	3.5	43.3	10.7	1.7
Ocean, Low Fat, Ross*	1 Crumble/300g	219	2.4	73	5.1	11.4	0.8	0.4
Rhubarb, Average	1 Portion/150g	330	11.1	220	2.7	35.5	7.4	1.9
Rhubarb, Devondale*	1 Cake/80g	316	13.2	395	3.5	57.0	16.5	9.0
Rhubarb, with Custard, Sainsbury's*	1 Serving/120g	288	13.9	240	2.4	31.4	11.6	2.3
Salmon, Youngs*	1 Pie/360g	367	14.4	102	5.4	11.1	4.0	1.0
CRUMBLE MIX								
Luxury, Tesco*	¼ Pack/55g	243	9.0	441	5.7	67.9	16.3	3.2
Luxury, Wholegrain, GF, Hale & Hearty*	1 Serving/100g	447	17.0	447	2.5	71.0	17.0	3.6
CRUMBLE TOPPING								
Morrisons*	1 Serving/40g	179	6.6	448	5.4	69.5	16.5	2.8
Sainsbury's*	1 Serving/47g	188	9.2	401	5.9	50.3	19.6	5.3
CRUMPETS								
Asda*	1 Crumpet/45g	85	0.4	188	6.0	39.0	0.9	2.1
Fruit, from Bakery, Tesco*	1 Crumpet/73g	161	1.7	220	6.2	43.2	2.3	1.1
Gluten, Wheat & Milk Free, Free From, Livwell*	1 Crumpet/55g	83	1.7	151	3.6	26.9	3.1	2.0
Golden Sun*	1 Crumpet/43g	83	0.7	193	7.8	37.1	1.6	1.6
Kingsmill*	1 Crumpet/55g	99	0.4	180	5.8	37.5	0.8	1.7
Less Than 2% Fat, M & S*	1 Crumpet/61g	116	0.8	190	8.0	36.9	1.3	2.1
Morning Fresh*	1 Crumpet/20g	36	0.3	180	7.3	34.8	1.3	5.2
Mother's Pride*	1 Crumpet/43g	80	0.4	185	5.6	38.3	1.0	2.3
Perfectly Balanced, Waitrose*	1 Crumpet/55g	94	0.2	171	6.1	36.1	0.3	4.4
Premium, Sainsbury's*	1 Crumpet/50g	96	0.7	191	6.1	38.6	1.4	1.7
Rowan Hill Bakery, Lidl*	1 Crumpet/44g	78	0.5	178	5.5	34.5	1.2	0.0
Scottish, Nick Nairn's*	1 Serving/100g	186	9.6	186	5.3	43.0	9.6	1.5
Smart Price, Asda*	1 Crumpet/36g	67	0.3	188	6.0	39.0	0.9	2.1
Soldier, Mother's Pride*	1 Crumpet/30g	58	0.5	193	7.8	37.1	1.6	1.6
Square, Spongebob Squarepants*	1 Crumpet/50g	93	0.5	186	7.0	37.2	1.0	1.0
Square, Tesco*	1 Crumpet/60g	101	0.5	168	6.3	33.8	0.8	2.7
Toasted, Average	1 Crumpet/40g	80	0.4	199	6.7	43.4	1.0	2.0
Toaster, Organic, Waitrose*	1 Crumpet/55g	95	0.3	172	7.3	34.4	0.6	4.6
Warburton's*	1 Crumpet/55g	98	0.4	178	5.6	36.1	0.7	2.3
CRUNCHIE								
Blast, Cadbury*	1 Serving/42g	199	8.3	480	4.7	69.6	20.1	0.7
Cadbury*	1 Bar/40g	185	7.5	465	4.0	69.5	18.9	0.5
Nuggets, Cadbury*	1 Bag/125g	569	20.5	455	3.8	73.1	16.4	0.0
Treat Size, Cadbury*	1 Bar/17g	80	3.1	470	4.0	71.5	18.4	0.0
CRUNCHY STICKS								
Ready Salted, M & S*	1 Pack/75g	398	24.8	530	5.6	52.2	33.0	3.8
Ready Salted, Tesco*	1 Serving/25g	119	5.9	475	5.6	60.3	23.5	3.0
Salt & Vinegar, Shapers, Boots*	1 Pack/21g	96	3.8	457	5.7	66.7	18.1	2.4
CUCUMBER								
Average	***1 Serving/80g***	***8***	***0.1***	***10***	***0.7***	***1.5***	***0.1***	***0.6***
CUMIN								
Seeds, Ground, Schwartz*	1 Tsp/5g	22	1.2	446	19.0	40.3	23.2	0.0
Seeds, Whole, Average	***1 Tsp/2g***	***8***	***0.5***	***375***	***17.8***	***44.2***	***22.7***	***10.5***
CUPCAKES								
Assorted, Sainsbury's*	1 Cake/38g	130	2.3	341	2.2	69.3	6.1	0.4

	Measure INFO/WEIGHT	per Measure KCAL	FAT	Nutrition Values per 100g / 100ml KCAL	PROT	CARB	FAT	FIBRE
CUPCAKES								
Carrot, Average	1 Cake/40g	157	8.6	392	3.6	45.4	21.6	0.6
Chocolate, 5% Fat, Sainsbury's*	1 Cake/38g	133	1.7	349	2.5	74.8	4.4	1.7
Chocolate, Average	1 Cake/40g	159	6.4	398	3.5	59.9	16.0	1.2
Chocolate, BGTY, Sainsbury's*	1 Cake/38g	121	1.7	318	2.5	66.5	4.6	0.8
Chocolate, COU, M & S*	1 Cake/45g	130	1.3	290	4.6	62.2	2.8	4.3
Chocolate, Fabulous Bakin' Boys*	1 Cake/34g	152	8.1	448	4.0	54.0	24.0	1.0
Chocolate, Healthy Option, Average	1 Cake/40g	128	1.6	319	3.2	67.8	3.9	2.3
Chocolate, Lyons*	1 Cake/39g	125	1.8	321	2.4	67.5	4.6	0.8
Chocolate, Mini, Weight Watchers*	1 Cake/20g	87	4.3	426	6.1	52.0	21.1	1.8
Cookies & Cream, Secret Chocolate Centre, Tesco*	1 Cake/69g	335	20.0	485	2.7	52.2	29.0	1.0
Jam Splatter, Tesco*	1 Cake/47g	221	10.2	470	2.3	65.6	21.8	0.5
Lemon, Average	1 Cake/40g	184	10.1	461	3.0	55.5	25.3	1.1
Lemon, COU, M & S*	1 Cake/43g	130	0.9	305	3.3	68.1	2.1	2.0
Lemon, Healthy Option, Average	1 Cake/40g	131	1.5	328	2.7	68.9	3.7	5.2
Lemon, Mini, Weight Watchers*	1 Cake/17g	56	0.8	333	2.4	63.3	4.9	12.1
Pink, M & S*	1 Cake/39g	160	3.3	410	2.5	81.3	8.5	0.6
Vanilla Iced, Jack O' Lantern, Mini, The Cookieman Ltd*	1 Cake/25g	105	3.8	419	2.4	66.8	15.3	2.0
CURACAO								
Average	***1 Shot/35ml***	***109***	***0.0***	***311***	***0.0***	***28.3***	***0.0***	***0.0***
CURLY WURLY								
Cadbury*	1 Bar/26g	115	4.5	442	3.5	69.2	17.3	0.8
Squirlies, Cadbury*	1 Squirl/3g	13	0.5	442	3.5	69.2	17.3	0.8
CURRANTS								
Average	***1oz/28g***	***75***	***0.1***	***267***	***2.3***	***67.8***	***0.4***	***1.9***
CURRY								
Aubergine	1oz/28g	33	2.8	118	1.4	6.2	10.1	1.5
Beef, Hot, Canned, M & S*	1 Can/425g	446	21.7	105	12.2	2.8	5.1	1.0
Beef, Sainsbury's*	1 Serving/400g	552	32.8	138	10.7	5.4	8.2	0.9
Beef, Smart Price, Asda*	1 Serving/392g	223	2.0	57	4.0	9.0	0.5	1.0
Beef, with Rice, Asda*	1 Pack/406g	548	15.8	135	6.0	19.0	3.9	1.2
Beef, with Rice, Birds Eye*	1 Pack/388g	524	10.9	135	6.9	20.8	2.8	0.8
Beef, with Rice, Weight Watchers*	1 Pack/328g	249	3.3	76	4.2	12.5	1.0	0.3
Blackeye Bean, Gujerati	1oz/28g	36	1.2	127	7.2	16.1	4.4	2.8
Butternut Squash, Bombay, Veg Pot, Innocent*	1 Pot/380g	296	4.2	78	2.6	12.5	1.1	4.1
Cabbage	1oz/28g	23	1.4	82	1.9	8.1	5.0	2.1
Cauliflower & Chickpea, Lovely Vegetables, M & S*	1 Serving/390g	351	13.6	90	2.9	11.2	3.5	3.7
Cauliflower & Potato	1oz/28g	17	0.7	59	3.4	6.6	2.4	1.8
Chana Dahl, Curry Special*	1 Pack/350g	434	22.8	124	6.0	10.5	6.5	5.9
Chick Pea, Whole, Average	1oz/28g	50	2.1	179	9.6	21.3	7.5	4.5
Chick Pea, Whole, Basic, Average	1oz/28g	30	1.0	108	6.0	14.2	3.6	3.3
Chicken, Asda*	1 Can/200g	210	10.0	105	10.0	5.0	5.0	0.0
Chicken, Canned, Sainsbury's*	1 Serving/100g	136	6.1	136	11.1	9.1	6.1	1.0
Chicken, Chinese, with Rice, Ready Meal, Average	1 Serving/450g	490	11.5	109	7.2	14.1	2.6	1.3
Chicken, Diet Chef Ltd*	1 Portion/300g	342	13.2	114	9.1	9.5	4.4	1.0
Chicken, Extra Strong, M & S*	1oz/28g	28	1.1	100	13.8	2.5	3.9	1.4
Chicken, Green Thai, BGTY, Sainsbury's*	1 Pack/400g	316	10.4	79	10.6	3.4	2.6	1.9
Chicken, Green Thai, Birds Eye*	1 Pack/450g	536	19.8	119	4.7	15.2	4.4	0.3
Chicken, Green Thai, Breasts, Finest, Tesco*	1 Serving/200g	292	16.0	146	16.5	2.0	8.0	0.7
Chicken, Green Thai, Charlie Bigham's*	½ Pack/300g	402	26.7	134	9.9	3.6	8.9	0.8
Chicken, Green Thai, Jasmine Rice, Weight Watchers*	1 Pack/320g	291	3.2	91	6.1	14.3	1.0	0.5
Chicken, Green Thai, Sainsbury's*	½ Pack/200g	264	13.6	132	13.0	4.8	6.8	0.9
Chicken, Green Thai Style & Sticky Rice, Asda*	1 Pack/450g	585	10.8	130	7.0	20.0	2.4	0.1
Chicken, Healthy Options, Birds Eye*	1 Pack/350g	336	3.2	96	5.1	16.8	0.9	0.5

	Measure INFO/WEIGHT	per Measure KCAL	FAT	Nutrition Values per 100g / 100ml KCAL	PROT	CARB	FAT	FIBRE
CURRY								
Chicken, Hot, Can, Tesco*	1 Can/418g	514	26.3	123	9.7	6.9	6.3	0.9
Chicken, Hot, Canned, Asda*	1 Can/398g	501	23.9	126	11.0	7.0	6.0	0.5
Chicken, Hot, Iceland*	1 Can/392g	492	20.4	126	10.0	9.8	5.2	0.7
Chicken, Kashmiri, Waitrose*	1 Serving/400g	640	36.4	160	14.5	5.0	9.1	0.6
Chicken, Malaysian, Chosen By You, Asda*	1 Serving/375g	390	9.8	104	6.1	13.3	2.6	1.5
Chicken, Malaysian, Finest, Tesco*	1 Pack/375g	375	8.3	100	7.4	12.2	2.2	0.8
Chicken, Medium Hot, M & S*	1 Serving/200g	310	14.2	155	7.8	14.3	7.1	0.8
Chicken, Mild, Asda*	½ Can/190g	239	11.4	126	11.0	7.0	6.0	0.5
Chicken, Mild, BGTY, Sainsbury's*	1 Serving/200g	184	5.2	92	10.0	7.2	2.6	0.5
Chicken, Mild, Canned, Bilash, Aldi*	½ Can/200g	180	7.6	90	9.5	4.5	3.8	0.7
Chicken, Mild, Iceland*	½ Can/200g	234	9.0	117	10.6	8.5	4.5	0.7
Chicken, Mild, Sainsbury's*	1 Can/400g	472	27.6	118	10.5	3.5	6.9	1.3
Chicken, Mild, Tinned, Sainsbury's*	1 Serving/200g	214	7.0	107	12.7	6.1	3.5	1.1
Chicken, Mild & Fruity, Breasts, HE, Tesco*	2 Breasts/345g	321	5.2	93	15.8	4.1	1.5	0.5
Chicken, Red Thai, & Fragrant Rice, Charlie Bigham's*	½ Pack/418g	602	28.4	144	6.7	14.0	6.8	0.0
Chicken, Red Thai, 97% Fat Free, Birds Eye*	1 Pack/366g	425	7.0	116	5.7	19.0	1.9	0.5
Chicken, Red Thai, Asda*	1 Pack/360g	461	27.7	128	9.1	5.5	7.7	1.0
Chicken, Red Thai, COU, M & S*	1 Pack/400g	420	9.2	105	7.1	13.4	2.3	1.4
Chicken, Red Thai, Tesco*	1 Serving/175g	215	11.6	123	10.5	5.5	6.6	1.4
Chicken, Red Thai, with Jasmine Rice, Weight Watchers*	1 Pack/400g	344	3.2	86	6.5	12.9	0.8	0.8
Chicken, Red Thai, with Rice, Tesco*	1 Serving/475g	746	32.3	157	7.2	16.8	6.8	1.1
Chicken, Reduced Fat, Asda*	1 Pack/400g	476	10.4	119	6.0	18.0	2.6	0.9
Chicken, Rendang, Sainsbury's*	1 Pack/350g	690	53.6	197	9.6	5.1	15.3	1.7
Chicken, Smart Price, Asda*	1 Can/392g	282	5.1	72	4.0	11.0	1.3	1.0
Chicken, with Naan Bread, Iceland*	1 Portion/260g	484	16.4	186	10.1	22.3	6.3	1.4
Chicken, with Potato Wedges, HE, Tesco*	1 Pack/450g	428	12.2	95	7.6	10.3	2.7	1.1
Chicken, with Potatoes, Diet Chef Ltd*	1 Pack/300g	291	13.2	97	7.5	6.9	4.4	2.8
Chicken, with Rice, Average	1 Serving/400g	465	11.0	116	5.1	17.8	2.8	0.8
Chicken, with Rice, Birds Eye*	1 Pack/400g	468	11.2	117	4.5	18.4	2.8	0.6
Chicken, with Rice, Dunnes Stores*	1 Pack/375g	400	6.3	107	4.2	20.2	1.7	0.8
Chicken, with Rice, Fresh, Co-Op*	1 Pack/300g	270	9.0	90	3.0	13.0	3.0	1.0
Chicken, with Rice, Frozen, Tesco*	1 Pack/400g	488	15.6	122	4.6	17.2	3.9	0.7
Chicken, with Rice, Fruity, HL, Tesco*	1 Pack/450g	495	5.4	110	6.5	18.2	1.2	1.2
Chicken, with Rice, Malaysian, Bernard Matthews*	1 Pack/400g	512	15.6	128	6.1	17.0	3.9	0.0
Chicken, with Rice, Ross*	1 Serving/320g	275	3.8	86	3.7	14.8	1.2	0.5
Chicken, Yellow Thai Style, HL, Tesco*	1 Pack/450g	504	12.2	112	9.3	12.6	2.7	0.5
Chicken & Vegetable, Big Eat, Heinz*	1 Pot/350g	392	18.2	112	5.4	10.9	5.2	4.3
Chicken Katsu, City Kitchen, Tesco*	1 Pack/385g	465	13.2	121	6.0	16.3	3.4	1.3
Chinese Chicken, Morrisons*	1 Pack/340g	347	15.6	102	10.3	5.0	4.6	0.8
Courgette & Potato	1oz/28g	24	1.5	86	1.9	8.7	5.2	1.2
Dudhi, Kofta	1oz/28g	32	2.1	113	2.6	9.4	7.4	2.8
Fish, Bangladeshi, Average	1oz/28g	35	2.2	124	12.2	1.5	7.9	0.3
Fish, Red Thai, Waitrose*	1 Pack/500g	275	11.0	55	5.2	3.7	2.2	1.0
Fish & Vegetable, Bangladeshi, Average	1oz/28g	33	2.4	117	9.1	1.4	8.4	0.5
Gobi Aloo Sag, Retail	1oz/28g	27	1.9	95	2.2	7.1	6.9	1.4
Green Thai, & Rice, GFY, Asda*	1 Pack/400g	356	7.6	89	7.0	11.0	1.9	1.6
Green Thai, with Sticky Rice, HL, Tesco*	1 Pack/450g	518	12.2	115	7.7	14.9	2.7	0.6
Indian Daal, Tasty Veg Pot, Innocent*	1 Pot/380g	319	9.9	84	2.8	9.7	2.6	5.3
King Prawn, Coconut & Lime, Sainsbury's*	½ Pack/351g	207	8.8	59	3.7	5.4	2.5	1.0
King Prawn, Goan, M & S*	1 Pack/400g	680	44.4	170	5.1	11.6	11.1	1.5
King Prawn, Malay with Rice, Sainsbury's*	1 Pack/400g	608	20.4	152	5.0	21.5	5.1	1.4
King Prawn, Red Thai, City Kitchen, Tesco*	1 Pack/385g	460	14.4	119	4.5	16.7	3.7	1.0
King Prawn Malay, Waitrose*	1 Pack/350g	364	19.2	104	6.6	7.1	5.5	0.9

	Measure INFO/WEIGHT	per Measure KCAL	FAT	Nutrition Values per 100g / 100ml KCAL	PROT	CARB	FAT	FIBRE
CURRY								
Lamb, Hot, M & S*	½ Can/213g	320	19.6	150	14.9	6.0	9.2	2.3
Lamb, Kefthedes, Waitrose*	½ Pack/200g	294	17.6	147	9.0	8.0	8.8	2.1
Lamb & Potato, 385, Wiltshire Farm Foods*	1 Serving/210g	334	23.0	159	8.9	6.2	11.0	1.7
Masala, Aubergine, TTD, Sainsbury's*	½ Pack/115g	135	11.4	117	2.9	4.1	9.9	5.8
Masala, Indian, Veg Pot, Innocent*	1 Pot/380g	331	10.3	87	2.9	11.6	2.7	3.6
Matar Paneer, Peas & Cheese, Ashoka*	½ Pack/150g	183	10.0	122	5.3	10.0	6.7	2.0
Medium, with Long Grain Rice, Rice Time, Uncle Ben's*	1 Pot/300g	396	9.0	132	2.3	23.2	3.0	1.2
Monkfish, & King Prawn, Gastropub, M & S*	½ Pack/285g	270	15.3	95	8.5	2.3	5.4	1.4
Mushroom & Pea, Masala, Indian, Sainsbury's*	1 Pack/300g	264	14.7	88	3.3	5.2	4.9	5.1
Potato & Pea	1oz/28g	26	1.1	92	2.9	13.0	3.8	2.4
Prawn, & Mushroom	1oz/28g	47	4.0	168	7.3	2.5	14.4	1.0
Prawn, Red Thai, Sainsbury's*	1 Pack/300g	546	39.6	182	6.3	9.4	13.2	1.7
Prawn, Red Thai Sauce, Youngs*	1 Pack/255g	197	8.7	77	4.8	6.5	3.4	0.8
Prawn, Spicy, Kashmiri, Sizzler, Tesco*	1 Pack/380g	266	9.5	70	5.7	4.6	2.5	2.3
Prawn, Thai, with Jasmine Rice, BGTY, Sainsbury's*	1 Serving/401g	353	6.0	88	4.2	14.5	1.5	2.0
Prawn, with Rice, Asda*	1 Pack/400g	420	10.4	105	3.5	17.0	2.6	1.1
Prawn, with Rice, Birds Eye*	1 Pack/375g	442	0.0	118	3.5	20.6	0.0	0.0
Prawn, with Rice, Frozen, Sainsbury's*	1 Pack/400g	552	7.6	138	3.9	26.4	1.9	2.1
Prawn, with Rice, Iceland*	1 Pack/450g	468	14.4	104	3.2	16.4	3.2	1.5
Prawn, with Rice, Light & Easy, Youngs*	1 Pack/310g	248	3.4	80	3.3	14.2	1.1	0.9
Red Kidney Bean, Punjabi	1oz/28g	30	1.6	106	4.7	10.1	5.6	3.8
Red Thai, Vegetarian, Tesco*	1 Pack/429ml	588	21.9	137	5.4	17.3	5.1	1.6
Red Thai, with Rice, Finest, Tesco*	1 Pack/500g	660	15.5	132	8.0	17.8	3.1	0.6
Salmon, Green, Waitrose*	1 Pack/401g	581	40.5	145	9.1	4.5	10.1	2.7
Spicy Paneer, Lovely Vegetables, M & S*	1 Pot/300g	330	12.0	110	4.3	11.9	4.0	4.0
Vegetable, & Rice, Microwaveable, M & S*	1 Pot/325g	390	7.2	120	2.3	22.3	2.2	2.2
Vegetable, Asda*	1 Pack/350g	329	21.0	94	1.9	8.0	6.0	1.9
Vegetable, Canned, Sainsbury's*	½ Can/200g	200	12.2	100	1.4	9.8	6.1	1.8
Vegetable, Diet Chef Ltd*	1 Pack/300g	153	3.6	51	2.0	8.0	1.2	2.1
Vegetable, Frozen, Mixed Vegetables, Average	1oz/28g	25	1.7	88	2.5	6.9	6.1	0.0
Vegetable, in Sweet Sauce, Average	1 Serving/330g	162	6.9	49	1.4	6.7	2.1	1.3
Vegetable, Indian, Canned, Tesco*	1 Can/400g	320	18.0	80	2.0	6.7	4.5	1.1
Vegetable, Indian, Sainsbury's*	½ Pack/200g	206	14.6	103	2.5	6.8	7.3	4.6
Vegetable, Indian Meal for One, Tesco*	1 Serving/200g	218	14.4	109	2.0	9.0	7.2	1.2
Vegetable, LC, Tesco*	1 Pack/350g	350	4.2	100	2.3	19.4	1.2	1.5
Vegetable, Medium, Tesco*	1 Pack/350g	326	21.7	93	2.3	7.1	6.2	1.9
Vegetable, Mild, Tesco*	1 Can/425g	314	10.6	74	2.1	10.7	2.5	1.7
Vegetable, Mixed, Organic, Pure & Pronto*	1 Pack/400g	368	11.6	92	4.2	12.4	2.9	4.8
Vegetable, Pakistani, Average	1oz/28g	17	0.7	60	2.2	8.7	2.6	2.2
Vegetable, Sabzi Tarkari, Patak's*	1 Pack/400g	500	31.2	125	2.5	11.1	7.8	2.2
Vegetable, Smart Price, Asda*	½ Can/203g	132	1.0	65	2.0	13.0	0.5	1.7
Vegetable, Takeaway, Average	1 Serving/330g	346	24.4	105	2.5	7.6	7.4	0.0
Vegetable, Tinned, Asda*	½ Can/200g	206	12.0	103	2.2	10.0	6.0	2.5
Vegetable, with Pilau Rice, Linda McCartney*	1 Pack/339g	224	2.0	66	1.6	13.5	0.6	0.5
Vegetable, with Pilau Rice, Weight Watchers*	1 Pack/400g	296	3.2	74	1.6	15.1	0.8	1.9
Vegetable, with Rice, Asda*	1 Pack/393g	432	12.2	110	2.6	18.0	3.1	1.4
Vegetable, with Rice, Birds Eye*	1 Pack/414g	455	9.5	110	2.3	19.6	2.3	1.1
Vegetable, with Rice, Healthy Range, Average	1 Serving/400g	351	4.6	88	2.3	16.8	1.1	1.9
Vegetable, with Rice, Tesco*	1 Pack/400g	440	12.0	110	2.1	18.7	3.0	1.0
Vegetable, with Yoghurt, Average	1oz/28g	17	1.1	62	2.6	4.6	4.1	1.4
Vegetable, WTF, Sainsbury's*	½ Pack/344g	227	3.8	66	2.5	11.6	1.1	1.4
Vegetable, Yellow, Tesco*	1 Pack/356g	324	17.4	91	1.9	9.9	4.9	1.4
Vegetable, Yellow Thai, Sainsbury's*	1 Pack/400g	624	48.8	156	2.2	9.4	12.2	1.1

	Measure INFO/WEIGHT	per Measure KCAL	FAT	Nutrition Values per 100g / 100ml KCAL	PROT	CARB	FAT	FIBRE
CURRY								
Vegetable Masala, LC, Tesco*	1 Pack/350g	298	6.0	85	3.8	13.6	1.7	3.4
CURRY LEAVES								
Fresh	***1oz/28g***	***27***	***0.4***	***97***	***7.9***	***13.3***	***1.3***	***0.0***
CURRY PASTE								
Balti, Asda*	1 Tube/100g	164	9.8	164	4.2	11.6	9.8	6.3
Balti, Sharwood's*	¼ Pack/73g	328	28.7	453	5.0	19.2	39.6	3.1
Balti, Tomato & Coriander, Original, Patak's*	1 Tbsp/15g	58	5.1	388	4.0	14.6	34.0	3.7
Bhuna, Tomato & Tamarind, Patak's*	1 Serving/10g	40	5.6	397	4.3	17.5	56.2	6.3
Garam Masala, Cinnamon & Ginger, Hot, Patak's*	1 Serving/30g	121	10.6	403	3.2	17.9	35.4	0.6
Green Thai, Average	1 Tsp/5g	6	0.4	128	2.1	11.7	7.9	3.1
Hot, Sharwood's*	1oz/28g	123	10.7	439	5.1	18.6	38.3	2.6
Jalfrezi, Patak's*	1 Serving/30g	96	8.1	320	3.7	14.2	26.9	5.6
Korma, Asda*	1 Tube/100g	338	23.5	338	5.1	26.6	23.5	1.2
Korma, Coconut & Coriander, Original, Patak's*	1 Serving/30g	124	11.7	415	3.5	11.6	39.0	5.2
Madras, Cumin & Chilli, Hot, Patak's*	¼ Jar/70g	202	18.1	289	4.7	7.6	25.9	10.8
Medium, Asda*	1 Tsp/5ml/5g	18	1.6	364	5.0	14.0	32.0	5.0
Medium, Barts Spices*	1 Serving/30g	88	6.4	295	4.5	19.2	21.5	5.5
Medium, M & S*	1oz/28g	64	5.5	230	2.5	10.7	19.5	4.9
Medium, Sharwood's*	1oz/28g	122	10.9	434	4.5	16.8	38.8	2.7
Mild, Asda*	¼ Jar/46g	206	18.9	448	3.8	16.0	41.0	7.0
Mild, Coriander & Cumin, Original, Patak's*	1 Serving/35g	99	8.6	283	4.8	9.1	24.6	10.7
Mild, Sharwood's*	1oz/28g	78	6.0	279	3.6	17.7	21.5	3.4
Red Thai, Average	1 Tsp/5g	7	0.5	132	2.3	9.5	9.1	3.0
Rogan Josh, Tomato & Paprika, Patak's*	1 Serving/30g	119	11.0	397	4.1	12.7	36.7	5.9
Tamarind & Ginger, Original, Patak's*	1 Tbsp/15g	20	0.3	133	3.4	23.1	2.0	2.9
Tandoori, Sharwood's*	1oz/28g	64	4.4	228	5.9	15.5	15.8	1.9
Tandoori, Tamarind & Ginger, Patak's*	1 Serving/30g	33	0.5	110	3.1	20.4	1.8	2.6
Tikka, Asda*	½ Tube/50g	118	8.5	235	4.5	16.1	17.0	1.6
Tikka Masala, Coriander & Lemon, Medium, Patak's*	1 Serving/30g	111	9.5	369	3.8	16.9	31.8	2.9
Tikka Masala, Sharwood's*	1oz/28g	53	4.3	191	3.2	9.9	15.4	2.6
Tikka Masala, Spice, Patak's*	1 Tbsp/15g	46	3.4	305	3.4	17.8	22.8	5.6
Tom Yum, Thai Taste*	1 Tsp/13g	35	2.0	269	5.4	30.8	15.4	7.7
Yellow, Thai, Barts*	1 Serving/30g	84	3.8	281	2.7	30.4	12.8	8.3
Yellow Thai, Tesco*	1 Tbsp/15g	15	0.6	100	1.9	13.6	4.1	4.9
CURRY POWDER								
Average	***1 Tsp/2g***	***6***	***0.3***	***325***	***12.7***	***41.8***	***13.8***	***0.0***
CURRY SAUCE								
Asda*	1 Tbsp/15g	62	2.1	414	13.0	59.0	14.0	1.3
Balti, Asda*	¼ Jar/125g	155	12.5	124	1.6	7.0	10.0	1.7
Balti, Loyd Grossman*	½ Jar/175g	180	11.7	103	1.3	8.4	6.7	1.7
Basics, Sainsbury's*	¼ Jar/110g	70	2.8	64	0.7	9.7	2.5	0.9
Dopiaza, Finest, Tesco*	1 Jar/350g	234	10.5	67	1.3	8.5	3.0	3.7
Green Thai, Asda*	1 Jar/340g	309	27.2	91	0.5	4.3	8.0	0.2
Green Thai, Express, Uncle Ben's*	1 Pack/170g	131	9.9	77	1.1	5.4	5.8	0.0
Green Thai, Stir Fry, Blue Dragon*	1 Sachet/120g	74	4.8	62	0.9	5.7	4.0	0.5
Jalfrezi, Average	1 Sm Jar/350g	326	23.7	93	1.3	6.7	6.8	1.6
Jalfrezi, Loyd Grossman*	½ Jar/175g	159	10.3	91	1.4	7.3	5.9	1.6
Jalfrezi, Piri Piri, Finest, Tesco*	1 Serving/175g	145	10.8	83	1.2	5.7	6.2	1.5
Korma, Average	1 Sm Jar/350g	584	42.3	167	2.3	11.7	12.1	1.3
Korma, Loyd Grossman*	½ Jar/175g	224	14.5	128	1.5	11.3	8.3	0.8
Korma, Uncle Ben's*	1 Jar/500g	630	42.0	126	1.4	11.1	8.4	0.0
Madras, Average	1 Sm Jar/350g	355	24.2	102	1.7	8.0	6.9	1.7
Madras, Cooking, Chosen By You, Asda*	¼ Jar/125g	76	4.4	61	3.2	2.5	3.5	0.0

	Measure INFO/WEIGHT	per Measure KCAL	FAT	Nutrition Values per 100g / 100ml KCAL	PROT	CARB	FAT	FIBRE
CURRY SAUCE								
Madras, Cooking, Sharwood's*	1 Tsp/2g	2	0.1	86	1.5	6.9	5.8	1.3
Madras, Cumin & Chilli, Original, in Glass Jar, Patak's*	1 Jar/540g	648	38.3	120	2.1	11.9	7.1	1.8
Madras, Indian, Sharwood's*	1 Jar/420g	433	26.5	103	1.8	9.7	6.3	1.9
Madras, Sharwood's*	1 Jar/420g	466	28.1	111	1.8	10.9	6.7	2.5
Makhani, Sharwood's*	1 Jar/420g	399	29.0	95	0.9	7.2	6.9	0.4
Malaysian Rendang, Loyd Grossman*	1 Serving/100g	143	10.1	143	2.6	10.4	10.1	1.4
Masala, Red Pepper & Mango, Sainsbury's*	½ Jar/175g	142	8.6	81	1.4	7.8	4.9	1.1
Medium, Uncle Ben's*	1 Jar/500g	330	10.0	66	0.9	10.9	2.0	0.0
Moglai Pasanda, Asda*	½ Jar/170g	277	21.0	163	2.9	10.0	12.4	1.1
Red Thai, Stir Fry, Blue Dragon*	1 Sachet/120g	112	9.6	93	0.9	4.4	8.0	0.5
Rogan Josh, Worldwide Sauces*	1 Jar/500g	255	1.5	51	1.1	11.0	0.3	0.0
Sri Lankan Devil Curry, Sharwood's*	1 Jar/380g	220	11.4	58	0.5	7.2	3.0	2.1
Tikka, Cooking, Tesco*	1 Jar/500g	617	42.2	123	1.7	10.1	8.4	2.0
Tikka Masala, Cooking, HL, Tesco*	¼ Jar/125g	78	3.1	62	0.4	9.0	2.5	0.7
Tikka Masala, COU, M & S*	½ Pack/100g	80	2.6	80	4.5	9.9	2.6	1.7
Tikka Masala, Ready Made, Average	1 Sm Jar/350g	422	28.8	121	2.0	9.6	8.2	1.2
Vindaloo, Cooking, Chosen By You, Asda*	½ Jar/160g	128	5.4	80	1.5	10.4	3.4	1.0
Vindaloo, Hot, Patak's*	1 Jar/540g	643	46.4	119	1.7	8.5	8.6	2.1
CUSTARD								
Banana Flavour, Ambrosia*	1 Pot/135g	139	3.9	103	2.9	16.1	2.9	0.0
Banana Flavour, Pot, Average	1 Pot/135g	138	3.9	102	2.9	16.0	2.9	0.0
Chocolate, COU, M & S*	1 Pot/140g	147	3.1	105	3.1	18.6	2.2	1.0
Chocolate, Ready to Eat, Tesco*	1 Pot/150g	150	3.4	100	3.2	16.2	2.3	0.3
Chocolate Flavour, Ambrosia*	1 Pot/150g	177	4.4	118	3.0	20.0	2.9	0.7
Chocolate Flavour, Pot, Average	1 Pot/125g	138	3.4	111	3.1	18.2	2.7	0.6
Dairy Free, Sainsbury's*	1 Serving/250g	210	4.2	84	3.0	14.2	1.7	0.2
Instant, Just Add Water, Weight Watchers*	1 Sachet/145g	93	0.6	64	1.2	13.9	0.4	0.9
Low Fat, Average	***1/3 Pot/141g***	***116***	***1.6***	***82***	***2.9***	***15.0***	***1.2***	***0.0***
Pot, Forest Fruits Flavour, Hot 'n' Fruity, Bird's*	1 Pot/174g	171	4.2	98	0.9	18.5	2.4	0.1
Powder	***1 Tsp/5g***	***18***	***0.0***	***354***	***0.6***	***92.0***	***0.7***	***0.1***
Ready to Serve, Average	***1 Serving/50g***	***59***	***2.3***	***118***	***3.3***	***16.1***	***4.6***	***0.2***
Strawberry Flavour, Pot, Average	1 Pot/125g	130	3.3	104	2.7	17.3	2.7	0.0
Strawberry Style, Shapers, Boots*	1 Pot/148g	83	1.2	56	4.0	8.2	0.8	0.1
Summer, Ambrosia*	1 Pack/500g	490	15.0	98	2.7	15.0	3.0	0.0
Toffee Flavour, Ambrosia*	1 Pot/150g	156	4.2	104	2.8	17.0	2.8	0.0
Vanilla, COU, M & S*	1 Pot/140g	147	3.5	105	4.3	16.6	2.5	0.6
Vanilla, Low Fat, Fresh, Waitrose*	1/5 Pot/100g	104	2.4	104	3.5	17.1	2.4	0.0
Vanilla, Madagascan, Simply Creamy, Fresh, Waitrose*	1/5 Pot/100g	208	14.4	208	3.4	16.3	14.4	1.1
Vanilla, TTD, Sainsbury's*	1 Pot/150g	312	23.2	208	2.5	14.7	15.5	0.1
Vanilla Bean, Dollop*	1 Dollop/100g	127	3.0	127	20.2	27.7	3.0	0.0
Vanilla Flavour, Pot, Average	1 Pot/125g	128	3.5	102	2.8	16.4	2.8	0.0
CUSTARD APPLE								
Cherimoya, Weighed without Skin & Seeds, Average	1 Piece/312g	234	2.1	75	1.6	17.7	0.7	3.0
CUTLETS								
Nut, Goodlife*	1 Cutlet/88g	283	19.4	322	9.1	21.8	22.0	3.4
Nut, Meat Free, Tesco*	1 Cutlet/70g	240	16.2	340	8.0	22.7	23.0	3.8
Nut, Retail, Fried in Vegetable Oil, Average	1 Cutlet/90g	260	20.1	289	4.8	18.7	22.3	1.7
Nut, Retail, Grilled, Average	1 Cutlet/90g	191	11.7	212	5.1	19.9	13.0	1.8
Vegetable & Nut, Asda*	1 Cutlet/88g	296	20.3	335	10.0	22.0	23.0	4.6
CUTTLEFISH								
Raw	***1oz/28g***	***20***	***0.2***	***71***	***16.1***	***0.0***	***0.7***	***0.0***

	Measure INFO/WEIGHT	per Measure KCAL	FAT	Nutrition Values per 100g / 100ml KCAL	PROT	CARB	FAT	FIBRE
DAB								
Fillets, Lightly Dusted, M & S*	1 Fillet/112g	190	9.7	170	12.8	9.7	8.7	0.5
Raw	***1oz/28g***	***21***	***0.3***	***74***	***15.7***	***0.0***	***1.2***	***0.0***
DAIRYLEA DUNKERS								
Baked Crisps, Dairylea, Kraft*	1 Pack/45g	101	4.0	225	9.2	26.0	9.0	1.1
Jumbo Munch, Dairylea, Kraft*	1 Serving/50g	150	9.2	300	7.2	26.5	18.5	1.2
Salt & Vinegar, Dairylea, Kraft*	1 Tub/42g	116	8.2	275	6.7	17.5	19.5	0.3
with Jumbo Tubes, Kraft*	1 Pack/43g	108	5.1	255	9.1	27.0	12.0	0.9
with Ritz Crackers, Dairylea, Kraft*	1 Tub/46g	143	7.6	310	13.5	26.0	16.5	1.4
DAIRYLEA LUNCHABLES								
Cheese & Pizza Crackers, Dairylea, Kraft*	1oz/28g	105	7.6	375	10.5	24.5	27.0	1.4
Ham & Cheese Pizza, Dairylea, Kraft*	1 Pack/97g	247	10.7	255	11.5	26.0	11.0	1.6
Harvest Ham, Dairylea, Kraft*	1 Pack/110g	314	18.7	285	16.5	16.5	17.0	0.3
Tasty Chicken, Dairylea, Kraft*	1 Pack/110g	314	18.2	285	17.0	17.5	16.5	0.3
DAMSONS								
Raw, Weighed with Stones, Average	***1oz/28g***	***10***	***0.0***	***34***	***0.5***	***8.6***	***0.0***	***1.6***
Raw, Weighed without Stones, Average	***1oz/28g***	***11***	***0.0***	***38***	***0.5***	***9.6***	***0.0***	***1.8***
DANDELION & BURDOCK								
Barr*	1 Bottle/250ml	40	0.0	16	0.0	4.0	0.0	0.0
Fermented, Botanical, Fentiman's*	1 Bottle/275ml	130	0.0	47	0.0	11.6	0.0	0.0
Original, Ben Shaws*	1 Can/440ml	128	0.0	29	0.0	7.0	0.0	0.0
Sparkling, Diet, Morrisons*	1 Glass/200ml	2	0.0	1	0.0	0.3	0.0	0.0
DANISH PASTRY								
Apple, Bar, Sara Lee*	1/6 Bar/70g	160	4.0	229	4.3	42.1	5.7	1.7
Apple, Fresh Cream, Sainsbury's*	1 Pastry/67g	248	14.6	368	3.1	40.2	21.6	0.4
Apple & Cinnamon, Danish Twist, Entenmann's*	1 Serving/52g	150	1.0	288	5.6	62.0	1.9	1.5
Apple Danish, Bakery, Waitrose*	1 Pastry/123g	400	22.2	325	5.1	35.7	18.0	2.4
Average	1 Pastry/110g	411	19.4	374	5.8	51.3	17.6	1.6
Cherry & Custard, Bar, Tesco*	1 Bar/350g	910	49.0	260	3.5	29.9	14.0	7.7
Custard, Bar, Sara Lee*	¼ Bar/100g	228	6.4	228	6.6	36.1	6.4	0.8
Fruit Filled, Average	1 Pastry/94g	335	15.9	356	5.1	47.9	17.0	0.0
Pecan, M & S*	1 Serving/67g	287	17.4	428	6.2	45.0	26.0	1.3
Toasted Pecan, Danish Twist, Entenmann's*	1 Slice/48g	171	7.6	351	7.0	47.2	15.6	1.4
DATES								
Bite Size, Snack Pack, Whitworths*	1 Pack/35g	119	0.6	340	2.0	74.7	1.8	8.2
Deglet Nour, Graze*	1 Pack/60g	181	0.3	301	2.1	72.0	0.5	0.0
Deglet Nour, Love Life, Waitrose*	1 Portion/50g	144	0.1	287	3.3	68.0	0.2	8.0
Dried, Average	***1 Date/20g***	***54***	***0.1***	***272***	***2.8***	***65.4***	***0.4***	***4.2***
Dried, Medjool, Average	***1 Date/20g***	***56***	***0.1***	***279***	***2.2***	***69.3***	***0.3***	***4.3***
Fresh, Raw, Yellow, Average	***1 Date/20g***	***23***	***0.0***	***116***	***1.4***	***29.1***	***0.1***	***1.6***
Hadrawi, Love Life, Waitrose*	5 Dates/50g	144	0.1	288	3.4	68.0	0.2	8.0
Halawi, Tesco*	6 Dates/60g	165	0.1	275	2.3	65.5	0.2	4.3
Medjool, Love Life, Waitrose*	1 Date/20g	58	0.0	291	3.3	68.0	0.2	6.7
Medjool, Stuffed with Walnuts, Tesco*	2 Dates/40g	98	2.3	245	4.4	44.0	5.7	3.4
Medjool, TTD, Sainsbury's*	1 Serving/50g	148	0.0	296	1.9	72.0	0.1	6.7
Soft, Dried, Whitworths*	1 Serving/25g	85	0.4	340	2.0	74.7	1.8	8.2
Stoned, Wholefoods, Tesco*	1 Pack/500g	1600	13.0	320	4.4	69.2	2.6	8.4
DELIGHT								
Butterscotch Flavour, No Added Sugar, Tesco*	1 Pack/49g	225	10.0	460	4.8	63.3	20.5	0.0
Chocolate Flavour, Dry, Tesco*	1 Pack/49g	220	9.0	450	6.2	64.2	18.4	2.3
Raspberry, Ravishing, Made Up, Asda*	1/3 Pack/100g	112	3.9	112	3.2	16.0	3.9	0.0
Strawberry, No Added Sugar, Dry, Tesco*	1 Pack/49g	51	1.8	105	3.4	13.7	3.7	0.1
Strawberry, Shapers, Boots*	1 Pot/122g	96	1.2	79	4.5	13.0	1.0	0.1
Vanilla, No Added Sugar, Dry, Tesco*	1 Pack/49g	51	1.8	105	3.4	13.7	3.7	0.1

	Measure INFO/WEIGHT	per Measure KCAL	FAT	Nutrition Values per 100g / 100ml KCAL	PROT	CARB	FAT	FIBRE
DESSERT								
Baked Lemon, COU, M & S*	1 Serving/100g	140	2.5	140	6.8	22.0	2.5	0.8
Banana Split	1 Serving/175g	368	25.5	210	2.2	18.0	14.6	0.2
Banoffee, Sainsbury's*	1 Pot/140g	360	19.1	257	2.7	30.9	13.6	1.3
Banoffee, Shape, Danone*	1 Pot/120g	175	2.8	146	3.3	28.0	2.3	0.5
Banoffee, Weight Watchers*	1 Dessert/81g	170	3.6	210	4.9	37.7	4.4	1.4
Black Cherry, & Chocolate, COU, M & S*	1 Pack/115g	132	1.6	115	3.6	22.6	1.4	1.2
Black Cherry, Dragana, Waitrose*	1 Pot/125g	236	11.4	189	2.1	24.7	9.1	0.5
Black Forest, LC, Tesco*	1 Pot/145g	188	2.3	130	3.2	25.8	1.6	0.9
Black Forest, Tesco*	1 Pot/100g	287	14.4	287	3.5	35.8	14.4	2.4
Bounty, Mars*	1 Pot/110g	253	15.0	230	5.3	23.2	13.6	0.0
Buttons, Milk Chocolate, Cadbury*	1 Pot/100g	280	14.9	280	6.2	30.8	14.9	0.0
Cappuccino, Italian, Co-Op*	1 Pack/90g	256	10.8	285	5.0	39.0	12.0	0.1
Caramel, Delights, Shape, Danone*	1 Pot/110g	109	2.5	99	3.3	16.3	2.3	0.1
Caramel, Pots of Joy, Dairy Milk, Cadbury*	1 Pot/70g	150	7.3	215	2.5	27.1	10.5	0.1
Caramel Crunch, Weight Watchers*	1 Serving/89g	174	2.6	196	4.6	37.9	2.9	1.7
Caramel Shortcake, Luxury, Weight Watchers*	1 Pot/100ml	103	3.5	103	1.9	17.9	3.5	0.8
Catalan Cream, Sainsbury's*	1 Pot/95g	375	35.2	395	4.2	11.2	37.0	0.1
Cheeky & Saucy, Little Pots Au Chocolat, Gu*	1 Pot/45g	199	16.6	443	3.3	24.1	36.9	2.3
Cherry & Vanilla, BGTY, Sainsbury's*	1 Pot/115g	225	7.6	196	1.6	32.6	6.6	1.0
Chocolate, Campina*	1 Pot/125g	186	8.6	149	3.2	18.5	6.9	0.0
Chocolate, Delights, Shape, Danone*	1 Pot/110g	109	2.4	99	3.3	16.3	2.2	0.6
Chocolate, Frappe, Skinny, COU, M & S*	1 Pot/100g	115	2.0	115	5.7	18.3	2.0	0.5
Chocolate, HL, Tesco*	1 Pot/95g	87	2.2	92	3.7	14.1	2.3	1.1
Chocolate, M & S*	1 Serving/120g	168	2.5	140	5.6	26.4	2.1	1.1
Chocolate, Triple Delight, Weight Watchers*	1 Dessert/110g	183	2.9	166	4.9	30.8	2.6	2.6
Chocolate, Weight Watchers*	1 Serving/82g	145	2.5	177	5.2	32.3	3.0	2.9
Chocolate Banoffee, Gu*	1 Pot/85g	325	21.5	382	3.9	35.0	25.3	1.0
Chocolate Brownie, M & S*	¼ Pack/144g	610	39.5	425	4.7	39.6	27.5	1.0
Chocolate Buttons, Cadbury*	1 Pack/100g	275	14.5	275	5.0	30.5	14.5	0.0
Chocolate Desire, Magnum, Wall's Ice Cream*	1 Dessert/85g	374	24.0	440	5.3	40.0	28.2	0.0
Chocolate Dream, Co-Op*	1 Pot/110g	184	7.7	167	4.1	22.0	7.0	0.0
Chocolate Duetto, Weight Watchers*	1 Pot/85g	99	2.4	117	4.4	18.4	2.8	0.0
Chocolate Fudge Brownie, Tesco*	1 Pot/125g	374	16.6	299	4.6	40.2	13.3	1.3
Chocolate Hazelnut, Charolait, Aldi*	1 Serving/200g	270	11.0	135	3.3	18.1	5.5	0.0
Chocolate Honeycomb Crisp, COU, M & S*	1 Serving/71g	110	2.1	155	4.6	27.6	2.9	1.0
Chocolate Marshmallow, Weight Watchers*	1 Serving/50g	97	2.4	194	3.2	34.5	4.7	1.3
Chocolate Muffin, COU, M & S*	1 Pot/110g	154	2.8	140	6.1	26.1	2.5	1.5
Chocolate Toffee, Weight Watchers*	1 Dessert/89g	177	4.0	197	4.3	34.9	4.5	2.2
Chocolate Truffle, Triple, Entenmann's*	1 Serving/100g	304	19.1	304	4.5	28.4	19.1	2.2
Creme Caramel, Sainsbury's*	1 Pot/100g	116	1.6	116	2.6	22.9	1.6	0.0
Crunchie, Dairy Milk, Cadbury*	1 Pot/100g	260	12.2	260	4.4	33.4	12.2	0.0
Flake, Milk Chocolate, Cadbury*	1 Pot/90g	216	11.3	240	4.4	26.6	12.6	0.0
Fruit & Nut, Cadbury*	1 Pot/100g	285	12.5	285	6.4	36.3	12.5	0.0
Fudge, Cadbury*	1 Pot/90g	216	11.2	240	4.1	28.5	12.4	0.0
Galaxy, Mars*	1 Pot/75g	166	9.2	221	4.9	22.7	12.3	0.0
Gulabjam Indian, Waitrose*	1 Pot/180g	479	15.5	266	4.8	42.9	8.6	0.6
Key Lime Pie	1 Serving/125g	431	25.0	344	4.1	37.9	20.0	1.4
Lemon, Sainsbury's*	1 Pot/115g	136	1.7	118	2.8	23.2	1.5	0.9
Lemon Meringue, Weight Watchers*	1 Pot/85g	161	0.4	189	2.4	43.1	0.5	0.6
Lemoncello, Italian, Co-Op*	1 Pot/90g	266	14.4	295	3.0	34.0	16.0	0.1
Mandarin, COU, M & S*	1 Serving/150g	195	5.7	130	1.0	22.0	3.8	0.1
Maple & Pecan, American Style, Sainsbury's*	1 Pot/110g	287	15.6	261	2.6	30.6	14.2	1.2
Mars, Mars*	1 Pot/110g	214	7.4	195	6.0	28.2	6.7	0.7

	Measure INFO/WEIGHT	per Measure KCAL	FAT	Nutrition Values per 100g / 100ml KCAL	PROT	CARB	FAT	FIBRE
DESSERT								
Millionaire's Shortbread, M & S*	1 Dessert/120g	440	27.8	365	3.2	35.5	23.1	1.0
Mississippi Mud Pie	1 Serving/125g	480	32.0	384	5.3	33.1	25.6	1.8
Peach & Raspberry, COU, M & S*	1 Pot/90g	135	1.4	150	2.6	30.5	1.6	1.0
Pineapple & Passionfruit, M & S*	1 Pot/100g	130	3.8	130	0.8	21.7	3.8	0.3
Raspberry, Frappe, Skinny, COU, M & S*	1 Pot/95g	109	1.3	115	3.1	22.0	1.4	0.5
Raspberry Royale, Essential, Waitrose*	1 Pot/150g	216	10.6	144	1.1	18.9	7.1	0.5
Rocky Road, Sainsbury's*	1 Pot/110g	328	21.6	298	3.6	26.8	19.6	2.1
Rolo, Nestle*	1 Pot/70g	170	8.3	243	3.3	30.8	11.9	0.5
Strawberries & Cream, BFY, Morrisons*	1 Serving/200g	244	2.2	122	2.2	26.0	1.1	0.1
Strawberry, BGTY, Sainsbury's*	1 Pot/115g	133	1.6	116	2.7	23.1	1.4	1.3
Strawberry, HL, Tesco*	1 Pot/122g	94	2.3	77	2.7	12.3	1.9	1.1
Strawberry & Rhubarb, COU, M & S*	1 Pot/110g	104	0.8	95	1.5	20.1	0.7	0.9
Summer Berry, HL, Tesco*	1 Pot/93g	120	2.1	130	2.8	24.5	2.3	1.5
Summer Fruits, COU, M & S*	1 Serving/105g	110	1.2	105	2.1	21.6	1.1	1.2
Summer Fruits, Marbled Cream, Waitrose*	1 Serving/125g	214	11.4	171	2.1	20.2	9.1	1.1
Tiramisu	1 Serving/150g	420	20.8	280	4.4	34.0	13.9	0.8
Toffee, with Biscuit Pieces, Iced, Weight Watchers*	1 Pot/57g	93	2.7	163	2.7	26.2	4.8	0.2
Toffee, with Biscuit Pieces, Weight Watchers*	1 Pot/57g	93	2.7	163	2.7	26.2	4.8	0.2
Toffee & Vanilla, Weight Watchers*	1 Pot/67g	107	0.5	159	3.1	34.8	0.8	3.9
Toffee Chocolate, Weight Watchers*	1 Pot/100g	197	4.5	197	4.3	34.9	4.5	2.2
Toffee Flavour Custard, Ambrosia*	1 Pack/135g	139	3.9	103	2.7	16.4	2.9	0.1
Toffee Muffin, COU, M & S*	1 Serving/100g	180	2.2	180	3.7	35.8	2.2	0.3
Vanilla, Exquisa*	1 Serving/100g	103	0.2	103	5.2	20.0	0.2	0.0
Vanilla, Luxury, Charolait*	1 Serving/200g	248	10.2	124	3.0	16.6	5.1	0.0
Vanilla, with Strawberries Swirl, Weight Watchers*	1 Pot/57g	46	1.3	81	1.5	13.3	2.2	0.2
Vanilla Flavour, Soya, Dairy Free, Organic, Provamel*	1 Pot/125g	105	2.2	84	3.2	13.4	1.8	0.5
Vanilla Supreme, Sainsbury's*	1 Pot/95g	116	3.8	122	3.0	18.0	4.0	0.0
Zabaglione	1 Serving/100g	278	18.3	278	3.6	24.3	18.3	2.3
DHAL								
Black Gram, Average	1oz/28g	21	1.0	74	4.2	7.0	3.4	1.7
Blackeye Bean, Patak's*	1oz/28g	29	1.3	102	3.6	12.4	4.6	1.8
Chick Pea	1oz/28g	42	1.7	149	7.4	17.7	6.1	3.8
Lentil, Patak's*	1 Can/283g	156	2.8	55	2.8	9.3	1.0	1.0
Lentil, Red, WTF, Sainsbury's*	½ Pack/273g	254	4.1	93	5.5	14.4	1.5	1.4
Lentil, Red Masoor, Punjabi, Average	1oz/28g	39	1.3	139	7.2	19.2	4.6	2.0
Lentil, Red Masoor & Tomato with Butter, Average	1oz/28g	26	1.4	94	4.0	9.7	4.9	0.9
Lentil, Red Masoor & Vegetable, Average	1oz/28g	31	1.1	110	5.8	14.7	3.8	1.8
Lentil, Red Masoor with Vegetable Oil, Average	1oz/28g	48	2.2	172	7.6	19.2	7.9	1.8
Lentil, Red Masoorl & Mung Bean, Average	1oz/28g	32	1.9	114	4.8	9.9	6.7	1.6
Makhani, Curry Collection, Veetee*	1 Pack/300g	306	17.4	102	4.2	11.1	5.8	2.8
Mung Bean, Bengali	1oz/28g	20	0.9	73	4.2	7.4	3.3	1.7
Mung Beans, Dried, Boiled in Unsalted Water	1oz/28g	26	0.1	92	7.8	15.3	0.4	0.0
Mung Beans, Dried, Raw	1oz/28g	81	0.3	291	26.8	46.3	1.1	0.0
Split Peas, Yellow, Chana, Asda*	1 Serving/275g	300	19.2	109	2.6	9.0	7.0	1.8
Tarka, Asda*	½ Pack/150g	216	12.0	144	6.0	12.0	8.0	6.0
DHANSAK								
Chicken, Ready Meals, M & S*	1oz/28g	50	3.2	180	12.4	6.6	11.5	1.6
Chicken, with Bagara Rice, Waitrose*	1 Pack/450g	549	8.1	122	8.2	18.2	1.8	1.2
Vegetable, Sainsbury's*	1 Serving/200g	148	5.6	74	3.1	8.9	2.8	2.8
DILL								
Dried, Average	***1 Tsp/1g***	***3***	***0.0***	***253***	***19.9***	***42.2***	***4.4***	***13.6***
Fresh, Average	***1 Tbsp/3g***	***1***	***0.0***	***25***	***3.7***	***0.9***	***0.8***	***2.5***

D

	Measure INFO/WEIGHT	per Measure KCAL	FAT	Nutrition Values per 100g / 100ml KCAL	PROT	CARB	FAT	FIBRE
DIM SUM								
Dumplings, Chicken, Spicy, Zao, Taiko Foods*	1 Dumpling/18g	31	0.4	166	14.1	21.4	2.1	1.5
From Restaurant, Average	1 Piece/12g	50	2.4	433	28.9	31.3	20.4	0.0
Steamed, Prawn, M & S*	6 Dim Sum/120g	222	3.2	185	1.1	39.0	2.7	1.5
DIME								
Terry's*	1oz/28g	154	9.5	550	4.6	68.5	33.8	0.6
DIP								
Aubergine, Fresh, Waitrose*	1 Serving/85g	159	12.8	187	2.5	10.5	15.0	1.7
Bean & Cheese, Asda*	1 Serving/50g	78	4.5	157	7.0	12.0	9.0	1.7
Beetroot & Sesame, Sainsbury's*	¼ Pot/45g	65	3.7	145	4.2	11.8	8.3	3.1
Blue Cheese, Fresh, Sainsbury's*	1/5 Pot/34g	115	11.7	337	3.6	3.1	34.5	0.1
Cheddar & Spring Onion, M & S*	1 Pack/125g	581	60.4	465	3.6	4.7	48.3	0.5
Cheddar Cheese, Mature, & Chive, Fresh, Waitrose*	½ Pot/85g	393	40.5	462	5.8	2.4	47.7	1.7
Cheese & Chive, 50% Less Fat, Asda*	1 Pot/125g	261	21.5	209	4.5	9.0	17.2	0.0
Cheese & Chive, Asda*	1 Serving/43g	190	19.6	447	4.9	3.4	46.0	0.0
Chilli, M & S*	1 Pot/35g	103	0.1	295	0.4	73.2	0.2	0.4
Chilli Cheese, Max, Walkers*	1 Jar/300g	390	27.3	130	3.3	9.4	9.1	0.3
Chillimole, Tesco*	1 Serving/50g	142	11.9	285	4.2	13.0	23.8	3.9
Frijolemole, Cannellini Bean & Chick Pea, Waitrose*	¼ Pot/50g	104	7.6	208	4.3	12.2	15.2	2.6
Frijolemole, Tesco*	¼ Pot/50g	105	8.1	210	3.6	12.3	16.2	2.0
Garlic, Olive Oil & Butter, Pizza Express*	½ Pot/17g	106	11.5	621	1.5	2.8	67.4	0.5
Garlic & Herb	1 Serving/100g	584	62.4	584	1.4	4.1	62.4	0.2
Garlic & Herb, Reduced Fat, M & S*	1 Serving/10g	10	0.4	95	6.0	8.1	4.0	0.5
Garlic & Herb, Tesco*	¼ Pack/43g	257	27.8	604	0.9	3.2	65.4	0.3
Guacamole, Reduced Fat, BGTY, Sainsbury's*	¼ Pot/43g	62	5.7	146	1.3	2.9	13.5	4.0
Guacamole, Supreme, Waitrose*	½ Pot/85g	105	10.3	124	1.6	2.1	12.1	4.3
Guacamole Style, Topping, Discovery*	1 Serving/37g	29	2.1	79	1.2	6.0	5.6	1.2
Mexican Bean, Doritos, Walkers*	1 Tbsp/20g	18	0.7	89	2.7	12.1	3.3	2.4
Moroccan, Spicy, BGTY, Sainsbury's*	½ Pot/85g	56	1.7	66	2.1	10.0	2.0	1.7
Nacho Cheese, Average	1 Serving/50g	175	17.2	350	6.3	3.4	34.4	0.9
Nacho Cheese, Doritos, Walkers*	1 Serving/40g	92	8.1	231	3.4	8.5	20.2	0.6
Nacho Cheese, Primula*	1 Serving/57g	144	14.2	253	2.7	3.6	24.9	2.1
Onion & Garlic, 50% Less Fat, Asda*	1oz/28g	59	4.8	209	4.5	9.0	17.2	0.0
Onion & Garlic, Average	1 Tbsp/15g	62	6.4	410	1.7	4.8	42.7	0.4
Pea, Yoghurt & Mint, Sainsbury's*	¼ Pack/50g	119	10.8	238	3.4	7.5	21.6	2.1
Peanut, Satay Selection, Occasions, Sainsbury's*	1 Serving/2g	4	0.2	186	7.1	13.8	11.4	1.1
Pecorino, Basil & Pine Nut, Fresh, Waitrose*	½ Pot/85g	338	33.7	398	5.1	5.1	39.7	0.0
Pepper, Red, Nando's*	1 Serving/260g	490	7.2	188	5.2	35.2	2.8	1.6
Pepper, Red, Sainsbury's*	1 Pot/100g	103	4.0	103	2.3	14.6	4.0	0.0
Pepper, Smoky Red, Gazpacho, Graze*	1 Punnet/23g	54	1.3	242	5.7	40.1	5.9	3.7
Raita, Indian, Asda*	1 Pot/70g	120	11.5	172	2.6	3.6	16.4	0.5
Salmon, Smoked, & Dill, Fresh, Waitrose*	½ Pot/85g	373	38.0	439	5.1	4.1	44.7	0.1
Salmon, Smoked, & Dill, Reduced Fat, Waitrose*	½ Pot/85g	184	16.7	217	3.9	6.1	19.7	1.1
Salsa, Chunky, Fresh, Sainsbury's*	1 Serving/100g	51	1.7	51	1.1	7.8	1.7	1.2
Salsa, Chunky Tomato, Tesco*	1 Pot/170g	68	2.2	40	1.1	5.9	1.3	1.1
Salsa, GFY, Asda*	1 Pot/170g	68	0.7	40	1.2	8.0	0.4	1.5
Salsa, Hot, Doritos, Walkers*	1 Jar/300g	99	0.3	33	1.1	6.4	0.1	0.9
Salsa, Mild, Doritos, Walkers*	1 Tbsp/30g	9	0.1	30	0.8	6.0	0.3	1.5
Salsa Mild, Asda*	1 Portion/100g	47	0.3	47	1.4	8.7	0.3	1.8
Sour Cream, Co-Op*	1oz/28g	137	14.6	490	2.0	3.0	52.0	0.0
Sour Cream, Tesco*	1 Serving/38g	111	11.2	297	3.4	3.9	29.8	0.2
Sour Cream & Chive, Average	1 Tbsp/15g	48	4.8	317	3.2	4.0	32.0	0.3
Sour Cream & Chive, BGTY, Sainsbury's*	1oz/28g	46	4.1	165	4.9	3.4	14.6	0.7
Sour Cream & Chive, Doritos, Walkers*	1 Tbsp/20g	52	4.9	258	1.9	6.9	24.7	1.9

	Measure INFO/WEIGHT	per Measure KCAL	FAT	Nutrition Values per 100g / 100ml KCAL	PROT	CARB	FAT	FIBRE
DIP								
Sour Cream & Chive, Half Fat, Waitrose*	½ Pot/85g	133	9.9	157	5.5	7.6	11.6	0.1
Sour Cream & Chive, Mexican Style, Morrisons*	¼ Pack/25g	68	7.0	274	2.2	3.4	27.9	0.4
Sour Cream & Chive, Primula*	1 Serving/57g	169	17.4	297	4.3	1.3	30.5	1.0
Soured Cream & Chive, 95% Fat Free, M & S*	1oz/28g	25	0.8	90	6.5	9.6	2.8	0.5
Soured Cream & Chive, BGTY, Sainsbury's*	1 Serving/170g	253	17.5	149	4.2	9.9	10.3	0.1
Soured Cream & Chive, for Skins, Tesco*	1 Serving/12g	36	3.6	297	3.4	3.9	29.8	0.2
Soured Cream & Chive, HL, Tesco*	1 Serving/31g	45	3.3	145	3.8	7.5	10.6	0.2
Soured Cream & Chive, LC, Tesco*	¼ Pot/50g	65	4.5	130	4.3	7.4	9.0	0.1
Sweet & Sour, M & S*	1oz/28g	36	0.0	130	0.7	31.4	0.1	0.5
Sweet & Sour, Primula*	1 Serving/57g	76	0.1	133	0.4	32.8	0.2	0.0
Sweet Chilli, Chinese Snack Selection, Morrisons*	½ Pot/20g	64	0.0	320	0.1	79.4	0.2	0.6
Sweet Chilli, Oriental Selection, Waitrose*	½ Pot/35g	88	0.3	250	1.3	59.4	0.8	0.4
Sweet Chilli Mango, Encona*	1 Tbsp/15ml	22	0.1	148	0.4	35.4	0.6	0.0
Thousand Island, HL, Tesco*	1 Serving/31g	57	4.6	183	2.5	9.6	14.9	0.3
Thousand Island, M & S*	1oz/28g	69	6.2	245	2.1	9.4	22.2	0.7
Tomato Ketchup, Asda*	1 Pack/25g	18	0.0	71	1.6	16.0	0.1	1.0
Yoghurt & Cucumber Mint, Tesco*	1oz/28g	34	2.0	121	7.0	7.2	7.1	0.6
DISCOS								
Beef, KP Snacks*	1 Pack/28g	145	8.2	518	5.1	58.7	29.3	2.4
Cheese & Onion, KP Snacks*	1 Pack/28g	146	8.2	520	5.1	59.1	29.3	2.5
Salt & Vinegar, KP Snacks*	1 Bag/28g	145	8.3	517	4.7	58.3	29.5	2.3
DOLLY MIXTURES								
M & S*	1 Pack/115g	431	1.6	375	1.8	89.2	1.4	0.0
Sainsbury's*	1 Serving/10g	40	0.2	401	1.4	94.4	1.9	0.1
Tesco*	1 Pack/100g	376	1.5	376	1.6	88.9	1.5	0.0
DOPIAZA								
Chicken, M & S*	1 Pack/350g	402	21.4	115	11.5	3.7	6.1	2.5
Chicken, Sainsbury's*	½ Pack/200g	272	15.8	136	13.2	3.1	7.9	0.8
Chicken, Tesco*	1 Pack/350g	448	24.8	128	10.8	5.3	7.1	0.6
Chicken, with Pilau Rice, Sharwood's*	1 Pack/375g	472	17.2	126	5.3	15.8	4.6	0.8
Chicken, with Pilau Rice, Tesco*	1 Pack/400g	424	15.2	106	5.7	12.3	3.8	1.5
Mushroom, Retail	1oz/28g	19	1.6	69	1.3	3.7	5.7	1.1
Mushroom, Waitrose*	½ Pack/150g	81	4.6	54	2.2	4.3	3.1	2.3
DORADA								
Whole	1 Serving/100g	92	5.9	92	18.0	1.0	5.9	0.0
DORITOS								
Chargrilled BBQ, Walkers*	1 Bag/35g	170	8.8	485	5.5	59.0	25.0	3.5
Cheesy 3d's, Doritos, Walkers*	1 Pack/20g	89	3.2	445	7.0	68.0	16.0	3.0
Chilli Heatwave, Walkers*	1 Bag/30g	150	7.8	500	7.0	60.0	26.0	3.0
Cool, Ranch Chips, Walkers*	1 Pack/50g	250	13.0	504	8.1	64.5	26.2	4.0
Cool Original, Walkers*	1 Bag/40g	200	10.8	500	7.5	58.0	27.0	3.0
Cool Spice 3ds, Walkers*	1 Bag/24g	108	4.3	450	8.0	64.0	18.0	4.4
Dippas, Hint of Chilli, Dipping Chips, Walkers*	1 Bag/35g	173	8.8	495	7.0	61.0	25.0	3.5
Dippas, Hint of Garlic, Dipping Chips, Walkers*	1 Serving/35g	175	8.8	500	7.0	61.0	25.0	3.5
Dippas, Hint of Lime, Walkers*	1 Bag/35g	173	8.8	495	7.0	60.0	25.0	3.5
Dippas, Lightly Salted, Dipping Chips, Walkers*	1 Serving/35g	178	9.4	510	6.5	60.0	27.0	3.0
Latinos, Chargrilled BBQ, Walkers*	1 Serving/35g	170	8.8	485	5.5	59.0	25.0	3.5
Latinos, Mexican Grill, Walkers*	1 Serving/35g	170	8.8	485	6.5	59.0	25.0	3.5
Latinos, Sour Cream & Sweet Pepper, Walkers*	1 Pack/40g	194	10.0	485	5.5	60.0	25.0	3.5
Lighly Salted, Corn Chips, Doritos*	1 Bag/30g	149	7.1	497	6.9	62.9	23.6	3.3
Mexican Hot, Walkers*	1 Bag/40g	202	10.8	505	8.0	57.0	27.0	3.5
Tangy Cheese, Walkers*	1 Bag/40g	200	10.8	500	7.0	57.0	27.0	3.0

D

	Measure INFO/WEIGHT	per Measure KCAL	FAT	Nutrition Values per 100g / 100ml KCAL	PROT	CARB	FAT	FIBRE
DOUBLE DECKER								
Cadbury*	1 Bar/55g	251	10.3	460	4.4	68.4	18.9	0.6
Snack Size, Cadbury*	1 Bar/36g	165	7.4	465	4.8	64.5	20.9	0.0
with Nuts, Cadbury*	1 Bar/60g	291	14.7	485	7.9	58.6	24.5	0.0
DOUGH BALLS								
Cheese & Garlic, Occasions, Sainsbury's*	1 Ball/12g	41	2.2	341	10.3	33.4	18.5	2.1
Garlic, GFY, Asda*	1 Ball/8g	21	0.2	250	9.0	49.0	2.0	2.0
Garlic, Tesco*	1 Serving/10g	40	2.3	400	7.0	40.0	23.0	1.0
Garlic, Waitrose*	1 Ball/11g	38	1.8	347	8.5	41.4	16.4	3.3
Garlic & Herb, Asda*	4 Balls/48g	173	8.5	361	9.2	40.9	17.8	3.6
Garlic & Herb, Occasions, Sainsbury's*	1 Ball/12g	41	2.1	343	8.4	38.7	17.2	2.2
Sainsbury's*	1 Ball/12g	41	2.1	343	8.4	38.7	17.2	2.2
Supermarket, Pizza Express*	8 Balls/100g	363	1.7	363	14.3	72.9	1.7	3.3
with Garlic & Herb Butter, Aldi*	1 Ball/12g	45	2.2	365	7.7	46.7	18.2	1.8
with Garlic & Herb Butter, Sainsbury's*	½ Pack/100g	362	14.8	362	9.6	47.7	14.8	2.9
DOUGHNUTS								
Apple, & Custard, Finger, Sainsbury's*	1 Serving/65g	136	6.0	210	4.4	27.5	9.2	1.9
Apple, & Fresh Cream, Sainsbury's*	1 Doughnut/79g	216	11.4	273	5.4	30.5	14.4	1.9
Baked, HL, Tesco*	1 Doughnut/67g	166	3.9	248	6.4	42.2	5.9	1.4
Chocolate Topped, Mini, Chosen By You, Asda*	1 Serving/100g	393	19.5	393	5.2	49.1	19.5	2.0
Cream & Jam, Assorted Box, Sainsbury's*	1 Doughnut/71g	229	12.7	322	6.2	34.2	17.9	2.2
Cream & Jam, Tesco*	1 Doughnut/90g	288	14.1	320	5.4	39.4	15.7	2.0
Custard Filled, Average	1 Doughnut/75g	268	14.2	358	6.2	43.3	19.0	0.0
Finger, Co-Op*	1 Doughnut/82g	299	14.8	365	4.0	45.0	18.0	2.0
Jam, American Style, Budgens*	1 Doughnut/46g	126	3.1	275	7.1	46.5	6.7	0.0
Jam, American Style, Sainsbury's*	1 Doughnut/65g	220	20.6	339	4.9	49.6	31.8	3.5
Jam, Fresh Cream, Sweet Fresh, Tesco*	1 Doughnut/74g	248	12.1	335	5.5	40.7	16.4	1.9
Jam, Mini, Frozen, Party, Tesco*	2 Doughnuts/25g	101	5.5	405	5.3	45.0	22.1	2.0
Jam Filled, Average	1 Doughnut/75g	252	10.9	336	5.7	48.8	14.5	0.0
Mini, Sainsbury's*	1 Doughnut/14g	53	2.7	379	5.2	47.9	18.9	2.1
Ring, Iced, Average	1 Doughnut/70g	268	12.2	383	4.8	55.1	17.5	0.0
Ring, Plain, Average	1 Doughnut/60g	238	13.0	397	6.1	47.2	21.7	0.0
Strawberry Jam & Cream, Sainsbury's*	1 Doughnut/80g	299	18.5	374	5.3	36.2	23.2	1.3
Toffee, Tesco*	1 Doughnut/75g	235	8.7	313	8.0	44.2	11.6	1.6
Yum Yums, Glazed, Sweet, Waitrose*	1 Doughnut/45g	172	10.0	382	4.0	41.6	22.2	2.0
Yum Yums, Tesco*	1 Doughnut/50g	220	13.2	440	4.7	43.7	26.4	3.1
DOVER SOLE								
Fillet, Raw, Average	***1oz/28g***	***25***	***0.5***	***89***	***18.1***	***0.0***	***1.8***	***0.0***
DR PEPPER*								
Coca-Cola*	1 Bottle/500ml	210	0.0	42	0.0	10.9	0.0	0.0
Z, Coca-Cola*	1 Glass/250ml	10	0.0	4	0.0	0.0	0.0	0.0
Zero, Coca-Cola*	1 Can/330ml	2	0.0	0	0.0	0.0	0.0	0.0
DRAGON FRUIT								
Raw, Edible Portion, Average	1 Serving/100g	41	0.5	41	0.7	9.6	0.5	3.6
DRAMBUIE								
39% Volume	***1 Shot/35ml***	***125***	***0.0***	***358***	***0.0***	***23.0***	***0.0***	***0.0***
DREAM								
Double Fudge, Cadbury*	1oz/28g	139	7.1	495	6.3	61.4	25.2	0.0
Snowbites, Cadbury*	1 Serving/31g	170	10.2	545	3.1	59.7	32.7	0.0
White Chocolate, Cadbury*	1 Piece/8g	44	2.7	555	4.5	59.7	33.3	0.0
DREAM TOPPING								
Dry, Bird's*	1oz/28g	193	16.4	690	6.7	32.5	58.5	0.5
Made Up, Skimmed Milk, Bird's*	1oz/28g	21	1.5	75	2.0	4.8	5.3	0.0
Sugar Free, Dry, Bird's*	1oz/28g	195	16.9	695	7.3	30.5	60.5	0.5

	Measure INFO/WEIGHT	per Measure KCAL	FAT	Nutrition Values per 100g / 100ml KCAL	PROT	CARB	FAT	FIBRE
DRESSING								
Balsamic, Fresh Olive Co*	1 Tbsp/15g	42	0.1	282	1.5	67.8	0.5	0.6
Balsamic, Italian, Loyd Grossman*	1 Serving/10g	36	3.4	357	0.9	13.1	33.5	0.1
Balsamic, Italian, The English Provender Co.*	1 Serving/30ml	20	0.8	67	0.8	9.9	2.7	0.2
Balsamic, LC, Tesco*	1 Tbsp/14g	12	0.2	85	0.3	16.7	1.5	0.2
Balsamic, M & S*	1 Tbsp/15g	74	7.2	490	0.3	9.7	48.0	0.5
Balsamic, New, Sainsbury's*	1 Tbsp/15g	58	5.2	389	0.6	18.3	34.8	0.8
Balsamic, Sainsbury's*	1 Tbsp/15ml	47	4.3	316	0.4	13.8	28.8	0.4
Balsamic, Schwartz*	1 Tbsp/15ml	12	0.3	77	0.5	14.2	2.0	0.0
Balsamic, Sweet, Finest, Tesco*	1 Serving/10ml	16	0.0	155	0.4	36.9	0.1	0.4
Balsamic, Vinaigrette, Newman's Own*	1 Tbsp/15ml	56	5.7	372	0.1	7.2	38.2	0.5
Balsamic, Weight Watchers*	1 Serving/15ml	12	0.3	81	0.1	16.0	1.8	0.5
Balsamic Vinegar, Asda*	1 Pack/44ml	121	11.9	275	0.9	7.0	27.0	0.0
Balsamic Vinegar, Light, Kraft*	1 Serving/15ml	15	0.9	100	0.3	9.6	6.3	0.5
Balsamic Vinegar, Morrisons*	1 Serving/15ml	17	0.2	111	0.1	22.9	1.6	0.1
Balsamic Vinegar, Olives & Herb, COU, M & S*	1 Serving/30g	22	0.6	75	0.5	14.3	2.0	0.5
Basil & Pesto, COU, M & S*	1 Serving/50ml	30	1.1	60	0.6	8.3	2.2	0.8
Blue Cheese, 60% Less Fat, BGTY, Sainsbury's*	1 Tbsp/15ml	26	2.3	172	1.9	7.3	15.1	0.2
Blue Cheese, Chunky, Lite, Marie's*	2 Tbsp/31g	72	7.2	233	3.3	3.3	23.3	0.0
Blue Cheese, Fresh, Sainsbury's*	1 Dtsp/10ml	42	4.6	423	2.3	0.5	45.7	0.1
Blue Cheese, HE, Tesco*	1 Tsp/5g	4	0.2	82	4.4	9.0	3.1	0.1
Blue Cheese, Hellmann's*	1 Tbsp/15g	69	7.1	459	0.7	6.3	47.2	1.1
Blue Cheese, Low Fat, Weight Watchers*	1oz/28g	17	1.0	59	1.5	5.8	3.4	0.0
Blue Cheese, Sainsbury's*	1 Serving/20g	64	6.0	321	2.3	10.6	29.9	0.4
Blue Cheese, Salad, Waitrose*	1 Serving/50g	265	25.2	530	2.1	17.3	50.3	4.1
Blue Cheese, Tesco*	1 Serving/15ml	75	7.7	500	2.5	6.9	51.4	0.2
Caesar, Asiago, Briannas*	1 Tbsp/15ml	70	7.5	467	3.3	3.3	50.0	0.0
Caesar, Classic, Sainsbury's*	1 Tsp/5ml	22	2.3	442	2.7	4.6	45.9	0.5
Caesar, Creamy, Get Dressed, Kraft*	1 Serving/67g	68	2.3	102	2.1	15.0	3.5	0.1
Caesar, Creamy, Waistline, Crosse & Blackwell*	1 Dtsp/11g	15	1.0	135	1.5	11.1	9.2	0.3
Caesar, Fat Free, Average	1 Tsp/5g	4	0.2	84	4.6	11.0	4.1	0.2
Caesar, Finest, Tesco*	1 Tbsp/15ml	72	7.6	477	1.9	2.8	50.9	0.2
Caesar, Fresh, Asda*	1 Dtsp/10ml	45	4.8	454	2.4	3.2	48.0	0.0
Caesar, Fresh, M & S*	1 Tsp/6g	32	3.4	525	2.0	1.8	56.4	0.2
Caesar, Hellmann's*	1 Tsp/6g	30	3.1	499	2.5	4.5	51.7	0.3
Caesar, Light, Kraft*	1 Serving/15g	22	1.6	148	0.5	11.5	11.0	0.2
Caesar, Low Fat, Average	1 Tsp/5g	4	0.1	77	2.3	11.1	2.6	0.2
Caesar, Loyd Grossman*	1 Dtsp/10g	34	3.4	342	2.1	7.0	33.9	0.0
Caesar, Luxury, Hellmann's*	1 Tsp/4g	20	2.1	498	2.5	4.4	51.7	0.3
Caesar, Mary Berry*	1 Serving/100g	573	56.9	573	2.4	12.8	56.9	0.1
Caesar, Original, Cardini's*	1 Serving/10g	56	6.0	555	2.3	1.5	60.0	0.2
Caesar, Tesco*	1 Tbsp/15ml	65	6.8	435	0.9	5.4	45.1	0.3
Caesar, Waitrose*	1 Serving/15ml	72	7.6	479	4.5	0.9	50.8	0.2
Caesar Style, GFY, Asda*	1 Sachet/44ml	34	1.0	77	5.0	9.0	2.3	0.0
Champagne, For Smoked Haddock Tian, Waitrose*	½ Pack/38g	195	21.1	513	1.1	2.3	55.5	0.8
Cream Cheese & Chive, Creamy Ranch, Kraft*	1 Serving/15ml	31	2.6	205	1.2	11.0	17.0	0.0
Creamy, Waistline, 93% Fat Free, Crosse & Blackwell*	1 Tsp/6g	7	0.4	120	1.0	14.4	6.4	0.2
Creme Fraiche, Salad, Kraft*	1 Tbsp/15ml	12	0.4	78	0.8	12.5	2.5	0.0
French, BGTY, Organic, Sainsbury's*	1 Tbsp/15ml	11	0.6	71	0.2	8.3	4.1	0.5
French, BGTY, Sainsbury's*	1 Tbsp/15ml	12	0.7	79	1.1	8.8	4.4	0.5
French, Chilled, Tesco*	1 Tbsp/15ml	63	5.9	421	1.1	15.1	39.6	0.0
French, Cider Vinegar & Mustard, Tesco*	1 Tbsp/15ml	45	4.2	300	0.7	9.9	28.1	0.3
French, Classic, Fat Free, Kraft*	1 Tsp/5ml	2	0.0	39	0.1	8.7	0.0	0.5
French, Classic, Sachet, The English Provender Co.*	1 Sachet/25g	21	0.6	84	0.8	14.7	2.4	0.0

	Measure INFO/WEIGHT	per Measure KCAL	FAT	Nutrition Values per 100g / 100ml KCAL	PROT	CARB	FAT	FIBRE
DRESSING								
French, Classic, Sainsbury's*	1 Tbsp/15ml	71	7.4	473	1.0	5.7	49.6	0.5
French, Classics, M & S*	1 Tbsp/15ml	77	8.0	516	0.6	8.2	53.1	0.2
French, COU, M & S*	1/3 Bottle/105g	74	2.7	70	0.7	11.5	2.6	0.7
French, Fresh, Florette*	1 Bottle/175ml	763	73.1	436	0.8	14.1	41.8	0.0
French, Fresh, Organic, Sainsbury's*	1 Tbsp/15ml	45	4.6	301	0.4	5.5	31.0	0.4
French, Fresh, Sainsbury's*	1 Tbsp/15ml	64	6.7	429	0.6	6.6	44.6	0.6
French, Light, Heinz*	1 Sachet/12g	13	0.6	111	0.7	15.4	5.4	0.0
French, Luxury, Hellmann's*	1 Tbsp/15g	45	3.9	297	0.4	14.9	25.9	0.3
French, Oil Free, French, Waitrose*	1 Tsp/5ml	4	0.1	76	1.5	13.1	2.0	0.6
French, Organic, M & S*	1 Tbsp/15g	98	10.4	655	0.2	7.5	69.4	0.3
French, Organic, Tesco*	1 Tsp/5ml	23	2.2	451	0.6	11.0	44.9	0.2
French, Reduced Fat, M & S*	1 Tbsp/15g	10	0.4	70	0.7	11.5	2.8	0.7
French, Sainsbury's*	1 Tbsp/15ml	33	2.9	219	0.6	9.8	19.1	0.5
French, Vinaigrette, TTD, Sainsbury's*	1 Tbsp/15ml	69	6.7	460	0.6	13.9	44.5	0.5
French, Virtually Fat Free, Aldi*	1 Serving/10g	3	0.0	33	0.9	6.7	0.3	1.1
French Herb, Mary Berry*	1 Serving/100g	504	49.3	504	0.8	14.2	49.3	0.3
French Salad, M & S*	1 Serving/25ml	156	16.8	625	0.5	3.8	67.3	0.1
French Style, Oil Free, HE, Tesco*	1 Tbsp/15g	4	0.0	30	0.3	6.0	0.2	1.4
Garlic, Fire Roasted, & Thyme, Tesco*	1 Serving/10ml	45	4.7	447	0.9	4.7	47.2	0.0
Garlic, Roasted, Creamy, GFY, Asda*	1 Tbsp/15g	10	0.6	70	0.8	8.0	3.9	0.6
Garlic & Herb, Perfectly Balanced, Waitrose*	1 Serving/50ml	68	0.7	135	0.6	29.9	1.4	0.8
Garlic & Herb, Reduced Calorie, Hellmann's*	1 Tbsp/15ml	35	2.9	232	0.6	12.8	19.3	0.4
Garlic & Herb, Tesco*	1 Tbsp/15g	32	3.0	210	0.9	5.8	20.2	0.8
Green Olive, M & S*	1oz/28g	40	4.0	144	1.5	2.2	14.4	1.3
Green Thai, Coconut & Lemon Grass, Loyd Grossman*	1oz/28g	49	3.0	174	0.2	19.3	10.6	0.5
Green Thai, Finest, Tesco*	1 Bottle/250ml	940	81.8	376	0.3	19.1	32.7	0.3
Honey & Mustard, BGTY, Sainsbury's*	1 Tbsp/20g	14	0.1	71	0.4	16.1	0.5	0.2
Honey & Mustard, Finest, Tesco*	1 Serving/25ml	72	5.6	288	1.7	19.6	22.5	0.7
Honey & Mustard, Fresh, M & S*	1 Serving/10ml	43	4.2	430	1.7	9.7	42.4	0.5
Honey & Mustard, GFY, Asda*	1 Tbsp/15g	13	0.5	89	1.5	13.0	3.4	0.8
Honey & Mustard, Hellmann's*	1 Serving/15ml	27	0.2	182	0.7	13.7	1.6	0.3
Honey & Mustard, M & S*	1 Tbsp/15ml	64	6.4	427	1.7	9.7	42.4	0.6
Honey & Mustard, Sainsbury's*	1 Serving/10ml	37	3.3	366	1.0	15.4	33.0	0.1
Honey & Mustard, The English Provender Co.*	1 Tbsp/15ml	17	0.2	111	2.5	21.8	1.5	1.0
Italian, Light, Low Fat, Newman's Own*	1 Serving/15g	9	0.4	58	0.1	6.7	2.8	0.5
Italian, Low Fat, Heinz*	1 Pot/30ml	26	1.9	86	0.9	6.3	6.3	2.7
Italian, M & S*	1 Tbsp/15ml	62	6.2	415	0.9	8.9	41.5	1.0
Italian, Reduced Calorie, Hellmann's*	1 Serving/25ml	67	5.2	269	0.5	19.5	20.8	0.3
Italian, Waistline, 99% Fat Free, Crosse & Blackwell*	1 Tsp/6g	2	0.1	39	0.7	7.0	0.9	0.3
Lemon, Feta & Oregano, M & S*	1 Tbsp/15ml	24	2.0	160	1.3	8.2	13.4	0.6
Lemon & Cracked Black Pepper, GFY, Asda*	1 Tbsp/15g	9	0.0	57	0.2	14.0	0.0	0.3
Lemon & Tarragon, HE, Tesco*	1 Serving/10ml	11	0.2	113	1.1	21.6	2.4	0.0
Lemon & Watercress, COU, M & S*	1 Serving/28g	14	0.5	50	0.4	8.5	1.8	0.5
Lime & Coriander, Oil Free, Waitrose*	1 Tsp/5ml	3	0.1	65	1.5	11.9	1.3	0.4
Lime & Coriander, Sainsbury's*	1 Tbsp/15ml	61	6.1	409	0.4	10.0	40.8	0.5
Lime & Coriander, The English Provender Co.*	1 Serving/50g	28	0.2	57	0.3	13.3	0.3	0.0
Mayonnaise Style, 90% Fat Free, Weight Watchers*	1 Tsp/11g	14	1.0	125	1.7	8.9	9.2	0.0
Mint & Tomato, Mary Berry*	1 Serving/100g	399	37.1	399	0.8	14.8	37.1	0.3
Mustard, Mild, Low Fat, Weight Watchers*	1 Tbsp/10g	6	0.4	63	2.0	5.7	3.6	0.0
Mustard & Dill, Perfectly Balanced, Waitrose*	1 Tbsp/15ml	24	0.5	159	1.1	31.5	3.2	1.1
Oil & Lemon	1 Tbsp/15g	97	10.6	647	0.3	2.8	70.6	0.0
Olive Oil, Pizza Express*	1 Tbsp/15g	86	9.4	573	1.4	3.4	63.0	0.0
Orange & Cracked Pepper, Tesco*	1 Tbsp/15ml	17	0.0	114	0.5	27.8	0.1	0.3

	Measure INFO/WEIGHT	per Measure KCAL	FAT	Nutrition Values per 100g / 100ml KCAL	PROT	CARB	FAT	FIBRE
DRESSING								
Orange & Honey, Luxury, Hellmann's*	1 Serving/15ml	16	0.5	110	0.8	17.5	3.5	0.8
Parmesan & Peppercorn, Loyd Grossman*	1oz/28g	98	9.9	349	2.1	5.9	35.2	0.5
Passion Fruit & Mango, HE, Tesco*	1 Tbsp/15ml	25	0.3	169	0.6	36.7	2.2	0.4
Ranch, Creamy, 95% Fat Free, Kraft*	1 Tsp/6ml	7	0.3	111	1.4	14.5	5.0	0.3
Ranch, Texas, Frank Cooper*	1 Pot/28g	128	12.8	457	1.9	9.4	45.8	0.2
Ranch Style, Asda*	1 Serving/44ml	37	1.7	85	3.5	9.0	3.9	0.0
Red Pepper, BGTY, Sainsbury's*	1 Bottle/250g	108	0.8	43	0.2	9.8	0.3	0.2
Red Pepper, Fire Roasted, M & S*	1 Serving/30g	14	0.0	45	0.5	10.7	0.1	0.9
Red Pepper, M & S*	1 Tbsp/15ml	58	5.9	385	0.6	7.6	39.2	0.5
Salad, Blue Cheese, Heinz*	1 Serving/15g	55	5.5	369	1.2	7.8	36.9	0.2
Salad, Caesar, Light, Fry Light*	1 Spray/0.2ml	1	0.1	321	0.4	9.2	30.7	0.1
Salad, Catalina, Kraft*	1 Serving/34g	100	6.0	294	0.0	29.4	17.6	0.0
Salad, HE, Tesco*	1 Tbsp/15g	22	1.4	144	0.7	14.0	9.5	0.5
Salad, Honey & Mustard, Light, Kraft*	1 Tbsp/15ml	19	0.7	126	1.2	19.0	4.6	1.1
Salad, Italian, Hellmann's*	1 Serving/50g	103	8.4	206	0.7	12.8	16.7	0.0
Salad, Italian, Light, Kraft*	1 Tbsp/15ml	5	0.0	31	0.1	6.8	0.0	0.6
Salad, Italian, Newman's Own*	1 Tbsp/15g	82	9.0	545	0.2	1.0	59.8	0.0
Salad, Light, Heinz*	1 Serving/10g	24	2.0	244	1.8	13.5	19.9	0.0
Salad, Low Fat, Weight Watchers*	1 Tbsp/10g	10	0.4	106	1.5	15.4	4.3	0.0
Salad, Mary Berry*	1 Serving/15g	77	6.6	513	0.8	28.5	44.0	0.1
Salad, Pizza Express*	1 Serving/5g	29	3.2	573	1.4	3.4	63.0	0.0
Salad, Raspberry Balsamic, GFY, Asda*	1 Tbsp/15ml	6	0.1	40	0.7	9.3	0.7	1.3
Salad, Thousand Island, 95% Fat Free, Asda*	1 Tsp/6g	6	0.3	99	1.6	12.6	4.7	0.5
Salad, Thousand Island, Hellmann's*	1oz/28g	97	8.7	347	0.9	15.2	31.0	1.0
Salad, Thousand Island, Reduced Calorie, Hellmann's*	1oz/28g	73	5.4	259	1.0	19.0	19.4	0.9
Seafood, M & S*	1 Tsp/7g	39	4.2	555	0.9	4.9	59.3	0.9
Thai, Fragrant, Love Life, Waitrose*	1 Serving/16ml	9	0.0	57	1.8	12.0	0.1	0.6
Thai Lime & Coriander, The English Provender Co.*	1 Serving/25g	26	0.2	104	1.6	22.3	0.9	1.1
Thousand Island	1 Tsp/6g	19	1.8	323	1.1	12.5	30.2	0.4
Thousand Island, Light, Kraft*	1 Tbsp/15ml	16	0.0	105	0.6	23.0	0.2	3.0
Thousand Island, Original, Kraft*	1oz/28g	102	8.8	365	0.9	19.0	31.5	0.4
Thousand Island, Reduced Calorie	1 Tsp/6g	12	0.9	195	0.7	14.7	15.2	0.0
Tomato, Fire Roasted, Basil, COU, M & S*	1 Serving/30g	14	0.3	45	0.6	8.1	0.9	1.1
Tomato & Basil, HL, Tesco*	½ Pot/75ml	41	1.1	55	0.8	9.0	1.5	0.5
Tomato & Herb, Less Than 1% Fat, Asda*	1 Tbsp/15g	6	0.1	43	0.7	8.0	0.9	0.4
Tomato & Red Pepper, BGTY, Sainsbury's*	1 Serving/50ml	42	2.2	83	1.1	10.0	4.3	0.6
Vinaigrette, BGTY, Sainsbury's*	1 Dtsp/20g	13	0.5	64	1.1	9.3	2.4	2.5
Vinegar & Oil Based, Fat Free, Average	1 Tsp/5g	2	0.0	37	0.4	7.9	0.2	0.4
Waistline, Reduced Fat, Crosse & Blackwell*	1oz/28g	29	1.7	105	0.8	11.6	6.0	0.3
Yoghurt & Mint, HE, Tesco*	1 Tbsp/15g	20	0.4	135	1.5	26.2	2.7	0.0
Yoghurt & Mint, HL, Tesco*	1 Serving/50g	31	1.2	62	4.1	6.9	2.5	0.2
Yoghurt & Mint, Perfectly Balanced, Waitrose*	1 Serving/100ml	130	2.6	130	4.6	22.1	2.6	0.7
DRIED FRUIT								
Banana, Bites, Kiddylicious, Babylicious*	1 Serving/15g	43	2.9	285	10.8	43.6	19.3	6.1
Banana Chips, Honey Coated, Whitworths*	1 Serving/25g	132	7.8	526	1.0	59.9	31.4	1.7
Beach Bum, Graze*	1 Pack/28g	93	4.2	332	4.0	46.0	15.0	9.0
Blueberry Pieces, Jus Fruit, Yu!*	1 Pack/24g	84	0.1	350	0.8	80.8	0.4	0.0
Dragons Nest, Kids, Graze*	1 Punnet/33g	119	3.3	362	3.0	68.0	10.0	4.0
Exotic, Ready to Eat, Sainsbury's*	1/3 Pack/85g	241	0.1	284	0.2	70.6	0.1	2.4
Figgy Pop, Graze*	1 Pack/40g	100	0.4	251	2.5	61.6	1.1	0.0
Fruit Tumble, Kids, Graze*	1 Punnet/37g	111	0.4	299	2.0	71.0	1.0	3.0
Goji Berry, Graze*	1 Pack/45g	234	17.3	521	17.1	28.4	38.4	0.0
Jewel of the Nile, Graze*	1 Pack/45g	112	0.4	248	2.5	61.3	0.8	0.0

	Measure INFO/WEIGHT	per Measure KCAL	FAT	Nutrition Values per 100g / 100ml KCAL	PROT	CARB	FAT	FIBRE
DRIED FRUIT								
Juicy Sprinkle, Nature's Harvest*	1 Serving/20g	79	2.0	397	4.9	71.9	10.0	4.2
Mango, Sweetened, Whitworths*	1 Pack/30g	80	0.4	260	0.3	61.3	1.3	0.5
Mango Pieces, Jus Fruit, Yu!*	1 Pack/24g	87	0.1	364	1.0	84.7	0.4	0.0
Pineapple, Sweetened, Whitworths*	1 Bag/35g	122	0.1	350	0.4	86.3	0.2	0.5
Prunes, Juicy, Whitworths*	1 Pack/500g	740	2.0	148	2.5	34.0	0.4	5.7
Strawberry, Banana & Cherry, Sunshine Mix, Graze*	1 Pack/50g	78	0.2	157	9.7	37.2	0.4	0.0
Top Banana, Graze*	1 Serving/40g	115	0.4	287	2.6	70.1	0.9	0.0
Trail Mix, Kick Start, Wholefoods, Asda*	1 Serving/50g	194	10.2	387	10.9	40.0	20.4	10.7
Tropical Treasure, Kids, Graze*	1 Punnet/36g	134	2.9	373	3.0	76.0	8.0	5.8
DRIED FRUIT MIX								
5 Fruits, Ready to Eat, Sundora*	½ Pack/100g	233	0.4	233	1.6	58.4	0.4	6.8
Agadoo, Pineapple, Jumbo & Green Raisins, Graze*	1 Pack/40g	110	0.4	275	2.1	69.0	0.9	0.0
Albert Heijn*	1 Serving/50g	110	0.2	220	2.1	51.0	0.5	0.0
Apple Strudel, Graze*	1 Pack/40g	99	0.3	247	2.2	58.7	0.7	5.9
Average	1 Tbsp/25g	67	0.1	268	2.3	68.1	0.4	2.2
Eden, Graze*	1 Punnet/25g	69	0.2	275	2.0	63.7	1.0	8.1
Exotic Mix, Sundora*	1 Sm Pack/50g	138	1.4	276	2.3	60.6	2.7	3.8
Festival Fruits, Graze*	1 Punnet/32g	84	0.2	261	1.7	67.1	0.6	6.5
Fig & Cherry Preserve, Graze*	1 Pack/44g	116	0.4	263	2.9	64.6	0.9	7.6
Fruit Salad, Whitworths*	1 Serving/62g	113	0.3	183	2.9	41.8	0.5	6.6
Fruit Sangria, Graze*	1 Punnet/36g	110	0.6	306	3.8	70.3	1.8	2.6
Fruit Sundae, Graze*	1 Punnet/34g	98	0.3	287	2.1	70.1	1.0	4.1
Garden of England, Graze*	1 Punnet/25g	70	0.2	280	1.0	71.2	0.7	5.6
Hanging Gardens of Babylon, Graze*	1 Punnet/49g	114	0.2	232	3.2	57.1	0.5	7.6
Little Figgy Went to Market, Graze*	1 Punnet/36g	95	0.3	265	2.0	66.0	0.9	7.0
Medley, Shapers, Boots*	1 Serving/50g	131	0.3	262	3.2	61.0	0.6	5.5
Pear Tatin, Graze*	1 Punnet/35g	143	6.3	408	7.0	57.2	18.1	5.9
Scandinavian Forest, Graze*	1 Punnet/28g	79	0.2	282	2.0	71.0	0.6	8.0
Scrumptious Blueberry Swirl, Graze*	1 Punnet/40g	155	3.2	392	1.2	76.0	8.0	3.0
Sultanas, Currants, Raisins & Citrus Peel, Asda*	1 Serving/100g	283	0.5	283	2.6	67.0	0.5	1.7
Sultanas Raisins & Cranberries, Dunnes*	1 Sm Handful/15g	47	0.1	315	2.0	80.2	0.9	4.7
Taste of Hawaii, Extra Special, Asda*	1 Serving/100g	314	0.8	314	1.7	75.0	0.8	4.4
Tropical, Morrisons*	1 Pack/200g	368	1.0	184	1.7	50.6	0.5	6.3
Tropical Sundae, Graze*	1 Punnet/29g	86	0.3	299	2.7	72.7	1.0	8.5
DRIFTER								
Nestle*	1 Finger/20g	99	4.3	484	4.1	68.9	20.9	1.2
DRINKING CHOCOLATE								
Cadbury*	1 Heap Tbsp/16g	64	0.4	402	4.4	89.3	2.4	0.0
Dry, Asda*	1 Serving/30g	111	1.8	370	6.0	73.0	6.0	0.0
Dry, M & S*	3 Heap Tsp/20g	73	0.9	365	8.4	66.0	4.4	13.0
Dry Powder, Cocodirect*	1 Serving/18g	67	1.5	372	8.9	65.1	8.4	0.0
Fairtrade, Truly Irresistible, Co-Op*	1 Serving/20g	73	1.9	365	10.0	60.3	9.4	13.8
Made Up, BGTY, Sainsbury's*	1 Serving/178g	114	0.4	64	3.9	11.4	0.2	0.7
Made Up with Semi-Skimmed Milk, Average	1 Mug/227ml	129	4.3	57	3.5	7.0	1.9	0.2
Made Up with Skimmed Milk, Average	1 Mug/227ml	100	1.1	44	3.5	7.0	0.5	0.0
Made Up with Whole Milk, Average	1 Mug/227ml	173	9.5	76	3.4	6.8	4.2	0.2
Maxpax, Light, Suchard*	1 Serving/11g	37	0.6	355	20.0	56.0	5.5	9.3
Milk, Instant Break, Cadbury*	4 Tsp/28g	119	3.9	425	10.9	64.2	14.0	0.0
Orange, Mix, Clipper*	1 Pack/28g	98	0.4	350	14.6	69.7	1.5	0.0
Powder, Made Up with Skimmed Milk	1 Mug/227ml	134	1.4	59	3.5	10.8	0.6	0.0
Powder, Made Up with Whole Milk	1 Mug/227ml	204	9.3	90	3.4	10.6	4.1	0.0
DRIPPING								
Beef	***1oz/28g***	***249***	***27.7***	***891***	***0.0***	***0.0***	***99.0***	***0.0***

D

	Measure INFO/WEIGHT	per Measure KCAL	FAT	Nutrition Values per 100g / 100ml KCAL	PROT	CARB	FAT	FIBRE
DUCK								
Breast, Meat Only, Cooked, Average	***1oz/28g***	***48***	***2.0***	***172***	***25.3***	***1.8***	***7.0***	***0.0***
Breast, Meat Only, Raw, Average	***1 Serving/160g***	***206***	***6.8***	***128***	***22.6***	***0.0***	***4.2***	***0.2***
Fillets, Gressingham, Mini, TTD, Sainsbury's*	½ Pack/90g	127	2.4	141	29.0	0.0	2.7	0.6
Leg, Meat & Skin, Average	***1oz/28g***	***80***	***5.6***	***286***	***17.2***	***9.5***	***20.0***	***0.4***
Raw, Meat, Fat & Skin	***1oz/28g***	***109***	***10.4***	***388***	***13.1***	***0.0***	***37.3***	***0.0***
Raw, Meat Only, Weighed with Fat, Skin & Bone	1 Serving/100g	38	1.8	38	5.5	0.0	1.8	0.0
Roasted, Meat, Fat & Skin	***1oz/28g***	***118***	***10.7***	***423***	***20.0***	***0.0***	***38.1***	***0.0***
Roasted, Meat Only, Weighed with Fat, Skin & Bone	1 Serving/100g	41	2.2	41	5.3	0.0	2.2	0.0
Shredded, & Spring Onion, Rice Paper Rolls, Waitrose*	1 Pack/95g	101	0.7	104	6.6	17.7	0.8	0.7
DUCK &								
Plum Sauce, Roasted, Sainsbury's*	½ Pack/150g	174	3.8	116	6.9	16.0	2.5	1.8
DUCK A L' ORANGE								
Roast, M & S*	½ Pack/270g	554	42.1	205	12.5	4.1	15.6	0.6
DUCK AROMATIC								
Crispy, ¼ with Hoisin Sauce, & 6 Pancakes, Tesco*	1/6 Pack/40g	100	4.2	250	12.3	25.3	10.6	2.0
Crispy, Asda*	1/3 Pack/166g	469	24.9	283	19.0	18.0	15.0	0.8
Crispy, Half, with Hoisin Sauce, & 12 Pancakes, Tesco*	1/6 Pack/70g	162	7.4	232	18.3	15.9	10.6	1.1
Crispy, Half Duck & Pancakes, M & S*	½ Pack/311g	590	26.7	190	13.9	14.0	8.6	2.1
Crispy, with Hoisin Sauce, & 18 Pancakes, Tesco*	1/9 Pack/100g	280	17.2	280	18.9	12.0	17.2	0.4
with Plum Sauce, Tesco*	½ Pack/250g	350	11.5	140	9.3	15.2	4.6	0.3
DUCK CANTONESE								
Style, Roast, Tesco*	1 Pack/300g	375	6.9	125	8.2	17.9	2.3	0.5
DUCK IN								
Chinese Barbecue, Wings, Sainsbury's*	1 Serving/175g	430	25.0	246	19.4	9.7	14.3	0.0
Orange Sauce, Iceland*	1 Serving/200g	336	20.8	168	11.3	7.4	10.4	1.2
Orange Sauce, Legs, Extra Special, Asda*	1oz/28g	39	1.6	141	18.0	4.3	5.7	1.3
Oriental Sauce, Iceland*	1 Pack/201g	352	22.7	175	12.0	6.3	11.3	1.5
Plum & Chilli Sauce, Legs, Aldi*	½ Pack/200g	342	11.6	171	5.7	24.0	5.8	0.6
Plum Sauce, Crispy, M & S*	1 Pack/325g	569	31.2	175	10.7	11.2	9.6	0.9
Plum Sauce, Legs, Asda*	1 Leg/200g	452	23.0	226	24.1	6.4	11.5	0.5
Red Wine Sauce, Free Range Fillets, Waitrose*	½ Pack/250g	378	19.2	151	16.4	4.1	7.7	2.2
DUCK PEKING								
Crispy, Aromatic, Sainsbury's*	½ Pack/300g	1236	110.7	412	19.5	0.6	36.9	0.1
Crispy, Cherry Valley*	1 Serving/270g	702	35.9	260	17.5	17.8	13.3	0.7
DUCK WITH								
Hoisin & Noodles, Fuller for Longer, M & S*	1 Pack/370g	335	7.4	91	8.2	10.0	2.0	2.0
Noodles, Shanghai Roast, Sainsbury's*	1 Pack/450g	580	17.1	129	5.6	18.0	3.8	1.2
Pancakes, Shredded, Iceland*	1 Pack/220g	471	5.9	214	20.4	27.0	2.7	1.5
Pancakes & Hoisin Sauce, M & S*	1 Pack/80g	136	3.2	170	13.0	19.9	4.0	0.9
DUMPLINGS								
Average	1oz/28g	58	3.3	208	2.8	24.5	11.7	0.9
Dried Mix, Tesco*	1 Pack/137g	404	16.7	295	5.4	39.9	12.2	2.8
Farmhouse, Mix, Goldenfry Foods Ltd*	1 Serving/35g	148	5.3	422	9.1	62.0	15.1	1.0
Homestyle, Baked Weight, Frozen, Aunt Bessie's*	1 Dumpling/49g	188	8.6	384	9.7	44.4	17.6	2.8
Pork & Garlic Chive, Waitrose*	1 Pack/115g	215	8.1	187	9.4	20.4	7.0	1.1
Prawn, Cantonese, Crispy, Sainsbury's*	1 Dumpling/11g	27	1.5	241	9.3	20.9	13.4	1.1
Prawn, Siu Mai, Chinese, M & S*	8 Dumplings/170g	170	2.9	100	7.8	13.1	1.7	1.3

	Measure INFO/WEIGHT	per Measure KCAL	FAT	Nutrition Values per 100g / 100ml KCAL	PROT	CARB	FAT	FIBRE
EASTER EGG								
After Eight, Giant, Nestle*	¼ Egg/50g	268	16.2	536	5.0	50.3	32.3	8.0
Buttons, Chocolate Shell Only, Cadbury*	1 Egg/162g	859	48.6	530	7.5	56.8	30.0	0.7
Caramel, Chocolate Egg Shell Only, Cadbury*	1 Egg/343g	1801	102.9	525	7.5	56.8	30.0	0.7
Chocolate, Dark, 70%, Green & Black's*	1 Egg/165g	960	69.5	580	9.1	36.5	42.0	10.0
Chocolate, Dark, Thorncroft's*	1 Egg/360g	1890	134.6	525	6.8	39.4	37.4	9.8
Chocolate, Milk, Nestle*	½ Egg/42g	205	9.7	489	5.0	65.2	23.1	0.5
Chocolate, Milk, Swiss, Hollow, M & S*	1 Egg/18g	100	6.3	555	6.7	53.2	34.8	2.5
Chocolate, White, Thorntons*	1 Egg/360g	1958	109.1	544	5.5	62.2	30.3	2.1
Chocolate Orange, Terry's*	1 Egg/120g	636	36.6	530	7.4	57.0	30.5	2.4
Creme Egg, Shell Only, Cadbury*	1 Egg/178g	943	53.4	530	7.5	56.8	30.0	0.7
Crunchie, Cadbury*	1 Egg/167g	885	50.1	530	7.5	56.8	30.0	0.7
Disney, Nestle*	1 Egg/65g	342	18.9	526	6.3	59.7	29.1	0.6
Flake, Shell Only, Cadbury*	1 Shell/153g	811	45.9	530	7.5	56.8	30.0	0.7
Kit Kat, Chunky, Nestle*	1 Egg/235g	1250	67.7	532	5.5	61.7	28.8	1.7
Mars*	1 Serving/63g	281	10.9	449	4.2	69.0	17.4	0.0
Milky Bar, Nestle*	1 Egg/40g	182	6.9	454	4.2	70.8	17.2	0.0
Roses, Shell Only, Cadbury*	1 Egg/200g	1060	60.0	530	7.5	56.8	30.0	0.7
Shell Only, Dairy Milk, Cadbury*	1 Egg/178g	943	53.4	530	7.5	56.8	30.0	0.7
Smarties, Nestle*	1 Egg/258g	1367	74.0	530	5.3	62.2	28.7	1.7
Twirl, Shell Only, Cadbury*	1 Egg/325g	1722	97.5	530	7.5	56.8	30.0	0.7
Wispa, Shell Only, Cadbury*	1 Egg/313g	1643	93.9	525	7.5	56.8	30.0	0.7
ECLAIR								
Chocolate, 25% Less Fat, Sainsbury's*	1 Eclair/58g	171	9.3	295	6.8	31.1	16.0	1.2
Chocolate, Belgian, Weight Watchers*	1 Eclair/30g	81	3.5	271	3.9	37.6	11.7	6.6
Chocolate, Cream, Fresh, Tesco*	1 Eclair/66g	285	20.5	430	6.0	31.1	30.9	1.8
Chocolate, Cream filled, VLH Kitchens	1 Eclair/66g	286	44.2	434	7.0	36.4	29.2	1.8
Chocolate, Double, with Fresh Cream, Tesco*	1 Eclair/69g	275	18.6	400	5.9	33.4	27.0	1.6
Chocolate, Fresh Cream, M & S*	1 Eclair/44g	170	12.2	390	6.3	28.4	27.9	2.0
Chocolate, Fresh Cream, Sainsbury's*	1 Eclair/59g	212	13.9	360	4.2	32.7	23.6	0.5
Chocolate, Frozen, Morrisons*	1 Eclair/31g	116	9.6	374	5.0	18.8	31.0	1.3
Chocolate, HL, Tesco*	1 Serving/77g	192	9.7	249	6.8	27.1	12.6	0.9
Chocolate, Mini, Iceland*	1 Eclair/13g	55	4.6	426	4.9	21.5	35.6	0.4
EEL								
Cooked or Smoked, Dry Heat, Average	***1 Serving/100g***	***236***	***15.0***	***236***	***23.6***	***0.0***	***15.0***	***0.0***
Jellied, Average	***1oz/28g***	***27***	***2.0***	***98***	***8.4***	***0.0***	***7.1***	***0.0***
Raw, Average	***1oz/28g***	***47***	***3.2***	***168***	***16.6***	***0.0***	***11.3***	***0.0***
EGG SUBSTITUTE								
99% Real Eggs, The Crafty Cook*	¼ Cup/61g	30	0.0	49	10.0	2.0	0.0	0.0
Original, The Crafty Cook*	¼ Cup 1oz/28g	30	0.0	107	21.4	3.6	0.0	0.0
EGGS								
Dried, White, Average	***1 Tbsp/14g***	***41***	***0.0***	***295***	***73.8***	***0.0***	***0.0***	***0.0***
Dried, Whole, Average	***1oz/28g***	***159***	***11.6***	***568***	***48.4***	***0.0***	***41.6***	***0.0***
Duck, Boiled & Salted, Average, Weight with Shell	1 Egg/75g	169	13.2	225	16.6	0.0	17.6	0.0
Duck, Whole, Raw, Average, Weight with Shell	***1 Egg/75g***	***139***	***10.0***	***185***	***16.2***	***0.0***	***13.4***	***0.0***
Free Range, Large, Average, Weight with Shell	***1 Egg/68g***	***109***	***7.6***	***161***	***14.1***	***0.9***	***11.2***	***0.0***
Fried in Veg Oil, Average	1 Med/60g	107	8.3	179	13.6	0.0	13.9	0.0
Fried without Fat, Average	1 Med/60g	104	7.6	174	15.0	0.0	12.7	0.0
Goose, Whole, Fresh, Raw, Average, Weight with Shell	***1 Egg/144g***	***267***	***19.1***	***185***	***13.9***	***1.4***	***13.3***	***0.0***
Large, Average, Weight with Shell	1 Egg/68g	115	8.6	170	14.0	0.0	12.6	0.0
Medium, Average, Weight with Shell	1 Egg/58g	98	7.3	170	14.0	0.1	12.6	0.0
Medium, Boiled, Average, Weight with Shell	1 Egg/58g	96	7.0	165	14.0	0.6	12.1	0.1
Poached, Weight with Shell	1 Med/50g	83	6.1	165	14.0	0.6	12.1	0.6
Quail, Whole, Raw, Weight with Shell	***1 Egg/13g***	***21***	***1.6***	***164***	***14.0***	***0.4***	***12.1***	***0.0***

	Measure INFO/WEIGHT	per Measure KCAL	FAT	Nutrition Values per 100g / 100ml KCAL	PROT	CARB	FAT	FIBRE
EGGS								
Scrambled, Average	1 Serving/100g	160	11.6	160	13.8	0.0	11.6	0.0
Scrambled, with Milk, Average	1 Serving/100g	257	23.4	257	10.9	0.7	23.4	0.0
Turkey, Whole, Raw, Weight with Shell	***1 Egg/79g***	***154***	***10.9***	***194***	***15.5***	***1.3***	***13.9***	***0.0***
Very Large, Average, Weight with Shell	1 Egg/78g	125	8.7	161	14.1	0.9	11.2	0.0
White, Free Range, Liquid, Two Chicks*	3 Tbsp/45g	23	0.0	50	10.5	1.0	0.0	0.0
Whites, Liquid, Myprotein*	1 Egg White/32g	16	0.0	50	11.2	0.0	0.0	0.0
Whites Only, Raw, Average	***1 Egg/33g***	***12***	***0.0***	***36***	***9.0***	***0.0***	***0.0***	***0.0***
Yolks, Raw	***1 Yolk/14g***	***47***	***4.3***	***339***	***16.1***	***0.0***	***30.5***	***0.0***
ELDERBERRIES								
Average	***1oz/28g***	***10***	***0.1***	***35***	***0.7***	***7.4***	***0.5***	***0.0***
ELICHE								
Dry Weight, Buitoni*	1 Serving/80g	282	1.5	352	11.2	72.6	1.9	0.0
ELK								
Raw, Meat only	1 Serving/100g	111	1.4	111	23.0	0.0	1.4	0.0
Roasted, Meat only	1 Serving/100g	146	1.9	146	30.2	0.0	1.9	0.0
ENCHILADAS								
3 Bean, Ready Meal, Average	1 Pack/400g	505	16.6	126	4.4	16.9	4.2	3.2
Beef, LC, Tesco*	1 Pack/400g	440	11.2	110	5.4	13.4	2.8	3.1
Chicken, American, HL, Tesco*	1 Serving/240g	353	4.3	147	10.4	22.5	1.8	1.2
Chicken, Average	1 Serving/295g	483	18.8	164	11.6	16.0	6.4	1.7
Chicken, Diner Specials, M & S*	½ Pack/227g	340	12.0	150	9.9	15.4	5.3	2.0
Chicken, Perfectly Balanced, Waitrose*	1 Pack/450g	482	14.4	107	6.9	12.7	3.2	1.1
Chicken, Suiza, Smart Ones, Weight Watchers*	1 Pack/255g	290	5.0	114	4.3	18.0	2.0	1.2
Vegetable, GFY, Asda*	1 Pack/350g	399	15.8	114	4.4	14.0	4.5	1.3
Vegetable, Morrisons*	1 Pack/400g	468	18.4	117	4.5	14.4	4.6	1.8
Vegetable & Bean, Eat Smart, Morrisons*	1 Pack/380g	475	9.9	125	4.7	20.7	2.6	3.2
ENDIVE								
Raw	***1oz/28g***	***4***	***0.1***	***13***	***1.8***	***1.0***	***0.2***	***2.0***
ENERGY DRINK								
Average	1 Can/250ml	118	0.0	47	0.0	11.4	0.0	0.0
Blue Bolt, Sainsbury's*	1 Can/250ml	124	0.0	49	0.0	11.3	0.0	0.0
Burn, Coca-Cola*	1 fl oz/30ml	13	0.0	44	0.0	10.5	0.0	0.0
Cherry, Lucozade*	1 Bottle/500ml	345	0.0	69	0.0	17.1	0.0	0.0
Isostar Sport, Isostar*	1 Glass/250ml	74	0.0	30	0.0	7.0	0.0	0.0
Juiced Berry, Relentless*	1 Can/500g	230	0.0	46	0.0	10.7	0.0	0.0
Libertus, Blue, Sugar Free, Relentless*	1 Can/500ml	20	0.0	4	0.0	0.0	0.0	0.0
Monster*	1 Can/500ml	240	0.0	48	0.0	12.0	0.0	0.0
Orange, Isotonic, Myprotein*	1 Bottle/500ml	148	0.0	30	0.0	6.9	0.0	0.0
Original, Rockstar*	1 Can/500ml	290	0.0	60	0.4	13.6	0.0	0.0
Powerade, Aqua+*	1 Bottle/500ml	80	0.0	16	0.0	3.7	0.0	0.0
Red Devil, Britvic*	1 Can/250ml	160	0.0	64	0.4	15.1	0.0	0.0
Redcard, Britvic*	1 Can/330ml	96	0.0	29	0.1	7.0	0.0	0.0
Relentless, Original, Relentless*	1 Can/500ml	230	0.0	46	0.0	10.4	0.0	0.0
Relentless, Sugar Free, Coca-Cola*	1 Can/500ml	20	0.0	4	0.0	0.0	0.0	0.0
Revive, Cranberry with Acai, Light Sparkling, Lucozade*	1 Bottle/380ml	50	0.0	13	0.0	2.8	0.0	0.0
SoBe, Appleberry Burst, Britvic*	1 Can/250ml	135	0.0	54	0.4	12.0	0.0	0.0
Sparkling Orange, Dual Energy, Powerade*	1 Bottle/500ml	225	0.0	45	0.0	10.5	0.0	0.0
Sugar Free, Boost Drinks Ltd*	1 Can/250ml	5	0.0	2	0.0	0.0	0.0	0.0
Sugar Free, Diet, Mountain Dew, Britvic*	1 Can/440ml	3	0.0	1	0.0	0.0	0.0	0.0
Tropical, Emerge, Cott Beverages Ltd*	1 Can/250ml	115	0.0	46	0.0	10.7	0.0	0.0
V, Frucor Beverages*	1 Can/250ml	112	0.0	45	0.0	11.2	0.0	0.0
X8 Exhilarate, Berry Flavour, Sugar Free, X8 Exhilarate*	1 Shot/60ml	0	0.0	0	0.0	0.0	0.0	0.0

	Measure INFO/WEIGHT	per Measure KCAL	FAT	Nutrition Values per 100g / 100ml KCAL	PROT	CARB	FAT	FIBRE
FAGGOTS								
in Rich Gravy, Iceland*	1 Faggot/81g	116	5.2	143	6.5	15.9	6.4	1.1
Mushy Peas & Mash, Sainsbury's*	1 Pack/450g	576	19.4	128	6.0	16.3	4.3	1.6
Pork & Onion Gravy, 222, Oakhouse Foods Ltd*	1 Meal/360g	299	9.0	83	4.9	10.9	2.5	1.6
FAJITA								
Beef, GFY, Asda*	½ Pack/208g	354	9.8	170	11.0	21.0	4.7	1.6
Chicken, Average	1 Serving/275g	409	14.7	149	10.2	15.0	5.4	2.3
Chicken, BGTY, Sainsbury's*	1 Pack/172g	256	4.3	149	10.8	20.9	2.5	1.7
Chicken, COU, M & S*	1 Pack/230g	288	5.3	125	10.0	16.5	2.3	1.5
Chicken, Crispy, Old El Paso*	1 Fajita/70g	183	5.4	263	7.6	41.0	7.8	1.8
Chicken, GFY, Asda*	½ Pack/225g	233	4.1	104	9.3	12.9	1.8	2.0
Chicken, Just Cook, Sainsbury's*	½ Pack/200g	200	3.0	100	18.5	3.1	1.5	2.0
Chicken, Mexican, No Mayo, Foo-Go*	1 Pack/198g	360	11.1	182	9.6	23.3	5.6	2.4
Chicken, Salt Balanced, COU, M & S*	1 Pack/230g	253	5.3	110	9.5	13.2	2.3	1.7
Gammon Steaks, Tesco*	1 Serving/250g	368	15.5	147	17.5	5.3	6.2	0.0
Meal Kit, Tesco*	1 Serving/100g	210	3.4	210	6.1	38.2	3.4	2.1
Steak, M & S*	1oz/28g	53	2.5	190	8.9	17.2	9.1	0.6
Vegetable	1 Serving/275g	472	14.9	172	4.9	25.6	5.4	1.9
FALAFEL								
12 pack, Sainsbury's*	1 Falafel/17g	44	2.5	259	7.3	20.6	14.8	7.2
Asda*	½ Pack/50g	140	9.6	281	8.3	18.9	19.1	8.2
Balls, Meat Free, Tesco*	3 Balls/67g	135	5.3	205	7.1	21.7	8.1	6.3
Fried in Vegetable Oil, Average	1 Falafel/25g	45	2.8	179	6.4	15.6	11.2	3.4
Gourmet, Meat Free, Vegideli, The Redwood Co*	1 Patty/17g	26	1.4	159	6.1	20.5	8.5	8.1
Mini, M & S*	1 Falafel/14g	43	2.5	310	7.9	28.1	18.4	2.6
Mini, Sainsbury's*	1 Serving/168g	499	29.6	297	8.0	26.8	17.6	3.2
Mix, Asda*	1 Packet/120g	313	15.0	261	6.4	30.8	12.5	2.6
Mix, Authentic, Al'fez*	1 Serving/100g	235	13.8	235	7.1	26.3	13.8	8.8
Mix, Lebanese Style, Al'fez*	½ Pack/200g	470	27.6	235	7.1	26.3	13.8	0.0
Mix, Organic, Quick & Easy, Hale & Hearty*	1 Pack/200g	646	11.0	323	19.2	43.8	5.5	10.7
Organic, Cauldron Foods*	1 Falafel/25g	51	2.4	203	8.4	20.3	9.8	7.2
Vegetarian, Organic, Waitrose*	1 Falafel/25g	55	2.6	220	8.0	23.3	10.5	7.6
FANTA								
Apple, Z, Coca-Cola*	1 Can/330ml	13	0.0	4	0.0	0.6	0.0	0.0
Fruit Twist, Coca-Cola*	1 Serving/250ml	132	0.0	53	0.0	13.0	0.0	0.0
Lemon, Coca-Cola*	1 Can/330ml	165	0.0	50	0.0	12.0	0.0	0.0
Lemon, Icy, Coca-Cola*	1 Can/330ml	112	0.0	34	0.0	8.3	0.0	0.0
Lemon, Icy, Zero, Coca-Cola*	1 Can/330ml	7	0.0	2	0.0	0.2	0.0	0.0
Light, Coca-Cola*	1 Glass/250ml	5	0.0	2	0.0	0.5	0.0	0.0
Orange, Coca-Cola*	1 Glass/250ml	75	0.0	30	0.0	7.1	0.0	0.0
Orange, Zero, Coca-Cola*	1 Can/330ml	11	0.0	3	0.0	0.5	0.0	0.0
Peach, Singapore, Coca-Cola*	1 Bottle/500ml	230	0.0	46	0.0	11.0	0.0	0.0
Red Fruits, Coca-Cola*	1 Serving/100ml	37	0.0	37	0.0	9.0	0.0	0.0
Summer Fruits, Z, Coca-Cola*	1 fl oz/30ml	1	0.0	3	0.0	0.6	0.0	0.0
FARFALLE								
Bows, Dry, Average	***1 Serving/75g***	***265***	***1.4***	***353***	***11.4***	***72.6***	***1.9***	***1.9***
FENNEL								
Florence, Boiled in Salted Water	***1oz/28g***	***3***	***0.1***	***11***	***0.9***	***1.5***	***0.2***	***2.3***
Florence, Raw, Unprepared, Average	***1 Bulb/250g***	***30***	***0.5***	***12***	***0.9***	***1.8***	***0.2***	***2.4***
Florence, Steamed	***1 Serving/80g***	***9***	***0.2***	***11***	***9.0***	***1.5***	***0.2***	***2.3***
FENUGREEK								
Leaves, Raw, Fresh, Average	***1 Serving/80g***	***28***	***0.2***	***35***	***4.6***	***4.8***	***0.2***	***1.1***
FETTUCINI								
Cajun Chicken, Chosen By You, Asda*	1 Pack/400g	360	5.2	90	6.3	12.6	1.3	1.4

F

	Measure INFO/WEIGHT	per Measure KCAL	FAT	Nutrition Values per 100g / 100ml KCAL	PROT	CARB	FAT	FIBRE
FETTUCINI								
Chicken, Cajun, GFY, Asda*	1 Pack/400g	384	7.6	96	8.9	9.7	1.9	2.4
Chicken, Cajun Spiced, COU, M & S*	1 Pack/400g	400	8.0	100	8.0	12.3	2.0	1.3
Chicken Mushroom, GFY, Asda*	1 Pack/400g	359	7.0	90	7.2	11.2	1.8	0.7
Dry Weight, Buitoni*	1 Serving/90g	326	1.5	362	12.2	74.4	1.7	0.0
with Tomato & Mushroom, Easy Cook, Napolina*	1 Pack/120g	461	8.6	384	11.8	67.9	7.2	0.0
FIG ROLLS								
Asda*	1 Biscuit/19g	71	1.7	372	4.8	68.0	9.0	0.0
Bolands*	1 Biscuit/17g	63	1.4	372	4.1	68.3	8.0	5.0
Go Ahead, McVitie's*	1 Biscuit/15g	55	0.7	365	4.2	76.8	4.6	2.9
Jacob's*	1 Biscuit/18g	68	1.5	380	4.0	71.4	8.5	3.3
Sainsbury's*	1 Biscuit/19g	67	1.6	360	4.3	64.5	8.7	3.4
Vitalinea, Jacob's*	1 Biscuit/18g	61	1.0	339	3.7	68.2	5.8	3.8
FIGS								
Dried, Average	***1 Fig/14g***	***32***	***0.1***	***232***	***3.6***	***53.2***	***1.1***	***8.6***
Dried, Organic, Love Life, Waitrose*	1 Fig/30g	66	0.4	221	3.3	48.6	1.5	9.8
Dried, Ready to Eat, Chosen By You, Asda*	1 Serving/30g	70	0.4	234	3.3	48.4	1.5	6.9
Fresh, Black Bursa, Morrisons*	1 Fig/54g	119	0.8	221	3.3	48.6	1.5	6.9
In Light Syrup, Asda*	1 Serving/100g	75	0.1	75	0.4	18.0	0.1	0.7
Raw, Fresh, Average	***1 Fig/35g***	***16***	***0.1***	***45***	***1.3***	***9.8***	***0.2***	***1.5***
FISH								
Balls, Gefilte, M & S*	1 Pack/200g	280	7.8	140	14.1	11.9	3.9	1.0
Battered, Portion, Ross*	1 Serving/110g	223	11.9	203	10.4	16.1	10.8	0.8
Battered, White, Skinless & Boneless, Farmfoods*	1 Serving/122g	238	12.3	195	9.3	16.7	10.1	2.3
Breaded, Asda*	1 Serving/150g	351	21.0	234	15.0	12.0	14.0	0.5
Crumbed, Pak-N-Save*	2 Pieces/140g	298	17.8	213	10.8	13.9	12.7	0.0
Dried, Small, Ogura*	1 Serving/10g	32	0.3	320	69.0	0.3	3.0	0.0
Fillets, Garlic & Herb, Youngs*	1 Fillet/118g	261	14.8	222	11.0	16.2	12.6	1.4
Fillets, Lemon & Pepper, Youngs*	1 Fillet/130g	283	16.7	218	10.3	15.3	12.9	4.3
Fillets, Lime & Chilli, Fish Fusions, Birds Eye*	1 Portion/160g	270	10.1	169	15.0	12.9	6.3	0.5
Fillets, Pollack, Breaded, Cooked, Tesco*	1 Fillet/125g	315	12.2	250	15.0	24.4	9.7	2.0
Fillets, White, Breaded, Tesco*	1 Piece/95g	198	10.4	208	10.6	16.9	10.9	1.0
Fillets, White, Breaded, Value, Tesco*	1 Serving/100g	192	9.7	192	10.6	15.6	9.7	2.2
Fillets, White, Natural, Tesco*	1 Fillet/100g	72	0.6	72	16.6	0.0	0.6	0.0
Goujons, Asda*	1 Serving/125g	240	8.0	192	12.8	20.8	6.4	0.2
Grouper	1 Serving/100g	92	1.0	92	19.4	0.0	1.0	0.0
Melts, with Tomato & Mozzarella Filling, Birds Eye*	1 Fillet/100g	255	15.0	255	13.0	17.0	15.0	0.6
Portion, Chip Shop, Youngs*	1 Portion/135g	315	19.7	233	11.0	15.1	14.6	0.6
Portion, in Oven Crisp Batter, Value, Tesco*	1 Serving/100g	209	11.0	209	11.0	16.4	11.0	2.6
Pouting, Fillet, Tesco*	1 Serving/100g	85	0.3	85	19.7	0.3	0.3	0.0
River Cobbler, Smoked, Tesco*	1 Fillet/165g	124	3.5	75	13.9	0.0	2.1	1.5
River Cobbler, Value, Tesco*	½ Pack/133g	133	5.3	100	15.1	0.1	4.0	0.1
Salted, Chinese, Steamed	1oz/28g	43	0.6	155	33.9	0.0	2.2	0.0
Seaside Shapes, Birds Eye*	2 Pieces/80g	197	11.2	246	11.0	19.0	14.0	1.1
Steaks, Chip Shop, Youngs*	1 Serving/100g	198	10.4	198	11.0	14.9	10.4	0.9
Sushi, Medium Pack, Tesco*	1 Pack/224g	336	3.8	150	4.0	29.4	1.7	1.0
White, Breaded, Fillets, Ocean Pure*	1 Fillet/113g	276	11.5	245	20.8	16.9	10.2	1.2
White, Smoked, Average	1 Serving/100g	108	0.9	108	23.4	0.0	0.9	0.0
White, Tesco*	1 Med Fillet/100g	78	0.6	78	16.6	0.0	0.6	0.0
FISH & CHIPS								
Cod, Asda*	1 Serving/280g	450	14.0	161	8.0	21.0	5.0	1.1
Cod, HL, Tesco*	1 Pack/400g	492	7.2	123	5.3	21.4	1.8	1.7
Co-Op*	1 Pack/250g	388	15.0	155	6.0	18.0	6.0	2.0
Mini Meal, 093, Wiltshire Farm Foods*	1 Serving/185g	255	8.3	138	6.9	17.7	4.5	2.8

	Measure INFO/WEIGHT	per Measure KCAL	FAT	Nutrition Values per 100g / 100ml KCAL	PROT	CARB	FAT	FIBRE
FISH & CHIPS								
Ross*	1 Serving/250g	415	19.0	166	6.2	18.1	7.6	1.6
Tesco*	1 Serving/300g	489	18.6	163	5.5	21.2	6.2	1.6
with Mushy Peas, Kershaws*	1 Pack/315g	450	18.3	143	6.4	16.4	5.8	1.6
FISH CAKES								
Breaded, Sainsbury's*	1 Cake/42g	75	3.4	179	10.0	16.2	8.1	0.7
Bubbly Batter, Youngs*	1 Cake/44g	109	6.7	247	7.1	20.5	15.1	1.4
Captain's Coins, Mini, Captain Birds Eye, Birds Eye*	1 Cake/20g	38	1.7	188	9.5	18.7	8.3	1.1
Cod, Big Time, Birds Eye*	1 Cake/114g	223	11.6	196	8.3	17.8	10.2	1.0
Cod, Birds Eye*	1 Cake/51g	93	4.4	182	10.0	16.0	8.7	1.1
Cod, Cheese & Chive, Finest, Tesco*	1 Cake/100g	212	11.5	212	9.7	18.3	11.5	1.7
Cod, Chunky, Breaded, Chilled, Youngs*	1 Cake/90g	192	11.5	213	9.5	14.9	12.8	1.2
Cod, Fresh, Asda*	1 Cake/75g	164	8.2	219	7.0	23.0	11.0	1.6
Cod, Homemade, Average	1 Cake/50g	120	8.3	241	9.3	14.4	16.6	0.7
Cod, King Prawn & Pancetta, Extra Special, Asda*	1 Cake/115g	202	7.7	176	11.0	17.8	6.7	15.0
Cod, Line Caught, Sainsbury's*	1 Cake/90g	161	6.9	179	10.4	17.1	7.7	1.3
Cod, M & S*	1 Cake/85g	153	7.8	180	8.9	15.4	9.2	1.3
Cod, Macfisheries*	1 Cake/85g	164	7.0	192	7.6	22.1	8.2	1.1
Cod, Tesco*	1 Cake/90g	202	9.4	224	8.9	23.8	10.4	0.2
Cod & Pancetta, Cafe Culture, M & S*	1 Cake/85g	166	13.2	195	9.2	7.2	15.5	2.0
Cod & Parsley, Waitrose*	1 Cake/85g	147	6.5	173	9.2	16.9	7.6	1.1
Crab & Prawn, Thai, Tesco*	1 Cake/115g	269	16.6	234	8.8	17.4	14.4	1.2
Fried in Blended Oil	1 Cake/50g	109	6.7	218	8.6	16.8	13.4	0.0
Frozen, Average	1 Cake/85g	112	3.3	132	8.6	16.7	3.9	0.0
Great Value, Iceland*	1 Cake/42g	74	2.7	175	9.1	20.3	6.4	1.6
Grilled, Average	1 Cake/50g	77	2.2	154	9.9	19.7	4.5	0.0
Haddock, Breaded, Asda*	1 Cake/90g	187	7.6	208	10.0	22.8	8.5	1.2
Haddock, Fresh Tastes, Asda*	1 Cake/75g	141	5.0	188	9.6	22.2	6.7	1.8
Haddock, Sainsbury's*	1 Cake/135g	253	10.0	188	10.8	18.7	7.4	1.5
Haddock, Smoked, Asda*	1 Cake/90g	185	9.0	206	10.0	19.0	10.0	1.4
Haddock, Smoked, Breaded, Asda*	1 Cake/90g	202	11.7	225	9.0	18.0	13.0	1.6
Haddock, Smoked, Extra Special, Asda*	1 Cake/115g	218	10.9	190	12.8	13.2	9.5	1.3
Haddock, Smoked, Frozen, Waitrose*	1 Cake/85g	186	10.3	219	9.6	17.8	12.1	0.8
Haddock, Smoked, M & S*	1 Cake/85g	153	8.0	180	10.6	13.4	9.4	2.6
Haddock, Smoked, Sainsbury's*	1 Cake/63g	127	6.0	201	11.0	17.8	9.5	2.1
Haddock, Smoked, Tesco*	1 Cake/135g	236	9.3	175	7.7	19.9	6.9	2.8
M & S*	1 Cake/80g	180	10.6	225	8.0	18.0	13.2	0.0
Prawn, Battered, Asda*	1 Cake/90g	182	10.0	202	10.0	15.6	11.1	1.0
Prawn, Sainsbury's*	1 Cake/90g	184	7.8	204	9.6	21.7	8.7	1.2
Prawn, Tesco*	1 Cake/90g	209	8.2	232	8.2	29.2	9.1	1.8
Prawn, Thai Style, Finest, Tesco*	1 Cake/145g	305	13.5	210	6.7	24.2	9.3	1.0
Ross*	1 Cake/52g	83	3.8	160	7.4	15.9	7.4	1.2
Salmon, & Hollandaise Sauce, Saucy Fish Co*	1 Cake/135g	270	13.0	200	9.2	19.2	9.6	1.4
Salmon, Asda*	1 Cake/86g	215	12.0	250	8.0	23.0	14.0	1.4
Salmon, Birds Eye*	1 Cake/50g	84	4.5	168	9.5	12.2	9.0	1.4
Salmon, Breaded, Crispy, Frozen, Sainsbury's*	1 Cake/60g	140	8.7	234	12.2	13.7	14.5	1.9
Salmon, Chunky, Sainsbury's*	1 Cake/84g	192	10.5	228	13.2	15.8	12.5	2.9
Salmon, Ginger & Chilli, Sainsbury's*	1 Cake/150g	332	17.0	221	11.1	17.7	11.3	2.3
Salmon, Homemade, Average	1 Cake/50g	136	9.8	273	10.4	14.4	19.7	0.7
Salmon, in Crunch Crumb, Birds Eye*	1 Cake/50g	107	6.4	216	9.7	15.0	13.0	1.4
Salmon, M & S*	1 Cake/86g	180	10.9	210	9.1	15.1	12.7	1.7
Salmon, Melting Middle, Lochmuir, M & S*	1 Pack/290g	551	30.4	190	9.1	14.3	10.5	1.5
Salmon, Spinach & Sicilian Lemon, Finest, Tesco*	1 Cake/145g	290	16.2	200	9.9	14.3	11.2	1.4
Salmon, Tesco*	1 Cake/90g	239	13.5	266	11.4	21.3	15.0	0.0

	Measure INFO/WEIGHT	per Measure KCAL	FAT	Nutrition Values per 100g / 100ml KCAL	PROT	CARB	FAT	FIBRE
FISH CAKES								
Salmon, VLH Kitchens	1 Serving/56g	156	35.7	278	10.5	14.4	20.0	0.6
Salmon, with Lemon Butter Sauce, Gastropub, M & S*	1 Cake/107g	188	13.3	175	7.8	8.5	12.4	1.2
Salmon, with Parsley Sauce, Finest, Tesco*	½ Pack/170g	350	23.6	206	8.6	11.7	13.9	1.0
Salmon & Asparagus, Finest, Tesco*	1 Cake/115g	300	17.8	261	10.7	19.6	15.5	0.4
Salmon & Broccoli, Morrisons*	1 Cake/110g	211	10.3	191	9.0	16.7	9.3	2.2
Salmon & Dill, Cook*	1 Cake/95g	144	5.3	152	11.3	14.2	5.6	1.5
Salmon & Haddock with Lemon & Dill Sauce, Waitrose*	1 Cake/187g	304	18.1	163	9.2	9.7	9.7	1.5
Salmon & Leek, Northern Catch, Aldi*	1 Cake/114g	212	9.0	186	9.5	19.3	7.9	0.9
Salmon & Tarragon, Waitrose*	1 Cake/85g	179	10.0	211	11.9	14.3	11.8	2.2
Smart Price, Asda*	1 Cake/42g	78	3.3	188	7.0	22.0	8.0	0.9
Thai, Finest, Tesco*	1 Cake/65g	150	8.6	230	7.5	20.3	13.2	1.6
Thai, Frozen, Sainsbury's*	1 Cake/15g	28	1.1	187	21.3	9.3	7.3	0.7
Thai, Oriental Selection, Waitrose*	1 Cake/11g	18	0.3	161	17.8	15.8	3.0	1.5
Thai Style, Sainsbury's*	1 Cake/49g	69	2.1	141	12.0	13.8	4.2	1.7
Tuna, Asda*	1 Cake/75g	185	10.1	247	14.9	16.5	13.5	1.4
Tuna, Lime & Coriander, BGTY, Sainsbury's*	1 Cake/91g	200	10.7	220	10.7	17.7	11.8	2.6
Tuna, Sainsbury's*	1 Cake/90g	183	7.5	203	13.7	18.4	8.3	2.1
Tuna & Red Pepper, Waitrose*	1 Cake/85g	175	10.0	206	9.5	15.4	11.8	1.6
FISH FINGERS								
Atlantis*	1 Finger/30g	52	2.2	172	12.0	14.0	7.5	0.4
Chip Shop, Youngs*	1 Finger/30g	75	4.9	251	9.3	16.6	16.4	1.2
Chunky, Cooked, Tesco*	2 Fingers/98g	230	10.0	235	13.2	21.6	10.2	1.3
Cod, 100% Cod Fillet, Tesco*	1 Finger/30g	53	2.2	177	12.4	14.9	7.5	1.4
Cod, Chunky, Tesco*	1 Finger/40g	70	3.0	175	12.3	14.3	7.6	1.6
Cod, Fillet, Asda*	1 Finger/31g	66	3.1	214	13.0	18.0	10.0	0.0
Cod, Fillet, Chunky, M & S*	1 Finger/40g	70	2.4	175	12.0	17.2	6.0	1.0
Cod, Fillet, Chunky, TTD, Sainsbury's*	2 Fingers/120g	274	13.2	228	13.4	18.3	11.0	1.2
Cod, Fillet, Iceland*	1 Finger/30g	62	2.5	205	13.0	19.5	8.3	1.4
Cod, Fillet, Waitrose*	1 Finger/30g	55	2.2	183	11.9	16.9	7.5	0.7
Cod, Fried in Blended Oil, Average	1 Finger/28g	67	3.9	238	13.2	15.5	14.1	0.6
Cod, Frozen, Average	1 Finger/28g	48	2.2	170	11.6	14.2	7.8	0.6
Cod, Grilled, Average	1 Finger/28g	56	2.5	200	14.3	16.6	8.9	0.7
Free From, Sainsbury's*	1 Finger/30g	56	2.3	188	11.4	18.0	7.8	0.7
Haddock, Fillet, Asda*	1 Finger/30g	62	2.7	205	14.0	17.0	9.0	0.0
Haddock, in Crispy Batter, Birds Eye*	1 Finger/30g	56	2.3	188	14.3	15.1	7.8	0.7
Haddock, in Crunchy Crumb, Morrisons*	1 Finger/30g	57	2.4	190	13.1	16.3	8.0	1.1
Hoki, Fillet, Birds Eye*	1 Finger/30g	58	2.7	193	12.6	15.6	8.9	0.7
Iceland*	1 Finger/23g	44	2.0	192	11.5	17.3	8.5	1.3
in Batter, Crispy, Jumbo, Morrisons*	1 Finger/71g	146	8.9	205	11.3	12.2	12.5	0.6
Omega 3, Grilled, Tesco*	3 Fingers/71g	150	6.8	210	12.4	17.8	9.5	1.3
Ross*	1 Finger/26g	50	2.3	193	10.7	17.7	8.8	0.8
Sainsbury's*	1 Finger/27g	52	2.3	194	13.4	16.0	8.5	0.7
Salmon, Birds Eye*	1 Finger/28g	63	2.7	225	13.2	21.7	9.5	0.9
Smart Price, Asda*	1 Finger/25g	46	2.0	184	12.0	16.0	8.0	1.1
Value, Tesco*	1 Finger/25g	42	2.0	170	11.5	11.9	8.1	1.7
FISH IN								
Batter, Light, Iceland*	1 Fillet/120g	230	12.1	192	13.6	11.6	10.1	0.7
Batter, Morrisons*	1 Fish/140g	235	8.1	168	14.0	15.0	5.8	0.2
Batter, Youngs*	1 Serving/100g	315	19.7	315	14.9	20.4	19.7	0.8
Butter Sauce, Steaks, Ross*	1 Serving/140g	111	4.0	84	10.6	3.6	3.0	0.3
Butter Sauce, Steaks, Youngs*	1 Steak/140g	102	2.9	73	9.6	3.7	2.1	0.5
Parsley Sauce, Steaks, Ross*	1 Serving/150g	123	5.6	82	9.1	3.1	3.7	0.1

F

	Measure INFO/WEIGHT	per Measure KCAL	FAT	Nutrition Values per 100g / 100ml KCAL	PROT	CARB	FAT	FIBRE
FISH WITH								
Mushrooms, Carrots & Broccoli, Parcel, Birds Eye*	1 Pack/250g	235	14.0	94	7.9	3.1	5.6	0.8
FIVE SPICE								
Powder, Sharwood's*	1 Tsp/2g	3	0.2	172	12.2	11.6	8.6	23.4
FLAKE								
Dipped, Cadbury*	1 Bar/41g	215	12.5	530	7.6	56.1	30.8	0.8
Luxury, Cadbury*	1 Bar/45g	240	13.6	533	7.3	57.8	30.2	0.0
Praline, Cadbury*	1 Bar/38g	201	12.9	535	7.7	49.5	34.3	0.0
Snow, Cadbury*	1 Bar/36g	198	11.1	550	7.2	60.1	30.9	0.0
FLAN								
Cauliflower, Cheese & Broccoli, Hot, Sainsbury's*	¼ Flan/100g	303	19.8	303	6.4	24.7	19.8	1.2
Cheese & Onion, M & S*	1oz/28g	81	5.2	290	6.1	25.1	18.7	1.4
Cheese & Potato, Hot, Tesco*	¼ Flan/100g	282	19.7	282	6.0	20.0	19.7	2.3
Chicken & Smoked Bacon, Hot, Sainsbury's*	¼ Flan/100g	293	18.5	293	10.2	21.5	18.5	1.2
Mediterranean Vegetable, Co-Op*	¼ Flan/88g	188	10.5	215	4.0	22.0	12.0	3.0
Pastry, with Fruit	1oz/28g	33	1.2	118	1.4	19.3	4.4	0.7
Sponge, with Fruit	1oz/28g	31	0.4	112	2.8	23.3	1.5	0.6
FLAN CASE								
Sponge, Average	***1oz/28g***	***90***	***1.5***	***320***	***7.0***	***62.5***	***5.4***	***0.7***
FLAPJACK								
90% Fat Free, Cookie Coach*	1 Flapjack/75g	287	7.4	383	7.0	66.2	9.9	0.0
All Butter, Blackcurrant Jam, M & S*	1 Serving/65g	280	12.1	430	4.8	60.5	18.6	2.2
All Butter, Organic, Sainsbury's*	1 Serving/35g	156	8.0	446	5.3	54.5	23.0	2.7
All Butter, Sainsbury's*	1 Flapjack/35g	156	8.0	446	5.7	54.5	22.8	2.7
All Butter, Squares, M & S*	1 Flapjack/34g	150	7.2	441	6.2	56.2	21.2	4.4
All Butter, Waitrose*	1 Flapjack/34g	126	9.0	376	3.8	52.4	26.8	1.2
Almond, Hazlenut & Almond, Seriously Nutty, Waitrose*	1 Square/26g	133	8.4	517	9.2	46.7	32.6	3.1
Apple & Raisin, Lite, Crazy Jack*	1 Flapjack70g	227	1.5	324	9.8	72.0	2.1	0.0
Apple & Raspberry, Fox's*	1 Flapjack/26g	105	5.0	403	4.8	52.5	19.4	3.7
Apple & Sultana, Blackfriars*	1 Flapjack/110g	507	24.2	461	5.5	61.0	22.0	0.0
Apple & Sultana, Mr Kipling*	1 Flapjack/27g	123	6.0	456	4.6	59.0	22.4	3.6
Apple Strudel, Devondale*	1 Flapjack/95g	413	22.5	435	4.1	50.8	23.7	3.2
Apricot, The Handmade Flapjack Company*	1 Flapjack/90g	321	4.8	357	5.5	71.6	5.4	0.0
Apricot & Raisin, Waitrose*	1 Flapjack/38g	143	4.2	376	4.7	64.3	11.1	5.8
Average	1 Serving/50g	242	13.3	484	4.5	60.4	26.6	2.7
Banana, The Handmade Flapjack Company*	1 Flapjack/90g	379	13.1	421	5.3	67.2	14.6	0.0
Banoffee, Iced, Devondale*	1 Flapjack/95g	428	24.7	450	3.6	51.0	26.0	2.5
Black Cherry, Blackfriars*	1 Serving/110g	529	25.3	481	5.0	63.0	23.0	0.0
Brazil Nut Cluster, The Handmade Flapjack Company*	1 Flapjack/90g	353	9.1	392	6.6	68.7	10.2	0.0
Butter, Kate's Cakes Ltd*	1 Serving/100g	425	22.2	425	5.4	51.4	22.2	3.3
Butter, Mr Kipling*	1 Flapjack/75g	337	15.9	450	5.4	59.6	21.2	3.2
Cappuccino, Blackfriars*	1 Flapjack/110g	481	27.5	437	5.0	61.0	25.0	0.0
Cappuccino, Iced, Devondale*	1 Flapjack/95g	442	23.2	465	3.9	53.6	24.4	2.8
Caramel Bake, The Handmade Flapjack Company*	1 Flapjack/90g	375	13.0	417	6.0	65.6	14.5	0.0
Cherry & Coconut, Blackfriars*	1 Flapjack/110g	490	23.1	445	5.0	58.0	21.0	0.0
Cherry & Sultana, Cookie Coach*	1 Pack/90g	373	15.6	414	6.2	58.2	17.3	0.0
Cherry Bakewell, Iced, Devondale*	1 Flapjack/95g	432	21.9	455	3.7	54.0	23.1	2.6
Cherry Sultana, Devondale*	1 Flapjack/95g	412	21.8	434	4.0	51.0	23.0	3.0
Chocoholic, Iced, Devondale*	1 Flapjack/95g	439	23.9	462	3.8	51.8	25.2	3.2
Chocolate, Chunky, M & S*	1 Flapjack/80g	348	15.1	435	5.8	59.9	18.9	2.2
Chocolate, McVitie's*	1 Flapjack/85g	422	23.0	496	6.6	56.6	27.1	3.2
Chocolate, The Handmade Flapjack Company*	1 Flapjack/90g	392	17.6	435	6.0	58.6	19.6	0.0
Chocolate & Hazelnut, M & S*	1 Flapjack/71g	330	18.1	465	7.3	55.6	25.5	3.8
Chocolate Chip, Boots*	1 Flapjack/75g	313	11.2	417	5.6	65.0	15.0	3.5

	Measure INFO/WEIGHT	per Measure KCAL	FAT	Nutrition Values per 100g / 100ml KCAL	PROT	CARB	FAT	FIBRE
FLAPJACK								
Chocolate Chip, Devondale*	1 Flapjack/95g	434	24.7	457	4.3	49.0	26.0	3.6
Chocolate Chunk, Boots*	1 Slice/75g	351	18.8	468	5.7	55.0	25.0	3.0
Chocolate Dipped, Belgian, Asda*	1 Serving/67g	321	16.8	477	6.0	57.0	25.0	3.2
Chocolate Dipped, M & S*	1 Flapjack/96g	442	21.5	460	6.1	61.3	22.4	3.0
Chocolate Special, The Handmade Flapjack Company*	1 Flapjack/90g	392	17.8	436	5.7	58.7	19.8	0.0
Cranberry, Apple & Raisin, LC, Tesco*	1 Flapjack/30g	98	1.7	325	5.7	63.1	5.6	5.7
Crazy Raizin, Fabulous Bakin' Boys*	1 Pack/90g	378	15.3	420	6.0	60.0	17.0	4.0
Date & Apple, Multigrain, Devondale*	1 Flapjack/80g	338	16.8	422	3.5	53.6	21.0	2.7
Date & Walnut, The Handmade Flapjack Company*	1 Flapjack/90g	360	13.5	400	6.1	60.2	15.0	0.0
Fingers, GFY, Asda*	1 Finger/37g	130	3.7	350	5.0	60.0	10.0	3.5
Fruit, GFY, Asda*	1 Flapjack/45g	173	3.6	384	6.0	72.0	8.0	3.4
Fruit, Kate's Cakes Ltd*	1 Serving/100g	425	16.7	425	7.3	58.2	16.7	4.7
Fruit, Mr Kipling*	1 Flapjack/75g	306	13.6	408	4.8	56.7	18.1	3.0
Fruit, Weight Watchers*	1 Serving/30g	106	1.9	353	6.0	68.3	6.3	4.7
Fruit, with Raisins, Boots*	1 Pack/75g	329	15.8	439	5.4	57.0	21.0	3.5
Fruit & Nut, Organic, Evernat*	1oz/28g	136	7.4	484	4.5	60.4	26.6	0.0
Fruity, Waitrose*	1 Serving/50g	199	6.8	398	6.1	62.9	13.5	3.9
Fudge, Blackfriars*	1 Serving/110g	528	26.4	480	5.0	60.0	24.0	0.0
Hobnobs, Chocolate, Milk, McVitie's*	1 Flapjack/35g	155	6.0	443	5.8	64.2	17.2	4.2
Honey & Clotted Cream, Devondale*	1 Flapjack/95g	419	23.8	441	4.6	48.0	25.0	3.5
Jaffa Cake, Graze*	1 Punnet/53g	242	12.7	457	6.0	53.0	24.0	5.0
Lemon, Multigrain, Devondale*	1 Flapjack/80g	341	18.2	426	3.9	51.0	22.8	2.9
Lemon Curd, Graze*	1 Punnet/53g	248	12.7	468	6.0	60.0	24.0	6.0
M & S*	1 Flapjack/53g	228	10.1	430	6.0	59.1	19.0	3.5
Millionaire, Anytime, Gu*	1 Flapjack/19g	87	4.8	465	4.9	54.2	25.4	2.2
Oat, GF, Hale & Hearty*	1 Cake/36g	165	9.1	457	6.8	55.1	25.2	8.9
Oats, Butter & Syrup, McVitie's*	1 Bar/79g	356	17.7	454	4.9	57.9	22.5	3.7
Oaty, Fingers, Golden, Tesco*	1 Finger/25g	112	5.3	450	5.7	59.6	21.1	3.4
Organic, Wholebake*	1 Bar/90g	388	18.7	431	6.0	59.4	20.8	0.0
Plain, Devondale*	1 Flapjack/95g	400	25.1	421	3.4	42.0	26.4	2.5
Plain, The Handmade Flapjack Company*	1 Flapjack/90g	398	19.2	442	5.4	57.1	21.3	0.0
Raspberry, Devondale*	1 Flapjack/95g	406	21.7	427	4.0	51.0	22.8	3.0
Snickers, McVitie's*	1 Flapjack/65g	315	18.5	484	7.9	49.0	28.5	6.0
Strawberries & Cream, Iced, Devondale*	1 Flapjack/95g	427	24.1	449	3.3	53.2	25.4	2.3
Strawberry, Multigrain, Devondale*	1 Flapjack/80g	341	18.2	426	3.9	51.6	22.8	2.9
Sultana, Tesco*	1 Flapjack/50g	173	10.0	346	5.0	36.2	20.1	3.7
Summer Berry, Graze*	1 Punnet/52g	230	10.9	442	5.0	56.0	21.0	5.0
Sunflower & Raisin, Devondale*	1 Flapjack/95g	426	25.0	448	5.2	47.9	26.3	3.2
Toffee, Finest, Tesco*	1 Flapjack/35g	156	6.7	446	4.9	63.6	19.1	1.3
Toffee Apple, Iced, Devondale*	1 Flapjack/95g	427	24.1	449	3.6	53.2	25.4	2.7
Toffeemac, The Handmade Flapjack Company*	1 Flapjack/90g	411	19.7	457	6.1	59.0	21.9	0.0
Triple Choc, Iced, Devondale*	1 Flapjack/95g	439	23.8	462	3.8	51.0	25.0	3.2
Tropical Mix, Reduced Fat, Fabulous Bakin' Boys*	1 Flapjack/90g	346	10.8	385	6.0	63.0	12.0	3.0
Walnut & Maple, Devondale*	1 Flapjack/95g	445	27.6	468	4.0	45.2	29.0	3.2
Weight Watchers*	1 Slice/30g	109	1.8	363	6.7	71.0	6.0	4.0
with Sultanas, Tesco*	1 Flapjack/49g	217	10.3	442	5.3	57.9	21.0	3.7
Yoghurt & Apricot, Iced, Devondale*	1 Flapjack/95g	443	25.6	466	4.5	51.0	27.0	3.3
Yoghurt Flavour, Blackfriars*	1 Bar/110g	521	26.4	474	7.0	58.0	24.0	0.0
FLATBREAD								
Caesar, Chicken, Shapers, Boots*	1 Serving/160g	254	3.4	159	13.0	22.0	2.1	2.0
Cajun Style Chicken, GFY, Asda*	1 Wrap/176g	231	2.1	131	9.0	21.0	1.2	0.9
Cheese & Onion Swedish Style, Shapers, Boots*	1 Flatbread/127g	265	10.3	209	10.0	24.0	8.1	1.3
Cheese & Tomato, Tesco*	¼ Pack/54g	160	3.5	295	11.6	45.7	6.4	1.9

F

	Measure INFO/WEIGHT	per Measure KCAL	FAT	Nutrition Values per 100g / 100ml KCAL	PROT	CARB	FAT	FIBRE
FLATBREAD								
Chicken, Mediterranean, Ginsters*	1 Pack/168g	302	6.7	180	10.6	25.5	4.0	0.0
Chicken, Mexican, Stonebaked, Finest, Tesco*	1 Pack/155g	280	5.1	180	11.7	25.1	3.3	1.6
Chicken, Mexican Style, GFY, Asda*	1 Pack/161g	241	3.2	150	13.0	20.0	2.0	2.5
Chicken, Spicy, Shapers, Boots*	1 Pack/181g	292	4.5	161	11.0	23.0	2.5	0.0
Chicken, Sticky BBQ Style, Shapers, Boots*	1 Pack/158g	274	7.3	173	10.0	23.0	4.6	2.8
Chicken & Mango, Spiced, Love Life, Waitrose*	1 Pack/174g	298	4.7	171	9.7	26.1	2.7	1.9
Chicken & Mango Salad, Sainsbury's*	1 Pack/100g	251	2.5	251	16.9	40.4	2.5	2.5
Chicken & Salsa, Spicy, HL, Tesco*	1 Serving/183g	251	2.6	137	10.1	21.1	1.4	1.2
Chicken Tikka, Shapers, Boots*	1 Flatbread/164g	269	4.1	164	11.0	24.0	2.5	1.5
Chinese Chicken, COU, M & S*	1 Flatbread/156g	281	4.4	180	13.9	24.3	2.8	2.2
Chinese Chicken, Shapers, Boots*	1 Pack/159g	274	2.1	172	11.0	29.0	1.3	1.8
Gluten, Wheat & Milk Free, 4 Pack, Free From, Livwell*	1 Flatbread/55g	148	2.9	269	6.4	53.6	5.3	4.6
Greek Feta Salad, Boots*	1 Pack/158g	241	5.7	153	6.4	24.0	3.6	1.2
Greek Style, GFY, Asda*	1 Flatbread/165g	256	7.1	155	7.0	22.0	4.3	2.1
Greek Style Salad, Waitrose*	1 Pack/172g	280	8.4	163	7.4	22.3	4.9	3.3
King Prawn Tikka, Waitrose*	1 Pack/165g	257	3.3	156	9.4	25.1	2.0	1.5
Peking Duck, Less Than 3% Fat, Shapers, Boots*	1 Pack/156g	246	3.7	158	7.2	27.0	2.4	1.9
Rancher's Chicken, COU, M & S*	1 Pack/174g	270	3.5	155	10.9	23.0	2.0	1.5
Salsa Chicken, Shapers, Boots*	1 Pack/191g	328	8.4	172	11.0	22.0	4.4	1.6
Spicy Mexican, New, Shapers, Boots*	1 Pack/184g	281	5.0	153	8.0	24.0	2.7	1.9
Steak, & Jalapeño, Melt	1 Flatbread/256g	349	9.5	136	9.7	16.4	3.7	1.6
Tomato & Chilli, Sainsbury's*	¼ Bread/65g	155	3.1	238	11.9	36.9	4.7	2.8
Tuna, Mediterranean, Ginsters*	1 Pack/167g	297	6.3	178	10.3	25.6	3.8	0.0
FLAXSEED								
Milled, Organic, Linwoods*	2 Dtsp/30g	170	13.9	568	21.9	1.7	46.2	28.9
Organic, Premium Ground, Prewett's*	1 Tbsp/15g	73	6.0	489	24.0	2.0	40.0	23.0
FLOUR								
00 Grade, Pasta, TTD, Sainsbury's*	1 Bag/1000g	3390	13.0	339	11.5	70.3	1.3	3.0
Arrowroot, Average	***1oz/28g***	***100***	***0.0***	***357***	***0.3***	***88.2***	***0.1***	***3.4***
Bread, Brown, Strong, Average	***1 Serving/100g***	***311***	***1.8***	***311***	***14.0***	***61.0***	***1.8***	***6.4***
Bread, White, Strong, Average	***1oz/28g***	***94***	***0.4***	***336***	***11.8***	***68.4***	***1.5***	***3.4***
Brown, Chapati, Average	***1 Tbsp/20g***	***67***	***0.2***	***333***	***11.5***	***73.7***	***1.2***	***0.0***
Brown, Wheat	***1oz/28g***	***90***	***0.5***	***323***	***12.6***	***68.5***	***1.8***	***6.4***
Chick Pea	***1oz/28g***	***88***	***1.5***	***313***	***19.7***	***49.6***	***5.4***	***10.7***
Coconut, Organic, Sukrin*	1 Serving/100g	320	12.0	320	19.0	9.0	12.0	50.0
GF, Alternative, Wellfoods*	1 Serving/100g	351	1.3	351	1.5	83.1	1.3	2.1
Millet	***1oz/28g***	***99***	***0.5***	***354***	***5.8***	***75.4***	***1.7***	***0.0***
Peanut, Protein Plus*	¼ Cup/30g	110	4.0	367	53.3	26.7	13.3	13.3
Plain, Average	***1oz/28g***	***98***	***0.4***	***349***	***10.3***	***73.8***	***1.5***	***2.2***
Potato	***1oz/28g***	***92***	***0.3***	***328***	***9.1***	***75.6***	***0.9***	***5.7***
Quinoa	1 Serving/100g	349	5.2	349	14.1	61.4	5.2	3.4
Rice	***1 Tsp/5g***	***18***	***0.0***	***366***	***6.4***	***80.1***	***0.8***	***2.0***
Rye, Whole	***1oz/28g***	***94***	***0.6***	***335***	***8.2***	***75.9***	***2.0***	***11.7***
Sauce, Dry, Sainsbury's*	1 Serving/20g	69	0.3	343	9.8	73.0	1.3	3.0
Soya, Full Fat, Average	***1oz/28g***	***118***	***6.1***	***422***	***37.9***	***19.8***	***21.8***	***11.6***
Soya, Low Fat, Average	***1oz/28g***	***99***	***2.0***	***352***	***45.3***	***28.2***	***7.2***	***13.5***
Speciality GF, Dove's Farm*	1 Serving/100g	353	1.8	353	4.7	85.2	1.8	2.7
Spelt, Average	***1 Serving/57g***	***216***	***1.7***	***381***	***14.3***	***74.5***	***3.0***	***6.4***
Strong, Wholemeal, Average	***1 Serving/100g***	***315***	***2.2***	***315***	***13.2***	***60.6***	***2.2***	***9.0***
White, Average	***1oz/28g***	***89***	***0.3***	***319***	***9.8***	***66.8***	***1.0***	***2.9***
White, Chapati, Average	***1 Tbsp/20g***	***67***	***0.1***	***335***	***9.8***	***77.6***	***0.5***	***0.0***
White, Self Raising, Average	***1oz/28g***	***94***	***0.4***	***336***	***9.9***	***71.8***	***1.3***	***2.9***
White, Self Raising, Gluten & Wheat Free, Dove's Farm*	1 Serving/100g	344	1.0	344	5.5	78.1	1.0	1.4

	Measure INFO/WEIGHT	per Measure KCAL	FAT	Nutrition Values per 100g / 100ml KCAL	PROT	CARB	FAT	FIBRE
FLOUR								
White, Wheat, Average	***1oz/28g***	***95***	***0.4***	***341***	***10.4***	***76.5***	***1.4***	***3.1***
Wholemeal, Average	***1oz/28g***	***87***	***0.6***	***312***	***12.6***	***61.9***	***2.2***	***9.0***
Wholemeal, Seed & Grain, Allinson*	1 Serving/100g	340	2.1	340	14.6	58.3	2.1	14.6
Wholemeal, Self Raising, Tesco*	1oz/28g	89	0.6	317	11.5	62.9	2.2	9.0
FLYTE								
Mars*	1 Bar/23g	99	3.2	441	3.4	74.8	14.2	0.0
Snacksize, Mars*	1 Bar/23g	98	3.3	436	3.8	72.5	14.5	0.0
FOOL								
Apricot, Fruit, Tesco*	1 Pot/113g	200	12.7	177	2.6	16.4	11.2	0.3
Blackcurrant, Asda*	1 Pot/114g	89	3.0	78	3.6	10.0	2.6	0.6
Blackcurrant, BGTY, Sainsbury's*	1 Pot/113g	89	2.9	79	3.5	10.4	2.6	0.6
Fruit, Average	1 Pot/120g	196	11.2	163	1.0	20.2	9.3	1.2
Gooseberry, BFY, Morrisons*	1 Pot/114g	99	3.9	87	3.4	10.7	3.4	0.4
Gooseberry, Fruit, BGTY, Sainsbury's*	1 Pot/121g	93	3.4	77	2.9	10.0	2.8	0.8
Gooseberry, Fruit, Co-Op*	1 Pot/114g	211	11.4	185	3.0	22.0	10.0	1.0
Gooseberry, Perfectly Balanced, Waitrose*	1 Pot/113g	125	2.9	111	3.6	18.3	2.6	0.7
Gooseberry, Sainsbury's*	1 Pot/113g	214	12.9	189	2.6	19.1	11.4	1.1
Gooseberry, Tesco*	1 Pot/112g	225	14.1	200	3.0	17.8	12.5	0.7
Lemon, Fruit, BGTY, Sainsbury's*	1 Pot/113g	94	3.8	83	3.4	9.7	3.4	0.3
Lemon, Signature, Morrisons*	1 Pot/114g	213	11.8	187	3.0	20.0	10.4	0.5
Raspberry, Fruit, Tesco*	1 Pot/113g	234	12.8	207	2.6	23.6	11.3	0.3
Rhubarb, Fruit, BGTY, Sainsbury's*	1 Pot/120g	91	3.1	76	3.5	9.5	2.6	0.3
Rhubarb, Fruit, Waitrose*	1 Pot/114g	182	12.9	160	2.7	11.9	11.3	0.3
Rhubarb, Perfectly Balanced, Waitrose*	1 Pot/113g	101	2.9	89	3.5	13.0	2.6	0.3
Rhubarb, Sainsbury's*	1 Pot/113g	180	12.9	159	2.6	11.5	11.4	0.4
Strawberry, Fruit, BGTY, Sainsbury's*	1 Pot/120g	100	3.1	83	3.7	11.1	2.6	0.8
Strawberry, Fruit, Co-Op*	1 Pot/114g	188	10.3	165	2.0	18.0	9.0	0.8
Strawberry, GFY, Asda*	1 Pot/114g	95	3.0	83	3.8	11.0	2.6	0.8
FRANKFURTERS								
Average	***1 Frankfurter/42g***	***123***	***11.2***	***292***	***12.0***	***1.3***	***26.6***	***0.0***
FRANKFURTERS VEGETARIAN								
Asda*	1 Frankfurter/27g	54	3.4	199	18.0	3.5	12.5	2.5
Tivall*	1 Sausage/30g	73	4.8	244	18.0	7.0	16.0	3.0
FRAZZLES								
Bacon, Smith's, Walkers*	1 Bag/23g	113	5.3	488	7.5	62.0	23.0	1.3
FRENCH FRIES								
Cheese & Onion, Walkers*	1 Pack/22g	95	3.5	430	5.0	66.0	16.0	5.0
Ready Salted, Walkers*	1 Bag/22g	83	3.0	377	4.5	56.4	13.6	4.5
Salt & Vinegar, BGTY, Sainsbury's*	1 Bag/15g	51	0.2	340	6.0	80.1	1.5	4.1
Salt & Vinegar, Walkers*	1 Bag/22g	95	3.5	430	5.0	66.0	16.0	5.0
Worcester Sauce, Walkers*	1 Bag/22g	96	3.5	435	5.0	65.0	16.0	5.0
FRENCH TOAST								
Asda*	1 Toast/8g	30	0.4	381	10.0	74.0	5.0	4.0
Co-Op*	1 Toast/8g	31	0.5	385	10.0	72.0	6.0	5.0
Sainsbury's*	1 Toast/8g	31	0.5	382	10.0	72.0	6.6	5.0
FRIDGE RAIDERS								
Chicken, Barbeque Flavour, Bites, Mattessons*	1 Bag/60g	134	7.5	223	20.5	6.5	12.5	1.1
Chicken, Chilli & Lime Flavour, Bites, Mattessons*	1 Bag/60g	129	7.4	215	20.3	5.2	12.4	0.8
Chicken, Hot And Spicy, Bites, Mattessons*	1 Bag/60g	131	7.3	218	21.1	5.4	12.2	1.1
Chicken, Piri Piri, Bites, Mattessons*	1 Bag/60g	122	7.0	203	19.5	4.9	11.6	0.7
Chicken, Southern Fried, Bites, Mattessons*	1 Bag/60g	133	8.5	221	18.8	4.2	14.2	0.8
Chicken, Tikka Flavour, Bites, Mattessons*	1 Bag/60g	110	6.2	184	19.9	2.0	10.4	1.3

	Measure INFO/WEIGHT	per Measure KCAL	FAT	Nutrition Values per 100g / 100ml KCAL	PROT	CARB	FAT	FIBRE
FRIES								
9/16" Straight Cut Home, Deep Fried, McCain*	1oz/28g	65	2.8	233	3.2	32.7	9.9	0.0
9/16" Straight Cut Home, Oven Baked, McCain*	1oz/28g	53	1.5	188	3.2	31.5	5.5	0.0
American Style, Frozen, Thin, Tesco*	1 Serving/125g	208	10.1	166	2.2	21.1	8.1	1.9
American Style, Slim, Iceland*	1 Serving/100g	187	6.1	187	2.4	30.6	6.1	2.4
Crispy French, Weighed Deep Fried, McCain*	1 Serving/100g	193	8.5	193	1.9	27.4	8.5	0.9
Curly, Cajun, Weighed Frozen, McCain*	1 Portion/100g	156	8.7	156	1.6	17.7	8.7	1.8
Curly, Southern Style, Tesco*	1 Serving/50g	124	3.6	248	3.8	41.7	7.3	3.8
Curly, Twisters, Frozen, Conagra Foods*	1 Serving/150g	273	14.0	182	2.5	22.0	9.3	2.2
Extra Chunky, Oven Baked, Homefries, McCain*	1 Serving/200g	306	6.2	153	3.2	28.0	3.1	2.3
Oven, American Style, Frozen, Asda*	1 Serving/180g	407	14.4	226	3.9	34.6	8.0	4.0
Oven, Straight Cut, Morrisons*	1 Serving/100g	149	4.3	149	2.8	24.6	4.3	2.6
Seasoned, Conagra Foods*	1 Serving/150g	248	12.0	165	2.4	20.8	8.0	1.9
Southern, Oven Cook, Baked, Potato Winners, McCain*	1 Serving/100g	232	8.3	232	3.6	35.7	8.3	2.4
Southern, Oven Cook, Frozen, Potato Winners, McCain*	1 Serving/100g	176	6.7	176	2.4	26.5	6.7	1.6
Southern Spicy Spiral, Deep Fried, McCain*	1oz/28g	58	2.9	208	2.7	26.4	10.2	0.0
Southern Spicy Spiral, Oven Baked, McCain*	1oz/28g	46	1.8	165	1.7	24.6	6.6	0.0
FRISPS								
Tangy Salt & Vinegar, KP Snacks*	1 Bag/30g	160	10.0	532	5.0	52.6	33.5	2.9
Tasty Cheese & Onion, KP Snacks*	1 Bag/28g	150	9.4	537	5.5	53.2	33.6	3.2
FRITTATA								
Vegetable, Chosen By You, Asda*	1 Serving/150g	183	7.8	122	6.2	12.1	5.2	1.0
FROG								
Legs, Raw, Meat Only	***1oz/28g***	***20***	***0.1***	***73***	***16.4***	***0.0***	***0.3***	***0.0***
FROMAGE FRAIS								
0% Fat, Vitalinea, Danone*	1 Tbsp/28g	14	0.0	50	7.4	4.7	0.1	0.0
Apple Pie, Low Fat, Sainsbury's*	1 Pot/90g	108	2.3	120	6.7	17.3	2.6	0.3
Apricot, Summer Fruit, Layered, Weight Watchers*	1 Pot/100g	46	0.1	46	5.4	5.8	0.1	0.2
Apricot, Tesco*	1 Pot/100g	77	3.0	77	6.5	6.0	3.0	1.3
Bakewell Tart Flavour, BGTY, Sainsbury's*	1 Pot/100g	54	0.2	54	7.6	5.5	0.2	1.1
Banana, Organic, Yeo Valley*	1 Pot/90g	118	5.4	131	6.6	12.6	6.0	0.2
Black Cherry, Asda*	1 Pot/100g	113	5.0	113	4.1	13.0	5.0	0.0
Blackberry, Berry Fruits, Layered, Weight Watchers*	1 Pot/100g	49	0.2	49	5.5	5.7	0.2	0.4
Blackcurrant, GFY, Asda*	1 Pot/100g	43	0.2	43	6.0	4.2	0.2	0.0
Cherries & Chocolate, Finest, Tesco*	1 Serving/165g	299	14.5	181	5.4	20.1	8.8	0.7
Cherry, 0% Fat, Vitalinea, Danone*	1 Serving/150g	88	0.2	59	6.1	8.0	0.2	1.6
Fat Free, Average	***1 Pot/60g***	***35***	***0.1***	***58***	***7.7***	***6.8***	***0.2***	***0.0***
Forest Fruit, Layered, Weight Watchers*	1 Pot/100g	47	0.2	47	5.5	5.7	0.2	0.4
Fruit, Balanced Lifestyle, Aldi*	1 Pot/100g	52	0.2	52	5.4	7.1	0.2	0.7
Fruit on the Bottom, BFY, Morrisons*	1 Pot/100g	66	0.2	66	5.6	10.6	0.2	0.0
Kids, Yeo Valley*	1 Serving/90g	111	4.8	123	6.6	12.6	5.3	0.0
Lemon, Balanced Lifestyle, Aldi*	1 Serving/100g	52	0.3	52	5.6	6.6	0.3	0.6
Lemon Pie, Low Fat, Sainsbury's*	1 Pot/90g	108	2.4	120	6.7	17.3	2.7	0.2
Low Fat, Aldi*	1 Pot/100g	52	0.3	52	5.4	7.1	0.3	0.7
Mandarin & Orange, HL, Tesco*	1 Pot/100g	55	0.2	55	6.2	7.0	0.2	0.3
Morello Cherries, Perfectly Balanced, Waitrose*	½ Pot/250ml	260	4.8	104	2.5	19.1	1.9	1.8
Morrisons*	1 Serving/28g	17	0.0	59	9.8	4.8	0.0	0.0
Munch Bunch, Nestle*	1 Pot/42g	44	1.3	105	6.7	12.6	3.0	0.0
Natural, Creamy, Co-Op*	1 Pot/200g	204	14.6	102	6.1	2.9	7.3	0.0
Natural, GFY, Asda*	½ Pot/100g	52	0.3	52	7.3	5.0	0.3	0.0
Natural, HL, Tesco*	1 Serving/65g	30	0.1	46	7.8	3.3	0.2	0.0
Natural, Virtually Fat Free, French, Waitrose*	1 Tub/500g	260	1.5	52	7.3	5.0	0.3	0.0
Normandy, LC, Tesco*	1 Serving/100g	46	0.2	46	7.8	3.3	0.2	0.0
Normandy, Sainsbury's*	1 Serving/25g	29	2.0	116	7.7	3.4	8.1	0.0

	Measure	per Measure		Nutrition Values per 100g / 100ml				
	INFO/WEIGHT	KCAL	FAT	KCAL	PROT	CARB	FAT	FIBRE
FROMAGE FRAIS								
Organic, Vrai*	1 Serving/100g	83	3.6	83	8.1	4.5	3.6	0.0
Peach, BGTY, Sainsbury's*	1 Pot/100g	53	0.2	53	7.2	5.5	0.2	0.5
Peach, Summer Fruit, Layered, Weight Watchers*	1 Pot/100g	46	0.1	46	5.0	8.0	0.1	0.0
Petit Dessert, Co-Op*	1 Pot/60g	74	2.6	123	6.3	14.5	4.4	0.0
Pineapple & Passion Fruit, HL, Tesco*	1 Pot/100g	55	0.2	55	6.2	7.1	0.2	0.1
Plain, Average	***1oz/28g***	***32***	***2.0***	***113***	***6.8***	***5.7***	***7.1***	***0.0***
Raspberry, Berry Fruits, Layered, Weight Watchers*	1 Pot/100g	47	0.2	47	5.5	5.7	0.2	0.4
Raspberry, COU, M & S*	1 Pot/100g	60	0.2	60	7.0	8.1	0.2	0.5
Raspberry, GFY, Asda*	1 Pot/100g	43	0.2	43	6.0	4.2	0.2	0.0
Raspberry, Healthy Choice, Asda*	1 Pot/100g	41	0.2	41	6.0	3.8	0.2	0.0
Raspberry, Little Stars, Muller*	1 Pot/60g	66	2.4	110	5.0	12.7	4.0	0.4
Raspberry, Low Fat, Sainsbury's*	1 Pot/90g	96	2.3	107	5.8	15.1	2.6	0.1
Raspberry, Organic, Yeo Valley*	1 Pot/100g	127	6.5	127	6.1	11.1	6.5	0.4
Raspberry & Redcurrant, BGTY, Sainsbury's*	1 Pot/100g	51	0.1	51	7.4	5.4	0.1	1.6
Real Fruit, Tesco*	1 Pot/100g	54	0.1	54	5.6	7.6	0.1	0.1
Red Cherry, Tesco*	1 Pot/100g	75	3.0	75	6.5	5.5	3.0	2.3
Rhubarb & Crumble, Low Fat, Sainsbury's*	1 Pot/90g	96	2.3	107	6.7	14.1	2.6	0.4
Strawberry, 0% Fat, Vitalinea, Danone*	1 Serving/150g	82	0.2	55	6.0	7.4	0.2	1.6
Strawberry, 99.9% Fat Free, Onken*	1 Serving/50g	46	0.0	91	6.9	15.3	0.1	0.0
Strawberry, Balanced Lifestyle, Aldi*	1 Serving/100g	52	0.2	52	5.4	7.1	0.2	0.7
Strawberry, COU, M & S*	1 Pot/100g	60	0.2	60	6.5	8.0	0.2	0.5
Strawberry, GFY, Asda*	1 Pot/100g	58	0.2	58	6.0	8.0	0.2	0.0
Strawberry, Langley Farm*	1 Pot/125g	189	9.8	151	7.0	13.3	7.8	0.0
Strawberry, Low Fat, St Ivel*	1 Pot/100g	69	1.2	69	6.9	6.8	1.2	0.0
Strawberry, Organic, Yeo Valley*	1 Pot/90g	116	5.4	129	6.3	12.5	6.0	0.2
Strawberry, Petits Filous, Yoplait*	1 Pot/50g	52	1.4	104	6.7	12.6	2.9	0.2
Strawberry, Tesco*	1 Pot/100g	75	3.0	75	6.5	5.5	3.0	2.5
Strawberry, Thomas the Tank Engine, Yoplait*	1 Pot/50g	50	0.6	101	6.8	15.4	1.3	0.0
Strawberry & Raspberry, Organic, Yeo Valley*	1 Pot/90g	118	5.4	131	6.3	12.9	6.0	0.2
Strawberry Tart, Sainsbury's*	1 Pot/100g	54	0.2	54	7.6	5.5	0.2	1.1
Toffee & Pecan Pie, Smooth & Creamy, Tesco*	1 Pot/100g	148	6.8	148	6.9	14.8	6.8	0.2
Tropical Fruit, COU, M & S*	1 Pot/100g	60	0.2	60	6.5	8.4	0.2	0.5
Vanilla, Danone*	1 Serving/200g	274	8.2	137	5.3	19.6	4.1	0.0
Virtually Fat Free, Tesco*	1 Pot/100g	56	0.1	56	5.6	8.2	0.1	0.0
FROZEN YOGHURT								
Angelmoo, Yoomoo*	1 Serving/100g	162	2.7	162	3.9	28.7	2.7	3.8
Black Cherry, M & S*	1 Pot/125g	164	1.4	131	3.1	27.1	1.1	0.5
Blood Orange, Pinkberry*	1 Small Pot/140g	154	0.0	110	3.0	23.0	0.0	0.0
Cherry Garcia, Low Fat, Ben & Jerry's*	1 Serving/100g	143	2.4	143	3.0	26.0	2.4	1.0
Chocmoo, Yoomoo*	1 Serving/100g	142	1.7	142	3.5	26.0	1.7	4.1
Chocolate, Average	1 Portion/100g	120	1.9	120	4.3	22.0	1.9	2.1
Chocolate, Pinkberry*	1 Small Pot/140g	168	2.1	120	5.0	23.0	1.5	2.0
Chocolate, Snog*	1 Serving/100g	109	1.6	109	4.5	19.9	1.6	1.7
Chocolate Fudge Brownie, Low Fat, Ben & Jerry's*	1 Serving/100g	180	3.0	180	4.0	34.0	3.0	1.5
Coconut, Pinkberry*	1 Small Pot/140g	196	0.0	140	4.0	30.0	0.0	0.0
Devilmoo, Yoomoo*	1 Serving/100g	167	2.6	167	3.6	30.4	2.6	3.8
Frae*	1 Small/83ml	56	0.0	67	2.4	12.0	0.0	0.0
Green Tea, Pinkberry*	1 Small Pot/100g	110	0.0	110	4.0	25.0	0.0	0.0
Lychee, Pinkberry*	1 Small Pot/140g	154	0.0	110	3.0	23.0	0.0	0.0
Mango, Pinkberry*	1 Small Cup/140g	140	0.0	100	3.0	23.0	0.0	0.0
Nakedmoo, Yoomoo*	1 Serving/125g	168	2.0	134	3.3	24.5	1.6	4.1
Natural, Average	1 Portion/100g	101	0.8	101	3.8	19.9	0.8	0.9
Natural, Snog*	1 Serving/100g	89	0.2	89	3.3	18.4	0.2	0.5

F

	Measure INFO/WEIGHT	per Measure KCAL	FAT	Nutrition Values per 100g / 100ml KCAL	PROT	CARB	FAT	FIBRE
FROZEN YOGHURT								
Original, Pinkberry*	1 Small Pot/140g	140	0.0	100	3.0	21.0	0.0	0.0
Passionfruit, Pinkberry*	1 Small Pot/140g	140	0.0	100	3.0	22.0	0.0	0.0
Peppermint, Pinkberry*	1 Small Pot/140g	154	0.0	110	4.0	24.0	0.0	0.0
Phish Food, Lower Fat, Ben & Jerry's*	½ Pot/211g	464	10.6	220	4.0	40.0	5.0	1.5
Pomegranate, Pinkberry*	1 Small Pot/140g	168	0.0	120	3.0	26.0	0.0	0.0
Pumpkin, Pinkberry*	1 Small Pot/140g	154	0.0	110	3.0	23.0	0.0	0.0
Raspberry, Handmade Farmhouse, Sainsbury's*	1 Serving/100g	132	3.8	132	2.7	21.8	3.8	2.2
Raspberry, Orchard Maid*	1 Serving/80ml	89	1.7	111	2.8	19.9	2.1	0.0
Salted Caramel, Pinkberry*	1 Small Pot/140g	168	0.0	120	4.0	26.0	0.0	0.0
Strawberry, Average	1 Portion/100g	114	2.2	114	2.6	21.2	2.2	0.5
Strawberry Cheesecake, Low Fat, Ben & Jerry's*	1 Serving/100g	170	3.0	170	4.0	31.0	3.0	1.0
Strawbmoo, Yoomoo*	1 Serving/100g	133	1.5	133	3.2	24.7	1.5	4.1
Tropicoolmoo, Yoomoo*	1 Pot/92g	134	1.2	146	2.9	28.9	1.3	3.6
Vanilla, Less Than 5% Fat, Tesco*	1 Pot/120g	179	2.9	149	8.1	23.8	2.4	0.7
Vanilla Bean & Honey, Yog*	1 Serving/100g	93	1.9	93	3.1	14.3	1.9	0.5
Watermelon, Pinkberry*	1 Small Pot/140g	140	0.0	100	3.0	22.0	0.0	0.0
FRUIT								
Apple, Pineapple & Grape, Ready to Eat, Sainsbury's*	1 Pack/180g	94	0.2	52	0.5	8.3	0.1	1.3
Apple & Pear, Snack Pack, Great Stuff, Asda*	1 Pack/80g	42	0.1	52	0.4	11.0	0.1	2.6
Baked, Nibbles, Cherry Berry, We Are Bear*	1 Packet/30g	87	0.0	290	1.2	76.0	0.2	10.3
Baked, Nibbles, Mango Pineapple, We Are Bear*	1 Bag/30g	85	0.0	285	1.4	73.0	0.2	11.0
Bananito, Fresh, Raw, Tesco*	1 Fruit/40g	38	0.1	95	1.2	23.2	0.3	1.1
Berry Medley, Freshly Prepared, M & S*	1 Pack/180g	90	0.4	50	0.7	10.9	0.2	2.9
Bites, Raspberry, Mini, HL, Tesco*	1 Bag/25g	88	0.7	350	4.5	76.8	2.7	4.4
Black Forest, Frozen, Tesco*	1 Serving/80g	37	0.0	46	0.8	10.5	0.0	1.8
Cempedak	1 Serving/100g	116	0.4	116	3.0	28.6	0.4	0.0
Citrus Selection, Fresh, Sainsbury's*	1 Pack/240g	79	0.2	33	0.9	7.1	0.1	1.6
Deluxe, Fresh, Rindless, Shapers, Boots*	1 Pack/168g	64	0.3	38	0.7	8.3	0.2	0.7
Exotic, M & S*	1 Pack/425g	212	1.3	50	0.7	11.8	0.3	0.0
Exotic Fruit Frenzy, Freshly Prepared, Tesco*	1 Pack/300g	132	0.6	44	0.6	9.8	0.2	1.6
Fabulous Fruity Fingers, Melon & Mango, M & S*	1 Pack/240g	96	0.5	40	0.6	8.2	0.2	1.0
Fingers, Melon & Pineapple, Sainsbury's*	1 Pack/240g	74	0.2	31	0.5	6.5	0.1	0.8
Fingers, Sun-Maid*	1 Pack/50g	162	2.2	325	3.5	68.3	4.3	4.3
Frozen, Garden, M & S*	1 Serving/30g	8	0.1	25	0.7	4.6	0.2	1.8
Grape, Sweet, Snack, Shapers, Boots*	1 Pack/80g	53	0.1	66	0.4	15.0	0.1	1.0
Grapefruit & Orange Segments, Breakfast, Del Monte*	1 Can/411g	193	0.4	47	1.0	10.2	0.1	1.0
Melon, Kiwi, & Strawberry, Fully Prepared, Sainsbury's*	1 Pack/245g	74	0.5	30	0.8	6.3	0.2	1.3
Melon, Kiwi Fruit & Strawberries, Fresh Tastes, Asda*	1 Pack/240g	96	0.5	40	0.8	7.7	0.2	2.1
Melon & Grape, Munchies, Eat Well, M & S*	½ Pack/200g	70	0.2	35	0.5	8.3	0.1	0.7
Melon & Grape, Pot, Co-Op*	1 Pot/125g	44	0.1	35	0.6	7.0	0.1	0.9
Melon & Grape, Sainsbury's*	½ Pack/200g	66	0.2	33	0.5	7.1	0.1	0.7
Melon & Grapes, Morrisons*	1 Pack/360g	112	0.4	31	0.6	6.4	0.1	0.8
Mix for Pie or Crumble, Frozen, Sainsbury's*	1 Pack/400g	128	0.8	32	0.8	5.7	0.2	2.1
Mixed, Fresh, 5 a Day, Tesco*	1 Pack/400g	136	0.8	34	0.8	7.4	0.2	1.4
Mixed, Fresh, Tesco*	1 Pack/200g	70	0.4	35	0.8	7.4	0.2	1.4
Mixed, Fruitime, Pieces, Tesco*	1 Can/140g	84	0.0	60	0.4	14.0	0.0	1.0
Mixed, in Fruit Juice, Pieces, Fruitini, Del Monte*	1 Serving/120g	61	0.1	51	0.4	12.0	0.1	0.5
Mixed, Pieces, in Orange Jelly, Fruitini, Del Monte*	1 Can/140g	94	0.1	67	0.3	15.8	0.1	0.0
Mixed, Tropical, Fruit Express, Del Monte*	1 Pot/185g	89	0.2	48	0.2	11.2	0.1	1.2
Mixed, Vine, Crazy Jack*	1 Serving/10g	31	0.0	309	2.8	74.0	0.3	4.7
Mount Pleasant, Graze*	1 Pack/21g	87	5.1	415	2.5	46.9	24.2	9.2
Pineapple, Grape & Kiwi, Asda*	1 Serving/200g	98	0.6	49	0.6	11.0	0.3	1.7
Pineapple, Grape & Kiwi, Fresh Tastes, Asda*	1 Pack/200g	106	0.6	53	0.6	11.0	0.3	1.8

F

	Measure INFO/WEIGHT	per Measure KCAL	FAT	Nutrition Values per 100g / 100ml KCAL	PROT	CARB	FAT	FIBRE
FRUIT								
Pineapple, Mango & Nectarine, Fresh Tastes, Asda*	1 Pack/240g	127	0.5	53	0.8	11.0	0.2	2.1
Pineapple & Mango Tango, Eat Well, M & S*	1 Pack/200g	100	0.8	50	1.0	22.2	0.4	2.6
Rolls, Peach, Yo Yo, Bear*	1 Roll/10g	28	0.0	275	1.4	72.0	0.2	10.0
Snack Pack, Fresh, Sainsbury's*	1 Serving/120g	54	0.1	45	0.1	11.0	0.1	1.3
Strawberries, Apple & Grapes, Fresh Tastes, Asda*	1 Pot/190g	91	0.2	48	0.5	10.6	0.1	0.0
Strawberries, Coconut & Chocolate, Pret a Manger*	1 Serving/125g	194	15.8	155	2.0	8.2	12.6	4.6
Summer Berries, M & S*	1 Pack/160g	80	0.3	50	0.7	10.0	0.2	3.0
to Go, Del Monte*	1 Can/113g	80	0.0	71	0.0	17.7	0.0	0.0
Topper, Frozen, Sainsbury's*	1 Bag/400g	168	0.4	42	0.7	8.8	0.1	1.5
Tropical, in Juice, Dole*	1 Pot/113g	59	0.0	52	0.3	14.2	0.0	1.8
Tropical, Tesco*	1 Pack/180g	85	0.4	47	0.6	10.8	0.2	1.9
Tropical Shaker, with Coulis, Morrisons*	1 Pot/250g	168	1.0	67	0.8	14.6	0.4	0.9
Tutti Frutti Collection, Freshly Prepared, Tesco*	1 Pack/200g	86	0.4	43	0.6	9.1	0.2	1.4
FRUIT & NUT MIX								
After Dinner Mint, Graze*	1 Pack/42g	203	12.2	483	10.0	42.0	29.0	7.0
Almond, Raisin & Berry, Sainsbury's*	1 Bag/50g	188	7.2	377	6.1	57.6	14.3	4.2
Almonds & Raisins, Love Life, Waitrose*	1 Pack/150g	681	42.6	454	11.6	38.1	28.4	4.7
Bakewell Tart, Graze*	1 Pack/37g	154	8.1	416	8.9	48.3	21.8	4.7
Banana Split, Graze*	1 Punnet/36g	145	7.2	402	9.0	50.0	20.0	5.0
Banoffee Pie, Graze*	1 Punnet/34g	149	9.2	438	7.0	42.0	27.0	5.0
Billionaire's Shortbread, Graze*	1 Punnet/41g	192	10.2	469	8.0	53.0	25.0	5.0
Bounty Hunter, Graze*	1 Punnet/31g	147	8.3	474	4.0	54.4	26.8	5.6
Cacao Vine, Graze*	1 Punnet/45g	187	9.4	416	8.5	51.4	20.8	0.0
Cheeky Monkey, Graze*	1 Punnet/30g	130	6.4	435	6.4	54.7	21.2	0.0
Cherish, Graze*	1 Punnet/40g	148	9.3	369	4.4	35.8	23.2	6.6
Cherries, Raisins & Nuts, Love Life, Waitrose*	1 Serving/30g	132	7.5	439	7.7	45.8	25.0	3.4
Cinnamon & Prailine, Christmas, Finest, Tesco*	¼ Pot/106g	470	26.7	442	8.2	45.9	25.1	11.5
Date & Banana Loaf, Graze*	1 Punnet/41g	132	1.8	327	3.3	68.3	4.4	6.3
Dried, Bear Necessities, Graze*	1 Pack/35g	126	8.1	361	4.6	34.9	23.2	6.5
Dried, Selection, Wholesome, Love Life, Waitrose*	1 Serving/30g	144	9.6	479	9.8	38.0	32.0	4.4
Eleanor's Apple Crumble, Graze*	1 Pack/32g	115	4.0	356	6.4	62.0	12.5	8.0
Eton Mess, Graze*	1 Punnet/33g	140	4.6	420	5.4	67.5	13.9	4.5
Exotic, Waitrose*	1 Serving/50g	207	8.8	414	9.0	54.6	17.7	4.6
Fajita, Graze*	1 Box/55g	255	17.0	463	15.1	38.0	30.9	0.0
Flapjack, Fruit & Seed, Graze*	1 Punnet/53g	226	11.1	426	6.0	54.0	21.0	5.0
Fruit & Nut Case, Graze*	1 Punnet/40g	168	8.8	420	5.8	52.1	22.1	2.9
Fruit Squash, Graze*	1 Pack/41g	183	9.7	451	13.4	47.5	23.8	6.4
Fruitabulous, You Are What You Eat*	1 Bag/40g	155	7.8	388	7.2	46.0	19.5	5.5
Grandma's Apple Crumble, Graze*	1 Punnet/40g	154	7.8	385	0.0	48.9	19.6	4.0
Hazelnut Espresso, Natural Treats, Graze*	1 Punnet/39g	191	12.3	490	8.4	42.9	31.6	4.2
Himalayas & Beyond, Graze*	1 Pack/30g	140	9.2	465	5.0	44.1	30.7	6.7
Honeycomb Crunch, Graze*	1 Punnet/40g	181	9.7	446	9.0	50.0	24.0	4.0
Jaffa Cake, Graze*	1 Punnet/44g	208	13.7	472	7.0	43.0	31.0	6.0
Jam Doughnut, Graze*	1 Punnet/31g	131	4.7	422	7.0	65.0	15.0	6.0
Johnny Come Lately, Graze*	1 Pack/65g	262	14.8	403	10.0	41.4	22.8	0.0
Jungle Fever, Graze*	1 Pack/30g	135	8.3	449	7.4	42.3	27.8	6.8
Jungle Trekker, Kids, Graze*	1 Punnet/32g	137	5.8	427	10.0	56.0	18.0	5.0
Lemon Meringue Pie, Graze*	1 Punnet/45g	177	6.0	393	5.0	66.3	13.4	2.0
Limoncello, Graze*	1 Punnet/41g	162	8.4	396	6.3	50.6	20.6	4.3
Lost, Coconut, Banana & Raisins, Graze*	1 Punnet/30g	115	5.8	382	3.5	51.0	19.2	5.8
Luxury, Asda*	1 Serving/50g	226	15.2	451	9.0	33.5	30.5	7.4
M & S*	1 Pack/75g	338	19.0	450	12.4	44.3	25.3	6.0
Macadamias & Dried Cranberries, Love Life, Waitrose*	1 Serving/30g	143	9.2	477	3.3	47.1	30.8	6.2

F

	Measure INFO/WEIGHT	per Measure KCAL	FAT	Nutrition Values per 100g / 100ml KCAL	PROT	CARB	FAT	FIBRE
FRUIT & NUT MIX								
Marvellous Macaroon, Graze*	1 Punnet/28g	157	10.9	562	11.0	41.0	39.0	6.0
Mayan Mocha, Graze*	1 Punnet/40g	185	11.1	462	10.4	46.4	27.8	6.0
New World, Graze*	1 Serving/50g	206	11.7	413	16.8	45.2	23.4	0.0
Nuts & Raisins, Mixed, Natural, Love Life, Waitrose*	1 Serving/50g	258	16.4	515	16.5	38.4	32.8	7.2
Ooh La La, Graze*	1 Punnet/45g	181	7.2	402	5.0	63.6	15.9	1.0
Organic, Love Life, Waitrose*	1 Serving/30g	115	6.1	383	9.8	40.4	20.2	5.8
Organic, Waitrose*	1 Pack/100g	489	32.6	489	15.0	33.8	32.6	5.4
Papaya & Cranberry, Sainsbury's*	1 Serving/75g	300	11.0	400	4.1	63.1	14.6	7.3
Peanuts, Cashews & Mango, Fair Trade, Tesco*	1/6 Pack25g	130	8.7	520	16.4	33.2	34.8	4.8
Peanuts & Flame Raisins, Wholefoods, Tesco*	1 Serving/30g	142	8.3	475	18.6	34.7	27.8	4.5
Pure Vitality, Graze*	1 Punnet/45g	151	6.4	337	11.2	46.0	14.3	9.5
Seed, Nut & Sultana Sprinkle, Love Life, Waitrose*	1 Serving/30g	177	15.4	591	17.2	15.4	51.2	4.3
Shangri-la, Graze*	1 Punnet/29g	132	8.3	454	15.7	38.2	28.5	8.5
Strawberry Milkshake, Graze*	1 Pack/39g	148	3.9	380	2.0	72.0	10.0	2.0
Sun Dance, Graze*	1 Punnet/38g	136	3.8	358	4.3	67.2	9.9	4.5
Swallows & Amazons, Graze*	1 Pack/60g	252	11.8	420	6.3	56.3	19.7	0.0
The Mix, Whitworths*	1 Pot/90g	341	13.1	379	4.1	63.1	14.6	7.3
The Waldorf, Graze*	1 Punnet/28g	109	6.2	389	6.0	43.5	22.1	5.7
Trail Mix, Average	1oz/28g	121	8.0	432	9.1	37.2	28.5	4.3
Trail Mix, Classic, Penn State*	1 Serving/30g	160	10.7	533	17.0	33.0	35.7	5.3
Trail Mix, Love Life, Waitrose*	1 Portion/30g	126	9.3	506	14.2	28.5	37.2	6.3
Tropical Praline, Graze*	1 Punnet/35g	121	4.2	347	4.2	59.2	12.1	2.0
Unsalted, Tesco*	1 Serving/25g	112	4.6	449	12.6	58.1	18.5	12.2
Vanilla, Cherry, Frangipane, Graze*	1 Punnet/39g	201	13.2	516	15.0	38.0	34.0	6.0
Walnut & Vanilla Truffle, Graze*	1 Punnet/38g	187	12.1	496	10.0	43.9	32.2	6.0
Walnut Whip, Graze*	1 Pack/38g	187	12.2	495	10.0	43.9	32.2	6.0
White Chocolate & Raspberry Cheesecake, Graze*	1 Punnet/39g	204	13.7	524	7.5	44.7	35.1	4.5
Ying & Yang, Graze*	1 Pack/60g	296	19.5	493	6.8	41.2	32.5	0.0
FRUIT COCKTAIL								
Fresh, Morrisons*	1oz/28g	12	0.1	44	0.6	11.3	0.2	1.0
Fresh & Ready, Sainsbury's*	1 Pack/300g	117	0.3	39	0.6	9.0	0.1	1.2
in Apple Juice, Asda*	1/3 Can/80g	40	0.1	50	0.3	12.0	0.1	1.6
in Fruit Juice, Heinz*	1 Pot/125g	78	0.0	62	0.5	15.0	0.0	1.0
in Fruit Juice, Morrisons*	1 Can/140g	64	0.0	46	0.4	11.0	0.0	0.0
in Fruit Juice, Sainsbury's*	1 Serving/198g	97	0.2	49	0.3	11.9	0.1	1.3
in Fruit Juice, Waitrose*	1 Can/142g	71	0.0	50	0.4	12.0	0.0	1.0
in Grape Juice, Tesco*	1oz/28g	12	0.0	43	0.4	10.0	0.0	1.0
in Juice, Del Monte*	1 Can/415g	203	0.4	49	0.4	11.2	0.1	0.0
in Light Syrup, Princes*	1 Serving/206g	64	0.0	31	0.4	7.3	0.0	1.0
in Light Syrup, Sainsbury's*	½ Can/125g	72	0.1	58	0.4	14.0	0.1	1.3
in Light Syrup, Valfrutta*	1 Serving/206g	95	0.0	46	0.2	11.4	0.0	1.5
in Syrup, Del Monte*	1 Can/420g	315	0.4	75	0.4	18.0	0.1	0.0
in Syrup, Morrisons*	½ Can/205g	129	0.2	63	0.3	14.9	0.1	0.0
in Syrup, Smart Price, Asda*	1 Can/411g	173	0.4	42	0.3	10.0	0.1	1.6
in Syrup, Tesco*	1 Serving/135g	85	0.0	63	0.4	15.0	0.0	1.0
in Very Light Syrup, Value, Tesco*	1 Can/410g	123	0.0	30	0.4	7.3	0.0	1.0
No Added Sugar, Asda*	1 Serving/134g	67	0.1	50	0.3	12.0	0.1	1.6
Tropical, Asda*	½ Can/135g	81	0.0	60	0.0	15.0	0.0	1.6
Tropical, Canned, Asda*	½ Can/200g	120	0.0	60	0.0	15.0	0.0	1.6
Tropical, Heinz*	1 Pot/113g	61	0.0	54	0.5	13.0	0.0	1.0
Tropical, in Juice, Morrisons*	1 Serving/100g	56	0.0	56	0.0	14.0	0.0	0.0
Tropical, in Syrup, Sainsbury's*	½ Can/130g	95	0.1	73	0.5	17.6	0.1	1.4

	Measure INFO/WEIGHT	per Measure KCAL	FAT	Nutrition Values per 100g / 100ml KCAL	PROT	CARB	FAT	FIBRE
FRUIT GUMS								
Fruit Salad, Tesco*	6 Sweets/30g	100	0.2	335	8.3	73.4	0.5	0.3
No Added Sugar, Boots*	1 Sweet/2g	1	0.0	88	0.0	22.0	0.0	0.0
Rowntree's*	1 Tube/49g	170	0.1	344	4.8	81.3	0.2	0.0
Sugar Free, Sainsbury's*	1 Serving/30g	63	0.1	209	7.7	71.3	0.2	0.1
FRUIT MIX								
Apple Cosmo, Graze*	1 Punnet/34g	100	0.2	292	1.5	69.8	0.7	4.6
Apple Strudel, Graze*	1 Punnet/55g	172	0.4	312	2.6	63.5	0.7	0.0
Apricot, Torte, Graze*	1 Punnet/45g	151	3.6	335	3.3	63.0	8.0	4.0
Banana, Coconut & Mango, Dried, Graze*	1 Punnet/45g	144	3.7	320	18.7	57.1	8.2	0.0
Berry, Sainsbury's*	1 Serving/20g	64	0.4	319	1.0	78.1	1.9	5.5
Caribbean, Dried, Graze*	1 Punnet/50g	187	6.4	374	1.2	67.6	12.8	0.0
Cherish, Graze*	1 Punnet/50g	222	10.0	443	5.2	52.5	20.0	0.0
Date To Remember, Graze*	1 Punnet/40g	131	1.8	327	3.3	68.3	4.4	6.3
Fig & Cherry Fruit Bake, Graze*	1 Punnet/44g	116	0.4	263	2.9	64.6	0.9	7.6
Fig Roll, Graze*	1 Punnet/35g	110	0.6	313	1.6	23.1	1.7	2.0
Forest Fruit, Dried, Graze*	1 Punnet/50g	160	0.4	319	1.8	76.0	0.8	0.0
Frozen, Blueberries & Strawberries, Sainsbury's*	1 Serving/75g	26	0.2	34	0.7	6.5	0.2	1.5
Go Goji Go Go Go, Graze*	1 Punnet/40g	112	0.3	279	2.2	69.0	0.8	0.0
Golden Pineapple Rings, Graze*	1 Punnet/20g	53	0.1	263	0.6	72.0	0.6	8.1
Italian Stallion, Graze*	1 Punnet/40g	118	0.4	296	1.7	71.0	0.9	2.6
Loco in Acapulco, Graze*	1 Punnet/30g	123	6.4	410	4.0	53.2	21.4	0.0
Love Mix, Graze*	1 Punnet/40g	99	0.4	245	4.0	58.0	0.9	5.9
Luxury, Sainsbury's*	1 Serving/30g	78	0.2	261	1.8	62.3	0.5	2.7
Mango & Cranberry, WTF, Sainsbury's*	1 Serving/50g	166	0.4	331	1.8	79.4	0.7	4.8
Melon, Strawberry & Grape, Sainsbury's*	1 Pack/180g	58	0.4	32	0.5	7.0	0.2	0.4
Nectarine, Raspberry & Blueberry, Seasonal, M & S*	1 Pack/160g	72	0.3	45	1.3	8.3	0.2	2.7
Pineapple, Kiwi, Mango & Blueberry, Waitrose*	1 Pack/330g	208	1.0	63	0.7	14.5	0.3	1.9
Pineapple, Melon, Mango, Tesco*	1 Pack/440g	242	0.9	55	1.1	11.4	0.2	1.3
Pumpkin Pie, Graze*	1 Punnet/65g	274	11.2	422	11.4	48.2	17.2	0.0
Raisins & Apricots, Great Stuff, Asda*	1 Pack/40g	112	0.1	281	2.6	66.9	0.3	6.0
Rocky Mountain, Graze*	1 Punnet/50g	264	19.3	529	3.2	38.2	38.6	0.0
Scandi Berries, Graze*	1 Punnet/23g	61	0.1	270	1.6	65.3	0.6	6.6
Sour Mango Tangtastic, Graze*	1 Punnet/34g	110	0.2	323	1.3	79.8	0.6	2.0
Strawberries & Cream, Graze*	1 Punnet/70g	303	11.4	433	3.7	66.9	16.3	0.0
Strawberry Fields Forever, Graze*	1 Punnet/40g	117	0.4	292	1.9	70.9	0.9	2.5
Summer Fruits, British, Frozen, Waitrose*	1 Pack/380g	99	0.8	26	1.0	5.2	0.2	5.5
Summer Pudding, Graze*	1 Punnet/32g	109	0.4	342	1.6	81.2	1.2	4.2
Super Dried, Graze*	1 Punnet/55g	176	0.9	320	5.6	76.4	1.6	0.0
Super Wholefood with Blueberries & Mango, M & S*	1 Pack/215g	260	7.7	121	4.4	17.0	3.6	8.7
Tropical, Fresh, Waitrose*	1 Pack/240g	122	0.5	51	0.6	11.6	0.2	1.9
Tutti Frutti, Graze*	1 Punnet/41g	120	0.4	292	1.9	72.3	0.9	4.0
FRUIT SALAD								
Apple, Orange, Pineapple & Grape, Morrisons*	1 Serving/64g	40	0.1	62	0.8	13.1	0.1	2.6
Apple, Pineapple & Grape, Sweet & Tangy, Sainsbury's*	1 Pack/180g	70	0.2	39	0.5	8.3	0.1	1.3
Autumn, Fresh, M & S*	½ Pack/160g	64	0.2	40	0.7	9.4	0.1	2.9
Berry, Asda*	1 Pack/250g	122	0.2	49	0.6	10.9	0.1	0.0
Berry, Seasonal, Asda*	1 Pack/300g	93	0.3	31	0.6	7.0	0.1	2.1
Chunky, in Fruit Juice, Canned, John West*	1 Can/411g	193	0.8	47	0.4	11.0	0.2	0.8
Citrus, Asda*	1 Serving/265g	88	0.3	33	0.9	7.2	0.1	1.5
Citrus, Fresh, M & S*	½ Pack/225g	79	0.2	35	0.9	7.7	0.1	1.5
Classic, Co-Op*	1 Box/285g	142	0.3	50	0.6	11.0	0.1	2.3
Classic, Fresh, Prepared, Sainsbury's*	1 Pack/320g	157	0.3	49	0.6	10.3	0.1	2.0
Classic, Shapers, Boots*	1 Pack/200g	75	0.2	38	0.7	8.5	0.1	1.3

F

	Measure INFO/WEIGHT	per Measure KCAL	FAT	Nutrition Values per 100g / 100ml KCAL	PROT	CARB	FAT	FIBRE
FRUIT SALAD								
Dried, M & S*	½ Pack/125g	269	0.5	215	1.8	51.4	0.4	5.9
Exotic, Fresh, Tesco*	1 Serving/225g	86	0.4	38	0.7	8.4	0.2	1.5
Exotic, Fully Prepared, Sainsbury's*	1 Serving/200g	74	0.4	37	0.6	8.3	0.2	1.3
Exotic, Morrisons*	1 Serving/150g	78	0.3	52	0.6	12.2	0.2	0.0
Exotic, Waitrose*	1 Pack/300g	126	0.6	42	0.6	9.5	0.2	1.1
Exotic, with Melon, Mango, Kiwi Fruit & Grapes, Asda*	1 Pot/300g	141	0.9	47	0.6	10.5	0.3	1.4
Fresh, Budgens*	1 Pack/250g	105	0.2	42	0.7	9.6	0.1	1.3
Fresh, Morrisons*	1 Tub/350g	150	0.4	43	0.7	9.9	0.1	0.0
Fresh, Sweet, Ripe & Moist, Tesco*	1 Serving/750g	345	0.8	46	0.7	10.6	0.1	1.6
Fresh, Tesco*	1 Pack/200g	84	0.4	42	0.7	9.3	0.2	1.5
Fresh, Washed, Ready to Eat, Tesco*	1 Pack/200g	92	0.2	46	0.7	10.6	0.1	1.6
Fresh for You, Tesco*	1 Pack/160g	59	0.3	37	0.6	8.2	0.2	1.1
Freshly Prepared, M & S*	1 Pack/350g	140	0.7	40	0.5	9.3	0.2	1.0
Frozen, Basics, Sainsbury's*	1 Serving/100g	38	0.1	38	0.5	8.8	0.1	1.1
Fruit, Mediterranean Style, Shapers, Boots*	1 Pack/142g	61	0.1	43	0.6	10.0	0.1	1.5
Golden, Fresh, Asda*	1 Pot/147g	69	0.1	47	0.6	11.0	0.1	1.6
Grapefruit & Orange, Fresh, M & S*	1 Serving/250g	88	0.2	35	0.9	7.4	0.1	1.6
Green, M & S*	1 Pack/400g	200	0.8	50	0.6	10.9	0.2	1.2
Homemade, Unsweetened, Average	1 Serving/140g	77	0.1	55	0.7	13.8	0.1	1.5
Juicy Melon, Pineapple & Grapes, Asda*	1 Pot/300g	111	0.3	37	0.5	8.4	0.1	0.9
Kiwi, Pineapple & Grape, Fresh Tastes, Asda*	1 Pack/200g	106	0.6	53	0.6	11.0	0.3	1.8
Layered, Tropical Rainbow, Freshly Prepared, M & S*	1 Pack/375g	206	1.1	55	0.7	12.6	0.3	1.7
Luxury, Fresh, Tesco*	1 Serving/400g	164	0.8	41	0.7	9.2	0.2	1.6
Luxury, Frozen, Boylans*	1 Serving/100g	54	0.2	54	0.8	12.7	0.2	0.0
Luxury, Frozen, Tesco*	½ Pack/250g	115	0.2	46	0.7	10.7	0.1	1.3
Mango, Kiwi, Blueberry & Pomegranate, Fresh, M & S*	1 Pack/350g	210	1.0	60	0.9	13.4	0.3	2.4
Mediterranean Style, Budgens*	1 Serving/250g	95	0.5	38	0.6	8.5	0.2	0.8
Melon, Kiwi, Grapes & Pomegranate Seeds, Morrisons*	1 Pack/400g	152	1.2	38	0.7	8.2	0.3	1.2
Melon, Pineapple & Grapes, Fresh, Tesco*	1 Pack/300g	120	0.3	40	0.5	9.2	0.1	1.0
Melon & Mango, Shapers, Boots*	1 Pack/80g	29	0.1	36	0.6	7.8	0.1	1.2
Melon & Red Grape, Freshly Prepared, M & S*	1 Pack/450g	158	0.4	35	0.5	8.4	0.1	0.7
Mixed, Average	1 Bowl/100g	42	0.2	42	0.6	9.4	0.2	1.5
Oranges, Apple, Pineapple & Grapes, Fresh, Asda*	1 Pack/260g	120	0.3	46	0.6	10.5	0.1	2.1
Peaches & Pears, Fruit Express, Del Monte*	1 Serving/185g	87	0.2	47	0.4	10.8	0.1	0.9
Pineapple, Apple & Strawberries, Tesco*	1 Pack/190g	80	0.2	42	0.4	9.8	0.1	1.4
Pineapple, Mandarin & Grapefruit, Asda*	1 Serving/200g	86	0.2	43	0.6	10.0	0.1	0.0
Pineapple, Mango, Apple & Grape, Waitrose*	1 Pack/300g	186	0.6	62	0.5	14.7	0.2	1.7
Pineapple, Melon, Kiwi & Blueberry, Shapers, Boots*	1 Pack/179g	75	0.4	42	0.6	8.7	0.2	1.4
Plum, Blackberries, & Fig, Tesco*	1 Pot/260g	109	0.5	42	0.8	8.2	0.2	2.5
Radiant Rainbow, Layered, Eat Well, M & S*	1 Pack/350g	140	0.7	40	0.5	9.1	0.2	0.9
Rainbow, Asda*	1 Pack/350g	140	1.0	40	0.6	8.8	0.3	1.4
Rainbow Layers, Tesco*	1 Pack/270g	122	0.5	45	0.5	9.8	0.2	1.1
Seasonal, Fresh, Asda*	1 Pack/125g	55	0.1	44	0.5	10.4	0.1	1.2
Seasonal, M & S*	1 Serving/200g	100	0.4	50	0.5	11.8	0.2	2.1
Sharing, Fresh Tastes, Asda*	1 Pack/450g	220	0.9	49	0.4	10.4	0.2	0.0
Strawberry & Blueberry, Asda*	1 Pack/240g	86	0.2	36	0.9	7.0	0.1	1.5
Summer, Red, Fresh, M & S*	1 Pack/400g	160	0.8	40	0.0	10.0	0.2	1.2
Summer, Sainsbury's*	1 Pack/240g	84	0.5	35	0.7	7.8	0.2	1.3
Sunshine, Fresh, M & S*	1 Serving/200g	70	0.2	35	0.0	8.3	0.1	1.3
Tropical, Australian Gold*	1 Pot/130g	92	0.1	71	0.6	17.2	0.1	0.0
Tropical, Fresh, Asda*	1 Pack/400g	164	0.8	41	0.7	9.0	0.2	1.8
Tropical, Fruit Snacks, Frozen, Sainsbury's*	1 Serving/175g	79	0.2	45	0.7	10.4	0.1	1.6
Tropical, Tropical Harvest*	1 Serving/100g	52	0.0	52	0.3	12.8	0.0	1.4

	Measure INFO/WEIGHT	per Measure KCAL	FAT	Nutrition Values per 100g / 100ml KCAL	PROT	CARB	FAT	FIBRE
FRUIT SALAD								
Virgin Trains*	1 Serving/140g	56	0.1	40	0.4	10.0	0.1	0.8
Weight Watchers*	1 Serving/135g	50	0.1	37	0.2	9.0	0.1	0.7
FRUIT SHOOT								
Apple, Low Sugar, Robinson's*	1 Bottle/200ml	14	0.0	7	0.0	1.2	0.0	0.0
Apple & Blackcurrant, Robinson's*	1 Bottle/200ml	10	0.0	5	0.1	0.8	0.0	0.0
Hydro Orange & Pineapple, Spring Water, Robinson's*	1 Bottle/350ml	4	0.0	1	0.0	0.0	0.0	0.0
Orange, Pure, Robinson's*	1 Bottle/250ml	115	0.2	46	0.5	9.9	0.1	0.2
FRUIT SPREAD								
Apricot, Pure, Organic, Whole Earth*	1 Serving/20g	33	0.1	167	0.8	40.0	0.4	0.9
Blackcurrant, Carb Check, Heinz*	1 Tbsp/15g	8	0.0	54	0.5	12.8	0.1	2.7
Blackcurrant, Weight Watchers*	1 Tsp/6g	6	0.0	106	0.2	26.3	0.0	0.9
Cherries & Berries, Organic, Meridian Foods*	1 Tbsp/15g	16	0.0	109	0.5	26.0	0.3	1.1
High, Blueberry, St Dalfour*	1 Tsp/15g	34	0.0	228	0.5	56.0	0.2	2.2
Raspberry, Weight Watchers*	1 Tsp/6g	7	0.0	111	0.4	27.1	0.1	0.9
Raspberry & Cranberry, No Added Sugar, Superjam*	1 Spread/10g	22	0.0	216	2.1	47.0	0.3	0.0
Seville Orange, Weight Watchers*	1 Tsp/15g	17	0.0	111	0.2	27.5	0.0	0.3
Strawberry, Weight Watchers*	1 Tbsp/15g	23	0.0	156	0.7	39.8	0.1	1.8
FU YUNG								
Egg, Average	1oz/28g	67	5.8	239	9.9	2.2	20.6	1.3
FUDGE								
All Butter, Finest, Tesco*	1 Sweet/10g	43	1.4	429	1.3	73.4	14.5	0.0
Butter, Milk, Thorntons*	1 Sweet/13g	60	2.5	462	3.7	68.5	19.2	0.0
Cadbury*	1 Bar/25g	115	4.0	440	2.4	73.7	15.3	0.4
Cherry & Almond, Thorntons*	1 Bag/100g	464	19.1	464	3.2	70.5	19.1	0.4
Chocolate, Average	1 Sweet/30g	132	4.1	441	3.3	81.1	13.7	0.0
Chocolate, Thorntons*	1 Bag/100g	459	19.1	459	3.1	69.0	19.1	0.6
Chunks, for Baking	1 Serving/100g	428	12.2	428	1.7	77.2	12.2	0.6
Chunks, Mini, Sainsbury's*	1 Pack/100g	409	11.3	409	1.9	74.8	11.3	0.0
Clotted Cream, Sainsbury's*	1 Sweet/8g	35	0.9	430	1.9	81.5	10.7	0.7
Dairy, Co-Op*	1 Sweet/9g	39	1.2	430	2.0	76.0	13.0	0.0
Pure Indulgence, Thorntons*	1 Bar/45g	210	9.9	466	1.8	65.9	21.9	0.0
Vanilla, Bar, M & S*	1 Bar/43g	205	10.0	476	3.7	63.0	23.3	0.4
Vanilla, Diabetic, Bar, Thorntons*	1 Bar/34g	121	6.7	356	3.2	69.7	19.7	0.6
Vanilla, Thorntons*	1 Bag/100g	465	21.9	465	1.8	65.9	21.9	0.0
Vanilla, Whipped, M & S*	1 Serving/43g	210	10.3	490	3.8	65.4	23.9	0.3
FUSE								
Cadbury*	1 Bar/49g	238	12.2	485	7.6	58.2	24.8	0.0
FUSILLI								
Carb Check, Heinz*	1 Serving/75g	219	1.7	292	52.7	15.2	2.3	20.8
Chickpea, Dell'ugo*	1 Serving/100g	275	2.4	275	19.2	38.1	2.4	12.1
Cooked, Average	***1 Serving/210g***	***248***	***1.4***	***118***	***4.2***	***23.8***	***0.6***	***1.2***
Dry, Average	***1 Serving/90g***	***316***	***1.4***	***352***	***12.3***	***72.0***	***1.6***	***2.2***
Fresh, Cooked, Average	***1 Serving/200g***	***329***	***3.6***	***164***	***6.4***	***30.6***	***1.8***	***1.8***
Fresh, Uncooked, Average	***1 Serving/75g***	***208***	***2.0***	***277***	***10.9***	***53.4***	***2.7***	***2.1***
Tricolore, Dry, Average	***1 Serving/75g***	***264***	***1.3***	***351***	***12.2***	***71.8***	***1.7***	***2.7***
Twists, Quick Cook, Morrisons*	1 Serving/75g	265	1.5	353	12.0	72.0	2.0	3.1
Whole Wheat, Dry Weight, Average	***1 Serving/90g***	***290***	***2.1***	***322***	***13.1***	***62.3***	***2.3***	***9.0***
FYBOGEL								
Lemon, Reckitt Benckiser*	1 Serving/4g	4	0.0	95	2.4	11.3	1.1	64.8
Orange, Reckitt Benckiser*	1 Serving/4g	5	0.0	106	2.4	12.7	1.1	64.4

	Measure INFO/WEIGHT	per Measure KCAL	per Measure FAT	KCAL	PROT	CARB	FAT	FIBRE
				Nutrition Values per 100g / 100ml				
GALANGAL								
Raw, Root, Average	1 Serving/100g	71	0.6	71	1.2	15.3	0.6	2.4
GALAXY								
Amicelli, Mars*	1 Serving/13g	66	3.5	507	6.2	59.7	27.1	0.0
Bubbles Filled, Chocolate Egg, Galaxy, Mars*	1 Egg/28g	155	9.5	555	6.5	54.7	34.1	1.5
Caramel, Mars*	1 Bar/49g	254	13.0	518	5.8	64.2	26.4	0.0
Caramel Crunch, Promises, Mars*	1 Bar/100g	540	31.8	540	6.1	57.5	31.8	0.0
Cookie Crumble, Mars*	1 Bar/114g	627	37.6	550	6.2	56.0	33.0	1.9
Fruit & Hazelnut, Milk, Mars*	1 Bar/47g	235	13.2	501	7.1	55.2	28.0	0.0
Hazelnut, Mars*	1 Piece/6g	37	2.5	582	7.8	49.4	39.2	0.0
Hazelnut, Roast, Promises, Mars*	1 Bar/100g	544	32.9	544	6.4	55.6	32.9	0.0
Liaison, Mars*	1 Bar/48g	233	11.9	485	5.4	60.3	24.7	0.0
Swirls, Mars*	1 Bag/150g	747	39.8	498	4.9	60.2	26.5	0.0
GAMMON								
Breaded, Average	1oz/28g	34	0.9	120	22.5	1.0	3.0	0.0
Dry Cured, Ready to Roast, M & S*	½ Joint/255g	255	3.8	100	20.5	0.5	1.5	0.5
Honey & Mustard, Average	½ Pack/190g	294	13.5	155	19.1	3.6	7.1	0.1
Joint, Applewood Smoked, Tesco*	1 Serving/100g	152	9.0	152	17.5	0.2	9.0	0.0
Joint, Boiled, Average	***1 Serving/60g***	***122***	***7.4***	***204***	***23.3***	***0.0***	***12.3***	***0.0***
Joint, Raw, Average	***1 Serving/100g***	***138***	***7.5***	***138***	***17.5***	***0.0***	***7.5***	***0.0***
Joint, Unsmoked, Tesco*	2 Slices/150g	248	15.6	165	16.8	0.2	10.4	0.0
Joint, with Sweet Maple Syrup Glaze, As Sold, Waitrose*	1 Serving/100g	211	12.6	211	14.1	10.2	12.6	0.9
Steaks, Cooked, Average	***1 Steak/97g***	***157***	***7.1***	***161***	***23.3***	***0.4***	***7.4***	***0.0***
Steaks, Healthy Range, Average	***1 Serving/110g***	***107***	***3.5***	***97***	***18.0***	***0.4***	***3.2***	***0.2***
Steaks, Honey Roast, Average	***1 Steak/100g***	***142***	***5.3***	***142***	***21.5***	***2.3***	***5.3***	***0.0***
Steaks, Smoked, Average	***1 Steak/110g***	***150***	***5.5***	***137***	***22.7***	***0.1***	***5.0***	***0.1***
Unsmoked, Dry Cured, TTD, Sainsbury's*	1 Serving/100g	214	11.2	214	27.7	0.5	11.2	0.8
GAMMON &								
Parsley Sauce, Steak, Tesco*	½ Pack/140g	217	7.3	155	23.7	2.9	5.2	0.5
Pineapple, 228, Oakhouse Foods Ltd*	1 Meal/360g	284	4.0	79	7.1	10.9	1.1	1.7
Pineapple, Roast, Dinner, Iceland*	1 Pack/400g	360	6.4	90	6.2	12.7	1.6	1.7
GAMMON IN								
Cheddar Sauce, Creamy, Steaks, Fresh Tastes, Asda*	½ Pack/143g	270	14.4	189	19.1	5.4	10.1	1.5
GAMMON WITH								
Cheese Sauce & Crumb, Steaks, Simply Cook, Tesco*	½ Pack/156g	218	12.0	140	14.2	3.1	7.7	1.0
Egg & Fries, Steaks	1 Serving/540g	684	26.9	127	10.3	10.1	5.0	0.0
Pineapple, Steaks, Asda*	½ Pack/195g	254	2.7	130	17.8	11.5	1.4	0.7
GARAM MASALA								
Dry, Ground, Average	***1 Tbsp/15g***	***57***	***2.3***	***379***	***15.6***	***45.2***	***15.1***	***0.0***
GARLIC								
Crushed, Frozen, Taj*	1 Block/18g	18	0.1	102	7.5	14.0	0.6	4.0
Minced, Nishaan*	1 Tsp/5g	5	0.0	97	6.0	16.2	0.9	0.0
Pickled, Bevellini*	1 Serving/12g	5	0.0	42	2.5	0.8	0.1	0.0
Powder, Average	***1 Tsp/3g***	***7***	***0.0***	***246***	***18.7***	***42.7***	***1.2***	***9.9***
Raw, Average	***1 Clove/3g***	***3***	***0.0***	***98***	***7.9***	***16.3***	***0.6***	***2.1***
Spice Blend, Gourmet Garden*	1 Squeeze/10ml	32	2.4	210	4.5	10.8	16.2	10.3
Very Lazy, The English Provender Co.*	1 Tsp/3g	3	0.0	111	6.0	20.9	0.4	3.0
Wild	1 Clove/3g	1	0.0	23	2.8	1.7	0.6	1.9
GARLIC & GINGER								
Minced, Paste, Nishaan*	1 Tsp/5g	4	0.1	71	2.4	8.5	1.6	0.0
GARLIC PUREE								
Average	***1 Tbsp/18g***	***68***	***6.0***	***380***	***3.5***	***16.9***	***33.6***	***0.0***
in Vegetable Oil, GIA*	1 Tsp/5g	12	0.9	248	3.6	18.8	17.7	0.0

G

	Measure INFO/WEIGHT	per Measure KCAL	FAT	Nutrition Values per 100g / 100ml KCAL	PROT	CARB	FAT	FIBRE
GATEAU								
Au Fromage Blanc, Ligne Et Plaisir*	1 Serving/80g	128	2.1	160	8.0	26.0	2.6	0.0
Black Forest, 500g Size, Tesco*	1 Cake/500g	1125	55.0	225	4.0	27.1	11.0	1.8
Black Forest, Family Size, 860g, Tesco*	1 Cake/860g	1978	113.5	230	3.4	24.8	13.2	0.9
Black Forest, Mini, Tesco*	1 Serving/55g	136	5.1	247	5.7	35.3	9.2	1.0
Black Forest, Sara Lee*	1 Serving/80g	221	9.8	276	3.6	37.9	12.3	1.2
Blackforest, Sainsbury's*	1/8 Cake/63g	163	10.8	259	3.9	27.7	17.1	3.5
Chocolate, Asda*	1 Serving/100g	176	10.0	176	2.4	19.0	10.0	0.4
Chocolate, Double, Frozen, Tesco*	1/5 Gateau/70g	119	4.7	265	5.0	35.8	10.4	4.0
Chocolate, Double, Light, Sara Lee*	1/5 Cake/59g	139	2.7	237	5.7	43.3	4.6	2.0
Chocolate, Swirl, Tesco*	1 Serving/83g	230	13.3	277	3.8	29.3	16.0	0.2
Chocolate, Triple, Heinz*	¼ Cake/85g	209	9.5	245	5.1	31.2	11.1	2.4
Chocolate Layer, M & S*	1 Serving/86g	278	15.7	323	4.2	35.9	18.3	0.9
Chocolate Orange, Co-Op*	1 Serving/97g	320	17.5	330	5.0	37.0	18.0	1.0
Coffee, Tesco*	1 Serving/100g	300	17.0	300	4.2	32.5	17.0	0.6
Ice Cream, Chocolate & Vanilla, Iceland*	1 Serving/130g	252	12.2	194	3.3	24.1	9.4	0.6
Lemon & Lime, M & S*	1 Serving/100g	295	15.6	295	3.2	35.0	15.6	0.3
Orange & Lemon, Iceland*	1 Serving/90g	220	9.9	245	2.6	33.8	11.0	0.3
Strawberry, Co-Op*	1 Serving/77g	222	12.9	288	5.1	29.2	16.7	1.0
Strawberry, Double, Sara Lee*	1/8 Cake/199g	533	24.3	268	3.2	36.2	12.2	0.6
Strawberry, Frozen, Tesco*	1/5 Gateau/75g	155	6.3	205	2.8	28.8	8.3	0.9
GELATINE								
Average	***1 Tsp/3g***	***10***	***0.0***	***338***	***84.4***	***0.0***	***0.0***	***0.0***
GEMELLI								
Durum Wheat, Tesco*	1 Serving/100g	354	2.0	354	13.2	68.5	2.0	2.9
GHEE								
Butter	***1oz/28g***	***251***	***27.9***	***898***	***0.0***	***0.0***	***99.8***	***0.0***
Palm	***1oz/28g***	***251***	***27.9***	***897***	***0.0***	***0.0***	***99.7***	***0.0***
Vegetable	***1oz/28g***	***251***	***27.8***	***895***	***0.0***	***0.0***	***99.4***	***0.0***
GHERKINS								
Pickled, Average	***1 Gherkin/36g***	***5***	***0.0***	***14***	***0.9***	***2.6***	***0.1***	***1.2***
Pickled, with Dill Flower, Drained, Waitrose*	1 Serving/25g	10	0.1	39	1.7	6.0	0.5	1.1
GIN								
& Diet Tonic, Can, Greenalls*	1 Can/250ml	95	0.0	38	0.0	0.0	0.0	0.0
37.5% Volume	***1 Shot/35ml***	***72***	***0.0***	***207***	***0.0***	***0.0***	***0.0***	***0.0***
40% Volume	***1 Shot/35ml***	***78***	***0.0***	***224***	***0.0***	***0.0***	***0.0***	***0.0***
Gordons & Bitter Lemon, Premixed, Canned, Gordons*	1 Can/250ml	170	0.0	68	0.0	7.1	0.0	0.0
London Dry, Bombay Sapphire*	1 Serving/25ml	59	0.0	236	0.0	0.0	0.0	0.0
GINGER								
Chunks, Crystallised, Julian Graves*	1 Serving/10g	28	0.0	283	0.2	70.1	0.2	1.5
Crystallised, Suma*	1 Serving/30g	104	0.0	348	0.2	82.0	0.1	0.3
Ground, Average	***1 Tsp/2g***	***5***	***0.1***	***258***	***7.4***	***60.0***	***3.3***	***0.0***
Root, Raw, Pared, Average	***1 Tsp/2g***	***2***	***0.0***	***86***	***2.0***	***19.1***	***0.8***	***2.2***
Root, Raw, Unprepared, Average	***1 Tsp Chopped/2g***	***2***	***0.0***	***80***	***1.8***	***17.8***	***0.8***	***2.0***
Very Lazy, The English Provender Co.*	1 Tsp/5g	3	0.0	52	0.7	10.9	0.8	0.8
GINGER ALE								
1870, Siver Spring*	1 Serving/100ml	18	0.0	18	0.0	4.2	0.0	0.0
American, Low Calorie, Tesco*	1 fl oz/30ml	0	0.0	1	0.0	0.0	0.0	0.0
American, Tesco*	1 Glass/250ml	58	0.0	23	0.0	5.5	0.0	0.0
Dry	1 Glass/250ml	38	0.0	15	0.0	3.9	0.0	0.0
Dry, Asda*	1 Serving/150ml	56	0.0	37	0.0	9.0	0.0	0.0
Dry, Sainsbury's*	1 Glass/250ml	95	0.2	38	0.1	9.1	0.1	0.1
GINGER BEER								
Alcoholic, Crabbies*	1 Bottle/500ml	254	0.0	51	0.0	7.1	0.0	0.0

	Measure INFO/WEIGHT	per Measure KCAL	FAT	Nutrition Values per 100g / 100ml KCAL	PROT	CARB	FAT	FIBRE
GINGER BEER								
Asda*	1 Can/330ml	144	0.0	44	0.0	10.9	0.0	0.0
Classic, Schweppes*	1 Can/330ml	115	0.0	35	0.0	8.4	0.0	0.0
D & G Old Jamaican*	1 Can/330ml	211	0.0	64	0.0	16.0	0.0	0.0
Diet, Crabbies*	1 Bottle/700ml	7	0.0	1	0.0	0.0	0.0	0.0
Fiery, Canned, Waitrose*	1 Can/330ml	178	0.0	54	0.0	13.3	0.0	0.0
Fiery, Low Calorie, Waitrose*	1 Can/330ml	3	0.0	1	0.1	0.0	0.0	0.0
Gastropub, M & S*	1 Bottle/1038ml	675	0.0	65	0.0	15.4	0.0	0.0
Jamaican, Boots*	1 Bottle/500ml	5	0.0	1	0.0	0.0	0.0	0.0
Light, Waitrose*	1 Glass/250ml	2	0.2	1	0.0	0.0	0.1	0.1
No Added Sugar, Aldi*	1 Glass/250ml	5	0.0	2	0.0	0.0	0.0	0.0
Sainsbury's*	1 Can/330ml	69	0.0	21	0.0	5.1	0.0	0.0
Sparkling, Organic, Whole Earth*	1 Can/330ml	116	0.0	35	0.0	8.2	0.0	0.0
Tesco*	1 Serving/200ml	70	0.2	35	0.1	8.2	0.1	0.0
Traditional, Fentiman's*	1 Bottle/275ml	130	0.0	47	0.0	11.3	0.0	0.0
Traditional Style, Tesco*	1 Can/330ml	218	0.0	66	0.0	16.1	0.0	0.0
GINGER WINE								
Green, & Scots Whisky, Crabbies*	1 Glass/125ml	192	0.0	153	14.3	14.3	0.0	0.0
GINGERBREAD								
Average	1oz/28g	106	3.5	379	5.7	64.7	12.6	1.2
Decorate Your Own, Chosen By You, Asda*	1 Serving/100g	414	12.6	414	4.8	70.4	12.6	2.3
Hansel the Snowman, Pret a Manger*	1 Gingerbread/48g	206	7.6	429	7.3	64.6	15.8	2.3
Men, Mini, M & S*	1 Biscuit/17g	78	3.1	470	6.2	63.9	18.6	1.7
Men, Mini, Sainsbury's*	1 Biscuit/12g	56	1.4	463	5.7	83.4	11.8	1.5
GNOCCHI								
Aldi*	1 Serving/100g	160	0.3	160	3.8	35.6	0.3	0.0
Di Patate, Italfresco*	½ Pack/200g	296	0.4	148	3.3	33.2	0.2	0.0
Fresh, Italian, Chilled, Sainsbury's*	¼ Pack/125g	190	0.4	152	3.8	33.6	0.3	1.4
Potato, Cooked, Average	***1 Serving/150g***	***200***	***0.0***	***133***	***0.0***	***33.2***	***0.0***	***0.0***
GOAT								
Meat, Uncooked	1 Portion/100g	109	2.3	109	20.0	0.0	2.3	0.0
Raw	***1oz/28g***	***31***	***0.6***	***109***	***20.6***	***0.0***	***2.3***	***0.0***
GOJI BERRIES								
Average	***1 Serving/100g***	***287***	***0.7***	***287***	***6.6***	***65.1***	***0.7***	***6.8***
Dried, Love Life, Waitrose*	1 Sm Handful/30g	91	0.5	302	13.6	57.8	1.8	12.2
GOOSE								
Leg with Skin, Fire Roasted	***1 Leg/174g***	***482***	***29.8***	***277***	***28.8***	***0.0***	***17.1***	***0.0***
Meat, Fat & Skin, Raw	***1oz/28g***	***101***	***9.2***	***361***	***16.5***	***0.0***	***32.8***	***0.0***
Meat, Raw	***1 Portion/185g***	***298***	***13.0***	***161***	***23.0***	***0.0***	***7.0***	***0.0***
Meat, Roasted	***1 Portion/143g***	***340***	***18.6***	***238***	***29.0***	***0.0***	***13.0***	***0.0***
Meat & Skin, Roasted	***½ Goose/774g***	***2361***	***169.5***	***305***	***25.2***	***0.0***	***21.9***	***0.0***
GOOSEBERRIES								
Dessert, Raw, Tops & Tails Removed	***1oz/28g***	***11***	***0.1***	***40***	***0.7***	***9.2***	***0.3***	***2.4***
Stewed with Sugar	***25g***	***14***	***0.1***	***54***	***0.7***	***12.9***	***0.3***	***4.2***
Stewed without Sugar	***25g***	***4***	***0.1***	***16***	***0.9***	***2.5***	***0.3***	***4.4***
GOULASH								
Beef, 114, Oakhouse Foods Ltd*	1 Meal/380g	410	20.1	108	7.5	7.4	5.3	1.7
Beef, Average	1 Serving/300g	310	9.5	103	8.1	10.4	3.2	0.9
Beef, Weight Watchers*	1 Pack/330g	241	5.6	73	4.8	9.5	1.7	0.6
Beef with Tagliatelle, COU, M & S*	1 Pack/360g	414	8.3	115	8.5	14.5	2.3	1.0
GRAPEFRUIT								
in Juice, Average	***1oz/28g***	***13***	***0.0***	***46***	***0.5***	***10.6***	***0.0***	***0.4***
in Syrup, Average	***1oz/28g***	***19***	***0.0***	***69***	***0.5***	***16.8***	***0.1***	***0.5***
Raw, Flesh Only, Average	***½ Fruit/160g***	***48***	***0.2***	***30***	***0.8***	***6.8***	***0.1***	***1.3***

	Measure INFO/WEIGHT	per Measure KCAL	FAT	Nutrition Values per 100g / 100ml KCAL	PROT	CARB	FAT	FIBRE
GRAPEFRUIT								
Raw, Weighed with Skin & Seeds, Average	***1 Lge/340g***	***109***	***0.3***	***32***	***0.6***	***8.1***	***0.1***	***1.1***
Ruby Red in Juice, Average	***1 Serving/135g***	***54***	***0.1***	***40***	***0.6***	***9.4***	***0.0***	***0.5***
GRAPES								
Green, Average	***1 Grape/5g***	***3***	***0.0***	***62***	***0.4***	***15.2***	***0.1***	***0.7***
Red, Average	***1 Grape/5g***	***3***	***0.0***	***65***	***0.4***	***15.8***	***0.1***	***0.6***
Red & Green Selection, Average	***1 Grape/5g***	***3***	***0.0***	***62***	***0.4***	***15.2***	***0.1***	***0.8***
Seedless, Black, Asda*	1 Serving/80g	51	0.1	64	0.4	15.4	0.1	0.7
GRAPPA								
	1 Serving/30ml	85	0.0	283	0.0	6.7	0.0	0.0
GRATIN								
Cauliflower, Findus*	1 Pack/400g	340	20.0	85	3.5	7.0	5.0	0.0
Dauphinoise, Budgens*	½ Pack/218g	277	15.7	127	3.0	12.5	7.2	2.5
Leek & Carrot, Findus*	1 Pack/400g	440	26.0	110	3.5	9.5	6.5	0.0
Potato, Creamy, M & S*	½ Pack/225g	360	25.0	160	2.2	11.9	11.1	0.9
Potato, HL, Tesco*	1 Serving/225g	169	5.0	75	2.3	11.4	2.2	0.6
Potato, Sainsbury's*	½ Pack/225g	448	34.0	199	4.4	11.4	15.1	1.0
GRAVLAX								
Salmon, Cured with Salt, Sugar & Herbs	1 Serving/100g	119	3.3	119	18.3	3.1	3.3	0.4
GRAVY								
Beef, Aunt Bessie's*	1 Serving/100g	73	5.3	73	1.0	5.3	5.3	0.5
Beef, Fresh, Sainsbury's*	1 Serving/83ml	47	2.7	56	2.4	4.5	3.2	0.6
Beef, Heat & Serve, Morrisons*	1 Serving/150g	27	0.4	18	0.3	3.9	0.3	0.5
Beef, Home Style, Savoury, Heinz*	¼ Cup/60g	30	1.0	50	1.7	6.7	1.7	0.0
Beef, with Winter Berry & Shallot, Made Up, Oxo*	1 Serving/105ml	24	0.3	23	0.6	4.3	0.3	0.1
Chicken, Granules For, Dry Weight, Bisto*	1 Serving/20g	80	3.2	400	1.9	62.5	15.8	0.2
Chicken, Rich, Ready to Heat, Schwartz*	½ Pack/100g	27	1.2	27	0.8	3.3	1.2	0.5
Favourite, Granules, Made Up, Bisto*	1 Serving/50ml	15	0.6	30	0.2	4.4	1.2	0.0
Granules, Beef, Dry, Tesco*	1 Serving/6g	29	2.1	480	5.5	36.4	34.7	1.5
Granules, Beef, Made Up, Tesco*	1 Serving/140ml	48	3.6	35	0.3	2.6	2.5	0.1
Granules, Chicken, Dry, Average	1 Tsp/4g	17	0.9	428	4.5	49.4	23.6	1.2
Granules, Chicken, Dry, Oxo*	1oz/28g	83	1.4	296	11.1	54.2	4.9	0.7
Granules, Chicken, Made Up, Oxo*	1 fl oz/30ml	5	0.1	18	0.7	3.3	0.3	0.0
Granules, Chicken & Hint of Sage & Onion, Oxo*	1 Serving/30g	95	1.8	316	11.1	54.2	6.1	0.7
Granules, Dry, Bisto*	1 Serving/10g	38	1.6	384	3.1	56.4	16.2	1.5
Granules, Instant, Dry	***1oz/28g***	***129***	***9.1***	***462***	***4.4***	***40.6***	***32.5***	***0.0***
Granules, Instant, Made Up	***1oz/28g***	***10***	***0.7***	***34***	***0.3***	***3.0***	***2.4***	***0.0***
Granules, Lamb, Dry, Average	1 Tsp/4g	14	0.3	344	10.8	56.2	8.4	2.8
Granules, Lamb, Hint of Mint, Made Up, Oxo*	1 Serving/100ml	25	0.5	25	0.7	4.3	0.5	0.0
Granules, Made Up, Bisto*	1 Serving/50ml	15	0.6	30	0.2	4.4	1.2	0.2
Granules, Made Up, Oxo*	1 Serving/150ml	28	0.4	19	0.6	3.4	0.3	0.0
Granules, Onion, Dry, Morrisons*	1 Serving/25g	124	8.7	495	3.4	44.0	34.7	0.0
Granules, Onion, Dry, Oxo*	1oz/28g	92	1.3	328	8.2	62.3	4.8	0.8
Granules, Onion, Made Up, Oxo*	1 fl oz/30ml	6	0.1	20	0.5	3.7	0.3	0.0
Granules, Original, Dry, Oxo*	1oz/28g	88	1.3	313	10.2	57.2	4.8	1.0
Granules, Vegetable, Dry, Oxo*	1oz/28g	88	1.4	316	8.4	59.5	4.9	0.9
Granules, Vegetable, Dry, Tesco*	½ Pint/20g	94	6.7	470	3.8	38.5	33.4	3.7
Onion, Caramelised, Made Up, Bisto*	1 Serving/70ml	20	0.3	29	0.1	6.1	0.4	0.1
Onion, Fresh, Asda*	1/6 Pot/77g	30	1.6	39	1.7	3.3	2.1	0.4
Onion, Granules, Made Up, Bisto*	1 Serving/50ml	14	0.3	28	0.2	5.6	0.6	0.0
Onion, Granules For, Dry Weight, Bisto*	4 Tsp/20g	78	2.9	391	2.4	62.3	14.7	2.3
Onion, Rich, M & S*	½ Pack/150g	60	1.8	40	2.0	5.9	1.2	0.3
Onion, Rich, Ready to Heat, Schwartz*	½ Sachet/100g	24	0.6	24	0.4	4.3	0.6	0.5
Paste, Beef, Antony Worrall Thompson's*	1 Portion/31g	104	5.7	334	11.8	30.3	18.4	0.6

	Measure INFO/WEIGHT	per Measure KCAL	FAT	Nutrition Values per 100g / 100ml KCAL	PROT	CARB	FAT	FIBRE
GRAVY								
Paste, Onion, Antony Worrall Thompson's*	1 Tsp/10g	26	0.4	262	7.0	48.7	4.4	1.4
Poultry, Fresh, Sainsbury's*	1 Serving/100g	46	1.2	46	3.5	4.9	1.2	0.5
Powder, GF, Dry, Allergycare*	1 Tbsp/10g	26	0.0	260	0.3	63.8	0.4	0.0
Powder, Made Up, Sainsbury's*	1 Serving/100ml	15	0.1	15	0.4	3.2	0.1	0.1
Powder, Vegetarian, Organic, Marigold*	1 Serving/22g	79	1.7	361	10.6	61.5	7.7	1.3
Turkey, Granules, Made Up, Bisto*	1 Serving/50ml	14	0.6	28	0.2	4.0	1.2	0.2
Turkey, Granules For, Dry Weight, Bisto*	4 Tsp/20g	75	3.1	377	2.4	57.2	15.5	1.0
Turkey, Pour Over, Bisto*	1 Pack/100g	23	0.6	23	0.4	4.1	0.6	0.1
Turkey, Rich, Ready to Heat, Schwartz*	1 Pack/200g	62	2.4	31	1.9	3.1	1.2	0.5
Vegetable, Granules For, Dry Weight, Bisto*	1 Tsp/4g	15	0.5	380	2.1	63.0	13.3	4.5
Vegetable, Granules For, Made Up, Bisto*	1 Serving/50ml	14	0.2	28	0.2	5.6	0.4	0.2
GREENGAGES								
Raw, Average	***1 Fruit/23g***	***9***	***0.0***	***38***	***0.8***	***9.4***	***0.1***	***2.0***
GREENS								
Spring, Boiled, Average	***1 Serving/80g***	***16***	***0.6***	***20***	***1.9***	***1.6***	***0.7***	***2.6***
Spring, Raw, Average	***1 Serving/80g***	***26***	***0.8***	***33***	***3.0***	***3.1***	***1.0***	***3.4***
GRILLS								
Bacon & Cheese, Tesco*	1 Grill/78g	222	14.7	284	15.0	13.4	18.9	1.2
Cheese & Bacon, Danepak*	1 Grill/85g	241	16.0	284	15.0	13.4	18.9	1.2
Tikka, Organic, Waitrose*	1 Grill/100g	185	9.3	185	6.9	18.5	9.3	3.4
Vegetable, Dalepak*	1 Grill/83g	125	4.1	151	4.0	22.5	5.0	1.6
Vegetable, Mediterranean, Cauldron Foods*	1 Grill/88g	145	10.4	166	5.3	15.8	11.9	6.5
Vegetable, Ross*	1 Grill/114g	252	12.9	221	4.3	25.5	11.3	0.9
Vegetable, Tesco*	1 Grill/72g	129	7.2	179	4.2	18.0	10.0	2.2
Vegetarian, Mushroom & Oregano, Organic, Waitrose*	1 Grill/100g	200	10.0	200	7.9	19.5	10.0	4.3
GRITS								
Hominy, White, Enriched, Old Fashioned, Quaker Oats*	¼ Cup/41g	140	0.5	341	7.3	78.0	1.2	4.9
GROUSE								
Meat Only, Roasted	***1oz/28g***	***36***	***0.6***	***128***	***27.6***	***0.0***	***2.0***	***0.0***
GUACAMOLE								
Average	1 Tbsp/17g	33	3.3	194	1.6	3.4	19.2	2.4
Avocado, Reduced Fat, The Fresh Dip Company*	1 Serving/113g	128	9.8	113	2.5	6.1	8.7	2.3
Chunky, M & S*	1 Pot/170g	221	19.2	130	1.5	5.1	11.3	1.7
Doritos, Walkers*	1 Tbsp/20g	32	3.2	159	1.2	2.6	16.0	0.1
Fresh, VLH Kitchens	1 Serving/17g	27	85.9	158	1.5	3.0	14.6	2.5
Fresh, Waitrose*	½ Pack/100g	190	18.4	190	1.9	4.1	18.4	2.5
GFY, Asda*	1 Pack/113g	144	12.4	127	2.8	4.3	11.0	2.2
Reduced Fat Average	1 Serving/100g	129	10.8	129	2.4	5.2	10.8	3.0
GUAVA								
Canned in Syrup	***1oz/28g***	***17***	***0.0***	***60***	***0.4***	***15.7***	***0.0***	***3.0***
Raw, Flesh Only, Average	***1 Fruit/55g***	***37***	***0.6***	***68***	***3.0***	***14.0***	***1.0***	***5.0***
GUINEA FOWL								
Boned & Stuffed, Fresh, Fayrefield Foods*	1 Serving/325g	650	39.3	200	19.1	3.3	12.1	0.5
Fresh, Free Range, Waitrose*	1 Portion/193g	258	11.9	134	19.5	0.0	6.2	0.3
GUMBO								
Cajun Vegetable, Sainsbury's*	1 Serving/450g	266	11.2	59	1.4	7.7	2.5	1.5
Louisiana Chicken, Perfectly Balanced, Waitrose*	1 Serving/235g	207	6.6	88	12.2	3.5	2.8	1.3
GUMS								
American Hard, Sainsbury's*	1 Sweet/6g	22	0.0	360	0.1	90.0	0.1	0.0
American Hard, Tesco*	1 Serving/200g	646	0.0	323	0.0	80.8	0.0	0.0
Milk Bottles, Bassett's*	1 Pack/25g	88	0.4	353	6.2	78.3	1.6	0.0
Milk Bottles, Milk Flavour, Asda*	1 Pack/100g	369	2.3	369	7.0	80.0	2.3	0.4

	Measure INFO/WEIGHT	per Measure KCAL	FAT	Nutrition Values per 100g / 100ml KCAL	PROT	CARB	FAT	FIBRE
HADDOCK								
Fillets, Battered, Average	1oz/28g	64	3.4	228	13.4	16.3	12.2	1.1
Fillets, Raw, Average	***1 Fillet/140g***	***112***	***1.2***	***80***	***18.0***	***0.2***	***0.8***	***0.0***
Fillets, Smoked, Cooked, Average	***1 Pack/300g***	***337***	***7.7***	***112***	***21.9***	***0.4***	***2.6***	***0.1***
Fillets, Smoked, in Mustard & Dill, The Saucy Fish Co.*	2 Fillets/270g	262	9.7	97	15.5	0.1	3.6	0.0
Fillets, Smoked, Raw, Average	***1 Pack/227g***	***194***	***1.0***	***86***	***20.3***	***0.1***	***0.5***	***0.2***
Flour, Fried in Blended Oil	1oz/28g	39	1.1	138	21.1	4.5	4.1	0.2
Goujons, Batter, Crispy, M & S*	1 Serving/100g	250	14.1	250	11.7	18.5	14.1	0.8
Loins, TTD, Sainsbury's*	1 Serving/100g	108	0.7	108	25.5	0.0	0.7	0.0
HADDOCK IN								
Breadcrumbs, Fillets, Average	1 Fillet/125g	253	12.4	203	13.5	14.9	9.9	1.2
Butter Sauce, Steaks, Youngs*	1 Serving/150g	134	5.6	89	9.9	4.0	3.7	0.5
Cheese & Chive Sauce, Smoked Fillets, Seafresh*	1 Serving/170g	201	10.4	118	14.7	1.2	6.1	0.1
Tomato Herb Sauce, Fillets, BGTY, Sainsbury's*	½ Pack/165g	150	4.6	91	12.9	3.6	2.8	0.1
Watercress Sauce, GFY, Asda*	1 Pack/400g	268	6.8	67	6.0	7.0	1.7	1.4
HADDOCK WITH								
Rich Cheese Crust, Smoked, Sainsbury's*	1 Serving/199g	295	18.9	148	13.0	2.5	9.5	0.9
Broccoli & Cheese, Lakeland*	1 Serving/150g	280	10.5	187	10.4	20.6	7.0	0.0
Cheese & Chive Sauce, Atlantic, Youngs*	½ Pack/180g	184	8.6	102	13.0	1.7	4.8	0.2
Creme Fraiche & Chive Sauce, Smoked, Tesco*	1 Serving/150g	154	4.6	103	16.8	2.1	3.1	0.3
HAGGIS								
Hall's*	1 Haggis/454g	1053	64.5	232	9.7	15.1	14.2	2.5
Neeps & Tatties, M & S*	1 Pack/300g	330	14.4	110	3.8	12.3	4.8	0.8
Traditional, Average	***1 Serving/454g***	***1119***	***66.5***	***246***	***12.4***	***17.2***	***14.6***	***1.0***
Traditional, Macsween*	1 Haggis/454g	1149	70.8	253	11.1	19.1	15.6	2.1
Vegetarian, Macsween*	1 Serving/100g	208	11.5	208	5.9	25.9	11.5	2.4
HAKE								
Fillets, Herby Mediterranean Glaze, Sensations, Youngs*	½ Pack/120g	106	2.6	88	16.8	0.4	2.2	0.0
Fillets, in Breadcrumbs, Average	1oz/28g	66	3.7	234	12.9	16.0	13.4	1.0
Goujons, Average	1 Serving/150g	345	17.8	230	12.4	18.6	11.9	1.3
Raw, Average	***1oz/28g***	***29***	***0.6***	***102***	***20.4***	***0.0***	***2.2***	***0.0***
HALIBUT								
Cooked, Dry Heat, Average	***1oz/28g***	***38***	***1.1***	***135***	***24.6***	***0.4***	***4.0***	***0.0***
Raw	***1oz/28g***	***29***	***0.5***	***103***	***21.5***	***0.0***	***1.9***	***0.0***
with Roasted Pepper Sauce, Fillets, M & S*	1 Serving/145g	218	14.4	150	12.7	2.4	9.9	0.6
HALVA								
Average	***1oz/28g***	***107***	***3.7***	***381***	***1.8***	***68.0***	***13.2***	***0.0***
HAM								
Applewood Smoked, Average	***1 Slice/28g***	***31***	***0.8***	***112***	***21.2***	***0.6***	***2.8***	***0.2***
Baked, Average	***1 Slice/74g***	***98***	***3.7***	***133***	***21.0***	***1.0***	***5.0***	***0.0***
Boiled, Average	***1 Pack/113g***	***154***	***6.5***	***136***	***20.6***	***0.6***	***5.8***	***0.0***
Breaded, Average	***1 Slice/37g***	***57***	***2.3***	***155***	***23.1***	***1.8***	***6.3***	***1.6***
Breaded, Dry Cured, Average	***1 Slice/33g***	***47***	***1.8***	***142***	***22.2***	***1.4***	***5.4***	***0.0***
Brunswick, Average	***1 Slice/20g***	***32***	***1.8***	***160***	***19.5***	***0.6***	***8.8***	***0.0***
Cooked, Sliced, Average	***1 Slice/17g***	***18***	***0.5***	***109***	***19.0***	***1.0***	***3.2***	***0.1***
Cooked, Wafer Thin, Weight Watchers*	1 Serving/60g	58	1.1	97	18.2	1.8	1.8	0.1
Crumbed, Sliced, Average	***1 Slice/28g***	***33***	***0.9***	***117***	***21.5***	***0.9***	***3.1***	***0.0***
Crumbed, Wafer Thin, Denny*	8 Slices/100g	112	2.3	112	21.8	2.4	2.3	0.0
Danish, Average	***1 Slice/11g***	***14***	***0.6***	***125***	***18.4***	***1.0***	***5.4***	***0.0***
Danish, Lean, Average	***1 Slice/15g***	***14***	***0.3***	***92***	***17.8***	***1.0***	***1.8***	***0.0***
Dry Cured, Average	***1 Slice/18g***	***26***	***1.0***	***144***	***22.4***	***1.0***	***5.6***	***0.2***
Extra Lean, Average	***1 Slice/11g***	***10***	***0.2***	***90***	***18.0***	***1.4***	***1.4***	***0.0***
Gammon, Breaded, Average	***1 Serving/25g***	***31***	***0.8***	***122***	***22.0***	***1.5***	***3.1***	***0.0***
Gammon, Dry Cured, Sliced, Average	***1 Slice/33g***	***43***	***1.4***	***131***	***22.9***	***0.4***	***4.2***	***0.0***

	Measure INFO/WEIGHT	per Measure KCAL	FAT	Nutrition Values per 100g / 100ml KCAL	PROT	CARB	FAT	FIBRE
HAM								
Gammon, Honey Roast, Average	***1 Serving/60g***	***81***	***2.8***	***134***	***22.4***	***0.4***	***4.8***	***0.0***
Gammon, Mustard, Cured, Waitrose*	1 Slice/45g	54	1.8	120	21.4	0.1	4.0	0.0
Gammon, Peppered, Waitrose*	1/3 Pack/36g	51	2.3	142	20.7	0.3	6.4	0.0
Gammon, Smoked, Average	***1 Slice/43g***	***59***	***2.1***	***137***	***22.3***	***0.7***	***4.9***	***0.2***
German Black Forest, Average	***½ Pack/35g***	***93***	***6.0***	***267***	***27.2***	***1.3***	***17.0***	***0.5***
Honey & Mustard, Average	***1oz/28g***	***39***	***1.2***	***140***	***20.8***	***4.6***	***4.3***	***0.0***
Honey Roast, Average	***1 Slice/20g***	***25***	***0.8***	***123***	***20.3***	***1.6***	***3.8***	***0.1***
Honey Roast, Dry Cured, Average	***1 Slice/33g***	***46***	***1.5***	***140***	***22.7***	***2.3***	***4.4***	***0.2***
Honey Roast, Lean, Average	***1 Serving/25g***	***28***	***0.8***	***111***	***18.2***	***2.7***	***3.1***	***0.0***
Honey Roast, Wafer Thin, Average	***1 Slice/10g***	***11***	***0.3***	***113***	***17.4***	***3.7***	***3.2***	***0.3***
Honey Roast, Wafer Thin, Premium, Average	***1 Slice/10g***	***15***	***0.6***	***149***	***22.0***	***1.6***	***6.0***	***0.0***
Jamon de Trevelez, Antonio Alvarez Jamones*	1 Slice/10g	19	0.9	192	35.6	0.0	8.6	0.0
Joint, Cured, Roasted, Average	1 Serving/100g	138	5.2	138	21.7	1.0	5.2	0.1
Lean, Average	***1 Slice/18g***	***19***	***0.4***	***104***	***19.5***	***1.1***	***2.4***	***0.3***
Oak Smoked, Average	***1 Slice/20g***	***26***	***0.9***	***130***	***21.0***	***1.0***	***4.7***	***0.3***
Parma, Average	***1 Slice/10g***	***21***	***1.1***	***213***	***29.3***	***0.0***	***10.6***	***0.0***
Parma, Premium, Average	***1 Slice/14g***	***36***	***2.3***	***258***	***27.9***	***0.3***	***16.1***	***0.0***
Peppered, Average	***1 Slice/12g***	***13***	***0.3***	***110***	***18.5***	***2.0***	***2.7***	***0.0***
Peppered, Dry Cured, Average	***1 Slice/31g***	***43***	***1.5***	***140***	***23.1***	***1.3***	***4.7***	***0.2***
Prosciutto, Average	***1 Slice/12g***	***27***	***1.5***	***226***	***28.7***	***0.0***	***12.4***	***0.4***
San Daniele, Finest, Tesco*	1 Slice/10g	24	1.3	242	30.5	0.5	13.1	0.0
Serrano, Average	***1 Slice/20g***	***46***	***2.4***	***230***	***30.5***	***0.4***	***11.8***	***0.0***
Smoked, Average	***1 Slice/18g***	***21***	***0.7***	***117***	***19.7***	***0.9***	***3.7***	***0.0***
Smoked, Dry Cured, Average	***1 Slice/28g***	***38***	***1.2***	***137***	***23.0***	***1.4***	***4.4***	***0.2***
Smoked, Wafer Thin, Average	***1 Serving/40g***	***41***	***1.2***	***102***	***17.7***	***1.2***	***2.9***	***0.2***
Suffolk Black, TTD, Sainsbury's*	1 Slice/42g	58	1.7	139	22.3	3.5	4.0	0.0
Thick Cut, Average	***1 Slice/74g***	***94***	***2.9***	***127***	***22.4***	***0.6***	***3.9***	***0.1***
Tinned, Average	***½ Can/100g***	***136***	***8.8***	***136***	***12.2***	***2.0***	***8.8***	***0.0***
Tinned, Lean, Average	***½ Can/100g***	***94***	***2.3***	***94***	***18.1***	***0.2***	***2.3***	***0.4***
Wafer Thin, Average	***1 Slice/10g***	***10***	***0.3***	***101***	***17.9***	***1.4***	***2.6***	***0.1***
Wiltshire, Average	***1oz/28g***	***41***	***1.7***	***148***	***23.1***	***0.0***	***6.0***	***0.0***
Wiltshire, Breaded, Average	***1oz/28g***	***41***	***1.4***	***145***	***23.9***	***1.0***	***5.0***	***0.0***
HARE								
Raw, Lean Only, Average	***1oz/28g***	***35***	***1.0***	***125***	***23.5***	***0.2***	***3.5***	***0.0***
Stewed, Lean Only, Average	***1oz/28g***	***48***	***1.5***	***170***	***29.5***	***0.2***	***5.5***	***0.0***
HARIBO*								
American Hard Gums, Haribo*	1 Pack/175g	630	3.3	360	0.3	85.5	1.9	0.2
Build a Burger, Haribo*	1oz/28g	96	0.1	344	6.6	79.0	0.2	0.3
Chamallows, Haribo*	1oz/28g	92	0.0	330	2.0	80.0	0.0	0.0
Cola Bottles, Fizzy, Haribo*	1 Pack/175g	595	0.4	340	6.3	78.3	0.2	0.3
Cola Bottles, Haribo*	1 Pack/16g	56	0.0	348	7.7	78.9	0.2	0.3
Dinosaurs, Haribo*	1oz/28g	95	0.1	340	6.3	78.3	0.2	0.5
Dolly Mixtures, Haribo*	1 Pack/175g	719	8.4	411	1.8	90.2	4.8	0.2
Fantasy Mix, Haribo*	1 Pack/100g	344	0.2	344	6.6	79.0	0.2	0.3
Fried Eggs/eggstras, Haribo*	1oz/28g	96	0.1	344	6.6	79.0	0.2	0.0
Gold Bears, Haribo*	1 Pack/100g	348	0.2	348	7.7	78.9	0.2	0.3
Happy Cherries, Haribo*	1 Serving/40g	139	0.1	348	7.7	78.9	0.2	0.3
Horror Mix, Haribo*	1 Pack/100g	344	0.2	344	6.6	79.0	0.2	0.3
Jelly Babies, Haribo*	1oz/28g	97	0.1	348	4.5	82.1	0.2	0.5
Jelly Beans, Haribo*	1 Pack/100g	379	0.2	379	0.6	93.8	0.2	0.1
Kiddies Super Mix, Haribo*	1 Pack/100g	344	0.2	344	6.6	79.0	0.2	0.3
Liquorice Cream Rock, Haribo*	1oz/28g	107	1.5	382	2.3	81.2	5.3	0.3
Liquorice Favourites, Haribo*	1 Serving/40g	143	1.2	357	2.8	78.8	3.0	2.3

	Measure INFO/WEIGHT	per Measure KCAL	FAT	Nutrition Values per 100g / 100ml KCAL	PROT	CARB	FAT	FIBRE
HARIBO*								
Magic Mix, Haribo*	1oz/28g	102	0.5	366	5.4	82.0	1.9	0.3
Maoam Stripes, Haribo*	1 Chew/7g	27	0.4	384	1.2	81.7	6.1	0.3
Mega Roulette, Haribo*	1oz/28g	97	0.1	348	7.7	78.9	0.2	0.3
Mega Roulette Sour, Haribo*	1oz/28g	95	0.1	340	6.3	78.3	0.2	0.5
Micro Mix, Haribo*	1oz/28g	106	0.7	379	4.7	84.5	2.5	0.4
Milky Mix, Haribo*	1 Pack/175g	607	0.4	347	7.1	79.6	0.2	0.4
Mint Imperials, Haribo*	1 Pack/175g	695	0.9	397	0.4	98.8	0.5	0.1
Peaches, Haribo*	1oz/28g	98	0.0	350	4.3	82.1	0.0	0.0
Pontefract Cakes, Haribo*	1 Serving/40g	118	0.1	296	5.3	68.2	0.2	0.5
Shrimps, Haribo*	1oz/28g	99	0.1	352	6.1	81.5	0.2	0.1
Snakes, Haribo*	1 Snake/8g	28	0.0	348	7.7	78.9	0.2	0.3
Starmix, Haribo*	1 Pack/100g	344	0.2	344	6.6	79.0	0.2	0.3
Tangfastics, Haribo*	1 Pack/100g	359	2.3	359	6.3	78.3	2.3	0.5
Tropifruit, Haribo*	1oz/28g	97	0.1	348	4.5	82.1	0.2	0.5
HARISSA PASTE								
Average	1 Tsp/5g	6	0.3	123	2.9	12.9	6.7	2.8
Barts*	1 Tbsp/15g	11	0.3	76	4.0	10.7	1.9	0.0
Easy, M & S*	1 Tbsp/15g	16	0.8	105	2.5	11.2	5.5	4.4
Moroccan Style, Al'fez*	1 Tsp/10g	19	1.1	190	4.0	18.2	11.2	3.4
HASH								
Barbecue Beef, COU, M & S*	1 Pack/400g	360	1.6	90	7.0	14.0	0.4	1.4
Corned Beef, Apetito*	1 Pack/380g	423	23.6	111	3.8	10.3	6.2	1.3
Corned Beef, Asda*	1 Pack/400g	416	14.4	104	6.0	12.0	3.6	1.1
Corned Beef, Canned, Princes*	1 Can/410g	726	45.1	177	11.5	7.1	11.0	1.9
Corned Beef, Chilled, Co-Op*	1 Pack/300g	345	18.0	115	9.0	5.0	6.0	1.0
Corned Beef, Frozen, Tesco*	1 Serving/400g	348	10.4	87	5.7	10.3	2.6	0.7
Corned Beef, M & S*	½ Pack/321g	385	20.2	120	8.1	7.4	6.3	1.3
Farmhouse, HE, Tesco*	1 Serving/300g	264	8.1	88	2.2	13.6	2.7	1.1
Vegetable & Lentil, Asda*	1 Pack/289g	254	6.1	88	3.2	14.0	2.1	0.0
HASH BROWNS								
Homestyle, Aunt Bessie's*	2 Hash Brown/98g	182	9.2	186	1.6	23.0	9.4	1.9
Oven Baked, Weighed Cooked, McCain*	1 Piece/38g	80	4.3	214	2.1	25.7	11.4	2.2
Oven Baked, Weighed Frozen, McCain*	1 Hash Brown/40g	75	4.1	187	1.7	21.8	10.3	2.1
Uncooked, Average	1 Hash Brown/45g	78	3.7	173	2.0	22.5	8.3	1.9
HAZELNUTS								
Blanched, Average	1 Serving/25g	164	15.9	656	15.4	5.8	63.5	6.5
Chopped, Average	***1 Serving/10g***	***67***	***6.4***	***666***	***16.8***	***5.6***	***64.0***	***6.6***
Whole, Average	***10 Whole/10g***	***66***	***6.4***	***655***	***15.4***	***5.8***	***63.5***	***6.5***
HEART								
Lambs, Average	***1 Heart/75g***	***92***	***4.5***	***122***	***16.0***	***1.0***	***6.0***	***0.0***
Ox, Raw	***1oz/28g***	***29***	***1.0***	***104***	***18.2***	***0.0***	***3.5***	***0.0***
Ox, Stewed	***1oz/28g***	***44***	***1.4***	***157***	***27.8***	***0.0***	***5.1***	***0.0***
Pig, Raw	***1oz/28g***	***27***	***0.9***	***97***	***17.1***	***0.0***	***3.2***	***0.0***
Pig, Stewed	***1oz/28g***	***45***	***1.9***	***162***	***25.1***	***0.0***	***6.8***	***0.0***
HERMESETAS								
Powdered, Hermes*	1 Tsp/0.78g	3	0.0	387	1.0	96.8	0.0	0.0
The Classic Sweetener, Hermes*	1 Tablet/0.5g	0	0.0	294	14.2	59.3	0.0	0.0
HERRING								
Canned in Tomato Sauce, Average	1oz/28g	57	4.3	204	11.9	4.1	15.5	0.1
Dried, Salted, Average	***1oz/28g***	***47***	***2.1***	***168***	***25.3***	***0.0***	***7.4***	***0.0***
Fillets, in Mustard & Dill Sauce, John West*	1 Can/190g	332	26.6	175	9.4	2.9	14.0	0.1
Fillets, in Olive Oil, Succulent, Princes*	1 Serving/50g	108	7.5	215	20.0	0.0	15.0	0.0
Fillets, Raw, Average	***1 Herring/100g***	***185***	***12.6***	***185***	***18.4***	***0.0***	***12.6***	***0.0***

H

	Measure INFO/WEIGHT	per Measure KCAL	FAT	Nutrition Values per 100g / 100ml KCAL	PROT	CARB	FAT	FIBRE
HERRING								
Grilled, Average	***1oz/28g***	***51***	***3.1***	***181***	***20.1***	***0.0***	***11.2***	***0.0***
Pickled, Average	1oz/28g	73	5.0	262	14.2	9.6	18.0	0.0
Pickled, in Mustard Sauce, Abba*	1 Serving/58g	150	10.9	260	7.0	16.0	19.0	0.0
Rollmops, Tesco*	1 Rollmop/65g	110	5.5	170	12.0	10.4	8.4	0.4
Rollmops, with Onion, Asda*	1 Rollmop/65g	89	3.1	137	13.2	10.3	4.8	0.8
Whole, Raw, Average	1 Serving/100g	190	13.2	190	17.8	0.0	13.2	0.0
HIGHLIGHTS								
Caffe Latte, Made Up, Cadbury*	1 Serving/200g	40	1.4	20	1.0	2.5	0.7	0.0
Choc Mint, Made Up, Cadbury*	1 Serving/200ml	40	1.4	20	1.0	2.5	0.7	0.3
Chocolate, Dairy Fudge, Dry Weight, Cadbury*	1 Serving/11g	40	1.1	363	17.0	50.0	10.0	0.0
Chocolate, Dark, Cadbury*	1 Sachet/11g	35	0.9	315	23.1	37.3	8.1	0.0
Chocolate Orange, Made Up, Cadbury*	1 Serving/200ml	40	1.4	20	1.0	2.3	0.7	0.3
Dairy Fudge, Made Up, Cadbury*	1 Serving/200ml	40	1.0	20	1.0	2.7	0.5	0.2
Dark, Bournville, Made Up, Cadbury*	1 Serving/200ml	35	0.9	18	1.2	2.0	0.4	0.0
Espresso, Made Up, Cadbury*	1 Serving/200ml	35	0.9	18	1.2	2.0	0.4	0.0
Hot Chocolate, Instant, Cadbury*	1 Sachet/22g	80	2.8	364	17.3	44.6	12.7	0.0
Hot Chocolate Drink, Instant, Dry Weight, Cadbury*	1 Sachet/11g	42	1.4	380	16.8	46.9	13.1	3.4
Hot Chocolate Drink, Instant, Made Up, Cadbury*	1 Serving/200ml	40	1.4	20	1.0	2.5	0.7	0.3
Mint, Cadbury*	1 Serving/200ml	40	1.4	20	1.0	2.5	0.7	0.0
Toffee Flavour, Made Up, Cadbury*	1 Serving/200ml	40	1.4	20	1.0	2.6	0.7	0.0
HOKI								
Grilled	***1oz/28g***	***34***	***0.8***	***121***	***24.1***	***0.0***	***2.7***	***0.0***
in Breadcrumbs, Average	1 Piece/156g	298	13.8	191	14.5	13.9	8.9	1.2
Raw	***1oz/28g***	***24***	***0.5***	***85***	***16.9***	***0.0***	***1.9***	***0.0***
Steaks in Batter, Crispy, Birds Eye*	1 Steak/123g	320	17.1	260	12.4	21.3	13.9	0.8
HONEY								
Acacia, Tesco*	1 Tsp/4g	12	0.0	307	0.4	76.4	0.0	0.0
Acacia Blossom, Sainsbury's*	1 Serving/24g	81	0.0	339	0.1	84.7	0.1	0.3
Australian Eucalyptus, Finest, Tesco*	1 Tsp/4g	12	0.0	307	0.4	76.4	0.0	0.0
Bio Active, New Zealand Honey Co*	1 Serving/10g	32	0.0	325	1.0	80.0	0.0	0.0
Clear, Basics, Sainsbury's*	1 Tsp/15g	46	0.0	307	0.4	76.4	0.1	0.0
Clear, Runny, Sainsbury's*	1 Serving/15g	51	0.0	339	0.1	84.7	0.1	0.3
Clear, Value, Tesco*	1 Serving/27g	86	0.0	320	1.0	78.0	0.0	0.0
Clover, Canadian, TTD, Sainsbury's*	1 Tbsp/15g	50	0.0	336	0.2	83.6	0.1	0.1
Florida Orange, Extra Special, Asda*	1 Tbsp/15g	50	0.0	334	0.5	83.0	0.0	0.0
Greek, Waitrose*	1 Tsp/6g	18	0.0	307	0.4	76.4	0.0	0.0
Pure, Clear, Average	***1 Tbsp/20g***	***63***	***0.0***	***315***	***0.5***	***78.5***	***0.0***	***0.0***
Pure, Clear, Squeezy, Oak Lane*	1 Tsp/5ml	16	0.0	330	0.5	81.0	0.0	0.0
Pure, Set, Average	***1 Tbsp/20g***	***62***	***0.0***	***312***	***0.4***	***77.6***	***0.0***	***0.0***
Scottish Heather, Waitrose*	1 Serving/20g	61	0.0	307	0.4	76.4	0.0	0.0
Spanish Orange Blossom, Sainsbury's*	1 Tbsp/15g	51	0.0	339	0.1	84.7	0.0	0.3
HONEYCOMB								
Natural, Epicure*	1 Serving/100g	290	4.6	290	0.4	74.4	4.6	0.0
HOOCH*								
Vodka, Calculated Estimate, Hooch*	1 Bottle/330ml	145	0.0	44	0.3	5.1	0.0	0.0
HORLICKS*								
Malted Drink, Extra Light, Instant, Dry Weight, Horlicks*	1 Serving/11g	35	0.7	319	8.4	57.4	6.2	10.5
Malted Drink, Light, Dry Weight, Horlicks*	1 Serving/32g	116	1.2	364	14.8	72.2	3.8	1.9
Malted Drink, Light, Made Up, Horlicks*	1 Mug/200ml	116	1.2	58	2.4	11.6	0.6	0.3
Powder, Made Up with Semi-Skimmed Milk	1 Mug/227ml	184	4.3	81	4.3	12.9	1.9	0.0
Powder, Made Up with Skimmed Milk	1 Mug/227ml	159	1.1	70	4.3	12.9	0.5	0.0
Powder, Made Up with Whole Milk	1 Mug/227ml	225	8.9	99	4.2	12.7	3.9	0.0
Snoozoo, Chocolate, Horlicks*	1 Sachet/20g	74	0.9	370	8.6	74.2	4.3	4.3

	Measure INFO/WEIGHT	per Measure KCAL	FAT	Nutrition Values per 100g / 100ml KCAL	PROT	CARB	FAT	FIBRE
HORSE								
Meat, Raw, Average	***1 Serving/110g***	***146***	***5.1***	***133***	***21.4***	***0.0***	***4.6***	***0.0***
HORSERADISH								
Prepared, Average	***1 Tsp/5g***	***3***	***0.0***	***62***	***4.5***	***11.0***	***0.3***	***6.2***
HOT CHOCOLATE								
Balanced Lifestyle, Camelot*	1 Sachet/11g	40	1.6	363	18.5	40.6	14.1	0.5
Cadbury*	1 Serving/12g	44	0.7	370	6.3	73.3	5.9	0.0
Caramel, Whittards of Chelsea*	1 Serving/20g	71	1.5	355	7.5	64.5	7.5	13.0
Caramel Flavoured, Instant, Dry, Aldi*	1 Serving/11g	40	1.6	363	18.5	40.6	14.1	8.5
Chococino, Dulce Gusto, Nescafe*	1 Serving/34g	149	5.5	437	14.6	58.6	16.1	4.6
Chocolate Break, Dry, Tesco*	1 Serving/21g	110	6.0	524	7.9	58.9	28.5	1.7
Cocoa, Lidl*	1 Serving/20g	77	1.2	386	6.1	74.1	6.2	0.0
Dreamtime, Whittards of Chelsea*	5 Tsps/20g	72	1.0	361	6.6	72.4	5.1	8.7
Drink, Organic, Green & Black's*	1 Tsp/4g	13	0.3	374	9.1	63.5	9.3	0.1
Drink, Twinings*	3 Tbsp/21g	81	0.7	387	5.0	82.0	3.3	6.0
Dry Weight, Tassimo, Suchard*	1 Cup/27g	88	2.4	325	3.2	58.0	8.9	2.6
Fairtrade, Whittards of Chelsea*	4 Tsp/20g	68	0.8	342	7.8	69.0	3.9	10.9
From Coffee Shop, Waitrose*	1 Serving/298ml	217	5.9	73	3.6	10.9	2.0	0.0
Galaxy, Mars*	1 Sachet/25g	97	1.9	386	4.8	71.9	7.7	4.7
Horlicks*	1 Serving/32g	128	2.6	400	8.8	72.5	8.1	3.8
Impress*	1 Serving/25g	90	0.9	360	5.6	76.0	3.6	6.0
Instant, BGTY, Made Up, Sainsbury's*	1 Sachet/28g	16	0.2	56	2.1	10.6	0.6	0.3
Instant, Skinny Cow*	1 Sachet/10g	37	1.5	370	19.7	39.3	14.6	0.0
Instant, Tesco*	1 Serving/32g	155	10.3	485	10.5	38.1	32.3	5.0
Instant Break, Cadbury*	1 Sachet/28g	119	3.9	425	10.9	64.2	14.0	0.0
Light, Caramel Flavour, Kruger*	1 Sachet/10g	37	1.4	370	13.0	41.4	14.2	6.8
Light, Hazelnut Flavour, Kruger*	1 Sachet/10g	37	1.4	370	13.0	41.4	14.2	6.8
Luxury, Skinny, Whittards of Chelsea*	1 Serving/28g	92	0.8	328	12.9	67.1	2.8	13.5
Made Up, Tassimo, Suchard*	1 Serving/280ml	88	2.4	31	0.3	5.5	0.9	0.2
Milk Drink, Low Calorie, You Count, Love Life, Waitrose*	1 Serving/11g	37	0.3	339	21.2	57.1	2.9	5.5
Slim Fast*	1 Serving/59g	203	2.8	347	22.2	53.8	4.8	8.4
Velvet, Cadbury*	1 Serving/28g	136	6.9	487	8.6	57.8	24.6	2.0
Wispa, Hot Frothy, Cadbury*	1 Sachet/27g	107	1.4	395	11.0	74.0	5.3	2.9
HOT DOG								
American Style, Hunters*	1 Sausage/23g	50	3.4	220	12.5	8.7	15.0	0.1
Sausage, American Style, Average	1 Sausage/75g	180	14.3	241	11.6	6.2	19.0	0.0
Sausage, Average	1 Sausage/23g	40	3.0	175	10.8	4.3	12.8	0.3
HOT DOG VEGETARIAN								
Meat Free, Sainsbury's*	1 Sausage/30g	71	4.5	237	18.0	7.6	15.0	1.0
Tesco*	1 Sausage/30g	66	4.5	220	18.0	2.7	15.0	2.0
HOT POT								
Beef, Healthy Options, Birds Eye*	1 Pack/350g	294	7.0	84	4.5	12.0	2.0	1.2
Beef, Minced, Sainsbury's*	1 Pack/450g	464	22.0	103	5.3	9.5	4.9	2.2
Beef, Ross*	1 Pack/310g	255	11.2	82	2.2	9.4	3.6	1.5
Beef, Weight Watchers*	1 Pack/320g	231	7.7	72	3.6	8.4	2.4	1.6
Chicken, Chunky, Weight Watchers*	1 Pack/320g	275	9.0	86	4.7	10.4	2.8	0.6
Chicken, Co-Op*	1 Pack/340g	289	10.2	85	6.0	9.0	3.0	0.7
Chicken, Frozen, Asda*	1 Pack/400g	300	6.0	75	5.5	9.9	1.5	0.8
Chicken, LC, Tesco*	1 Pack/347g	260	5.2	75	4.9	8.7	1.5	1.4
Chicken, Sainsbury's*	1 Pack/400g	340	11.0	85	5.2	9.8	2.8	1.3
Chicken & Cider, Ready Meals, Waitrose*	1 Pack/400g	500	20.4	125	6.8	12.9	5.1	1.1
Lamb, Cumbrian, Look What We Found*	1 Pack/300g	276	5.4	92	8.9	10.1	1.8	3.0
Lamb, Diet Chef Ltd*	1 Pack/300g	276	5.4	92	8.9	10.1	1.8	3.0
Lamb, Heinz*	1 Pack/340g	337	10.5	99	4.9	12.7	3.1	1.7

	Measure INFO/WEIGHT	per Measure KCAL	FAT	Nutrition Values per 100g / 100ml KCAL	PROT	CARB	FAT	FIBRE
HOT POT								
Lamb, Minced, Mini Classics, Asda*	1 Pack/300g	222	10.5	74	5.3	5.4	3.5	3.3
Lamb Shank, Extra Special, Asda*	1 Pack/450g	508	20.2	113	10.2	7.8	4.5	1.3
Lancashire, Asda*	1 Pack/401g	269	5.2	67	3.8	10.0	1.3	0.9
Lancashire, M & S*	1 Pack/454g	431	15.0	95	10.1	6.7	3.3	1.0
Lancashire, Weight-Away*	1 Pack/250g	214	5.3	85	8.8	7.2	2.1	1.5
Liver & Bacon, Tesco*	1 Pack/550g	693	31.4	126	6.4	12.3	5.7	1.5
Sausage, Aunt Bessie's*	¼ Pack/200g	212	9.2	106	3.6	12.6	4.6	1.9
Sausage, Smart Price, Asda*	1 Pack/300g	239	7.0	80	3.7	11.0	2.3	0.4
Sausage, with Baked Beans, Heinz*	1 Can/340g	354	10.9	104	4.6	14.3	3.2	2.4
Vegetable, Chunky, & Tomato, Big Eat, Heinz*	1 Pot/355g	213	1.4	60	2.5	11.7	0.4	4.1
Vegetable, Ready Meal, Average	1 Serving/400g	261	7.4	65	1.9	10.7	1.9	1.9
Vegetable, Vegetable Recipes, Ross*	1 Pack/300g	159	5.4	53	1.5	9.4	1.8	1.6
Vegetable, Weight Watchers*	1 Pack/335g	228	6.4	68	2.6	9.9	1.9	1.5
Vegetarian Sausage & Vegetable, Linda McCartney*	1 Pot/400g	516	20.4	129	6.4	15.7	5.1	2.3
HOUMOUS								
40% Less fat, Eat Smart, Morrisons*	½ Pack/85g	209	15.0	246	7.9	13.8	17.7	2.7
Aubergine, Roasted, M & S*	½ Pot/85g	132	10.3	155	4.9	6.9	12.1	5.1
Avocado, Fresh, San Amvrosia*	1 Serving/50g	172	16.0	344	5.4	8.5	32.1	2.5
Broad Bean, Asparagus & Mint, Tesco*	¼ Pot/42g	120	9.7	285	7.1	9.7	23.0	3.7
Caramelised Onion, Tesco*	¼ Pack/50g	125	9.7	250	5.5	13.0	19.4	4.2
Chilli & Red Pepper, Topped, Tesco*	½ Pack/100g	281	25.1	281	7.1	6.6	25.1	8.1
Feta, Fresh, Sainsbury's*	1 Serving/100g	292	27.4	292	8.0	3.5	27.4	6.7
Fresh, Waitrose*	1 Serving/75g	219	19.8	292	7.2	6.3	26.4	7.6
Garlic & Pesto, Asda*	1 Serving/34g	107	8.8	314	8.0	12.0	26.0	0.0
GFY, Asda*	1 Serving/50g	136	10.0	272	9.0	14.0	20.0	3.8
Indian Spiced, Glorious!*	1 Serving/100g	78	3.9	78	5.2	14.0	3.9	3.0
Jalapeno, Asda*	1 Serving/50g	166	14.5	331	7.0	10.6	29.0	4.5
Lemon & Coriander, BGTY, Sainsbury's*	½ Tub/100g	145	9.0	145	6.3	9.7	9.0	5.9
Lemon & Coriander, Sainsbury's*	¼ Tub/50g	146	12.6	291	7.0	9.1	25.1	6.0
Mediterranean Deli, M & S*	¼ Pack/70g	203	17.7	290	7.8	8.0	25.3	6.5
Moroccan, Tesco*	¼ Pot/50g	144	12.8	289	6.8	8.1	25.5	7.3
Olive & Sun Dried Tomato, Tesco*	1 Serving/50g	118	9.8	235	6.5	8.0	19.5	7.4
Olive & Tomato, Mixed, Sainsbury's*	¼ Tub/50g	136	12.6	272	6.0	5.3	25.2	7.4
Organic, M & S*	¼ Pack/25g	82	7.4	330	6.9	9.1	29.7	3.3
Organic, Sainsbury's*	¼ Pot/43g	139	12.1	326	6.8	10.7	28.4	3.5
Red Pepper, Roasted, 50% Less Fat, Tesco*	½ Pot/85g	156	10.5	184	7.3	10.9	12.4	9.5
Red Pepper, Roasted, Sainsbury's*	½ Pot/100g	317	27.2	317	6.2	9.0	27.2	5.7
Red Pepper, Roasted, VLH Kitchens	1 Serving/17g	31	49.4	183	6.5	15.6	8.4	6.2
Reduced Fat, Average	1 Tbsp/30g	72	5.0	241	9.2	13.3	16.8	3.6
Sea Salt & Cracked Black Pepper, Tesco*	¼ Pot/50g	148	13.6	295	7.0	4.8	27.2	9.5
Sweet Chilli, Tesco*	¼ Pot/50g	120	8.4	240	6.9	15.2	16.7	5.4
Three Bean, Reduced Fat, BGTY, Sainsbury's*	¼ Tub/50g	92	6.0	183	7.3	11.4	12.0	6.0
HULA HOOPS								
Bacon & Ketchup Flavour, KP Snacks*	1 Bag/27g	140	8.3	517	3.4	56.3	30.9	2.0
BBQ Beef, 55% Less Saturated Fat, KP Snacks*	1 Pack/34g	172	9.0	505	3.7	61.8	26.4	2.2
Cheese & Onion 55% Less Saturated Fat, KP Snacks*	1 Bag/34g	175	9.7	515	3.6	61.0	28.5	1.9
Chilli Salsa,Tortilla, KP Snacks*	1 Bag/25g	124	6.8	494	4.9	57.2	27.3	5.3
Multigrain, KP Snacks*	1 Pack/23g	113	5.9	491	5.6	60.0	25.6	4.4
Original, 55% Less Saturated Fat, KP Snacks*	1 Bag/34g	175	9.7	515	3.2	61.6	28.4	1.8
Original, Minis, KP Snacks*	1 Tub/140g	752	48.7	537	3.0	52.9	34.8	1.7
Salt & Vinegar, 50% Less Saturated Fat, KP Snacks*	1 Bag/25g	128	7.0	510	3.1	60.9	28.2	1.8

	Measure INFO/WEIGHT	per Measure KCAL	FAT	Nutrition Values per 100g / 100ml KCAL	PROT	CARB	FAT	FIBRE
ICE CREAM								
After Dinner, Mint, Dairy, Asda*	1 Serving/100g	182	8.0	182	3.4	24.0	8.0	0.4
After Eight, Nestle*	1 Serving/55g	114	5.2	207	3.6	27.1	9.4	0.3
Almond Indulgence, Sainsbury's*	1 Serving/120g	286	18.8	238	2.8	21.4	15.7	0.6
Baked Alaska, Ben & Jerry's*	1 Serving/100g	260	15.0	260	4.0	29.0	15.0	0.1
Banana Split, Tesco*	1 Scoop/53g	115	4.5	215	2.8	30.9	8.4	0.8
Bananas Foster, Haagen-Dazs*	1 Serving/125ml	260	15.0	208	3.2	22.4	12.0	0.0
Banoffee, Haagen-Dazs*	1 Serving/120ml	274	15.6	228	4.0	23.0	13.0	0.0
Banoffee Fudge, Sainsbury's*	1/8 Pot/67g	119	4.0	178	2.8	28.7	5.9	0.2
Billionaire Shortcake, Chokablok*	1 Scoop/100ml	225	11.4	225	2.8	27.0	11.4	0.7
Bourbon Biscuit, Asda*	1 Dessert/37g	120	4.5	324	5.9	48.6	12.2	1.6
Brandy, Luxurious, M & S*	1 Serving/100g	228	13.3	228	3.8	19.1	13.3	0.2
Cappuccino, Thorntons*	1oz/28g	61	3.6	218	4.4	20.7	12.9	0.0
Caramel & Cinnamon Waffle, Carte d'Or*	2 Scoops/55g	121	6.0	220	3.0	27.0	11.0	0.0
Caramel Chew Chew, Ben & Jerry's*	1 Tub/150ml	305	18.1	270	3.0	29.0	16.0	0.0
Caramel Craze, Organic, Tesco*	1 Serving/100g	253	15.3	253	3.3	25.5	15.3	0.0
Caramella, Tesco*	1 Serving/51g	120	5.5	235	2.6	32.0	10.7	1.1
Cheeky Choc, Brownie, Skinny Cow*	1 Tub/500ml	590	5.5	118	3.0	23.9	1.1	4.1
Cheesecake Brownie, Ben & Jerry's*	1 Serving/100g	260	16.0	260	4.0	26.0	16.0	0.0
Cherry Bomb Brownie, Chokablok*	1 Scoop/87g	191	8.3	220	3.3	29.9	9.5	1.4
Cherry Garcia, Ben & Jerry's*	1 Serving/100g	250	15.0	250	3.0	26.0	15.0	0.0
Chilli Red, Purbeck*	1 Serving/50g	99	5.8	198	4.8	18.7	11.5	0.0
Choc Chip, Cookie Dough, Haagen-Dazs*	1oz/28g	74	4.7	266	3.8	24.9	16.9	0.0
Choc Chip, Haagen-Dazs*	1oz/28g	80	5.2	286	4.7	24.8	18.7	0.0
Chocolate, Belgian, Haagen-Dazs*	1 Tub/100ml	249	16.2	318	4.6	28.4	20.7	0.0
Chocolate, Double, Nestle*	1 Serving/78g	248	14.3	320	4.8	33.7	18.4	0.0
Chocolate, Haagen-Dazs*	1 Serving/120ml	269	18.0	224	4.0	19.0	15.0	0.0
Chocolate, Organic, Green & Black's*	1 Serving/125g	310	17.6	248	5.0	25.3	14.1	1.1
Chocolate, Soft Scoop, Asda*	1 Scoop/47g	84	3.8	179	3.7	23.0	8.0	0.0
Chocolate, Swirl Pot, Skinny Cow*	1 Pot/100ml	98	0.6	98	2.9	20.2	0.6	2.7
Chocolate, Thorntons*	1oz/28g	67	3.6	238	4.6	25.1	12.9	0.0
Chocolate, Triple, Brownie, Skinny Cow*	1 Ice Cream/65g	93	1.7	144	3.5	24.1	2.6	5.3
Chocolate, Triple, Carte d'Or*	1 Serving/58g	122	5.7	210	3.7	27.0	9.8	0.0
Chocolate, Triple, Centenary, Cadbury*	1 Serving/100ml	255	15.6	255	2.5	27.1	15.6	0.0
Chocolate, Weight Watchers*	1 Serving/100ml	140	1.2	140	4.3	28.7	1.2	0.0
Chocolate & Nut, Creamy, Co-Op*	1oz/28g	66	3.6	235	4.0	25.0	13.0	0.5
Chocolate & Orange, Organic, Green & Black's*	1 Serving/100g	248	14.1	248	5.0	25.3	14.1	0.1
Chocolate Chip, Baskin Robbins*	1 Serving/75g	170	10.0	227	4.0	24.0	13.3	0.0
Chocolate Chip, Cornetto Soft, Wall's Ice Cream*	1 Serving/80g	256	13.6	320	3.5	37.0	17.0	1.5
Chocolate Chip, Mint, Cornetto Soft, Wall's Ice Cream*	1 Serving/80g	240	13.6	300	4.0	33.0	17.0	1.0
Chocolate Flavour, Average	1 Serving/70g	149	7.9	212	4.1	23.7	11.3	0.6
Chocolate Flavour, Healthy Option, Average	1 Serving/70g	89	1.2	127	3.5	25.9	1.7	0.3
Chocolate Fudge Brownie, Ben & Jerry's*	1 Mini Tub 150ml	285	14.8	250	4.0	32.0	13.0	1.5
Chocolate Fudge Swirl, Haagen-Dazs*	1oz/28g	77	4.8	276	4.6	25.6	17.2	0.0
Chocolate Honeycomb, Co-Op*	¼ Pot/81g	186	10.5	230	4.0	26.0	13.0	0.3
Chocolate Honeycomb, COU, M & S*	1 Serving/100ml	150	2.6	150	3.5	31.5	2.6	0.7
Chocolate Macadamia, Ben & Jerry's*	1 Serving/100g	260	18.0	260	4.0	22.0	18.0	0.8
Chocolate Midnight Cookies, Haagen-Dazs*	1oz/28g	81	4.8	289	4.9	28.7	17.2	0.0
Chocolate Orange, Deliciously Dairy, Co-Op*	1oz/28g	55	2.0	195	4.0	29.0	7.0	0.8
Chocolate Ripple, Perfectly Balanced, Waitrose*	1 Serving/125ml	205	3.1	164	4.8	30.5	2.5	4.1
Chocolate Sandwich, Skinny Cow*	1 Portion/36g	101	2.8	280	6.0	46.0	7.9	2.9
Chocolatino, Sundae, Tesco*	1 Tub/80g	160	5.9	200	4.4	29.0	7.4	2.4
Chocolatino, Tesco*	1 Serving/56g	115	3.8	205	3.4	31.4	6.8	1.8
Chunky Monkey, Ben & Jerry's*	1 Serving/100g	290	17.0	290	4.0	27.0	17.0	1.0

I

	Measure INFO/WEIGHT	per Measure KCAL	FAT	Nutrition Values per 100g / 100ml KCAL	PROT	CARB	FAT	FIBRE
ICE CREAM								
Coconut, Carte d'Or*	1 Serving/100ml	125	7.1	125	1.8	14.0	7.1	0.5
Coffee, Haagen-Dazs*	1 Serving/120ml	271	18.4	226	4.1	17.9	15.3	0.0
Coffee, Waitrose*	¼ Tub/125ml	292	16.4	234	3.6	25.4	13.1	0.0
Cookie Dough, Ben & Jerry's*	1 Serving/100g	270	14.0	270	4.0	31.0	14.0	0.0
Cookie Dough Mon Star, Chokablok*	1 Serving/100g	285	17.1	285	3.3	29.5	17.1	0.6
Cookies & Cream, Haagen-Dazs*	1 Sm Tub/100ml	226	14.7	226	4.0	19.5	14.7	0.0
Cornish, Dairy, Tesco*	1 Serving/49g	112	6.0	228	3.2	24.7	12.3	0.1
Cornish, Full Fat, Asda*	1 Serving/100g	204	11.6	204	3.5	21.4	11.6	0.1
Cornish Blackberry, Traditional, M & S*	1oz/28g	61	3.0	218	2.3	28.0	10.8	0.3
Cornish Strawberry, Traditional, M & S*	1oz/28g	64	3.1	229	2.3	29.7	11.2	0.2
Crema Di Mascarpone, Carte d'Or*	1 Serving/100g	207	8.9	207	2.8	29.0	8.9	0.0
Dairy, Flavoured	1oz/28g	50	2.2	179	3.5	24.7	8.0	0.0
Dairy Milk, Orange, Cadbury*	1 Serving/120ml	259	13.9	216	3.5	26.0	11.6	0.0
Date & Almond Cream, Haagen-Dazs*	1 Serving/120ml	254	15.6	212	5.0	19.0	13.0	0.0
Fig & Orange Blossom Honey, Waitrose*	1 Serving/100g	219	11.8	219	3.9	24.3	11.8	0.4
Fruit & Fresh Tropical, Carte d'Or*	1 Serving/83g	154	7.1	185	2.5	24.5	8.5	0.0
Fun-Illa, Skinny Cow*	1 Serving/100ml	97	1.6	97	3.1	17.6	1.6	2.4
Gelato, Vanilla	1 Serving/100g	162	7.2	162	2.4	22.6	7.2	0.3
Gold Digger Dynamite, Chokablok*	¼ Tub/125ml	288	14.0	230	3.2	28.2	11.2	0.9
Greek Yoghurt & Honey, Carte d'Or*	1 Serving/55g	114	4.8	207	2.7	29.0	8.8	0.0
Half Baked, Ben & Jerry's*	1 Serving/100g	270	13.0	270	5.0	32.0	13.0	1.0
Heavenly Vanilla, Cadbury*	1 Serving/250ml	355	23.2	142	2.5	12.8	9.3	0.0
Honeycomb Harvest, Mackies*	1 Serving/100g	209	10.0	209	4.0	25.0	10.0	0.0
Hunky Punky Chocolate, Booja-Booja*	1 Tub/500ml	685	33.0	137	3.3	17.5	6.6	0.0
Knickerbocker Glory	1oz/28g	31	1.4	112	1.5	16.4	5.0	0.2
Lactose Free, Hacendado*	1 Serving/100g	141	4.9	141	4.0	27.6	4.9	6.6
Lavazza, Carte d'Or*	1 Serving/55g	120	5.4	218	3.5	29.0	9.9	0.0
Lemon, Haagen-Dazs*	1 Serving/120ml	144	0.2	120	0.3	29.3	0.2	0.0
Lemon & White Chocolate, Crackpots, Iceland*	1 Serving/100g	202	8.4	202	1.7	29.9	8.4	0.3
Lemon Cream, Dairy, Sainsbury's*	1 Serving/100g	199	9.3	199	3.0	25.9	9.3	0.1
Lemon Curd Swirl, Duchy Originals*	¼ Pot/101g	247	14.2	245	3.7	25.8	14.1	0.0
Lemon Pie, Haagen-Dazs*	1oz/28g	73	4.6	262	3.9	24.5	16.3	0.0
Lychee Cream & Ginger, Haagen-Dazs*	1 Serving/120ml	258	12.7	215	3.6	26.1	10.6	0.0
Macadamia Nut, Baskin Robbins*	1 Serving/113g	270	18.0	239	4.4	22.1	15.9	0.9
Madly Deeply, Skinny Cow*	1 Serving/100g	149	2.2	149	4.2	28.3	2.2	3.4
Magnum Moments, Wall's Ice Cream*	1 Serving/18ml	58	3.7	323	4.0	30.0	20.8	0.0
Mango, 98% Fat Free, Bulla*	1 Serving/70g	94	1.1	134	4.2	25.4	1.6	0.0
Maple & Walnut, American, Sainsbury's*	1/8 Pot/68g	121	4.9	179	3.1	25.6	7.2	0.2
Maple Brazil, Thorntons*	1oz/28g	66	3.8	236	4.1	24.4	13.6	0.0
Mascarpone Forest Fruits, Taste Sensation, Aldi*	1 Pot/73g	159	7.4	217	1.8	29.6	10.1	0.6
Mince Pie, Finest, Tesco*	¼ Pack/188g	476	22.1	254	3.9	33.0	11.8	1.1
Mint, Majestic Luxury, Iceland*	1 Serving/80g	269	14.6	337	3.8	39.3	18.3	1.3
Mint, Thorntons*	1oz/28g	66	3.8	237	4.0	25.0	13.4	0.0
Mint & Chocolate Flavour, Average	1 Serving/70g	129	6.3	184	3.0	22.6	9.0	1.2
Mint & Chocolate Flavour, Healthy Option, Average	1 Serving/70g	101	1.8	144	4.1	29.9	2.6	4.1
Mint Crisp, Nestle*	1 Serving/75ml	232	16.4	309	2.9	25.5	21.9	0.9
Mint Crunch, Dairy Milk, Cadbury*	1 Serving/60ml	162	13.3	270	3.0	29.0	22.2	0.0
Mint Ripple, Good Choice, Iceland*	1 Scoop/50g	58	1.0	117	3.0	21.7	2.1	0.1
Mojito, Appassionato, YSCO*	1 Serving/100g	150	2.9	150	0.3	30.2	2.9	0.2
My Carte D'or, Caramel, Carte d'Or*	1 Tub/200ml	210	8.0	105	1.5	16.0	4.0	0.2
My Carte D'or, Chocolate, Carte d'Or*	1 Tub/200ml	220	11.0	110	1.8	12.5	5.5	0.4
Neapolitan, Average	1 Serving/70g	111	4.6	158	3.1	21.9	6.5	0.6
Neapolitan, Soft Scoop, Asda*	1 Scoop/47g	82	3.8	175	2.8	23.0	8.0	0.2

	Measure INFO/WEIGHT	per Measure KCAL	FAT	Nutrition Values per 100g / 100ml KCAL	PROT	CARB	FAT	FIBRE
ICE CREAM								
Neapolitan Sandwich, Gelatelli*	1 Sandwich/106g	233	9.5	220	4.9	29.0	9.0	1.9
Non-Dairy, Mixes	1oz/28g	51	2.2	182	4.1	25.1	7.9	0.0
Non-Dairy, Reduced Calorie	1oz/28g	33	1.7	119	3.4	13.7	6.0	0.0
Nuts About Caramel, Cadbury*	1 Ice/100ml	290	17.1	290	4.3	28.1	17.1	2.6
Panna Cotta, & Raspberry Swirl, Haagen-Dazs*	1 Serving/120ml	250	14.9	208	3.2	21.0	12.4	0.0
Panna Cotta, Haagen-Dazs*	1 Serving/120ml	248	16.0	207	3.4	18.4	13.3	0.0
Peach Melba, Soft Scoop, M & S*	1oz/28g	46	2.1	165	2.8	21.4	7.6	0.3
Pistachio, Haagen-Dazs*	1 Serving/120ml	276	18.8	230	4.4	17.7	15.7	0.0
Praline, Green & Black's*	1 Sm Pot/100g	191	10.8	191	3.5	20.0	10.8	0.9
Praline & Chocolate, Thorntons*	1oz/28g	87	6.4	309	4.6	21.3	22.9	0.6
Pralines & Cream, Baskin Robbins*	1 Serving/100g	252	13.6	252	4.5	27.7	13.6	0.3
Pralines & Cream, Haagen-Dazs*	1 Tub 100ml	213	12.9	272	3.9	27.2	16.5	0.0
Raspberries, Clotted Cream, Waitrose*	1 Tub/500ml	790	39.5	158	2.9	18.9	7.9	0.1
Raspberry, Easy Serve, Co-Op*	1oz/28g	43	1.7	152	2.5	22.3	5.9	0.0
Raspberry, Haagen-Dazs*	1 Serving/120ml	127	0.2	106	0.2	25.9	0.2	0.0
Raspberry, Swirl Pot, Skinny Cow*	1 Pot/100ml	86	0.3	86	2.5	18.4	0.3	2.2
Raspberry & Shortcake, Co-Op*	1oz/28g	64	3.9	230	3.0	23.0	14.0	0.3
Raspberry Ripple, Average	1 Serving/70g	93	3.3	134	1.9	20.8	4.7	0.1
Raspberry Ripple, Soft Scoop, Sainsbury's*	1 Serving/75g	128	5.2	170	2.6	24.2	7.0	0.3
Rocky Road, M & S*	1 Tub/500g	1475	88.5	295	4.2	29.5	17.7	1.2
Rolo, Nestle*	½ Tub/500ml	1180	52.5	236	3.4	31.9	10.5	0.2
Rum & Raisin, Carte d'Or*	2 Scoops/50g	100	4.0	200	2.5	24.0	8.0	1.0
Rum & Raisin, Haagen-Dazs*	1 Serving/120ml	264	17.6	220	3.4	18.6	14.7	0.0
Rum & Raisin, Organic, Iceland*	1oz/28g	55	2.0	195	4.5	28.1	7.2	0.0
Rum & Raisin, TTD, Sainsbury's*	¼ Pot/100g	220	10.4	220	3.8	27.7	10.4	1.0
Screwball, Asda*	1 Screwball/60g	122	6.0	203	3.3	25.0	10.0	1.5
Smarties, Nestle*	1 Serving/50g	125	6.0	250	3.6	32.3	11.9	0.2
Smarties, Pot, Nestle*	1 Pot/69g	151	5.7	218	4.4	33.6	8.2	0.0
Spagnola, Carte d'Or*	1 Serving/100g	187	5.7	187	2.0	32.0	5.7	0.0
Stem Ginger, with Belgian Chocolate, Waitrose*	1 Lolly/110g	255	14.4	232	2.9	25.5	13.1	1.7
Sticky Toffee, Cream O' Galloway*	1 Serving/30g	80	4.4	266	4.7	28.7	14.7	0.0
Strawberries & Cream, Deliciously Dairy, Co-Op*	1oz/28g	46	1.7	165	3.0	24.0	6.0	0.3
Strawberry, Cornetto Soft, Wall's Ice Cream*	1 Serving/80g	208	8.0	260	2.5	38.0	10.0	1.0
Strawberry, Get Fruit, Solero*	1 Serving/100ml	120	4.5	120	1.5	18.8	4.5	1.3
Strawberry, Haagen-Dazs*	1oz/28g	67	4.3	241	4.0	21.5	15.5	0.0
Strawberry, Soft Scoop, Tesco*	1 Serving/46g	78	3.4	170	2.8	23.1	7.4	0.1
Strawberry, Swirl Pot, Skinny Cow*	1 Pot/100ml	89	0.3	89	2.5	19.0	0.3	2.2
Strawberry, Thorntons*	1oz/28g	52	2.6	185	3.2	22.5	9.3	0.1
Strawberry, Weight Watchers*	1 Pot/57g	81	2.2	142	2.5	23.4	3.9	0.2
Strawberry & Cream, Mivvi, Nestle*	1 Serving/60g	118	4.6	196	2.6	29.4	7.6	0.2
Strawberry & Cream, Organic, Sainsbury's*	1 Serving/100g	193	9.8	193	3.6	22.6	9.8	0.4
Strawberry & Yoghurt Delice, Carte d'Or*	1 Portion/54g	95	2.0	175	1.5	34.0	3.6	0.0
Strawberry Cheesecake, Ben & Jerry's*	1 Serving 100g	240	14.0	240	3.0	27.0	14.0	0.0
Strawberry Cheesecake, Co-Op*	1/6 Pot/86g	163	6.0	190	3.0	29.0	7.0	0.2
Strawberry Cheesecake, Haagen-Dazs*	¼ Tub/125ml	295	17.0	236	3.3	25.1	13.6	0.3
Terry's Chocolate Orange, Carte d'Or*	1 Serving/100g	182	7.1	182	2.8	27.0	7.1	0.0
Tiramisu, COU, M & S*	¼ Tub/86g	120	2.5	140	2.1	26.4	2.9	3.0
Tiramisu, Haagen-Dazs*	1 Serving/120ml	303	19.6	253	3.8	22.7	16.3	0.0
Toblerone, Carte d'Or*	1 Serving/100g	211	9.1	211	3.7	29.0	9.1	0.0
Toffee, Dark, Organic, Green & Black's*	¼ Pot/125ml	192	9.9	154	2.8	18.1	7.9	0.1
Toffee, Deliciously Dairy, Co-Op*	1oz/28g	45	2.0	160	3.0	21.0	7.0	0.2
Toffee, Farmhouse, TTD, Sainsbury's*	¼ Pot/100g	293	18.6	293	3.2	28.3	18.6	0.6
Toffee, Swirl Pot, Skinny Cow*	1 Pot/66g	92	0.4	140	3.8	29.8	0.6	4.5

	Measure INFO/WEIGHT	per Measure KCAL	FAT	Nutrition Values per 100g / 100ml KCAL	PROT	CARB	FAT	FIBRE
ICE CREAM								
Toffee, Tantilising, COU, M & S*	¼ Pot/125ml	125	3.5	100	0.6	18.0	2.8	0.0
Toffee, Thorntons*	1oz/28g	61	3.2	218	4.1	24.5	11.6	0.0
Toffee & Biscuit, Weight Watchers*	1 Pot/100ml	93	2.7	93	1.5	14.9	2.7	0.1
Toffee & Honeycomb Sundaes, Weight Watchers*	1 Pot/98g	119	1.8	122	1.7	18.1	1.8	5.9
Toffee & Vanilla, Sainsbury's*	1 Serving/71g	146	6.8	205	3.1	26.7	9.5	0.1
Toffee Creme, Haagen-Dazs*	1oz/28g	74	4.4	265	4.5	26.7	15.6	0.0
Toffee Fudge, Soft Scoop, Asda*	1 Serving/50g	92	3.5	185	2.6	28.0	7.0	0.0
Toffee Ripple, Tesco*	1 Serving/100g	173	7.2	173	2.7	24.4	7.2	0.1
Toffee Vanilla, HE, Tesco*	1 Serving/73g	106	1.8	145	2.5	28.1	2.5	0.5
Truffle Berry Fling, Skinny Cow*	1 Serving/100g	156	2.0	156	4.0	30.5	2.0	3.3
Truly Lovin' Toffee, Skinny Cow*	1 Tub/352g	510	3.5	145	3.5	30.5	1.0	6.6
Vanilla, Ben & Jerry's*	1 Tub 150ml	258	16.8	230	4.0	20.0	15.0	0.1
Vanilla, Carte d'Or*	1 Serving/50g	105	4.8	210	3.0	26.0	9.5	0.0
Vanilla, Cornish, Organic, Iceland*	1oz/28g	60	3.5	214	4.1	21.4	12.4	0.0
Vanilla, Cornish, Soft Scoop, M & S*	1oz/28g	56	3.0	199	3.9	21.8	10.7	0.2
Vanilla, COU, M & S*	¼ Pot/79g	111	2.2	140	1.7	25.9	2.8	0.8
Vanilla, Criminally Creamy, Co-Op*	1oz/28g	60	4.2	215	3.0	18.0	15.0	0.1
Vanilla, Dairy, Average	1 Scoop/40g	80	4.4	201	3.5	23.6	11.0	0.7
Vanilla, Dairy, Organic, Yeo Valley*	1 Serving/100g	206	11.2	206	4.9	21.3	11.2	0.0
Vanilla, Dairy Milk, Cadbury*	1 Serving/120g	259	13.9	216	3.5	26.0	11.6	0.1
Vanilla, Fairtrade, Ben & Jerry's*	1 Serving/100g	230	15.0	230	4.0	20.0	15.0	0.1
Vanilla, Haagen-Dazs*	1oz/28g	70	4.8	250	4.5	19.7	17.1	0.0
Vanilla, Light, Carte d'Or*	1 Serving/100g	136	4.4	136	2.4	22.0	4.4	4.0
Vanilla, Light Soft Scoop, 25% Less Fat, Morrisons*	1 Scoop/50g	75	2.5	150	2.9	23.2	5.0	0.2
Vanilla, Low Fat, Average	1 Scoop/50g	59	1.7	118	2.3	19.4	3.4	0.6
Vanilla, Low Fat, Weight Watchers*	1 Scoop/125ml	75	2.1	60	1.1	9.7	1.7	0.1
Vanilla, Mackies*	1 Serving/100g	193	11.0	193	4.0	18.0	11.0	0.0
Vanilla, Non-Dairy, Average	1 Serving/60g	107	5.2	178	3.2	23.1	8.7	0.0
Vanilla, Organic, Iceland*	1oz/28g	61	3.4	217	4.5	22.2	12.2	0.0
Vanilla, Organic, Sainsbury's*	1 Serving/85g	176	10.2	207	4.3	20.5	12.0	0.1
Vanilla, Organic, Tesco*	1 Serving/100g	237	17.2	237	3.7	16.8	17.2	0.0
Vanilla, Organic, Waitrose*	1 Serving/125g	178	11.2	142	2.7	12.4	9.0	0.0
Vanilla, Pecan, Haagen-Dazs*	1 Serving/120ml	316	23.5	263	4.3	17.1	19.6	0.0
Vanilla, Pizza Express*	1 Serving/100g	119	6.8	119	0.9	13.8	6.8	0.0
Vanilla, Really Creamy, Asda*	1 Serving/50g	98	5.0	196	3.5	23.0	10.0	0.1
Vanilla, Sandwich, Skinny Cow*	1 Portion/36g	100	3.0	277	5.4	45.1	8.2	2.1
Vanilla, Smart Price, Asda*	1 Scoop/40g	55	2.4	137	2.8	19.0	6.0	0.2
Vanilla, Soft, Non Milk Fat, Waitrose*	1 Serving/125ml	78	3.4	62	1.3	8.0	2.7	0.1
Vanilla, Soft Scoop, 25% Less Fat, Asda*	1oz/28g	42	1.4	149	2.9	23.0	5.0	0.0
Vanilla, Soft Scoop, BGTY, Sainsbury's*	1 Serving/75g	88	1.3	117	3.1	22.2	1.7	0.2
Vanilla, Soft Scoop, GFY, Asda*	1 Serving/100g	117	1.7	117	3.1	22.0	1.7	0.2
Vanilla, Soft Scoop, Light, Wall's*, Wall's Ice Cream*	1 Scoop/50ml	31	1.3	62	1.3	7.0	2.6	0.9
Vanilla, Soft Scoop, Tesco*	1oz/28g	46	2.0	164	3.1	21.8	7.1	0.1
Vanilla, Soft Scoop, Value, Tesco*	1 Scoop/42g	57	2.4	137	2.8	18.7	5.7	0.2
Vanilla, Soft Slice, Wall's Ice Cream*	1 Serving/100ml	90	4.4	90	1.4	11.2	4.4	0.1
Vanilla, Thorntons*	1oz/28g	63	3.8	225	4.9	20.5	13.6	0.0
Vanilla, Toffee Crunch, Ben & Jerry's*	1 Tub/407g	1099	65.1	270	4.0	29.0	16.0	0.5
Vanilla, Too Good to Be True, Wall's Ice Cream*	1 Serving/50ml	35	0.2	70	2.0	14.9	0.4	0.1
Vanilla, Waitrose*	1 Serving/100ml	156	10.8	156	2.6	12.0	10.8	0.0
Vanilla, with Strawberry Swirl, Weight Watchers*	1 Mini Tub/57g	81	2.2	142	2.5	23.4	3.9	0.2
Vanilla, with Vanilla Pods, Sainsbury's*	1 Serving/100g	195	10.1	195	3.5	22.5	10.1	0.1
Vanilla & Cinnamon, Finest, Tesco*	1 Serving/50g	114	7.4	229	3.9	20.2	14.7	0.4
Vanilla & Cinnamon, Spar*	1 Serving/120g	247	10.3	206	3.8	28.0	8.6	0.0

	Measure INFO/WEIGHT	per Measure KCAL	FAT	Nutrition Values per 100g / 100ml KCAL	PROT	CARB	FAT	FIBRE
ICE CREAM								
Vanilla & Strawberry, Weight Watchers*	1 Serving/100ml	81	2.2	81	1.4	13.3	2.2	0.1
Vanilla Bean, Light, Deluxe*	1 Serving/64g	110	2.5	172	4.7	26.6	3.9	0.0
Vanilla Bean, Purbeck*	1 Serving/100g	198	11.5	198	4.8	18.7	11.5	0.0
Vanilla Caramel Brownie, Haagen-Dazs*	1 Serving/150g	410	24.8	273	4.5	26.8	16.5	0.0
Vanilla Choc Fudge, Haagen-Dazs*	1oz/28g	75	4.8	267	4.3	23.5	17.2	0.0
Vanilla Chocolate, Taste Sensation, Frosty's, Aldi*	1 Pot/73g	164	7.0	224	2.1	32.4	9.6	0.7
Vanilla Flavour, Budgens*	1oz/28g	45	1.9	159	3.0	21.7	6.7	0.1
Vanilla Flavour, Soft, VLH Kitchens	1 Serving/100g	235	15.0	235	4.0	22.1	15.0	0.2
Vanilla Flavour, Soft Scoop, Sainsbury's*	1 Serving/71g	96	3.9	136	2.9	18.8	5.5	0.2
Vanilletta, Tesco*	1 Serving/47g	82	3.8	175	4.0	21.6	8.1	0.0
ICE CREAM BAR								
Bailey's, Haagen-Dazs*	1oz/28g	86	5.9	307	4.1	24.8	21.2	0.0
Choc Chip, Haagen-Dazs*	1oz/28g	90	6.0	320	4.3	27.4	21.5	0.0
Chocolate, Chunky, Co-Op*	1 Bar/60g	204	12.0	340	5.0	35.0	20.0	1.0
Chocolate Covered	1 Bar/40g	128	9.3	320	5.0	24.0	23.3	0.0
Dairy Milk, Caramel, Cadbury*	1 Bar/60ml	175	10.3	290	3.6	30.2	17.1	0.0
Dairy Milk, Fruit & Nut, Cadbury*	1 Bar/90ml	243	15.3	270	3.5	26.1	17.0	0.0
Dairy Milk, Fudge, Cadbury*	1 Bar/60g	165	10.3	275	3.0	27.6	17.2	0.0
Dream, Cadbury*	1 Serving/118g	260	14.0	220	3.6	26.0	11.9	0.0
Galaxy, Mars*	1 Bar/60ml	203	13.4	339	4.7	29.7	22.4	0.0
Lion, Nestle*	1 Bar/45g	166	9.9	370	4.2	39.1	21.9	1.0
Maltesers, Mars*	1 Bar/45ml	113	7.0	252	2.9	25.0	15.6	0.7
Mars, Mars*	1 Bar/65g	182	10.5	280	3.4	29.7	16.2	0.8
Peanut, Farmfoods*	1 Bar/60ml	216	12.8	360	5.3	36.6	21.4	1.2
Racer, Aldi*	1 Bar/59g	194	11.0	328	6.0	34.2	18.6	0.0
Red Fruits, Solero*	1 Bar/80g	99	2.2	124	1.6	25.0	2.7	0.0
Snickers, Mars*	1 Bar/67g	250	15.0	373	6.0	37.3	22.4	0.0
Toffee, Chunky, Co-Op*	1 Bar/60g	204	12.6	340	4.0	34.0	21.0	1.0
Toffee Crunch, English, Weight Watchers*	1 Bar/40g	110	6.0	275	2.5	32.5	15.0	5.0
Twix, Mars*	1 Serving/43ml	128	7.3	301	4.0	32.0	17.1	1.2
Vanilla & Raspberry, Weight Watchers*	1 Serving/100g	81	0.3	81	2.0	23.0	0.3	0.0
Viennetta, Biscuit Caramel, Wall's Ice Cream*	1/6 Serving/58g	183	12.1	315	3.3	27.8	20.9	0.0
Viennetta, Cappuccino, Wall's Ice Cream*	1 Serving/75g	191	12.8	255	3.5	22.0	17.0	0.0
Viennetta, Chocolate, Wall's Ice Cream*	¼ Pot/80g	200	12.2	250	4.1	24.0	15.2	0.0
Viennetta, Forest Fruit, Wall's Ice Cream*	1 Serving/98g	265	15.9	270	3.4	27.2	16.2	0.0
Viennetta, Mint, Wall's Ice Cream*	1 Serving/80g	204	13.3	255	3.4	23.0	16.6	0.0
Viennetta, Selection Brownie, Wall's Ice Cream*	1 Serving/70g	194	11.3	277	4.2	28.5	16.2	0.0
Viennetta, Strawberry, Wall's Ice Cream*	1 Serving/80g	204	13.4	255	3.4	22.1	16.8	0.0
ICE CREAM CONE								
After Eight, Nestle*	1 Cone/100ml	174	8.0	174	2.4	23.0	8.0	0.9
Average	1 Cone/75g	140	6.4	186	3.5	25.5	8.5	0.0
Blackcurrant, GFY, Asda*	1 Cone/67g	162	6.0	241	3.0	37.0	9.0	0.1
Carousel Wafer Company*	1 Cone/5g	19	0.2	392	9.8	78.6	4.2	0.0
Choc 'n' Nut, Farmfoods*	1 Cone/120ml	334	16.8	278	5.0	33.0	14.0	1.0
Chocolate, Mini, Cornetto, Wall's Ice Cream*	1 Cone/36g	110	5.9	300	3.5	34.0	16.0	2.0
Chocolate, Vanilla & Hazelnut, Sainsbury's*	1 Cone/62g	190	10.5	306	4.5	33.9	16.9	0.6
Chocolate & Caramel, Skinny Cow*	1 Cone/110ml	121	2.8	110	2.5	19.3	2.5	2.7
Chocolate & Nut, Co-Op*	1 Cone/110g	307	17.0	279	3.9	31.0	15.5	0.6
Chocolate & Vanilla, Good Choice, Iceland*	1 Cone/110ml	161	7.2	146	2.7	22.9	6.5	0.8
Classico, Mini, Cornetto, Wall's Ice Cream*	1 Cone/36g	120	6.8	320	3.5	35.0	18.0	1.0
Cornet, Wafer Cone, Askeys*	1 Cone/4g	13	0.1	376	10.7	77.6	2.5	0.0
Cornetto, Classico, Wall's Ice Cream*	1 Cone/98g	200	12.6	205	2.7	19.7	12.9	0.0
Cornetto, Frutti Disc, Wall's Ice Cream*	1 Cone/80g	200	8.8	250	2.5	35.0	11.0	0.0

	Measure INFO/WEIGHT	per Measure KCAL	FAT	Nutrition Values per 100g / 100ml KCAL	PROT	CARB	FAT	FIBRE
ICE CREAM CONE								
Cornetto, GFY, Asda*	1 Cone/67g	162	6.0	241	3.0	37.0	9.0	0.1
Cornetto, Mint, Wall's Ice Cream*	1 Cone/75g	190	9.9	250	4.0	31.0	13.0	0.8
Cornetto, Wall's Ice Cream*	1 Cone/75g	195	9.7	260	3.7	34.5	12.9	0.0
Creme Egg, Cadbury*	1 Cone/115ml	270	13.3	235	2.9	29.3	11.6	0.0
Cup Cornet, Wafer Cone, Askeys*	1 Cone/4g	13	0.1	376	10.7	77.6	2.5	0.0
Dairy Milk, Mint, Cadbury*	1 Cone/115mll	190	8.9	165	2.4	21.5	7.7	0.0
Flake 99, Cadbury*	1 Cone/125ml	244	12.5	195	2.6	23.2	10.0	0.0
Mini, Sainsbury's*	1 Cone/18g	66	3.8	366	4.4	39.8	21.0	3.4
Mini, Tesco*	1 Cone/48g	152	9.3	316	4.1	31.5	19.3	0.8
Picnic, Cadbury*	1 Cone/125ml	258	11.7	207	3.4	28.9	9.4	0.3
Raspberry & Vanilla, Refreshing, Skinny Cow*	1 Cone/110ml	122	2.8	111	1.7	20.4	2.5	1.5
Smarties, Nestle*	1 Cone/100g	177	8.1	177	2.4	23.6	8.1	0.7
Strawberry, BGTY, Sainsbury's*	1 Cone/69g	151	4.5	219	2.6	37.5	6.5	1.3
Strawberry, Co-Op*	1 Cone/110g	283	13.3	257	3.5	33.6	12.1	0.5
Strawberry & Vanilla, Asda*	1 Cone/115ml	193	9.0	168	1.8	22.6	7.8	0.1
Strawberry & Vanilla, HL, Tesco*	1 Serving/69g	149	4.3	216	3.4	36.4	6.3	1.4
Tropical, GFY, Asda*	1 Cone/100g	135	5.0	135	2.6	20.0	5.0	0.3
Vanilla & Chocolate, Everyday Value, Tesco*	1 Cone/58g	170	7.4	285	3.8	38.9	12.4	1.3
ICE CREAM ROLL								
Arctic, Average	1 Serving/70g	140	4.6	200	4.1	33.3	6.6	0.0
Mini, Cadbury*	1 Roll/45ml	99	5.9	220	3.4	24.3	13.1	0.0
ICE CREAM SANDWICH								
Mint, Skinny Cow*	1 Sandwich/71g	140	2.0	197	4.2	39.4	2.8	1.4
Vanilla, Chocolate Coated, Lidl*	1 Serving/51g	145	9.5	284	1.8	21.6	18.6	0.0
Wich, Ben & Jerry's*	1 Pack/117g	398	19.9	340	4.0	44.0	17.0	1.0
ICE CREAM STICK								
Berry Blast, Smoothie, Skinny Cow*	1 Stick/110ml	71	0.1	65	0.9	15.1	0.1	1.9
Chocolate, Milk, Mini, Weight Watchers*	1 Stick/32g	95	5.1	296	3.7	33.8	15.9	1.6
Chocolate, Triple, Skinny Cow*	1 Stick/68g	87	1.5	128	4.3	22.8	2.2	2.8
Chocolate Cookies, Haagen-Dazs*	1 Stick/43g	162	10.9	376	4.9	31.8	25.4	0.0
Cookies 'n' Cream, Skinny Cow*	1 Stick/67g	89	1.0	133	4.8	25.3	1.5	3.6
Mint, Double Chocolate, Skinny Cow*	1 Stick/110ml	94	1.8	85	2.7	15.1	1.6	2.4
Strawberries & Cream, Skinny Cow*	1 Stick/110ml	82	1.0	75	2.8	13.6	0.9	2.3
Toffee, Skinny Cow*	1 Stick/72g	87	0.4	121	3.9	25.2	0.5	4.2
Tropical Moment, Asda*	1 Stick/75g	112	3.1	150	1.7	26.1	4.2	0.4
Vanilla Macadamia, Haagen-Dazs*	1 Stick/42g	161	11.6	383	4.6	28.7	27.7	0.0
ICE LOLLY								
Assorted, De Roma*	1 Lolly/55ml	48	0.2	87	0.2	20.9	0.4	0.2
Assorted, Iceland*	1 Lolly/51g	33	0.0	65	0.0	16.2	0.0	0.0
Baby, Tesco*	1 Lolly/32g	26	0.0	80	0.1	20.0	0.0	0.1
Blackcurrant, Dairy Split, Sainsbury's*	1 Lolly/73ml	88	2.6	121	1.8	20.4	3.6	0.1
Blackcurrant, Ribena*	1 Lolly/35ml	25	0.0	68	0.0	16.4	0.0	0.0
Blackcurrant Split, Iceland*	1 Lolly/75g	61	2.4	81	1.1	12.0	3.2	0.1
Bournville, Cadbury*	1 Lolly/110g	270	17.2	245	2.5	23.2	15.6	0.0
Calippo, Lemon Lime, Mini, Wall's Ice Cream*	1 Lolly/80g	68	0.0	85	0.0	21.0	0.0	0.2
Calippo, Orange, Mini, Wall's Ice Cream*	1 Lolly/78g	70	0.0	90	0.0	21.9	0.0	0.2
Calippo, Strawberry Tropical, Wall's Ice Cream*	1 Lolly/105g	89	0.1	85	0.1	21.0	0.1	0.0
Choc & Almond, Mini, Tesco*	1 Lolly/31g	103	7.4	331	4.4	24.8	23.8	0.9
Choc Lime Split, Morrisons*	1 Lolly/73ml	120	6.1	164	1.6	20.4	8.4	0.1
Chocolate, Mini Milk, Milk Time, Wall's Ice Cream*	1 Lolly/23g	31	0.7	135	4.3	22.0	3.1	1.0
Chocolate, Plain, Mini, Tesco*	1 Lolly/31g	94	6.6	304	3.1	24.8	21.4	1.2
Chocolate, Pooh Stick, Nestle*	1 Lolly/40g	36	1.4	89	2.1	12.9	3.6	0.0
Chocolate & Vanilla, Sainsbury's*	1 Lolly/40g	143	10.1	357	3.7	28.7	25.3	2.2

I

	Measure INFO/WEIGHT	per Measure KCAL	FAT	Nutrition Values per 100g / 100ml KCAL	PROT	CARB	FAT	FIBRE
ICE LOLLY								
Chocolate Wonderpops, Sainsbury's*	1 Lolly/43g	118	8.3	276	2.6	21.8	19.4	0.7
Fab, Nestle*	1 Lolly/64g	90	3.2	141	0.5	23.4	5.0	0.4
Fab, Orange, Nestle*	1 Lolly/58g	81	2.7	140	0.6	24.0	4.7	0.0
Feast, Chocolate, Mini, Wall's Ice Cream*	1 Lolly/52g	165	11.9	318	3.3	24.0	23.0	0.0
Feast, Toffee, Mini, Wall's Ice Cream*	1 Lolly/52g	163	12.0	313	3.0	24.0	23.0	0.0
Fruit, Assorted, Waitrose*	1 Lolly/73g	59	0.0	81	0.0	20.0	0.0	0.1
Fruit, Red, Tesco*	1 Lolly/32g	40	0.6	128	1.8	25.6	2.0	0.6
Fruit Luxury, Mini, Co-Op*	1 Lolly/45g	58	2.7	130	2.0	18.0	6.0	0.2
Fruit Pastilles, Rowntree's*	1 Lolly/65ml	61	0.0	94	0.2	23.2	0.0	0.0
Fruit Split, Asda*	1 Lolly/74g	85	2.7	115	1.7	19.0	3.6	0.0
Fruit Split, BFY, Morrisons*	1 Lolly/73g	50	0.5	69	1.6	13.9	0.7	0.1
Fruit Split, Waitrose*	1 Lolly/73g	91	2.6	124	2.5	21.7	3.6	0.4
Funny Foot, Wall's Ice Cream*	1 Lolly/81ml	83	4.9	102	2.0	12.5	6.0	0.0
Icicles, All Flavours, Freezepops, Calypso*	1 Lolly/50ml	1	0.0	1	0.0	0.3	0.0	0.0
Lemon & Lime, Mini Bar, M & S*	1 Lolly/50g	48	0.0	95	0.1	23.6	0.1	0.2
Lemon & Lime, Rocket Split, De Roma*	1 Lolly/60ml	65	2.6	108	1.0	16.0	4.3	0.2
Lemon Sorbet, Mercadona*	1 Lolly/63g	38	0.2	61	0.5	32.4	0.3	8.0
Lemonade & Cola, Morrisons*	1 Lolly/55ml	36	0.0	65	0.0	16.2	0.0	0.0
Lemonade Flavour, R White*	1 Lolly/75ml	56	1.1	75	0.5	15.1	1.5	0.1
Lemonade Sparkle, Wall's Ice Cream*	1 Lolly/55g	40	0.0	73	0.0	18.2	0.0	0.0
Mango & Lemon, BGTY, Sainsbury's*	1 Lolly/72g	84	0.2	116	0.3	28.1	0.3	0.5
Mango & Passion Fruit Smoothie, Waitrose*	1 Lolly/73g	60	0.3	82	0.7	18.9	0.4	0.7
Milk Flavour, Farmfoods*	1 Lolly/50ml	91	5.0	182	2.8	20.1	10.1	0.1
Mint Chocolate, Tesco*	1 Lolly/70g	234	13.9	334	3.6	35.4	19.8	1.2
No Added Sugar, Tesco*	1 Lolly/32g	26	0.0	80	0.1	20.0	0.0	0.1
Nobbly Bobbly, Nestle*	1 Lolly/70ml	219	11.6	312	2.9	38.1	16.5	0.6
Orange, Average	1 Lolly/72g	66	0.0	92	0.4	22.4	0.0	0.1
Orange, Real Juice, Sainsbury's*	1 Lolly/72ml	63	0.1	88	0.7	21.0	0.1	0.1
Orange, Ribena*	1 Lolly/110ml	95	0.0	86	0.1	21.4	0.0	0.0
Orange, Water, Iceland*	1 Lolly/75g	74	0.0	98	0.2	24.4	0.0	0.2
Orange & Lemon Splits, Farmfoods*	1 Lolly/56ml	69	2.4	124	1.6	19.8	4.3	0.2
Orange Juice, Asda*	1 Lolly/70g	58	0.0	83	0.7	20.0	0.0	0.0
Orange Juice, Bar, M & S*	1 Lolly/75g	64	0.0	86	0.5	21.0	0.0	0.1
Orange Juice, Milfina*	1 Lolly/79g	69	0.0	87	0.5	23.3	0.0	0.0
Orange Juice, Tropicana*	1 Lolly/50g	42	0.0	85	0.5	20.7	0.0	0.0
Orange Maid, Nestle*	1 Lolly/73ml	66	0.0	91	0.5	21.6	0.0	0.0
Orange 'n' Cream, Tropicana*	1 Lolly/65g	83	2.9	129	1.4	20.5	4.5	0.3
Pineapple, Dairy Split, Sainsbury's*	1 Lolly/72ml	84	2.6	116	1.8	19.0	3.6	0.1
Pineapple, Real Fruit Juice, Sainsbury's*	1 Lolly/73ml	55	0.1	76	0.1	19.0	0.1	0.1
Polar Snappers, Double, Farmfoods*	1 Lolly/60ml	40	0.0	66	0.0	16.5	0.0	0.0
Pop Up, Chosen By You, Asda*	1 Lolly/80ml	65	0.0	81	0.0	20.1	0.0	0.3
Raspberry, Real Fruit Juice, Sainsbury's*	1 Lolly/72g	62	0.1	86	0.3	21.0	0.1	0.1
Raspberry, Smoothie, Iced, Del Monte*	1 Lolly/90ml	84	0.0	94	0.3	22.8	0.0	0.8
Raspberry & Apple, Sainsbury's*	1 Lolly/57ml	39	0.1	68	0.1	17.1	0.1	0.1
Refresher, Fruit Flavour, Bassett's*	1 Lolly/45g	56	0.7	125	1.6	26.0	1.6	0.3
Rocket, Co-Op*	1 Lolly/60g	42	0.0	70	0.0	17.0	0.0	0.0
Rocket, Sainsbury's*	1 Lolly/58g	42	0.1	72	0.1	17.8	0.1	0.1
Rolo, Nestle*	1 Lolly/75ml	243	14.1	324	3.8	36.5	18.8	0.0
Scooby Doo, Freezepops, Calypso*	1 Lolly/45ml	13	0.0	28	0.0	7.0	0.0	0.0
Skinny Dippers, Caramel & Chocolate, Skinny Cow*	1 Lolly/38ml	62	1.9	162	3.4	24.3	5.0	3.3
Solero, Exotic, Wall's Ice Cream*	1 Lolly/70g	94	1.1	134	1.5	28.0	1.5	0.5
Solero, Orange Fresh, Wall's Ice Cream*	1 Lolly/96g	78	0.0	81	0.2	20.0	0.0	0.0
Solero, Red Fruits, Wall's Ice Cream*	1 Lolly/95g	99	2.1	104	1.3	21.0	2.2	0.0

	Measure INFO/WEIGHT	per Measure KCAL	FAT	Nutrition Values per 100g / 100ml KCAL	PROT	CARB	FAT	FIBRE
ICE LOLLY								
Spotty Dotty, Sainsbury's*	1 Lolly/47g	111	6.5	236	1.8	25.5	13.8	1.3
Sprinkle Tops, Sainsbury's*	1 Lolly/40g	51	1.2	126	0.2	24.8	2.9	0.1
Strawberries & Cream, Cadbury*	1 Lolly/100ml	225	11.7	225	2.9	27.0	11.7	0.0
Strawberries 'n' Cream, Tropicana*	1 Lolly/50g	58	0.6	117	1.6	25.0	1.2	0.0
Strawberry, Fruit Split, Iceland*	1 Lolly/73g	77	2.4	105	0.9	17.8	3.3	0.5
Strawberry, Mini Milk, Milk Time, Wall's Ice Cream*	1 Lolly/23g	30	0.7	131	4.0	22.0	2.9	0.5
Strawberry, Orange & Pineapple, Rocket, Iceland*	1 Lolly/47g	38	0.0	81	0.0	20.2	0.0	0.1
Strawberry, So-Lo, Good Choice, Iceland*	1 Lolly/66g	85	1.2	128	2.4	25.6	1.8	0.1
Strawberry & Banana, Smoothies, Sainsbury's*	1 Lolly/60g	100	3.2	166	1.5	28.0	5.3	0.2
Strawberry & Vanilla, 99% Fat Free, So-Lo, Iceland*	1 Lolly/92g	98	0.4	107	2.3	23.5	0.4	2.2
Strawberry Fruit, Double, Del Monte*	1 Lolly/76g	84	2.0	111	1.8	20.1	2.6	0.0
Strawberry Split, Average	1 Lolly/72g	78	2.3	108	1.5	18.5	3.2	0.2
Sugar Free, Simpkins*	1 Lolly/15g	51	0.0	340	0.0	88.0	0.0	0.0
Tip Top, Calypso*	1 Lolly/20ml	6	0.0	30	0.1	7.1	0.1	0.0
Traffic Light, Co-Op*	1 Lolly/52g	55	0.4	105	0.4	25.0	0.8	0.0
Tropical, Mmmm, Tesco*	1 Lolly/73g	109	3.1	150	1.2	26.6	4.3	0.4
Tropical Fruit, Starburst, Mars*	1 Lolly/93ml	94	0.1	101	0.3	24.8	0.1	0.0
Tropical Fruit Sorbet, Waitrose*	1 Lolly/110g	90	2.2	82	1.5	14.5	2.0	0.2
Twister, Choc, Wall's Ice Cream*	1 Lolly/27g	40	1.6	150	3.5	22.0	6.0	0.9
Twister, Wall's Ice Cream*	1 Lolly/80ml	76	1.5	95	0.6	18.4	1.9	0.0
Vanilla, Mini Milk, Milk Time, Wall's Ice Cream*	1 Lolly/23g	29	0.7	127	3.8	21.0	2.9	0.3
Vimto Soft Drinks*	1 Lolly/73ml	84	3.0	115	1.3	18.2	4.1	0.1
Wonka Super Sour Tastic, Nestle*	1 Lolly/60ml	84	2.2	140	0.0	26.1	3.6	0.0
Zoom, Nestle*	1 Lolly/58ml	54	0.4	93	0.9	20.6	0.7	0.0
ICED DESSERT								
Cafe Latte, BGTY, Sainsbury's*	1 Serving/75g	104	2.7	139	2.9	23.7	3.6	3.3
Chocolate, Honeycomb Pieces, Weight Watchers*	1 Pot/58g	92	2.5	159	3.1	26.2	4.3	0.8
Chocolate & Mallow, GFY, Asda*	1 Pot/150ml	142	1.8	95	2.0	19.0	1.2	2.3
Chocolate Mint Crisp, COU, M & S*	¼ Pot/85g	115	2.5	135	5.4	21.9	2.9	1.0
Greek Style, Yoghurt, Tesco*	1 Serving/56g	90	1.8	160	2.6	29.7	3.3	1.4
Raspberry Swirl, Weight Watchers*	1 Scoop/60g	74	1.5	124	1.7	23.4	2.5	0.3
Strawberry Swirl, Weight Watchers*	1 Pot/100ml	92	1.7	92	1.1	18.1	1.7	0.5
Summer Fruits, Yoghurt, BGTY, Sainsbury's*	¼ Pot/85g	105	0.8	124	3.3	25.6	0.9	0.5
Toffee & Walnut, Free From, Sainsbury's*	¼ Tub/81g	203	10.0	251	3.3	31.6	12.4	0.3
Toffee Flavoured, Dairy, BGTY, Sainsbury's*	1 Serving/70g	103	3.2	147	2.7	24.0	4.5	0.2
Vanilla, Dairy, BGTY, Sainsbury's*	1 Serving/65g	78	1.0	120	3.0	23.6	1.5	0.6
Vanilla, Non Dairy, Soft, Swedish Glace*	1 Serving/100g	200	10.0	200	2.5	25.0	10.0	1.0
Vanilla & Chocolate, HL, Tesco*	1 Pot/73g	104	1.9	143	3.0	26.9	2.6	0.7
Vanilla Flavour, HE, Tesco*	1 Serving/50g	67	1.2	134	3.9	24.1	2.4	4.6
INDIAN MEAL								
for One, Asda*	1 Pack/550g	834	25.3	152	6.7	20.9	4.6	1.4
for One, GFY, Asda*	1 Serving/495g	644	23.3	130	8.0	14.0	4.7	1.0
for One, Vegetarian, Asda*	1 Pack/499g	789	44.9	158	3.2	16.0	9.0	1.4
for Two, Hot, Takeaway, Tesco*	1 Pack/825g	1215	60.6	147	6.6	13.6	7.4	1.9
for Two, Peshwari Naan, Finest, Tesco*	½ Pack/200g	612	17.8	306	8.3	48.3	8.9	5.2
INSTANT WHIP								
Chocolate Flavour, Dry, Bird's*	1oz/28g	109	1.7	390	3.8	80.5	5.9	0.7
Strawberry Flavour, Dry, Bird's*	1oz/28g	112	1.5	400	2.5	85.0	5.4	0.4
IRN BRU								
Diet, Barr's*	1 Can/330ml	2	0.0	1	0.1	0.1	0.0	0.0
Original, Barr's*	1 Bottle/500ml	214	0.0	43	0.0	10.5	0.0	0.0

I

	Measure INFO/WEIGHT	per Measure KCAL	FAT	Nutrition Values per 100g / 100ml KCAL	PROT	CARB	FAT	FIBRE
JACKFRUIT								
Raw, Average, Flesh Only	***1 Portion/162g***	***155***	***0.5***	***95***	***1.5***	***24.4***	***0.3***	***1.6***
JALFREZI								
Chicken, & Coriander Rice, TTD, Sainsbury's*	1 Pack/473g	501	15.1	106	6.2	13.2	3.2	3.1
Chicken, & Pilau Rice, Sainsbury's*	1 Pack/500g	600	20.5	120	6.9	13.9	4.1	1.5
Chicken, & Pilau Rice, Takeaway, Asda*	1 Pack/558g	792	23.4	142	7.0	19.0	4.2	1.3
Chicken, & Rice, Serves 1, Tesco*	1 Serving/475g	589	38.0	124	7.4	5.7	8.0	1.6
Chicken, Asda*	1 Pack/340g	415	20.4	122	10.0	7.0	6.0	1.6
Chicken, Budgens*	1 Serving/200g	210	6.4	105	9.8	9.2	3.2	0.9
Chicken, Canned, Tesco*	½ Can/200g	190	6.8	95	10.8	4.1	3.4	1.4
Chicken, Finest, Tesco*	1 Pack/350g	402	16.4	115	10.4	6.9	4.7	1.2
Chicken, GFY, Asda*	1 Pack/350g	238	3.2	68	9.0	6.0	0.9	1.8
Chicken, Hot & Spicy, Sainsbury's*	½ Pack/200g	228	11.4	114	12.8	2.9	5.7	1.0
Chicken, Indian Takeaway, Tesco*	1 Serving/350g	245	8.7	70	7.4	4.3	2.5	1.8
Chicken, Medium, GFY, Asda*	1 Pack/644g	972	27.7	151	6.0	22.0	4.3	0.9
Chicken, with Basmati Rice, Weight Watchers*	1 Pack/330g	238	1.6	72	5.0	11.8	0.5	0.5
Chicken, with Lemon Pilau Rice, Finest, Tesco*	1 Pack/493g	665	21.7	135	6.9	16.4	4.4	1.8
Chicken, with Pilau Basmati Rice, Frozen, Patak's*	1 Pack/400g	556	18.4	139	9.8	14.7	4.6	0.9
Chicken, with Pilau Rice, GFY, Asda*	1 Pack/446g	495	11.1	111	8.0	14.0	2.5	1.2
Chicken, with Pilau Rice, Tesco*	1 Pack/460g	506	17.5	110	5.3	13.6	3.8	0.9
Chicken, with Rice, Tesco*	1 Pack/550g	732	26.4	133	5.5	17.0	4.8	1.0
Vegetable, Co-Op*	1 Pack/400g	320	16.0	80	1.0	9.0	4.0	2.0
Vegetable, Eastern Indian, Sainsbury's*	1 Pack/400g	208	13.6	52	3.4	2.0	3.4	1.7
Vegetable, Indian, Sainsbury's*	½ Pack/200g	156	9.0	78	2.0	5.3	4.5	4.2
Vegetable, Waitrose*	1 Pack/400g	256	16.0	64	2.2	4.7	4.0	3.7
Vegetable, with Rice, Birds Eye*	1 Pack/350g	354	3.9	101	2.5	20.2	1.1	1.0
JAM								
Apricot, Average	***1 Tbsp/15g***	***37***	***0.0***	***248***	***0.2***	***61.6***	***0.0***	***1.5***
Apricot, Reduced Sugar, Average	***1 Serving/20g***	***37***	***0.1***	***186***	***0.4***	***46.0***	***0.3***	***0.4***
Apricot, Reduced Sugar, Weight Watchers*	1 Tsp/15g	23	0.0	153	0.5	37.5	0.1	1.2
Black Cherry, Average	***1 Tsp/5g***	***12***	***0.0***	***247***	***0.4***	***61.2***	***0.3***	***0.4***
Blackberry, Wild, Jelly, Baxters*	1 Tsp/15g	32	0.0	210	0.0	53.0	0.0	1.2
Blackcurrant, Average	***1 Tbsp/15g***	***38***	***0.0***	***250***	***0.2***	***62.3***	***0.0***	***1.0***
Blackcurrant, Reduced Sugar, Average	***1 Tsp/6g***	***10***	***0.0***	***178***	***0.4***	***44.4***	***0.2***	***1.0***
Blackcurrant, Reduced Sugar, Weight Watchers*	1 Heap Tsp/15g	22	0.0	144	0.5	35.3	0.1	3.1
Blueberry, Best, Hartley's*	1 Tsp/20g	49	0.0	244	0.3	60.6	0.1	0.0
Blueberry, St Dalfour*	1 Serving/20g	46	0.0	228	0.5	56.0	0.2	2.2
Blueberry & Blackberry, Baxters*	1 Tsp/15g	38	0.0	252	0.0	63.0	0.0	1.2
Country Berries, Luxury, Baxters*	1 Tsp/15g	37	0.0	247	0.5	60.0	0.1	2.0
Damson, Extra Fruit, Best, Hartley's*	1 Tsp/5g	12	0.0	244	0.2	60.8	0.0	0.0
Fig	1 Tsp/15g	36	0.0	242	0.5	60.0	0.0	0.0
Grape, Concorde, Jelly, Organic, Smucker's*	1 Tbsp/20g	50	0.0	250	0.0	65.0	0.0	0.0
Grape, Concorde, Sugar Free, Smucker's*	1 Serving/17g	0	0.0	0	0.0	29.4	0.0	0.0
Kiwi & Gooseberry, 66% Fruit, Asda*	1 Serving/30g	56	0.2	187	0.5	45.0	0.5	0.0
Mixed Fruit, Average	***1 Tbsp/15g***	***38***	***0.0***	***252***	***0.3***	***63.5***	***0.0***	***0.5***
Peach, Golden, Rhapsodie De Fruit, St Dalfour*	1 Tsp/10g	23	0.0	227	0.5	56.0	0.1	1.3
Plum, Tesco*	1 Serving/50g	130	0.0	261	0.2	64.4	0.0	0.6
Raspberry, Average	***1 Tbsp/15g***	***36***	***0.0***	***239***	***0.6***	***58.6***	***0.1***	***0.9***
Raspberry, Reduced Sugar, Average	***1 Tsp/6g***	***10***	***0.0***	***160***	***0.5***	***39.3***	***0.2***	***0.6***
Raspberry, Reduced Sugar, Baxters*	½ Tsp/5g	10	0.0	197	0.7	48.0	0.2	1.5
Raspberry, Reduced Sugar, Weight Watchers*	1 Tsp/15g	22	0.0	149	0.7	36.1	0.2	2.9
Raspberry, Seedless, Average	***1 Tsp/10g***	***26***	***0.0***	***257***	***0.4***	***63.6***	***0.0***	***0.3***
Rhubarb & Ginger, Baxters*	1 Tsp/15g	40	0.0	264	0.4	65.0	0.1	0.8
Strawberry, Average	***1 Tsp/10g***	***24***	***0.0***	***243***	***0.3***	***60.2***	***0.1***	***0.7***

	Measure INFO/WEIGHT	per Measure KCAL	FAT	Nutrition Values per 100g / 100ml KCAL	PROT	CARB	FAT	FIBRE
JAM								
Strawberry, Reduced Sugar, Average	***1 Tbsp/15g***	***28***	***0.0***	***187***	***0.4***	***45.8***	***0.3***	***0.2***
Strawberry, Reduced Sugar, Weight Watchers*	1 Serving/15g	23	0.0	154	0.5	37.5	0.2	1.2
Strawberry, Smooth, Squeezy, Hartley's*	1 Tsp/5g	10	0.0	196	0.4	48.6	0.0	0.0
Strawberry & Redcurrant, Reduced Sugar, Streamline*	1 Tbsp/15g	29	0.0	192	0.4	46.8	0.3	0.0
Strawberry & Vanilla, Best, Hartley's*	1 Tsp/5g	12	0.0	244	0.4	60.6	0.0	0.0
JAMBALAYA								
American, HE, Tesco*	1 Pack/450g	477	9.0	106	6.4	15.5	2.0	0.9
Chicken, Cajun, Cooked, BGTY, Sainsbury's*	1 Pack/400g	392	6.5	103	6.6	14.6	1.7	1.6
Chicken, Spicy, Eat Smart, Morrisons*	1 Pack/400g	384	4.8	96	7.4	13.9	1.2	2.7
Chicken & Prawn, Love Life, Waitrose*	1 Pack/390g	417	10.9	107	5.2	14.3	2.8	1.9
COU, M & S*	1 Pack/400g	340	8.0	85	6.5	10.8	2.0	0.9
Ready Meal, Average	1 Pack/450g	569	18.2	126	6.4	15.7	4.0	1.3
JELLY								
Apple & Blackcurrant, Crystals, Weight Watchers*	1 Packet/204g	14	0.2	7	0.1	1.4	0.1	0.1
Apple & Watermelon, Low Calorie, Hartley's*	1 Serving/175g	5	0.0	3	0.0	0.3	0.0	0.3
Blackcurrant, Made Up, Rowntree's*	¼ Jelly/140ml	100	0.1	71	1.4	16.4	0.1	0.0
Blackcurrant, Sugar Free, Unprepared, Rowntree's*	1 Pack/24g	73	0.0	305	50.0	25.0	0.0	25.0
Blackcurrant, Tesco*	1 Serving/100g	84	0.1	84	0.2	20.5	0.1	0.4
Bramble, Tesco*	1 Serving/100g	257	0.1	257	0.3	63.7	0.1	1.3
Fruit, Exotic, M & S*	1 Pot/175g	140	0.4	80	0.1	18.9	0.2	0.9
Fruit, Fresh, M & S*	1 Pot/175g	131	0.2	75	0.2	18.4	0.1	0.3
Fruitini, Del Monte*	1 Serving/120g	78	0.1	65	0.3	15.3	0.1	0.5
Lemon, Unprepared, Co-Op*	1 Pack/135g	412	0.0	305	5.0	71.0	0.0	0.0
Lime, Made Up, Rowntree's*	¼ Jelly/140ml	100	0.1	71	1.4	16.4	0.1	0.0
Lime, Unprepared, Co-Op*	1 Pack/135g	397	0.1	294	5.5	68.1	0.0	1.0
Lime Flavour, Cubes, Hartley's*	1 Cube/12g	36	0.0	296	5.1	68.9	0.0	0.0
Made Up, with Water, Average	***1oz/28g***	***17***	***0.0***	***61***	***1.2***	***15.1***	***0.0***	***0.0***
Mandarin & Pineapple, Sainsbury's*	1 Pot/125g	95	0.1	76	0.2	18.9	0.1	1.2
Orange, Sugar Free, Crystals, Bird's*	1 Sachet/12g	39	0.1	335	62.5	6.4	0.9	0.0
Orange, Sugar Free, Crystals, Dry Weight, Hartley's*	1 Pack/26g	66	0.0	254	57.4	6.1	0.0	0.0
Orange, Sugar Free, Made Up, Hartley's*	1 Serving/140ml	9	0.0	6	1.3	0.3	0.0	0.0
Orange, Sugar Free, Rowntree's*	1 Serving/140ml	8	0.0	6	1.4	0.1	0.0	0.0
Orange, Sugar Free, Unprepared, Asda*	1 Serving/12g	36	0.0	303	63.6	12.0	0.1	0.2
Orange, Unprepared, Rowntree's*	1 Square/11g	33	0.0	296	4.4	69.6	0.0	0.0
Peach Melba, Eat Well, M & S*	1 Pot/175g	114	0.4	65	0.2	15.9	0.2	0.2
Pineapple, with Pineapple Pieces, Tesco*	1 Serving/120g	96	0.1	80	1.2	18.6	0.1	0.7
Raspberry, Crystals, Vegetarian, Just Wholefoods*	1 Packet/85g	293	0.0	345	0.5	85.7	0.0	0.0
Raspberry, Unprepared, Co-Op*	1 Pack/135g	402	0.1	298	5.5	68.9	0.0	0.0
Raspberry, Unprepared, Rowntree's*	1 Serving/135g	405	0.5	300	5.6	67.3	0.4	0.0
Raspberry Flavour, Sugar Free, Made Up, Rowntree's*	1 Serving/140ml	9	0.0	6	1.4	0.1	0.0	0.0
Redcurrant, Average	***1oz/28g***	***70***	***0.0***	***250***	***0.2***	***64.4***	***0.0***	***0.0***
Strawberry, Goodness for Kids, Tesco*	1 Pot/75g	45	0.3	60	1.7	11.1	0.4	0.5
Strawberry, Made Up, Crystals, Tesco*	1 Serving/145g	9	0.0	6	1.3	0.3	0.0	0.0
Strawberry, No Added Sugar, Hartley's*	1 Pot/115g	4	0.0	4	0.0	0.4	0.0	0.3
Strawberry, Sugar Free, Crystals, Dry Weight, Hartley's*	1 Sachet/26g	73	0.0	280	56.8	13.1	0.0	0.0
Strawberry, Unprepared, Co-Op*	1 Pack/135g	402	0.1	298	5.5	69.1	0.0	0.0
Strawberry & Raspberry, Sainsbury's*	½ Pot/280g	230	0.0	82	0.2	20.2	0.0	1.2
Strawberry Flavour, Sugar Free, Made Up, Rowntree's*	1 Serving/140ml	10	0.0	7	1.5	0.1	0.0	0.0
Sugar Free, Dry, Tesco*	1 Pack/13g	36	0.0	285	55.4	15.6	0.0	0.2
Tangerine, Unprepared, Rowntree's*	1 Serving/33g	99	0.1	300	5.6	67.3	0.4	0.0
Tropical Fruit, WTF, Sainsbury's*	1 Serving/160g	144	1.6	90	0.3	19.9	1.0	0.9
JELLY BABIES								
Bassett's*	1 Sweet/6g	20	0.0	335	3.5	79.7	0.0	0.0

	Measure INFO/WEIGHT	per Measure KCAL	FAT	Nutrition Values per 100g / 100ml KCAL	PROT	CARB	FAT	FIBRE
JELLY BABIES								
M & S*	1 Pack/125g	418	0.0	334	5.2	78.0	0.0	0.0
Mini, Rowntree's*	1 Small Bag/35g	128	0.0	366	4.6	86.9	0.0	0.0
Mini, Waitrose*	1 Bag/125g	370	0.5	296	4.3	68.7	0.4	0.0
Sainsbury's*	1 Serving/70g	247	0.5	353	4.1	82.5	0.7	0.3
JELLY BEANS								
	1 Serving/100g	365	0.1	365	0.1	91.2	0.1	0.1
Jelly Belly*	35 Beans/40g	140	0.0	350	0.0	90.0	0.0	0.0
No Added Sugar, Jelly Belly*	1 Serving/40g	80	0.0	200	0.0	50.0	0.0	20.0
Rowntree's*	1 Pack/35g	128	0.0	367	0.0	91.8	0.0	0.0
JELLY TOTS								
Rowntree's*	1 Pack/42g	145	0.0	346	0.1	86.5	0.0	0.0
JERKY								
Beef, Peppered, Jack Link's*	1 Serving/28g	80	0.5	286	53.6	14.3	1.8	0.0
Beef, with Tomato Relish, Graze*	1 Pack/36g	91	1.0	253	22.2	30.6	2.8	2.5
Soy, Cajun Chick'n, Vegan, Tasty Eats*	1 Pack/28g	90	3.0	321	42.9	14.3	10.7	7.1
JUICE								
Apple, Cloudy, Pressed, Copella*	1 Glass/100ml	46	0.0	46	0.2	10.7	0.0	0.7
Apple, Concentrate, Average	***1 Tbsp/15ml***	***45***	***0.0***	***302***	***0.0***	***73.6***	***0.2***	***0.0***
Apple, Peach & Pear, Innocent*	1 Serving/100ml	45	0.1	45	0.4	10.0	0.1	1.4
Apple, Pressed, Not from Concentrate, Co-Op*	1 Glass/100ml	45	0.1	45	0.1	10.4	0.1	0.0
Apple, Pure, Average	1 Glass/100ml	47	0.0	47	0.1	11.2	0.0	0.0
Apple, Pure, Organic, Average	***1 Serving/200ml***	***92***	***0.1***	***46***	***0.0***	***11.2***	***0.0***	***0.0***
Apple, Raspberry & Grape, Pressed, Sainsbury's*	1 Serving/200ml	92	0.2	46	0.3	11.2	0.1	0.5
Apple, Vitafit, Lidl*	1 Carton/250ml	110	0.2	44	0.1	10.0	0.1	0.1
Apple, with Ginger, Waitrose*	1 Glass/150ml	72	0.0	48	0.3	11.0	0.0	0.5
Apple & Cherry, Sainsbury's*	1 Serving/200ml	96	0.0	48	0.3	10.8	0.0	0.8
Apple & Cranberry, Average	***1 Glass/250ml***	***114***	***0.0***	***46***	***0.1***	***10.2***	***0.0***	***0.0***
Apple & Elderflower, Copella*	1 Glass/250ml	108	0.2	43	0.4	10.2	0.1	0.0
Apple & Lychee, Cracker Drinks Co*	1 Serving/200ml	92	0.0	46	0.1	11.2	0.0	0.2
Apple & Mango, Average	***1 Glass/200ml***	***108***	***0.1***	***54***	***0.3***	***12.6***	***0.0***	***0.1***
Apple & Orange, Fresh Up*	1 Serving/250ml	105	0.0	42	0.0	10.3	0.0	0.0
Apple & Pomegranate, Pommy, Sparky*	1 Serving/250ml	125	0.5	50	0.4	10.0	0.2	0.5
Apple & Raspberry, Average	***1 Serving/200ml***	***89***	***0.1***	***44***	***0.4***	***10.2***	***0.0***	***0.2***
Apple & Raspberry, Tropicana*	1 Glass/150ml	72	0.0	48	0.2	10.5	0.0	0.9
Apple & Rhubarb, Caxton Vale*	1 Glass/250ml	115	1.0	46	0.2	9.7	0.4	0.0
Apple & Rhubarb, Pressed, Cawston Press*	1 Serving/200ml	92	0.8	46	0.2	9.7	0.4	0.0
Beetroot, Organic, James White*	1 Glass/250ml	105	0.2	42	0.9	9.3	0.1	0.0
Blackberry, Vita, Co-Op*	1 Glass/200ml	110	0.0	55	0.0	13.0	0.0	0.5
Breakfast, Ruby, Tropicana*	1 Glass/200ml	90	0.0	45	0.8	9.7	0.0	0.7
Breakfast, Sainsbury's*	1 Serving/200ml	94	0.2	47	0.7	11.3	0.1	0.3
Carrot, & Wild Strawberry, Kubus*	1 Glass/200ml	93	0.3	47	0.0	11.3	0.2	1.0
Carrot, Average	***1 Glass/200ml***	***48***	***0.2***	***24***	***0.5***	***5.7***	***0.1***	***0.0***
Citrus Fruit & Veg, V8*	1 Serving/150ml	56	0.3	37	0.3	8.4	0.2	0.0
Clementine, Morrisons*	1 Serving/100ml	48	0.1	48	0.5	10.9	0.1	0.1
Coconut, Foco*	1 Can/520ml	182	1.1	35	0.1	8.2	0.2	0.0
Cranberry, Average	***1 Bottle/250ml***	***139***	***0.2***	***56***	***0.1***	***13.4***	***0.1***	***0.3***
Cranberry, No Added Sugar, Average	***1 Glass/200ml***	***11***	***0.1***	***6***	***0.1***	***0.8***	***0.0***	***0.0***
Cranberry & Apple, No Added Sugar, Sainsbury's*	1 Glass/250ml	15	0.0	6	0.0	1.5	0.0	0.0
Cranberry & Raspberry, Low Sugar, Sainsbury's*	1 Glass/250ml	10	0.2	4	0.1	0.7	0.1	0.1
Fibre, Tropicana*	1 Serving/200ml	130	0.0	65	0.4	15.8	0.0	3.4
Fruit, Exotic, Pure, Del Monte*	1 Glass/200ml	96	0.0	48	0.3	11.3	0.0	0.0
Fruit, Tropical, Pure Premium, Tropicana*	1 Glass/200ml	98	0.0	49	0.5	11.0	0.0	0.8
Go!, Tropicana*	1 Bottle/200ml	80	0.0	40	0.3	9.7	0.0	0.0

	Measure INFO/WEIGHT	per Measure KCAL	per Measure FAT	Nutrition Values per 100g / 100ml KCAL	PROT	CARB	FAT	FIBRE
JUICE								
Grape, Concord, Kedem*	1 Bottle/946ml	587	0.0	62	0.0	15.4	0.0	0.0
Grape, Purple, Light, Welch's*	1 Serving/100ml	27	0.3	27	0.2	6.1	0.3	0.3
Grape, Purple, Welch's*	1 Serving/200ml	136	0.0	68	0.1	16.5	0.0	0.0
Grape, Red, Average	***1 Serving/100ml***	***62***	***0.0***	***62***	***0.2***	***15.2***	***0.0***	***0.0***
Grape, White, Average	***1 Can/160ml***	***95***	***0.1***	***60***	***0.2***	***14.3***	***0.1***	***0.1***
Grape & Peach, Don Simon*	1 Serving/200ml	94	0.0	47	0.4	11.3	0.0	0.0
Grape & Raspberry, Pressed, M & S*	1 Carton/330ml	182	0.3	55	0.4	12.9	0.1	0.1
Grapefruit, Pink, Average	***1 Glass/200ml***	***81***	***0.1***	***40***	***0.6***	***9.0***	***0.0***	***0.2***
Grapefruit, Pure, Average	***1 Glass/200ml***	***77***	***0.2***	***38***	***0.5***	***8.5***	***0.1***	***0.1***
Lime, Fresh, Average	***1 Tsp/5ml***	***0***	***0.0***	***9***	***0.4***	***1.6***	***0.1***	***0.1***
Lime, from Concentrate, Asda*	1 Tbsp/17g	1	0.0	6	0.3	0.8	0.1	0.2
Mandarin Orange, Tropicana*	1 Serving/200ml	94	0.0	47	0.6	10.0	0.0	0.8
Mango, Peach, Papaya, Pure, Premium, Tropicana*	1 Glass/200ml	88	0.0	44	0.5	9.8	0.0	0.1
Mango, Pure, Canned	***1 Glass/250ml***	***98***	***0.5***	***39***	***0.1***	***9.8***	***0.2***	***0.0***
Mango Veggie, Naked Juice Co*	1 Serving/240ml	150	1.0	62	1.2	15.8	0.4	2.1
Orange, Apple & Mango, Calypso*	1 Carton/200ml	92	0.4	46	0.0	11.0	0.2	0.1
Orange, C, No Added Sugar, Libby's*	1 Serving/250ml	32	0.0	13	0.1	2.7	0.0	0.0
Orange, Freshly Squeezed, Average	1 Serving/200ml	66	0.0	33	0.6	8.1	0.0	1.0
Orange, No Bits, Innocent*	1 Glass/250ml	120	0.0	48	0.8	10.9	0.0	0.2
Orange, Pulp Free, Napolina*	1 Serving/264ml	110	0.0	42	0.8	9.9	0.0	0.0
Orange, Pure, Premium, Smooth, No Bits, Tropicana*	1 Glass/200ml	96	0.0	48	0.8	10.0	0.0	0.4
Orange, Pure, Smooth, Average	***1 Glass/200ml***	***88***	***0.1***	***44***	***0.7***	***9.8***	***0.0***	***0.2***
Orange, Pure, Smooth, from Concentrate, Sainsbury's*	1 Serving/200ml	84	0.2	42	0.5	9.1	0.1	0.1
Orange, Pure, with Bits, Average	***1 Glass/200ml***	***90***	***0.1***	***45***	***0.6***	***10.2***	***0.1***	***0.1***
Orange, Red, Average	***1 Glass/250ml***	***115***	***0.1***	***46***	***0.4***	***10.7***	***0.0***	***0.2***
Orange, Smooth, Freshly Squeezed, TTD, Sainsbury's*	1 Serving/249g	132	0.0	53	0.7	11.4	0.0	0.2
Orange, Smooth, Happy Shopper*	1 Serving/150ml	63	0.2	42	0.5	9.1	0.1	0.2
Orange, Sparkling, 55, Britvic*	1 Bottle/275ml	135	0.3	49	0.3	11.3	0.1	0.1
Orange, with Bits, Freshly Squeezed, TTD, Sainsbury's*	1 Serving/249g	132	0.0	53	0.7	11.4	0.0	0.2
Orange, with Bits, Innocent*	1 Glass/250ml	120	0.0	48	0.8	10.9	0.0	0.3
Orange, with Bits, Not from Concentrate, Tesco*	1 Glass/250ml	110	0.0	44	0.4	10.6	0.0	0.0
Orange & Banana, Pure, Average	***1 Glass/150ml***	***79***	***0.1***	***53***	***0.7***	***12.1***	***0.1***	***0.2***
Orange & Carrot, Love Life, Waitrose*	1 Serving/150ml	57	0.3	38	0.6	8.5	0.2	1.2
Orange & Grapefruit, Average	***1 Glass/200ml***	***84***	***0.2***	***42***	***0.8***	***9.2***	***0.1***	***0.4***
Orange & Kiwi Fruit, Tropicana*	1 Serving/175ml	90	0.0	51	0.5	12.0	0.0	0.0
Orange & Lime, Tropicana*	1 Serving/250ml	115	0.0	46	1.1	9.4	0.0	0.6
Orange & Mango, Average	***1 Bottle/375ml***	***176***	***0.4***	***47***	***0.5***	***10.7***	***0.1***	***0.2***
Orange & Passionfruit, Tropicana*	1 Serving/200ml	94	0.0	47	0.8	10.0	0.0	0.7
Orange & Pineapple, Average	***1 Glass/120ml***	***56***	***0.6***	***46***	***0.4***	***10.5***	***0.5***	***0.5***
Orange & Raspberry, Average	***1 fl oz/30ml***	***15***	***0.0***	***50***	***0.6***	***11.4***	***0.1***	***0.2***
Orange & Raspberry, Tropicana*	1 Bottle/330ml	139	0.0	42	0.4	9.0	0.0	0.8
Orange & Strawberry, Average	***1 Serving/125ml***	***64***	***0.5***	***51***	***0.6***	***10.9***	***0.4***	***0.8***
Passion Fruit, Average	***1 Glass/200ml***	***94***	***0.2***	***47***	***0.8***	***10.7***	***0.1***	***0.0***
Pear, Pure, Heinz*	1 Serving/100ml	41	0.1	41	0.1	9.8	0.1	0.0
Pear, with a Hint of Ginger, Pressed, M & S*	1 Glass/250ml	125	0.2	50	0.3	11.7	0.1	0.0
Pineapple, Average	***1 Glass/200ml***	***100***	***0.1***	***50***	***0.3***	***11.7***	***0.1***	***0.2***
Pineapple & Coconut, Waitrose*	1 Serving/250ml	125	0.8	50	0.2	11.5	0.3	0.2
Pineapple & Guava, Tropicana*	1 Glass/200ml	106	0.0	53	0.3	12.3	0.0	1.2
Pomegranate, Grape & Apple, Tropicana*	1 Bottle/330ml	211	0.0	64	0.2	15.5	0.0	0.6
Pomegranate, Pomegreat*	1 Glass/200ml	88	0.0	44	0.1	11.1	0.0	0.0
Pomegranate, with Cherry, Pomegreat*	1 Serving/200ml	75	0.0	38	0.1	8.8	0.0	0.1
Pomegranate & Blueberry, Sainsbury's*	1oz/28g	14	0.0	49	0.0	11.7	0.0	0.1
Prune, Average	***1 Serving/200ml***	***123***	***0.1***	***61***	***0.6***	***15.3***	***0.1***	***1.8***

	Measure INFO/WEIGHT	per Measure KCAL	per Measure FAT	Nutrition Values per 100g / 100ml KCAL	PROT	CARB	FAT	FIBRE
JUICE								
Tomato, Average	***1 Glass/200ml***	***40***	***0.1***	***20***	***0.8***	***4.0***	***0.0***	***0.4***
Tomato, Tangy, Princes*	1 Serving/200ml	34	0.0	17	0.8	3.1	0.0	0.6
Tropical, Fruit & Vegetable, V8*	1 Serving/150ml	0	0.0	35	0.4	8.1	0.1	1.1
Tropical, Pure, Sainsbury's*	1 Glass/200ml	104	0.2	52	0.5	12.0	0.1	0.1
Tropical Fruit, Plenty*	1 Glass/200ml	120	0.2	60	0.5	13.7	0.1	0.0
Vegetable, 100%, V8*	1 Bottle/354ml	71	1.1	20	0.8	3.2	0.3	0.5
Vegetable, Organic, Evernat*	1 Glass/200ml	36	0.2	18	0.9	3.5	0.1	0.2
JUICE DRINK								
Apple, Juiceburst, Purity*	1 Bottle/500ml	220	0.0	44	0.0	11.0	0.0	0.0
Apple, Libby's*	1 Serving/100ml	43	0.0	43	0.0	10.3	0.0	0.0
Apple, No Added Sugar, Asda*	1 Glass/200ml	10	0.0	5	0.0	1.0	0.0	0.0
Apple, No Added Sugar, LC, Tesco*	1 Glass/250ml	12	0.0	5	0.0	0.9	0.0	0.0
Apple, Sparkling, Zing*	1 Can/250ml	92	0.0	37	0.1	8.5	0.0	0.0
Apple & Blackcurrant, Sparkling, Shapers, Boots*	1 Serving/500ml	26	0.1	5	0.0	0.9	0.0	0.0
Apple & Blueberry, The Feel Good Drinks Co*	1 Serving/375ml	163	0.4	44	0.1	10.6	0.1	0.0
Apple & Elderflower, Tesco*	1 Serving/200ml	76	0.0	38	0.0	9.4	0.0	0.0
Apple & Mango, Chosen By You, Asda*	1 Carton/250ml	115	0.0	46	0.0	11.0	0.0	0.0
Apple & Pomegranate, Sparkling Water, Sainsbury's*	1 Serving/200ml	4	0.0	2	0.0	0.3	0.0	0.0
Apple & Raspberry, Dr Gillian McKeith*	1 Bottle/200ml	86	0.1	43	0.1	10.6	0.0	0.0
Apple & Raspberry, Sainsbury's*	1 Serving/200ml	112	0.2	56	0.1	13.8	0.1	0.1
Apple & Strawberry, Sainsbury's*	1 Serving/250ml	13	0.1	5	0.0	1.0	0.0	0.0
Berry & Elderberry, Fusion, Oasis*	1 Bottle/375ml	11	0.0	3	0.0	0.4	0.0	0.0
Berry Blast, 5 Alive*	1 Glass/200ml	50	0.0	25	0.0	6.1	0.0	0.0
Blackcurrant, 45% High, No Added Sugar, Asda*	1 Serving/25ml	2	0.0	7	0.0	1.4	0.0	0.0
Blackcurrant, CVit*	1 Glass/200ml	4	0.0	2	0.0	0.2	0.0	0.0
Blackcurrant, Extra Light, Ribena*	1 Serving/200ml	8	0.0	4	0.0	0.5	0.0	0.0
Blackcurrant, Kids, Tesco*	1 Serving/250ml	128	0.0	51	0.0	12.4	0.0	0.0
Blackcurrant, Purity*	1 Bottle/500ml	265	0.0	53	0.0	13.2	0.0	0.0
Blackcurrant & Apple, Oasis*	1 Serving/500ml	90	0.0	18	0.0	4.1	0.0	0.0
Blackcurrant & Raspberry with Soya, Adez*	1 Glass/250ml	82	1.0	33	1.1	6.3	0.4	0.3
Blueberry, BGTY, Sainsbury's*	1 Serving/250ml	15	0.0	6	0.1	1.0	0.0	0.0
Cherry, No Added Sugar, Sainsbury's*	1 Carton/250ml	25	0.1	10	0.2	1.9	0.0	0.0
Citrus, Sainsbury's*	1 Serving/200ml	102	0.2	51	0.3	12.3	0.1	0.2
Citrus Burst, 5 Alive*	1 Carton/250ml	125	0.0	50	0.0	12.8	0.0	0.0
Cranberry, Classic, Ocean Spray*	1 Bottle/500ml	245	0.5	49	0.1	11.7	0.1	0.1
Cranberry, Grape & Apple, Ocean Spray*	1 Glass/200ml	108	0.0	54	0.1	12.9	0.0	0.0
Cranberry, Juice Burst, Purity*	1 Bottle/500ml	245	0.0	49	0.0	12.0	0.0	0.0
Cranberry, Light, Classic, Ocean Spray*	1 Glass/200ml	16	0.0	8	0.0	1.4	0.0	0.0
Cranberry, M & S*	1 Serving/100ml	60	0.0	60	0.1	14.3	0.0	0.0
Cranberry, No Added Sugar, BGTY, Sainsbury's*	1 Glass/200ml	4	0.0	2	0.0	0.3	0.0	0.0
Cranberry, Original, Concentrated, Ocean Spray*	1 Serving/15ml	27	0.0	183	0.2	44.1	0.0	0.0
Cranberry, Reduced Sugar, Sainsbury's*	1 Glass/200ml	72	0.0	36	0.1	8.4	0.0	0.0
Cranberry, Tropical, Ocean Spray*	1 Glass/200ml	96	0.0	48	0.1	11.5	0.0	0.0
Cranberry, Waitrose*	1 Serving/250ml	145	0.0	58	0.1	13.9	0.0	0.1
Cranberry & Apple, Ocean Spray*	1 Glass/200ml	92	0.0	46	0.0	11.1	0.0	0.0
Cranberry & Blackberry, Ocean Spray*	1 Glass/250ml	120	0.2	48	0.1	11.3	0.1	0.2
Cranberry & Blackcurrant, Ocean Spray*	1 Bottle/500ml	265	0.0	53	0.2	12.7	0.0	0.0
Cranberry & Blueberry, Ocean Spray*	1 Serving/100ml	48	0.0	48	0.0	11.6	0.0	0.0
Cranberry & Mango, Light, Ocean Spray*	1 Glass/250ml	22	0.0	9	0.0	2.0	0.0	0.1
Cranberry & Orange, No Added Sugar, Sainsbury's*	1 Glass/250ml	15	0.2	6	0.1	1.2	0.1	0.1
Cranberry & Pomegranate, Ocean Spray*	1 Glass/250ml	120	0.0	48	0.0	11.5	0.0	0.0
Cranberry & Raspberry, BGTY, Sainsbury's*	1 Glass/250ml	10	0.2	4	0.1	0.7	0.1	0.1
Cranberry & Raspberry, Ocean Spray*	1 Glass/200ml	96	0.0	48	0.0	11.6	0.0	0.0

	Measure INFO/WEIGHT	per Measure KCAL	FAT	Nutrition Values per 100g / 100ml KCAL	PROT	CARB	FAT	FIBRE
JUICE DRINK								
Cranberry Blend, Ocean Spray*	1 Glass/250ml	148	0.0	59	0.1	13.9	0.0	0.0
Exotic, Tesco*	1 Serving/250ml	128	0.0	51	0.1	12.3	0.0	0.0
Fruit Cocktail, Sainsbury's*	1 Glass/200ml	90	0.0	45	0.2	10.6	0.0	0.1
Grape, Apple & Raspberry, Asda*	1 Glass/200ml	90	0.0	45	0.2	11.0	0.0	0.0
Grape, Red, Sparkling, Shloer*	1 Glass/200ml	84	0.0	42	0.0	10.4	0.0	0.0
Grape, White, Sparkling, Shloer*	1 Serving/120ml	59	0.0	49	0.0	11.6	0.0	0.0
Grape & Elderflower, White, Sparkling, Shloer*	1 Glass/200ml	74	0.0	37	0.0	9.2	0.0	0.0
Grapefruit & Cranberry, M & S*	1 Serving/250ml	125	0.2	50	0.2	11.9	0.1	0.0
Grapefruit & Lime, Quest, M & S*	1 Bottle/330ml	53	0.0	16	0.0	4.0	0.0	0.0
Guava Exotic, Rubicon*	1 Carton/288ml	150	0.3	52	0.2	12.9	0.1	0.0
J2O, Apple & Blueberry, Britvic*	1 Bottle/275g	124	0.0	45	0.1	11.0	0.0	0.2
J2O, Apple & Mango, Britvic*	1 Bottle/275ml	83	0.0	30	0.1	6.8	0.0	0.2
J2O, Apple & Raspberry, Britvic*	1 Bottle/275ml	88	0.0	32	0.1	7.3	0.0	0.3
J2O, Glitterberry, Britvic*	1 Bottle/275ml	110	0.0	40	0.2	9.4	0.0	0.0
J2O, Orange & Passion Fruit, Britvic*	1 Bottle/275ml	88	0.0	32	0.3	7.2	0.0	0.2
J2O, White Blend, White Grape & Kiwi, Britvic*	1 Bottle/275ml	91	0.0	33	0.2	7.7	0.0	0.0
Lemon, The Feel Good Drinks Co*	1 Bottle/171ml	78	0.2	46	0.1	10.8	0.1	0.0
Lemon & Lime, Light, Oasis*	1 Bottle/250ml	6	0.0	3	0.0	0.2	0.0	0.0
Lemon & Mandarin, Diet, Quest, M & S*	1 Bottle/330ml	13	0.0	4	0.0	1.0	0.0	0.0
Lemonade, Asda*	1 Glass/200ml	88	0.0	44	0.1	11.0	0.0	0.0
Lychee, Sparkling, Rubicon*	1 Can/330g	182	0.0	55	0.0	13.6	0.0	0.0
Mango, Rubicon*	1 Serving/100ml	54	0.1	54	0.1	13.1	0.1	0.0
Mango, Sparkling, Rubicon*	1 Can/330ml	172	0.0	52	0.0	12.8	0.0	0.0
Mango & Passionfruit, Shot, Big Shotz*	1 Shot/120ml	67	0.5	56	0.0	12.1	0.4	3.4
Orange, Caprisun*	1 Pouch/200ml	89	0.0	45	0.0	10.8	0.0	0.0
Orange, Carrot & Lemon, Pago*	1 Serving/200g	90	0.2	45	0.2	10.5	0.1	0.0
Orange, Juice Burst, Purity*	1 Bottle/500ml	220	0.0	44	1.0	10.2	0.0	0.0
Orange, Mango & Lime, Fruit Crush, Shapers, Boots*	1 Bottle/330ml	150	0.6	45	0.4	10.6	0.2	0.4
Orange, Sainsbury's*	1 Serving/250ml	18	0.2	7	0.1	1.4	0.1	0.1
Passion Fruit, Exotic, Rubicon*	1 Serving/200ml	110	0.0	55	0.1	13.6	0.0	0.0
Peach, Fruit Float, Frubob*	1 Can/250ml	150	0.0	60	0.2	14.8	0.0	0.0
Peach, Passion Fruit, Extra Light, Oasis*	1 Bottle/500ml	18	0.0	4	0.0	0.6	0.0	0.0
Pear & Plum, Shapers, Boots*	1 Bottle/500ml	10	0.0	2	0.0	0.2	0.0	0.0
Pineapple, Mango & Passionfruit, Sainsbury's*	1 Serving/200ml	74	0.0	37	0.1	8.7	0.0	0.2
Pineapple & Grapefruit, Shapers, Boots*	1 Bottle/500ml	10	0.5	2	0.1	0.2	0.1	0.0
Pink Grapefruit, Juice Burst, Purity*	1 Bottle/500ml	210	0.0	42	0.4	10.0	0.0	0.0
Pomegranate, Rubicon*	1 Can/330mll	108	0.0	54	0.0	13.5	0.0	0.0
Pomegranate & Blueberry, Weight Watchers*	1 Bottle/500ml	15	0.0	3	0.0	0.5	0.0	0.0
Pomegranate & Raspberry, Still, Shapers, Boots*	1 Bottle/500ml	45	0.0	9	0.0	2.0	0.0	0.0
Raspberry, Ribena*	1 Bottle/500ml	215	0.0	43	0.0	10.4	0.0	0.0
Raspberry & Apple, No Added Sugar, Ribena*	1 Serving/200ml	8	0.0	4	0.0	0.5	0.0	0.0
Raspberry & Pear, Tesco*	1 Serving/250ml	118	0.0	47	0.0	11.3	0.0	0.0
Summer Fruits, Fresh, Tesco*	1 Glass/250ml	112	0.2	45	0.1	10.8	0.1	0.3
Summer Fruits, Oasis*	1 Bottle/500ml	90	0.0	18	0.0	4.2	0.0	0.0
Tropical, Be Light, Aldi*	1 Glass/250ml	62	0.2	25	0.2	5.4	0.1	0.2
Tropical, No Added Sugar, Tesco*	1 Carton/250ml	12	0.0	5	0.0	1.1	0.0	0.0
Tropical Fruit, Tesco*	1 Glass/250ml	118	0.0	47	0.0	11.4	0.0	0.0
Tropical Fruit, Waitrose*	1 Glass/250ml	118	0.0	47	0.2	11.2	0.0	0.0
Tropical Hit, 5 Alive*	1 Carton/250ml	92	0.0	37	0.0	9.3	0.0	0.0
JUNIPER								
Berries, Dried, Average	1 Tsp/2g	6	0.3	292	4.0	33.0	16.0	0.0

J

	Measure	per Measure		Nutrition Values per 100g / 100ml				
	INFO/WEIGHT	KCAL	FAT	KCAL	PROT	CARB	FAT	FIBRE
KALE								
Curly, Boiled in Salted Water, Average	***1 Sm Serving/60g***	***14***	***0.7***	***24***	***2.4***	***1.0***	***1.1***	***2.8***
Curly, Raw, Average	***1 Serving/90g***	***30***	***1.4***	***33***	***3.4***	***1.4***	***1.6***	***3.1***
KANGAROO								
Raw, Average	***1 Serving/200g***	***196***	***2.0***	***98***	***22.0***	***1.0***	***1.0***	***0.0***
Steak, Grilled, Average*	***1 Fillet/150g***	***198***	***1.8***	***132***	***30.0***	***0.0***	***1.2***	***0.0***
KEBAB								
BBQ Pork, Sainsbury's*	1 Serving/90g	65	2.2	72	11.0	1.4	2.4	0.9
Beef, Hot & Spicy, Tesco*	1 Kebab/41g	111	8.4	270	15.7	4.4	20.6	1.6
Beef, Kofta, Uncooked, Tesco*	1 Kebab/73g	163	12.5	225	14.0	3.2	17.3	1.2
Beef, with Onion, Dulano, Lidl*	1 Serving/100g	224	16.0	224	18.0	2.0	16.0	0.0
Beef, with Sweet Chilli Seasoning, Cooked, Sainsbury's*	1 Kebab/54g	118	7.0	219	20.2	5.3	12.9	0.5
Beef & Pepper, Kofta, Waitrose*	1 Kebab/138g	223	13.9	162	14.8	2.9	10.1	0.6
Chicken, & Pineapple, Aldi*	1 Kebab/85g	89	2.6	105	13.9	5.3	3.1	0.0
Chicken, & Pineapple, Caribbean Style, Iceland*	1 Kebab/44g	41	0.6	93	11.6	8.7	1.4	1.4
Chicken, & Sausage with Teriyaki Sauce, Asda*	1 Serving/110g	257	15.4	234	17.0	10.0	14.0	1.0
Chicken, Barbecue, Sainsbury's*	1 Pack/200g	238	3.4	119	24.4	1.5	1.7	1.8
Chicken, Breast, Mediterranean, Sainsbury's*	1 Kebab/65g	73	2.1	113	16.5	4.6	3.2	0.6
Chicken, Breast, Salsa, Sainsbury's*	1 Kebab/80g	94	0.9	118	20.1	6.5	1.1	0.6
Chicken, Breast, Sweet, Oriental, COU, M & S*	½ Pack/200g	220	2.0	110	20.8	4.3	1.0	0.1
Chicken, Caribbean, Iceland*	1 Kebab/44g	36	0.1	82	12.0	8.0	0.2	0.5
Chicken, Chilli & Lime, Breast Fillet, Sainsbury's*	1 Kebab/77g	120	0.7	156	29.9	6.2	0.9	0.3
Chicken, Chinese, Mini, M & S*	1 Kebab/11g	24	1.4	215	19.5	5.1	12.9	0.6
Chicken, Citrus Tikka, Mini, Sainsbury's*	1 Serving/48g	72	1.1	151	30.3	2.7	2.3	0.2
Chicken, Fillet, Mini, M & S*	1 Serving/150g	210	8.7	140	20.2	2.0	5.8	0.3
Chicken, Fillet, with a Tikka Marinade, Mini, Sainsbury's*	1 Kebab/25g	41	0.8	164	33.4	0.6	3.1	0.1
Chicken, Lemon & Ginger, Delicatezze, Waitrose*	1 Kebab/25g	50	2.8	201	24.5	0.3	11.3	2.7
Chicken, Mango & Lime, Perfectly Balanced, Waitrose*	1 Kebab/83g	103	1.3	125	26.0	1.2	1.6	1.1
Chicken, Red Pepper, Mini, Sainsbury's*	1 Kebab/52g	79	1.0	152	30.1	3.5	2.0	0.2
Chicken, Shish, in Pitta Bread with Salad	1 Kebab/250g	388	10.2	155	13.5	17.2	4.1	1.0
Chicken, Shish, Meat Only, Average	1 Kebab/250g	312	5.2	125	25.7	0.9	2.1	0.1
Chicken, Sweet Chilli, Perfectly Balanced, Waitrose*	1 Kebab/83g	111	0.9	135	28.6	1.7	1.1	0.5
Chicken, Thigh, Sticky Barbecue, M & S*	1 Kebab/100g	160	7.5	160	15.6	7.4	7.5	0.8
Chicken, Thin Sliced, Heat 'n' Eat, Asda*	½ Pack/50g	92	6.0	184	15.0	3.9	12.0	1.1
Chicken, with Sweet Chilli Sauce, M & S*	1 Serving/165g	228	1.3	138	17.9	14.7	0.8	1.2
Chicken Tikka, with Red Pepper & Pineapple, Tesco*	1 Kebab/80g	92	1.9	115	16.5	6.7	2.4	0.5
Doner, Heat 'n' Eat Thin Sliced, Asda*	1 Pack/100g	196	10.6	196	16.7	8.4	10.6	1.7
Doner, Iceland*	1 Serving/152g	268	7.1	176	9.2	24.4	4.6	2.4
Doner, Lidl*	1 Kebab/170g	509	31.3	300	14.7	15.3	18.4	0.0
Halloumi & Vegetable, Waitrose*	1 Kebab/127g	235	21.6	185	5.6	2.2	17.0	2.4
Lamb, Greek Style, Sainsbury's*	1 Serving/70g	196	15.3	282	16.1	4.9	22.0	1.8
Lamb, Kofta, Citrus Tikka, Sainsbury's*	1 Kebab/84g	199	11.6	235	18.1	9.8	13.7	2.6
Lamb, Kofta, Indian Style, Waitrose*	1 Kebab/125g	266	19.8	213	12.3	5.5	15.8	1.6
Lamb, Shami, with a Mint Raita Dip, M & S*	½ Pack/90g	189	12.1	210	12.8	9.7	13.4	3.5
Lamb, Shish, Sainsbury's*	1 Kebab/85g	178	11.3	210	19.7	2.8	13.3	0.7
Lamb, Shish, Waitrose*	1 Kebab/56g	114	7.1	203	15.3	6.8	12.7	1.1
Lamb, Shoulder, M & S*	½ Pack/250g	312	10.8	125	20.4	0.9	4.3	1.7
Lamb, with Halloumi Cheese & Olives, Waitrose*	1 Kebab/75g	123	6.2	164	20.0	2.4	8.3	0.2
Lamb, with Mint, Tesco*	1 Serving/80g	192	13.4	240	16.0	5.5	16.7	0.4
Pork & Pepper, BBQ, Sainsbury's*	1 Kebab/41g	65	2.2	158	24.1	3.1	5.4	1.9
Pork & Pepper, Co-Op*	1 Kebab/74g	78	3.0	105	17.0	1.0	4.0	0.5
Salmon, Cajun, Tesco*	1 Kebab/75g	100	3.2	133	19.8	3.9	4.2	1.3
Salmon, Chinese, Iceland*	1 Kebab/75g	115	3.4	153	23.8	4.1	4.6	1.6
Salmon, Hot & Spicy, Tesco*	1 Kebab/75g	88	2.2	118	22.0	1.1	2.9	0.0

	Measure INFO/WEIGHT	per Measure KCAL	FAT	Nutrition Values per 100g / 100ml KCAL	PROT	CARB	FAT	FIBRE
KEBAB								
Shish, with Onions & Peppers	1oz/28g	59	4.5	212	12.9	3.9	16.2	1.2
Sweetcorn, Tesco*	1 Kebab/130g	74	1.3	57	2.0	9.9	1.0	0.9
Tandoori, M & S*	1oz/28g	34	0.7	120	23.3	1.0	2.5	0.0
Tiger Prawn, Asda*	1oz/28g	17	0.0	59	14.6	0.0	0.1	0.0
Tikka, Mini, M & S*	1 Kebab/11g	23	1.4	205	18.4	4.0	12.7	0.6
Turkey, with Chinese Style Dressing, Sainsbury's*	1 Kebab/54g	84	2.7	157	21.4	6.4	5.1	1.7
Vegetable, Asda*	1 Kebab/40g	25	1.7	63	1.8	4.5	4.3	2.4
Vegetable, Mini, Sainsbury's*	1 Kebab/36g	22	0.8	61	2.5	7.4	2.3	2.4
KEDGEREE								
356, Oakhouse Foods Ltd.*	1 Meal/400g	432	15.6	108	8.2	9.8	3.9	0.6
Average	1oz/28g	48	2.4	171	15.9	7.8	8.7	0.1
COU, M & S*	1 Pack/370g	388	8.1	105	7.6	13.7	2.2	2.1
Smoked Haddock, Big Dish, M & S*	1 Pack/450g	585	22.5	130	8.5	13.0	5.0	1.9
KETCHUP								
Barbeque, Asda*	1 Tbsp/15g	20	0.0	136	0.9	33.0	0.0	0.0
BBQ, Heinz*	1 Serving/10g	14	0.0	137	1.3	31.3	0.3	0.3
Chilli, Mild, Twisted, Heinz*	1 Tbsp/15g	16	0.0	108	1.0	24.9	0.2	0.7
Tomato, Average	***1 Tsp/5g***	***6***	***0.0***	***120***	***1.5***	***28.1***	***0.2***	***0.8***
Tomato, Reduced Salt & Sugar, HP*	1 Tbsp/17g	15	0.0	86	0.7	19.5	0.1	0.4
Tomato, Reduced Sugar, Average	***1 Tbsp/10g***	***9***	***0.1***	***87***	***2.0***	***16.9***	***1.2***	***0.9***
Tomato, with Balsamic Vinegar, Basil & Oregano, Heinz*	1 Tsp/15g	17	0.0	110	1.4	25.3	0.1	1.3
Tomato, with Indian Spices, Heinz*	1 Tbsp/15g	17	0.1	114	1.1	24.8	0.4	0.8
Tomato, with Roasted Garlic, Thyme & Honey, Heinz*	1 Serving/15g	17	0.0	114	1.4	26.0	0.2	1.3
KIDNEY								
Lamb, Raw, Average	***1oz/28g***	***25***	***0.7***	***91***	***17.0***	***0.0***	***2.6***	***0.0***
Ox, Raw	***1oz/28g***	***25***	***0.6***	***88***	***17.2***	***0.0***	***2.1***	***0.0***
Ox, Stewed	***1oz/28g***	***39***	***1.2***	***138***	***24.5***	***0.0***	***4.4***	***0.0***
Pig, Fried	***1oz/28g***	***57***	***2.7***	***202***	***29.2***	***0.0***	***9.5***	***0.0***
Pig, Raw	***1oz/28g***	***24***	***0.8***	***86***	***15.5***	***0.0***	***2.7***	***0.0***
Pig, Stewed	***1oz/28g***	***43***	***1.7***	***153***	***24.4***	***0.0***	***6.1***	***0.0***
Veal, Raw, Average	1 Serving/100g	99	3.1	99	15.8	0.8	3.1	0.0
KIEV								
Cheese & Herb, Mini, Bernard Matthews*	1 Kiev/23g	46	2.3	199	15.7	12.1	9.8	0.0
Chicken, 370, Wiltshire Farm Foods*	1 Meal/350g	496	24.4	142	4.7	16.1	7.0	1.6
Chicken, Bernard Matthews*	1 Kiev/125g	374	27.9	299	10.6	13.9	22.3	2.7
Chicken, BFY, Morrisons*	1 Kiev/134g	304	17.4	227	16.1	11.5	13.0	1.0
Chicken, Breast, Hand Filled, Birds Eye*	1 Kiev/172g	330	17.2	192	15.5	9.9	10.0	2.0
Chicken, Cheesy Bean, Asda*	1 Kiev/94g	202	10.3	215	12.0	17.0	11.0	1.9
Chicken, Cooked, M Kitchen, Fresh Ideas, Morrisons*	1 Kiev/145g	359	20.8	248	17.5	12.0	14.4	0.9
Chicken, COU, M & S*	1 Kiev/150g	188	2.7	125	15.8	10.8	1.8	0.5
Chicken, Fillets, Whole, Frozen, Cooked, Birds Eye*	1 Portion/150g	300	16.0	200	14.7	11.3	10.7	1.4
Chicken, Finest, Tesco*	1 Kiev/237g	504	26.6	212	19.5	8.2	11.2	2.6
Chicken, Garlic, 25% Less Fat, GFY, Asda*	1 Kiev/134g	296	15.7	221	17.0	11.9	11.7	0.5
Chicken, Garlic, Creamy, Chilled, Tesco*	½ Pack/143g	285	17.1	200	12.9	9.7	12.0	1.3
Chicken, Garlic, M & S*	1 Kiev/150g	370	24.8	247	15.6	8.2	16.5	2.9
Chicken, Garlic, Morrisons*	1 Kiev/122g	289	19.2	237	14.3	9.8	15.7	0.0
Chicken, Garlic, Whole Breast, Asda*	1 Pack/290g	638	38.0	220	15.2	10.4	13.1	0.0
Chicken, Garlic & Herb, Reduced Fat, Sainsbury's*	1 Kiev/142g	317	18.0	223	15.1	12.1	12.7	0.6
Chicken, Garlic & Herb, Sainsbury's*	1 Kiev/134g	319	19.6	239	15.0	11.7	14.7	1.3
Chicken, Garlic & Mushroom, Sainsbury's*	1 Kiev/142g	346	19.1	243	16.2	14.5	13.4	1.4
Chicken, Garlic & Parsley, BGTY, Sainsbury's*	1 Kiev/126g	289	15.3	229	14.0	15.9	12.1	1.1
Chicken, Garlic & Parsley, Sainsbury's*	1 Kiev/120g	365	25.6	304	11.1	17.1	21.3	0.8
Chicken, Garlic Butter, HL, Tesco*	1 Kiev/143g	285	16.4	200	14.3	9.9	11.5	0.6

	Measure INFO/WEIGHT	per Measure KCAL	FAT	Nutrition Values per 100g / 100ml KCAL	PROT	CARB	FAT	FIBRE
KIEV								
Chicken, Good Choice, Iceland*	1 Kiev/120g	366	27.2	305	12.7	12.6	22.7	0.8
Chicken, Ham & Cheese, BGTY, Sainsbury's*	1 Kiev/132g	264	10.2	200	13.2	19.5	7.7	0.8
Chicken, Ham & Cheese, Tesco*	1 Serving/143g	307	18.6	215	14.4	9.3	13.0	1.3
Chicken, in Crispy Breadcrumbs, Sainsbury's*	1 Kiev/117g	310	22.4	266	12.8	10.6	19.2	1.1
Chicken, Italian Style, Sainsbury's*	1 Kiev/135g	341	21.7	253	14.3	12.8	16.1	1.3
Chicken, Maitre Jean-Pierre*	1 Kiev/140g	385	26.7	275	13.3	12.7	19.1	0.8
Chicken, Peppercorn, Creamy, Sun Valley*	1 Kiev/140g	382	25.9	273	13.3	13.5	18.5	0.0
Chicken, Peppercorn, Creamy, Tesco*	1 Kiev/132g	290	17.3	220	13.1	12.1	13.1	0.6
Chicken, Roast Garlic & Parsley, Sainsbury's*	1 Kiev/143g	369	21.3	258	14.5	16.5	14.9	0.8
Chicken, Tomato & Mozzarella, Tesco*	1 Kiev/143g	285	17.4	200	13.4	9.0	12.2	1.4
Chicken, Value, Tesco*	1 Serving/125g	355	27.1	284	10.4	11.7	21.7	1.8
Salmon, Fillet, Tesco*	1 Kiev/160g	376	19.5	235	13.3	18.0	12.2	2.5
Turkey, Mini, Baked, Bernard Matthews*	1 Kiev/23g	50	2.7	221	17.5	11.2	11.8	1.1
KIEV VEGETARIAN								
Aduki Bean, Cauldron Foods*	1 Kiev/110g	223	5.4	203	6.2	30.0	4.9	7.0
Garlic, Cheesy, Meat Free, Sainsbury's*	1 Kiev/123g	274	15.1	223	13.8	14.3	12.3	3.5
Garlic, Meat Free, Asda*	1 Kiev/125g	239	11.2	191	15.0	12.5	9.0	2.6
Garlic, Meat Free, Tesco*	1 Kiev/125g	244	11.2	195	15.0	12.5	9.0	2.6
Garlic Butter, Tivall*	1 Kiev/125g	366	26.2	293	15.1	10.8	21.0	2.6
Sweet Potato, Spinach & Quinoa, Linda McCartney*	1 Kiev/145g	319	13.5	220	3.8	28.7	9.3	3.4
Vegetable, M & S*	1 Kiev/155g	279	16.6	180	4.2	17.2	10.7	3.7
KIPPER								
Baked, Average	***1oz/28g***	***57***	***3.2***	***205***	***25.5***	***0.0***	***11.4***	***0.0***
Fillets, in Brine, John West*	1 Can/140g	269	16.8	192	21.0	0.0	12.0	0.0
Fillets, in Sunflower Oil, John West*	1 Can/140g	321	23.8	229	19.0	0.0	17.0	0.0
Fillets, Raw, Average	***1 Serving/200g***	***451***	***34.3***	***226***	***17.0***	***0.0***	***17.1***	***0.0***
Fillets, Smoked, TTD, Sainsbury's*	1 Serving/100g	255	19.4	255	20.1	0.1	19.4	0.0
Grilled, Average	***1oz/28g***	***71***	***5.4***	***255***	***20.1***	***0.0***	***19.4***	***0.0***
Smoked, Average	***1 Serving/150g***	***322***	***23.0***	***214***	***18.9***	***0.0***	***15.4***	***0.0***
KIT KAT								
2 Finger, Nestle*	2 Fingers/21g	107	5.3	512	6.0	63.5	25.5	2.1
4 Finger, Nestle*	4 Fingers/45g	233	11.7	513	5.9	63.3	25.7	2.1
Caramac, 4 Finger, Nestle*	4 Fingers/49g	259	14.1	532	5.9	61.9	29.0	0.6
Chunky, Caramel, Nestle*	1 Bar/48g	259	15.3	539	5.2	58.6	31.8	0.0
Chunky, Double Caramel, Nestle*	½ Bar/21g	109	5.8	520	6.5	61.0	27.6	1.0
Chunky, Nestle*	1 Bar/48g	248	12.6	516	5.9	62.5	26.3	2.1
Chunky, Orange, Nestle*	1 Bar/48g	247	12.5	515	5.8	62.0	26.1	0.0
Chunky, Peanut, Nestle*	1 Bar/50g	268	15.8	537	8.4	54.9	31.5	0.0
Chunky, Snack Size, Nestle*	1 Bar/26g	133	7.1	513	6.6	60.4	27.2	1.1
Cookies & Cream, Nestle*	2 Bar/21g	107	5.2	510	6.3	64.0	25.0	1.4
Editions, Mango & Passionfruit, Nestle*	1 Bar/45g	225	10.5	499	4.7	69.0	23.4	0.0
Editions, Seville Orange, Nestle*	1 Bar/45g	223	10.4	496	4.6	69.3	23.0	0.8
Kubes, Nestle*	1 Pack/50g	258	13.8	515	5.9	60.9	27.5	1.0
Kubes, Orange, Nestle*	4 Kubes/13g	66	3.5	514	5.7	61.1	27.4	1.0
Lemon & Yoghurt, Nestle*	1 Pack/45g	240	13.4	533	7.3	58.0	29.8	0.4
Low Carb, 2 Finger, Nestle*	2 Fingers/21g	92	6.6	438	9.2	28.3	31.3	1.3
Low Carb, 4 Finger, Nestle*	1 Finger/11g	46	3.3	438	9.2	28.3	31.3	1.3
Mini, Nestle*	1 Bar/15g	75	3.9	502	7.5	59.4	26.0	0.0
Mint, 4 Finger, Nestle*	4 Fingers/48g	244	12.7	508	6.0	61.5	26.4	1.1
Orange, 2 Finger, Nestle*	2 Fingers/21g	107	5.6	507	5.5	61.7	26.5	0.0
Senses, Nestle*	1 Bar/31g	165	9.5	531	7.5	56.3	30.7	0.0
White, Chunky, Nestle*	1 Bar/53g	276	14.6	521	8.3	60.3	27.5	0.7

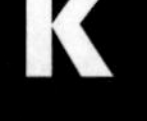

	Measure INFO/WEIGHT	per Measure KCAL	FAT	Nutrition Values per 100g / 100ml KCAL	PROT	CARB	FAT	FIBRE
KIWI FRUIT								
Fresh, Raw, Flesh & Seeds, Average	***1 Kiwi/60g***	***29***	***0.3***	***49***	***1.1***	***10.6***	***0.5***	***1.9***
Hayward, Perfectly Ripe, Waitrose*	1 Kiwi/85g	45	0.4	53	1.1	10.6	0.5	3.0
Weighed with Skin, Average	***1 Kiwi/60g***	***29***	***0.3***	***49***	***1.1***	***10.6***	***0.5***	***1.9***
KOHLRABI								
Boiled in Salted Water	***1oz/28g***	***5***	***0.1***	***18***	***1.2***	***3.1***	***0.2***	***1.9***
Raw	***1oz/28g***	***6***	***0.1***	***23***	***1.6***	***3.7***	***0.2***	***2.2***
KORMA								
Chicken, & Basmati Rice, Tesco*	1 Pot/350g	588	32.6	168	4.3	16.9	9.3	2.3
Chicken, & Pilau Rice, BGTY, Sainsbury's*	1 Pack/400g	404	5.2	101	8.0	14.3	1.3	0.6
Chicken, & Pilau Rice, Indian, Asda*	1 Pack/456g	643	22.8	141	8.0	16.0	5.0	2.4
Chicken, & Pilau Rice, Saint Agur*	1 Serving/367g	367	5.5	100	6.4	14.1	1.5	2.2
Chicken, & Pilau Rice, Tesco*	1 Serving/460g	722	45.1	157	5.6	11.5	9.8	1.3
Chicken, & Rice, 323, Oakhouse Foods Ltd*	1 Meal/400g	552	23.6	138	7.1	14.2	5.9	0.6
Chicken, & Rice, 95% Fat Free, Birds Eye*	1 Pack/370g	444	7.0	120	6.2	19.6	1.9	1.1
Chicken, & Rice, Good Choice, Iceland*	1 Pack/400g	464	8.4	116	5.8	18.4	2.1	0.8
Chicken, & Rice, Healthy Living, Co-Op*	1 Pack/400g	480	8.0	120	8.0	17.0	2.0	1.0
Chicken, & Rice, Organic, Tesco*	1 Pack/450g	922	47.7	205	6.0	21.5	10.6	0.4
Chicken, & Rice, World Flavours*	1 Pack/500g	705	23.5	141	8.7	16.0	4.7	0.0
Chicken, & White Rice, BGTY, Frozen, Sainsbury's*	1 Pack/375g	341	3.8	91	5.6	14.9	1.0	0.5
Chicken, & Yellow Pilau Rice, Chilled, Tesco*	1 Pack/550g	698	20.9	127	8.2	15.0	3.8	1.2
Chicken, Breast, Chunks, Sainsbury's*	1 Serving/227g	354	9.3	156	28.0	1.7	4.1	0.8
Chicken, Fresh, Chilled, Tesco*	1 Pack/350g	819	60.9	234	13.1	6.3	17.4	2.3
Chicken, HL, Tesco*	1 Pack/350g	371	4.2	106	7.7	15.9	1.2	0.8
Chicken, Indian, Takeaway, Tesco*	½ Pack/175g	222	13.5	127	9.0	5.5	7.7	1.8
Chicken, Indian Takeaway, Iceland*	1 Pack/400g	656	44.0	164	11.8	4.5	11.0	1.4
Chicken, Indian Takeaway for One, Sainsbury's*	1 Serving/300g	498	30.9	166	13.0	5.3	10.3	1.6
Chicken, Less Than 3% Fat, Birds Eye*	1 Pack/358g	440	6.8	123	6.5	20.4	1.9	0.8
Chicken, Less Than 3% Fat, Frozen, GFY, Asda*	1 Pack/401g	405	6.8	101	5.3	16.2	1.7	1.2
Chicken, Morrisons*	1 Pack/350g	707	46.6	202	13.6	7.0	13.3	0.7
Chicken, Plumrose*	1 Can/392g	431	22.0	110	8.0	6.9	5.6	0.0
Chicken, Rice, Ready Meal, Healthy Range, Average	1 Serving/400g	450	8.2	112	7.3	16.1	2.1	1.2
Chicken, Tesco*	1 Pack/350g	620	41.3	177	10.8	6.8	11.8	0.6
Chicken, Tinned, Asda*	½ Can/197g	321	21.7	163	8.0	8.0	11.0	2.3
Chicken, Waitrose*	1 Pack/400g	680	46.8	170	13.7	2.4	11.7	1.9
Chicken, with Peshwari Coriander Rice, Finest, Tesco*	1 Pack/550g	908	48.4	165	7.5	13.9	8.8	0.9
Chicken, with Pilau Rice, Asda*	1 Serving/350g	735	49.0	210	12.0	9.0	14.0	2.0
Chicken, with Pilau Rice, Perfectly Balanced, Waitrose*	1 Pack/400g	452	6.8	113	8.9	15.4	1.7	1.3
Chicken, with Pilau Rice, Sharwood's*	1 Pack/375g	489	16.2	130	5.2	17.1	4.3	1.2
Chicken, with Rice, Ready Meal, Average	1 Sm Pack/350g	648	30.4	185	8.4	18.1	8.7	1.7
Vegetable, & Rice, Tesco*	1 Pack/450g	621	26.6	138	2.9	18.3	5.9	1.6
Vegetable, Ready to Cook, Fresh, Sainsbury's*	½ Pack/255g	263	17.3	103	2.8	7.7	6.8	2.1
Vegetable, Sainsbury's*	1 Serving/200g	302	25.2	151	2.7	6.6	12.6	2.2
KRISPROLLS								
Cracked Wheat, Original, Pagen*	1 Krisproll/13g	48	0.9	380	12.0	67.0	7.0	9.0
Golden, Swedish Toasts, Pagen*	1 Krisproll/12g	48	1.0	400	11.0	69.0	8.5	5.0
Organic, Bio, Pagen*	1 Krisproll/12g	46	0.8	380	12.0	67.0	7.0	8.0
Swedish Toasts, Wholegrain, Pagen*	1 Toast/13g	51	0.8	390	11.0	67.0	6.5	8.5
KULFI								
Average	***1oz/28g***	***119***	***11.2***	***424***	***5.4***	***11.8***	***39.9***	***0.6***
KUMQUATS								
Raw	***1oz/28g***	***12***	***0.1***	***43***	***0.9***	***9.3***	***0.5***	***3.8***

	Measure INFO/WEIGHT	per Measure KCAL	FAT	Nutrition Values per 100g / 100ml KCAL	PROT	CARB	FAT	FIBRE
LAGER								
Alcohol Free, Becks*	1 Serving/275ml	55	0.0	20	0.7	5.0	0.0	0.0
Amstel, Heineken*	1 Pint/568ml	227	0.0	40	0.5	3.0	0.0	0.0
Average	1 Pint/568ml	233	0.0	41	0.3	3.1	0.0	0.0
Becks*	1 Can/275ml	113	0.0	41	0.0	3.0	0.0	0.0
Blanc, Kronenbourg*	½ Pint/284ml	119	0.0	42	0.0	3.3	0.0	0.0
Boston, Samuel Adams*	1 Bottle/355ml	160	0.0	45	0.0	0.0	0.0	0.0
Bottled, Brahma*	1 Bottle/330ml	125	0.0	38	0.0	0.0	0.0	0.0
Budweiser, 66, Anheuser-Busch*	1 Bottle/330ml	102	0.0	31	0.0	0.0	0.0	0.0
C2, Carling*	½ Pint/284ml	80	0.0	28	0.0	3.5	0.0	0.0
Can, Carlsberg*	1 Can/440ml	141	0.0	32	0.0	2.0	0.0	0.0
Draught, Carling*	1 Pint/568ml	189	0.0	33	0.0	1.4	0.0	0.0
Edge, Carlsberg*	1 Can/300ml	126	0.0	42	0.0	4.3	0.0	0.0
Export, Carlsberg*	1 Can/440ml	185	0.0	42	0.4	2.8	0.0	0.4
Export, Foster's*	1 Pint/568ml	210	0.0	37	0.0	2.2	0.0	0.0
Foster's*	1 Pint/568ml	193	0.0	34	0.0	3.1	0.0	0.0
German, Low Alcohol, Sainsbury's*	1 Bottle/330ml	92	0.3	28	0.4	5.9	0.1	0.1
Gold, Foster's*	1 Can/440ml	145	0.0	33	0.3	1.2	0.0	0.0
Grolsch*	1 Can/330ml	145	0.0	44	0.0	2.2	0.0	0.0
Heineken, 5%, Heineken*	1 Bottle/250ml	110	0.0	44	0.4	3.4	0.0	0.0
Kaliber, Guinness*	1 Can/440ml	110	0.0	25	0.2	6.0	0.0	0.0
Light, Coors*	1 Pint/500ml	150	0.0	30	0.3	1.5	0.0	0.0
Light, Corona*	1 Bottle/330ml	105	0.0	32	1.5	0.0	0.0	0.0
Light, Michelob*	1 Serving/340ml	113	0.0	33	0.3	2.0	0.0	0.0
Lite, Carlsberg*	1 Bottle/330ml	89	0.0	27	0.1	0.5	0.0	0.0
Low Alcohol	1 Can/440ml	44	0.0	10	0.2	1.5	0.0	0.0
Organic, Tesco*	1 Bottle/500ml	215	0.0	43	0.2	3.5	0.0	0.0
Pils, Holsten*	1 Can/440ml	167	0.0	38	0.3	2.4	0.0	0.0
Pilsner, Efes*	1 Can/500ml	226	0.0	45	0.0	7.6	0.0	0.0
Polish, Tyskie*	1 Can/550ml	236	0.0	43	0.0	0.0	0.0	0.0
Premier, Kronenbourg*	½ Pint/284ml	136	0.0	48	0.0	0.0	0.0	0.0
Premium	1 Can/440ml	260	0.0	59	0.3	2.4	0.0	0.0
Premium, French, Biere Speciale, Tesco*	1 Serving/250ml	105	0.0	42	0.3	3.3	0.0	0.0
Premium, Light, Amstel*	1 Can/355ml	95	0.0	27	0.0	1.4	0.0	0.0
Premium, San Miguel*	1 Bottle/330ml	148	0.0	45	0.3	3.7	0.0	0.0
Shandy, Traditional Style, Asda*	1 Serving/200ml	44	0.0	22	0.0	4.6	0.0	0.0
Tuborg Green, Carlsberg*	1 Serving/200ml	78	0.0	39	0.5	2.5	0.0	0.0
Ultra Low Carb, Michelob*	1 Bottle/275ml	88	0.0	32	0.2	0.9	0.0	0.0
Vier, Becks*	1 Bottle/275ml	110	0.0	40	0.0	3.0	0.0	0.0
LAKSA								
Chicken, COU, M & S*	1 Pack/450g	360	9.9	80	7.5	7.0	2.2	1.1
Thai Noodle, with Chicken, M & S*	1 Pack/400g	460	21.6	115	7.0	9.8	5.4	1.1
LAMB								
Breast, Lean, Roasted, Average	1 Serving/100g	273	18.5	273	26.7	0.0	18.5	0.0
Chops, Average	***1 Chop/82g***	***190***	***13.4***	***231***	***20.6***	***0.4***	***16.4***	***0.0***
Chops, Leg, De-boned, Grilled, Simply Cook, Tesco*	1 Chop/105g	330	17.7	314	39.2	0.0	16.9	0.0
Chops, Minted, Average	***1 Chop/100g***	***260***	***15.1***	***260***	***25.9***	***5.1***	***15.1***	***0.3***
Cutlets, Neck, Raw, Lean & Fat, Weighed with Bone	***1 Pack 210g***	***485***	***42.8***	***231***	***11.9***	***0.0***	***20.4***	***0.0***
Diced, From Supermarket, Healthy Range, Average	***½ Pack/200g***	***277***	***8.9***	***138***	***24.6***	***0.1***	***4.5***	***0.0***
Escalope, Asda*	1 Serving/100g	173	5.0	173	32.0	0.0	5.0	0.0
Fillet, Neck, Lean, Raw	1 Serving/100g	232	17.6	232	18.4	0.0	17.6	0.0
Grill Steak, Average	***1oz/28g***	***70***	***4.7***	***250***	***20.2***	***4.4***	***16.9***	***0.4***
Grill Steak, Prime, Average	***1 Steak/63g***	***197***	***16.1***	***312***	***18.5***	***2.0***	***25.5***	***0.1***
Grill Steak, Rosemary & Mint, Tesco*	1 Steak/62g	172	10.9	277	24.4	5.6	17.6	1.8

	Measure INFO/WEIGHT	per Measure KCAL	FAT	Nutrition Values per 100g / 100ml KCAL	PROT	CARB	FAT	FIBRE
LAMB								
Leg, Joint, Raw, Average	***1 Joint/510g***	***858***	***45.5***	***168***	***20.9***	***1.4***	***8.9***	***0.2***
Leg, Roasted, Lean, Average	***1oz/28g***	***58***	***2.7***	***206***	***29.9***	***0.0***	***9.6***	***0.0***
Leg, Roasted, Lean & Fat, Average	***1oz/28g***	***66***	***3.8***	***237***	***28.6***	***0.0***	***13.6***	***0.0***
Loin, Chop, Grilled, Lean & Fat, Weighed with Bone	1 Serving/100g	247	17.9	247	21.5	0.0	17.9	0.0
Loin, Chops, Raw, Lean & Fat, Weighed with Bone	1 Serving/100g	216	17.9	216	13.7	0.0	17.9	0.0
Mince, Average	***1oz/28g***	***58***	***4.2***	***207***	***17.6***	***0.5***	***14.8***	***0.0***
Mince, Extra Lean, Sainsbury's*	1 Serving/225g	324	11.9	144	24.1	0.0	5.3	0.1
Rack, Raw, Lean & Fat	***1oz/28g***	***79***	***6.7***	***283***	***17.3***	***0.0***	***23.8***	***0.0***
Rack, Raw, Lean Only, Weighed with Bone	***1 oz/28g***	***48***	***2.6***	***169***	***20.0***	***0.0***	***9.2***	***0.0***
Rack, Roasted, Lean	***1oz/28g***	***63***	***3.6***	***225***	***27.1***	***0.0***	***13.0***	***0.0***
Rack, Roasted, Lean & Fat	***1oz/28g***	***102***	***8.4***	***363***	***23.0***	***0.0***	***30.1***	***0.0***
Shank, Just Cook, Sainsbury's*	1 Shank/225g	394	18.7	175	22.9	1.8	8.3	0.0
Shoulder, Cooked, Lean & Fat	***1oz/28g***	***84***	***6.3***	***301***	***24.4***	***0.0***	***22.5***	***0.0***
Shoulder, Fillet, Average	***1oz/28g***	***66***	***5.1***	***235***	***17.6***	***0.0***	***18.3***	***0.0***
Shoulder, Raw, Average	***1oz/28g***	***70***	***5.7***	***248***	***16.8***	***0.0***	***20.2***	***0.0***
Shoulder, Roasted, Whole, Lean	***1oz/28g***	***61***	***3.4***	***218***	***27.2***	***0.0***	***12.1***	***0.0***
Steak, Leg, Raw, Average	***1 Steak/150g***	***169***	***5.5***	***112***	***20.0***	***0.0***	***3.6***	***0.0***
Steak, Minted, Average	***1 Steak/125g***	***212***	***9.0***	***170***	***22.7***	***3.4***	***7.2***	***0.9***
Steak, Raw, Average	***1 Steak/140g***	***190***	***7.6***	***136***	***21.7***	***0.2***	***5.4***	***0.0***
Stewing, Raw, Lean & Fat	***1oz/28g***	***57***	***3.5***	***203***	***22.5***	***0.0***	***12.6***	***0.0***
Stewing, Stewed, Lean	***1oz/28g***	***67***	***4.1***	***240***	***26.6***	***0.0***	***14.8***	***0.0***
Stewing, Stewed, Lean & Fat	***1oz/28g***	***78***	***5.6***	***279***	***24.4***	***0.0***	***20.1***	***0.0***
Trimmed Fat, Raw, Average	1 Serving/100g	518	51.6	518	13.3	0.0	51.6	0.0
LAMB BRAISED								
& Mash, Tesco*	1 Serving/450g	413	12.2	92	6.1	10.7	2.7	0.8
Shanks, with Chunky Vegetables, M & S*	½ Pack/425g	808	38.2	190	24.7	2.0	9.0	0.7
LAMB DINNER								
Roast, Birds Eye*	1 Dinner/340g	370	14.0	109	5.9	12.1	4.1	1.5
LAMB IN								
Garlic & Rosemary Gravy, Shank, Asda*	1 Shank/280g	451	23.2	161	19.8	1.7	8.3	0.5
Gravy, Minted, Roast, M & S*	1 Pack/200g	140	3.0	70	6.8	6.6	1.5	0.9
Gravy, Roast, Birds Eye*	1 Pack/239g	160	5.3	67	8.1	3.8	2.2	0.1
Mint Gravy, Sliced, Sainsbury's*	1 Pack/125g	134	4.8	107	15.3	2.9	3.8	0.8
Rich Minted Gravy, Shank, Morrisons*	1 Pack/400g	612	26.4	153	18.8	5.2	6.6	0.0
LAMB MEDITERRANEAN								
Shanks, Finest, Tesco*	1 Serving/404g	671	35.6	166	15.0	6.6	8.8	2.0
LAMB TAGINE								
Moroccan Style, with Cous Cous, COU, M & S*	1 Pack/400g	340	5.6	85	8.9	8.3	1.4	1.6
LAMB WITH								
Carrot & Swede Mash, Braised, Eat Smart, Morrisons*	1 Pack/400g	304	9.2	76	5.2	8.2	2.3	1.5
Cous Cous, Moroccan Style, Tesco*	1 Pack/550g	710	14.9	129	6.6	19.6	2.7	1.3
Gravy, Joint, Tesco*	1 Serving/225g	277	13.0	123	14.9	2.8	5.8	0.0
Gravy, Rosemary, Shank, Sainsbury's*	1 Serving/200g	204	8.2	102	13.2	3.1	4.1	0.3
Honey Roast Vegetables, Extra Special, Asda*	1 Pack/400g	400	14.8	100	9.9	6.7	3.7	2.5
Mango & Mint, Shoulder Chops, Waitrose*	1 Chop/250g	555	40.5	222	16.7	2.3	16.2	0.5
Mint, Leg Chops, Morrisons*	2 Chops/350g	858	45.2	245	29.4	2.4	12.9	0.9
Mint Butter, Leg Steaks, Waitrose*	1 Serving/155g	270	16.3	174	19.6	0.4	10.5	0.0
Mint Glaze & Redcurrant Sauce, Steaks, Leg, Asda*	½ Pack/145g	247	8.7	170	18.0	11.0	6.0	0.5
Mint Gravy, Joint, Tesco*	1 Serving/100g	88	1.7	88	16.6	1.8	1.7	0.1
Mint Gravy, Shanks, Frozen, Tesco*	1 Shank/200g	420	26.4	210	20.1	1.6	13.2	0.7
Redcurrant & Rosemary Sauce, Chops, Leg, Tesco*	1 Pack/325g	604	36.1	186	17.6	4.0	11.1	0.5
Rosemary, Joint, Tesco*	1 Serving/125g	250	17.6	200	17.5	0.8	14.1	0.5
Vegetables, Roasted, Shank, M & S*	½ Pack/420g	660	30.6	157	14.9	8.3	7.3	0.7

	Measure	per Measure		Nutrition Values per 100g / 100ml				
	INFO/WEIGHT	KCAL	FAT	KCAL	PROT	CARB	FAT	FIBRE
LARD								
Average	***1oz/28g***	***249***	***27.7***	***891***	***0.0***	***0.0***	***99.0***	***0.0***
LASAGNE								
Al Forno, Beef, with a Chianti Classico Ragu, M & S*	1 Pack/400g	640	38.0	160	8.2	10.7	9.5	2.8
Al Forno, Finest, Tesco*	1 Pack/400g	700	38.4	175	8.4	13.3	9.6	1.0
Asda*	1 Pack/398g	502	23.9	126	7.3	10.6	6.0	1.1
Beef, & Chunky Vegetable, HL, Tesco*	1 Pack/340g	354	9.5	104	5.9	13.8	2.8	1.2
Beef, BGTY, Sainsbury's*	1 Pack/390g	376	8.5	102	6.2	13.2	2.3	1.7
Beef, Frozen, Co-Op*	1 Pack/340g	388	15.6	114	7.5	10.7	4.6	1.4
Beef, Frozen, Tesco*	1 Pack/450g	608	25.2	135	7.5	12.6	5.6	0.8
Beef, Less Than 3% Fat, Frozen, GFY, Asda*	1 Pack/400g	369	10.0	92	7.3	8.9	2.5	2.5
Beef, Less Than 5% Fat, Asda*	1 Pack/400g	460	17.2	115	5.0	14.0	4.3	0.6
Beef, Little Dish*	1 Pack/200g	349	20.8	174	9.3	10.7	10.4	0.8
Beef, Ready Meal, Average	1 Serving/400g	553	24.0	138	8.2	12.7	6.0	1.4
Bolognese, & Vegetable, Weight Watchers*	1 Pack/300g	279	7.8	93	5.0	12.4	2.6	0.0
Bolognese, Lidl*	1 Serving/200g	336	18.0	168	8.0	13.7	9.0	0.0
Charlie Bigham's*	½ Pack/344g	557	29.2	162	8.5	11.3	8.5	0.7
Chicken, Italian, Sainsbury's*	1 Pack/450g	549	18.9	122	8.4	12.6	4.2	0.5
Chicken, LC, Tesco*	1 Pack/400g	344	6.8	86	7.1	10.5	1.7	1.8
Chicken, Mushroom & Asparagus, Finest, Tesco*	½ Pack/300g	360	16.2	120	7.6	10.2	5.4	0.8
Chicken, Ready Meals, Waitrose*	1 Pack/300g	411	19.8	137	6.3	13.0	6.6	0.9
Classic, Deep Filled, M & S*	1 Pack/400g	760	47.6	190	10.0	11.2	11.9	0.6
Diet Chef Ltd*	1 Pack/270g	288	13.8	107	5.6	9.6	5.1	1.9
Family, Big Value Pack, Iceland*	¼ Pack/237g	322	14.0	136	5.0	15.9	5.9	1.4
Family, M & S*	¼ Pack/225g	281	14.0	125	10.3	6.9	6.2	1.1
Fresh, Findus*	1 Pack/350g	402	15.8	115	6.2	11.7	4.5	0.0
Frozen, You Count, Love Life, Waitrose*	1 Pack/380g	359	10.3	94	5.0	12.2	2.7	0.6
Good Choice, Iceland*	1 Pack/400g	444	15.2	111	7.7	11.6	3.8	0.2
Italian, Family, Asda*	¼ Pack/185	306	18.5	166	8.0	11.0	10.0	1.7
Italian, Fresh, Chilled, Sainsbury's*	1 Pack/400g	480	22.0	120	10.1	7.5	5.5	1.4
Less Than 5% Fat, BFY, Morrisons*	½ Pack/350g	227	8.8	65	5.9	8.2	2.5	0.7
Low Fat, Co-Op*	1 Pack/300g	255	9.0	85	6.0	10.0	3.0	1.0
Low Saturated Fat, Waitrose*	1 Pack/400g	312	6.0	78	4.7	11.4	1.5	0.4
Mushroom & Spinach, Waitrose*	1 Pack/400g	373	14.0	93	3.1	12.3	3.5	1.3
Reduced Calorie, Chosen By You, Asda*	1 Pack/400g	332	10.0	83	6.0	8.4	2.5	1.3
Salmon, King Prawn & Spinach, Finest, Tesco*	1 Pack/400g	600	29.6	150	10.6	9.6	7.4	0.8
Salmon, Smoked, & Asparagus, Sainsbury's*	1 Pack/350g	665	37.4	190	7.9	15.6	10.7	0.7
Sheets, Boiled, Average	***1 Sheet/20g***	***20***	***0.1***	***100***	***3.0***	***22.0***	***0.6***	***0.9***
Sheets, Dry, Average	***1 Sheet/20g***	***70***	***0.3***	***349***	***11.9***	***72.1***	***1.5***	***2.9***
Sheets, Fresh, Dry, Average	***1 Sheet/21g***	***56***	***0.4***	***271***	***10.9***	***52.7***	***2.1***	***1.9***
Sheets, Verdi, Dry, Average	***1 Sheet/20g***	***71***	***0.4***	***356***	***12.6***	***71.1***	***2.2***	***2.8***
Sheets, Wholewheat, Cooked, Chosen By You, Asda*	1 Sheet/21g	31	0.2	148	4.8	28.3	0.9	3.7
Spinach & Cheese, Italian, Sainsbury's*	1 Pack/450g	666	30.6	148	6.0	15.5	6.8	0.5
Spinach & Ricotta, Asda*	1 Pack/400g	488	24.0	122	4.9	12.0	6.0	1.5
Spinach & Ricotta, Finest, Tesco*	1 Pack/350g	584	37.1	167	6.1	11.7	10.6	1.2
Spinach & Ricotta, Giovanni Rana*	1 Pack/350g	728	39.6	208	7.4	19.2	11.3	0.0
Value, Tesco*	1 Pack/300g	330	15.0	110	3.3	12.9	5.0	0.8
Vegetable, 254, Oakhouse Foods Ltd*	1 Meal/400g	344	17.6	86	3.4	8.0	4.4	1.4
Vegetable, Findus*	1 Pack/330g	314	8.2	95	4.0	13.0	2.5	0.0
Vegetable, Healthy Range, Average	1 Serving/400g	318	8.2	80	3.5	11.8	2.1	1.5
Vegetable, Italian, Frozen, Cooked, Sainsbury's*	1 Pack/378g	442	18.9	117	4.6	13.5	5.0	1.1
Vegetable, Low Saturated Fat, Waitrose*	1 Pack/400g	340	11.6	85	2.9	11.9	2.9	0.9
Vegetable, Mini, Classics, Co-Op*	1 Pack/300g	315	12.6	105	4.4	13.0	4.2	2.0
Vegetable, Ready Meal, Average	1 Serving/400g	408	17.6	102	4.1	12.4	4.4	1.0

	Measure INFO/WEIGHT	per Measure KCAL	FAT	Nutrition Values per 100g / 100ml KCAL	PROT	CARB	FAT	FIBRE
LASAGNE								
Vegetable, Roasted, M & S*	1 Pack/400g	440	20.4	110	3.4	12.8	5.1	1.7
Vegetable, Ross*	1 Pack/300g	270	8.4	90	2.9	13.3	2.8	1.2
Vegetable, Three Layer, Italian, Sainsbury's*	1 Pack/450g	554	23.4	123	4.8	14.3	5.2	0.5
Vegetable, Weight Watchers*	1 Pack/330g	251	5.6	76	3.6	11.8	1.7	0.7
Vegetable, You Count, Love Life, Waitrose*	1 Pack/400g	319	28.3	80	3.2	11.9	7.1	1.5
You Count, Love Life, Waitrose*	1 Pack/400g	306	6.4	76	6.7	8.1	1.6	1.2
LASAGNE VEGETARIAN								
Linda McCartney*	1 Pack/360g	451	20.2	125	6.3	12.4	5.6	1.4
Tesco*	1 Pack/450g	630	34.6	140	6.0	11.6	7.7	1.6
LAVERBREAD								
Average	***1oz/28g***	***15***	***1.0***	***52***	***3.2***	***1.6***	***3.7***	***0.0***
LEEKS								
Boiled, Average	***1oz/28g***	***6***	***0.2***	***21***	***1.2***	***2.6***	***0.7***	***1.7***
Creamed, Frozen, Waitrose*	1 Serving/225g	115	5.4	51	1.8	5.5	2.4	0.0
Frozen, Sliced, Asda*	1 Serving/100g	27	0.5	27	1.6	2.9	0.5	2.2
Raw, Unprepared, Average	***1 Leek/166g***	***64***	***1.5***	***39***	***2.8***	***5.1***	***0.9***	***3.9***
LEMON								
Extract	¼ Tsp/1ml	5	0.0	400	0.0	0.0	0.0	0.0
Fresh, Raw, Average	1 Slice/5g	1	0.0	20	1.0	3.2	0.3	2.4
Peel, Raw, Average	***1 Tbsp/6g***	***3***	***0.0***	***47***	***1.5***	***16.0***	***0.3***	***10.6***
LEMON CURD								
Average	***1 Tbsp/15g***	***44***	***0.7***	***294***	***0.7***	***62.9***	***4.7***	***0.1***
Luxury, Average	***1 Tsp/7g***	***23***	***0.6***	***326***	***2.8***	***59.7***	***8.4***	***0.1***
LEMON GRASS								
Easy, Asda*	1 Tsp/10g	5	0.1	52	0.4	7.4	1.2	5.2
Stalks, Tesco*	1 Stalk/13g	12	0.1	99	1.8	25.3	0.5	0.0
LEMON SOLE								
Fillets, Raw, Average	***1 Serving/220g***	***180***	***2.8***	***82***	***17.3***	***0.2***	***1.3***	***0.3***
Goujons, Average	1 Serving/150g	359	18.3	239	13.9	18.5	12.2	1.0
Grilled, Average	***1oz/28g***	***27***	***0.5***	***97***	***20.2***	***0.0***	***1.7***	***0.0***
in Breadcrumbs, Average	1 Fillet/142g	322	17.4	228	13.7	15.7	12.3	1.0
in White Wine & Herb Butter, Fillets, M & S*	1 Pack/220g	385	27.7	175	15.1	0.1	12.6	0.0
Steamed, Average	***1oz/28g***	***25***	***0.3***	***91***	***20.6***	***0.0***	***0.9***	***0.0***
with Lemon Mayonnaise, Goujons, Finest, Tesco*	1 Pack/230g	713	52.4	310	10.6	15.6	22.8	1.0
LEMONADE								
7 Up, Light, Britvic*	1 Can/330ml	4	0.0	1	0.1	0.2	0.0	0.0
7 Up, Zero, Britvic*	1 Can/330ml	6	0.0	2	0.1	0.1	0.0	0.0
Average	1 Glass/250ml	52	0.2	21	0.1	5.0	0.1	0.1
Cloudy, Diet, Sainsbury's*	1 Can/330ml	7	0.3	2	0.1	0.2	0.1	0.3
Cloudy, Gastropub, M & S*	1 Bottle/500ml	25	0.0	5	0.0	0.0	0.0	0.0
Cloudy, Shapers, Boots*	1 Bottle/500ml	15	0.0	3	0.0	0.3	0.0	0.0
Cloudy, Waitrose*	1 Glass/250ml	125	0.0	50	0.0	12.2	0.0	0.0
Diet, Average	1 Glass/250ml	4	0.1	2	0.1	0.2	0.0	0.0
Diet, Traditional Style, Tesco*	1 Glass/200ml	6	0.0	3	0.0	0.8	0.0	0.0
Low Calorie, Smart Price, Asda*	1 Glass/250ml	1	0.0	0	0.0	0.1	0.0	0.0
Organic, Tesco*	1 Can/142ml	61	0.0	43	0.0	10.6	0.0	0.0
Pink, Still, Pure Premium, Tropicana*	1 Serving/200ml	90	0.0	45	0.2	10.0	0.0	0.7
Premium, Freeway*	1 Glass/250ml	42	0.0	17	0.0	4.2	0.0	0.0
Premium, Pure, Still, Tropicana*	1 Glass/200ml	86	2.0	43	0.2	9.5	1.0	0.7
R White*	1 Glass/250ml	65	0.0	26	0.1	6.2	0.0	0.0
Schweppes*	1 Glass/250ml	45	0.0	18	0.0	4.2	0.0	0.0
Sicilian, Sainsbury's*	1 Glass/200ml	98	0.2	49	0.1	11.5	0.1	0.1
Sparkling, Co-Op*	1 Can/330ml	25	0.0	8	0.0	1.5	0.0	0.0

	Measure	per Measure		Nutrition Values per 100g / 100ml				
	INFO/WEIGHT	KCAL	FAT	KCAL	PROT	CARB	FAT	FIBRE
LEMONADE								
Sparkling, with Spanish Lemon Juice, Waitrose*	1 Glass/250ml	85	0.0	34	0.0	8.3	0.0	0.0
Still, Freshly Squeezed, M & S*	½ Bottle/250ml	100	0.5	40	0.1	9.0	0.2	0.5
Traditional Style, Tesco*	1 Glass/200ml	100	0.0	50	0.0	12.3	0.0	0.0
TTD, Sainsbury's*	1 Serving/248g	159	0.0	64	0.1	14.8	0.0	0.2
Victorian, Fentiman's*	1 Bottle/275ml	130	0.0	47	0.0	11.3	0.0	0.0
LEMSIP								
Beechams*	1 Sachet/3g	11	0.0	387	0.0	100.0	0.0	0.0
LENTILS								
Black Beluga, Ready to Eat, Merchant Gourmet*	1 Serving/63g	92	0.8	147	10.9	20.5	1.2	5.2
Campo Largo, Lidl*	1 Jar/400g	304	2.4	76	6.0	8.0	0.6	0.0
Green, Organic, Love Life, Waitrose*	1 Serving/40g	125	0.8	313	24.3	48.8	1.9	8.9
Green & Brown, Dried, Boiled in Salted Water, Average	***1 Tbsp/30g***	***32***	***0.2***	***105***	***8.8***	***16.9***	***0.7***	***3.8***
Green or Brown, Dried, Average	***1 Serving/50g***	***150***	***0.8***	***301***	***22.8***	***49.8***	***1.5***	***9.6***
Green or Brown in Water, Tinned, Average	***½ Can/132g***	***131***	***0.8***	***99***	***8.1***	***15.4***	***0.6***	***3.8***
Puy, Green, Dry, Average	1 Serving/100g	306	1.4	306	24.7	49.5	1.4	10.3
Red, Boiled in Unsalted Water, Average	***1oz/28g***	***28***	***0.1***	***102***	***7.6***	***17.5***	***0.4***	***2.6***
Red, Dried, Average	***1oz/28g***	***88***	***0.4***	***315***	***23.8***	***53.8***	***1.3***	***4.9***
Red, Split, Dried, Great Scot*	1 Serving/50g	152	0.5	304	23.8	53.2	1.0	0.0
Red, Split, Wholesome, Love Life, Waitrose*	1 Serving/80g	270	1.0	337	23.8	56.3	1.3	4.9
LETTUCE								
Average, Raw	½ Cup/28g	4	0.1	14	1.1	1.8	0.3	1.2
Crest, Sainsbury's*	1 Serving/80g	11	0.4	14	0.8	1.7	0.5	0.0
Curly Leaf, Sainsbury's*	1 Serving/80g	11	0.4	14	0.8	1.7	0.5	0.0
Iceberg, Average	***1 Serving/80g***	***11***	***0.3***	***13***	***0.8***	***1.8***	***0.3***	***0.5***
Lamb's, Average	***1 Serving/80g***	***12***	***0.2***	***14***	***1.4***	***1.6***	***0.2***	***1.0***
Radicchio, Red, Raw, Average	***1 Head/220g***	***29***	***0.2***	***13***	***1.4***	***1.6***	***0.1***	***3.0***
Red Gem, Tesco*	½ Lettuce/45g	7	0.2	15	0.8	1.7	0.5	0.9
Romaine, Average	***1 Serving/80g***	***12***	***0.4***	***15***	***0.9***	***1.7***	***0.5***	***0.7***
Romaine, Hearts, Average	***1 Serving/80g***	***12***	***0.4***	***16***	***0.9***	***1.7***	***0.6***	***1.0***
Romaine, Sweet, Average	***1 Serving/80g***	***12***	***0.4***	***16***	***0.9***	***1.6***	***0.6***	***0.8***
Round, Average	1 Serving/80g	10	0.2	13	1.4	2.2	0.2	1.1
LILT								
Fruit Crush, Coca-Cola*	1 Can/330ml	66	0.0	20	0.0	4.6	0.0	0.0
Fruit Crush, Zero, Coca-Cola*	1 Can/330ml	12	0.0	4	0.0	0.3	0.0	0.0
Z, Coca-Cola*	1 Can/330ml	10	0.0	3	0.0	0.4	0.0	0.0
LIME								
Peel, Raw	***1 Tbsp/6g***	***3***	***0.0***	***47***	***1.5***	***16.0***	***0.3***	***10.6***
Raw, Flesh Only, Average	***1 Lime/71g***	***18***	***0.1***	***25***	***0.6***	***8.8***	***0.2***	***2.4***
Raw, Weighed with Peel & Seeds, Average	***1 Lime/85g***	***26***	***0.2***	***30***	***0.7***	***10.5***	***0.2***	***2.8***
LINGUINE								
Cooked	1 Serving/100g	133	0.7	133	5.1	26.3	0.7	1.1
Crab, Rocket & Chilli, Italian, Finest, Tesco*	1 Pack/350g	718	36.4	205	6.5	20.7	10.4	1.7
Crab & Chilli, Waitrose*	1 Pack/350g	770	45.0	220	7.7	18.0	12.9	1.8
Dry, Average	***1 Serving/100g***	***352***	***2.2***	***352***	***13.1***	***70.0***	***2.2***	***2.8***
Dry, Parioli, Cucina*	1 Serving/75g	270	1.0	360	12.5	73.0	1.4	2.6
Dry Weight, De Cecco*	1 Serving/100g	350	1.5	350	13.0	71.0	1.5	2.9
Fresh, Dry, Average	***1 Pack/250g***	***681***	***6.5***	***272***	***12.3***	***51.7***	***2.6***	***4.0***
Garlic & Basil, Asda*	1 Serving/75g	108	0.4	144	5.4	29.5	0.5	2.5
King Prawn, Asda*	1 Pack/400g	380	10.4	95	6.4	11.5	2.6	1.5
Pomodoro, M & S*	1 Pack/300g	360	10.5	120	4.1	17.6	3.5	1.2
Salmon & Prawn, Iceland*	1 Meal/450g	540	19.8	120	4.5	15.8	4.4	1.5
Tomato & Mushroom, Perfectly Balanced, Waitrose*	1 Pack/350g	294	13.3	84	2.2	10.6	3.8	1.0
Vegetable & Ham, BGTY, Sainsbury's*	1 Pack/450g	410	13.5	91	4.4	11.7	3.0	0.9

	Measure INFO/WEIGHT	per Measure KCAL	FAT	Nutrition Values per 100g / 100ml KCAL	PROT	CARB	FAT	FIBRE
LINGUINE								
with Chicken & Basil Dressing, HL, Tesco*	1 Pack/359g	503	15.4	140	8.6	16.6	4.3	2.2
with Mushrooms, Vegelicious, Tesco*	1 Bowl/380g	399	12.5	105	4.3	13.7	3.3	2.0
with Prawns & Scallops, BGTY, Sainsbury's*	1 Pack/400g	320	2.0	80	6.2	12.7	0.5	0.8
with Salmon, Hot Smoked, GFY, Asda*	1 Pack/400g	348	9.2	87	6.0	10.6	2.3	1.6
LINSEEDS								
Average	***1 Tsp/5g***	***23***	***1.7***	***464***	***21.7***	***18.5***	***33.5***	***26.3***
Brown, Wholefoods, Tesco*	1 Portion/10g	52	4.2	515	18.3	1.6	42.2	27.3
LION BAR								
Mini, Nestle*	1 Bar/16g	80	3.6	486	4.6	67.7	21.7	0.0
Nestle*	1 Bar/52g	248	11.2	478	6.5	64.6	21.6	0.0
Peanut, Nestle*	1 Bar/40g	195	10.0	488	8.1	57.1	25.0	2.3
LIQUEURS								
Amaretto, Average	***1 Shot/25ml***	***97***	***0.0***	***388***	***0.0***	***60.0***	***0.0***	***0.0***
Cointreau, Specialite De France	***1 Serving/37ml***	***80***	***0.0***	***215***	***0.0***	***0.0***	***0.0***	***0.0***
Cream, Average	***1 Shot/25ml***	***81***	***4.0***	***325***	***0.0***	***22.8***	***16.1***	***0.0***
Grand Marnier*	***1 Shot/35ml***	***94***	***0.0***	***268***	***0.0***	***22.9***	***0.0***	***0.0***
High Strength, Average	***1 Shot/25ml***	***78***	***0.0***	***314***	***0.0***	***24.4***	***0.0***	***0.0***
Kirsch, Average	***1 Shot/25ml***	***67***	***0.0***	***267***	***0.0***	***20.0***	***0.0***	***0.0***
Marula Fruit & Cream Cocktail, Amarula*	1 fl oz/30ml	103	0.0	343	0.0	36.7	0.0	0.0
LIQUORICE								
Allsorts, Average	1 Sm Bag/56g	195	2.9	349	3.7	76.7	5.2	2.0
Allsorts, Bassett's*	1 Pack/225g	855	11.0	380	5.6	77.8	4.9	1.6
Allsorts, Fruit, Bassett's*	1 Serving/50g	160	0.2	320	1.8	76.9	0.4	0.0
Allsorts, Julian Graves*	1 Serving/30g	113	2.2	376	3.4	78.7	7.2	1.2
Assorted, Filled, Panda*	1 Sweet/4g	15	0.4	385	3.7	68.0	11.0	0.0
Bars, Panda*	1 Bar/32g	99	0.1	308	3.7	72.0	0.4	0.9
Catherine Wheels, Barratt*	1 Wheel/22g	65	0.1	290	3.8	67.2	0.3	0.7
Comfits, M & S*	1oz/28g	100	0.1	357	2.4	86.2	0.3	0.7
Organic, Laidback Liquorice*	1 Bar/28g	90	0.3	320	4.7	75.0	1.0	3.0
Panda*	1 Bar/32g	109	0.2	340	3.8	78.0	0.5	0.0
Red, Fresh, 98% Fat Free, RJ's Licorice Ltd*	1oz/28g	96	0.5	342	3.0	75.0	1.7	0.0
Shapes, Average	1oz/28g	78	0.4	278	5.5	65.0	1.4	1.9
Soft Eating, Australia, Darrell Lea*	1 Piece/20g	68	0.4	338	2.8	76.1	1.9	0.0
Sweets, Blackcurrant, Tesco*	1 Sweet/8g	32	0.3	410	0.0	92.3	3.8	0.0
Torpedos, Panda*	1 Serving/25g	92	0.0	366	1.9	88.0	0.2	1.4
Twists, Tesco*	1 Serving/63g	186	0.2	297	2.7	71.0	0.3	0.7
LIVER								
Calves, Fried	***1oz/28g***	***49***	***2.7***	***176***	***22.3***	***0.0***	***9.6***	***0.0***
Calves, Raw	***1oz/28g***	***29***	***1.0***	***104***	***18.3***	***0.0***	***3.4***	***0.0***
Calves, with Fresh Sage Butter, M & S*	1 Serving/117g	210	12.5	180	12.8	10.1	10.7	1.5
Calves, with Garlic Butter, M & S*	1oz/28g	56	3.8	200	13.3	7.3	13.5	0.4
Chicken, Cooked, Simmered, Average	***1 Serving/100g***	***167***	***6.5***	***167***	***24.5***	***0.9***	***6.5***	***0.0***
Chicken, Fried, Average	***1oz/28g***	***47***	***2.5***	***169***	***22.1***	***0.0***	***8.9***	***0.0***
Chicken, Raw, Average	***1oz/28g***	***26***	***0.6***	***92***	***17.7***	***0.0***	***2.3***	***0.0***
Lamb's, Braised, Average	***1 Serving/100g***	***220***	***8.8***	***220***	***30.6***	***2.5***	***8.8***	***0.0***
Lamb's, Fried, Average	***1oz/28g***	***66***	***3.6***	***237***	***30.1***	***0.0***	***12.9***	***0.0***
Lamb's, Raw, Average	***1 Serving/125g***	***171***	***7.8***	***137***	***20.3***	***0.0***	***6.2***	***0.0***
Ox, Raw	***1oz/28g***	***43***	***2.2***	***155***	***21.1***	***0.0***	***7.8***	***0.0***
Ox, Stewed	***1oz/28g***	***55***	***2.7***	***198***	***24.8***	***3.6***	***9.5***	***0.0***
Pig's, Raw	***1oz/28g***	***32***	***0.9***	***113***	***21.3***	***0.0***	***3.1***	***0.0***
Pig's, Stewed	***1 Serving/70g***	***132***	***5.7***	***189***	***25.6***	***3.6***	***8.1***	***0.0***
LIVER & BACON								
with Mash, Cooked, British Classics, Tesco*	1 Pack/450g	562	20.2	125	11.9	7.6	4.5	1.0

	Measure INFO/WEIGHT	per Measure KCAL	FAT	Nutrition Values per 100g / 100ml KCAL	PROT	CARB	FAT	FIBRE
LIVER & BACON								
with Mash, Creamy, GFY, Asda*	1 Pack/386g	282	5.4	73	5.5	9.6	1.4	2.2
with Mash, M Kitchen, Morrisons*	1 Pack/450g	463	16.6	103	7.4	9.3	3.7	1.4
with Mashed Potato, Fresh, Waitrose*	1 Pack/400g	416	17.2	104	7.3	9.0	4.3	1.3
LIVER & ONIONS								
British Classics, Tesco*	1 Pack/250g	265	12.0	106	9.7	5.9	4.8	0.5
M & S*	1 Serving/200g	250	12.0	125	7.6	10.5	6.0	0.9
LIVER SAUSAGE								
Average	***1 Slice/10g***	***22***	***1.5***	***216***	***15.3***	***4.4***	***15.2***	***0.2***
LLAMA								
Steak, Average	1 Steak/150g	158	2.0	105	23.0	0.2	1.3	0.0
LOBSTER								
Boiled, Average	***1oz/28g***	***29***	***0.4***	***103***	***22.1***	***0.0***	***1.6***	***0.0***
Dressed, John West*	1 Can/43g	45	2.2	105	13.0	2.0	5.0	0.0
Dressed, M & S*	1oz/28g	76	6.6	273	14.3	0.8	23.6	0.1
Half, M & S*	1oz/28g	66	5.5	235	12.1	2.4	19.6	0.2
Raw, Average	1 Serving/100g	92	1.4	92	18.7	0.3	1.4	0.0
Squat, Tails, Youngs*	½ Pack/125g	246	10.8	197	9.8	20.1	8.6	1.1
Thermidor, Finest, Tesco*	½ Pack/140g	381	25.2	272	15.3	12.1	18.0	1.0
Thermidor, M & S*	1 Serving/140g	287	19.2	205	10.7	9.7	13.7	0.0
LOGANBERRIES								
Raw	***1oz/28g***	***5***	***0.0***	***17***	***1.1***	***3.4***	***0.0***	***2.5***
LOLLIPOPS								
Assorted, Co-Op*	1 Lolly/10g	40	0.0	400	0.0	97.0	0.0	0.0
Assorted Flavours, Asda*	1 Lolly/7g	27	0.0	380	0.0	95.0	0.0	0.0
Blackcurrant, Sugar Free, Rowntree's*	1 Lolly/15g	35	0.0	233	0.1	89.4	0.0	0.0
Chocolate Lolly, M & S*	1 Lolly/45g	248	15.8	550	6.8	54.0	35.1	2.7
Chupa Chups*	1 Lolly/18g	44	0.2	247	0.0	96.5	1.3	0.0
Cremosa, Sugar Free, Chupa Chups*	1 Lolly/10g	28	0.5	275	0.2	92.5	5.4	0.0
Cuore Di Frutta, Chupa Chups*	1 Lolly/10g	25	0.1	247	0.0	96.5	1.3	0.0
Orange, Sugar Free, Rowntree's*	1 Lolly/15g	35	0.0	235	0.1	89.5	0.0	0.6
Refreshers, Bassett's*	1 Lolly/6g	25	0.0	417	0.0	108.3	0.0	0.0
Super Sour, Tesco*	1 Lolly/8g	32	0.0	385	0.1	95.6	0.2	0.5
LOQUATS								
Raw	***1oz/28g***	***8***	***0.1***	***28***	***0.7***	***6.3***	***0.2***	***0.0***
LOZENGES								
Blackcurrant Flavour, Fishermans Friend*	1 Lozenge/1g	3	0.0	251	0.1	97.2	1.3	0.0
Original, Extra Strong Lozenge, Fisherman's Friend*	1 Lozenge/1g	4	0.0	382	0.3	94.9	0.0	0.5
Original, Victory V*	1 Lozenge/3g	9	0.0	350	0.0	91.0	0.0	0.0
LUCOZADE								
Apple, Energy Drink, GlaxoSmithKline UK Limited*	1 Bottle/380ml	262	0.0	69	0.0	17.1	0.0	0.0
Caribbean Crush, Energy, Lucozade*	1 Bottle/380ml	217	0.0	57	0.0	13.9	0.0	0.0
Cherry, Sport, Lite, GlaxoSmithKline UK Limited*	1 Bottle/500ml	50	0.0	10	0.0	2.0	0.0	0.0
Citrus Clear, Energy, GlaxoSmithKline UK Limited*	1 Bottle/380ml	266	0.0	70	0.1	17.0	0.0	0.0
Citrus Fruits, Hydro Active, Sport, Lucozade*	1 Bottle/500ml	50	0.0	10	0.0	2.0	0.0	0.0
Energy, Original, GlaxoSmithKline UK Limited*	1 Bottle/380ml	266	0.0	70	0.0	17.2	0.0	0.0
Orange Energy Drink, GlaxoSmithKline UK Limited*	1 Bottle/500ml	350	0.0	70	0.0	17.2	0.0	0.0
LUNCHEON MEAT								
Pork, Average	***1oz/28g***	***81***	***6.8***	***288***	***13.3***	***4.0***	***24.3***	***0.0***
LYCHEES								
Fresh, Raw, Flesh Only	***1oz/28g***	***16***	***0.0***	***58***	***0.9***	***14.3***	***0.1***	***0.7***
in Juice, Amoy*	1oz/28g	13	0.0	46	0.4	10.9	0.0	0.0
in Syrup, Average	***1oz/28g***	***19***	***0.0***	***69***	***0.4***	***17.7***	***0.0***	***0.4***
Raw, Weighed with Skin & Stone	***1oz/28g***	***10***	***0.0***	***36***	***0.5***	***8.9***	***0.1***	***0.4***

	Measure INFO/WEIGHT	per Measure KCAL	FAT	Nutrition Values per 100g / 100ml KCAL	PROT	CARB	FAT	FIBRE
M&M'S								
Crispy, Mars*	1 Serving/36g	179	8.8	498	4.1	63.9	24.4	2.7
Mars*	1 Pack/45g	218	9.7	485	5.0	68.0	21.5	0.0
Mini, Mars*	1 Sm Pack/36g	176	8.4	489	6.3	63.6	23.2	0.0
Peanut, Mars*	1 Pack/45g	228	11.4	506	9.4	60.1	25.4	2.7
Peanut Butter, Mars*	1 Pack/46g	240	14.0	520	8.7	56.3	30.3	2.2
MACADAMIA NUTS								
Plain, Average	***1 Pack/100g***	***750***	***77.6***	***750***	***7.9***	***4.8***	***77.6***	***5.3***
Roasted, Salted, Average	***6 Nuts/10g***	***75***	***7.8***	***748***	***7.9***	***4.8***	***77.6***	***5.3***
MACARONI								
Dry, Average	***1oz/28g***	***99***	***0.5***	***354***	***11.9***	***73.5***	***1.7***	***2.6***
MACARONI CHEESE								
& Spinach, TTD, Sainsbury's*	1 Pack/500g	1025	57.5	205	6.5	18.9	11.5	1.3
Bettabuy, Morrisons*	1 Serving/205g	229	11.7	112	4.3	10.8	5.7	0.4
Birds Eye*	1 Pack/300g	470	15.0	157	5.7	22.3	5.0	0.8
Canned	1oz/28g	39	1.8	138	4.5	16.4	6.5	0.4
Charlie Bigham's*	½ Pack/335g	771	36.9	230	10.5	21.8	11.0	0.2
Chilled, GFY, Asda*	1 Pack/443g	469	12.8	106	6.0	14.0	2.9	1.6
Combino, Lidl*	1 Can/410g	472	25.8	115	4.5	10.1	6.3	0.3
COU, M & S*	1 Pack/360g	360	8.6	100	5.8	13.9	2.4	1.2
Diet Chef Ltd*	1 Pouch/250g	247	7.8	99	7.3	12.7	3.1	0.4
Four Cheese, Extra Special, Asda*	1 Pack/400g	664	30.8	166	7.7	16.4	7.7	1.1
HE, Tesco*	1 Pack/340g	252	8.5	74	6.6	6.2	2.5	0.6
Kids, Sainsbury's*	1 Pack/300g	336	7.2	112	4.6	17.9	2.4	1.7
LC, Tesco*	1 Pack/385g	465	7.3	121	7.0	18.7	1.9	1.5
Pasta, Fresh, Findus*	1 Pack/360g	360	7.2	100	5.0	16.0	2.0	0.5
Ready Meal, Average	1 Serving/300g	435	19.1	145	6.0	15.8	6.4	1.0
Red Leicester, Heinz*	1 Can/400g	332	10.8	83	3.5	11.1	2.7	0.3
Ross*	1 Pack/300g	327	9.3	109	4.2	16.2	3.1	1.3
MACAROONS								
Butterscotch, Picard*	1 Macaroon/20g	85	3.6	424	9.7	55.1	18.2	0.0
Coconut, Sainsbury's*	1 Macaroon/33g	146	6.1	441	4.7	63.7	18.6	0.8
Coconut, Tesco*	1 Macaroon/33g	140	6.1	425	4.4	59.0	18.6	5.7
French, Average	1 Serving/60g	225	11.0	375	6.7	46.7	18.3	3.3
MACKEREL								
Atlantic, Raw, Average	***1 Fillet/75g***	***154***	***10.4***	***205***	***18.6***	***0.0***	***13.9***	***0.0***
Fillets, Honey Roast Smoked, Sainsbury's*	1 Serving/100g	349	27.3	349	21.5	4.5	27.3	12.4
Fillets, in a Hot Chilli Dressing, Princes*	1 Pack/125g	370	33.8	296	13.3	0.0	27.0	0.0
Fillets, in Brine, Average	***1 Can/88g***	***206***	***15.3***	***234***	***19.4***	***0.0***	***17.4***	***0.0***
Fillets, in Curry Sauce, John West*	1 Can/125g	275	20.8	220	14.2	3.5	16.6	0.2
Fillets, in Green Peppercorn Sauce, John West*	1 Can/125g	329	26.2	263	14.0	4.5	21.0	0.1
Fillets, in Hot Smoked Peppered, Asda*	1 Fillet/100g	341	28.0	341	19.0	3.3	28.0	0.6
Fillets, in Mustard Sauce, Average	1 Can/125g	274	19.4	219	14.1	5.4	15.5	0.0
Fillets, in Olive Oil, Average	1 Serving/50g	149	12.2	298	18.5	1.0	24.4	0.0
Fillets, in Spicy Tomato Sauce, Average	1oz/28g	56	3.9	199	14.3	3.8	14.0	0.0
Fillets, in Sunflower Oil, Average	1 Can/94g	262	20.6	279	20.2	0.2	21.9	0.2
Fillets, in Teriyaki Sauce, Boneless & Skinless, Tesco*	1 Can/125g	320	20.3	255	12.6	13.4	16.2	2.0
Fillets, in Tomato Sauce, Average	1 Can/125g	251	18.3	200	14.3	2.7	14.7	0.0
Fillets, in White Wine & Spices, Connetable*	1 Can/120g	169	9.8	141	15.5	1.2	8.2	0.0
Fillets, Lemon & Parsley, Smoked, Fishmonger, Aldi*	1 Pack/200g	658	53.0	329	19.6	2.9	26.5	0.0
Fillets, Smoked, Average	***1 Fillet/75g***	***251***	***21.2***	***335***	***19.8***	***0.5***	***28.2***	***0.3***
Fillets, with Red Pepper & Onion, Smoked, Asda*	1 Serving/90g	319	27.9	354	18.0	0.8	31.0	1.2
Fried in Blended Oil	***1oz/28g***	***76***	***5.5***	***272***	***24.0***	***0.0***	***19.5***	***0.0***
Grilled	***1oz/28g***	***67***	***4.8***	***239***	***20.8***	***0.0***	***17.3***	***0.0***

	Measure INFO/WEIGHT	per Measure KCAL	FAT	Nutrition Values per 100g / 100ml KCAL	PROT	CARB	FAT	FIBRE
MACKEREL								
King, Raw	1 Fillet/198g	208	4.0	105	20.3	0.0	2.0	0.0
Raw, with Skin, Weighed with Bone, Average	***1oz/28g***	***67***	***4.9***	***238***	***19.9***	***0.0***	***17.6***	***0.0***
Roasted, with Piri-piri, Tesco*	1 Fillet/80g	240	19.0	300	20.7	0.0	23.8	1.0
Smoked, Lemon & Parsley, Morrisons*	½ Pack/100g	282	20.0	282	20.9	4.6	20.0	1.0
Smoked, Peppered, Average	***1oz/28g***	***87***	***7.0***	***310***	***20.4***	***0.3***	***25.2***	***0.2***
Spanish, Raw, Average	1 Fillet/100g	139	6.3	139	19.3	0.0	6.3	0.0
Whole, Raw, Average	1 Serving/100g	220	16.1	220	18.7	0.0	16.1	0.0
MADRAS								
Beef, Canned, BGTY, Sainsbury's*	1 Can/400g	344	14.4	86	9.5	4.0	3.6	0.9
Beef, Indian, Takeaway, Chosen By You, Asda*	½ Pack/200g	246	14.2	123	8.9	4.7	7.1	2.5
Beef, Tesco*	1 Pack/460g	616	37.7	134	10.6	4.5	8.2	1.2
Beef, Weight Watchers*	1 Pack/320g	317	4.8	99	5.6	15.8	1.5	0.3
Chicken, & Pilau Rice, Asda*	1 Pack/400g	588	28.0	147	8.0	13.0	7.0	1.7
Chicken, & Rice, Hot & Spicy, Sainsbury's*	1 Pack/500g	670	25.5	134	7.1	14.9	5.1	2.2
Chicken, Frozen, GFY, Asda*	1 Pack/400g	448	5.2	112	5.6	19.4	1.3	1.2
Chicken, Iceland*	1 Pack/400g	376	19.2	94	7.7	4.9	4.8	1.1
Chicken, Indian Take Away, Tesco*	1 Serving/175g	254	17.7	145	8.2	4.8	10.1	1.7
Chicken, Sainsbury's*	1 Pack/400g	468	27.2	117	11.7	2.2	6.8	2.8
Chicken, Waitrose*	1 Pack/400g	672	42.0	168	14.6	3.7	10.5	1.8
MAGNUM								
Almond, Wall's Ice Cream*	1 Bar/82g	270	17.2	330	5.0	30.0	21.0	1.5
Caramel & Almond, Temptation, Wall's Ice Cream*	1 Lolly/68g	239	15.0	351	5.4	34.0	22.0	0.0
Caramel & Nuts Bar, Wall's Ice Cream*	1 Bar/60g	132	9.0	220	4.0	19.0	15.0	0.0
Chocolate, Double, Wall's Ice Cream*	1 Bar/92g	346	22.0	378	4.5	36.0	24.0	0.0
Classic, Mini, Wall's Ice Cream*	1 Lolly/50g	170	11.0	340	4.0	30.0	22.0	0.0
Classic, Wall's Ice Cream*	1 Lolly/86g	239	15.0	278	3.5	26.7	17.4	1.2
Gluttony, Wall's Ice Cream*	1 Lolly/110ml	425	29.0	386	4.6	32.7	26.4	0.0
Greed, Wall's Ice Cream*	1 Bar/110ml	307	18.0	279	3.6	29.1	16.4	0.0
Pistachio, Wall's Ice Cream*	1 Bar/86g	275	18.9	320	4.0	30.0	22.0	0.0
White, Wall's Ice Cream*	1 Lolly/77g	250	16.0	325	3.9	29.9	20.8	0.0
MAKHANI								
Chicken, Sainsbury's*	½ Pack/199g	313	21.3	157	12.2	2.9	10.7	2.5
Chicken Tikka, BGTY, Sainsbury's*	1 Pack/251g	186	4.8	74	11.3	3.0	1.9	1.7
Chicken Tikka, Waitrose*	1 Pack/400g	560	30.4	140	14.0	3.8	7.6	2.1
King Prawns, Finest, Tesco*	1 Pack/350g	514	38.8	147	6.0	6.0	11.1	1.3
Paneer, Ashoka*	½ Pouch/150g	283	23.0	189	4.7	8.0	15.3	1.0
MALTESERS*								
MaltEaster, Chocolate Bunny, Mars*	1 Bunny/29g	156	9.2	538	6.9	57.0	31.7	0.0
Mars*	1 Reg Bag/37g	187	9.3	505	8.0	61.8	25.0	0.9
Mini Bunnies, Mars*	1 Bunny/12g	64	3.6	534	8.0	53.5	30.2	0.0
White Chocolate, Mars*	1 Pack/37g	186	9.4	504	7.9	61.0	25.4	0.0
MANDARIN ORANGES								
Broken, Segments in Fruit Juice, Basics, Sainsbury's*	½ Can/149g	51	0.0	34	0.7	7.7	0.0	0.3
in Juice, Average	***1oz/28g***	***11***	***0.0***	***39***	***0.7***	***9.0***	***0.0***	***0.5***
in Light Syrup, Average	***1 Can/298g***	***201***	***0.1***	***68***	***0.6***	***16.0***	***0.0***	***0.1***
in Orange Gel, Del Monte*	1 Can/128g	60	0.0	47	0.0	10.9	0.0	0.0
Weighed with Peel, Average	***1 Sm/50g***	***18***	***0.0***	***36***	***0.9***	***8.4***	***0.1***	***1.2***
MANGE TOUT								
& Sugar Snap Peas, Tesco*	1 Pack/150g	102	0.6	68	7.0	9.2	0.4	3.8
Boiled in Salted Water	***1oz/28g***	***7***	***0.0***	***26***	***3.2***	***3.3***	***0.1***	***2.2***
Raw, Average	***1 Serving/80g***	***26***	***0.2***	***32***	***3.6***	***4.2***	***0.2***	***1.2***
Stir-Fried in Blended Oil	***1oz/28g***	***20***	***1.3***	***71***	***3.8***	***3.5***	***4.8***	***2.4***

	Measure INFO/WEIGHT	per Measure KCAL	FAT	Nutrition Values per 100g / 100ml KCAL	PROT	CARB	FAT	FIBRE
MANGO								
Chunks, Fresh, Morrisons*	1 Serving/80g	53	0.2	66	0.7	14.1	0.2	2.6
Dried, Average	***1 Serving/50g***	***174***	***0.5***	***347***	***1.4***	***83.1***	***1.0***	***4.9***
Dried, Organic, Love Life, Waitrose*	1 Serving/50g	148	0.4	297	3.4	68.7	0.9	12.0
Dried, with Chilli, King Henry's*	1 Bag/120g	300	0.0	250	0.0	62.5	0.0	1.0
in Syrup, Average	***1oz/28g***	***22***	***0.0***	***80***	***0.3***	***20.5***	***0.0***	***0.9***
Pineapple & Passionfruit, M & S*	1 Pack/400g	200	0.8	50	0.6	10.9	0.2	1.7
Ripe, Raw, Weighed with Skin & Stone, Average	***1 Mango/225g***	***88***	***0.2***	***39***	***0.5***	***9.6***	***0.1***	***1.8***
Ripe, Raw, without Peel & Stone, Flesh Only, Average	***1 Mango/207g***	***81***	***1.0***	***39***	***0.5***	***9.6***	***0.5***	***1.8***
Slices, in Juice, SPC Nature's Finest*	1 Pot/400g	224	0.8	56	5.0	12.3	0.2	1.5
MANGOSTEEN								
Raw, Fresh, Average*	***1 Serving/80g***	***50***	***0.5***	***63***	***0.6***	***15.6***	***0.6***	***5.1***
MARGARINE								
Average	***1 Thin Spread/7g***	***51***	***5.7***	***726***	***0.1***	***0.5***	***81.0***	***0.0***
Baking, Average	***1 Thin Spread/7g***	***42***	***4.7***	***607***	***0.2***	***0.4***	***67.2***	***0.0***
Butter Style, Average	***1 Thin Spread/7g***	***44***	***4.8***	***627***	***0.7***	***1.1***	***68.9***	***0.0***
Buttery, Pro Activ, Flora*	1 Serving/10g	55	6.0	550	0.0	0.0	60.0	0.0
No Salt, Flora*	1 Thin Spread/7g	37	4.1	531	0.0	0.0	59.0	0.0
Omega 3 Plus, Flora*	1 Thin Spread/7g	24	2.7	350	0.1	3.0	38.0	0.0
Pro Activ, Extra Light, Flora*	1 Thin Spread/7g	15	1.6	218	0.1	2.9	23.0	0.2
Pro Activ, Light, Flora*	1 Thin Spread/7g	23	2.4	331	0.1	4.0	35.0	0.0
Pro Activ with Olive Oil, Flora*	1 Thin Spread/7g	23	2.4	331	0.1	4.0	35.0	0.0
Pro Active, Becel*	1 Serving/7g	22	1.8	320	0.0	0.0	25.0	0.0
Reduced Fat, Average	***1 Thin Spread/7g***	***25***	***2.7***	***356***	***0.6***	***3.0***	***38.0***	***0.0***
Soya, Granose*	1 Thin Spread/7g	52	5.7	745	0.1	0.1	82.0	0.0
Utterly Butterly*	1 Thin Spread/7g	32	3.4	452	0.3	2.5	49.0	0.0
White, Flora*	1 Thin Spread/7g	60	6.6	855	0.0	0.0	95.0	0.0
MARGARITA								
Sainsbury's*	1 Serving/100ml	53	0.1	53	0.1	12.8	0.1	0.1
MARINADE								
Barbecue, COU, M & S*	1 Serving/35g	52	0.1	150	1.2	35.5	0.2	1.0
Barbecue, Hot & Spicy, M & S*	1 Serving/18g	23	0.1	130	1.0	31.1	0.3	0.8
Barbeque, Sticky, Sainsbury's*	¼ Jar/77g	112	2.8	145	0.8	26.7	3.6	1.0
BBQ, Sticky, Newman's Own*	1/3 Jar/83ml	139	0.7	167	0.9	39.0	0.8	2.5
Cajun Spice, The English Provender Co.*	1 Serving/50g	94	6.7	187	1.3	15.3	13.4	1.6
Chinese, Classic, Sharwood's*	1oz/28g	32	1.3	113	1.8	16.1	4.8	1.0
Hickory Dickory Smokey, Ainsley Harriott*	1 Pot/300ml	360	0.3	120	0.6	28.1	0.1	0.0
Lemon & Rosemary, Nando's*	1fl oz/30ml	44	3.9	147	1.0	11.8	13.0	0.2
Lime & Coriander, with Peri Peri, Nando's*	1 Tsp/5g	9	0.8	182	0.0	13.1	16.6	0.2
Peri Peri, Hot, Nando's*	1 Serving/40g	46	2.2	115	1.4	15.2	5.4	0.9
Peri Peri, Portuguese Bbq, Nando's*	1 Serving/40g	36	0.6	90	1.1	17.7	1.6	1.0
Sun Dried Tomato & Basil, with Peri-Peri, Nando's*	1 Bottle/270g	319	25.6	118	0.1	15.3	9.5	0.8
Tequila Chilli Lime, M & S*	1 Serving/75ml	116	1.2	155	0.6	34.0	1.6	0.5
MARJORAM								
Dried	***1 Tsp/1g***	***2***	***0.0***	***271***	***12.7***	***42.5***	***7.0***	***0.0***
MARLIN								
Smoked, H Forman & Son*	1 Pack/200g	240	0.2	120	29.8	0.0	0.1	0.0
Steaks, Chargrilled, Sainsbury's*	1 Steak/240g	367	14.6	153	23.6	0.8	6.1	0.6
Steaks, Raw, Sainsbury's*	1 Steak/110g	109	0.2	99	24.3	0.0	0.2	0.0
MARMALADE								
3 Fruit, Thick Cut, Waitrose*	1 Tsp/15g	39	0.0	262	0.4	64.8	0.1	0.7
Blood Orange, Grandessa*	1 Serving/15g	36	0.0	240	0.4	59.0	0.1	0.7
Blood Orange, TTD, Sainsbury's*	1 Tbsp/15g	40	0.0	264	0.3	65.7	0.0	0.8

M

	Measure INFO/WEIGHT	per Measure KCAL	FAT	Nutrition Values per 100g / 100ml KCAL	PROT	CARB	FAT	FIBRE
MARMALADE								
Five Fruit, Tesco*	1 Serving/10g	28	0.0	278	0.2	68.2	0.1	0.9
Fresh Fruit, Three Fruits, TTD, Sainsbury's*	1 Tbsp/15g	40	0.0	268	0.3	66.7	0.0	0.8
Grapefruit, Fine Cut, Duerr's*	1 Tsp/15g	39	0.0	261	0.2	65.0	0.0	0.0
Grapefruit & Cranberry, M & S*	1 Tsp/15g	36	0.0	240	0.3	60.3	0.0	1.5
Lemon, with Shred, Average	***1 Serving/20g***	***50***	***0.0***	***248***	***0.2***	***61.6***	***0.0***	***0.6***
Lemon & Lime, Average	***1 Tbsp/20g***	***53***	***0.0***	***267***	***0.2***	***66.4***	***0.1***	***0.4***
Lemon Jelly, No Peel, Tesco*	1 Tsp/15g	39	0.0	263	0.1	65.0	0.0	0.4
Lime, with Shred, Average	***1 Tbsp/15g***	***39***	***0.0***	***261***	***0.2***	***65.0***	***0.1***	***0.4***
Onion, Organic, Antony Worrall Thompson's*	1 Serving/11g	20	0.1	191	1.1	44.9	0.8	1.8
Onion, Organic, Duchy Originals*	1 Serving/40g	103	1.0	257	1.0	57.8	2.4	2.6
Orange, Lemon & Grapefruit, Baxters*	1 Tsp/15g	38	0.0	252	0.0	63.0	0.0	0.1
Orange, Reduced Sugar, Average	***1 Tbsp/15g***	***26***	***0.0***	***170***	***0.4***	***42.0***	***0.1***	***0.6***
Orange, Reduced Sugar, Thin Cut, Streamline*	1 Serving/10g	18	0.0	178	0.5	43.0	0.3	0.0
Orange, Shredless, Average	***1 Tsp/10g***	***26***	***0.0***	***261***	***0.2***	***65.0***	***0.0***	***0.1***
Orange, with Drambuie, Finest, Tesco*	1 Serving/10g	33	0.0	329	0.3	82.0	0.0	0.7
Orange, with Shred, Average	***1 Tsp/5g***	***13***	***0.0***	***263***	***0.2***	***65.2***	***0.0***	***0.3***
Orange & Ginger, Average	***1 Tbsp/15g***	***40***	***0.0***	***264***	***0.2***	***65.7***	***0.1***	***0.3***
Orange & Lemon, Reduced Sugar, Zest*	1 Tsp/6g	12	0.0	195	0.3	47.1	0.2	0.0
Orange & Tangerine, Tiptree, Wilkin & Sons*	1 Tsp/15g	40	0.0	268	0.0	67.0	0.0	0.0
Orange & Whisky, Christmas, M & S*	1oz/28g	67	0.1	240	0.3	59.5	0.2	1.9
Pink Grapefruit, Thin Cut, Waitrose*	1 Serving/10g	26	0.0	261	0.2	65.0	0.0	0.4
Seville, Thick Cut, Organic, Fair Trade, Tesco*	1 Tbsp/15g	37	0.0	245	0.3	60.3	0.1	0.7
Three Fruit, Diabetic, Thursday Cottage*	1 Serving/5g	8	0.0	154	0.4	38.0	0.0	1.0
Three Fruit, Finest, Tesco*	1 Serving/15g	39	0.0	262	0.5	63.6	0.2	1.6
Three Fruits, Fresh Fruit, Sainsbury's*	1 Tsp/15g	38	0.0	250	0.0	61.3	0.0	0.0
MARMITE*								
XO, Marmite*	1 Serving/4g	10	0.0	250	37.5	25.0	0.2	0.2
Yeast Extract, Marmite*	1 Tsp/9g	22	0.0	250	39.0	24.0	0.1	3.5
Yeast Extract, with Gold Coloured Flecks, Marmite*	1 Serving/4g	10	0.0	250	39.0	24.0	0.1	3.5
MARROW								
Boiled, Average	***1oz/28g***	***3***	***0.1***	***9***	***0.4***	***1.6***	***0.2***	***0.6***
Raw	***1oz/28g***	***3***	***0.1***	***12***	***0.5***	***2.2***	***0.2***	***0.5***
MARS*								
Bar, 5 Little Ones, Mars*	1 Piece/8g	38	1.5	477	4.5	73.6	18.3	0.0
Bar, Duo, Mars*	1 Bar/42g	191	7.6	450	4.4	67.5	18.0	1.2
Bar, Funsize, Mars*	1 Bar/18g	80	3.0	446	3.5	70.1	16.8	1.1
Bar, Mars*	1 Std Bar/51g	229	8.7	449	4.0	69.0	17.0	1.0
Bar, Medium, 58g, Mars*	1 Bar/58g	263	10.5	453	4.6	67.9	18.1	0.0
Bar, Minis, Mars*	1 Bar/18g	80	11.6	444	3.3	0.0	64.4	1.1
Delight, Mars*	1 Bar/20g	110	6.7	552	4.5	57.8	33.6	1.3
Triple Choc, Bar, Limited Edition, Mars*	1 Bar/52g	233	9.0	448	4.5	67.7	17.3	2.0
MARSHMALLOWS								
Average	1 Mallow/5g	16	0.0	327	3.9	83.1	0.0	0.0
Chocolate Mallows, Cadbury*	1 Mallow/13g	56	2.2	435	4.7	64.7	17.4	0.8
Fat Free, Tesco*	1 Mallow/7g	24	0.0	339	3.4	80.8	0.2	0.5
Haribo*	1 Mallow/5g	16	0.0	330	3.0	80.0	0.0	0.0
No Added Sugar, Sainsbury's*	1 Mallow/2g	5	0.0	206	3.3	77.0	0.1	0.0
Pascall*	1 Mallow/5g	15	0.0	335	2.6	80.0	0.0	0.0
Pink & White, Co-Op*	1 Mallow/7g	24	0.0	340	3.0	82.0	0.0	0.0
Princess*	1 Mallow/5g	16	0.0	314	3.4	80.0	0.0	0.0
Raspberry & Cream, Sainsbury's*	1 Mallow/7g	23	0.0	330	4.1	78.5	0.0	0.5
MARZIPAN								
Dark Chocolate, Thorntons*	1 Serving/46g	207	8.0	451	5.2	69.4	17.4	2.1

	Measure INFO/WEIGHT	per Measure KCAL	FAT	Nutrition Values per 100g / 100ml KCAL	PROT	CARB	FAT	FIBRE
MARZIPAN								
Plain, Average	***1oz/28g***	***115***	***4.0***	***412***	***5.8***	***67.5***	***14.2***	***1.7***
MASALA								
Chicken, Tandoori, M & S*	½ Pack/175g	210	11.6	120	11.3	4.3	6.6	4.5
Dal, with Channa & Toor Lentils, Waitrose*	½ Pack/150g	166	6.2	111	6.6	12.0	4.1	5.0
Prawn, & Rice, Tesco*	1 Pack/475g	656	24.7	138	5.2	17.9	5.2	1.2
Prawn, King, Waitrose*	1 Pack/350g	385	25.9	110	7.1	3.8	7.4	1.8
Vegetable, Waitrose*	1 Serving/400g	288	19.2	72	2.2	4.9	4.8	2.5
Vegetable, with Rice, Feeling Great, Findus*	1 Pack/350g	350	7.0	100	3.0	18.0	2.0	1.7
MASH								
Carrot, Parsnip & Turnip, Mash Direct*	1 Serving/100g	63	2.0	63	1.0	10.2	2.0	2.8
Carrot & Swede, Creamy, Weight Watchers*	½ Pack/125g	91	2.1	73	1.4	11.8	1.7	2.4
Carrot & Swede, M Kitchen, Morrisons*	½ Pack/250g	155	4.8	62	0.9	9.0	1.9	2.6
Cheddar, Davidstow, Extra Special, Asda*	1 Serving/225g	292	16.9	130	5.3	10.4	7.5	2.6
Parsnip & Parmesan, Finest, Tesco*	½ Packet/250g	245	12.2	98	1.6	11.9	4.9	2.4
Potato, Carrot, Swede, Parsnip, Cream & Butter, Asda*	½ Pack/200g	94	3.0	47	1.0	7.2	1.5	3.3
Root, Asda*	½ Pack/200g	142	8.0	71	0.7	8.0	4.0	3.1
Root, Winter, Sainsbury's*	1 Serving/140g	157	2.1	112	2.7	22.0	1.5	0.9
Root Vegetable, Finest, Tesco*	½ Pack/250g	225	12.5	90	1.1	9.1	5.0	3.4
MAYONNAISE								
50% Less Fat, GFY, Asda*	1 Tbsp/10g	32	3.1	322	0.8	10.0	31.0	0.0
60% Less Fat, BGTY, Sainsbury's*	1 Tbsp/15ml	42	4.1	277	0.4	7.3	27.3	0.0
Aioli, Finest, Tesco*	1 Tsp/5g	20	2.1	408	0.8	8.5	41.2	0.0
Average	***1 Tsp/5g***	***35***	***3.8***	***690***	***0.9***	***1.6***	***75.5***	***0.0***
Branston, with a Twist, Petri Peri, Crosse & Blackwell*	1 Serving/15g	64	5.6	430	0.9	21.4	37.5	0.2
Branston, with a Twist, Sweet Chilli, Crosse & Blackwell*	1 Tbsp/15g	64	5.6	430	0.9	21.4	37.5	0.2
Branston, with a Twist of Pesto, Crosse & Blackwell*	1 Tbsp/30ml	124	11.6	412	1.2	14.1	38.6	0.2
Egg, Dairy & GF, Solesse*	1 Serving/100g	319	29.7	319	0.4	11.7	29.7	0.0
Egg & Dairy Free, Life Free From*	1 Serving/15g	76	8.0	508	0.9	5.6	53.3	0.2
Extra Light, Average	***1 Tbsp/33g***	***34***	***2.0***	***102***	***0.7***	***10.5***	***6.2***	***0.8***
Extra Light, Heinz*	1 Tbsp/12ml	9	0.4	75	0.6	11.4	3.0	0.6
Extra Light, Now Only 3% Fat, Hellmann's*	1 Serving/16g	12	0.5	73	0.6	11.0	3.0	0.6
Extra Light, Weight Watchers*	1 Serving/15g	15	0.9	97	1.1	9.6	5.9	3.2
French, Light, Sainsbury's*	1 Serving/15ml	46	4.7	307	0.4	6.1	31.1	0.2
French Style, BGTY, Sainsbury's*	1 Tbsp/15ml	55	5.5	366	0.6	7.5	36.9	0.0
Garlic, Retail, Average	1 Tsp/11g	44	4.4	403	1.2	8.6	40.3	0.0
Garlic, Toasted, Atkins & Potts*	1 Serving/30g	207	22.3	691	2.2	2.8	74.4	0.2
Garlic & Herb, M & S*	1 Tsp/6g	43	4.6	712	3.4	2.4	76.9	0.9
Garlic & Herb, Reduced Calorie, Hellmann's*	1 Serving/25ml	58	4.8	233	0.7	13.1	19.3	0.4
Garlic Flavoured, Frank Cooper*	1 Tsp/6g	28	2.8	460	2.2	8.8	46.2	0.1
Heinz*	1 Tbsp/15g	99	10.8	663	0.9	3.0	71.8	0.0
Lemon, Waitrose*	1 Tsp/8ml	56	6.1	694	1.2	1.3	76.0	5.4
Light, & Squeezy, Co-Op*	1 Tbsp/15ml	45	4.2	315	1.0	11.4	29.6	0.0
Light, BGTY, Sainsbury's*	1 Tbsp/15g	44	4.4	296	0.5	7.2	29.3	0.0
Light, Dijon, Benedicta*	1 Tbsp/15g	44	4.4	292	0.7	6.7	29.2	0.0
Light, Hellmann's*	1 Serving/10g	30	3.0	298	0.7	6.5	29.8	0.1
Light, Kraft*	1 Serving/25g	61	5.0	245	0.6	15.0	20.0	0.0
Light, Reduced Calorie, Hellmann's*	1 Tsp/10g	30	3.0	297	0.7	6.5	29.8	0.0
Light, Reduced Fat, Heinz*	1 Tbsp/15g	42	4.0	279	1.1	7.7	26.8	0.5
Light, Squeezable, Hellmann's*	1 Tbsp/15g	44	4.4	293	0.7	6.4	29.4	0.0
Light, Squeezy, Oak Lane*	1 Serving/15ml	46	4.4	305	0.5	9.1	29.4	0.0
Lighter than Light, Bramwells, Aldi*	1 Tbsp/15ml	10	0.4	67	0.4	10.4	2.6	0.0
Low Fat, Belolive*	1 Serving/15ml	45	4.4	298	0.8	11.1	29.0	0.0
Made with Free Range Eggs, M & S*	1 Tbsp/15g	108	11.8	720	1.1	1.2	78.5	0.0

M

	Measure INFO/WEIGHT	per Measure KCAL	FAT	Nutrition Values per 100g / 100ml KCAL	PROT	CARB	FAT	FIBRE
MAYONNAISE								
Mild Dijon Mustard, Frank Cooper*	1 Pot/28g	114	11.1	406	3.3	9.3	39.5	0.1
Organic, Evernat*	1 Tsp/11g	83	8.9	752	1.3	2.8	81.0	0.0
Organic, Whole Foods*	1 Tbsp/14g	100	11.0	714	0.0	7.1	78.6	0.0
Original, Egg, Dairy & GF, Tiger Tiger*	1 Tbsp/15g	66	6.8	440	1.4	5.8	45.6	0.3
Real, Asda*	1 Serving/10g	72	7.9	721	1.3	1.2	79.0	0.1
Real, Hellmann's*	1 Tsp/5g	36	4.0	720	1.1	1.5	79.1	0.0
Real, The Big Squeeze, Hellmann's*	1 Tbsp/15ml	101	11.1	676	1.0	1.2	74.0	0.0
Reduced Calorie, Average	***1 HeapTsp/11g***	***33***	***3.2***	***301***	***0.7***	***8.9***	***29.0***	***0.1***
Squeezy, Oak Lane*	1 Tbsp/15ml	112	12.3	750	0.6	1.2	82.3	0.0
Vegetarian, Tesco*	1 Tsp/12g	89	9.7	738	1.5	0.8	81.0	0.0
MEAT LOAF								
Beef & Pork, Co-Op*	¼ Loaf/114g	314	25.1	275	13.0	7.0	22.0	1.0
Iceland*	1 Serving/150g	332	23.6	221	10.8	9.3	15.7	0.9
in Onion Gravy, M & S*	¼ Pack/140g	203	11.9	145	11.3	6.3	8.5	1.2
Turkey & Bacon, Tesco*	1 Serving/225g	400	22.3	178	14.7	7.4	9.9	1.1
MEATBALLS								
Beef, Aberdeen Angus, 12 Pack, Waitrose*	1 Meatball/36g	93	7.1	259	18.0	2.3	19.8	0.1
Beef, Aberdeen Angus, with Tomato Sauce, Tesco*	½ Pack/250g	362	19.5	145	10.7	7.1	7.8	1.2
Beef, Diet Chef Ltd*	1 Pack/300g	408	18.6	136	11.3	8.7	6.2	2.7
Beef, in Tomato Sauce, Diet Chef Ltd*	1 Pack/300g	408	18.6	136	11.3	8.7	6.2	2.7
Beef, Italian Style, As Consumed, Morrisons*	3 Meatballs/104g	235	14.7	226	19.7	4.5	14.1	0.9
Beef, Sainsbury's*	1 Meatball/24g	59	4.0	251	19.6	4.8	16.9	0.5
Beef, TTD, Sainsbury's*	1 Meatball/35g	73	5.2	208	16.7	1.5	15.0	0.1
Beef, with Italian Herbs, British, Finest, Tesco*	1oz/28g	63	4.7	225	15.4	2.1	16.8	1.7
Chicken, in Tomato Sauce, Average	1 Can/392g	580	32.9	148	7.7	10.4	8.4	0.0
Chicken, Lemon, with Rice, BGTY, Sainsbury's*	1 Pack/400g	388	8.4	97	6.8	12.8	2.1	1.4
Greek, M & S*	1 Serving/350g	402	18.9	115	7.7	9.1	5.4	1.5
in Bolognese Sauce, Fray Bentos*	½ Can/204g	188	5.9	92	4.8	11.6	2.9	0.7
in Gravy, Campbell's*	½ Can/205g	164	5.3	80	5.6	8.6	2.6	0.0
in Gravy, Fray Bentos*	1 Meatball/21g	17	0.6	79	4.6	8.7	2.9	0.6
in Onion Gravy, Tesco*	½ Pack/200g	310	17.0	155	8.4	11.3	8.5	0.8
in Rich Gravy, Westlers*	½ Can/200g	170	6.8	85	4.1	9.5	3.4	0.4
in Sherry Sauce, Tapas, Waitrose*	1 Serving/185g	272	7.4	147	18.8	5.9	4.0	1.2
in Tomato & Basil Sauce, Global Cuisine*	1oz/28g	37	3.4	131	15.0	7.0	12.0	0.4
in Tomato & Basil Sauce, Go Cook, Asda*	½ Pack/270g	526	38.3	195	12.4	4.4	14.2	2.4
in Tomato Sauce, Canned, Average	1 Can/410g	387	15.1	94	5.6	9.8	3.7	0.0
in Tomato Sauce, Fray Bentos*	½ Can/206g	183	6.0	89	4.7	11.1	2.9	0.7
in Tomato Sauce, Mighty, Westlers*	1 Can/400g	424	19.0	106	5.8	10.2	4.8	0.0
in Tomato Sauce, Tapas, Waitrose*	1 Pack/185g	285	16.8	154	10.8	7.2	9.1	1.3
Italian Pork, Al Forno, Sainsbury's*	1 Pack/450g	644	23.8	143	6.1	17.6	5.3	1.4
Lamb, Asda*	1 Pack/340g	928	71.4	273	16.0	5.1	21.0	0.6
Lion's Head, M & S*	1 Serving/300g	435	27.9	145	10.4	5.1	9.3	1.0
M & S*	1oz/28g	58	3.8	208	10.9	10.7	13.5	2.4
Pork, British, Simply, M & S*	½ Pack/180g	396	27.2	220	17.0	4.3	15.1	0.5
Pork, Diet Chef Ltd*	1 Pack/300g	273	5.1	91	9.4	9.4	1.7	3.2
Pork & Beef, Swedish Style, Tesco*	1 Meatball/14g	34	2.5	245	14.3	6.5	17.7	2.0
Pork & Chorizo, with Paprika Potatoes, Finest, Tesco*	½ Pack/425g	527	25.9	124	7.5	9.8	6.1	2.8
Roman-Style, with Basil Mash, COU, M & S*	1 Pack/430g	344	9.5	80	3.7	10.9	2.2	1.9
Spaghetti, Tesco*	1 Pack/385g	377	16.0	98	5.4	9.8	4.2	1.2
Spicy, Deli Melt, Sainsbury's*	1 Pack/200g	338	21.4	169	12.7	5.5	10.7	2.9
Spicy, M & S*	1 Pack/400g	540	24.0	135	8.8	12.0	6.0	1.4
Swedish, Average	¼ Pack/88g	198	13.8	224	14.0	7.4	15.7	1.3
Turkey, GFY, Asda*	½ Pack/330g	333	12.2	101	10.0	7.0	3.7	0.0

	Measure INFO/WEIGHT	per Measure KCAL	FAT	Nutrition Values per 100g / 100ml KCAL	PROT	CARB	FAT	FIBRE
MEATBALLS								
Venison, Uncooked, Tesco*	1 Ball/30g	62	3.7	205	17.8	5.4	12.3	0.5
MEATBALLS VEGETARIAN								
Swedish Style, Sainsbury's*	1 Ball/27g	53	2.6	194	21.5	5.5	9.5	4.0
with Penne, Tesco*	1 Serving/460g	414	10.6	90	5.9	11.4	2.3	2.1
MEDLAR								
Raw, Flesh Only	***1 Fruit/28g***	***11***	***0.1***	***40***	***0.5***	***10.6***	***0.4***	***10.0***
MELBA TOAST								
Average	1 Serving/3g	13	0.2	396	12.0	76.0	4.9	4.6
Buitoni*	1 Serving/33g	130	1.6	395	12.1	75.5	4.9	4.6
Dutch, LC, Tesco*	1 Pack/20g	75	0.5	375	13.1	75.0	2.4	4.6
Organic, Trimlyne*	2 Toasts/7g	28	0.5	407	13.7	71.6	6.8	5.3
Organic Spelt, Amisa*	2 Slices/24g	95	1.9	395	12.4	68.5	7.9	0.0
Original, Van Der Meulen*	1 Slice/3g	12	0.1	399	12.8	80.5	2.9	3.9
Thinly Sliced Toasted Wheat Bread, Sainsbury's*	1 Slice/3g	12	0.1	374	13.1	75.1	2.4	4.6
Tomato & Basil, Morrisons*	1 Pack/20g	77	0.6	383	13.6	75.7	2.9	2.4
Wholegrain, HL, Tesco*	1 Pack/20g	74	1.0	370	16.8	63.8	4.9	8.9
Wholegrain, Morrisons*	6 Toasts/20g	73	1.0	367	16.8	63.8	4.9	8.9
with Sesame, Tesco*	1 Slice/3g	11	0.2	370	12.8	61.7	8.0	3.8
MELON								
& Blueberry, Snack Pot, Great Stuff, Asda*	1 Pack/80g	25	0.1	31	0.6	6.8	0.1	1.2
Cantaloupe, Flesh Only, Average	***½ Melon/255g***	***87***	***0.5***	***34***	***0.8***	***8.2***	***0.2***	***0.9***
Cantaloupe, Weighed with Rind, Average	***1 Wedge/100g***	***35***	***0.3***	***35***	***0.8***	***8.3***	***0.3***	***0.8***
Galia, Average	1 Serving/240g	60	0.1	25	0.8	5.8	0.0	0.2
Honeydew, Raw, Flesh Only, Average	***1oz/28g***	***8***	***0.0***	***30***	***0.7***	***7.0***	***0.1***	***0.5***
Medley, Pre Packed, Average	1 Pack/240g	66	0.3	27	0.6	6.0	0.1	0.5
Piel de Sapo, Waitrose*	1 Pack/200g	80	0.4	40	0.8	8.2	0.2	0.9
Pineapple & Strawberry, Fully Prepared, Sainsbury's*	1 Serving/245g	86	0.2	35	0.6	7.8	0.1	0.9
MENTOS								
Cola, Mentos*	1 Packet/38g	146	0.8	390	0.0	93.0	2.0	0.0
MERINGUE								
Average	***1 Meringue/8g***	***30***	***0.0***	***379***	***5.3***	***95.4***	***0.0***	***0.0***
Belgian Chocolate, Mini, Extra Special, Asda*	1 Meringue/6g	28	0.9	459	6.0	75.0	15.0	0.7
Bombe, Raspberry & Vanilla, M & S*	1 Bombe/100g	155	1.8	155	3.4	33.3	1.8	2.6
Chocolate, Waitrose*	1 Meringue/77g	341	11.3	444	2.6	75.3	14.7	0.5
Coffee Fresh Cream, Asda*	1 Meringue/28g	109	4.7	396	3.8	57.0	17.0	0.3
Cream, Fresh, Sainsbury's*	1 Meringue/35g	142	5.1	407	3.5	65.4	14.6	0.5
Cream, M & S*	1 Meringue/34g	145	7.6	425	4.1	52.6	22.2	1.4
Layered, Tesco*	1/5 Meringue/52g	146	0.8	280	3.5	63.2	1.5	1.4
Lemon, Morrisons*	1 Serving/120g	295	14.4	246	2.5	32.0	12.0	0.5
Mini, Extra Special, Asda*	1 Meringue/4g	14	0.0	394	5.0	93.0	0.2	0.5
Mini, M & S*	1 Meringue/4g	15	0.0	395	6.1	91.6	0.0	0.2
Nests, Average	1 Nest/16g	63	0.0	397	4.8	93.3	0.1	0.1
Nests, Tropical Fruit, Sainsbury's*	1 Nest/95g	234	7.4	246	2.0	42.0	7.8	2.4
Raspberry, M & S*	1 Serving/105g	215	13.8	205	1.8	20.6	13.1	3.1
Shells, Sainsbury's*	2 Shells/24g	93	0.0	387	3.9	92.8	0.0	0.0
Strawberry, COU, M & S*	1 Meringue/5g	20	0.0	385	6.4	90.0	0.1	1.4
Strawberry, Mini, Extra Special, Asda*	1 Meringue/4g	15	0.0	387	5.0	91.0	0.3	0.5
Summer Fruits, 90% Fat Free, Sara Lee*	1 Meringue/135g	308	11.5	228	2.5	35.7	8.5	2.2
Toffee, COU, M & S*	1 Mini/5g	20	0.1	395	5.0	95.3	1.7	0.7
Toffee, M & S*	1 Meringue/30g	124	6.3	415	4.1	52.2	20.9	0.8
Tropical, M & S*	1 Serving/53g	212	14.3	400	3.1	37.0	26.9	0.0
MIDGET GEMS								
M & S*	1 Bag/113g	367	0.1	325	6.3	75.1	0.1	0.0

M

	Measure INFO/WEIGHT	per Measure KCAL	per Measure FAT	Nutrition Values per 100g / 100ml KCAL	PROT	CARB	FAT	FIBRE
MIDGET GEMS								
Smart Price, Asda*	1 Pack/178g	586	0.2	329	6.0	76.0	0.1	0.0
MILK								
1% Fat, Fresh, Arla*	1 Glass/202ml	83	2.0	41	3.3	4.8	1.0	0.0
2% Low Fat, Dunkley's*	1 Cup/240ml	120	5.0	50	2.9	4.2	2.1	0.0
Alternative, Original, Good Hemp*	1 Glass/250ml	90	6.0	36	1.3	2.2	2.4	0.2
Condensed, Caramel, Carnation, Nestle*	1 Serving/50g	148	3.0	296	5.5	55.1	6.0	0.0
Condensed, Semi Skimmed, Sweetened	***1oz/28g***	***75***	***0.1***	***267***	***10.0***	***60.0***	***0.2***	***0.0***
Condensed, Skimmed, Unsweetened, Average	***1oz/28g***	***30***	***1.1***	***108***	***7.5***	***10.5***	***4.0***	***0.0***
Condensed, Whole, Sweetened, Average	***1oz/28g***	***93***	***2.8***	***333***	***8.5***	***55.5***	***10.1***	***0.0***
Dried, Skimmed, Average	***1oz/28g***	***99***	***0.3***	***355***	***35.4***	***52.3***	***0.9***	***0.0***
Dried, Skimmed, Powder, Value, Tesco*	1 Serving/50g	180	0.3	361	36.1	52.9	0.6	0.0
Dried, Whole, Average	***1oz/28g***	***137***	***7.4***	***490***	***26.3***	***39.4***	***26.3***	***0.0***
Evaporated, Average	***1 Serving/85g***	***136***	***7.6***	***160***	***8.2***	***11.6***	***9.0***	***0.0***
Evaporated, Reduced Fat, Average	***1oz/28g***	***33***	***1.5***	***118***	***7.4***	***10.5***	***5.2***	***0.0***
Evaporated, Sainsbury's*	1 Serving/50g	80	4.5	161	8.4	11.7	9.0	0.0
Goats, Pasteurised	***1 fl oz/30ml***	***18***	***1.0***	***60***	***3.1***	***4.4***	***3.5***	***0.0***
Goats, Semi Skimmed, St Helen's Farm*	1 Serving/250ml	109	4.0	44	3.0	4.3	1.6	0.0
Goats, Skimmed, St Helen's Farm*	1 Serving/125ml	38	0.1	30	3.0	4.3	0.1	0.0
Low Fat, Calcia Extra Calcium, Unigate*	1 fl oz/30ml	14	0.2	45	4.3	6.3	0.5	0.0
Powder, Instant, Skimmed, Basics, Sainsbury's*	1 Serving/60g	209	0.4	349	35.6	50.4	0.6	0.0
Semi Skimmed, Advance with Omega 3, St Ivel*	1 Glass/250ml	122	4.2	49	3.4	5.0	1.7	0.0
Semi Skimmed, Average	***1 fl oz/30ml***	***15***	***0.5***	***49***	***3.4***	***5.0***	***1.7***	***0.0***
Semi Skimmed, Long Life, Average	***1 fl oz/30ml***	***15***	***0.5***	***49***	***3.4***	***5.0***	***1.7***	***0.0***
Semi Skimmed, Low Lactose, Lactofree, Arla*	1 Glass/125ml	50	1.9	40	3.6	3.0	1.5	0.0
Semi Skimmed, Low Lactose, UHT, Lactofree, Arla*	1 Serving/100ml	38	1.7	38	3.2	2.6	1.7	0.0
Semi Skimmed, Organic, Country Life*	1 fl oz/30ml	15	0.5	49	3.4	5.0	1.7	0.0
Skimmed, Albert Heijn*	1 Glass/250ml	80	0.0	32	3.0	5.0	0.0	0.0
Skimmed, Average	***1 Pint/568ml***	***194***	***0.5***	***34***	***3.3***	***5.0***	***0.1***	***0.0***
Skimmed, Lactofree, Arla*	1 Serving/200ml	78	0.8	39	3.8	3.6	0.4	0.0
Skimmed, Uht, Average	***1 fl oz/30ml***	***10***	***0.0***	***34***	***3.4***	***5.0***	***0.1***	***0.0***
Skimmed 1% Fat, Waitrose*	1 Serving/200ml	70	0.2	35	3.4	5.0	0.1	0.0
Super Milk Low Fat 1%, Avonmore*	1 Litre/1000ml	420	10.0	42	3.4	5.0	1.0	0.0
Whole, Advance with Omega 3, St Ivel*	1 Serving/250ml	162	9.2	65	3.3	4.7	3.7	0.0
Whole, Average	***1 Serving/200ml***	***134***	***7.8***	***67***	***3.3***	***4.7***	***3.9***	***0.0***
Whole, Buffalo, Laverstoke Park Farm*	1 Serving/200ml	220	16.0	110	4.5	4.9	8.0	0.0
Whole, Lactose Free, Lactofree, Arla*	1 Serving/200ml	116	7.0	58	3.9	2.7	3.5	0.0
Whole, with Vitamin D, Oak Farms*	1 Container/236ml	150	8.0	64	3.4	4.7	3.4	0.0
MILK DRINK								
Banana Flavour, Sterilised, Low Fat, Gulp*	1 Bottle/500ml	425	9.0	85	5.2	11.9	1.8	0.0
Chocolate, Break Time, Arla*	1 Bottle/500ml	290	1.5	58	3.6	10.2	0.3	0.0
Chocolate, Spar*	1 Serving/500ml	290	1.5	58	3.6	10.2	0.3	0.0
Chocolate Coconut, Free From, Tesco*	1 Serving/250ml	125	5.4	49	0.4	6.8	2.1	0.7
Chocolate Flavoured, Goodness for Kids, Tesco*	1 Bottlel/330ml	248	5.9	75	3.8	10.3	1.8	0.7
Chocolate Sterilised Skimmed, Happy Shopper*	1 Bottle/500ml	295	1.5	59	3.6	10.4	0.3	0.0
Chocolatte, Cafe Met*	1 Bottle/290ml	174	4.1	60	3.7	9.1	1.4	0.3
Colombian Coffee Flavoured, Waitrose*	1 Serving/250ml	232	9.5	93	4.3	10.5	3.8	0.0
Family Fuel, Mars*	1 Serving/200ml	172	4.0	86	3.1	13.7	2.0	0.0
Hazelnut, Free From, Tesco*	1 Serving/250ml	85	2.5	34	0.2	5.2	1.0	1.5
Mocalatte, Cafe Met*	1 Bottle/290ml	160	3.8	55	2.9	8.0	1.3	0.0
No Added Sugar, Mars*	1 Serving/200ml	108	3.4	54	3.4	6.2	1.7	0.5
Original, Mars*	1 Serving/330g	284	6.9	86	3.1	13.7	2.1	0.0
Refuel, Mars*	1 Bottle/388ml	299	5.8	77	3.1	13.5	1.5	0.0
Semi Skimmed, Cholesterol Lowering, Pro Activ, Flora*	1 Serving/250ml	125	4.5	50	3.6	4.8	1.8	0.0

	Measure INFO/WEIGHT	per Measure KCAL	per Measure FAT	Nutrition Values per 100g / 100ml KCAL	PROT	CARB	FAT	FIBRE
MILK DRINK								
Strawberry Flavoured, Goodness for Kids, Tesco*	1 Bottle/330ml	248	5.6	75	4.0	9.9	1.7	0.4
MILK SHAKE								
Banana, Diet Chef Ltd*	1 Drink/330ml	225	3.0	68	4.2	10.5	0.9	1.5
Banana, Yazoo, Campina*	1 Bottle/200ml	120	2.4	60	3.1	9.6	1.2	0.0
Banana Flavour, Frijj*	1 Bottle/500ml	325	4.5	65	3.7	10.5	0.9	0.0
Banana Flavour, Shapers, Boots*	1 Bottle/250ml	201	1.9	80	5.6	12.8	0.8	1.9
Banana Flavour, Spar*	1 Bottle/500ml	250	0.5	50	3.3	9.1	0.1	0.0
Cafe Latte, Diet Chef Ltd*	1 Carton/330ml	218	3.3	66	4.2	8.9	1.0	2.0
Chocolate, Asda*	1 Serving/250ml	198	9.2	79	4.4	7.0	3.7	0.4
Chocolate, Extreme, Frijj*	1 Bottle/500g	425	10.5	85	3.9	12.7	2.1	0.0
Chocolate Flavour, BGTY, Sainsbury's*	1 Bottle/500ml	290	2.5	58	5.3	8.0	0.5	0.9
Chocolate Flavour, Diet Chef Ltd*	1 Drink/330ml	210	2.3	64	4.1	8.5	0.7	1.9
Chocolate Flavoured, Fresh, Thick, Frijj*	1 Bottle/500ml	350	5.0	70	3.5	11.7	1.0	0.0
Honeycomb Choc Swirl Flavour, The Incredible, Frijj*	1 Bottle/500ml	450	12.5	90	4.0	13.0	2.5	0.2
Measure Up, Asda*	1 Glass/250ml	200	2.4	80	6.0	12.0	1.0	2.4
Milky Way, Thick, Mars*	1 Bottle/440ml	282	4.8	64	3.4	10.0	1.1	0.7
Mount Caramel, Frijj*	1 Bottle/500ml	360	4.5	72	3.4	12.7	0.9	0.0
Peachy Banana, Syrup, Robinson's*	1 Serving/50ml	79	0.0	158	0.0	39.0	0.0	0.0
Powder, Made Up with Semi-Skimmed Milk	1 Serving/250ml	172	4.0	69	3.2	11.3	1.6	0.0
Powder, Made Up with Whole Milk	1 Serving/250ml	218	9.2	87	3.1	11.1	3.7	0.0
Sticky Toffee Pudding Flavour, The Incredible, Frijj*	1 Bottle/500ml	445	10.0	89	4.0	13.7	2.0	0.1
Strawberry, Diet Chef Ltd*	1 Drink/330g	225	3.0	68	4.2	10.5	0.9	1.5
Strawberry, Yazoo, Campina*	1 Bottle/475ml	300	6.0	60	3.1	9.5	1.2	0.0
Strawberry & Raspberry, Syrup, Robinson's*	1 Serving/50ml	20	0.7	39	2.9	4.0	1.4	0.0
Strawberry Flavour, Thick, Low Fat, Frijj*	1 Bottle/250ml	155	2.0	62	3.4	10.1	0.8	0.0
Vanilla, Diet Chef Ltd*	1 Pack/330ml	225	3.0	68	4.2	10.5	0.9	1.5
Vanilla, Frijj*	1 Bottle/500ml	320	4.0	64	3.4	10.7	0.8	0.0
Vanilla Flavour, BGTY, Sainsbury's*	1 Bottle/500ml	230	0.5	46	5.3	5.9	0.1	0.4
MILKY BAR								
Buttons, Nestle*	1 Std Pack/30g	164	9.5	547	7.3	58.4	31.7	0.0
Choo, Nestle*	1 Bar/25g	116	4.3	464	4.2	73.1	17.2	0.0
Chunky, Nestle*	¼ Bar/38g	207	12.0	547	7.3	58.4	31.7	0.0
Crunchies, Nestle*	1 Pack/30g	168	10.4	560	7.0	54.9	34.7	0.0
Eggs, Mini, Nestle*	1 Pack/100g	500	23.3	500	4.2	68.4	23.3	0.0
Funsize (17g), Mars*	1 Bar/17g	75	2.7	449	3.8	71.8	16.3	0.6
Munchies, Nestle*	1 Serving/70g	392	24.3	560	7.0	54.9	34.7	0.1
Nestle*	1 Sm Bar/13g	68	4.0	547	7.3	58.4	31.7	0.0
MILKY WAY								
Fun Size, Mars*	1 Bar/17g	75	2.7	447	3.8	71.6	16.2	0.0
Mars*	1 Single Bar/22g	96	3.4	448	3.7	72.4	15.9	0.6
MINCEMEAT								
Average	***1oz/28g***	***77***	***1.2***	***274***	***0.6***	***62.1***	***4.3***	***1.3***
Organic, Waitrose*	1oz/28g	81	0.7	290	0.9	65.8	2.6	2.0
Traditional, Robertson*	1 Tbsp/17g	49	0.6	286	0.6	62.5	3.4	2.5
Traditional, Sainsbury's*	1 Tbsp/23g	65	0.7	282	0.9	62.4	3.2	1.4
with Cherries, Almonds & Brandy, Tesco*	¼ Jar/103g	295	5.0	287	1.4	58.8	4.9	1.4
MINSTRELS								
Galaxy, Mars*	1 Serving/100g	503	22.3	503	5.2	70.3	22.3	1.1
MINT								
Dried, Average	***1 Tsp/5g***	***14***	***0.2***	***279***	***24.8***	***34.6***	***4.6***	***0.0***
Fresh, Average	***2 Tbsp/3g***	***1***	***0.0***	***43***	***3.8***	***5.3***	***0.7***	***0.0***
MINTS								
After Dinner, Dark, Elizabeth Shaw*	1 Sweet/9g	42	2.1	469	2.8	62.5	23.1	0.0

M

	Measure INFO/WEIGHT	per Measure KCAL	FAT	Nutrition Values per 100g / 100ml KCAL	PROT	CARB	FAT	FIBRE
MINTS								
After Dinner, Sainsbury's*	1 Mint/7g	32	1.5	456	4.1	62.1	21.2	4.1
Assortment, M & S*	1 Sweet/7g	26	0.5	375	0.4	78.2	6.9	0.0
Butter Mintoes, M & S*	1 Sweet/9g	35	0.6	391	0.0	84.0	6.8	0.0
Butter Mintoes, Tesco*	1 Sweet/7g	24	0.5	349	0.0	71.3	7.1	0.0
Clear, Co-Op*	1 Sweet/6g	24	0.0	395	0.0	98.0	0.0	0.0
Cream, Luxury, Thorntons*	1 Sweet/13g	62	3.1	477	4.2	62.3	23.8	2.3
Creams, Bassett's*	1 Sweet/11g	40	0.0	365	0.0	91.8	0.0	0.0
Curiously Strong, M & S*	1 Sweet/1g	4	0.0	390	0.4	97.5	0.0	0.0
Everton, Co-Op*	1 Sweet/6g	25	0.2	410	0.6	92.0	4.0	0.0
Extra, Peppermint Coolburst, Wrigleys*	1 Pack/22g	53	0.2	240	0.0	98.0	1.0	0.0
Extra, Spearmint, Sugar Free, Wrigleys*	1 Sweet/1g	3	0.0	244	0.0	98.5	0.8	0.0
Extra, Wrigleys*	1 Sweet/1g	3	0.0	240	0.0	64.0	1.0	0.0
Extra Strong, Peppermint, Trebor*	1 Roll/46g	180	0.1	395	0.4	98.1	0.2	0.0
Extra Strong, Spearmint, Trebor*	1 Pack/44g	174	0.0	395	0.4	98.7	0.0	0.0
Favourites, Bassett's*	1 Sweet/6g	22	0.4	367	0.9	77.4	5.9	0.0
Glacier, Fox's*	1 Sweet/5g	19	0.0	386	0.0	96.4	0.0	0.0
Humbugs, Co-Op*	1 Sweet/8g	34	0.6	425	0.6	89.9	7.0	0.0
Humbugs, M & S*	1 Sweet/9g	37	0.4	407	0.6	91.1	4.4	0.0
Humbugs, Thorntons*	1 Sweet/9g	31	0.4	340	1.0	87.8	4.4	0.0
Imperials, M & S*	1 Sweet/3g	12	0.0	391	0.0	97.8	0.0	0.0
Imperials, Sainsbury's*	1 Sweet/3g	10	0.0	374	0.0	92.1	0.0	0.0
Mento, Sugar Free, Mentos*	1 Sweet/2g	5	0.1	260	1.0	87.0	5.5	0.0
Peppermints, Strong, Altoids*	1 Sweet/1g	3	0.0	385	0.5	96.0	0.0	0.0
Smooth, Weight Watchers*	1 Tube/25g	58	0.0	231	0.2	61.6	0.0	0.0
Soft, Trebor*	1 Pack/48g	182	0.0	380	0.0	94.9	0.0	0.0
Softmints, Peppermint, Trebor*	1 Pack/48g	170	0.0	355	0.0	88.9	0.0	0.0
Softmints, Spearmint, Trebor*	1 Pack/45g	170	0.0	375	0.0	94.3	0.0	0.0
Thins, Chocolate, Waitrose*	1 Thin/5g	27	1.3	509	4.2	69.6	23.8	0.2
MIRIN								
Rice Wine, Sweetened, Average	***1 Tbsp/15ml***	***35***	***0.0***	***231***	***0.2***	***41.6***	***0.0***	***0.0***
MISO								
Average	***1oz/28g***	***57***	***1.7***	***203***	***13.3***	***23.5***	***6.2***	***0.0***
MIXED HERBS								
Average	***1 Tsp/5g***	***13***	***0.4***	***260***	***13.0***	***37.5***	***8.5***	***6.7***
Herbes De Provence, Dried, Schwartz*	1 Tsp/2g	7	0.1	364	12.9	65.0	5.8	0.0
MIXED SPICE								
Rub, Moroccan, Schwartz*	1 Serving/3g	9	0.3	309	15.0	36.4	11.4	19.5
Schwartz*	1 Tsp/2g	8	0.2	390	10.4	65.8	9.5	2.0
MIXED VEGETABLES								
Baby, Iceland*	1 Serving/100g	20	0.0	20	1.2	3.9	0.0	2.7
Baby, Steam, Fresh, Tesco*	1 Pack/160g	72	1.3	45	2.7	6.7	0.8	3.8
Baby Corn, Mange Tout & Baby Carrots, Tesco*	1 Pack/220g	64	0.9	29	2.3	4.3	0.4	2.2
Bag, M & S*	1 Serving/200g	70	0.4	35	2.9	5.6	0.2	0.0
Broccoli, Peas & Green Beans, Co-Op*	1 Serving/80g	36	0.3	45	4.8	3.8	0.4	3.6
Broccoli & Cauliflower Florets, Baby Carrots, Asda*	1 Serving/113g	28	0.7	25	2.2	2.6	0.6	2.4
Canned, Drained, Sainsbury's*	1 Can/200g	114	0.6	57	3.0	10.6	0.3	2.3
Canned, Re-Heated, Drained	1oz/28g	11	0.2	38	1.9	6.1	0.8	1.7
Carrot, Batons, Cauliflower & Broccoli, Steamed, Asda*	1 Bag/120g	28	0.7	23	1.8	2.6	0.6	3.1
Carrot, Cauliflower & Broccoli, Prepared, Co-Op*	1 Pack/250g	100	1.5	40	2.4	5.0	0.6	2.7
Carrot, Swede, Leek & Onion for Casserole, M & S*	1 Serving/100g	35	0.4	35	0.8	5.6	0.4	2.6
Carrots, Broccoli & Sweetcorn, Steam Veg, Tesco*	1 Sachet/160g	80	1.8	50	2.5	7.5	1.1	3.0
Carrots, Cauliflower & Broccoli, Waitrose*	1 Serving/100g	35	0.6	35	2.4	4.9	0.6	2.9
Carrots & Peas, 386, Wiltshire Farm Foods*	1 Serving/160g	72	1.1	45	3.0	7.2	0.7	3.5

	Measure INFO/WEIGHT	per Measure KCAL	per Measure FAT	KCAL	PROT	CARB	FAT	FIBRE
MIXED VEGETABLES								
Casserole, Frozen, Tesco*	1 Serving/100g	26	0.4	26	0.8	4.8	0.4	2.0
Casserole, Ready to Cook, Sainsbury's*	½ Pack/240g	74	0.7	31	0.9	6.2	0.3	1.4
Casserole, Tesco*	1 Pack/440g	176	1.3	40	1.2	8.0	0.3	2.3
Casserole, with Baby Potatoes, Fresh, M & S*	½ Pack/350g	140	1.0	40	1.2	7.8	0.3	2.1
Chef's Style, Ready Prepared, M & S*	1 Pack/240g	72	1.2	30	2.6	4.5	0.5	2.9
Chunky, Frozen, Sainsbury's*	1 Serving/85g	31	0.6	37	2.9	4.7	0.7	3.1
Country Selection, Budgens*	1 Serving/113g	27	0.4	24	1.6	3.6	0.4	2.9
Crunchy, Tesco*	1 Pack/210g	63	0.8	30	1.7	5.0	0.4	2.4
Farmhouse, Four Seasons*	1 Serving/100g	26	0.7	26	2.2	2.7	0.7	0.0
Farmhouse, Frozen, Waitrose*	1 Serving/90g	22	0.5	25	1.9	3.1	0.6	2.4
Fresh, Asda*	1oz/28g	7	0.2	26	1.9	3.0	0.7	1.0
Freshly Frozen, Asda*	1 Serving/80g	42	0.6	52	3.2	8.0	0.8	3.0
Frozen, Aldi*	1 Serving/100g	34	0.7	34	2.8	4.3	0.7	0.0
Frozen, Boiled in Salted Water	1oz/28g	12	0.1	42	3.3	6.6	0.5	0.0
Frozen, Waitrose*	1 Serving/80g	43	0.6	54	3.1	8.7	0.8	3.5
Green, Microwave, Aldi*	1 Serving/300g	189	9.0	63	3.5	5.6	3.0	4.1
in Salted Water, Canned, Asda*	1 Serving/65g	31	0.1	48	2.6	9.0	0.2	1.7
in Salted Water, Nisa Heritage*	1 Serving/100g	39	0.8	39	1.9	6.1	0.8	1.7
Layered, Classics, M & S*	½ Pack/160g	112	6.2	70	1.2	7.3	3.9	1.2
Organic, Waitrose*	1oz/28g	19	0.4	69	4.4	10.0	1.3	2.7
Oriental, M & S*	1 Serving/250g	50	0.8	20	1.6	3.4	0.3	1.6
Peas, Carrots, & Baby Leeks, Prepared, Tesco*	½ Pack/130g	57	1.2	44	3.1	5.8	0.9	3.5
Peas & Carrots, Crinkle Cut, D'Aucy*	1 Serving/265g	138	1.3	52	3.2	6.5	0.5	4.3
Potatoes, Broad Beans & Peas, M & S*	1 Pack/245g	147	3.2	60	2.9	12.9	1.3	3.4
Ready to Roast, Asda*	½ Pack/362g	315	11.6	87	1.6	13.0	3.2	2.4
Red Peppers & Courgette, Tesco*	1 Pack/250g	68	1.2	27	1.7	3.8	0.5	2.0
Roast, Four Seasons*	1 Serving/187g	79	0.4	42	1.2	8.8	0.2	0.0
Sainsbury's*	1 Serving/230g	55	1.4	24	2.1	2.5	0.6	0.0
Seasonal Selection, Tesco*	1 Serving/100g	37	0.4	37	1.1	7.2	0.4	2.2
Special, Freshly Frozen, Morrisons*	1 Serving/100g	48	0.8	48	3.2	7.2	0.8	0.0
Special, Sainsbury's*	1 Serving/120g	68	1.2	57	3.2	8.9	1.0	2.9
Summer, Tesco*	1 Pack/167g	55	0.8	33	2.6	4.5	0.5	2.8
Tenderstem Broccoli, Carrots & Mange Tout, M & S*	½ Pack/100g	35	0.2	35	2.9	5.6	0.2	2.1
Thai Style in a Herb Marinade, Straight to Wok, Amoy*	1 Pouch/400g	74	0.8	19	0.7	3.5	0.2	0.0
MOLASSES								
Average	***1 Tsp/5g***	***13***	***0.0***	***266***	***0.0***	***68.8***	***0.1***	***0.0***
MONKEY NUTS								
without Shell, Average	***1oz/28g***	***158***	***13.4***	***565***	***25.6***	***8.2***	***48.0***	***6.3***
MONKFISH								
Grilled	***1oz/28g***	***27***	***0.2***	***96***	***22.7***	***0.0***	***0.6***	***0.0***
Raw	***1oz/28g***	***18***	***0.1***	***66***	***15.7***	***0.0***	***0.4***	***0.0***
MONSTER MUNCH								
Flamin' Hot, Walkers*	1 Bag/22g	108	5.5	490	7.0	59.0	25.0	1.5
Pickled Onion, Walkers*	1 Bag/22g	108	5.5	490	6.0	60.0	25.0	1.7
Roast Beef, Walkers*	1 Bag/22g	108	5.5	490	7.0	59.0	25.0	1.7
Spicy, Walkers*	1 Bag/25g	125	7.2	500	5.0	55.0	29.0	1.3
MORNAY								
Cod, Fillets, Sainsbury's*	1 Serving/153g	236	14.4	154	15.2	2.2	9.4	0.9
Cod, Gratin, Cooked, Just Cook, Sainsbury's*	1 Pack/320g	518	32.2	185	13.3	6.9	11.5	0.5
Cod, Nutritionally Balanced, M & S*	1 Pack/400g	320	10.4	80	6.8	7.2	2.6	1.6
Cod, Sainsbury's*	1 Serving/180g	277	16.9	154	15.2	2.2	9.4	0.9
Haddock, COU, M & S*	½ Pack/194g	165	3.9	85	14.5	2.6	2.0	0.6
Haddock, Perfectly Balanced, Waitrose*	1 Pack/360g	310	5.4	86	16.6	1.6	1.5	0.5

Nutrition Values per 100g / 100ml apply to columns KCAL, PROT, CARB, FAT, FIBRE (right group).

M

	Measure INFO/WEIGHT	per Measure KCAL	FAT	Nutrition Values per 100g / 100ml KCAL	PROT	CARB	FAT	FIBRE
MORNAY								
Haddock, Youngs*	½ Pack/190g	236	14.8	124	12.1	1.3	7.8	0.6
Salmon, with Broccoli, Weight Watchers*	1 Pack/320g	231	9.6	72	4.5	6.5	3.0	0.5
Spinach, Waitrose*	½ Pack/125g	112	8.6	90	3.3	3.6	6.9	1.6
MOUSSAKA								
Aubergine & Lentil, Asda*	1 Pack/451g	370	17.1	82	3.9	8.1	3.8	2.9
Beef, BGTY, Sainsbury's*	1 Pack/400g	300	10.4	75	6.1	6.8	2.6	1.2
Beef, GFY, Asda*	1 Pack/400g	300	8.4	75	7.0	7.0	2.1	0.7
Charlie Bigham's*	½ Pack/328g	396	24.2	121	7.0	7.0	7.4	0.9
COU, M & S*	1 Pack/340g	272	9.9	80	5.3	8.5	2.9	1.4
Lamb, Sainsbury's*	1 Pack/329g	497	32.3	151	8.4	7.2	9.8	1.0
Low Saturated Fat, Waitrose*	1 Pack/350g	304	10.8	87	6.3	8.4	3.1	3.1
TTD, Sainsbury's*	1 Pack/399g	546	35.9	137	8.1	5.8	9.0	0.6
Vegetable, COU, M & S*	1 Pack/400g	280	10.8	70	2.7	9.1	2.7	2.4
Vegetarian, Tesco*	1 Pack/300g	489	31.2	163	6.4	11.0	10.4	0.9
MOUSSE								
Aero, Chocolate, Nestle*	1 Pot/58g	101	3.0	174	4.8	27.3	5.1	1.1
Aero, Twist Cappuccino & Chocolate, Nestle*	1 Pot/75g	135	8.1	180	4.2	16.8	10.8	0.2
Apricot, Lite, Onken*	1 Pot/150g	156	2.2	104	4.6	18.0	1.5	0.3
Banoffee, COU, M & S*	1 Pot/70g	102	1.5	145	2.9	28.8	2.1	1.5
Black Cherry, Lite, Onken*	1 Pot/150g	156	2.2	104	4.6	17.9	1.5	0.2
Blackcurrant, HL, Tesco*	1 Pot/113g	80	2.9	71	3.7	8.3	2.6	1.8
Blackcurrant, Onken*	1 Pot/150g	210	10.2	140	5.2	14.6	6.8	0.0
Cappuccino, Essential, Waitrose*	1 Pot/100g	279	16.7	279	4.2	27.7	16.7	0.5
Caramel, Meringue, Cadbury*	1 Pot/65g	181	6.7	277	4.6	42.4	10.3	1.0
Chocolate	1 Pot/60g	83	3.2	139	4.0	19.9	5.4	0.0
Chocolate, Belgian, & Vanilla, Weight Watchers*	1 Pot/80g	106	2.2	132	4.4	22.2	2.8	0.9
Chocolate, Belgian, Finest, Tesco*	1 Pot/120g	360	22.7	300	5.1	26.6	18.9	1.1
Chocolate, BGTY, Sainsbury's*	1 Pot/63g	83	1.8	133	4.9	21.8	2.9	0.5
Chocolate, Cadbury*	1 Pot/55g	107	4.5	195	6.1	24.6	8.2	0.0
Chocolate, COU, M & S*	1 Pot/70g	84	1.9	120	5.2	20.3	2.7	1.0
Chocolate, Dairy Milk, Mini Chunks, Cadbury*	1 Pot/100g	215	9.9	215	6.1	25.7	9.9	0.0
Chocolate, Finest, Tesco*	1 Pot/82g	321	26.4	391	3.7	21.7	32.2	0.0
Chocolate, GFY, Asda*	1 Pot/60g	70	1.7	117	4.8	17.9	2.9	3.5
Chocolate, Italian Style, Tesco*	1 Pot/90g	243	11.9	270	5.0	32.8	13.2	2.4
Chocolate, Light, Cadbury*	1 Pot/55g	60	1.9	110	4.6	14.2	3.4	0.0
Chocolate, Low Fat, Danette, Danone*	1 Pot/60g	73	1.1	121	5.1	20.8	1.9	1.5
Chocolate, Minty, Bubbly, Dessert, Aero, Nestle*	1 Pot/58g	108	5.9	186	4.6	18.9	10.2	0.3
Chocolate, Plain, Low Fat, Nestle*	1 Pot/120g	71	0.9	59	2.4	10.4	0.8	0.0
Chocolate, Shapers, Boots*	1 Pot/70g	97	1.9	138	5.3	23.0	2.7	1.7
Chocolate, White, Bubbly, Dessert, Aero, Nestle*	1 Pot/58g	99	4.4	170	4.3	21.0	7.5	0.2
Chocolate, White, Finest, Tesco*	1 Pot/92g	436	34.5	474	3.9	30.2	37.5	0.0
Chocolate, with Vanilla Layer, Cadbury*	1 Pot/100g	162	6.1	162	4.8	21.9	6.1	0.0
Chocolate & Hazelnut, Creamy, Dr Oetker*	1 Pot/115g	158	6.9	137	3.3	17.6	6.0	0.6
Chocolate & Hazelnut, Onken*	1 Pot/125g	171	7.5	137	3.3	17.8	6.0	0.0
Chocolate & Mint, COU, M & S*	1 Pot/70g	84	1.8	120	6.2	18.7	2.5	1.0
Chocolate & Orange, COU, M & S*	1 Pot/70g	77	1.8	110	5.9	16.0	2.6	0.9
Chocolate Orange, Low Fat, Cadbury*	1 Pot/100g	110	3.0	110	5.6	15.1	3.0	0.0
Dream, Cadbury*	1 Pot/53g	100	4.2	189	6.0	22.0	8.0	0.0
Fruit Juice, Shape, Danone*	1 Pot/100g	115	2.8	115	3.5	18.5	2.8	0.0
Lemon, Classic, Onken*	1 Pot/150g	210	9.4	140	5.1	15.8	6.3	0.0
Lemon, COU, M & S*	1 Pot/70g	91	1.8	130	3.1	23.7	2.5	0.6
Lemon, Dessert, Sainsbury's*	1 Pot/63g	114	5.9	182	3.6	20.7	9.4	0.6
Lemon, GFY, Asda*	1 Pot/63g	58	1.8	92	3.6	13.0	2.8	1.7

	Measure INFO/WEIGHT	per Measure KCAL	per Measure FAT	Nutrition Values per 100g / 100ml KCAL	PROT	CARB	FAT	FIBRE
MOUSSE								
Lemon, HL, Tesco*	1 Pot/113g	94	2.9	83	3.6	11.3	2.6	0.2
Lemon, Less Than 3% Fat, BGTY, Sainsbury's*	1 Pot/62g	70	1.7	113	4.5	17.6	2.8	0.3
Lemon, Less Than 3% Fat, HE, Tesco*	1 Pot/60g	57	1.6	95	3.4	14.3	2.7	0.7
Lemon, Lite, Onken*	1 Pot/150g	156	2.2	104	4.6	17.2	1.5	0.2
Lemon, Low Fat, Morrisons*	1 Pot/63g	99	5.8	158	3.7	15.4	9.3	0.3
Lemon, Perfectly Balanced, Waitrose*	1 Pot/95g	150	2.6	158	3.1	30.2	2.7	0.1
Lemon, Tesco*	1 Pot/60g	67	1.6	111	3.4	18.2	2.7	0.0
Orange, Mango & Lime, Onken*	1 Pot/150g	207	9.4	138	5.1	15.3	6.3	0.1
Orange & Nectarine, Shape, Danone*	1 Pot/100g	47	1.9	47	3.0	4.9	1.9	0.0
Peach, Onken*	1 Pot/150g	204	9.4	136	5.1	15.1	6.3	0.2
Peach, Shape, Danone*	1 Pot/100g	43	1.8	43	3.0	3.9	1.8	0.1
Peach & Passion Fruit, Perfectly Balanced, Waitrose*	1 Pot/95g	118	2.7	124	3.5	21.2	2.8	0.5
Pineapple, COU, M & S*	1 Pot/70g	84	1.7	120	3.3	20.7	2.4	3.5
Raspberry, Lite, Onken*	1 Pot/150g	156	2.2	104	4.6	17.3	1.5	0.1
Raspberry & Cranberry, Luxury, Weight Watchers*	1 Pot/80g	62	1.0	78	3.8	13.0	1.2	1.0
Raspberry Ripple, Value, Tesco*	1 Pot/47g	70	2.9	149	2.1	21.3	6.1	0.1
Rhubarb, COU, M & S*	1 Pot/70g	88	1.5	125	2.9	25.7	2.1	4.2
Rhubarb, Lite, Onken*	1 Pot/150g	154	2.2	103	4.6	17.8	1.5	0.3
Rhubarb & Vanilla, Onken*	1 Pot/150g	210	9.4	140	5.0	15.8	6.3	0.2
Strawberry, Asda*	1 Pot/64g	107	5.8	167	3.5	18.0	9.0	0.2
Strawberry, HL, Tesco*	1 Pot/114g	90	3.0	79	3.8	10.2	2.6	0.8
Strawberry, Light, Muller*	1 Pot/150g	147	0.6	98	4.3	19.4	0.4	0.0
Strawberry, Lite, Onken*	1 Pot/150g	152	2.2	101	4.6	17.2	1.5	0.2
Strawberry, Low Fat, Waitrose*	1 Pot/95g	112	2.7	118	3.2	20.0	2.8	0.6
Strawberry, Sainsbury's*	1 Pot/63g	106	5.9	168	3.4	17.5	9.4	0.1
Strawberry, Shape, Danone*	1 Pot/100g	44	1.8	44	3.0	4.0	1.8	0.0
Strawberry, Tesco*	1 Pot/63g	106	5.8	169	3.5	17.9	9.3	0.2
Strawberry, with Strawberry Sauce, Ski, Nestle*	1 Pot/60g	79	3.1	131	3.1	18.1	5.2	0.0
Strawberry & Vanilla, Weight Watchers*	1 Pot/80g	87	1.9	109	3.8	18.1	2.4	0.4
Strawberry Fruity, Organic, Sainsbury's*	1 Pot/125g	129	3.8	103	6.2	15.7	3.0	3.6
Summer Fruits, Light, Muller*	1 Pot/149g	143	0.6	96	4.3	18.7	0.4	0.0
Toffee, M & S*	1 Pot/90g	180	7.2	200	4.5	27.6	8.0	0.6
Vanilla, Finesse, Aero, Rowntree's*	1 Pot/57g	127	8.3	223	3.7	18.8	14.6	0.0
MUFFIN								
All Butter, M & S*	1 Muffin/65g	175	4.7	270	10.3	40.8	7.3	2.1
Apple, Sultana & Cinnamon, GFY, Asda*	1 Muffin/50g	134	1.8	268	6.0	53.0	3.5	3.9
Banana & Walnut, The Handmade Flapjack Company*	1 Muffin/135g	520	30.6	385	5.3	40.5	22.7	0.0
Banana Pecan, Organic, Honeyrose Bakery*	1 Muffin/110g	300	12.6	273	4.1	38.3	11.5	4.3
Berry Burst, Asda*	1 Muffin/60g	139	1.4	232	6.2	46.7	2.3	1.7
Blueberry, & Redcurrant, BGTY, Sainsbury's*	1 Muffin/65g	159	1.6	245	5.0	50.0	2.5	3.1
Blueberry, American Style, Aldi*	1 Muffin/85g	344	17.3	405	4.3	51.2	20.3	0.0
Blueberry, American Style, Sainsbury's*	1 Muffin/72g	256	13.1	355	5.1	42.7	18.2	1.9
Blueberry, Asda*	1 Muffin/77g	273	13.1	353	5.0	45.0	17.0	1.3
Blueberry, GFY, Asda*	1 Muffin/59g	146	1.3	249	6.0	51.0	2.3	3.0
Blueberry, Low Fat, David Powell*	1 Muffin/100g	246	3.8	246	6.0	47.9	3.8	0.0
Blueberry, M & S*	1 Muffin/75g	255	12.6	340	4.9	41.9	16.8	1.3
Blueberry, McVitie's*	1 Muffin/80g	328	18.6	405	4.7	47.9	23.0	1.3
Blueberry, Mini, Sainsbury's*	1 Muffin/28g	82	2.3	293	6.3	48.9	8.1	1.9
Blueberry, Perfectly Balanced, Waitrose*	1 Muffin/100g	225	2.2	225	4.6	46.5	2.2	1.8
Blueberry, The Handmade Flapjack Company*	1 Muffin/135g	479	26.6	355	4.7	39.9	19.7	0.0
Blueberry, Waitrose*	1 Muffin/65g	239	9.2	367	4.7	55.2	14.2	1.7
Blueberry, Weight Watchers*	1 Muffin/63g	156	2.0	247	4.8	46.4	3.1	7.0
Blueberry, Wild Canadian, Fabulous Bakin' Boys*	1 Muffin/40g	140	8.0	349	4.0	39.0	20.0	1.0

M

	Measure	per Measure		Nutrition Values per 100g / 100ml				
	INFO/WEIGHT	KCAL	FAT	KCAL	PROT	CARB	FAT	FIBRE
MUFFIN								
Bran, & Sultana, Weight Watchers*	1 Muffin/60g	144	1.3	240	4.5	50.7	2.1	2.3
Bran, Average	1 Muffin/57g	155	4.4	272	7.8	45.6	7.7	7.7
Caramel, Cadbury*	1 Muffin/116g	535	30.3	461	5.9	50.8	26.1	0.0
Caramel, Salted, TTD, Sainsbury's*	1 Muffin/113g	447	22.0	396	4.8	49.6	19.5	1.5
Carrot, Asda*	1 Muffin/59g	138	1.4	233	6.0	47.0	2.3	1.6
Carrot Cake, Entenmann's*	1 Muffin/105g	344	15.9	328	5.1	45.8	15.1	3.0
Carrot Cakelet, The Handmade Flapjack Company*	1 Muffin/135g	479	23.9	355	4.0	45.1	17.7	0.0
Cheese, Tesco*	1 Muffin/67g	150	1.9	224	13.0	36.4	2.9	3.0
Cherry, Cheeky, Fabulous Bakin' Boys*	1 Muffin/118g	446	21.0	378	5.5	51.0	17.8	0.7
Cherry, The Handmade Flapjack Company*	1 Muffin/135g	500	26.6	370	4.6	43.8	19.7	0.0
Cherry Bakewell, Mr Kipling*	1 Muffin/100g	355	19.6	355	5.0	55.0	19.6	1.4
Cherry Mega, The Handmade Flapjack Company*	1 Muffin/135g	506	26.7	375	4.4	44.8	19.8	0.0
Choc Chip, Double, Weight Watchers*	1 Muffin/65g	189	5.4	291	6.8	47.2	8.3	3.6
Choc Chip, Mini, Weight Watchers*	1 Muffin/15g	47	1.3	312	6.6	52.1	8.6	3.1
Chocolate, Double, 95% Fat Free, Entenmann's*	1 Muffin/58g	152	2.7	262	2.6	52.3	4.7	1.8
Chocolate, Double, Free From, Tesco*	1 Muffin/70g	281	12.7	402	4.7	54.8	18.2	1.7
Chocolate, Double, Mini, M & S*	1 Muffin/32g	133	6.9	416	5.4	49.8	21.7	1.1
Chocolate, Galaxy, McVitie's*	1 Muffin/88g	319	17.1	364	5.0	44.5	19.5	0.0
Chocolate, HL, Tesco*	1 Muffin/71g	204	6.2	288	5.5	46.9	8.7	5.5
Chocolate, The Handmade Flapjack Company*	1 Muffin/135g	526	30.8	390	5.3	41.5	22.8	0.0
Chocolate, Triple, Triumph, Fabulous Bakin' Boys*	1 Muffin/40g	160	9.6	400	4.5	42.0	24.0	0.0
Chocolate, Truly Madly, Fabulous Bakin' Boys*	1 Muffin/105g	405	23.1	386	5.0	41.0	22.0	2.0
Chocolate, White, & Strawberry Filled, Tesco*	1 Muffin/103g	415	20.3	405	5.2	51.3	19.8	1.3
Chocolate, White, Chunk Lemon, Mini, M & S*	1 Muffin/28g	130	6.7	464	6.4	55.4	23.9	2.1
Chocolate Chip, American Style, Sainsbury's*	1 Muffin/72g	284	14.4	395	5.0	48.8	20.0	2.1
Chocolate Chip, BGTY, Sainsbury's*	1 Muffin/75g	282	12.3	376	5.2	51.8	16.4	1.6
Chocolate Chip, Blackfriars*	1 Muffin/50g	218	11.5	435	6.0	51.0	23.0	4.0
Chocolate Chip, Double, American Style, Sainsbury's*	1 Muffin/72g	276	14.6	384	5.2	45.0	20.3	2.9
Chocolate Chip, Double, Co-Op*	1 Muffin/60g	246	12.6	410	6.0	49.0	21.0	3.0
Chocolate Chip, Double, Mini, Asda*	1 Muffin/19g	76	3.7	400	7.4	48.5	19.6	2.7
Chocolate Chip, Double, Mini, Weight Watchers*	1 Muffin/15g	45	1.3	300	7.0	48.5	8.7	3.5
Chocolate Chip, Double, Tesco*	1 Muffin/100g	360	17.9	360	6.1	44.9	17.9	5.4
Chocolate Indulgence, McVitie's*	1 Muffin/75g	254	6.9	338	5.8	57.9	9.2	1.3
Cinnamon & Sultana, Morrisons*	1 Muffin/75g	183	1.0	244	8.3	48.2	1.4	2.9
Cranberry & White Chocolate, Sainsbury's*	1 Muffin/72g	253	13.3	352	5.7	40.7	18.5	1.5
English	1 Muffin/57g	120	1.0	211	7.0	43.9	1.8	1.8
English, Gluten, Wheat & Milk Free, Free From, Livwell*	1 Muffin/50g	160	4.9	320	4.6	52.8	9.8	3.2
English, Kingsmill*	1 Muffin/75g	167	1.4	222	9.7	40.4	1.8	2.6
English, Plain, Oakrun Bakery*	1 Muffin/57g	139	1.0	244	8.4	47.4	1.8	1.4
Family, Irwin's Bakery*	1 Muffin/40g	116	2.5	291	8.9	50.0	6.2	0.0
Finger, Double Chocolate, Bakers Delight*	1 Muffin/25g	104	4.6	416	5.8	56.9	18.4	1.7
Fruit, Spiced, TTD, Sainsbury's*	1 Muffin/70g	181	3.6	259	10.1	43.1	5.1	2.1
Lemon, Boots*	1 Muffin/110g	424	20.9	385	3.6	50.0	19.0	1.3
Lemon & Blueberry, Tesco*	1 Muffin/110g	411	23.0	374	4.0	42.4	20.9	1.1
Lemon & Poppy Seed, Entenmann's*	1 Muffin/105g	417	20.3	397	5.6	52.8	19.3	2.5
Lemon & Poppy Seed, M & S*	1 Muffin/72g	281	14.3	390	6.3	46.1	19.8	1.5
Lemon & Sultana, BGTY, Sainsbury's*	1 Muffin/75g	211	3.4	281	4.5	55.6	4.5	1.4
Mini, Tesco*	1 Muffin/28g	120	6.3	428	6.4	50.0	22.6	1.2
Mixed Fruit, Low Fat, Abbey Bakery*	1 Muffin/35g	93	1.6	267	4.5	55.6	4.5	1.4
Morning Sunrise, Ryvita*	1 Muffin/110g	330	10.0	300	4.5	49.1	9.1	1.8
Muesli, Breakfast, Love Life, Waitrose*	1 Muffin/68g	216	6.2	318	9.1	50.0	9.1	3.4
Muesli, Sainsbury's*	1 Muffin/113g	447	25.7	396	6.5	41.5	22.7	1.4
Orange, Apricot & Almond, Organic, Honeyrose Bakery*	1 Muffin/110g	312	11.4	284	3.5	44.2	10.4	1.9

	Measure INFO/WEIGHT	per Measure KCAL	FAT	Nutrition Values per 100g / 100ml KCAL	PROT	CARB	FAT	FIBRE
MUFFIN								
Oven Bottom, Aldi*	1 Muffin/68g	173	1.0	255	10.0	50.4	1.5	2.2
Oven Bottom, Asda*	1 Muffin/68g	173	1.0	255	10.0	50.4	1.5	2.2
Oven Bottom, Mini, Morrisons*	1 Muffin/42g	107	0.6	255	10.0	50.4	1.5	2.2
Oven Bottom, Warburton's*	1 Muffin/69g	175	2.0	253	10.9	45.8	2.9	0.0
Plain, Co-Op*	1 Muffin/60g	135	1.1	225	11.2	41.3	1.9	2.4
Plain, Morrisons*	1 Muffin/70g	140	0.8	200	8.0	41.4	1.1	0.0
Plain, Prepared From Recipe, Average	1 Muffin/57g	169	6.5	296	6.9	41.4	11.4	2.7
Raspberry, Perfectly Balanced, Waitrose*	1 Muffin/101g	220	2.1	219	4.7	45.4	2.1	3.7
Raspberry Cream, Sainsbury's*	1 Muffin/90g	314	19.8	349	3.9	33.8	22.0	1.3
Raspberry Injected, The Handmade Flapjack Company*	1 Muffin/135g	564	27.3	418	4.5	54.7	20.2	0.0
Rolo, Nestle*	1 Muffin/80g	289	14.4	361	5.4	44.3	18.0	0.8
Sausage, Egg & Cheese, American Style, Tesco*	1 Muffin/155g	383	20.5	247	12.2	19.9	13.2	1.0
Spiced Fruit, Co-Op*	1 Muffin/60g	159	1.2	265	11.0	52.0	2.0	3.0
Spiced Fruit, Toasting, Finest, Tesco*	1 Muffin/77g	215	5.2	279	9.2	43.2	6.8	3.9
Spicy Fruit, Quality Bakers*	1 Muffin/65g	146	1.0	225	9.4	38.0	1.5	3.3
Strawberry Cakelet, The Handmade Flapjack Company*	1 Muffin/135g	526	29.6	390	4.5	43.6	21.9	0.0
Sunblest*	1 Muffin/72g	166	1.3	230	9.6	43.9	1.8	2.2
Toasting, Warburton's*	1 Muffin/64g	138	1.0	216	8.9	41.4	1.6	2.9
Toffee, GFY, Asda*	1 Muffin/90g	151	2.3	168	2.1	34.0	2.6	0.0
Toffee, The Handmade Flapjack Company*	1 Muffin/135g	533	31.6	395	4.4	41.2	23.4	0.0
Toffee & Pecan, Finest, Tesco*	1 Muffin/127g	551	29.0	434	5.4	51.8	22.8	0.9
Toffee Choo Choo, Tesco*	1 Muffin/95g	402	21.3	423	6.4	49.1	22.4	1.0
Toffee Mega, The Handmade Flapjack Company*	1 Muffin/135g	567	34.7	420	4.5	43.2	25.7	0.0
Toffee Temptation, McVitie's*	1 Muffin/86g	297	8.1	347	4.7	60.8	9.5	0.8
Vanilla & Choc Chip, GFY, Asda*	1 Muffin/59g	152	1.3	260	7.0	53.0	2.2	1.6
Wholemeal, Organic, Love Life, Waitrose*	1 Muffin/100g	245	3.6	245	11.7	40.8	3.6	6.3
Wholemeal, Tesco*	1 Muffin/65g	130	1.3	200	12.6	32.9	2.0	5.7
MULBERRIES								
Raw	***1oz/28g***	***10***	***0.0***	***36***	***1.3***	***8.1***	***0.0***	***0.0***
MULLET								
Grey, Grilled	***1oz/28g***	***42***	***1.5***	***150***	***25.7***	***0.0***	***5.2***	***0.0***
Grey, Raw	***1oz/28g***	***32***	***1.1***	***115***	***19.8***	***0.0***	***4.0***	***0.0***
Red, Grilled	***1oz/28g***	***34***	***1.2***	***121***	***20.4***	***0.0***	***4.4***	***0.0***
Red, Raw, Weighed Whole, Flesh Only	***1 Portion/100g***	***109***	***3.8***	***109***	***18.7***	***0.0***	***3.8***	***0.0***
MUNCHIES								
Mint, Nestle*	1 Pack/62g	267	10.1	432	3.8	67.5	16.4	0.0
Original, Tube, Nestle*	1 Pack/55g	266	12.3	487	5.4	64.6	22.5	1.4
MUSHROOMS								
Breaded, Average	***3 Mushrooms/51g***	***77***	***2.9***	***152***	***4.3***	***20.8***	***5.7***	***0.6***
Breaded, Garlic, Average	3 Mushrooms/50g	92	4.9	183	5.2	18.7	9.7	1.7
Buna Shimeji, Livesey Brothers*	½ Pack/75g	29	0.3	39	2.7	5.9	0.4	1.2
Button, Raw, Average	1 Serving/50g	7	0.2	15	2.3	0.5	0.4	1.2
Cheesey, Stuffed, Asda*	1 Serving/290g	322	17.4	111	4.3	10.0	6.0	0.0
Chestnut, Average	***1 Med/5g***	***1***	***0.0***	***13***	***1.8***	***0.4***	***0.5***	***0.6***
Chinese, Dried, Raw	***1oz/28g***	***80***	***0.5***	***284***	***10.0***	***59.9***	***1.8***	***0.0***
Closed Cup, Average	***1 Handfull/30g***	***4***	***0.2***	***14***	***1.8***	***0.4***	***0.5***	***1.1***
Common, Boiled in Salted Water, Average	***1oz/28g***	***3***	***0.1***	***11***	***1.8***	***0.4***	***0.3***	***1.1***
Common, Fried, Average	***1oz/28g***	***44***	***4.5***	***157***	***2.4***	***0.3***	***16.2***	***1.5***
Common, Raw, Average	***1 Serving/80g***	***10***	***0.4***	***13***	***1.9***	***0.3***	***0.5***	***1.1***
Creamed, Average	***1oz/28g***	***23***	***1.5***	***82***	***1.3***	***6.8***	***5.5***	***0.5***
Crispy, M & S*	1 Serving/130g	390	33.4	300	4.2	12.5	25.7	1.8
Dried	***1oz/28g***	***45***	***1.7***	***159***	***21.8***	***4.8***	***6.0***	***13.3***
Enoki, Average	***1 Serving/80g***	***34***	***0.0***	***42***	***3.0***	***7.0***	***0.0***	***3.0***

M

	Measure INFO/WEIGHT	per Measure KCAL	FAT	Nutrition Values per 100g / 100ml KCAL	PROT	CARB	FAT	FIBRE
MUSHROOMS								
Exotic Selection, Fresh, TTD, Sainsbury's*	1 Pack/140g	60	0.7	43	3.2	7.4	0.5	0.0
Flat, Large, Average	***1 Mushroom/52g***	***10***	***0.3***	***20***	***3.3***	***0.5***	***0.5***	***0.7***
Frozen, Cooks' Ingredients, Waitrose*	1 Portion/75g	14	0.2	18	2.1	1.8	0.3	2.5
Garlic, Average	½ Pack/150g	159	14.0	106	2.1	3.7	9.3	1.7
Giant, with Tomatoes & Mozzarella, M & S*	1 Serving/145g	218	15.8	150	6.3	7.1	10.9	5.5
Hon Shimeji, Sainsbury's*	1 Serving/80g	18	0.4	22	4.0	3.9	0.5	1.1
Medley, Asda*	½ Pack/100g	89	7.8	89	3.2	1.4	7.8	2.8
Oyster, Average	***1 Serving/80g***	***12***	***0.2***	***15***	***1.6***	***1.6***	***0.2***	***1.3***
Porcini, Dried, Asda*	1 Bag/25g	65	1.2	260	30.4	24.1	4.7	17.5
Porcini, Wild, Dried, Merchant Gourmet*	1 Pack/25g	66	0.8	265	27.9	30.6	3.4	18.7
Portobello, Mini, Sainsbury's*	1 Serving/100g	16	0.5	16	1.8	0.4	0.5	1.1
Shiitake, Cooked	***1oz/28g***	***15***	***0.1***	***55***	***1.6***	***12.3***	***0.2***	***0.0***
Shiitake, Dried, Raw	***1oz/28g***	***83***	***0.3***	***296***	***9.6***	***63.9***	***1.0***	***0.0***
Shiitake, Raw, Waitrose*	1 Serving/100g	32	0.5	32	2.2	48.0	0.5	25.0
Sliced, Average	***1oz/28g***	***3***	***0.1***	***12***	***1.8***	***0.4***	***0.3***	***1.1***
Straw, Canned, Drained	***1oz/28g***	***4***	***0.1***	***15***	***2.1***	***1.2***	***0.2***	***0.0***
Stuffed, Ready to Eat, Morrisons*	1oz/28g	29	1.1	104	3.5	10.8	4.1	2.6
Stuffed, Ready to Roast, Waitrose*	1 Serving/125g	94	4.6	75	3.9	6.5	3.7	1.5
MUSSELS								
Boiled, Flesh Only, Average	1 Mussel/2g	2	0.1	104	16.7	3.5	2.7	0.0
Boiled, Weighed in Shell, Average	***1 Mussel/7g***	***7***	***0.2***	***104***	***16.7***	***3.5***	***2.7***	***0.0***
Pickled, Drained, Average	***1oz/28g***	***32***	***0.6***	***112***	***20.0***	***1.5***	***2.2***	***0.0***
Raw, Weighed in Shell, Average	***1oz/28g***	***24***	***0.7***	***87***	***12.7***	***3.6***	***2.5***	***0.2***
Scottish, in Garlic Butter Sauce with Shells, Aldi*	1 Serving/113g	93	3.9	82	7.8	4.7	3.4	0.5
MUSSELS IN								
Garlic Butter Sauce, Average	½ Pack/225g	179	11.5	80	6.4	2.0	5.1	0.2
Garlic Butter Sauce, Creamy, Bantry Bay*	1 Serving/225g	198	7.9	88	9.0	5.2	3.5	0.6
Thai Sauce, Scottish, Waitrose*	1 Serving/250g	135	6.2	54	5.4	2.6	2.5	0.6
White Wine Sauce, Sainsbury's*	½ Pack/250g	221	9.2	88	8.0	5.8	3.7	0.0
White Wine Sauce, Seasoned, Bantry Bay*	1 Serving/450g	270	9.0	60	6.3	4.1	2.0	0.1
MUSTARD								
American, Average	***1 Tsp/5g***	***5***	***0.2***	***102***	***4.4***	***10.5***	***5.0***	***2.5***
Cajun, Colman's*	1 Tsp/6g	11	0.4	187	7.0	23.0	6.5	2.7
Coarse Grain, Average	***1 Tsp/5g***	***7***	***0.4***	***141***	***7.7***	***8.4***	***8.3***	***5.9***
Dijon, Average	***1 Tsp/5g***	***8***	***0.6***	***163***	***7.4***	***7.7***	***11.3***	***1.1***
English, Average	***1 Tsp/5g***	***9***	***0.4***	***173***	***6.8***	***19.2***	***7.6***	***1.2***
English, with Chillies, Sainsbury's*	1 Tsp/5g	10	0.5	204	8.3	18.1	10.9	6.4
French, Average	***1 Tsp/5g***	***5***	***0.3***	***106***	***5.4***	***8.1***	***5.6***	***1.8***
German Style, Sainsbury's*	1 Serving/10g	9	0.6	92	5.5	2.8	6.5	0.0
Honey, Colman's*	1 Tsp/6g	12	0.5	208	7.4	24.0	8.2	0.0
Powder, Average	***1 Tsp/3g***	***15***	***0.9***	***452***	***28.9***	***20.7***	***28.7***	***0.0***
Powder, Made Up, Average	***1oz/28g***	***63***	***4.0***	***226***	***14.5***	***10.4***	***14.4***	***0.0***
Smooth, Average	***1 Tsp/8g***	***11***	***0.7***	***139***	***7.1***	***9.7***	***8.2***	***0.0***
Sweet Peppers, Colman's*	1 Tsp/6g	13	0.7	218	7.9	20.0	11.0	4.9
Whole Grain, Average	***1 Tsp/8g***	***11***	***0.8***	***140***	***8.2***	***4.2***	***10.2***	***4.9***
Whole Grain, with Green Peppercorns, Finest, Tesco*	1 Serving/20g	41	1.9	205	7.9	22.0	9.5	3.3
Yellow, Prepared	***1 Tbsp/15ml***	***11***	***0.6***	***73***	***4.0***	***6.0***	***4.0***	***0.0***
MUSTARD CRESS								
Raw	***1oz/28g***	***4***	***0.2***	***13***	***1.6***	***0.4***	***0.6***	***1.1***
MUTTON								
Lean, Raw, Average*	1 Serving/100g	236	13.4	236	17.9	0.1	13.4	0.0

	Measure INFO/WEIGHT	per Measure KCAL	FAT	Nutrition Values per 100g / 100ml KCAL	PROT	CARB	FAT	FIBRE
NACHOS								
American Chilli Beef, Asda*	1 Serving/200g	208	10.0	104	10.0	4.7	5.0	0.8
Cheesy with Salsa & Soured Cream, Sainsbury's*	½ Pack/170g	449	26.9	264	8.8	21.5	15.8	1.4
Chilli, Sainsbury's*	½ Pack/250g	695	32.2	278	10.9	29.5	12.9	1.3
Kit, Old El Paso*	½ Pack/260g	598	26.0	230	4.0	31.0	10.0	0.0
NASI GORENG								
Indonesian, Asda*	1 Pack/360g	778	22.7	216	7.4	32.3	6.3	1.3
Vitasia, Lidl*	1 Bowl/250g	438	11.0	175	7.3	25.8	4.4	1.1
NECTARINES								
Fresh, Raw, Weighed with Stone, Average	***1 Med/140g***	***53***	***0.1***	***38***	***1.3***	***8.5***	***0.1***	***1.2***
White Flesh, Love Life, Waitrose*	1 Fruit/130g	60	0.1	46	1.4	9.0	0.1	1.6
NESQUIK*								
Strawberry Milk, Fresh, Nesquik, Nestle*	1 Glass/250g	175	4.0	70	3.3	10.4	1.6	0.3
NIK NAKS								
Cream 'n' Cheesy, KP Snacks*	1 Bag/34g	196	13.0	575	5.2	52.7	38.1	0.2
Nice 'n' Spicy, KP Snacks*	1 Bag/30g	171	11.5	571	4.6	51.6	38.4	1.6
Rib 'n' Saucy, Golden Wonder*	1 Bag/25g	143	9.4	571	4.5	53.7	37.6	0.5
Scampi 'n' Lemon, KP Snacks*	1 Bag/25g	143	9.4	573	4.9	53.1	37.5	0.1
NOODLES								
Beef, Oriental, GFY, Asda*	1 Pack/400g	372	6.8	93	7.4	12.1	1.7	1.7
Beef, Shanghai, COU, M & S*	1 Pack/400g	380	6.4	95	6.8	13.1	1.6	1.5
Beef Flavour, Instant, Prepared, Heinz*	1 Pack/384g	257	0.4	67	2.1	14.4	0.1	0.6
Buckwheat, Cold, Famima*	1 Pack/295g	163	3.0	55	4.8	9.5	1.0	0.7
Cellophane, Glass, Dry Weight	1 Serving/100g	351	0.1	351	0.1	86.1	0.1	0.5
Char Sui, Cantonese, Sainsbury's*	1 Pack/450g	378	7.2	84	6.8	10.5	1.6	1.5
Chicken, & Coconut & Lime, Fuller Longer, M & S*	1 Pack/390g	448	17.6	115	8.7	10.0	4.5	1.6
Chicken, Chinese Style, GFY, Asda*	1 Pack/393g	295	6.7	75	6.0	9.0	1.7	0.6
Chicken, Dry Weight, Heinz*	1 Pack/85g	257	0.3	302	9.5	65.3	0.4	2.7
Chicken, Instant, Less Than 1% Fat, Prepared, Heinz*	1 Pack/385g	258	0.4	67	2.1	14.4	0.1	0.6
Chicken, Instant, Weight Watchers*	1 Pack/385g	270	0.4	70	2.3	14.9	0.1	0.6
Chicken Curry Flavour, Instant, Sainsbury's*	1 Pack/85g	167	6.2	196	4.6	27.9	7.3	0.8
Chicken Flavour, 3 Minute, Dry, Blue Dragon*	1 Pack/85g	403	18.2	475	9.3	61.2	21.4	0.0
Chicken Flavour, Dry, Princes*	1 Pack/85g	395	16.0	465	10.0	63.8	18.8	0.0
Chicken Flavour, Instant, Made Up, Tesco*	½ Pack/168g	285	10.6	170	4.1	23.7	6.3	1.5
Chicken Flavour, Instant, Sainsbury's*	1 Pack/335g	549	21.4	164	4.4	22.3	6.4	1.3
Chilli Beef, Finest, Tesco*	1 Pack/450g	486	8.6	108	7.7	15.2	1.9	0.9
Chilli Chicken, GFY, Asda*	1 Pack/415g	461	3.3	111	6.0	20.0	0.8	1.0
Chilli Chicken, Tesco*	1 Pack/385g	545	15.7	142	6.4	19.5	4.1	1.4
Chilli Infused, Blue Dragon*	1 Serving/150g	286	1.0	191	6.1	33.6	0.7	0.3
Chinese, Stir Fry, Sainsbury's*	1 Serving/100g	185	4.8	185	6.0	29.5	4.8	1.5
Chinese Pork, Chosen By You, Asda*	1 Pack/400g	380	6.4	95	6.7	12.6	1.6	1.8
Chow Mein, Dry Weight, Snack in a Pot, HL, Tesco*	1 Pot/56g	202	0.8	360	13.4	72.2	1.4	5.0
Chow Mein, Instant, Made Up, Tesco*	1 Pack/168g	255	8.4	152	3.8	23.0	5.0	1.2
Chow Mein, Sainsbury's*	1 Pack/125g	136	2.2	109	3.9	19.2	1.8	0.8
Chow Mein, Snack in a Pot, LC, Tesco*	1 Pot/235g	235	1.2	100	3.7	19.4	0.5	1.8
Chow Mein, Stir Fry, Tesco*	1 Serving/200g	116	2.4	58	2.1	9.7	1.2	1.0
Chow Mein Flavour, Dry, Princes*	1 Pack/85g	396	15.8	466	10.1	64.6	18.6	0.0
Crab Flavour, Dry, 3 Minute, Blue Dragon*	1 Pack/85g	393	16.3	463	9.9	62.6	19.2	0.0
Crispy, Dry, Blue Dragon*	1 Box/125g	438	0.6	350	2.4	84.0	0.5	0.0
Curry, Instant, Dry, Heinz*	1 Serving/85g	261	0.3	307	9.5	66.4	0.4	2.7
Curry, Mealpack, All About Weight*	1 Pack/37g	152	7.5	416	35.0	22.4	20.6	5.0
Curry Flavour, Instant, from Heinz, Weight Watchers*	1 Pack/385g	266	0.4	69	2.2	14.8	0.1	0.6
Curry Flavour, Instant, Sainsbury's*	1 Pack/335g	412	15.4	123	2.6	17.8	4.6	0.1
Egg, Boiled	***1oz/28g***	***17***	***0.1***	***62***	***2.2***	***13.0***	***0.5***	***0.6***

	Measure INFO/WEIGHT	per Measure KCAL	FAT	Nutrition Values per 100g / 100ml KCAL	PROT	CARB	FAT	FIBRE
NOODLES								
Egg, Dry, Average	***1 Block/63g***	***218***	***1.2***	***348***	***12.1***	***70.1***	***1.9***	***2.6***
Egg, Fine, Blue Dragon*	1 Serving/100g	356	1.7	356	13.8	70.0	1.7	3.4
Egg, Fine, Dry Weight, Sharwood's*	1 Block/63g	216	1.3	346	12.0	70.0	2.1	2.5
Egg, Fine, Fresh, M & S*	1 Pack/275g	330	6.0	120	4.4	20.7	2.2	1.5
Egg, Fine, Waitrose*	¼ Pack/63g	221	1.6	353	15.0	67.3	2.6	3.8
Egg, Fine Thread, Dry, M & S*	1 Serving/63g	220	0.6	350	14.3	71.6	0.9	5.1
Egg, Free Range, Asda*	1 Serving/125g	205	4.9	164	5.1	27.0	3.9	1.8
Egg, Free Range, Fresh, Sainsbury's*	½ Pack/205g	340	7.0	166	5.0	28.0	3.4	1.8
Egg, Fresh, Just Stir Fry, Sainsbury's*	½ Pack/192g	314	6.5	163	5.0	28.1	3.4	1.8
Egg, Fresh, Tesco*	½ Pack/205g	287	3.9	140	4.9	25.3	1.9	2.0
Egg, Medium, Dry, Blue Dragon*	1 Serving/50g	158	1.2	317	10.1	62.3	2.4	3.1
Egg, Medium, Dry, Sharwood's*	1 Serving/63g	216	1.3	346	12.0	70.0	2.1	2.5
Egg, Medium, Sainsbury's*	1 Serving/122g	168	1.0	138	5.7	26.9	0.8	1.0
Egg, Ramen, Fresh, The Original Noodle Company*	1 Serving/63g	186	1.7	298	11.3	57.0	2.7	0.0
Egg, Raw, Medium, Waitrose*	¼ Pack/63g	221	1.6	353	15.0	67.3	2.6	3.8
Egg, Thread, Cooked Weight, Sharwood's*	1oz/28g	30	0.2	107	3.6	21.8	0.6	1.1
Egg, Tossed in Sesame Oil, Asda*	½ Pack/150g	174	10.5	116	2.3	11.0	7.0	0.6
Egg & Bean Sprouts, Cooked, Tesco*	1 Pack/250g	238	5.2	95	4.4	14.6	2.1	1.5
Fried, Average	***1oz/28g***	***43***	***3.2***	***153***	***1.9***	***11.3***	***11.5***	***0.5***
Instant, Dry, Sainsbury's*	1 Pack/100g	392	14.0	392	9.4	57.0	14.0	0.2
Instant, Express, Dry, Blue Dragon*	1 Serving/75g	338	12.8	450	10.0	65.0	17.0	2.0
Instant, Fat Free, Koka*	1 Piece/80g	143	0.0	179	6.2	38.5	0.0	1.0
Instant, Value, Tesco*	1 Packet/265g	334	9.0	126	3.2	20.7	3.4	0.9
Japanese Udon, Sainsbury's*	1 Serving/150g	210	2.7	140	3.9	27.1	1.8	1.2
Nest, Medium, Cooked, Waitrose*	1 Nest/63g	88	0.3	139	5.0	28.6	0.5	0.6
Oriental, Chinese, Tesco*	1 Pack/200g	184	5.0	92	2.8	14.7	2.5	1.0
Oriental, Snack Pot, Dry, HL, Tesco*	1 Pot/57g	210	1.0	369	14.0	74.4	1.7	2.0
Oriental, Snack Pot, Made Up, HL, Tesco*	1 Serving/238g	221	0.7	93	3.1	19.4	0.3	0.6
Pad Thai, Ribbon, Ready to Wok, Sharwood's*	1 Serving/150g	206	1.6	137	5.0	26.3	1.1	1.0
Peking Duck, Shapers, Boots*	1 Pack/280g	395	3.9	141	7.2	25.0	1.4	1.8
Plain, Boiled	***1oz/28g***	***17***	***0.1***	***62***	***2.4***	***13.0***	***0.4***	***0.7***
Plain, Dry	***1oz/28g***	***109***	***1.7***	***388***	***11.7***	***76.1***	***6.2***	***2.9***
Prawn, Instant, Made Up, Tesco*	1 Serving/168g	251	8.7	150	3.8	21.9	5.2	1.3
Ramen, with Chilli Beef, M & S*	1 Pack/484g	532	17.4	110	8.1	11.9	3.6	0.8
Ramen, with Wakame, The Original Noodle Company*	½ Pack/124g	304	1.0	245	7.4	51.8	0.8	1.8
Ribbon, Thai Style, Ready to Wok, Sharwood's*	1 Pack/150g	206	1.6	137	5.0	26.3	1.1	1.0
Rice, Brown, 100%, Organic, King Soba*	1 Pack/83g	252	2.0	303	6.0	64.4	2.4	0.0
Rice, Cooked	1 Cup/176g	192	0.4	109	0.9	24.9	0.2	1.0
Rice, Cooked, Sharwood's*	1 Serving/200g	239	0.6	120	2.0	27.2	0.3	0.8
Rice, Dry, Amoy*	1oz/28g	101	0.3	361	6.5	86.6	1.0	0.0
Rice, Dry, Blue Dragon*	1 Serving/30g	113	0.0	376	7.0	84.0	0.0	0.0
Rice, Medium, Blue Dragon*	1 Serving/63g	235	0.0	376	7.0	84.0	0.0	0.0
Rice, Oriental, Thai, Stir Fry, Dry Weight, Sharwood's*	1 Serving/63g	226	0.6	361	6.5	86.8	1.0	2.4
Rice, Stir Fry, Tesco*	½ Pack/190g	304	10.8	160	2.0	24.8	5.7	1.0
Rice, Straight to Wok, Amoy*	1 Pack/150g	174	0.2	116	1.6	27.4	0.1	0.0
Rice, Thai, Wheat & GF, King Soba*	1 Serving/55g	193	0.8	351	8.9	75.6	1.4	0.0
Rice, Thick, Thai, Dry, M & S*	1 Serving/100g	355	0.7	355	6.5	80.6	0.7	1.4
Singapore, BGTY, Sainsbury's*	1 Pack/369g	317	10.0	86	7.2	8.2	2.7	2.1
Singapore, LC, Tesco*	1 Pack/450g	338	7.6	75	4.8	9.8	1.7	1.2
Singapore, Sainsbury's*	1 Pack/400g	432	15.6	108	6.5	11.7	3.9	2.8
Singapore, Straight to Wok, Amoy*	1 Serving/150g	232	4.2	155	4.8	28.4	2.8	0.0
Singapore, Waitrose*	1 Pack/400g	476	17.6	119	7.3	12.6	4.4	2.1
Singapore, You Count, Love Life, Waitrose*	1 Pot/260g	243	5.0	97	5.4	13.3	2.0	2.2

	Measure INFO/WEIGHT	per Measure KCAL	FAT	Nutrition Values per 100g / 100ml KCAL	PROT	CARB	FAT	FIBRE
NOODLES								
Singapore Style, Asda*	1 Pack/400g	688	32.0	172	7.0	18.0	8.0	1.0
Spicy, Sainsbury's*	1 Serving/180g	182	8.3	101	10.4	4.5	4.6	0.9
Spicy Curry Flavour, Dry, Princes*	1 Pack/85g	395	16.0	465	9.6	64.1	18.8	0.0
Spicy Thai, Instant, Heinz*	1 Pack/385g	262	0.4	68	2.1	14.6	0.1	0.6
Stir Fry, Tesco*	1 Serving/150g	202	3.6	135	5.3	23.0	2.4	1.5
Straight to Wok, Medium, Amoy*	1 Pack/150g	240	2.2	160	5.8	31.7	1.5	0.0
Super, Bacon Flavour, Dry Weight, Batchelors*	1 Packet/100g	526	23.6	526	9.4	69.2	23.6	1.6
Super, Barbecue Beef, Made Up, Batchelors*	1 Serving/100g	156	6.7	156	3.2	20.9	6.7	1.1
Super, Chicken & Herb, Low Fat, Made Up, Batchelors*	1 Pack/170g	322	1.6	189	6.1	39.2	0.9	1.2
Super, Chicken Flavour, Dry Weight, Batchelors*	1 Serving/100g	449	19.2	449	8.7	60.3	19.2	2.5
Super, Chicken Flavour, Made Up, Batchelors*	1 Serving/150g	264	11.8	176	3.1	23.0	7.9	0.4
Super, Chow Mein Flavour, Made Up, Batchelors*	½ Pack/150g	262	11.8	175	3.0	23.0	7.9	0.4
Super, Mild Curry, Dry Weight, Batchelors*	½ Pack/50g	260	11.7	520	9.4	67.8	23.4	1.4
Super, Mild Curry Flavour, Made Up, Batchelors*	1 Serving/100g	157	6.7	157	3.2	20.9	6.7	1.0
Super, Mushroom Flavour, Made Up, Batchelors*	1 Serving/100g	157	6.8	157	3.2	20.9	6.8	1.0
Super, Roast Chicken, to Go, 98% Fat Free, Batchelors*	1 Serving/380g	308	0.8	81	2.6	17.2	0.2	0.5
Super, Southern Fried Chicken, Made Up, Batchelors*	1 Serving/100g	171	7.2	171	3.3	23.2	7.2	0.5
Super, Spicy Salsa, Dry Weight, Batchelors*	1 Pack/105g	474	19.5	451	7.0	63.8	18.6	1.7
Super, Sweet Thai Chilli, Dry Weight, Batchelors*	1 Pack/85g	292	1.0	343	10.6	72.5	1.2	3.0
Sweet & Sour, BGTY, Sainsbury's*	1 Serving/100g	112	3.1	112	2.3	18.6	3.1	0.0
Sweet Chilli, Sainsbury's*	½ Pack/110g	172	6.0	156	4.0	24.6	5.5	1.0
Sweet Chilli, Wok, Findus*	1 Pack/300g	300	1.5	100	3.0	20.0	0.5	0.0
Szechuan Beef Flavour, Dry, Blue Dragon*	½ Pack/100g	350	1.2	350	10.5	72.3	1.2	0.0
Thai, Spicy, Stir Fry, HL, Tesco*	½ Pack/250g	220	5.5	88	4.1	12.9	2.2	1.7
Thai, Waitrose*	1 Pack/300g	357	6.3	119	6.8	18.4	2.1	1.7
Thai Glass, Vermicelli, Wai Wai*	1oz/28g	112	0.3	400	7.3	89.1	0.9	1.8
Thai Style, Asda*	1 Pot/238g	226	0.7	95	3.0	20.0	0.3	0.8
Thai Style, Sainsbury's*	1 Pack/340g	381	7.8	112	3.3	19.4	2.3	0.7
Thread, Fine, Straight to Wok, Amoy*	1 Pack/150g	237	3.9	158	5.0	28.7	2.6	0.0
Tiger Prawn, Stir Fry, Tesco*	1 Pack/400g	596	14.8	149	6.0	23.0	3.7	2.7
Traditional, Medium, Straight to Wok, Amoy*	1 Serving/150g	243	2.2	162	4.3	34.3	1.5	1.3
Udon, Straight to Wok, Amoy*	1 Pack/150g	212	2.0	141	4.4	28.8	1.3	0.0
Vegetable, Savoury, COU, M & S*	1 Pack/450g	270	2.7	60	2.9	11.5	0.6	1.2
Vermicelli Rice, Mama*	1 Serving/45g	166	0.4	370	7.0	81.0	1.0	0.0
Whole Wheat, Add to Wok, Chef Kuo*	1 Serving/150g	236	0.6	157	4.6	28.6	0.4	2.6
Whole Wheat, Dry, Blue Dragon*	1 Serving/65g	208	1.3	320	12.5	63.0	2.0	8.0
Yaki Udan, Chicken & Prawn, M & S*	1 Pack/395g	434	14.2	110	8.1	11.9	3.6	0.8
Zero, Glow Nutrition Ltd*	1 Serving/100g	5	0.0	5	0.0	4.0	0.0	4.0
NOUGAT								
Almond & Cherry, M & S*	1 Sweet/7g	28	0.6	405	4.5	76.0	9.1	1.1
Average	1 Sm Bar/28g	108	2.4	384	4.4	77.3	8.5	0.9
Bassetts & Beyond, Cadbury*	1oz/28g	105	1.1	375	4.0	82.0	4.0	0.0
Raspberry & Orange Hazelnut, Thorntons*	1 Sweet/9g	39	1.8	433	4.8	60.0	20.0	2.2
Soft, Bar, Bassett's*	1 Bar/25g	94	1.0	375	4.0	82.0	4.0	0.0
NUT CLUSTERS								
Almond, Sweet Pecan & Peanut, Red Sky*	1 Serving/30g	182	13.9	607	17.9	32.1	46.4	7.1
Peanut, Red Sky*	1 Serving/30g	182	13.9	607	21.4	32.1	46.4	7.1
NUT ROAST								
Average	1 Serving/200g	704	51.4	352	13.3	18.3	25.7	4.2
Courgette & Spiced Tomato, Cauldron Foods*	1 Serving/100g	208	12.3	208	11.7	12.5	12.3	4.9
Leek, Cheese & Mushroom, Organic, Cauldron Foods*	½ Pack/143g	343	21.3	240	13.2	13.2	14.9	4.1
Lentil, Average	***1oz/28g***	***62***	***3.4***	***222***	***10.6***	***18.8***	***12.1***	***3.8***
Tomato & Courgette, Vegetarian, Organic, Waitrose*	½ Pack/142g	295	17.5	208	11.7	12.5	12.3	4.9

	Measure INFO/WEIGHT	per Measure KCAL	FAT	Nutrition Values per 100g / 100ml KCAL	PROT	CARB	FAT	FIBRE
NUTMEG								
Ground, Average	***1 Tsp/3g***	***16***	***1.1***	***525***	***5.8***	***45.3***	***36.3***	***0.0***
NUTS								
Almonds, Whole, Sainsbury's*	1 Serving/10g	59	4.9	588	25.8	10.2	49.3	8.5
Assortment, Eat Well, M & S*	1 Pack/70g	441	41.2	630	16.7	8.5	58.9	5.3
Bento Box, Mix, Graze*	1 Portion/30g	141	6.6	469	17.9	50.1	22.1	3.7
Fire, Graze*	1 Pack/40g	220	16.3	549	17.9	28.4	40.7	7.1
Honey Roasted, M & S*	1oz/28g	175	14.6	625	18.1	20.5	52.2	5.1
Luxury, Organic, M & S*	1oz/28g	179	15.8	640	21.1	11.6	56.6	6.1
Mixed	1 Pack/40g	243	21.6	607	22.9	7.9	54.1	6.0
Mixed, Almonds, Brazil, Hazel & Walnuts, M & S*	1 Serving/25g	168	16.0	670	16.0	4.8	64.0	5.4
Mixed, Americas, Graze*	1 Punnet/40g	263	25.6	658	15.5	5.2	64.0	5.6
Mixed, America's, Graze*	1 Punnet/40g	263	25.3	657	16.3	6.2	63.2	6.0
Mixed, Ancient Forest, Graze*	1 Pack/36g	229	21.9	636	17.4	8.3	60.7	7.0
Mixed, Black Forest, Graze*	1 Pack/55g	258	13.8	470	6.6	54.4	25.1	0.0
Mixed, Chocolate Orange Granola, Graze*	1 Punnet/41g	195	11.3	475	12.0	43.7	27.5	7.7
Mixed, Chopped, Julian Graves*	1 Pack/300g	1773	152.7	591	23.2	10.0	50.9	0.0
Mixed, Chopped, Sainsbury's*	1 Serving/100g	605	50.9	605	27.1	9.6	50.9	6.0
Mixed, Chopped, Tesco*	1 Serving/25g	149	12.6	595	23.5	10.5	50.6	6.0
Mixed, Cookies & Cream, Graze*	1 Punnet/38g	214	16.0	562	12.0	36.0	42.0	5.0
Mixed, Honey Monster, Graze*	1 Med Pack/50g	280	20.4	559	10.8	45.2	40.8	0.0
Mixed, Honey Roasted, Waitrose*	1 Serving/50g	292	22.5	583	17.1	27.5	45.0	5.3
Mixed, Island, Graze*	1 Pack/55g	354	33.0	643	15.1	10.5	60.0	0.0
Mixed, Natural, Asda*	1 Snack/30g	197	18.8	656	18.0	4.3	62.7	7.4
Mixed, Natural, Love Life, Waitrose*	1 Serving/50g	314	25.8	628	17.4	24.9	51.6	12.1
Mixed, Natural, Luxury, Tesco*	1oz/28g	179	16.2	639	22.6	6.9	57.9	5.6
Mixed, Natural Energy, Graze*	1 Punnet/36g	227	21.3	629	19.0	8.0	59.0	8.0
Mixed, Nature's Harvest*	1 Serving/25g	145	13.4	581	17.5	7.7	53.4	6.3
Mixed, Roasted, Salted, Waitrose*	1 Pack/200g	1252	116.8	626	13.7	11.3	58.4	4.4
Mixed, Roasted, Waitrose*	1 Serving/25g	166	16.0	662	15.2	6.2	64.0	8.2
Mixed, Sweet & Sour, Graze*	1 Pack/40g	222	17.4	556	19.1	23.7	43.4	0.0
Mixed, Unsalted, Sainsbury's*	1 Serving/50g	311	28.8	622	18.5	7.2	57.7	8.7
Mixed, Wholesome, Love Life, Waitrose*	1 Serving/30g	206	19.6	685	14.6	5.0	65.2	5.4
Oak Smoke Flavour Selection, Finest, Tesco*	1 Serving/25g	158	14.0	633	21.4	11.2	55.8	6.3
Peanuts, Roasted, Salted, Value, Tesco*	1/8 Pack/25g	151	12.4	604	25.5	13.8	49.6	6.8
Peanuts & Cashews, Honey Roast, Tesco*	1 Serving/25g	145	10.7	579	21.6	26.6	42.9	4.2
Pecan, Wholesome, Love Life, Waitrose*	1 Serving/30g	207	21.0	691	9.2	5.8	70.1	9.6
Pine, Tesco*	1 Pack/100g	699	68.6	699	16.5	4.0	68.6	1.9
Pine, Wholefoods, Tesco*	1 Serving/10g	69	6.9	690	14.0	4.0	68.6	1.9
Roast, Salted, Luxury, KP Snacks*	1oz/28g	181	16.1	646	21.9	10.1	57.6	5.9
Roasted, Salted, Assortment, Luxury, Tesco*	1 Serving/25g	161	14.5	643	21.1	9.4	57.9	8.1
Salted, Selection, Sainsbury's*	1 Serving/30g	190	17.1	634	20.6	9.7	56.9	8.2
Soya, Dry Roasted, The Food Doctor*	1 Serving/50g	203	10.7	406	37.5	15.9	21.4	16.1
Soya, Roast, Wholefoods, Tesco*	1/5 Pack/20g	80	3.8	400	38.0	19.1	19.0	13.4
Soya Beans, Roasted & Salted, Chinese Style, Tesco*	1 Serving/26g	100	5.0	385	46.1	6.9	19.2	21.8
Unsalted, Selection, Sainsbury's*	1 Serving/75g	491	48.0	655	14.7	5.0	64.0	6.7
Walnut Pieces, Morrisons*	7 Peices/6g	41	4.1	689	14.7	3.3	68.5	3.5
NUTS & RAISINS								
Mixed, Average	1 Serving/30g	144	10.2	481	14.1	31.5	34.1	4.5
Mixed, KP Snacks*	1 Serving/50g	273	20.2	546	21.4	24.4	40.3	5.2
Mixed, Nature's Harvest*	1 Serving/50g	232	16.8	463	12.4	32.9	33.7	3.4
Peanuts, Mixed, Average	1 Pack/40g	174	10.4	435	15.3	37.5	26.0	4.4
Yoghurt Coated, Waitrose*	1 Serving/50g	264	18.4	527	10.9	38.2	36.7	3.0

	Measure INFO/WEIGHT	per Measure KCAL	FAT	Nutrition Values per 100g / 100ml KCAL	PROT	CARB	FAT	FIBRE
OAT BAKES								
Cheese, Nairn's*	1 Bag/30g	130	4.7	432	15.0	57.4	15.8	1.3
Honey & Lemon, Graze*	1 Punnet/31g	124	3.0	400	6.1	70.0	9.8	4.9
Mediterranean Tomato & Herb, Nairn's*	1 Bag/30g	129	4.7	431	8.1	64.2	15.8	8.3
Sweet Chilli, Nairn's*	1 Bag/30g	128	4.0	426	8.1	68.4	13.3	7.2
OAT CAKES								
Bran, Paterson's*	1 Cake/13g	52	2.0	416	10.0	58.5	15.8	9.5
Cheese, Nairn's*	1 Cake/8g	39	2.3	471	13.2	43.3	27.2	6.8
Fine Milled, Nairn's*	1 Cake/8g	35	1.7	449	10.5	52.6	21.8	8.6
Herb & Pumpkin Seed, Nairn's*	1 Cake/10g	43	2.1	426	12.2	46.8	21.1	13.0
Highland, Organic, Sainsbury's*	1 Cake/13g	57	2.4	456	10.2	59.8	19.5	5.5
Highland, Walkers*	1 Cake/12g	54	2.5	451	10.3	56.0	20.6	6.7
Oatmeal, Rough, Nairn's*	1 Cake/11g	45	2.0	421	10.6	52.8	18.6	10.5
Oatmeal, Rough, Organic, Nairn's*	1 Cake/10g	43	1.7	418	10.2	57.7	16.3	7.5
Retail, Average	1 Cake/13g	57	2.4	441	10.0	63.0	18.3	0.0
Rough, Scottish, Sainsbury's*	1 Cake/11g	51	2.1	462	12.3	59.9	19.3	6.5
Rough, with Bran, Walkers*	1 Cake/13g	55	2.2	424	11.0	57.1	16.8	8.1
Rough, with Olive Oil, Paterson's*	1 Cake/13g	54	2.2	431	10.6	58.4	17.2	8.1
Scottish, Organic, Waitrose*	1 Cake/13g	58	2.5	447	11.2	57.0	19.4	6.6
Suncakes*	1 Serving/65g	164	1.9	252	10.8	44.6	2.9	7.7
Traditional, M & S*	1 Cake/11g	49	2.0	445	11.0	59.3	18.3	6.6
OAT DRINK								
Healthy, Enriched, Oatly*	1 Serving/250ml	112	3.8	45	1.0	6.5	1.5	0.8
Oat Milk, Organic, Healthy, Oatly*	1 Serving/250ml	88	1.8	35	1.0	6.5	0.7	0.8
OATMEAL								
Raw	***1oz/28g***	***112***	***2.4***	***401***	***12.4***	***72.8***	***8.7***	***6.8***
OCTOPUS								
Chunks in Olive Oil, Palacio De Oriente*	1 Tin/111g	148	4.0	133	21.6	4.5	3.6	0.0
Raw	***1oz/28g***	***23***	***0.4***	***83***	***17.9***	***0.0***	***1.3***	***0.0***
OIL								
Avocado, Olivado*	1 Tsp/5ml	40	4.4	802	0.0	0.0	88.0	0.0
Butter, Cooking Mist, Spray, Cook's Range, Lurpak*	1 Spray/0.2ml	2	0.2	792	0.3	0.2	87.9	0.0
Chilli, Average	***1 Tsp/5ml***	***41***	***4.6***	***824***	***0.0***	***0.0***	***91.5***	***0.0***
Coconut, Average	***1 Tsp/5ml***	***45***	***5.0***	***899***	***0.0***	***0.0***	***99.9***	***0.0***
Cod Liver, Average	***1 Capsule/1g***	***9***	***1.0***	***900***	***0.0***	***0.0***	***100.0***	***0.0***
Corn, Average	***1 Tsp/5ml***	***43***	***4.8***	***864***	***0.0***	***0.0***	***96.0***	***0.0***
Cuisine, Flora*	1 Tsp/5ml	32	3.5	630	0.1	1.0	70.3	0.0
Dipping, Herb, Italian Style, Finest, Tesco*	1 Serving/5g	44	4.8	877	0.4	0.9	96.9	0.4
Evening Primrose, Average	***1 Serving/1g***	***9***	***1.0***	***900***	***0.0***	***0.0***	***100.0***	***0.0***
Fish, Average	***1 Serving/1g***	***9***	***1.0***	***900***	***0.0***	***0.0***	***100.0***	***0.0***
Flax Seed, Average	***1 Tbsp/15ml***	***124***	***13.9***	***829***	***0.0***	***0.0***	***92.6***	***0.0***
Fry Light, Bodyline*	1 Spray/0.25ml	1	0.1	522	0.0	0.0	55.2	0.0
Grapeseed, Average	***1 Tsp/5ml***	***43***	***4.8***	***866***	***0.0***	***0.0***	***96.2***	***0.0***
Groundnut, Average	***1 Tsp/5ml***	***41***	***4.6***	***824***	***0.0***	***0.0***	***91.8***	***0.0***
Hazelnut, Average	***1 Tsp/5ml***	***45***	***5.0***	***899***	***0.0***	***0.0***	***99.9***	***0.0***
Linseed, Organic, Biona*	1 Serving/10ml	84	9.3	837	0.0	0.0	93.0	0.0
Macadamia Nut, Oz Tukka*	1 Tsp/5ml	40	4.6	805	0.0	0.0	91.0	0.0
Olive, Average	***1 Tsp/5ml***	***43***	***4.7***	***855***	***0.0***	***0.0***	***94.9***	***0.0***
Olive, Basil Infused, Tesco*	1 Serving/20ml	180	20.0	900	0.0	0.0	100.0	0.0
Olive, Extra Virgin, Average	***1 Tsp/5ml***	***42***	***4.7***	***848***	***0.0***	***0.0***	***94.5***	***0.0***
Olive, Extra Virgin, Mist Spray, Belolive*	1 Serving/5ml	25	2.8	500	0.0	0.0	55.0	0.0
Olive, Extra Virgin, Only 1 Cal, Spray, Fry Light*	1 Spray/0.2ml	1	0.1	498	0.0	0.0	55.2	0.0
Olive, Garlic, Average	***1 Tbsp/15ml***	***127***	***14.1***	***848***	***0.0***	***0.0***	***94.3***	***0.0***
Olive, Lemon Flavoured, Sainsbury's*	1 Tbsp/15ml	123	13.7	823	0.1	0.0	91.4	0.1

	Measure INFO/WEIGHT	per Measure KCAL	FAT	Nutrition Values per 100g / 100ml KCAL	PROT	CARB	FAT	FIBRE
OIL								
Olive, Mild, Average	***1 Tbsp/15ml***	***129***	***14.4***	***862***	***0.0***	***0.0***	***95.7***	***0.0***
Olive, Spray, Fry Light*	5 Sprays/1ml	5	0.5	520	0.0	0.0	54.2	0.0
Palm, Average	***1 Tsp/5ml***	***45***	***5.0***	***899***	***0.0***	***0.0***	***99.9***	***0.0***
Palm, Red, & Canola, Carotino*	1 Tsp/5ml	41	4.6	812	0.0	0.0	92.0	0.0
Peanut, Average	***1 Tsp/5ml***	***45***	***5.0***	***899***	***0.0***	***0.0***	***99.9***	***0.0***
Rapeseed, Average	***1 Tbsp/15ml***	***130***	***14.4***	***864***	***0.0***	***0.0***	***96.0***	***0.0***
Rice Bran, Average	1 Tbsp/14g	120	13.6	884	0.0	0.0	100.0	0.0
Safflower, Average	***1 Tsp/5ml***	***45***	***5.0***	***899***	***0.0***	***0.0***	***99.9***	***0.0***
Sesame, Average	***1 Tsp/5ml***	***45***	***5.0***	***892***	***0.1***	***0.0***	***99.9***	***0.0***
Soya, Average	***1 Tsp/5ml***	***45***	***5.0***	***899***	***0.0***	***0.0***	***99.9***	***0.0***
Stir Fry, Sharwood's*	1 fl oz/30ml	269	29.9	897	0.0	0.0	99.7	0.0
Sunflower, Average	***1 Tsp/5ml***	***43***	***4.8***	***869***	***0.0***	***0.0***	***96.6***	***0.0***
Sunflower, Cooking Spray, LC Spray*	1 Spray/10ml	21	2.2	210	0.0	0.0	22.0	0.0
Sunflower, Spray, Fry Light*	1 Spray/0.2ml	1	0.1	522	0.0	0.0	55.2	0.0
Truffle, Black, Grapeseed, Cuisine Perel*	1 Tsp/5ml	43	5.0	857	0.0	7.1	100.0	0.0
Ultimate Blend, Udo's Choice*	1 Capsule/1ml	9	1.0	900	1.3	0.0	96.8	0.0
Vegetable, Average	***1 Tbsp/15ml***	***129***	***14.3***	***858***	***0.0***	***0.0***	***95.3***	***0.0***
Walnut, Average	***1 Tsp/5ml***	***45***	***5.0***	***899***	***0.0***	***0.0***	***99.9***	***0.0***
Wheatgerm, Average	***1 Tsp/5ml***	***45***	***5.0***	***899***	***0.0***	***0.0***	***99.9***	***0.0***
OKRA								
Boiled in Unsalted Water, Average	***1 Serving/80g***	***22***	***0.7***	***28***	***2.5***	***2.7***	***0.9***	***3.6***
Canned, Drained, Average	***1 Serving/80g***	***17***	***0.6***	***21***	***1.4***	***2.5***	***0.7***	***2.6***
Raw, Average	***1 Serving/80g***	***25***	***0.8***	***31***	***2.8***	***3.0***	***1.0***	***4.0***
Stir-Fried in Corn Oil, Average	***1 Serving/80g***	***215***	***20.9***	***269***	***4.3***	***4.4***	***26.1***	***6.3***
OLIVES								
Black, Pitted, Average	***½ Jar/82g***	***135***	***13.3***	***164***	***1.0***	***3.5***	***16.2***	***3.1***
Black & Green, with Greek Feta Cheese, Tesco*	1 Pot/100g	200	20.1	200	3.4	0.3	20.1	4.6
Green, Garlic Stuffed, Asda*	1 Olive/3g	6	0.6	174	1.8	3.5	17.0	0.0
Green, Pitted, Average	***1 Olive/3g***	***4***	***0.4***	***130***	***1.1***	***0.9***	***13.3***	***2.5***
Green, Pitted, Stuffed with Anchovies, Sainsbury's*	1 Serving/50g	78	8.0	155	1.8	0.6	16.1	3.2
Green, Stuffed with Almonds, Pitted, Waitrose*	1 Serving/50g	90	8.4	180	3.8	3.2	16.9	2.5
Green, with Chilli & Garlic, Graze*	1 Punnet/44g	133	13.6	301	0.6	1.4	30.9	2.9
Green, with Lemon & Garlic, Lightly Flavoured, Attis*	1 Serving/50g	82	8.2	164	1.7	2.2	16.5	0.0
Kalamata, Kalamata*	***1 Olive/3g***	***9***	***0.9***	***300***	***1.0***	***6.7***	***30.0***	***0.0***
Kalamata, with Herbs, Graze*	1 Punnet/52g	144	15.3	277	0.6	1.7	29.4	3.1
Marinated, Mixed, M & S*	1 Serving/20g	33	3.0	165	1.6	6.5	14.9	3.0
Marinated, Selection, M & S*	4 Olives/20g	44	4.4	225	1.4	3.9	22.6	2.1
Mixed, Chilli & Garlic, Asda*	1 Serving/30g	43	4.7	144	0.9	0.0	15.6	6.1
Mixed, Marinated, Anti Pasti, Asda*	1 Serving/100g	215	22.0	215	1.8	0.7	22.0	3.1
Mixed, Marinated with Feta & Red Peppers, Asda*	1 Pot/120g	233	21.6	194	5.8	2.2	18.0	1.7
Pimento Stuffed, in Brine, Tesco*	1 Serving/25g	38	4.1	153	0.8	0.1	16.4	2.1
OMELETTE								
Cheese, 2 Egg, Average	1 Omelette/180g	479	40.7	266	15.9	0.0	22.6	0.0
Cheese, Asda*	1 Omelette/119g	268	22.6	225	12.0	1.5	19.0	0.0
Cheese, Findus*	1 Serving/200g	400	26.0	200	9.5	14.0	13.0	0.0
Cheese & Mushroom, Apetito*	1 Serving/320g	486	25.0	152	6.2	14.4	7.8	1.9
Ham & Mushroom, Farmfoods*	1 Omelette/120g	200	16.7	167	8.7	1.8	13.9	0.1
Plain, 2 Egg	1 Omelette/120g	229	19.7	191	10.9	0.0	16.4	0.0
Spanish	1oz/28g	34	2.3	120	5.7	6.2	8.3	1.4
Spanish, Potato, Rapido, Unearthed*	1 Pack/175g	273	13.6	156	4.6	15.8	7.8	2.2
ONION POWDER								
	1 Tsp/2g	7	0.0	341	10.4	79.1	1.0	15.2

	Measure INFO/WEIGHT	per Measure KCAL	FAT	Nutrition Values per 100g / 100ml KCAL	PROT	CARB	FAT	FIBRE
ONION RINGS								
Battered, Asda*	1 Serving/100g	343	22.7	343	3.8	31.0	22.7	1.7
Battered, Oven Baked, Tesco*	1 Serving/50g	110	5.0	219	3.9	28.4	10.0	3.5
Battered, Sainsbury's*	1 Ring/12g	26	1.2	219	3.9	28.4	10.0	3.5
Breadcrumbs, Tesco*	1 Serving/100g	294	15.6	294	4.3	34.1	15.6	2.3
Breaded, Asda*	1 Serving/10g	29	1.5	289	4.4	34.0	15.0	2.7
ONIONS								
Baked	***1oz/28g***	***29***	***0.2***	***103***	***3.5***	***22.3***	***0.6***	***3.9***
Boiled in Unsalted Water	***1oz/28g***	***5***	***0.0***	***17***	***0.6***	***3.7***	***0.1***	***0.7***
Borettane, Char-Grilled, Sacla*	1 Serving/100g	90	5.6	90	0.9	8.9	5.6	2.5
Brown, Value, Tesco*	1 Onion/100g	36	0.2	36	1.3	7.8	0.2	1.8
Dried, Raw, Average	***1oz/28g***	***88***	***0.5***	***313***	***10.2***	***68.6***	***1.7***	***12.1***
Fried, Average	***1oz/28g***	***46***	***3.1***	***164***	***2.3***	***14.1***	***11.2***	***3.1***
Pickled, Average	***1 Onion/15g***	***3***	***0.0***	***23***	***0.8***	***4.9***	***0.1***	***0.7***
Raw, Average	***1 Med/180g***	***69***	***0.4***	***38***	***1.2***	***7.9***	***0.2***	***1.3***
Red, Raw, Average	***1 Med/180g***	***66***	***0.4***	***37***	***1.2***	***7.9***	***0.2***	***1.5***
Sliced, Frozen, Farmfoods*	1 Serving/80g	29	0.2	36	1.2	7.9	0.2	1.4
Spring, Raw, Average	***1 Med/15g***	***4***	***0.1***	***25***	***2.0***	***3.0***	***0.5***	***1.5***
OPTIONS								
Choca Mocha Drink, Ovaltine*	1 Sachet/11g	39	1.3	359	14.1	50.1	11.4	7.0
Chocolate Au Lait, Ovaltine*	1 Sachet/10g	36	1.0	355	11.8	54.5	10.0	7.3
Coffee, Dreamy Cappuccion, Cafe, Ovaltine*	1 Sachet/25g	64	4.2	256	12.9	58.1	16.9	0.0
Dreamy Caramel, Hot Chocolate, Ovaltine*	1 Sachet/11g	39	0.9	354	12.3	48.5	7.8	0.0
Irish Cream, Ovaltine*	1 Sachet/11g	39	1.2	357	13.9	50.0	11.3	8.1
Mint Madness, Belgian, Ovaltine*	1 Sachet/11g	38	0.8	348	12.3	49.2	6.9	20.0
Outrageous Orange, Hot Chocolate, Ovaltine*	1 Sachet/11g	38	0.8	348	12.3	49.3	6.9	20.0
Tempting Toffee, Ovaltine*	1 Sachet/11g	43	1.0	391	13.6	66.4	9.1	0.0
Wicked White, Hot Chocolate, Ovaltine*	1 Sachet/11g	44	1.1	398	10.5	64.6	10.0	3.7
ORANGE CURD								
Baxters*	1 Tbsp/15g	51	1.1	343	2.0	67.0	7.4	0.1
Florida, Finest, Tesco*	1 Tbsp/15g	52	1.3	348	2.9	63.8	9.0	0.2
Jaffa, Luxury, Waitrose*	1 Tbsp/15g	54	1.5	357	3.0	63.5	10.1	0.1
Sainsbury's*	2 Tsps/12g	34	0.5	282	1.1	59.2	4.4	0.4
ORANGES								
Blood, Average	***1 Orange/140g***	***82***	***0.0***	***58***	***0.8***	***13.3***	***0.0***	***2.5***
Fresh, Weighed with Peel, Average	***1oz/28g***	***10***	***0.0***	***37***	***1.1***	***8.5***	***0.1***	***1.7***
Fresh, without Peel, Average	***1 Med/145g***	***54***	***0.1***	***37***	***1.1***	***8.5***	***0.1***	***1.7***
Peel Only, Raw, Average	***1 Tbsp/6g***	***6***	***0.0***	***97***	***1.5***	***25.0***	***0.2***	***10.6***
Ruby Red, Tesco*	1 Med/130g	51	0.1	39	1.1	8.5	0.1	1.7
OREGANO								
Dried,	***1 Tsp/1g***	***3***	***0.1***	***306***	***11.0***	***49.5***	***10.3***	***0.0***
Fresh	***1 Tsp/1g***	***1***	***0.0***	***66***	***2.2***	***9.7***	***2.0***	***0.0***
OVALTINE*								
Chocolate, Light, Ovaltine*	4 Tsps/20g	76	1.2	380	8.5	70.5	6.0	4.5
Chocolate, Light, Sachet, Ovaltine*	1 Sachet/25g	96	1.5	384	7.4	73.0	5.9	4.7
Hi Malt, Light, Instant Drink, Ovaltine*	1 Sachet/20g	72	1.2	358	9.1	67.1	5.9	2.8
Powder, Made Up with Semi-Skimmed Milk, Ovaltine*	1 Mug/227ml	179	3.9	79	3.9	13.0	1.7	0.0
Powder, Made Up with Whole Milk, Ovaltine*	1 Mug/227ml	220	8.6	97	3.8	12.9	3.8	0.0
OXTAIL								
Raw	***1oz/28g***	***48***	***2.8***	***171***	***20.0***	***0.0***	***10.1***	***0.0***
Stewed, Bone Removed	***1oz/28g***	***68***	***3.8***	***243***	***30.5***	***0.0***	***13.4***	***0.0***
OYSTERS								
in Vegetable Oil, Smoked, John West*	1oz/28g	64	3.9	230	16.0	10.0	14.0	0.0
Raw, Shelled, Shucked	***1 Oyster/14g***	***9***	***0.2***	***65***	***10.8***	***2.7***	***1.3***	***0.0***

	Measure INFO/WEIGHT	per Measure KCAL	FAT	Nutrition Values per 100g / 100ml KCAL	PROT	CARB	FAT	FIBRE
PAELLA								
Bistro, Waitrose*	1 Serving/300g	534	19.8	178	7.4	22.2	6.6	0.7
Chicken, & Chorizo, Asda*	1 Pack/390g	484	8.6	124	10.0	16.0	2.2	2.6
Chicken, & Chorizo, Big Dish, M & S*	1 Pack/450g	630	17.6	140	7.9	18.4	3.9	1.6
Chicken, & Chorizo, LowLow*	1 Pack/320g	333	3.8	104	5.6	17.1	1.2	1.2
Chicken, & King Prawn, BGTY, Sainsbury's*	1 Pack/400g	336	5.2	84	5.4	11.8	1.3	1.9
Chicken, & Prawn, Asda*	1 Pack/400g	352	4.4	88	5.8	13.7	1.1	1.4
Chicken, & Prawn, HL, Tesco*	1 Pack/380g	370	6.9	97	6.5	13.0	1.8	1.8
Chicken, & Vegetable, HL, Tesco*	1 Pack/450g	441	5.8	98	9.7	11.8	1.3	1.1
Chicken, King Prawns, British, Sainsbury's*	1 Pack/400g	380	4.8	95	7.6	13.3	1.2	0.9
Chicken, King Prawns & Chorizo, Fuller Longer, M & S*	1 Pack/390g	410	11.3	105	9.8	10.1	2.9	1.6
Chicken, Tesco*	1 Serving/475g	575	14.2	121	7.9	15.7	3.0	1.6
Diet Chef Ltd*	1 Packet/250g	355	3.0	142	11.2	21.7	1.2	0.4
Seafood, COU, M & S*	1 Pack/400g	400	7.2	100	6.2	13.8	1.8	1.4
Seafood, Espana, M & S*	1 Bowl/380g	565	12.1	150	5.5	25.2	3.2	0.5
Seafood, Finest, Tesco*	1 Pack/400g	756	23.6	189	6.8	27.2	5.9	1.0
Seafood, M & S*	1 Pack/450g	518	17.1	115	6.4	13.7	3.8	3.2
Seafood, Sainsbury's*	1 Pack/400g	504	5.2	126	8.3	20.3	1.3	0.6
Vegetable, Espana, M & S*	1 Pack/375g	505	13.5	135	2.8	22.4	3.6	1.3
Vegetable, Love Life, Waitrose*	1 Pack/400g	344	12.4	86	1.6	12.9	3.1	1.7
Vegetable, Lovely Vegetables, M & S*	1 Pack/430g	387	13.8	90	2.2	13.7	3.2	1.7
Vegetable, Waitrose*	1 Serving/174g	202	3.1	116	2.2	22.7	1.8	1.5
PAIN AU CHOCOLAT								
Average	1 Serving/60g	253	13.7	422	8.0	45.8	22.8	3.1
Chocolate Filled, Chosen By You, Asda*	1 Pain/45g	198	11.3	441	7.1	44.9	25.2	2.9
Mini, Asda*	1 Pastry/23g	96	5.5	420	8.0	43.0	24.0	3.3
Mini, Cafe Simple*	1 Pastry/27g	122	7.2	452	10.2	42.8	26.7	2.5
PAIN AU RAISIN								
Takeaway, Average	1 Pastry/100g	313	13.2	313	5.2	43.0	13.2	1.3
Twist, Extra Special, Asda*	1 Pastry/110g	421	20.9	383	7.0	46.0	19.0	2.5
PAK CHOI								
Raw, Average	***1 Leaf/14g***	***2***	***0.0***	***13***	***1.5***	***2.2***	***0.2***	***1.0***
PAKORA								
Bhaji, Onion, Fried in Vegetable Oil	1oz/28g	76	4.1	271	9.8	26.2	14.7	5.5
Bhajia, Potato Carrot & Pea, Fried in Vegetable Oil	1oz/28g	100	6.3	357	10.9	28.8	22.6	6.1
Bhajia, Vegetable, Retail	1oz/28g	66	4.1	235	6.4	21.4	14.7	3.6
Chicken, Tikka, Asda*	1 Pack/350g	696	38.5	199	16.0	9.0	11.0	1.1
Potato & Spinach, Waitrose*	1 Pakora/50g	120	8.2	240	5.5	17.3	16.5	4.7
Prawn, Indian Appetisers, Waitrose*	1 Pakora/21g	35	1.7	165	16.8	5.9	8.2	1.5
Sainsbury's*	1 Pakora/55g	166	10.1	302	7.3	26.8	18.3	1.1
Spinach, Sainsbury's*	1 Pakora/18g	35	1.9	195	5.1	19.4	10.8	3.8
Vegetable, Indian Selection, Party, Co-Op*	1 Pakora/23g	47	1.6	205	6.0	28.0	7.0	4.0
Vegetable, Indian Starter Selection, M & S*	1 Pakora/23g	61	4.2	265	6.3	19.6	18.1	2.9
Vegetable, Mini, Indian Snack Collection, Tesco*	1 Pakora/21g	36	1.9	173	6.0	16.8	9.1	4.9
PANCAKE								
Apple, GFY, Asda*	1 Pancake/74g	100	1.8	135	4.2	24.0	2.5	1.0
Apple & Sultana, M & S*	1 Serving/80g	160	6.3	200	2.2	30.2	7.9	1.2
Asda*	1 Pancake/23g	59	1.6	254	4.8	43.0	7.0	4.0
Big, Crafty, Genesis*	1 Pancake/71g	171	3.7	241	6.2	42.3	5.2	2.1
Blueberry, Tesco*	1 Pancake/75g	195	3.1	260	4.8	49.5	4.1	2.0
Cherry, GFY, Asda*	1 Serving/206g	206	3.8	100	1.9	18.9	1.8	1.8
Chinese Roll, Farmfoods*	1 Pancake/88g	125	3.8	142	4.3	21.6	4.3	1.0
Chinese Style, Cherry Valley*	1 Pancake/8g	25	0.5	310	9.2	54.7	6.0	0.0
Chocolate, M & S*	1 Pancake/80g	125	4.9	156	3.1	22.1	6.1	0.2

	Measure INFO/WEIGHT	per Measure KCAL	FAT	Nutrition Values per 100g / 100ml KCAL	PROT	CARB	FAT	FIBRE
PANCAKE								
for Duck, Sainsbury's*	1 Pancake/10g	33	0.9	333	10.9	51.7	9.3	2.4
Golden Syrup, Warburton's*	1 Pancake/26g	65	1.6	250	6.3	40.7	6.3	2.4
HL, Tesco*	1 Pancake/25g	60	0.5	240	5.8	48.8	2.0	1.9
Irish, Rankin Selection, Irwin's Bakery*	1 Pancake/40g	101	1.3	252	6.2	49.2	3.2	2.5
LC, Tesco*	1 Pancake/27g	66	0.7	243	6.9	47.7	2.6	0.0
Lemon, M & S*	1 Pancake/38g	90	2.8	235	4.5	38.5	7.2	2.8
Lemon & Raisin, Genius*	1 Pancake/56g	130	1.8	232	5.8	44.8	3.3	3.1
M & S*	1 Pancake/62g	170	7.7	275	5.7	33.9	12.5	1.5
Maple & Raisin, M & S*	1 Pancake/35g	102	2.4	290	5.6	50.4	6.9	2.2
Mini, Scotch, Tesco*	1 Pancake/16g	44	0.9	277	6.7	50.0	5.6	1.4
Morello Cherry, Iceland*	1 Pancake/129g	204	3.7	158	3.1	29.8	2.9	2.9
North Staffordshire Oatcakes Ltd*	1 Pancake/71g	166	4.3	234	5.0	40.9	6.1	1.0
Perfect, Kingsmill*	1 Pancake/27g	71	1.2	264	6.2	49.7	4.5	1.2
Plain, Sainsbury's*	1 Pancake/46g	102	2.4	221	6.9	36.1	5.3	1.2
Pockets, Strawberry, Kingsmill*	1 Pancake/44g	112	1.6	254	4.3	50.5	3.6	1.3
Raisin & Lemon, Asda*	1 Serving/30g	92	2.4	304	6.0	52.0	8.0	1.4
Raisin & Lemon, Sainsbury's*	1 Pancake/35g	95	1.5	272	6.3	51.8	4.4	2.2
Ready Made, Average	1 Small/30g	77	1.9	258	6.1	44.2	6.4	1.7
Savoury, Made with Skimmed Milk, Average	1 6"/77g	192	11.3	249	6.4	24.1	14.7	0.8
Savoury, Made with Whole Milk, Average	1 6"/77g	210	13.5	273	6.3	24.0	17.5	0.8
Scotch	1 Pancake/50g	146	5.8	292	5.8	43.6	11.7	1.4
Scotch, BGTY, Sainsbury's*	1 Pancake/30g	76	1.2	252	5.3	48.5	4.1	1.3
Scotch, Hovis*	1 Pancake/30g	88	2.5	295	5.5	48.1	8.4	2.3
Scotch, Low Fat, Asda*	1 Pancake/32g	87	0.7	272	6.0	57.0	2.2	1.3
Sultana & Syrup, Asda*	1 Pancake/34g	89	2.4	263	5.9	43.7	7.2	1.5
Sweet, Made with Skimmed Milk	1oz/28g	78	3.9	280	6.0	35.1	13.8	0.8
Sweet, Made with Whole Milk	1oz/28g	84	4.5	301	5.9	35.0	16.2	0.8
Sweet, Raspberry Ripple Sauce, Findus*	1 Pancake/38g	80	1.8	210	3.9	37.1	4.7	0.9
Syrup, Tesco*	1 Pancake/30g	80	2.5	265	4.7	42.1	8.2	1.5
Traditional, Aunt Bessie's*	1 Pancake/60g	90	1.9	150	6.1	24.6	3.1	1.1
Traditional, Tesco*	1 Pancake/62g	137	3.1	221	8.4	35.6	5.0	1.5
with Golden Syrup, Value, Tesco*	1 Pancake/24g	61	1.5	255	5.1	44.1	6.3	1.9
with Maple Sauce & Fromage Frais, BGTY, Sainsbury's*	1 Serving/100g	163	2.5	163	5.0	30.0	2.5	0.8
with Syrup, American Style, Large, Tesco*	1 Pancake/38g	102	1.3	268	5.1	54.2	3.4	0.9
PANCAKE MIX								
4 Grain, Wheat & GF, Organic, Hale & Hearty*	½ Pack/180g	562	2.9	312	7.8	66.6	1.6	5.7
Fresh, M & S*	1 Pancake/38g	90	5.0	235	7.5	22.4	13.1	0.5
Glutano*	1 Tbsp/15g	57	0.3	378	8.9	75.6	2.2	0.0
Traditional, Asda*	1 Pack/256g	545	23.0	213	6.0	27.0	9.0	1.8
PANCETTA								
Average	***½ Pack/65g***	***212***	***18.7***	***326***	***17.0***	***0.1***	***28.7***	***0.0***
PANINI								
Bacon, British Midland*	1 Serving/150g	273	9.9	182	9.1	21.6	6.6	0.0
Cheese, Tesco*	1 Panini/100g	249	9.1	249	10.5	31.3	9.1	3.1
Chicken Arrabiata, Ginsters*	1 Panini/200g	489	16.8	245	12.8	29.4	8.4	2.4
Ham & Cheese, Ginsters*	1 Panini/200g	567	25.6	283	13.3	28.7	12.8	1.6
Mozzarella & Tomato, Ginsters*	1 Panini/207g	536	21.9	259	12.3	28.5	10.6	2.1
Tuna & Sweetcorn, Tesco*	1 Serving/250g	559	16.4	224	12.0	29.3	6.6	1.4
Tuna Melt, Ginsters*	1 Panini/210g	479	15.8	228	13.1	26.9	7.5	1.9
PANNA COTTA								
BGTY, Sainsbury's*	1 Pot/150g	150	2.8	100	2.4	18.2	1.9	1.4
Caramel, Sainsbury's*	1 Pot/120g	335	15.7	279	2.5	34.6	13.1	3.3
Sainsbury's*	1 Pot/100g	304	15.7	304	3.0	41.5	15.7	4.0

	Measure INFO/WEIGHT	per Measure KCAL	FAT	Nutrition Values per 100g / 100ml KCAL	PROT	CARB	FAT	FIBRE
PANNA COTTA								
Strawberry, COU, M & S*	1 Pot/145g	145	3.8	100	2.6	15.7	2.6	0.8
PAPAYA								
Dried, Pieces, Nature's Harvest*	1 Serving/50g	178	0.0	355	0.2	85.4	0.0	2.6
Dried, Strips, Tropical Wholefoods*	1 Strip/10g	31	0.1	310	3.9	71.4	0.9	1.5
Dried, Sweetened, Tesco*	4 Pieces/25g	59	0.2	235	0.4	56.3	0.9	2.9
Raw, Flesh Only, Average	***1 Serving/140g***	***37***	***0.1***	***26***	***0.4***	***6.6***	***0.1***	***1.2***
Raw, Unripe, Flesh Only	1 Serving/100g	27	0.1	27	0.9	5.5	0.1	1.0
Raw, Weighed with Seeds & Skin	***1 Serving/140g***	***55***	***0.2***	***39***	***0.6***	***9.8***	***0.1***	***1.8***
PAPPARDELLE								
Basil, Fresh, Sainsbury's*	1 Serving/240g	281	3.4	117	5.0	21.2	1.4	2.0
Buitoni*	1 Serving/65g	242	3.1	373	15.0	67.5	4.8	0.0
Chilli, Fresh, Sainsbury's*	1 Serving/250g	302	4.2	121	5.7	20.7	1.7	2.0
Egg, Dry, Average	***1 Serving/100g***	***364***	***3.7***	***364***	***14.1***	***68.5***	***3.7***	***2.1***
Egg, Fresh, Waitrose*	¼ Pack/125g	350	3.4	280	12.9	51.0	2.7	1.9
Egg & Spinach, Extra Special, Asda*	½ Pack/200g	328	3.6	164	6.5	30.5	1.8	1.4
Saffron, Eat Well, M & S*	1 Serving/100g	360	2.5	360	14.0	69.0	2.5	3.2
PAPRIKA								
Average	***1 Tsp/2g***	***6***	***0.3***	***289***	***14.8***	***34.9***	***13.0***	***0.0***
PARATHA								
Average	***1 Paratha/80g***	***258***	***11.4***	***322***	***8.0***	***43.2***	***14.3***	***4.0***
PARSLEY								
Dried	***1 Tsp/1g***	***2***	***0.1***	***181***	***15.8***	***14.5***	***7.0***	***26.9***
Fresh, Average	***1 Tbsp/4g***	***1***	***0.0***	***34***	***3.0***	***2.7***	***1.3***	***5.0***
PARSNIP								
Boiled, Average	***1 Serving/80g***	***53***	***1.0***	***66***	***1.6***	***12.9***	***1.2***	***4.7***
Honey Glazed, Roasting, Cooked, Betty Smith's*	1 Serving/80g	177	11.9	221	1.4	18.7	14.9	3.4
Honey Roasted, Tesco*	½ Pack/125g	165	6.6	130	1.3	16.7	5.2	5.2
Raw, Unprepared, Average	***1oz/28g***	***19***	***0.3***	***66***	***1.8***	***12.5***	***1.1***	***4.6***
Roast, Honey Glazed, Baked, Aunt Bessie's*	1 Serving/80g	177	11.9	221	1.4	18.7	14.9	3.4
PARTRIDGE								
Breast, Fillets, Raw, Skinned, Abel & Cole*	1 Serving/100g	145	4.7	145	25.8	0.0	4.7	0.0
Meat Only, Roasted	***1oz/28g***	***59***	***2.0***	***212***	***36.7***	***0.0***	***7.2***	***0.0***
PASANDA								
Chicken, Sainsbury's*	1 Serving/200g	368	24.8	184	14.7	3.4	12.4	2.3
Chicken, Waitrose*	1oz/28g	52	3.4	185	14.8	3.8	12.3	1.1
Chicken, with Pilau Rice, HL, Tesco*	1 Pack/440g	466	11.0	106	5.7	15.2	2.5	0.9
PASSATA								
Basil, Del Monte*	1 Jar/500g	160	1.0	32	1.4	5.9	0.2	0.0
Classic, Italian with Onion & Garlic, Sainsbury's*	1oz/28g	10	0.0	37	1.4	7.7	0.1	1.3
Napolina*	1 Bottle/690g	172	0.7	25	1.4	4.5	0.1	0.0
Smart Price, Asda*	1 Serving/100g	25	0.1	25	1.4	4.5	0.1	0.2
So Organic, Sainsbury's*	¼ Jar/175g	38	0.7	22	0.9	3.8	0.4	0.9
with Fresh Leaf Basil, Waitrose*	¼ Jar/170g	44	0.2	26	1.0	5.2	0.1	0.8
with Garlic & Italian Herbs, Tesco*	1 Serving/165g	53	0.3	32	1.2	6.4	0.2	1.1
PASSION FRUIT								
Raw, Fresh, Average	***1 Fruit/30g***	***11***	***0.1***	***36***	***2.6***	***5.8***	***0.4***	***3.3***
Weighed with Skin, Average	***1 Fruit/30g***	***11***	***0.1***	***36***	***2.6***	***5.8***	***0.4***	***3.3***
PASTA								
Basilico, Pasta King*	1 Serving/100g	123	3.3	123	3.8	19.5	3.3	2.1
Bean & Tuna, BGTY, Sainsbury's*	1 Serving/200g	176	1.8	88	7.3	12.6	0.9	2.8
Blue Cheese, Bacon & Spinach, M & S*	1 Pack/400g	640	34.0	160	6.5	13.8	8.5	0.7
Boccoletti, Dried, Sainsbury's*	1 Serving/90g	321	1.5	357	12.3	73.1	1.7	2.5
Bolognese, Diet Chef Ltd*	1 Pack/300g	255	10.2	85	7.9	5.8	3.4	4.4

	Measure INFO/WEIGHT	per Measure KCAL	FAT	Nutrition Values per 100g / 100ml KCAL	PROT	CARB	FAT	FIBRE
PASTA								
Bolognese, Pasta King*	1 Serving/100g	121	2.6	121	5.1	19.3	2.6	1.9
Bolognese, Vegetarian, Pasta King*	1 Serving/100g	117	2.1	117	4.9	19.7	2.1	1.9
Cappalletti, Meat, Sainsbury's*	1 Pack/420g	816	23.9	195	10.0	25.8	5.7	2.3
Carbonara, Pasta King*	1 Serving/100g	122	2.9	122	5.1	19.3	2.9	1.2
Carbonara, Pasta Vita, Dolmio*	1 Pot/300g	372	13.8	124	4.5	15.8	4.6	0.0
Carbonara, with Cheese & Bacon, Slim Fast*	1 Serving/70g	240	4.4	343	22.7	48.9	6.3	5.7
Cheddar, Country, Bowl, Haribo*	1 Serving/269g	400	19.0	149	5.6	15.2	7.1	1.5
Cheese, Creamy, Big Eat, Heinz*	1 Pot/350g	438	32.2	125	3.7	7.0	9.2	1.8
Cheese, Pasta King*	1 Serving/100g	117	2.3	117	5.0	19.2	2.3	1.1
Cheese, Tomato & Pesto, Boots*	1 Pack/250g	355	11.0	142	5.9	20.0	4.4	2.0
Cheese & Broccoli, LC, Tesco*	1 Pack/348g	435	8.0	125	4.4	21.2	2.3	2.4
Cheese & Broccoli, Tubes, Tesco*	1 Serving/202g	319	13.9	158	5.0	19.1	6.9	2.3
Cheese & Ham, Shapers, Boots*	1 Pack/76g	220	4.9	289	23.7	34.2	6.4	6.4
Cheese & Tortellini in Tomato Sauce, Heinz*	1 Pack/250g	229	7.6	92	2.2	13.7	3.0	0.2
Cheesy Spirals, Curly Whirly, Asda*	1/3 Pack/200g	214	5.2	107	6.0	15.0	2.6	0.5
Cheesy Tubes, Pot, Goodness for Kids, Tesco*	1 Pot/200g	240	5.6	120	4.7	18.6	2.8	1.3
Chicken, Chargrilled, & Bacon, Tesco*	1 Pack/200g	420	23.6	210	6.7	18.8	11.8	1.3
Chicken, Chargrilled, Asda*	1 Serving/250g	538	27.5	215	7.0	22.0	11.0	1.7
Chicken, Sicilian, City Kitchen, Tesco*	1 Pack/385g	500	13.5	130	9.1	14.6	3.5	0.6
Chicken, Tomato & Basil, Asda*	1 Pack/400g	474	10.0	118	6.5	17.5	2.5	1.2
Chicken, Tomato & Basil, GFY, Asda*	1 Pack/400g	404	9.2	101	6.4	13.6	2.3	1.4
Chicken, Tomato & Herb, Easy Steam, Tesco*	1 Serving/400g	528	24.8	132	8.9	10.2	6.2	1.3
Chicken, Tomato & Mascarpone, Easy Steam, Tesco*	1 Pack/400g	468	16.4	117	9.7	10.3	4.1	0.9
Chicken, Tomato & Mascarpone, HL, Tesco*	1 Pack/450g	504	11.2	112	7.5	14.8	2.5	1.1
Chicken, Tomato & Mascarpone, Italiano, Tesco*	1 Pack/400g	572	24.8	143	7.4	14.3	6.2	1.3
Chicken & Asparagus, GFY, Asda*	1 Pack/400g	388	8.8	97	10.9	8.5	2.2	1.5
Chicken & Chorizo, Average	1 Pack/400g	174	5.7	174	10.1	20.3	5.7	1.5
Chicken & Chorizo, Quadrotti, TTD, Sainsbury's*	1 Pack/320g	675	28.8	211	11.8	20.6	9.0	2.7
Chicken & Green Pesto, HL, Tesco*	1 Serving/376g	440	4.5	117	8.3	18.5	1.2	1.4
Chicken & Ham, Easy Steam, Tesco*	1 Pack/400g	572	26.4	143	9.8	11.2	6.6	0.6
Chicken & Mushroom, Big Eat, Heinz*	1 Pot/350g	340	15.8	97	4.8	9.2	4.5	0.5
Chicken & Mushroom, Pasta & Sauce, Dry, Tesco*	1 Pack/120g	427	4.3	356	16.0	65.0	3.6	3.9
Chicken & Mushroom Flavour, Quick, Sainsbury's*	1 Pot/220g	235	6.2	107	3.3	16.1	2.8	1.9
Chicken & Pineapple, Shapers, Boots*	1 Pack/221g	210	3.3	95	5.4	15.0	1.5	0.9
Chicken & Roasted Tomato, HL, Tesco*	1 Serving/374g	426	7.1	114	7.4	16.7	1.9	1.3
Chicken & Vegetable, Mediterranean, Waitrose*	1 Serving/400g	375	9.2	94	7.5	10.5	2.3	2.2
Chicken Italiano, Pasta King*	1 Serving/100g	125	3.2	125	5.5	18.9	3.2	1.9
Chicken Penne, Weight Watchers*	1 Pot/261g	248	3.7	95	5.0	14.6	1.4	2.1
Chilli, Vegetable, Pasta King*	1 Serving/100g	121	2.1	121	5.2	20.9	2.1	2.3
Chilli Beef, Pasta King*	1 Serving/100g	125	2.6	125	5.4	20.5	2.6	2.2
Courgette, Green Bean & Basil Pappardelle, M & S*	1 Pack/270g	324	15.9	120	4.7	11.8	5.9	1.6
Dischi Volanti, Tesco*	1 Serving/50g	178	0.7	355	12.5	73.0	1.4	2.6
Elicoidali, Waitrose*	1 Serving/200g	682	2.6	341	11.5	70.7	1.3	3.7
Fagottini, Wild Mushroom, Sainsbury's*	½ Pack/125g	274	9.4	219	10.2	27.7	7.5	2.7
Feta & Black Olive Girasole, Extra Special, Asda*	½ Pack/150g	360	15.4	240	8.3	28.4	10.3	0.0
Filled, Garlic Mushroom, Extra Special, Asda*	1 Serving/125g	224	8.8	179	8.0	21.0	7.0	2.5
Filled, Tomato & Mozzarella Caramella, Jamie Oliver*	½ Pack/165g	294	9.2	178	8.9	24.9	5.6	2.0
Fiorelli, Egg, M & S*	1 Serving/100g	355	2.8	355	13.9	68.5	2.8	3.0
Fiorelli, Mozzarella, Tomato & Basil, Waitrose*	1 Serving/125g	352	11.6	282	10.8	38.9	9.3	1.7
Garlic & Tomato, Pasta Vita, Dolmio*	1 Pot/300g	336	5.7	112	4.4	18.4	1.9	1.4
Garlic Mushroom, Creamy, HL, Tesco*	1 Serving/100g	106	3.7	106	3.6	14.6	3.7	1.1
Girasole, Filled with Red Pepper & Goats Cheese, Asda*	½ Pack/150g	261	9.9	174	7.2	21.4	6.6	1.8
High Fibre, Uncooked, Fiber Gourmet*	1 Serving/56g	130	1.0	232	12.5	75.0	1.8	32.1

	Measure INFO/WEIGHT	per Measure KCAL	FAT	Nutrition Values per 100g / 100ml KCAL	PROT	CARB	FAT	FIBRE
PASTA								
Honey & Mustard Chicken, Tesco*	1 Pack/375g	865	48.3	231	6.7	22.0	12.9	0.0
Lumache, Tesco*	1 Serving/100g	345	2.0	345	13.2	68.5	2.0	2.9
Lumaconi, TTD, Sainsbury's*	1 Serving/90g	321	1.5	357	12.3	73.1	1.7	2.5
Macaroni Cheese, Meal in 5, Ainsley Harriott*	1 Pot/387g	467	16.0	121	3.8	17.3	4.1	1.0
Meat Feast, Italian, Sainsbury's*	1 Pack/450g	508	18.0	113	7.4	11.8	4.0	0.6
Medaglioni, Bolognese, Rich Red Wine, Waitrose*	½ Pack/125g	266	7.0	213	12.5	28.1	5.6	2.6
Mushroom, Creamy, LC, Tesco*	1 Pack/350g	455	4.9	130	4.3	25.0	1.4	1.3
Mushroom, Creamy, Sainsbury's*	1 Serving/63g	148	9.1	237	4.5	21.7	14.6	1.2
Mushroom & Emmental, Stuffed, Sainsbury's*	1 Pack/250g	650	23.0	260	11.3	33.5	9.2	3.7
Organic, GF, Dove's Farm*	1 Serving/100g	338	1.5	338	7.9	70.3	1.5	4.1
Orzo, Dry, Average	1 Serving/100g	348	1.5	348	12.4	71.9	1.5	3.0
Paccheri, Finest, Tesco*	1 Serving/100g	360	1.5	360	13.5	72.5	1.5	1.6
Penne, Creamy Mushroom, Prepared, Tesco*	½ Pack/200g	288	12.8	144	4.5	17.4	6.4	3.3
Penne, Mediterranean, HL, Tesco*	1 Pack/400g	296	10.8	74	2.9	9.6	2.7	1.5
Pennoni, TTD, Sainsbury's*	1 Serving/90g	321	1.5	357	12.3	73.1	1.7	2.5
Peperonata, Pasta King*	1 Serving/100g	104	1.4	104	3.5	19.4	1.4	1.8
Pepper, Zingy, Pasta King*	1 Serving/100g	106	1.5	106	3.6	19.6	1.5	1.8
Pepper & Tomato, Asda*	1 Serving/250g	340	17.5	136	3.2	15.0	7.0	2.4
Pomodoro, Pasta King*	1 Serving/100g	109	1.8	109	3.6	19.6	1.8	1.8
Pomodoro, with Tomato & Herbs, Slim Fast*	1 Serving/71g	235	3.1	331	21.5	51.5	4.3	6.0
Pumpkin & Sage, Mezze Lune, Whole Foods, Co-Op*	½ Pack/146g	256	6.3	175	6.8	26.0	4.3	2.6
Raviolini, Gorgonzola & Walnut, M & S*	½ Pack/125g	381	16.5	305	12.6	33.6	13.2	2.0
Riccioli, Dry Weight, Buitoni*	1 Serving/75g	264	1.4	352	11.2	72.6	1.9	0.0
Rigatoni, Tuna, Diet Chef Ltd*	1 Pack/300g	336	13.2	112	5.9	12.2	4.4	1.0
Sausage & Tomato, Italiano, Tesco*	1 Serving/450g	680	26.6	151	5.7	18.8	5.9	1.6
Seafood, Retail	1oz/28g	31	1.3	110	8.9	7.6	4.8	0.4
Shells, Tomato & Onion, Tesco*	1 Serving/193g	643	3.1	333	12.5	67.1	1.6	6.3
Spiralli, Tomato & Chicken, HL, Tesco*	1 Pack/350g	402	5.2	115	7.8	17.3	1.5	1.6
Spirals, in Cheese Sauce, Mini, Heinz*	1 Can/154g	120	3.5	78	3.9	10.4	2.3	0.3
Sun Dried Tomato, Sainsbury's*	1 Serving/50g	196	17.8	393	4.5	13.4	35.7	6.2
Sweet Pepper, Pasta Vita, Dolmio*	1 Pot/300g	327	5.7	109	4.4	17.9	1.9	1.4
Tomato, Spicy, Meal in 5, Ainsley Harriott*	1 Pot/387g	369	2.1	95	2.6	20.0	0.5	1.5
Tomato & Basil Chicken, Boots*	1 Serving/320g	621	28.8	194	9.0	19.0	9.0	1.4
Tomato & Chicken, Creamy, Great Stuff, Asda*	1 Pack/300g	351	11.7	117	7.0	13.5	3.9	2.3
Tomato & Chilli, Pasta Vita, Dolmio*	1 Pot/300g	330	5.4	110	4.4	18.4	1.8	1.5
Tomato & Mascarpone, GFY, Asda*	½ Can/200g	128	4.4	64	2.1	9.0	2.2	0.0
Tomato & Mascarpone, Tesco*	1 Pack/400g	468	16.4	117	9.7	10.3	4.1	0.9
Tomato & Pepper, GFY, Asda*	1 Pack/400g	344	7.6	86	3.1	14.0	1.9	1.1
Tomato & Pepperoni Sauce, Spicy, with Fusilli, Heinz*	1 Pack/250g	318	13.8	127	4.4	14.8	5.5	0.6
Tomato & Vegetable, Diet Chef Ltd*	1 Pack/300g	216	6.0	72	2.6	10.9	2.0	1.8
Tomato & Vegetable, Look What We Found*	1 Pouch/300g	216	6.0	72	2.6	10.9	2.0	1.8
Tortelloni, Spinach & Ricotta, Giovanni Rana*	½ Pack/125g	319	10.0	255	9.0	35.5	8.0	3.1
Twists, Tuna & Tomato, Canned, Be Light, Aldi*	1 Can/400g	264	6.8	66	4.8	7.8	1.7	1.7
Twists, with Tuna, Italian, Weight Watchers*	1 Can/385g	239	5.4	62	4.3	8.2	1.4	0.6
Vegetable, Creamy, BGTY, Sainsbury's*	1 Pack/400g	348	6.0	87	4.0	14.3	1.5	1.9
Vegetable, Creamy, Meal in 5, Ainsley Harriott*	1 Pot/387g	414	10.1	107	2.8	18.1	2.6	0.8
Vegetable, Mediterranean, Sainsbury's*	1 Pack/400g	504	11.6	126	4.0	20.9	2.9	1.8
Vegetable, Mediterranean, Weight Watchers*	1 Pack/400g	262	3.2	66	2.6	12.0	0.8	1.6
Vegetable Rice, Dry Weight, Orgran*	1 Serving/66g	233	1.3	353	6.8	80.0	2.0	4.8
Wheat Free, Delverde*	1 Serving/63g	229	1.2	366	0.5	86.9	1.9	1.2
Whole Wheat, Bella Terra*	1 Serving/100g	375	1.8	375	12.5	78.5	1.8	10.7
Wholewheat, Cooked, Tesco*	1 Serving/200g	284	1.8	142	5.7	27.9	0.9	4.5

	Measure INFO/WEIGHT	per Measure KCAL	FAT	Nutrition Values per 100g / 100ml KCAL	PROT	CARB	FAT	FIBRE
PASTA BAKE								
Aberdeen Angus Meatball, Waitrose*	½ Pack/350g	501	28.0	143	5.2	12.5	8.0	0.9
Bacon & Leek, Average	1 Serving/400g	633	32.3	158	6.7	14.8	8.1	1.3
Bolognese, Asda*	¼ Pack/375g	514	23.6	137	7.3	12.7	6.3	1.8
Bolognese, Finest, Tesco*	1 Serving/250g	375	15.8	150	7.3	16.1	6.3	1.1
Bolognese, GFY, Asda*	1 Pack/400g	376	8.4	94	5.8	13.1	2.1	0.9
Bolognese, Weight Watchers*	1 Pack/400g	324	8.0	81	6.1	9.6	2.0	1.3
Cheese & Bacon, Asda*	1 Serving/120g	168	14.4	140	3.0	5.2	12.0	0.3
Cheese & Tomato, Italiano, Tesco*	1 Bake/300g	354	12.6	118	3.9	16.1	4.2	1.0
Chicken, Bacon & Mushroom, Average	1 Serving/400g	632	29.2	158	7.8	15.1	7.3	2.3
Chicken, BGTY, Sainsbury's*	1 Pack/400g	348	8.0	87	9.7	7.5	2.0	0.8
Chicken, Italiano, Tesco*	1 Serving/190g	218	7.8	115	8.4	11.2	4.1	3.1
Chicken, Mozzarella & Tomato, Birds Eye*	1 Pack/360g	468	6.8	130	7.1	14.3	1.9	0.3
Chicken, Mushroom & Leek, HE, Tesco*	1 Pack/450g	468	11.2	104	8.6	11.9	2.5	1.4
Chicken, Tomato, & Mascarpone, Tesco*	1 Serving/400g	448	8.4	112	8.0	15.2	2.1	1.7
Chicken, Weight Watchers*	1 Pack/300g	249	2.7	83	6.0	12.1	0.9	1.1
Chicken & Bacon, Average	1 Serving/400g	627	28.7	157	9.0	13.7	7.2	1.6
Chicken & Bacon, Healthy Range, Average	1 Serving/400g	466	9.6	116	6.6	17.2	2.4	1.6
Chicken & Broccoli, Morrisons*	1 Pack/400g	452	16.0	113	6.1	13.3	4.0	0.6
Chicken & Broccoli, Pasta Presto, Findus*	1 Pack/321g	449	22.5	140	7.5	12.0	7.0	0.0
Chicken & Broccoli, Weight Watchers*	1 Bake/305g	290	4.6	95	6.0	14.2	1.5	0.9
Chicken & Courgette, Asda*	½ Pack/387g	519	23.2	134	6.0	14.0	6.0	0.6
Chicken & Leek, HL, Tesco*	1 Pack/400g	460	7.6	115	10.8	13.1	1.9	1.6
Chicken & Mushroom, Waitrose*	1 Pack/400g	532	30.8	133	6.7	9.1	7.7	0.8
Chicken & Spinach, GFY, Asda*	1 Pack/400g	374	6.0	94	5.0	15.0	1.5	1.2
Chicken & Spinach, Sainsbury's*	1 Pack/340g	286	9.2	84	4.9	10.0	2.7	0.6
Chilli & Cheese, American Style, Tesco*	1 Pack/425g	638	16.6	150	6.8	21.8	3.9	1.5
Chilli Beef, Asda*	1 Pack/1500g	2010	90.0	134	7.0	13.0	6.0	1.2
Conchiglie, Tuna, M & S*	1 Pack/400g	520	17.2	130	8.6	14.3	4.3	1.1
Findus*	1 Pack/320g	448	22.4	140	7.5	12.0	7.0	0.0
Ham & Broccoli, Asda*	1 Pack/340g	309	13.9	91	3.4	10.0	4.1	0.5
Ham & Mushroom, Italiano, Tesco*	1 Pack/425g	646	20.4	152	5.8	21.3	4.8	1.7
King Prawn & Salmon, GFY, Asda*	1 Pack/400g	420	11.6	105	6.9	12.7	2.9	1.2
Leek & Bacon, Morrisons*	1 Pack/401g	553	36.1	138	4.8	9.9	9.0	0.2
Meat Feast, Average	1 Serving/400g	601	21.4	150	5.8	19.2	5.4	1.4
Meatball, Tesco*	1 Pack/400g	576	19.2	144	5.9	19.3	4.8	0.5
Mediterranean, Weight Watchers*	1 Pack/397g	262	3.2	66	2.6	12.0	0.8	1.6
Mediterranean Style, Tesco*	1 Pack/450g	423	1.8	94	2.9	19.6	0.4	2.0
Mix, Tuna, Colman's*	1 Sachet/45g	145	2.3	323	9.2	60.0	5.2	4.7
Mozzarella & Tomato, Asda*	1 Pack/400g	532	19.2	133	4.4	18.1	4.8	1.8
Mushroom, Creamy, Asda*	¼ Jar/118g	204	20.1	173	1.8	3.3	17.0	0.5
Mushroom, Creamy, Dolmio*	½ Jar/245g	267	22.5	109	1.1	5.5	9.2	0.0
Penne Mozzarella, Tesco*	1 Pack/340g	408	8.5	120	4.7	19.7	2.5	0.6
Pepperoni & Ham, Tesco*	½ Pack/425g	502	2.6	118	8.9	19.3	0.6	2.5
Sausage, Average	1 Serving/400g	591	24.0	148	5.5	17.7	6.0	1.9
Tomato, Creamy, Dolmio*	1 Serving/125g	141	9.0	113	2.3	8.4	7.2	0.0
Tomato & Bacon, Italian, Creamy, Asda*	1 Serving/125g	131	11.2	105	2.0	3.9	9.0	0.6
Tomato & Cheese, LC, Tesco*	1 Pack/350g	385	4.6	110	3.2	20.9	1.3	1.5
Tomato & Herb, Asda*	1 Jar/436g	715	56.7	164	1.8	10.0	13.0	1.2
Tomato & Mozzarella, Average	1 Serving/400g	500	12.4	125	5.3	17.3	3.1	1.5
Tomato & Mozzarella, LC, Tesco*	1 Pack/400g	380	4.4	95	3.4	17.2	1.1	1.2
Tomato & Pepperoni, Spicy, Asda*	1 Pack/440g	431	26.4	98	1.1	10.0	6.0	1.2
Tuna, Co-Op*	1 Serving/340g	306	6.8	90	7.0	12.0	2.0	1.0
Tuna, COU, M & S*	1 Pack/360g	432	15.5	120	8.0	11.9	4.3	0.8

	Measure INFO/WEIGHT	per Measure KCAL	FAT	Nutrition Values per 100g / 100ml KCAL	PROT	CARB	FAT	FIBRE
PASTA BAKE								
Tuna, Lean Cuisine*	1 Pack/346g	380	8.6	110	5.0	16.0	2.5	1.5
Tuna, Weight Watchers*	1 Pack/400g	292	3.2	73	7.0	9.4	0.8	1.4
Tuna & Sweetcorn, Average	1 Pack/400g	423	22.4	106	5.0	8.6	5.6	1.9
Tuna & Tomato, BGTY, Sainsbury's*	1 Pack/450g	554	18.9	123	8.7	12.6	4.2	0.4
Vegetable, Asda*	1 Serving/300g	231	10.5	77	2.4	9.0	3.5	0.8
Vegetable, Findus*	1 Pack/331g	430	21.5	130	6.0	13.0	6.5	0.0
Vegetable, M & S*	½ Pack/175g	201	8.8	115	4.1	12.6	5.0	2.2
Vegetable, Mediterranean, HL, Tesco*	1 Serving/450g	374	3.6	83	2.9	16.0	0.8	1.5
Vegetable, Mediterranean, Tesco*	1 Serving/450g	495	20.7	110	4.3	12.9	4.6	1.3
Vegetable, Ready Meals, Waitrose*	1oz/28g	44	2.4	157	5.9	14.4	8.6	1.0
Vegetable, Tesco*	1 Pack/380g	467	21.3	123	5.6	12.6	5.6	1.6
Vegetables, Roasted Mediterranean, Dolmio*	1 Portion/125g	66	2.1	53	1.3	8.1	1.7	1.2
PASTA 'N' SAUCE								
Bolognese Flavour, Dry, Batchelors*	½ Pack/65g	228	1.7	353	15.1	67.2	2.6	3.9
Carbonara Flavour, Dry, Batchelors*	1 Pack/120g	463	6.0	386	14.3	71.0	5.0	3.1
Cheese, Leek & Ham, Batchelors*	1 Pack/120g	454	6.1	378	16.1	67.0	5.1	2.0
Cheese & Broccoli, Made Up, Smart Price, Asda*	1 Serving/120g	198	8.4	165	4.6	21.0	7.0	2.1
Chicken & Mushroom, Batchelors*	½ Pack/63g	227	1.1	361	14.1	72.3	1.7	2.8
Chicken & Mushroom, Made Up, Morrisons*	1 Pack/110g	166	6.2	151	5.0	20.3	5.6	2.1
Chicken & Mushroom, Made Up, Smart Price, Asda*	1 Pack/110g	183	6.6	166	5.0	23.0	6.0	2.2
Chicken & Roasted Garlic Flavour, Dry, Batchelors*	½ Pack/60g	223	1.7	372	12.6	73.8	2.9	3.4
Macaroni Cheese, Dry, Batchelors*	1 Pack/108g	402	5.1	372	17.2	65.2	4.7	2.7
Mild Cheese & Broccoli, Batchelors*	½ Pack/61g	221	2.4	363	15.0	67.0	3.9	4.0
Mushroom & Wine, Batchelors*	½ Pack/50g	242	2.8	483	18.5	89.9	5.5	4.4
Mushroom & Wine, Dry, Batchelors*	1 Pack/132g	498	6.5	377	12.0	71.3	4.9	2.5
Tikka Masala, Creamy, Dry, Batchelors*	1 Pack/122g	426	2.7	349	12.7	69.5	2.2	4.4
Tomato, Onion & Herb, Made Up, Morrisons*	1 Serving/110g	141	5.0	128	3.2	18.7	4.5	2.3
Tomato, Onion & Herbs, Dry, Batchelors*	1 Pack/135g	455	1.8	337	12.8	68.5	1.3	5.8
Tomato & Bacon Flavour, Dry, Batchelors*	1 Pack/134g	476	3.5	355	13.0	70.0	2.6	3.0
Tomato & Mascarpone, BGTY, Sainsbury's*	1 Pack/380g	555	7.2	146	6.6	25.6	1.9	1.3
Tomato & Mushroom, Creamy, Dry, Batchelors*	1 Pack/125g	458	4.1	366	13.0	71.0	3.3	3.2
PASTA QUILLS								
Dry, Average	***1 Serving/75g***	***256***	***0.9***	***342***	***12.0***	***72.3***	***1.2***	***2.0***
GF, Salute*	1 Serving/75g	269	1.4	359	7.5	78.0	1.9	0.0
PASTA SALAD								
Basil & Parmesan, Tesco*	1 Serving/50g	65	1.8	130	4.3	20.2	3.6	0.6
BBQ Bean, Tesco*	1 Pack/850g	1139	43.4	134	3.6	18.5	5.1	1.8
BBQ Chicken, Positive Eating, Scottish Slimmers*	1 Serving/240g	223	4.3	93	6.4	14.0	1.8	1.3
Caesar, & Santa Tomatoes, M & S*	1 Serving/220g	495	33.7	225	5.2	15.9	15.3	0.8
Caesar, Chicken, Asda*	1 Pack/297g	683	41.3	230	9.6	16.6	13.9	2.5
Caesar, Chicken, Ginsters*	1 Pack/220g	504	35.4	229	7.5	13.6	16.1	0.0
Caesar, Chicken, Shapers, Boots*	1 Pack/218g	288	8.3	132	6.7	18.0	3.8	1.8
Cheese, Average	1 Serving/370g	782	56.8	211	5.5	12.8	15.4	1.2
Cheese, with Mayonnaise & Vinaigrette, Sainsbury's*	¼ Pot/50g	124	8.6	249	6.1	17.0	17.3	1.7
Cheese Layered, Asda*	1 Pack/440g	471	21.6	107	5.2	10.4	4.9	2.0
Chicken, Asda*	1 Pot/250g	322	12.2	129	5.8	15.5	4.9	1.3
Chicken, Chargrilled, & Pesto Pasta, Sainsbury's*	1 Pack/240g	454	22.1	189	7.2	19.4	9.2	0.0
Chicken, Chargrilled, Italian Style, Fresh, Asda*	1 Pack/200g	318	14.0	159	7.0	17.0	7.0	0.4
Chicken, Chargrilled, M & S*	1 Serving/190g	285	5.5	150	9.6	23.6	2.9	1.6
Chicken, Lime & Coriander, M & S*	1 Serving/190g	370	23.2	195	7.6	14.4	12.2	0.6
Chicken, Mediterranean, Waitrose*	1 Serving/200g	314	13.6	157	7.0	16.9	6.8	2.1
Chicken, Mexican, Weight Watchers*	1 Pack/249g	284	4.2	114	7.8	16.9	1.7	3.6
Chicken, Spicy, Budgens*	1 Serving/213g	452	22.2	212	5.1	24.5	10.4	4.4

	Measure INFO/WEIGHT	per Measure KCAL	FAT	Nutrition Values per 100g / 100ml KCAL	PROT	CARB	FAT	FIBRE
PASTA SALAD								
Chicken, Spicy, Geo Adams*	1 Pack/230g	580	43.9	252	5.1	14.9	19.1	2.9
Chicken & Bacon, Tesco*	½ Pack/200g	450	29.0	225	6.3	16.8	14.5	3.2
Chicken & Smoked Bacon, M & S*	1 Pack/380g	817	46.7	215	7.5	19.0	12.3	1.9
Chilli & Cheese, Sainsbury's*	1 Serving/300g	384	16.8	128	4.3	15.5	5.6	0.3
Crayfish, Rocket & Lemon, Finest, Tesco*	1 Serving/250g	728	39.8	291	8.9	28.0	15.9	4.2
Crayfish, Shapers, Boots*	1 Pack/280g	269	6.4	96	6.0	13.0	2.3	0.7
Farfalle, Prawns Tomatoes & Cucumber, Sainsbury's*	1 Serving/260g	270	12.2	104	4.5	10.9	4.7	0.7
Goats Cheese & Mixed Pepper, Sainsbury's*	1 Pack/200g	366	18.8	183	6.4	18.2	9.4	1.5
Ham, Sainsbury's*	1 Pot/250g	610	48.2	244	4.1	13.4	19.3	0.8
Honey & Mustard Chicken, M & S*	1 Serving/190g	304	4.8	160	8.7	26.7	2.5	1.5
Honey & Mustard Chicken, Sainsbury's*	1 Pack/190g	344	16.9	181	7.1	18.0	8.9	0.0
Honey & Mustard Chicken, Shapers, Boots*	1 Serving/252g	350	5.5	139	8.4	22.0	2.2	2.8
Italian, Tesco*	½ Pack/225g	315	8.3	140	3.5	22.6	3.7	2.3
Italian Style, Sainsbury's*	1/3 Pot/84g	129	5.3	153	3.5	20.5	6.3	1.4
Italian Style, Snack, Asda*	1 Pack/150g	141	6.0	94	3.4	11.0	4.0	4.1
Kraft*	½ Cup/68g	183	11.0	269	4.0	26.5	16.2	0.0
Mediterranean Style, Layered, Waitrose*	1 Pot/275g	190	3.6	69	2.6	11.8	1.3	1.0
Mixed Bean, Diet Chef Ltd*	1 Packet/300g	300	3.6	100	4.7	17.5	1.2	2.8
Mushroom, Roasted, Spinach & Tarragon, Tesco*	1 Pot/200g	216	4.8	108	4.3	17.2	2.4	0.8
Pepper, Side, Tesco*	1 Serving/46g	56	3.0	122	2.4	13.0	6.5	1.3
Pepper & Tomato, Fire Roasted, Finest, Tesco*	1 Pack/200g	260	8.2	130	3.7	19.4	4.1	2.5
Pesto, Chilli, Spicy, Sainsbury's*	¼ Pot/63g	170	12.2	272	3.8	20.1	19.6	1.6
Prawn, Layered, Asda*	½ Pack/220g	279	11.4	127	5.2	14.2	5.2	2.0
Prawn, Tesco*	½ Pack/250g	488	27.8	195	4.9	18.9	11.1	2.0
Prawn Cocktail, Layered, Shapers, Boots*	1 Pot/210g	181	5.2	86	3.6	13.0	2.5	1.3
Prawns, King & Juicy Fresh Tomatoes, COU, M & S*	1 Serving/270g	256	4.0	95	5.1	16.4	1.5	0.9
Salmon, Hot Smoked, No Mayonnaise, Tesco*	1 Pack/275g	426	17.0	155	7.1	16.6	6.2	4.1
Salmon, M & S*	1 Serving/380g	817	57.8	215	6.8	12.7	15.2	0.7
Salmon, Poached, Sainsbury's*	1 Serving/200g	472	30.6	236	6.7	17.9	15.3	12.0
Sweetcorn & Pepper, GFY, Asda*	1 Serving/175g	68	0.7	39	1.9	7.0	0.4	0.0
Tiger Prawn, Waitrose*	1 Serving/225g	544	38.5	242	5.4	16.7	17.1	0.4
Tiger Prawn & Tomato, GFY, Asda*	1 Serving/200g	250	5.8	125	4.6	20.0	2.9	2.0
Tomato, Aldi*	1 Serving/50g	58	1.8	117	3.9	18.6	3.6	0.0
Tomato, Bacon & Cheese, Ginsters*	1 Pack/220g	381	19.8	173	7.4	15.6	9.0	0.0
Tomato, Diet Chef Ltd*	1 Pack/300g	264	5.4	88	2.3	15.6	1.8	1.2
Tomato & Basil, Chicken, Waitrose*	1 Pack/205g	434	24.6	212	8.3	17.7	12.0	1.1
Tomato & Basil, M & S*	1 Pot/225g	484	35.8	215	2.9	15.0	15.9	1.2
Tomato & Basil, Perfectly Balanced, Waitrose*	1 Serving/100g	97	1.7	97	3.7	16.8	1.7	0.0
Tomato & Basil, Pot, HL, Tesco*	1 Pot/200g	242	5.4	121	2.0	22.1	2.7	2.2
Tomato & Basil, Sainsbury's*	1 Serving/62g	87	4.3	141	3.2	16.4	6.9	3.8
Tomato & Mozzarella, Leaf, Shapers, Boots*	1 Pack/185g	356	22.3	192	5.1	16.0	12.0	2.5
Tomato & Mozzarella, Sainsbury's*	1 Pack/200g	440	22.6	220	7.5	22.2	11.3	1.3
Tomato & Pepper, HL, Tesco*	1 Serving/200g	162	3.2	81	2.6	13.9	1.6	1.4
Tomato & Tuna, Snack, Sainsbury's*	1 Serving/200g	238	2.4	119	5.3	21.7	1.2	0.0
Tuna, Mediterranean, Shapers, Boots*	1 Serving/239g	232	3.1	97	6.2	15.0	1.3	0.9
Tuna, Perfectly Balanced, Waitrose*	1 Tub/190g	180	4.4	95	7.0	11.5	2.3	1.1
Tuna, Tesco*	1 Pot/300g	399	21.9	133	6.2	10.5	7.3	0.0
Tuna & Spinach, COU, M & S*	1 Pack/270g	256	4.9	95	6.8	14.3	1.8	3.8
Tuna & Sweetcorn, Sainsbury's*	1 Serving/100g	111	1.2	111	7.1	18.3	1.2	1.2
Tuna Crunch, Shapers, Boots*	1 Pack/250g	352	6.8	141	9.8	19.0	2.7	2.8
Tuna Nicoise, Waitrose*	1 Pot/190g	306	17.1	161	5.1	14.9	9.0	1.1
Vegetable, Roasted, Waitrose*	1 Pack/190g	270	8.7	142	6.8	18.2	4.6	1.1
Vegetable & Bean, Mediterranean, BGTY, Sainsbury's*	1 Serving/66g	53	1.3	80	3.2	12.5	1.9	2.8

	Measure INFO/WEIGHT	per Measure KCAL	FAT	Nutrition Values per 100g / 100ml KCAL	PROT	CARB	FAT	FIBRE
PASTA SALAD								
Vegetables, Chargrilled, & Tomato, Shapers, Boots*	1 Pack/175g	187	5.4	107	2.8	17.0	3.1	1.5
Vegetables, Chargrilled, Sainsbury's*	1 Serving/178g	192	4.8	108	2.7	15.9	2.7	4.7
PASTA SAUCE								
Amatriciana, M & S*	1 Jar/340g	425	32.3	125	3.4	6.3	9.5	2.9
Arrabbiata, Barilla*	1 Serving/100g	47	3.0	47	1.5	3.5	3.0	0.0
Arrabbiata, Fresh, Morrisons*	1 Pot/350g	139	5.2	40	1.9	5.4	1.5	0.0
Arrabbiata, GFY, Asda*	1 Serving/350g	133	3.9	38	1.1	6.0	1.1	0.0
Arrabbiata, Italian, Waitrose*	1 Jar/320g	115	3.2	36	1.5	6.7	1.0	1.4
Arrabbiata, Romano*	1 Serving/100g	69	3.4	69	2.5	7.0	3.4	0.6
Arrabbiata, Stir in, BGTY, Sainsbury's*	1 Serving/75g	53	2.9	71	1.3	7.6	3.9	0.7
Aubergine & Pepper, Sacla*	½ Pot/95g	238	23.3	250	1.8	5.6	24.5	0.0
Bolognese, Carb Check, Heinz*	1 Serving/150g	80	3.9	53	3.8	3.6	2.6	0.4
Bolognese, Finest, Tesco*	1 Serving/175g	170	10.7	97	7.0	3.8	6.1	0.5
Bolognese, Fresh, Sainsbury's*	½ Pot/150g	120	6.2	80	6.0	4.7	4.1	1.2
Bolognese, GFY, Asda*	1 Jar/500g	210	1.5	42	0.7	7.9	0.3	2.4
Bolognese, Italiano, Tesco*	1 Serving/175g	194	13.1	111	5.9	4.8	7.5	0.8
Bolognese, Light, Original, Ragu, Knorr*	1 Jar/515g	196	0.5	38	1.4	8.2	0.1	1.2
Bolognese, Mediterranean Vegetable, Chunky, Dolmio*	½ Jar/250g	138	4.0	55	1.3	8.8	1.6	1.1
Bolognese, Organic, Seeds of Change*	1 Jar/500g	290	6.0	58	1.3	10.4	1.2	0.8
Bolognese, Original, Light, Low Fat, Dolmio*	1 Serving/125g	44	0.4	35	1.5	6.7	0.3	0.9
Bolognese, Seasonal, Dolmio*	1 Jar/500g	205	1.0	41	1.5	7.4	0.2	1.4
Bolognese, Spicy, Ragu, Knorr*	1 Jar/500g	260	1.0	52	1.9	9.7	0.2	1.4
Bolognese, Tomato, Beef & Red Wine, Fresh, Waitrose*	1 Pot/350g	301	17.2	86	5.4	5.3	4.9	2.0
Bolognese, Traditional, Ragu, Knorr*	1 Jar/320g	157	5.4	49	1.3	7.1	1.7	1.2
Bolognese, VLH Kitchens	1 Serving/380g	316	1.1	83	6.0	4.7	4.1	1.2
Bolognese, with Red Wine, Weight Watchers*	1 Jar/350g	98	0.4	28	1.4	5.3	0.1	1.3
Cacciatore, Fresh, Sainsbury's*	½ Pot/150g	152	8.8	101	5.4	8.1	5.9	1.5
Carbonara, 50% Less Fat, Asda*	½ Pot/175g	170	10.5	97	4.8	6.0	6.0	0.6
Carbonara, Asda*	½ Pot/175g	359	29.8	205	7.0	6.0	17.0	0.1
Carbonara, Bottled, Tesco*	1 Jar/315g	504	41.6	160	3.2	6.8	13.2	0.1
Carbonara, Chosen By You, Asda*	1 Serving/100g	162	12.6	162	7.3	4.5	12.6	0.5
Carbonara, Creamy, Dolmio Express, Dolmio*	1 Pack/150g	171	13.8	114	3.1	4.7	9.2	0.1
Carbonara, Creamy, Stir in Sauce, Dolmio*	1 Serving/75g	98	8.0	130	3.3	5.2	10.6	0.2
Carbonara, Fresh, BGTY, Sainsbury's*	1 Tub/300g	255	10.8	85	5.4	7.8	3.6	0.5
Carbonara, Reduced Fat, BFY, Morrisons*	½ Pot/175g	135	5.8	77	6.6	5.1	3.3	0.5
Carbonara, with Pancetta, Loyd Grossman*	½ Pack/170g	209	15.5	123	2.8	7.5	9.1	0.1
Cheese, Fresh, Perfectly Balanced, Waitrose*	½ Pot/175g	144	5.1	82	6.1	7.9	2.9	0.5
Chilli, Spicy Italian, Express, Dolmio*	1 Serving/170g	87	2.7	51	1.5	7.5	1.6	0.0
Fiorentina, Fresh, Sainsbury's*	½ Pot/157g	165	13.2	105	3.2	4.3	8.4	0.9
Five Cheese, Italiano, Tesco*	½ Tub/175g	271	20.1	155	6.8	6.0	11.5	0.0
Four Cheese, BGTY, Sainsbury's*	1 Serving/150g	104	6.0	69	2.9	5.5	4.0	0.1
Four Cheese, Fresh, Asda*	½ Pot/162g	309	28.8	191	5.4	2.2	17.8	0.5
Four Cheese, Loyd Grossman*	1 Jar/350g	476	41.6	136	2.6	4.6	11.9	0.0
Garlic, Perfectly Balanced, Waitrose*	1 Jar/440g	330	7.5	75	2.3	12.7	1.7	2.3
Garlic, Roasted, Spicy, Seeds of Change*	1 Serving/195g	123	3.9	63	1.5	9.7	2.0	1.2
Garlic & Chilli, Slow Roasted, Seeds of Change*	½ Jar/175g	158	9.3	90	1.7	8.7	5.3	2.0
Garlic & Herbs, Low Fat, LC, Tesco*	1 Jar/500g	200	1.5	40	1.6	6.8	0.3	1.9
Garlic & Onion, Finest, Tesco*	1 Serving/126g	43	0.5	34	0.8	6.9	0.4	1.3
Grilled Vegetables, Bertolli*	1 Jar/400g	215	10.0	43	1.4	4.9	2.0	1.1
Ham & Mushroom, Creamy, Stir & Serve, Homepride*	1 Serving/92g	124	10.8	135	1.8	5.5	11.7	0.0
Mediterranean, BGTY, Sainsbury's*	1oz/28g	23	1.2	82	1.9	9.0	4.3	1.4
Mediterranean, Fresh, Waitrose*	1 Pot/350g	214	13.6	61	1.4	5.0	3.9	2.4
Mushroom, Co-Op*	¼ Jar/125g	75	2.5	60	2.0	9.0	2.0	1.0

P

	Measure INFO/WEIGHT	per Measure KCAL	FAT	Nutrition Values per 100g / 100ml KCAL	PROT	CARB	FAT	FIBRE
PASTA SAUCE								
Mushroom, Creamy, Dolmio*	1 Pack/150g	166	15.0	111	1.3	3.7	10.0	0.0
Mushroom, for Bolognese, Country, Ragu, Knorr*	1 Jar/510g	347	10.7	68	2.0	9.5	2.1	1.2
Mushroom, Fresh, Waitrose*	1 Serving/175g	142	10.0	81	1.6	5.7	5.7	0.5
Mushroom, Garlic & Oregano, Rustico, Bertolli*	1 Serving/100g	90	7.5	90	1.9	3.8	7.5	0.0
Mushroom, GFY, Asda*	1 Serving/175g	112	4.9	64	2.7	7.0	2.8	0.0
Mushroom, Microwaveable, Dolmio*	1 Serving/150g	160	14.4	107	1.4	3.8	9.6	0.0
Mushroom, Perfectly Balanced, Waitrose*	1 Jar/440g	330	8.4	75	2.6	11.8	1.9	2.2
Mushroom, Sainsbury's*	1 Serving/100g	66	2.1	66	2.0	9.8	2.1	1.7
Mushroom & Garlic, 98% Fat Free, Homepride*	1 Jar/450g	230	6.3	51	1.1	8.9	1.4	0.5
Mushroom & Garlic, Deliciously Good, Homepride*	1/3 Jar/147g	109	7.1	74	0.9	6.9	4.8	0.3
Mushroom & Marsala Wine, Sacla*	½ Pot/85g	165	16.0	194	2.2	3.9	18.8	0.0
Mushroom & Mascarpone, HE, Tesco*	½ Jar/175g	86	3.9	49	2.1	5.3	2.2	0.3
Mushroom & Mascarpone, Morrisons*	½ Pot/175g	200	17.0	114	2.3	4.3	9.7	0.0
Mushroom & White Wine, Knorr*	1oz/28g	27	2.2	98	1.0	4.0	8.0	0.0
Napoletana, BGTY, Sainsbury's*	½ Pot/151g	71	3.8	47	1.2	5.0	2.5	1.3
Napoletana, Buitoni*	½ Jar/200g	146	8.2	73	1.6	7.3	4.1	2.2
Napoletana, Fresh, Sainsbury's*	1oz/28g	25	1.6	91	1.9	7.9	5.8	1.1
Napoletana, Fresh, Waitrose*	1 Serving/175g	82	3.0	47	1.3	6.6	1.7	1.0
Napoletana, GFY, Asda*	1 Serving/175g	58	1.8	33	1.0	5.0	1.0	0.0
Napoletana, Sainsbury's*	½ Pot/150g	126	8.4	84	1.9	6.6	5.6	0.9
Olive, Barilla*	1 Serving/100g	92	5.0	92	1.5	10.3	5.0	0.0
Olive & Tomato, Sacla*	1 Serving/95g	87	7.6	92	1.3	3.6	8.0	0.0
Onion & Garlic, Co-Op*	1 Serving/125g	106	3.8	85	2.0	12.0	3.0	0.7
Onion & Roasted Garlic, Knorr*	1 Jar/500g	210	0.0	42	1.3	9.2	0.0	1.1
Parmesan & Pesto, Weight Watchers*	½ Jar/175g	86	2.8	49	1.8	6.7	1.6	1.0
Pepper & Tomato, M & S*	1 Jar/320g	224	13.4	70	1.6	6.1	4.2	0.9
Pepper & Tomato, Spicy, Sacla*	½ Jar/95g	132	11.2	139	1.4	6.8	11.8	0.0
Pomodoro, Cirio*	1 Serving/200g	116	4.6	58	1.4	8.4	2.3	0.0
Porcini Mushroom & Pepperoni, Asda*	½ Jar/140g	158	8.4	113	3.8	11.0	6.0	0.0
Porcini Mushroom Stir in, BGTY, Sainsbury's*	½ Jar/75g	57	3.2	76	3.8	5.7	4.2	1.9
Primavera, Fresh, Morrisons*	½ Pot/175g	152	10.3	87	2.4	6.1	5.9	0.0
Primavera, Loyd Grossman*	1 Jar/350g	343	25.9	98	1.4	6.3	7.4	0.9
Puttanesca, Italian, Waitrose*	1 Jar/350g	195	9.8	56	1.5	6.1	2.8	1.3
Puttanesca, Loyd Grossman*	1 Jar/350g	315	21.7	90	1.7	6.8	6.2	0.9
Puttanesca, Sainsbury's*	1 Serving/110g	132	9.7	120	2.0	8.1	8.8	0.0
Red Pepper, & Italian Cheese, Stir Through, Asda*	½ Jar/95g	86	4.7	90	2.9	8.5	4.9	0.9
Red Pepper, & Plum, Finest, Tesco*	1 Serving/63g	109	7.2	173	3.7	14.0	11.4	5.4
Red Pepper, & Roasted Vegetable, Spicy, Asda*	1 Serving/175g	140	7.7	80	1.2	9.0	4.4	1.0
Red Wine, Traditional Recipe, Dolmio*	1 Serving/100g	64	0.8	64	1.5	10.3	0.8	0.0
Romano*	1 Serving/235g	141	4.7	60	1.7	8.8	2.0	1.1
Spicy, with Peppers, Tesco*	1 Jar/500g	240	4.5	48	2.2	7.8	0.9	1.8
Spinach & Ricotta, Asda*	½ Pot/175g	175	12.2	100	3.2	6.0	7.0	0.5
Spinach & Ricotta, BGTY, Sainsbury's*	1 Serving/150g	74	4.0	49	2.7	3.4	2.7	2.2
Spinach & Ricotta, Fresh, Perfectly Balanced, Waitrose*	½ Pot/175g	96	3.7	55	3.3	5.7	2.1	0.9
Spinach & Ricotta, Stir Through, Sacla*	½ Jar/95g	196	18.6	206	3.7	3.7	19.6	0.0
Stir & Serve, Homepride*	1 Jar/480g	187	5.8	39	1.2	6.0	1.2	0.0
Sun Dried Tomato, Asda*	½ Jar/159g	165	12.7	104	1.9	6.0	8.0	1.5
Sun Dried Tomato, Garlic & Basil, Finest, Tesco*	1 Jar/340g	493	39.1	145	1.8	7.7	11.5	2.3
Sun Dried Tomato, Heinz*	½ Jar/150g	56	0.3	37	1.5	7.3	0.2	1.1
Sun Dried Tomato, Stir In, Light, Dolmio*	1 Serving/75g	62	3.5	83	1.7	9.8	4.7	0.0
Sun Dried Tomato & Basil, Free From, Sainsbury's*	½ Jar/172g	124	4.8	72	2.9	8.7	2.8	1.5
Sun Dried Tomato & Basil, Organic, Seeds of Change*	½ Jar/100g	155	13.1	155	1.6	7.7	13.1	0.0
Sun Dried Tomato & Garlic, M & S*	½ Jar/95g	147	13.0	155	2.9	4.4	13.7	0.8

P

	Measure INFO/WEIGHT	per Measure KCAL	per Measure FAT	KCAL	PROT	CARB	FAT	FIBRE
				Nutrition Values per 100g / 100ml				
PASTA SAUCE								
Sun Dried Tomato & Garlic, Sacla*	1 Serving/95g	177	14.0	186	3.0	10.3	14.7	0.0
Sun Dried Tomato & Olive Oil, Loyd Grossman*	1oz/28g	52	4.4	187	0.8	10.3	15.8	0.3
Sun Ripened Tomato & Basil, Dolmio*	1 Serving/150g	117	6.9	78	1.3	7.9	4.6	0.0
Three Cheeses, Co-Op*	1 Pack/300g	405	27.0	135	6.0	6.0	9.0	0.1
Tomato, Bacon & Mushroom, Asda*	½ Pot/50g	33	1.8	66	2.5	6.0	3.6	0.0
Tomato, Basil & Parmesan Stir in, BGTY, Sainsbury's*	1 Serving/75g	69	4.1	92	2.9	7.8	5.5	1.0
Tomato, Chilli & Onion, Bertolli*	1 Serving/100g	49	1.7	49	1.8	6.7	1.7	1.8
Tomato, Creamy, Carb Check, Heinz*	1 Serving/150g	92	6.0	61	2.0	4.2	4.0	0.5
Tomato, Ginger & Basil, Cranks*	½ Jar/175g	130	8.2	74	1.7	6.3	4.7	1.1
Tomato, Low Price, Sainsbury's*	1 Jar/440g	220	3.1	50	0.6	10.1	0.7	0.4
Tomato, Pecorino Romano Cheese & Garlic, Bertolli*	1 Serving/125g	76	3.5	61	2.3	6.5	2.8	0.9
Tomato, Red Wine, Shallots, Bertolli*	½ Jar/250g	112	4.2	45	1.7	7.2	1.7	1.5
Tomato, Spicy, Asda*	1 Serving/155g	76	1.9	49	1.5	8.0	1.2	1.0
Tomato & Basil, Bertolli*	1 Jar/500g	215	5.0	43	1.2	7.3	1.0	0.4
Tomato & Basil, Carb Check, Heinz*	1 Serving/150g	84	5.4	56	1.5	4.4	3.6	0.6
Tomato & Basil, Classic, Sacla*	1 Serving/100g	137	11.1	137	2.0	7.2	11.1	2.8
Tomato & Basil, Dolmio*	1 Serving/170g	95	3.6	56	1.4	7.9	2.1	0.0
Tomato & Basil, Loyd Grossman*	½ Jar/175g	107	6.0	61	1.5	5.8	3.4	0.8
Tomato & Basil, M & S*	1 Jar/340g	119	7.1	35	2.0	2.1	2.1	0.9
Tomato & Basil, Organic, Simply Organic*	1 Pot/300g	183	12.9	61	1.5	4.2	4.3	0.6
Tomato & Black Olive, Carb Control, Tesco*	1 Serving/110g	74	4.7	67	1.3	6.0	4.3	2.3
Tomato & Garlic, Chosen By You, Asda*	½ Jar/160g	74	0.8	46	1.6	7.9	0.5	1.7
Tomato & Herb, for Bolognese, Lighter, Sainsbury's*	¼ Jar/125g	35	0.4	28	1.1	4.4	0.3	1.5
Tomato & Herb, M & S*	1 Jar/500g	400	15.5	80	2.6	10.1	3.1	1.7
Tomato & Herb, Organic, M & S*	1 Jar/550g	302	19.8	55	1.4	4.2	3.6	2.6
Tomato & Herb, Organic, Meridian Foods*	½ Jar/220g	141	6.2	64	1.6	8.1	2.8	1.1
Tomato & Herb, Perfectly Balanced, Waitrose*	½ Tub/176g	65	2.1	37	1.3	5.3	1.2	2.3
Tomato & Mascarpone, BGTY, Sainsbury's*	1 Pot/300g	150	9.0	50	2.0	3.6	3.0	3.6
Tomato & Mascarpone, Finest, Tesco*	1 Serving/175g	135	8.8	77	2.7	5.4	5.0	0.8
Tomato & Mascarpone, Italiano, Tesco*	½ Pot/175g	168	12.2	96	2.8	5.5	7.0	0.7
Tomato & Mascarpone, Pasta Reale*	1 Pack/300g	318	23.7	106	2.9	5.9	7.9	0.5
Tomato & Mascarpone, Sacla*	½ Jar/95g	161	14.2	169	2.2	6.2	15.0	0.0
Tomato & Mascarpone, Sainsbury's*	½ Pot/150g	137	9.9	91	2.1	5.9	6.6	1.2
Tomato & Mascarpone, So Organic, Sainsbury's*	1/3 Jar/146g	180	13.2	123	1.9	8.7	9.0	2.8
Tomato & Mushroom, Chosen By You, Asda*	½ Jar/160g	70	1.0	44	2.1	7.0	0.6	1.1
Tomato & Mushroom, Organic, Sainsbury's*	1 Serving/150g	87	3.9	58	1.6	7.1	2.6	1.5
Tomato & Olives, La Doria*	1 Jar/90g	76	5.9	84	1.2	5.0	6.6	0.0
Tomato & Parmesan, Seeds of Change*	1 Serving/150g	100	4.4	67	2.5	7.8	2.9	1.1
Tomato & Pesto, Planet Cook, Heinz*	1 Jar/300g	237	17.1	79	1.7	5.2	5.7	1.0
Tomato & Ricotta, Italian, Sainsbury's*	1 Pack/390g	238	11.7	61	2.5	6.1	3.0	1.2
Tomato & Roasted Garlic, Chosen By You, Asda*	1 Pot/350g	122	2.1	35	1.5	5.0	0.6	1.7
Tomato & Roasted Garlic, Loyd Grossman*	½ Jar/175g	107	5.4	61	1.5	6.3	3.1	0.8
Vegetable, Chunky, Asda*	1 Serving/250g	122	4.2	49	1.4	7.0	1.7	1.2
Vegetable, Chunky, Tesco*	1 Jar/500g	235	5.0	47	1.8	6.8	1.0	1.8
Vegetable, Mediterranean, Organic, Pasta Reale*	1 Pack/300g	183	13.8	61	1.0	3.9	4.6	0.3
Vegetable, Mediterranean, Organic, Seeds of Change*	1 Jar/350g	210	10.2	60	1.2	6.6	2.9	1.4
Vegetable, Mediterranean, Rustico, Bertolli*	½ Jar/160g	141	11.5	88	1.7	4.1	7.2	0.7
PASTA SHAPES								
Alphabetti, in Tomato Sauce, Heinz*	1 Can/200g	118	1.0	59	1.8	11.7	0.5	1.5
Bob The Builder, in Tomato Sauce, Heinz*	1 Can/205g	111	0.6	54	1.7	11.3	0.3	1.5
Cooked, Tesco*	1 Serving/260g	356	2.1	137	5.1	26.3	0.8	1.1
Disney Princess, in Tomato Sauce, Heinz*	1 Can/200g	114	0.6	57	1.8	11.9	0.3	1.5
Dried, Tesco*	1 Serving/100g	345	2.0	345	13.2	68.5	2.0	2.9

	Measure INFO/WEIGHT	per Measure KCAL	FAT	Nutrition Values per 100g / 100ml KCAL	PROT	CARB	FAT	FIBRE
PASTA SHAPES								
Durum Wheat, Dry, Basics, Sainsbury's*	1 Serving/75g	260	1.5	346	12.0	70.0	2.0	4.0
Postman Pat, HP*	1 Can/410g	279	1.6	68	1.8	14.3	0.4	0.7
Scooby Doo, HP*	1 Can/410g	279	1.6	68	1.8	14.3	0.4	0.7
Spiderman, in Tomato Sauce, Heinz*	½ Can/200g	114	1.0	57	1.7	11.4	0.5	1.5
Spiderman, Mini Sausages in Tomato Sauce, Heinz*	1 Can/200g	178	6.2	89	3.6	11.6	3.1	0.5
Teletubbies, in Tomato Sauce, Heinz*	1 Can/400g	244	1.6	61	2.0	12.3	0.4	0.6
Thomas Tank Engine, in Tomato Sauce, Heinz*	1 Can/205g	109	0.4	53	1.7	11.0	0.2	0.5
Tweenies, in Tomato Sauce, Heinz*	1 Can/205g	121	1.0	59	1.8	11.7	0.5	1.5
PASTA SHELLS								
Conchiglie, Dry Weight, Parioli, Cucina*	1 Serving/75g	266	1.0	355	12.5	73.0	1.4	2.6
Dry, Average	***1 Serving/75g***	***265***	***1.5***	***353***	***11.1***	***71.8***	***2.0***	***2.0***
Egg, Fresh, Average	***1 Serving/125g***	***344***	***3.6***	***275***	***11.5***	***49.8***	***2.8***	***3.4***
Wholewheat, Healthy Living, Co-Op*	1 Serving/75g	232	0.8	310	11.0	64.0	1.0	12.0
PASTA SPIRALS								
Co-Op*	1 Serving/100g	350	1.0	350	12.0	73.0	1.0	3.0
Glutenfree, Glutano*	1oz/28g	100	0.3	357	4.0	83.0	1.0	0.0
PASTA TWIRLS								
Dry, Asda*	1 Serving/50g	173	0.8	346	12.0	71.0	1.5	3.0
Tri-Colour, Sainsbury's*	1 Serving/75g	268	1.3	357	12.3	73.1	1.7	2.5
PASTA TWISTS								
Dry, Average	***1oz/28g***	***99***	***0.4***	***354***	***12.2***	***71.8***	***1.5***	***2.2***
Wheat & GF, Glutafin*	1 Serving/75g	262	1.5	350	8.0	75.0	2.0	0.1
PASTE								
Bacon & Tomato, Tesco*	1 Serving/20g	46	3.6	232	14.0	3.4	18.0	0.1
Beef, Asda*	1 Serving/37g	72	5.2	194	17.0	0.1	14.0	0.0
Beef, Princes*	1 Serving/18g	40	2.8	220	14.4	5.2	15.8	0.0
Beef, Sainsbury's*	1 Jar/75g	142	9.9	189	16.0	1.5	13.2	1.4
Chicken, Asda*	1 Thin Spread/7g	13	0.9	184	16.0	0.8	13.0	0.0
Chicken, Princes*	1 Thin Spread/9g	22	1.7	240	12.6	5.6	18.5	0.0
Chicken & Ham, Princes*	1 Jar/100g	233	18.6	233	13.6	2.8	18.6	0.0
Chicken & Ham, Sainsbury's*	1 Thin Spread/9g	14	0.9	158	16.0	1.1	10.0	1.1
Chicken & Mushroom, Princes*	1 Serving/50g	94	5.5	187	17.1	5.0	11.0	0.0
Chicken & Stuffing, Princes*	1 Jar/100g	229	17.0	229	15.7	3.3	17.0	0.0
Crab, Princes*	1 Pot/35g	36	1.2	104	13.4	4.8	3.5	0.0
Crab, Sainsbury's*	1 Thick Spread/5g	6	0.2	115	16.5	1.7	4.7	0.5
Curry, Keralan, Waitrose*	¼ Jar/50g	112	8.4	223	3.2	14.9	16.7	1.9
Salmon, Asda*	1 Serving/53g	76	3.7	143	15.0	5.0	7.0	0.0
Salmon, Princes*	1 Serving/30g	58	3.8	195	13.5	6.5	12.8	0.0
Salmon & Shrimp, Tesco*	1 Jar/75g	83	2.6	111	15.1	5.0	3.4	0.1
Sardine & Tomato, Princes*	1 Jar/75g	130	8.1	173	13.9	3.4	10.8	3.2
Sardine & Tomato, Sainsbury's*	1 Mini Pot/35g	60	3.8	170	16.9	1.2	10.8	1.3
Tuna & Mayonnaise, Princes*	1 Pot/75g	86	12.3	115	16.8	3.8	16.4	0.0
Tuna & Mayonnaise, Sainsbury's*	1 Tbsp/17g	41	3.1	242	19.2	0.6	18.1	1.6
PASTILLES								
Blackcurrant, Rowntree's*	1 Tube/53g	188	0.0	353	4.4	84.0	0.0	0.0
Fruit, Average	1 Tube/33g	108	0.0	327	2.8	84.2	0.0	0.0
Fruit, Rowntree's*	1 Tube/53g	186	0.0	351	4.4	83.7	0.0	0.0
Wine, Maynards*	1 Sweet/5g	15	0.0	325	6.1	75.0	0.0	0.0
PASTRAMI								
Beef, Average	***1 Serving/40g***	***51***	***1.4***	***128***	***23.1***	***1.1***	***3.6***	***0.2***
TTD, Sainsbury's*	1 Slice/10g	12	0.3	121	21.6	1.0	3.4	0.4
Turkey, Average	***½ Packet/35g***	***38***	***0.5***	***107***	***21.8***	***1.7***	***1.5***	***0.5***

	Measure INFO/WEIGHT	per Measure KCAL	FAT	Nutrition Values per 100g / 100ml KCAL	PROT	CARB	FAT	FIBRE
PASTRY								
Case, From Supermarket, Average	***1 Case/230g***	***1081***	***58.9***	***470***	***5.8***	***55.9***	***25.6***	***1.2***
Choux, Cooked, Average	***1oz/28g***	***91***	***5.5***	***325***	***8.5***	***29.8***	***19.8***	***1.2***
Choux, Raw, Average	***1oz/28g***	***59***	***3.6***	***211***	***5.5***	***19.4***	***12.9***	***0.8***
Filo, Average	***1 Sheet/45g***	***137***	***1.2***	***304***	***9.0***	***61.4***	***2.7***	***0.9***
Filo, Frozen, Jus-Rol*	1 Sheet/45g	123	1.2	273	8.1	52.1	2.7	2.1
Flaky, Chinese, Average	***1oz/28g***	***110***	***4.6***	***392***	***5.4***	***59.3***	***16.4***	***0.0***
Flaky, Cooked, Average	***1oz/28g***	***157***	***11.4***	***560***	***5.6***	***45.9***	***40.6***	***1.8***
Flaky, Raw, Average	***1oz/28g***	***119***	***8.6***	***424***	***4.2***	***34.8***	***30.7***	***1.4***
Flan Case, Average	***1 Case/113g***	***615***	***38.0***	***544***	***7.1***	***56.7***	***33.6***	***1.8***
Greek, Average	***1oz/28g***	***90***	***4.8***	***322***	***4.7***	***40.0***	***17.0***	***0.0***
Puff, Fresh, Sainsbury's*	½ Pack/250g	1112	85.8	445	5.4	28.8	34.3	1.3
Puff, Frozen, Average	***1 Serving/47g***	***188***	***12.0***	***400***	***5.0***	***29.2***	***25.6***	***0.0***
Puff, Light, Sheet, Jus-Rol*	1 Serving/50g	166	8.2	332	6.4	38.3	16.5	2.3
Shortcrust, Cooked, Average	***1oz/28g***	***146***	***9.0***	***521***	***6.6***	***54.2***	***32.3***	***2.2***
Shortcrust, Raw, Average	***1oz/28g***	***127***	***8.1***	***453***	***5.6***	***44.0***	***29.1***	***1.3***
Spring Roll Wrapper, TYJ Food Manufacturing*	1 Sheet/18g	54	0.0	300	0.0	73.0	0.0	0.0
Wholemeal, Cooked, Average	***1oz/28g***	***140***	***9.2***	***499***	***8.9***	***44.6***	***32.9***	***6.3***
Wholemeal, Raw, Average	***1oz/28g***	***121***	***8.0***	***431***	***7.7***	***38.5***	***28.4***	***5.4***
PASTY								
Beef, Port Royal*	1 Pattie/130g	299	13.3	230	10.2	24.4	10.2	0.0
Cheddar & Onion, Hand Crimped, Waitrose*	1 Pasty/200g	546	42.2	273	8.8	22.5	21.1	2.2
Cheddar & Onion, Westcountry, Multi Pack, Ginsters*	1 Pasty/130g	370	23.9	285	7.1	23.2	18.4	2.0
Cheese, & Onion, Three, Ginsters*	1 Pasty/180g	531	36.9	295	8.0	19.7	20.5	3.1
Cheese & Onion, Average	1 Pasty/150g	435	27.6	290	7.3	24.5	18.4	1.4
Chicken, Port Royal*	1 Pattie/130g	289	10.9	222	5.5	31.2	8.4	0.0
Chicken & Bacon, Ginsters*	1 Pasty/180g	457	29.0	254	8.0	19.3	16.1	2.8
Chicken & Vegetable, Proper Cornish Ltd*	1 Pasty/255g	671	34.7	263	7.4	30.2	13.6	2.4
Chicken Balti, Special Edition, Ginsters*	1 Pasty/180g	398	23.2	221	6.7	19.5	12.9	2.6
Corned Beef, Mega, M & S*	1oz/28g	87	5.7	310	9.5	22.3	20.2	0.9
Cornish, Average	1 Pasty/160g	450	27.7	281	7.0	24.2	17.3	1.6
Cornish, BGTY, Sainsbury's*	1 Pasty/135g	308	12.7	228	7.7	28.2	9.4	1.6
Cornish, Cheese & Onion, Ginsters*	1 Pasty/130g	511	33.0	393	10.4	30.7	25.4	2.3
Cornish, Chicken & Bacon, Ginsters*	1 Pasty/227g	574	34.5	253	6.9	22.2	15.2	0.8
Cornish, Crimped, TTD, Sainsbury's*	1 Pasty/200g	515	28.7	258	8.3	23.7	14.4	1.2
Cornish, Frozen, Oven Baked, Iceland*	1 Pasty/167g	501	29.2	300	7.5	22.0	17.5	0.0
Cornish, Mini, M & S*	1 Pasty/75g	244	17.6	325	7.3	21.9	23.4	1.8
Cornish, Mini, Sainsbury's*	1 Pasty/70g	280	20.1	400	7.3	28.1	28.7	1.5
Cornish, Multi Pack, Ginsters*	1 Pasty/130g	358	24.3	275	6.0	20.6	18.7	2.6
Cornish, Original, Ginsters*	1 Pasty/227g	549	32.2	242	5.3	23.2	14.2	3.1
Cornish, Pork Farms*	1 Pasty/250g	672	40.8	269	7.7	22.8	16.3	0.0
Cornish, Snack Pack, Six, Ginsters*	1 Pasty/40g	116	8.0	289	7.2	20.3	19.9	2.8
Cornish, Traditional Style, Geo Adams*	1 Pasty/165g	488	30.4	296	7.1	25.4	18.4	1.3
Cornish Roaster, Ginsters*	1 Pasty/130g	417	24.2	321	8.5	29.9	18.6	1.3
Lamb, Port Royal*	1 Pattie/130g	352	17.4	271	7.2	30.5	13.4	0.0
Olive & Cheese, Tapas, Waitrose*	1 Pack/130g	455	25.2	350	8.1	35.8	19.4	1.3
Salt Fish, Port Royal*	1 Pattie/130g	300	13.4	231	6.8	27.8	10.3	0.0
Tandoori & Vegetable, Holland & Barrett*	1 Pack/110g	232	9.4	211	4.3	29.4	8.5	1.8
Vegetable	1oz/28g	77	4.2	274	4.1	33.3	14.9	1.9
Vegetable, Hand Crimped, Waitrose*	1 Pasty/200g	454	22.6	227	4.5	26.8	11.3	2.2
Vegetarian, Country Slice, Linda McCartney*	1 Pasty/150g	373	20.2	249	5.6	26.5	13.5	2.9
Vegetarian, Port Royal*	1 Pattie/130g	315	13.8	242	12.5	24.1	10.6	0.0
PATE								
Apricot, Asda*	1 Serving/50g	156	14.0	312	12.0	3.0	28.0	0.0

	Measure INFO/WEIGHT	per Measure KCAL	FAT	Nutrition Values per 100g / 100ml KCAL	PROT	CARB	FAT	FIBRE
PATE								
Ardennes, Asda*	1 Serving/50g	143	12.0	286	13.9	3.6	24.0	1.3
Ardennes, BGTY, Sainsbury's*	¼ Pack/50g	90	5.7	180	16.6	2.9	11.4	0.0
Ardennes, Iceland*	1 Serving/70g	223	20.0	318	12.0	3.4	28.5	0.5
Ardennes, Reduced Fat, Waitrose*	¼ Pack/42g	94	7.1	224	15.4	2.6	16.9	0.5
Ardennes, Tesco*	1 Tbsp/15g	53	5.0	354	13.3	0.5	33.2	1.2
Ardennes, with Bacon, Tesco*	½ Pack/85g	241	20.6	284	11.4	5.1	24.2	1.1
Aubergine, Spiced, Waitrose*	¼ Pack/38g	71	5.2	186	4.9	10.9	13.6	2.4
Bean Feast, The Redwood Co*	1 Serving/60g	161	10.2	268	7.3	21.1	17.0	3.8
Brussels, 25% Less Fat, Morrisons*	¼ Pack/43g	106	8.8	249	14.2	0.7	20.6	0.0
Brussels, BGTY, 50% Less Fat, Sainsbury's*	1 Serving/100g	223	16.0	223	14.6	5.1	16.0	0.1
Brussels, HL, Tesco*	1 Serving/29g	66	4.4	229	14.4	8.4	15.3	1.8
Brussels, M & S*	1 Pot/170g	518	45.2	305	13.3	2.8	26.6	1.0
Brussels, Sainsbury's*	1 Pack/170g	663	64.9	390	10.6	1.1	38.2	0.1
Brussels, Smooth, 50% Less Fat, Tesco*	1 Pack/175g	350	26.8	200	14.1	1.2	15.3	1.8
Brussels, Smooth, Spreadable, Sainsbury's*	1 Serving/30g	97	8.7	323	10.7	4.7	29.0	0.0
Brussels, with Forest Mushroom, Co-Op*	1 Serving/57g	180	16.5	315	12.0	2.0	29.0	1.0
Brussels, with Garlic, Asda*	1 Serving/50g	170	15.6	340	10.7	4.0	31.3	2.5
Brussels, with Herbs, Tesco*	1 Serving/25g	87	8.2	347	8.4	6.4	32.6	1.5
Brussels & Garlic, Reduced Fat, Tesco*	1 Serving/65g	135	8.0	208	16.2	8.1	12.3	0.6
Brussels & Garlic, Tesco*	1 Serving/40g	145	13.5	363	8.7	6.0	33.8	0.0
Brussels & Mushroom, Mini, GFY, Asda*	1 Pack/40g	67	4.4	167	14.7	2.3	11.0	3.9
Brussels Style, Organic, The Redwood Co*	¼ Pack/30g	82	6.1	273	15.2	8.0	20.4	1.3
Carrot, Ginger & Spring Onion, Roasted, M & S*	1 Serving/50g	72	5.5	145	1.5	9.6	11.0	0.9
Celery, Stilton & Walnut, Waitrose*	1 Pot/115g	294	26.4	256	9.0	3.2	23.0	2.2
Chick Pea & Black Olive, Cauldron Foods*	1 Pot/113g	193	11.9	171	7.6	11.4	10.5	6.6
Chicken, with Sauternes, TTD, Sainsbury's*	1 Serving/30g	114	11.1	381	6.5	5.3	37.1	0.6
Chicken & Brandy, Morrisons*	1 Serving/44g	133	11.8	303	10.8	4.3	26.9	0.8
Chicken Liver, & Brandy, Asda*	1 Serving/50g	176	16.4	353	9.0	5.5	32.8	3.2
Chicken Liver, & Garlic, Smooth, Asda*	1 Serving/31g	119	11.1	388	9.0	7.0	36.0	3.2
Chicken Liver, Asda*	1 Serving/65g	131	10.4	202	13.0	4.0	16.0	0.8
Chicken Liver, BGTY, Sainsbury's*	1 Serving/30g	64	4.8	214	11.5	6.0	16.0	0.5
Chicken Liver, M & S*	1oz/28g	79	6.7	281	14.0	1.9	24.1	0.1
Chicken Liver, Parfait, Waitrose*	1 Pack/100g	258	22.9	258	7.5	4.8	22.9	1.1
Chicken Liver, with Brandy, Tesco*	1oz/28g	82	7.2	293	11.8	3.5	25.8	1.4
Chicken Liver, with Madeira, Sainsbury's*	1 Serving/30g	84	7.3	279	13.1	1.9	24.3	0.0
Chickpea, Moroccan, Organic, Cauldron Foods*	½ Pot/58g	119	7.9	207	6.8	16.3	13.7	4.9
Crab, M & S*	1oz/28g	63	4.8	225	12.1	5.9	17.3	0.0
Crab, Terrine, Orkney, Luxury, Castle MacLellan*	1 Tub/113g	250	21.4	221	7.3	5.5	18.9	0.9
De Campagne, Sainsbury's*	1 Serving/55g	129	10.0	235	16.3	1.4	18.2	0.0
Duck & Orange, Asda*	1 Serving/40g	94	7.2	235	16.0	2.2	18.0	0.0
Duck & Orange, Smooth, Tesco*	1 Serving/50g	188	17.7	377	10.5	4.0	35.4	0.5
Duck & Truffle, Medallions, M & S*	1 Serving/25g	91	8.8	365	9.0	4.8	35.0	1.4
Farmhouse, Coarse, Organic, Sainsbury's*	1 Serving/56g	138	11.0	246	13.3	3.7	19.7	0.8
Farmhouse, Simply, M & S*	¼ Pack/42g	113	9.7	265	11.4	3.4	22.8	0.4
Farmhouse, with Herbes De Provence, Tesco*	1 Serving/50g	136	10.8	273	13.9	5.4	21.6	1.0
Farmhouse, with Mushrooms & Garlic, Tesco*	1 Serving/90g	256	22.8	285	13.8	0.6	25.3	1.3
Farmhouse Style, Finest, Tesco*	1 Serving/28g	83	7.3	295	11.9	3.6	25.9	1.0
Farmhouse Style, Weight Watchers*	1 Serving/37g	49	2.1	133	14.8	5.5	5.7	0.5
Forestiere, M & S*	1 Serving/20g	61	5.3	305	11.5	4.2	26.6	1.4
Kipper, Waitrose*	¼ Tub/28g	105	9.2	370	16.8	2.0	32.7	0.6
Liver, Value, Tesco*	1 Serving/50g	151	13.0	302	13.0	4.1	26.0	0.5
Liver & Bacon, Spreading, Value, Tesco*	1 Roll/150g	423	37.2	282	12.7	2.1	24.8	1.4
Liver & Bacon, Tesco*	1 Serving/10g	28	2.3	276	12.9	4.3	23.0	0.4

P

	Measure INFO/WEIGHT	per Measure KCAL	FAT	Nutrition Values per 100g / 100ml KCAL	PROT	CARB	FAT	FIBRE
PATE								
Mackerel, Smoked	1oz/28g	103	9.6	368	13.4	1.3	34.4	0.0
Mousse De Canard, French, Weight Watchers*	1 Portion/50g	122	9.5	245	14.0	4.4	19.0	0.0
Mushroom, BGTY, Sainsbury's*	½ Pot/58g	29	0.3	50	4.6	6.7	0.5	3.0
Mushroom, COU, M & S*	1oz/28g	17	0.5	60	2.9	7.4	1.9	0.9
Mushroom, Farmhouse, Asda*	1 Serving/50g	126	10.0	252	13.0	5.0	20.0	0.7
Mushroom, M & S*	1 Pot/115g	224	20.1	195	4.2	4.8	17.5	1.5
Mushroom, Organic, Cauldron Foods*	1 Pot/113g	170	15.0	150	2.9	6.2	13.3	1.5
Mushroom & Tarragon, Cauldron Foods*	1 Pot/113g	118	9.4	104	2.7	5.9	8.3	1.2
Mushroom & Tarragon, Waitrose*	1 Serving/30g	46	4.0	155	2.8	5.5	13.5	1.4
Parsnip & Carrot, Roasted, Organic, Cauldron Foods*	1 Pot/115g	132	7.7	115	3.5	10.2	6.7	4.9
Parsnip & Carrot, Spiced, Organic, Asda*	½ Pot/58g	63	3.5	109	3.7	10.0	6.0	2.6
Pork, with Apple & Cider, Sainsbury's*	1 Serving/50g	152	12.6	303	12.5	6.3	25.3	1.1
Pork, with Peppercorns, Tesco*	1 Serving/28g	84	7.5	300	12.9	1.4	26.8	0.7
Pork, with Port & Cranberry, Tesco*	1 Serving/28g	83	7.2	296	12.1	4.3	25.6	0.6
Red Pepper, Oven Roasted, Castle MacLellan*	1oz/28g	46	3.8	163	3.3	8.2	13.5	0.8
Red Pepper, Roasted, & Houmous, Princes*	¼ Jar/27g	32	1.6	120	4.6	12.4	5.8	0.0
Red Pepper, Roasted, Princes*	1 Serving/35g	47	1.8	135	4.8	17.6	5.0	0.0
Ricotta, Sun Dried Tomato & Basil, Princes*	1 Jar/110g	343	31.6	312	5.2	8.3	28.7	0.0
Salmon, John West*	1 Serving/50g	136	11.8	272	14.9	0.0	23.5	0.2
Salmon, Organic, M & S*	1oz/28g	76	6.3	270	16.9	0.0	22.5	0.0
Salmon, Poached, & Watercress, Tesco*	1 Serving/25g	60	4.4	238	19.2	0.4	17.7	0.2
Salmon, Smoked, M & S*	1oz/28g	74	6.2	265	16.9	0.0	22.0	0.0
Salmon, Smoked, Scottish, Castle MacLellan*	¼ Tub/28g	76	6.4	271	9.0	7.0	22.9	0.0
Salmon, Smoked, Scottish, M & S*	1 Serving/30g	81	6.7	270	17.0	0.2	22.3	0.0
Salmon Dill, Princes*	1 Serving/70g	124	7.8	177	15.4	4.0	11.1	0.5
Soya & Mushroom, Cauldron Foods*	1 Pot/115g	199	10.8	173	8.8	6.4	9.4	6.5
Spicy Bean, BGTY, Sainsbury's*	½ Pot/58g	56	1.1	97	5.0	15.1	1.9	5.4
Spicy Bean, Princes*	½ Pot/55g	46	0.2	84	3.6	16.7	0.3	0.0
Spicy Bean, Weight Watchers*	1 Serving/37g	33	0.6	89	5.7	12.9	1.6	4.2
Spicy Mexican, Organic, Waitrose*	1 Serving/50g	58	3.1	115	6.2	8.6	6.2	3.5
Spinach, Cheese & Almond, Organic, Cauldron Foods*	½ Pot/58g	103	8.2	179	7.7	5.1	14.2	3.2
Sun-Dried Tomato & Basil, Cauldron Foods*	1 Pot/115g	189	11.7	164	6.9	11.1	10.2	4.6
Tofu, Spicy Mexican, Organic, GranoVita*	1 Serving/50g	108	10.0	216	6.0	3.0	20.0	0.0
Tomato, Lentil & Basil, Cauldron Foods*	1 Pot/115g	161	7.8	140	6.8	14.0	6.8	3.2
Trout, Smoked, Waitrose*	½ Pot/56g	130	10.3	232	15.8	0.9	18.4	0.6
Tuna, M & S*	1oz/28g	106	9.5	380	17.0	0.8	33.8	0.7
Tuna, Tesco*	1 Pack/115g	332	26.7	289	19.8	0.3	23.2	0.2
Vegetable	1oz/28g	48	3.8	173	7.5	5.9	13.4	0.0
Vegetable, Cauldron Foods*	1 Pack/113g	220	12.7	195	9.2	14.1	11.3	4.4
Vegetable, Chargrilled, BGTY, Sainsbury's*	½ Pot/57g	43	0.7	75	4.9	10.8	1.3	2.7
Vegetable, Mediterranean Roast, Tesco*	1 Serving/28g	31	2.6	112	2.4	4.3	9.4	1.2
Vegetable, Roasted, COU, M & S*	1 Pot/115g	86	1.7	75	6.2	9.1	1.5	1.4
Vegetarian, with Mushrooms, Organic, Tartex*	¼ Tube/50g	102	8.0	203	7.7	7.0	16.0	0.0
Yeast, Garlic & Herb, Tartex*	1 Serving/30g	69	5.4	230	7.0	10.0	18.0	0.0
Yeast, Pateole, GranoVita*	1 Portion/30g	66	5.3	219	10.2	4.5	17.8	0.0
Yeast, Wild Mushroom, GranoVita*	1oz/28g	60	4.8	213	10.0	5.0	17.0	0.0
PAVLOVA								
Mandarin, Mini, Iceland*	1 Pavlova/22g	59	2.6	268	2.1	37.9	12.0	1.7
Raspberry, Co-Op*	1/6 Pavlova/49g	147	5.9	300	3.2	44.8	12.0	1.1
Raspberry, M & S*	1 Serving/84g	193	8.1	230	2.3	33.3	9.6	0.3
Raspberry, Mini, Iceland*	1 Pavlova/21g	58	2.9	273	2.3	35.1	13.7	2.6
Raspberry, Sara Lee*	1/6 Pavlova/55g	168	8.5	303	2.7	38.5	15.3	1.1
Raspberry & Lemon, Asda*	1 Serving/43g	102	1.9	235	2.8	46.0	4.4	0.5

	Measure INFO/WEIGHT	per Measure KCAL	FAT	Nutrition Values per 100g / 100ml KCAL	PROT	CARB	FAT	FIBRE
PAVLOVA								
Sticky Toffee, Sainsbury's*	1/6 Pavlova/60g	249	9.8	415	3.7	63.1	16.4	0.9
Strawberry, Co-Op*	1 Serving/52g	177	7.3	340	3.0	50.0	14.0	0.4
Strawberry, COU, M & S*	1 Pot/95g	147	2.3	155	2.4	30.5	2.4	0.8
Strawberry, Farmfoods*	1/6 Pavlova/52g	152	7.8	292	2.3	36.9	15.0	2.2
Strawberry & Champagne, Mini, Co-Op*	1 Pavlova/19g	65	3.6	340	3.0	40.0	19.0	0.8
Toffee, Co-Op*	1/6 Pavlova/53g	193	8.5	365	3.0	52.0	16.0	0.6
Toffee, Mini, Iceland*	1 Pavlova/19g	68	2.9	353	3.0	51.5	15.0	1.9
Toffee Pecan, M & S*	1oz/28g	118	7.4	420	3.9	41.5	26.6	0.4
PAW-PAW								
Raw, Fresh	***1oz/28g***	***10***	***0.0***	***36***	***0.5***	***8.8***	***0.1***	***2.2***
Raw, Weighed with Skin & Pips	***1oz/28g***	***8***	***0.0***	***27***	***0.4***	***6.6***	***0.1***	***1.7***
PEACH								
Dried, Average	***1 Pack/250g***	***472***	***1.6***	***189***	***2.6***	***45.0***	***0.6***	***6.9***
in Fruit Juice, Average	***1oz/28g***	***13***	***0.0***	***47***	***0.5***	***11.2***	***0.0***	***0.7***
in Fruit Juice, Slices, Average	1 Serving/100g	49	0.0	49	0.6	11.6	0.0	0.5
in Light Syrup, Canned, As Sold	1 Serving/100g	66	0.0	66	0.4	15.9	0.0	1.0
in Syrup, Average	***1oz/28g***	***19***	***0.0***	***67***	***0.4***	***16.3***	***0.1***	***0.4***
Raw, Stoned, Average	1oz/28g	9	0.0	33	1.0	7.6	0.1	1.5
Raw, Weighed with Stone, Average	***1 Peach/125g***	***41***	***0.1***	***33***	***1.0***	***7.6***	***0.1***	***1.4***
PEANUT BRITTLE								
Thorntons*	2 Pieces/32g	163	8.6	509	12.4	54.3	26.9	2.6
PEANUT BUTTER								
30% Less Fat, Tesco*	1 Tbsp/15g	86	5.7	570	18.4	37.1	37.9	3.6
Chocolate Flavour, Nuts 'n More*	1 Serving/10g	59	3.8	588	43.8	18.8	37.5	15.6
Creamy, Smooth, Sun Pat*	1 Serving/15g	93	7.5	620	24.0	17.5	50.2	6.1
Crunchy, Basics, Sainsbury's*	1 Serving/10g	61	5.3	610	22.2	12.0	52.6	5.6
Crunchy, Chosen By You, Asda*	1 Serving/10g	60	4.9	603	24.5	15.5	49.2	6.6
Crunchy, Harvest Spread*	1 Serving/25g	148	12.4	592	23.6	12.5	49.7	6.9
Crunchy, No Added Sugar, Organic, Whole Earth*	1 Serving/25g	148	12.6	592	24.9	10.1	50.2	7.3
Crunchy, Organic, Evernat*	1 Tsp/10g	64	5.3	641	29.0	13.0	53.0	7.0
Crunchy, Organic, No Added Sugar, Waitrose*	1 Serving/12g	71	6.0	592	24.9	10.1	50.2	7.3
Crunchy, Organic, Tesco*	1 Serving/25g	149	12.4	595	23.6	12.5	49.7	6.9
Crunchy, Original Style, No Added Sugar, Whole Earth*	1 Serving/20g	129	10.9	643	27.7	7.4	54.3	6.7
Crunchy, Route 66*	1 Serving/10g	65	5.8	648	20.0	13.0	58.0	5.4
Crunchy, Sainsbury's*	1 Serving/10g	62	5.0	620	28.6	12.6	49.6	4.3
Crunchy, Sun Pat*	1 Serving/50g	308	24.4	615	25.3	15.1	48.9	6.8
Crunchy, Tesco*	1 Serving/20g	123	10.2	615	23.8	14.6	50.8	6.4
Crunchy, Whole Nut, Average	1 Tsp/10g	61	5.3	606	24.9	7.7	53.1	6.0
Crunchy, Whole Nut, Organic, Meridian Foods*	1 Serving/28g	171	13.6	612	31.2	12.2	48.7	6.5
Extra Crunch, Skippy*	2 Tbsps/40g	252	20.0	630	22.7	22.9	50.0	7.7
Extra Crunchy, Sun Pat*	1 Serving/20g	119	10.2	597	21.9	12.6	51.0	7.3
GFY, Asda*	1 Serving/15g	80	5.2	531	28.0	31.0	35.0	0.0
Organic, Rapunzel*	1 Serving/5g	31	2.6	613	29.0	4.5	53.0	0.0
Powdered, PB2, Bell Plantation*	2 Tbsp/12g	45	1.5	375	41.7	41.7	12.5	16.7
Smooth, 30% Reduced Fat, Duerr's*	1 Serving/20g	107	7.0	533	22.6	31.7	35.1	6.7
Smooth, 33% Less Fat, BGTY, Sainsbury's*	1 Serving/10g	53	3.5	533	22.6	31.7	35.1	6.7
Smooth, Average	1 Serving/20g	125	10.7	623	22.6	13.1	53.7	5.4
Smooth, Kernel King, Duerr's*	1 Serving/15g	89	7.5	596	23.3	12.4	50.3	6.8
Smooth, Kraft*	1 Serving/20g	127	10.7	636	23.1	17.6	53.5	0.0
Smooth, Light, Kraft*	1 Serving/20g	114	7.7	571	16.3	40.1	38.6	0.0
Smooth, No Added Sugar, Organic, Whole Earth*	1 Serving/20g	126	10.2	628	25.6	13.7	51.2	4.9
Smooth, Organic, Meridian Foods*	1 Serving/10g	61	4.9	612	31.2	12.2	48.7	6.5
Smooth, Organic, Waitrose*	1 Serving/20g	125	10.2	623	28.0	13.0	51.0	0.0

	Measure INFO/WEIGHT	per Measure KCAL	FAT	Nutrition Values per 100g / 100ml KCAL	PROT	CARB	FAT	FIBRE
PEANUT BUTTER								
Smooth, Original, No Added Sugar, Whole Earth*	1 Serving/10g	64	5.4	645	26.3	9.2	54.5	6.5
Smooth, Sun Pat*	1 Serving/20g	123	9.8	614	25.0	15.2	48.9	6.7
Stripy, Sun Pat*	1 Tsp/10g	62	4.7	617	13.0	35.0	47.0	3.0
Wholenut, Sainsbury's*	1 Serving/15g	90	7.7	598	24.2	9.8	51.3	7.0
Wholenut, Waitrose*	1 Serving/12g	70	6.0	587	24.9	9.3	50.0	6.3
PEANUTS								
Chilli, Average	½ Pack/50g	303	25.3	605	28.2	9.3	50.6	6.8
Chilli, Hot, Holland & Barrett*	1 Pack/100g	523	31.0	523	14.0	47.0	31.0	5.5
Chilli, Sweet, Nobby's*	1 Bag/40g	214	13.6	535	15.0	42.0	34.0	3.0
Chocolate Coated, White, Graze*	1 Pack/30g	166	11.8	553	14.7	37.8	39.3	0.0
Dry Roasted, Average	1 Serving/20g	117	9.8	587	25.7	11.5	48.8	6.5
Dry Roasted, Classic, Nobbys*	1 Bag/50g	302	24.0	603	25.0	12.0	48.0	9.0
Honey Roasted, Average	1oz/28g	169	13.2	605	26.8	23.6	47.0	5.5
Plain, Average	***10 Whole/10g***	***59***	***5.0***	***592***	***24.7***	***11.0***	***50.0***	***6.3***
Roast, Salted, Average	10 Whole/12g	74	6.3	614	27.8	7.9	52.4	4.9
Roasted, Love Life, Waitrose*	1 Serving/30g	170	13.8	567	25.6	12.5	46.1	8.0
Salted, Average	10 Whole/6g	37	3.1	609	27.0	8.3	52.0	5.4
Salted, Classic, Nobbys*	1 Bag/50g	315	26.0	630	27.0	11.0	52.0	7.0
Yoghurt Coated, Graze*	1 Pack/35g	189	12.3	540	9.9	48.1	35.1	0.0
PEARL BARLEY								
Boiled	***1oz/28g***	***34***	***0.1***	***123***	***2.3***	***28.2***	***0.4***	***3.8***
Raw, Average	***1oz/28g***	***99***	***0.3***	***352***	***9.9***	***77.7***	***1.2***	***15.6***
PEARS								
Abate Fetel, Average	***1 Med/133g***	***48***	***0.1***	***36***	***0.4***	***8.3***	***0.1***	***2.2***
Asian, Nashi, Raw, Average	***1 Lge/209g***	***88***	***0.5***	***42***	***0.5***	***10.6***	***0.2***	***3.6***
Comice, Raw, Weighed with Core	***1 Med/170g***	***56***	***0.0***	***33***	***0.3***	***8.5***	***0.0***	***2.0***
Conference, Average	***1 Lge/209g***	***88***	***0.2***	***42***	***0.3***	***10.1***	***0.1***	***2.0***
Dried, Average	***1 Pear Half/16g***	***33***	***0.1***	***204***	***1.9***	***48.4***	***0.5***	***9.7***
Dried, Williams, Love Life, Waitrose*	1 Serving/50g	110	0.2	221	1.6	52.4	0.5	8.3
Frozen, Diced, Asda*	1 Serving/50g	24	0.0	47	0.3	10.4	0.1	1.7
in Fruit Juice, Average	***1 Serving/225g***	***102***	***0.1***	***45***	***0.3***	***10.9***	***0.0***	***1.2***
in Syrup, Average	***1oz/28g***	***16***	***0.0***	***58***	***0.2***	***14.4***	***0.1***	***1.4***
Prickly, Raw, Fresh	***1oz/28g***	***14***	***0.1***	***49***	***0.7***	***11.5***	***0.3***	***0.0***
Raw, Weighed with Core, Average	***1 Med/166g***	***62***	***0.2***	***38***	***0.3***	***9.1***	***0.1***	***1.4***
William, Raw, Average	***1 Med/170g***	***58***	***0.2***	***34***	***0.4***	***8.3***	***0.1***	***2.2***
PEAS								
Dried, Boiled in Unsalted Water, Average	***1oz/28g***	***31***	***0.2***	***109***	***6.9***	***19.9***	***0.8***	***5.5***
Dried, Raw, Average	***1oz/28g***	***85***	***0.7***	***303***	***21.6***	***52.0***	***2.4***	***13.0***
Edible Podded, Raw	***1 Cup/63g***	***26***	***0.1***	***42***	***2.8***	***7.6***	***0.2***	***2.6***
Frozen, Average	***1 Serving/85g***	***62***	***0.8***	***73***	***6.0***	***9.7***	***1.0***	***4.5***
Frozen, Boiled, Average	***1 Serving/75g***	***51***	***0.7***	***68***	***6.0***	***9.4***	***0.9***	***5.1***
Garden, Canned, No Sugar Or Salt, Average	***1 Can/80g***	***36***	***0.3***	***45***	***4.4***	***6.0***	***0.4***	***2.8***
Garden, Canned with Sugar & Salt, Average	***1 Serving/90g***	***59***	***0.6***	***66***	***5.3***	***9.3***	***0.7***	***5.1***
Garden, Frozen, Average	***1 Serving/90g***	***66***	***1.0***	***74***	***6.3***	***9.8***	***1.1***	***3.3***
Garden, Minted, Average	***1 Serving/80g***	***59***	***0.9***	***74***	***6.3***	***9.7***	***1.1***	***5.9***
Marrowfat, Average	***1 Sm Can/160g***	***140***	***0.9***	***88***	***6.4***	***14.3***	***0.6***	***3.9***
Mushy, Average	1 Can/200g	173	1.0	86	6.2	14.4	0.5	2.2
Mushy, Frozen, Cooked, Chosen By You, Asda*	1 Serving/80g	75	0.6	94	6.5	11.8	0.8	7.2
Processed, Canned, Average	***1 Sm Can/220g***	***176***	***1.8***	***80***	***6.1***	***12.3***	***0.8***	***3.6***
Snow	***1 Serving/80g***	***24***	***0.2***	***29***	***3.3***	***3.9***	***0.2***	***2.1***
Sugar Snap, Average	***1 Serving/80g***	***27***	***0.2***	***34***	***3.3***	***4.9***	***0.2***	***1.4***
Wasabi, Average	1 Serving/28g	114	3.8	406	15.2	54.0	13.7	8.6
Wasabi, Delicious, Boots*	½ Bag/25g	98	2.4	393	19.0	51.0	9.6	15.0

	Measure INFO/WEIGHT	per Measure KCAL	FAT	Nutrition Values per 100g / 100ml KCAL	PROT	CARB	FAT	FIBRE
PEAS								
Wasabi, Roasted, Savoury Snack, Humdinger*	1 Portion/20g	81	2.4	404	15.8	50.3	12.0	15.9
PEASE PUDDING								
Canned, Re-Heated, Drained	1oz/28g	26	0.2	93	6.8	16.1	0.6	1.8
PECAN NUTS								
Average	***3 Nuts/6g***	***42***	***4.2***	***692***	***10.0***	***5.6***	***70.1***	***4.7***
Honey, Golden, Graze*	1 Pack/26g	168	15.4	647	7.6	23.4	59.4	0.0
PENNE								
Arrabbiata, BGTY, Sainsbury's*	1 Pack/450g	414	7.2	92	2.9	16.5	1.6	1.9
Brown Rice, GF, Organic, Dove's Farm*	1 Serving/100g	338	1.5	338	7.9	70.3	1.5	4.1
Cooked, Average	***1 Serving/185g***	***244***	***1.3***	***132***	***4.7***	***26.7***	***0.7***	***1.1***
Corn, Free From, Dry Weight, Sainsbury's*	1 Serving/100g	348	2.3	348	7.6	74.2	2.3	5.2
Dry, Average	***1 Serving/100g***	***352***	***1.9***	***352***	***12.4***	***71.3***	***1.9***	***2.7***
Dry Weight, Parioli, Cucina*	1 Serving/76g	270	1.1	355	12.5	73.0	1.4	2.6
Egg, Fresh, Average	***1 Serving/125g***	***352***	***4.0***	***282***	***11.1***	***52.2***	***3.2***	***2.0***
Free From, Tesco*	1 Serving/100g	340	2.0	340	8.0	72.5	2.0	2.5
Fresh, Dry, Average	***1 Serving/125g***	***222***	***2.4***	***178***	***7.3***	***32.2***	***1.9***	***1.6***
Organic, Dry, Average	***1 Serving/100g***	***352***	***1.8***	***352***	***12.4***	***71.6***	***1.8***	***1.9***
Rigate, Dry Weight, Average	***1 Serving/90g***	***318***	***1.6***	***353***	***12.3***	***72.1***	***1.8***	***1.8***
Whole Wheat, Asda*	1 Serving/100g	333	2.1	333	12.1	66.3	2.1	6.9
PEPERAMI*								
Firestick, Peperami*	1 Stick/25g	127	11.0	508	24.5	3.5	44.0	1.2
Hot, Peperami*	1 Stick/25g	126	11.0	504	24.5	2.5	44.0	1.2
Lunchbox Minis, 30% Less Fat, Peperami*	1 Stick/10g	38	3.0	379	25.0	1.5	30.0	3.0
Original, Peperami*	1 Stick/25g	126	11.0	504	24.0	2.5	44.0	0.1
Wideboy, Peperami*	1 Stick/40g	202	17.6	504	24.0	2.5	44.0	0.1
PEPPER								
Black, Freshly Ground, Average	***1 Tsp/2g***	***5***	***0.1***	***255***	***11.0***	***64.8***	***3.3***	***26.5***
Cayenne, Ground	***1 Tsp/2g***	***6***	***0.3***	***318***	***12.0***	***31.7***	***17.3***	***0.0***
White	***½ Tsp/1g***	***3***	***0.0***	***296***	***10.4***	***68.6***	***2.1***	***26.2***
PEPPERCORNS								
Black, Schwartz*	1 Tsp/2g	11	0.4	529	13.0	68.7	22.5	27.0
PEPPERS								
Chilli, Chopped, Stir Fry, Schwartz*	1 Tbsp/19g	24	1.2	130	2.2	15.6	6.5	0.0
Chilli, Crushed, Schwartz*	1 Tsp/0.5g	2	0.1	321	12.0	29.0	17.0	27.0
Chilli, Dried, Flakes, Average	1 Tsp/3g	13	0.4	425	16.0	56.0	15.0	44.0
Chilli, Dried, Whole, Red, Schwartz*	1 Tsp/0.5g	2	0.1	425	15.9	56.4	15.1	0.0
Chilli, Green, Raw, Unprepared, Average	***1 Med/13g***	***5***	***0.0***	***40***	***2.0***	***9.5***	***0.2***	***1.5***
Chilli, Green, Very Lazy, The English Provender Co.*	1 Serving/10g	11	0.4	114	4.2	15.3	4.0	0.5
Chilli, Red, Raw, Unprepared, Average	***1 Sm Pepper/13g***	***5***	***0.0***	***40***	***2.0***	***9.5***	***0.2***	***1.5***
Chilli, Red, Very Lazy, The English Provender Co.*	1 Serving/15g	17	0.6	114	4.2	15.3	4.0	0.5
Green, Boiled in Salted Water	***1oz/28g***	***5***	***0.1***	***18***	***1.0***	***2.6***	***0.5***	***1.8***
Green, Filled, Tesco*	1 Pepper/150g	117	5.2	78	2.6	9.0	3.5	0.7
Green, Raw, Unprepared, Average	***1 Med/160g***	***24***	***0.5***	***15***	***0.8***	***2.6***	***0.3***	***1.6***
Italian Style, Sainsbury's*	1 Serving/150g	160	7.5	107	3.5	14.1	5.0	2.1
Jalapeno, Crushed, Schwartz*	1 Tsp/0.5g	1	0.1	136	15.9	56.4	15.1	0.0
Jalapeno, Raw	***1 Cup, Sliced/90g***	***27***	***0.6***	***30***	***1.4***	***5.9***	***0.6***	***2.8***
Mixed Bag, From Supermarket, Average	***1oz/28g***	***7***	***0.1***	***25***	***1.0***	***4.4***	***0.4***	***1.7***
Orange, Sweet, Raw, Average	***1oz/28g***	***8***	***0.1***	***30***	***1.8***	***5.0***	***0.3***	***1.5***
Pickled, Hot, Turkish, Melis, Melis*	1 Serving/25g	9	0.0	35	1.0	7.9	0.0	1.0
Ramiro, Red, Sainsbury's*	1 Serving/100g	30	0.3	30	1.6	5.1	0.3	2.2
Red, Boiled in Salted Water	***1oz/28g***	***10***	***0.1***	***34***	***1.1***	***7.0***	***0.4***	***1.7***
Red, Filled, Halves, Vegetarian, M & S*	1 Pack/295g	280	10.3	95	2.9	12.3	3.5	1.1
Red, Filled with Feta, COU, M & S*	1 Pepper/154g	200	11.1	130	4.1	12.4	7.2	0.6

P

	Measure INFO/WEIGHT	per Measure KCAL	FAT	Nutrition Values per 100g / 100ml KCAL	PROT	CARB	FAT	FIBRE
PEPPERS								
Red, Raw, Unprepared, Average	1oz/28g	9	0.1	32	1.0	6.4	0.4	1.6
Red, Roasted, in Brine, Cooks & Co*	1 Serving/100g	23	0.3	23	1.6	4.5	0.3	0.0
Red, Roasted, Melis*	1 Serving/100g	90	1.0	90	1.1	18.8	1.0	0.2
Red, Sweet, Pointed, TTD, Sainsbury's*	1 Serving/100g	32	0.4	32	1.0	6.4	0.4	0.0
Stuffed, Fresh, Asda*	1 Pepper/150g	144	7.5	96	3.8	9.0	5.0	1.2
Stuffed, Perfectly Balanced, Waitrose*	1 Pack/300g	243	7.2	81	3.0	11.8	2.4	1.3
Stuffed, Sainsbury's*	1 Serving/137g	169	9.5	123	3.3	11.8	6.9	1.0
Stuffed, with Rice Based Filling, Average	1oz/28g	24	0.7	85	1.5	15.4	2.4	1.3
Stuffed, with Vegetables, Cheese Topping, Average	1oz/28g	31	1.9	111	3.4	9.8	6.7	1.5
Sweet, Pointed, Extra Special, Asda*	1 Serving/100g	36	0.4	36	1.0	6.4	0.4	1.6
Sweet, Raw, Average	***1 Serving/100g***	***16***	***0.3***	***16***	***0.8***	***2.6***	***0.3***	***1.6***
Sweet, Tinned, Sainsbury's*	½ Can/125g	45	0.5	36	1.1	7.0	0.4	1.7
Yellow, Raw, Unprepared, Average	***1 Med/160g***	***42***	***0.3***	***26***	***1.2***	***5.3***	***0.2***	***1.7***
PERCH								
Raw, Atlantic	***1oz/28g***	***26***	***0.5***	***94***	***18.6***	***0.0***	***1.6***	***0.0***
PERNOD*								
19% Volume, Pernod*	***1 Shot/35ml***	***46***	***0.0***	***130***	***0.0***	***0.0***	***0.0***	***0.0***
PESTO								
Sauce, Basil, M & S*	1 Serving/65g	348	30.5	535	7.5	20.7	46.9	1.4
Sauce, Dressing, Finest, Tesco*	1 Serving/30ml	108	11.1	360	3.5	2.9	37.1	0.9
Sauce, Fiery Chilli, Sacla*	½ Jar/95g	342	29.3	360	4.8	16.0	30.8	3.4
Sauce, Green, Average	¼ Jar/48g	246	22.6	517	20.4	2.0	47.5	0.0
Sauce, Green, Classic, Sacla*	1 Serving/40g	185	18.6	462	5.2	7.6	46.5	0.0
Sauce, Green, Fresh, Sainsbury's*	1 Serving/60g	328	31.7	546	9.4	8.3	52.8	0.1
Sauce, Green, Less Than 60% Fat, BGTY, Sainsbury's*	¼ Jar/48g	61	5.3	128	4.2	2.6	11.2	0.0
Sauce, Green, Verde, Bertolli*	¼ Jar/46g	266	27.5	575	5.7	4.3	59.5	0.0
Sauce, Mary Berry*	1 Serving/100g	528	49.3	528	1.1	19.4	49.3	1.1
Sauce, Red, Garlic & Chilli, Jamie Oliver*	1 Jar/190g	494	48.8	260	1.1	5.6	25.7	1.1
Sauce, Red, Italian, Tesco*	1 Serving/38g	128	11.5	340	8.2	8.2	30.6	1.2
Sauce, Red, M & S*	1oz/28g	93	9.3	331	3.6	6.9	33.2	3.5
Sauce, Red, Rosso, Bertolli*	1 Jar/185g	703	64.8	380	6.8	9.5	35.0	2.0
Sauce, Red, Tesco*	¼ Jar/50g	162	15.2	325	5.6	6.3	30.3	6.0
Sauce, Ricotta & Red Pepper, Chosen By You, Asda*	1 Jar/190g	486	37.2	256	4.2	14.4	19.6	2.4
Sauce, Spinach & Parmesan, Sainsbury's*	¼ Jar/46g	162	16.0	349	4.6	5.3	34.4	2.5
Sauce, Sun Dried Tomato, Sacla*	1 Serving/30g	87	8.4	289	4.2	5.2	27.9	0.0
Sauce, Verde, Traditional Italian, Sacla*	1 Serving/100g	454	45.4	454	5.3	6.0	45.4	0.0
PETIT POIS								
& Baby Carrots, Canned, Drained, Average	½ Can/122g	58	0.8	47	2.9	7.0	0.7	3.2
Canned, Drained, Average	1 Sm Can/200g	125	1.0	63	4.8	8.9	0.5	2.6
Fresh, Frozen, Average	1 Serving/80g	51	0.8	63	5.4	7.1	1.0	4.8
PHEASANT								
Breast, Fillets, Skinless, Cooked, Gressingham Foods*	1 Serving/100g	127	2.4	127	32.7	0.0	2.4	0.0
Meat Only, Roasted	***1oz/28g***	***62***	***3.4***	***220***	***27.9***	***0.0***	***12.0***	***0.0***
Meat Only, Roasted, Weighed with Bone	***1oz/28g***	***61***	***3.3***	***219***	***27.9***	***0.0***	***11.9***	***0.0***
Stuffed, Easy Carve, Finest, Tesco*	1 Serving/200g	540	37.4	270	23.2	2.2	18.7	0.9
Whole with Bacon, Cooked, Gressingham Foods*	1 Serving/100g	220	14.5	220	21.9	0.0	14.5	0.0
PHYSALIS								
Goldenberries, Dried, Neal's Yard*	1 Serving/20g	60	1.6	302	6.0	42.8	8.0	17.4
Raw, without Husk, Average	***5 Fruits/30g***	***16***	***0.2***	***53***	***1.9***	***11.2***	***0.7***	***0.4***
PICCALILLI								
Dijon, Sainsbury's*	1 Dtsp/15g	14	0.1	91	1.8	19.0	0.9	0.7
Haywards*	1 Serving/28g	18	0.1	66	1.4	13.9	0.5	0.0
Heinz*	1 Serving/10g	10	0.1	99	1.0	20.5	0.6	0.6

	Measure INFO/WEIGHT	per Measure KCAL	FAT	Nutrition Values per 100g / 100ml KCAL	PROT	CARB	FAT	FIBRE
PICCALILLI								
Sandwich, Tesco*	1 Serving/20g	16	0.0	80	0.4	18.5	0.0	1.6
Spicy, Sainsbury's*	1 Serving/15g	12	0.1	80	0.7	15.3	0.5	1.0
Sweet, Asda*	1 Tbsp/15g	17	0.0	112	0.5	27.0	0.2	0.6
Tesco*	1 Serving/50g	51	1.8	102	0.5	17.8	3.6	2.0
Three Mustard, Finest, Tesco*	1 Serving/30g	40	0.2	134	1.3	30.7	0.7	1.0
TTD, Sainsbury's*	1 Serving/19g	13	0.2	67	0.7	13.9	0.9	1.8
PICKLE								
Branston, Beetroot, Crosse & Blackwell*	1 Tsp/20g	25	0.1	123	1.2	28.2	0.3	1.6
Branston, Red Onion & Cranberry, Crosse & Blackwell*	1 Tbsp/14g	13	0.1	92	0.6	21.4	0.4	0.8
Branston, Red Pepper & Tomato, Crosse & Blackwell*	1 Tbsp/14g	12	0.0	84	1.2	17.7	0.3	1.1
Branston, Small Chunk, Squeezy, Crosse & Blackwell*	1 Serving/15g	19	0.0	127	0.9	29.8	0.2	1.1
Branston, Smooth, Squeezy, Crosse & Blackwell*	1 Serving/15g	19	0.0	127	0.9	29.8	0.2	1.1
Branston, Sweet, Original, Crosse & Blackwell*	1 Serving/15g	17	0.0	112	0.8	26.1	0.2	1.1
Branston, Sweet, Small Chunk, Crosse & Blackwell*	1 Serving/20g	22	0.0	109	0.8	26.1	0.2	1.1
Brinjal, Patak's*	1 Tsp/16g	59	3.9	367	2.2	34.6	24.4	0.9
Chilli, Patak's*	1 Tsp/16g	52	5.4	325	4.3	1.3	33.7	0.0
Cornichons, in Sweet & Sour Vinegar, Waitrose*	1 Serving/10g	3	0.0	28	0.6	6.1	0.1	0.6
Garlic, Patak's*	1 Tsp/16g	42	3.0	261	3.6	20.0	18.5	1.6
Ginger, Priya*	1 Tsp/10g	27	1.7	270	3.3	26.7	16.7	0.0
Green Chilli, Priya*	1 Tsp/10g	19	1.7	190	3.3	6.7	16.7	4.8
Hot Chilli Jam, What A Pickle*	1 Tsp/8g	14	0.0	178	0.6	44.0	0.1	1.2
Lime, Hot, Asda*	1 Dtsp/10g	12	1.0	123	2.2	6.0	10.0	1.0
Lime, Hot, Patak's*	1 Tsp/16g	31	3.0	194	2.2	4.0	18.7	0.4
Lime, M & S*	1 Tsp/16g	34	0.8	215	0.8	42.5	4.8	2.4
Lime, Sharwood's*	1 Tbsp/20g	28	2.0	142	1.7	11.5	9.9	1.3
Mango, Hot, Patak's*	1 Tsp/16g	43	4.1	270	2.3	7.4	25.7	1.9
Mixed, Drained	1 Serving/100g	14	0.2	14	1.0	1.9	0.2	1.0
Onion, Priya*	1 Tsp/10g	20	1.5	203	3.3	13.3	15.0	0.0
Red Cabbage, Asda*	1 Serving/50g	16	0.0	32	1.6	6.0	0.1	0.0
Red Chilli, Priya*	1 Tsp/10g	22	1.7	217	3.3	13.3	16.7	0.0
Sandwich, Tangy, Heinz*	1 Tsp/10g	13	0.0	134	0.7	31.4	0.2	0.9
Sandwich, Tesco*	1 Serving/5g	7	0.0	138	1.0	33.1	0.2	1.0
Sweet	***1 Tsp/10g***	***14***	***0.0***	***141***	***0.6***	***36.0***	***0.1***	***1.2***
Sweet, Frank Cooper*	1 Pot/20g	21	0.0	104	0.5	25.3	0.1	0.8
Sweet, Hartley's*	1 Tsp/16g	22	0.0	140	0.5	36.2	0.0	0.0
Tomato, Priya*	1 Tsp/10g	22	1.7	217	3.3	13.3	16.7	0.0
Tomato, Tangy, Heinz*	1 Tsp/10g	10	0.0	102	2.0	22.0	0.3	1.5
PICNIC								
Cadbury*	1 Bar/48g	230	10.9	475	7.3	60.9	22.6	2.1
PIE								
Admiral's, Light & Easy, Youngs*	1 Pack/360g	342	14.0	95	4.1	10.9	3.9	0.8
Admiral's, Ross*	1 Pie/340g	357	15.6	105	4.8	10.9	4.6	0.7
Apple, American, Iceland*	1 Serving/92g	258	10.7	280	4.8	39.2	11.6	2.2
Apple, Asda*	¼ Pack/107g	287	11.7	269	3.6	39.0	11.0	1.7
Apple, Bramley, & Blackberry, Aunt Bessie's*	¼ Pie/138g	344	12.5	250	2.1	40.1	9.1	2.6
Apple, Bramley, & Blackberry, M & S*	¼ Pie/146g	380	14.5	260	3.4	39.8	9.9	1.3
Apple, Bramley, & Custard, Lattice Topped, Mr Kipling*	1 Pie/64g	236	9.9	369	3.8	53.7	15.4	1.1
Apple, Bramley, & Damson, M & S*	¼ Pie/142g	370	13.9	260	3.3	39.7	9.8	2.1
Apple, Bramley, Aunt Bessie's*	¼ Pie/138g	351	15.1	255	2.8	36.2	11.0	1.2
Apple, Bramley, Deep Filled, Sainsbury's*	1/6 Pie/120g	329	14.3	274	3.7	38.0	11.9	1.9
Apple, Bramley, Free From, Sainsbury's*	1 Pie/60g	220	7.6	367	1.1	61.8	12.6	1.2
Apple, Bramley, Individual, Mr Kipling*	1 Pie/66g	228	8.6	346	3.4	53.8	13.0	1.4
Apple, Bramley, Large, Tesco*	1/8 Pie/87g	311	13.0	358	3.9	51.9	15.0	1.9

P

	Measure INFO/WEIGHT	per Measure KCAL	FAT	Nutrition Values per 100g / 100ml KCAL	PROT	CARB	FAT	FIBRE
PIE								
Apple, Bramley, Less Than 10% Fat, Sainsbury's*	1 Pie/54g	165	5.0	307	3.6	52.2	9.3	1.3
Apple, Bramley, M & S*	1 Pie/55g	184	6.4	335	2.9	57.6	11.7	1.6
Apple, Bramley, Rowan Hill Bakery*	1 Pie/64g	216	8.3	337	3.6	51.5	13.0	1.4
Apple, Deep Filled, Amanda Smith*	1/5 Pie/150g	420	19.8	280	2.8	37.4	13.2	1.2
Apple, Deep Filled, Iceland*	1 Serving/116g	332	15.3	286	2.5	39.2	13.2	1.1
Apple, Lattice, Tesco*	1 Serving/145g	325	13.3	224	2.2	33.2	9.2	1.4
Apple, Low Price, Sainsbury's*	¼ Pie/103g	291	15.0	283	4.4	33.5	14.6	1.3
Apple, McVitie's*	1 Serving/117g	316	12.9	270	3.0	39.0	11.0	2.0
Apple, Puff Pastry, M & S*	1 Pie/135g	338	17.1	250	2.4	31.3	12.7	1.0
Apple, Ready Baked, Sara Lee*	1/6 Pie/90g	249	12.4	277	2.8	35.4	13.8	1.2
Apple, Sainsbury's*	1/6 Pie/118g	314	13.6	266	3.4	37.1	11.5	0.6
Apple, Sultana & Cinnamon, Finest, Tesco*	1 Slice/83g	193	7.3	233	2.8	35.6	8.8	5.0
Apple, VLH Kitchens	1 Serving/50g	136	22.4	272	3.7	40.0	11.2	1.7
Apple, with Custard	1 Serving/217g	353	18.8	163	2.4	25.2	8.7	1.1
Apple & Blackberry, Co-Op*	1 Serving/138g	338	15.2	245	3.0	33.0	11.0	2.0
Apple & Blackberry, Fruit, Finest, Tesco*	1 Pie/95g	265	11.3	279	13.7	29.3	11.9	2.8
Apple & Blackberry, Lattice Topped, BGTY, Sainsbury's*	¼ Pie/100g	256	7.5	256	2.8	44.4	7.5	3.1
Apple & Blackberry, Shortcrust, M & S*	1 Serving/142g	469	17.8	330	4.3	50.2	12.5	1.1
Apple & Blackberry, Tesco*	1 Serving/106g	287	11.9	271	4.2	38.4	11.2	1.7
Apple & Blackcurrant, Mr Kipling*	1 Pie/66g	211	8.4	320	3.3	47.9	12.8	1.2
Apple Meringue, Frozen, Sara Lee*	1/6 Pie/74g	179	6.5	242	2.7	37.9	8.8	1.5
Apricot Fruit, GFY, Asda*	1 Serving/52g	162	5.2	311	3.3	52.0	10.0	0.0
Banoffee, Individual, Sainsbury's*	1 Pie/104g	365	21.0	351	3.2	39.2	20.2	2.2
Banoffee, Mini, Waitrose*	1 Pie/26g	115	5.8	444	3.3	57.0	22.5	1.2
Banoffee, Tesco*	1/6 Pie/94g	365	19.7	390	3.9	45.8	21.1	1.5
Banoffee Cream, American Dream, Heinz*	1/6 Pie/70g	239	15.0	342	3.7	33.7	21.4	3.9
Beef, Lean, BGTY, Sainsbury's*	1 Serving/212g	280	12.7	132	7.3	12.2	6.0	1.5
Beef, Sainsbury's*	1 Pie/210g	535	30.0	255	10.3	21.2	14.3	2.0
Beef, Shamrock, Pieminister*	1 Pie/270g	648	30.8	240	8.8	24.5	11.4	1.8
Beef & Kidney, 208, Oakhouse Foods Ltd*	1 Meal/360g	540	24.8	150	6.5	15.1	6.9	1.8
Beef & Onion, Pukka Pies Ltd*	1 Serving/231g	529	32.6	229	7.6	17.9	14.1	3.0
Beef & Vegetable, Macdougalls, McDougalls*	¼ Pie/114g	292	19.3	256	5.3	20.6	16.9	0.3
Beef Steak, Aberdeen Angus, Top Crust, Waitrose*	½ Pie/280g	476	24.1	170	10.0	13.4	8.6	4.1
Blackberry & Apple, Sara Lee*	1 Serving/100g	272	13.9	272	2.9	34.0	13.9	0.0
Blackcurrant, Deep Filled, Sainsbury's*	1 Slice/137g	440	19.3	321	5.8	42.6	14.1	2.2
Blackcurrant, Shortcrust, M & S*	1 Pie/142g	412	14.3	290	3.9	45.6	10.1	1.3
Butternut Squash, Skinny, & Red Pepper, Little, Higgidy*	1 Pie/180g	367	23.6	204	4.2	17.2	13.1	1.6
Cheese & Onion, Hollands*	1 Pie/200g	516	24.4	258	6.3	30.9	12.2	0.0
Cheese & Onion, Oven Baked, Average	1 Serving/200g	654	40.0	327	8.2	30.4	20.0	1.2
Cheese & Potato	1oz/28g	39	2.3	139	4.8	12.6	8.1	0.7
Cheese & Potato, Aunt Bessie's*	¼ Serving/200g	288	18.8	144	4.6	11.7	9.4	1.5
Cherry, & Custard, Diabetic, 903, Wiltshire Farm Foods*	1 Serving/150g	255	14.6	170	1.9	19.0	9.7	0.6
Cherry, Asda*	1/6 Pie/117g	337	14.5	289	3.1	41.2	12.4	1.8
Cherry, Sainsbury's*	1 Serving/117g	325	13.6	278	3.9	39.6	11.6	1.7
Chicken, Aunt Bessie's*	¼ Pie/200g	474	24.2	237	10.6	21.4	12.1	2.1
Chicken, Bacon & Cheddar Cheese, Lattice, Birds Eye*	1 Pie/155g	454	26.8	293	13.4	21.0	17.3	1.5
Chicken, Broccoli & White Wine, Waitrose*	1 Serving/200g	605	40.5	302	12.6	17.7	20.2	2.3
Chicken, Cheese & Bacon, HL, Tesco*	1 Pack/450g	382	9.9	85	5.9	9.4	2.2	1.6
Chicken, Cheese & Broccoli Lattice, Birds Eye*	1 Pie/155g	446	25.3	288	12.6	22.7	16.3	1.1
Chicken, Cheese & Leek Lattice, Sun Valley*	1 Lattice/125g	315	21.9	252	15.2	8.6	17.5	1.0
Chicken, Cottage, Frozen, Tesco*	1 Pack/450g	292	2.2	65	2.8	11.7	0.5	1.0
Chicken, Deep Filled, Puff Pastry, Sainsbury's*	1 Pie/210g	538	31.9	256	10.0	19.9	15.2	3.1
Chicken, Finest, Tesco*	1 Pie/250g	615	32.2	246	10.7	21.9	12.9	1.2

	Measure INFO/WEIGHT	per Measure KCAL	FAT	Nutrition Values per 100g / 100ml KCAL	PROT	CARB	FAT	FIBRE
PIE								
Chicken, Ginsters*	¼ Pie/136g	374	23.7	275	10.0	19.0	17.4	1.0
Chicken, Individual, Made with 100% Breast, Birds Eye*	1 Pie/154g	455	28.1	296	7.9	25.0	18.3	1.0
Chicken, Individual Shortcrust, Asda*	1 Pie/175g	534	29.8	305	10.0	28.0	17.0	1.0
Chicken, Leek & Ham, Morrisons*	1 Serving/113g	305	16.6	270	8.8	25.7	14.7	1.1
Chicken, Leek & Sweetcorn, Love Life, Waitrose*	1 Pie/421g	358	14.3	85	5.2	8.6	3.4	1.7
Chicken, Newgate*	1 Pie/142g	358	23.6	252	6.1	23.1	16.6	1.0
Chicken, Puff Pastry, Tesco*	¼ Pie/114g	250	12.7	220	8.6	21.3	11.2	1.4
Chicken, Roast, & Vegetable, Pot, M & S*	1/3 Pie/183g	366	22.9	200	7.7	13.5	12.5	4.5
Chicken, Roast, COU, M & S*	1 Pack/320g	272	3.2	85	9.4	9.7	1.0	0.8
Chicken, Roast, in Gravy, Deep Fill, Tesco*	1 Pie/700g	1540	68.6	220	11.2	20.2	9.8	2.0
Chicken, Roast, M & S*	1/3 Pie/182g	465	24.1	255	7.8	26.4	13.2	2.2
Chicken, Roast, Puff Pastry, Deep Fill, Asda*	½ Pie/259g	739	44.1	285	10.0	23.0	17.0	0.8
Chicken, Roast, Shortcrust, Sainsbury's*	1 Pie/200g	1012	56.0	506	19.2	44.4	28.0	2.4
Chicken, Short Crust, M & S*	1 Pie/170g	510	29.6	300	9.7	26.2	17.4	1.7
Chicken, Tomato & Basil Lattice, Birds Eye*	1 Serving/155g	340	19.6	220	10.8	15.7	12.7	1.4
Chicken & Asparagus, Lattice, Waitrose*	1 Serving/100g	295	19.6	295	7.4	22.3	19.6	1.8
Chicken & Asparagus, McDougalls*	1 Serving/170g	394	21.9	232	7.4	21.6	12.9	1.5
Chicken & Asparagus, Puff Pasty, John Bullers*	1 Pie/174g	477	29.6	274	11.0	19.0	17.0	2.0
Chicken & Asparagus, Tesco*	1 Serving/170g	468	28.7	275	8.3	22.4	16.9	0.8
Chicken & Bacon, Filo Pastry, Finest, Tesco*	1 Serving/160g	362	18.7	226	11.3	18.9	11.7	1.7
Chicken & Bacon, Puff Pastry, Deep Fill, Sainsbury's*	1/3 Pie/200g	532	34.0	266	9.1	19.1	17.0	1.3
Chicken & Bacon, with Cheese Sauce, Tesco*	1 Serving/200g	540	33.6	270	12.0	17.6	16.8	0.8
Chicken & Basil, M & S*	1oz/28g	59	3.3	210	8.9	17.0	11.9	1.1
Chicken & Broccoli, BGTY, Sainsbury's*	1 Pack/450g	297	3.6	66	5.9	8.9	0.8	1.8
Chicken & Broccoli, COU, M & S*	1 Serving/320g	272	6.1	85	8.1	8.8	1.9	1.3
Chicken & Broccoli, Lattice, Sainsbury's*	½ Pie/192g	520	30.7	271	9.3	22.4	16.0	0.9
Chicken & Broccoli, LC, Tesco*	1 Pack/450g	382	7.2	85	7.0	10.3	1.6	0.8
Chicken & Gravy, Deep Fill, Asda*	1 Serving/130g	370	22.1	285	10.0	23.0	17.0	0.8
Chicken & Gravy, LC, Tesco*	1 Pack/450g	410	10.9	90	5.9	10.6	2.4	1.4
Chicken & Gravy, Shortcrust Pastry, Large, Tesco*	1 Pie/600g	1578	91.2	263	8.2	23.4	15.2	1.0
Chicken & Gravy, Shortcrust Pastry, Sainsbury's*	1 Serving/250g	638	35.2	255	8.0	24.1	14.1	1.0
Chicken & Ham, Charlie Bigham's*	1 Pie/325g	679	39.6	209	10.0	14.2	12.2	0.9
Chicken & Ham, Deep Filled, Sainsbury's*	1 Pie/210g	594	37.2	283	8.0	23.0	17.7	1.0
Chicken & Ham, Family, Farmfoods*	1oz/28g	67	3.9	241	9.9	19.4	13.8	1.2
Chicken & Ham, Sainsbury's*	1 Pie/128g	461	28.7	360	11.0	28.5	22.4	2.0
Chicken & Ham, Tesco*	1 Serving/113g	293	17.6	259	9.4	20.2	15.6	1.2
Chicken & Leek, Deep Filled, Puff Pastry, Sainsbury's*	1/3 Pie/451g	1109	65.4	246	10.1	18.7	14.5	1.5
Chicken & Leek, LC, Tesco*	1 Pie/350g	298	5.6	85	6.6	10.3	1.6	1.3
Chicken & Leek, M & S*	1oz/28g	70	4.2	250	10.1	18.8	15.1	1.1
Chicken & Leek, Shortcrust, TTD, Sainsbury's*	½ Pie/300g	824	48.8	275	12.2	19.8	16.3	1.1
Chicken & Mushroom, & Potato, Filo, COU, M & S*	1 Pack/260g	273	7.0	105	7.5	12.1	2.7	1.5
Chicken & Mushroom, Average	1 Serving/200g	540	31.7	270	8.0	23.8	15.9	1.0
Chicken & Mushroom, Chilled, Weight Watchers*	1 Pack/400g	304	4.8	76	5.7	9.8	1.2	1.5
Chicken & Mushroom, Deep Filled, Frozen, Tesco*	¼ Pie/198g	465	22.2	235	9.0	23.8	11.2	1.2
Chicken & Mushroom, Dietary Specials*	1 Pie/140g	300	14.0	214	6.3	24.7	10.0	0.9
Chicken & Mushroom, Fray Bentos*	1 Pie/425g	684	40.4	161	6.7	11.5	9.5	0.0
Chicken & Mushroom, Ginsters*	1 Pie/180g	486	31.1	270	8.3	20.2	17.3	1.3
Chicken & Mushroom, Individual, Frozen, Tesco*	1 Pie/141.75	347	17.9	245	8.9	23.5	12.6	1.2
Chicken & Mushroom, Luxury, M & S*	½ Pie/275g	880	61.9	320	9.9	20.0	22.5	1.0
Chicken & Mushroom, Puff Pastry, Birds Eye*	1 Pie/152g	415	21.3	273	11.9	24.9	14.0	1.6
Chicken & Mushroom, Pukka Pies Ltd*	1 Pie/226g	475	29.2	210	7.6	15.7	12.9	3.5
Chicken & Mushroom, Weight Watchers*	1 Pie/136g	317	15.1	233	8.0	25.1	11.1	1.5
Chicken & Vegetable, Farmfoods*	1 Pie/128g	384	24.1	300	7.2	25.4	18.8	1.4

	Measure INFO/WEIGHT	per Measure KCAL	FAT	Nutrition Values per 100g / 100ml KCAL	PROT	CARB	FAT	FIBRE
PIE								
Chicken & Vegetable, Freshbake*	1 Pie/125g	319	19.6	255	6.5	21.8	15.7	2.7
Chicken & Vegetable, Kids, Tesco*	1 Serving/235g	235	10.6	100	5.9	9.1	4.5	0.7
Chicken & Vegetable, Perfectly Balanced, Waitrose*	1 Serving/375g	285	5.2	76	5.1	10.8	1.4	1.3
Chicken Balti, Ginsters*	1 Pie/180g	416	25.0	231	7.3	19.2	13.9	1.9
Chicken Curry, Iceland*	1 Pie/156g	440	23.7	282	10.2	26.2	15.2	2.0
Chicken Pot, with Ham & Leek, Higgidy*	1 Pie/250g	710	33.5	284	13.1	19.1	13.4	1.1
Chocolate, Mini, Waitrose*	1 Pie/24g	109	6.1	455	5.3	51.4	25.3	1.7
Cod & Smoked Haddock, COU, M & S*	1 Pack/400g	320	9.6	80	6.1	9.0	2.4	1.2
Cottage, Aberdeen Angus, Waitrose*	1 Pie/350g	340	12.2	97	5.3	11.0	3.5	0.9
Cottage, Aunt Bessie's*	1 Pack/350g	413	18.2	118	4.8	12.1	5.2	1.0
Cottage, Chicken, Tesco*	1 Pack/400g	340	2.8	85	6.0	12.8	0.7	1.7
Cottage, COU, M & S*	1 Pack/400g	340	8.0	85	6.0	11.0	2.0	1.5
Cottage, Diet Chef Ltd*	1 Pack/270g	235	9.7	87	3.7	9.8	3.6	1.7
Cottage, Disney, Tesco*	1 Pack/281g	250	7.0	89	4.9	11.8	2.5	1.9
Cottage, Family, Iceland*	¼ Pack/259g	262	10.6	101	4.2	11.8	4.1	0.8
Cottage, Fresh, M & S*	1 Pie/400g	460	22.4	115	6.8	9.9	5.6	0.6
Cottage, Frozen, Chosen By You, Asda*	1 Pack/400g	368	9.6	92	6.5	10.6	2.4	1.0
Cottage, Healthy Living, Co-Op*	1 Pack/400g	320	6.4	80	5.0	11.0	1.6	2.0
Cottage, LC, Tesco*	1 Pack/500g	400	8.5	80	4.5	11.4	1.7	1.7
Cottage, Lentil & Vegetable, Linda McCartney*	1 Pot/398g	374	10.3	94	2.8	13.5	2.6	2.5
Cottage, Luxury, M & S*	½ Pack/310g	403	21.7	130	7.9	8.3	7.0	1.8
Cottage, Meal for One, M & S*	1 Pack/445g	356	16.0	80	5.4	6.2	3.6	1.7
Cottage, Meatfree, Sainsbury's*	1 Pack/400g	364	12.0	91	4.4	11.7	3.0	0.7
Cottage, Mini, Waitrose*	1 Pack/250g	268	10.5	107	6.4	11.1	4.2	1.4
Cottage, Retail, Average	1 Pack/400g	399	15.7	100	5.5	10.5	3.9	1.3
Cottage, Ross*	1 Pack/320g	240	7.0	75	3.0	10.9	2.2	0.3
Cottage, Salmon, Sainsbury's*	1 Serving/299g	218	4.2	73	4.6	10.4	1.4	1.3
Cottage, Vegetarian, Sainsbury's*	1 Pack/450g	328	9.9	73	3.0	10.2	2.2	1.8
Cottage, Weight Watchers*	1 Pack/300g	186	3.9	62	3.6	9.0	1.3	0.3
Cottage, You Count, Love Life, Waitrose*	1 Pack/402g	291	7.0	82	4.4	10.9	2.0	1.2
Country, Vegetarian, Tesco*	1 Pie/142g	381	21.6	268	5.6	27.3	15.2	1.2
Cumberland, Asda*	1 Pack/400g	504	22.4	126	6.3	12.7	5.6	1.5
Cumberland, Beef, HL, Tesco*	1 Pack/500g	460	13.5	92	5.0	11.8	2.7	0.9
Cumberland, BGTY, Sainsbury's*	1 Pack/450g	360	9.0	80	5.3	10.1	2.0	1.6
Cumberland, Cod & Prawn, Tesco*	1 Pack/450g	428	11.2	95	7.9	9.5	2.5	1.3
Cumberland, GFY, Asda*	1 Pack/451g	469	9.9	104	11.4	11.4	2.2	2.1
Cumberland, HL, Tesco*	1 Pie/500g	430	13.5	86	4.5	10.8	2.7	1.2
Cumberland, M & S*	1 Pie/195g	312	20.3	160	6.9	10.1	10.4	1.1
Farmhouse, Vegetable, Linda McCartney*	1 Pie/146g	380	23.2	260	5.8	23.4	15.9	1.6
Fish	1 Serving/250g	262	7.5	105	8.0	12.3	3.0	0.7
Fish, BFY, Morrisons*	1 Pack/350g	301	10.2	86	5.0	10.0	2.9	0.9
Fish, Chilled, GFY, Asda*	1 Pie/450g	405	12.6	90	6.8	9.3	2.8	1.4
Fish, Creamy, Classics, Large, Finest, Tesco*	½ Pack/350g	402	19.6	115	6.4	8.6	5.6	0.9
Fish, Cumberland, BGTY, Sainsbury's*	1 Serving/450g	342	8.6	76	7.3	7.3	1.9	1.8
Fish, Extra Special, Asda*	1 Pack/400g	540	30.8	135	9.8	6.5	7.7	1.1
Fish, Frozen, GFY, Asda*	1 Pack/360g	342	8.6	95	5.8	12.5	2.4	0.9
Fish, Healthy Options, Birds Eye*	1 Pack/350g	238	2.8	68	3.7	11.6	0.8	0.7
Fish, HL, Tesco*	1 Pack/400g	316	8.8	79	4.0	10.8	2.2	1.7
Fish, Kids, Great Stuff, Asda*	1 Pack/300g	276	9.0	92	7.8	8.4	3.0	1.4
Fish, Large (700g), Extra Special, Asda*	1 Serving/350g	525	30.8	150	9.9	7.8	8.8	0.6
Fish, Luxury, M & S*	1 Pack/300g	330	16.8	110	7.3	7.6	5.6	1.5
Fish, Seasonal, Mix, Sainsbury's*	1 Pack/320g	480	28.2	150	17.7	0.0	8.8	0.0
Fish, The Best, Morrisons*	½ Pack/225g	250	11.9	111	6.6	9.3	5.3	0.8

	Measure INFO/WEIGHT	per Measure KCAL	FAT	Nutrition Values per 100g / 100ml KCAL	PROT	CARB	FAT	FIBRE
PIE								
Fish, TTD, Sainsbury's*	½ pack/390g	386	12.9	99	7.1	10.3	3.3	1.6
Fish, with Cheddar & Parsley Sauce, Go Cook, Asda*	½ Pack/450g	428	16.2	95	7.8	7.9	3.6	0.8
Fish, with Cheese, Ross*	1 Pack/300g	321	13.5	107	4.7	12.0	4.5	0.8
Fish, with Grated Cheddar, Asda*	¼ Pie/250g	262	12.5	105	7.0	8.0	5.0	1.0
Fish, with Vegetables, Ross*	1 Pack/300g	255	8.7	85	4.4	10.2	2.9	1.3
Fish, Yummy Pollock, Jamie Oliver, Youngs*	1 Pie/217g	204	7.2	94	6.8	8.6	3.3	1.5
Fish, Yummy Salmon, Jamie Oliver, Youngs*	1 Pie/207g	224	8.5	108	8.1	9.3	4.1	0.9
Fish, Yummy Salmon & Broccoli, Jamie Oliver, Youngs*	1 Pie/220g	211	7.5	96	6.5	9.3	3.4	1.3
Fish & Prawn, Perfectly Balanced, Waitrose*	1 Serving/375g	379	13.5	101	6.8	10.4	3.6	0.7
Fisherman's, British Recipe, Waitrose*	1 Pack/400g	408	16.4	102	7.7	8.5	4.1	1.2
Fisherman's, Chilled, Co-Op*	1 Pie/300g	345	18.0	115	4.0	11.0	6.0	0.7
Fisherman's, Famous, Chilled, Youngs*	1 Pack/400g	448	22.8	112	7.6	7.6	5.7	0.9
Fisherman's, HE, Tesco*	1 Pie/400g	308	8.8	77	5.1	9.2	2.2	1.3
Fisherman's, Healthy Options, Asda*	1 Pie/406g	337	10.2	83	5.0	10.0	2.5	0.9
Fisherman's, M & S*	1 Pie/248g	335	15.9	135	9.3	9.8	6.4	0.3
Fisherman's, Nisa Heritage*	1 Serving/550g	588	30.8	107	5.2	9.0	5.6	0.2
Fisherman's, Perfectly Balanced, Waitrose*	1 Pack/376g	380	13.5	101	6.8	10.4	3.6	0.7
Fisherman's, Sainsbury's*	1 Pack/300g	195	3.6	65	3.9	9.7	1.2	1.2
Fisherman's, Value, Tesco*	1 Pie/300g	195	3.0	65	3.3	9.1	1.0	1.6
Fruit, Pastry Top & Bottom	1oz/28g	73	3.7	260	3.0	34.0	13.3	1.8
Fruit, Selection, Mr Kipling*	1 Pie/66g	232	9.0	350	3.5	53.5	13.6	1.3
Gala, Tesco*	1 Serving/70g	241	17.6	344	10.6	24.5	25.2	0.0
Haddock & Broccoli, M & S*	1 Serving/250g	262	10.0	105	8.1	9.3	4.0	0.5
Key Lime, Sainsbury's*	¼ Pie/80g	280	11.2	350	4.2	51.8	14.0	0.7
Lamb & Mint, Shortcrust Pasty, Tesco*	¼ Pack/150g	412	26.1	275	5.9	23.6	17.4	1.6
Lemon Meringue	1 Portion/120g	383	17.3	319	4.5	45.9	14.4	0.7
Lemon Meringue, 90% Fat Free, Sara Lee*	1/6 Pie/75g	204	6.7	272	2.4	46.1	8.9	0.9
Lemon Meringue, Lyons*	1 Serving/100g	310	14.4	310	0.0	45.9	14.4	0.0
Lemon Meringue, Mini, Asda*	1 Pie/26g	101	3.3	396	3.7	66.0	13.0	1.8
Lemon Meringue, Mr Kipling*	1 Pie/51g	184	6.2	360	2.9	59.9	12.1	3.0
Lemon Meringue, Sainsbury's*	¼ Pie/110g	351	9.9	319	2.3	57.3	9.0	0.5
Lemon Meringue, Tesco*	1 Pie/385g	989	28.1	257	4.0	43.7	7.3	0.5
Lemon Meringue, Weight Watchers*	1 Serving/85g	161	0.4	189	2.4	43.1	0.5	0.6
Macaroni Cheese, Countryside*	1 Serving/144g	282	10.1	196	4.9	28.3	7.0	1.2
Mariner's, Light & Easy, Youngs*	1 Pack/350g	368	14.3	105	5.0	12.0	4.1	1.1
Mariner's, Ross*	1 Pie/340g	435	20.1	128	5.0	13.9	5.9	1.0
Meat, Freshbake*	1 Pie/49g	152	10.5	313	6.6	23.2	21.6	1.0
Meat & Potato, Hollands*	1 Pie/175g	410	19.2	234	6.1	27.5	11.0	0.0
Meat & Potato, Shortcrust, Co-Op*	¼ Pie/137g	403	26.2	294	7.3	23.3	19.1	1.4
Meat & Potato, Tesco*	1 Serving/150g	414	26.8	276	5.1	23.6	17.9	1.6
Mince, Deep, Morrisons*	1 Pie/65g	243	9.1	371	3.7	57.8	13.9	1.5
Mince, Deep Filled, Sainsbury's*	1 Pie/61g	251	9.0	406	4.1	63.6	14.5	2.5
Mince, Dusted, Mini, Finest, Tesco*	1 Pie/20g	76	2.4	379	7.3	62.9	12.2	5.0
Mince, Extra Special, Asda*	1 Pie/60g	225	8.3	378	3.9	59.0	14.0	2.2
Mince, Iced Top, Asda*	1 Pie/57g	221	6.7	391	2.7	67.3	11.9	1.9
Mince, Iceland*	1 Pie/39g	156	6.4	405	4.4	59.6	16.6	3.8
Mince, Individual, Average	1 Pie/48g	203	9.8	423	4.3	59.0	20.4	2.1
Mince, Individual, Mr Kipling*	1 Pie/66g	253	9.2	381	3.7	59.5	13.8	1.3
Mince, Lattice, Classics, M & S*	1 Pie/53g	210	8.0	400	4.0	61.7	15.2	2.4
Mince, Luxury, Deep Filled, M & S*	1 Pie/65g	234	9.0	360	4.3	55.0	13.8	3.8
Mince, Mini, Waitrose*	1 Pie/30g	150	9.1	501	5.7	51.3	30.3	1.7
Mince, Organic, Sainsbury's*	1 Pie/46g	177	7.5	384	5.0	54.5	16.2	5.6
Mince, Rowan Hill Bakery*	1 Pie/55g	202	8.2	370	3.8	54.8	15.1	0.0

	Measure INFO/WEIGHT	per Measure KCAL	FAT	Nutrition Values per 100g / 100ml KCAL	PROT	CARB	FAT	FIBRE
PIE								
Mince, Shortcrust, Waitrose*	1 Pie/55g	210	8.0	385	3.6	60.0	14.6	20.9
Mince, Star Motif, Mini, Finest, Tesco*	1 Pie/17g	62	2.1	365	3.8	59.9	12.1	3.8
Mince, Trufree*	1 Pie/60g	238	9.8	397	2.1	58.5	16.4	3.6
Mince Puff, Tesco*	1 Pie/25g	105	4.4	420	3.3	62.0	17.6	2.0
Minced Beef, Aberdeen Angus, Shortcrust, M & S*	1 Pie/171g	435	26.6	255	9.3	19.3	15.6	3.0
Minced Beef, Plate, M & S*	1oz/28g	71	4.5	253	7.6	20.7	16.0	2.0
Minced Beef & Onion, Birds Eye*	1 Pie/145g	419	25.1	289	7.1	26.3	17.3	0.7
Minced Beef & Onion, Denny*	1 Pie/140g	288	19.7	206	6.1	17.3	14.1	0.0
Minced Beef & Onion, Farmfoods*	1 Pie/128g	378	23.9	295	7.3	24.4	18.7	1.0
Minced Beef & Onion, Tesco*	1 Pie/150g	454	28.5	303	5.7	27.4	19.0	1.7
Minced Beef & Potato, Weight Watchers*	1 Pie/200g	328	12.4	164	6.7	20.2	6.2	3.6
Minced Beef & Vegetable, Pot, M & S*	1/3 Pie/183g	366	26.5	200	7.8	9.1	14.5	7.1
Mississippi Mud, Tesco*	1 Serving/104g	399	26.6	384	5.3	33.1	25.6	1.8
Mushroom & Leaf Spinach, Little, Higgidy*	1 Pie/180g	441	25.9	245	6.6	22.3	14.4	0.7
Ocean, Basics, Sainsbury's*	1 Serving/302g	196	3.6	65	3.9	9.7	1.2	1.2
Ocean, BGTY, Sainsbury's*	1 Pack/350g	285	4.7	81	6.3	11.1	1.3	0.8
Ocean, Frozen, BGTY, Sainsbury's*	1 Pack/350g	318	5.2	91	7.0	12.4	1.5	0.9
Ocean, M & S*	1 Pie/650g	618	22.8	95	8.2	7.6	3.5	0.9
Ocean, Original, Frozen, Youngs*	1 Pack/375g	420	21.4	112	7.6	7.6	5.7	0.9
Ocean, The Original, Light & Easy, Youngs*	1 Pack/415g	432	18.7	104	6.4	9.5	4.5	1.0
Ocean, Weight Watchers*	1 Pack/300g	196	3.3	65	4.2	9.2	1.1	0.8
Pork, Buffet, Bowyers*	1 Pie/60g	217	14.7	362	10.4	24.9	24.5	0.0
Pork, Buffet, Farmfoods*	1 Pie/65g	252	17.4	388	8.8	28.2	26.7	1.0
Pork, Cheddar & Pickle, Mini, Finest, Tesco*	1 Pie/50g	185	10.8	365	10.0	31.3	21.4	1.9
Pork, Cheese & Pickle, Mini, Tesco*	1 Pie/49g	191	12.8	389	9.2	29.3	26.1	1.2
Pork, Crusty Bake, Mini, Sainsbury's*	1 Pie/43g	165	11.2	384	11.5	26.0	26.0	1.5
Pork, Crusty Bake, Sainsbury's*	1 Pie/75g	292	20.0	390	10.5	27.0	26.7	1.0
Pork, Geo Adams*	1 Pie/125g	488	34.8	390	11.8	23.1	27.8	0.9
Pork, Individual	1 Pie/75g	272	19.3	363	10.8	23.7	25.7	0.9
Pork, Melton, Mini, Pork Farms*	1 Pie/50g	200	14.6	399	8.9	26.2	29.2	0.0
Pork, Melton Mowbray, Cured, M & S*	1 Pie/290g	1044	71.0	360	10.1	25.9	24.5	1.0
Pork, Melton Mowbray, Cured, Mini, M & S*	1 Pie/50g	192	12.2	385	9.8	32.6	24.4	1.0
Pork, Melton Mowbray, Individual, Sainsbury's*	1 Pie/75g	296	20.8	395	10.2	26.1	27.7	2.4
Pork, Melton Mowbray, Large, Co-Op*	¼ Pie/110g	418	35.2	380	11.0	12.0	32.0	5.0
Pork, Melton Mowbray, Lattice, Sainsbury's*	1 Serving/100g	342	23.6	342	10.8	21.7	23.6	1.2
Pork, Melton Mowbray, Mini, M & S*	1 Pie/50g	185	12.1	370	11.6	26.1	24.2	1.6
Pork, Melton Mowbray, Mini, Morrisons*	1 Pie/50g	197	12.5	393	10.9	31.3	24.9	0.9
Pork, Melton Mowbray, Tesco*	1 Sm Pie/148g	679	49.9	459	10.0	29.0	33.7	1.3
Pork, Melton Mowbray, Uncured, Small, Tesco*	1 Pie/140g	465	29.5	332	11.2	24.4	21.1	2.4
Pork, Mini	1 Pie/50g	196	13.9	391	10.6	26.3	27.8	1.0
Pork, Sliced	1 Slice/100g	380	29.9	380	10.2	18.7	29.9	0.0
Pork, VLH Kitchens	1 Serving/36g	168	100.0	466	11.0	26.0	36.0	2.5
Pork, with Cheese & Pickle, Waitrose*	1 Pack/150g	568	36.9	379	10.3	29.1	24.6	2.7
Pork & Egg, M & S*	¼ Pie/108g	379	28.0	351	9.7	19.8	25.9	0.8
Pork & Pickle, Bowyers*	1 Pie/150g	576	41.0	384	10.0	26.3	27.3	0.0
Potato & Meat, Farmfoods*	1 Pie/158g	416	26.9	263	5.4	22.0	17.0	1.0
Rhubarb, Sara Lee*	1 Serving/90g	224	12.4	250	2.9	28.7	13.8	1.3
Salmon, Crumble, Light & Easy, Youngs*	1 Pack/320g	282	6.4	88	5.7	11.8	2.0	1.0
Salmon, Value, Tesco*	1 Pack/300g	312	13.5	104	4.5	11.3	4.5	1.0
Salmon & Broccoli, Birds Eye*	1 Pie/351g	449	21.8	128	6.6	11.4	6.2	0.7
Salmon & Broccoli, Filo Pastry, Finest, Tesco*	1 Pie/170g	386	22.6	227	7.9	18.9	13.3	2.1
Salmon & Broccoli, Lattice Bar, Asda*	1/3 Bar/133g	360	20.0	271	6.0	28.0	15.0	0.8
Salmon & Broccoli, LC, Tesco*	1 Pack/400g	350	7.2	88	7.0	10.2	1.8	1.7

	Measure INFO/WEIGHT	per Measure KCAL	FAT	Nutrition Values per 100g / 100ml KCAL	PROT	CARB	FAT	FIBRE
PIE								
Salmon & Broccoli, Premium, Tesco*	1 Serving/170g	425	29.2	250	6.1	17.7	17.2	0.7
Sausage & Onion, Lattice, Puff Pastry, Tesco*	1/3 Pie/133g	480	22.5	361	9.1	20.6	16.9	4.6
Sausage & Onion, Tesco*	1 Pack/300g	333	18.3	111	2.3	11.7	6.1	0.5
Scotch, Co-Op*	1 Pie/132g	408	24.9	309	7.3	27.3	18.9	1.5
Scotch, Farmfoods*	1 Pie/151g	430	24.6	285	7.8	26.8	16.3	1.2
Shepherd's, 218, Oakhouse Foods Ltd*	1 Meal/390g	406	17.2	104	6.3	10.3	4.4	1.6
Shepherd's, Average	1oz/28g	31	1.7	112	6.0	9.3	5.9	0.7
Shepherd's, Baked Bean Cuisine, Heinz*	1 Pie/340g	299	9.5	88	4.1	11.6	2.8	1.5
Shepherd's, British Classic, Serves 1, Sainsbury's*	1 Pack/450g	454	22.0	101	6.2	7.9	4.9	1.7
Shepherd's, British Classics, Chilled, Tesco*	1 Pack/500g	500	20.5	100	4.8	10.6	4.1	1.2
Shepherd's, Charlie Bigham's*	½ Pack/324g	496	28.8	153	8.1	9.6	8.9	0.9
Shepherd's, Diet Chef Ltd*	1 Serving/270g	235	10.5	87	3.2	9.8	3.9	1.9
Shepherd's, Frozen, Tesco*	1 Pack/400g	270	9.1	68	4.1	7.6	2.3	1.2
Shepherd's, GFY, Asda*	1 Pack/399g	339	10.8	85	4.0	11.1	2.7	1.4
Shepherd's, Vegetarian, Average	1 Serving/400g	371	14.6	93	4.0	10.4	3.6	2.5
Shepherd's, Weight Watchers*	1 Pack/320g	211	5.8	66	3.2	8.8	1.8	1.1
Shepherd's, Welsh Hill Lamb, Gastropub, M & S*	½ Pack/330g	314	11.6	95	5.4	10.2	3.5	1.5
Steak, & Mash, Frozen, Oven Baked, Greggs, Iceland*	½ Pie/154g	339	17.7	220	10.5	17.5	11.5	0.0
Steak, Braised, Shortcrust Pastry, Asda*	½ Pack/260g	785	46.8	302	9.0	26.0	18.0	0.9
Steak, Deep Fill, Tesco*	¼ Pie/195g	468	25.5	240	9.7	20.0	13.1	1.5
Steak, Dietary Specials*	1 Pie/140g	328	14.4	234	9.8	25.7	10.3	0.4
Steak, in Rich Gravy, Aunt Bessie's*	¼ Pie/200g	440	20.6	220	9.6	22.0	10.3	1.5
Steak, Individual, British Classics, Tesco*	1 Pie/150g	450	27.6	300	9.1	23.3	18.4	2.5
Steak, Large, Glenfell*	¼ Pie/170g	445	27.9	262	6.8	21.8	16.4	1.0
Steak, M & S*	1oz/28g	64	3.6	230	10.0	19.0	12.7	1.2
Steak, Mini, Asda*	1 Serving/67g	117	5.3	176	9.0	17.0	8.0	0.9
Steak, Mushroom & Ale, Topcrust, Waitrose*	1 Pie/250g	500	29.5	200	11.1	12.2	11.8	1.1
Steak, Puff Pastry, Deep Filled, Sainsbury's*	1 Pie/210g	536	30.0	255	10.3	21.2	14.3	2.0
Steak, Scotch, Bell's Bakery*	1 Serving/150g	378	20.2	252	13.6	18.6	13.5	0.7
Steak, Short Crust, Sainsbury's*	½ Pie/118g	314	24.1	267	10.9	22.2	20.5	1.7
Steak, Shortcrust, 3½ Minute, Pukka Pies Ltd*	1 Pie/198g	586	32.5	296	9.4	28.6	16.4	2.1
Steak, Shortcrust Pastry, Finest, Tesco*	1 Pie/250g	660	37.8	264	10.9	21.2	15.1	0.8
Steak, Tesco*	1 Serving/205g	556	33.8	271	7.2	23.3	16.5	1.4
Steak, Top Crust, TTD, Sainsbury's*	½ Pie/299g	530	23.1	177	15.4	11.4	7.7	0.5
Steak, TTD, Sainsbury's*	½ Pie/300g	713	35.4	238	12.6	20.3	11.8	1.0
Steak & Ale, Average	1 Pie/200g	507	28.7	253	9.8	21.1	14.4	1.3
Steak & Ale, Charlie Bigham's*	1 Pie/300g	774	48.9	258	13.4	14.1	16.3	1.1
Steak & Ale, Deep Fill, Puff Pastry, Tesco*	¼ Pie/150g	324	19.6	216	8.0	16.6	13.1	2.3
Steak & Ale, Fray Bentos*	1 Pie/425g	697	38.7	164	7.6	13.0	9.1	0.0
Steak & Ale, Pub Style, Co-Op*	1 Pie/250g	538	30.0	215	9.0	17.0	12.0	2.0
Steak & Ale, Puff Pastry, Asda*	1/3 Pie/200g	520	30.2	260	10.6	20.4	15.1	1.6
Steak & Ale, with Chips & Gravy	1 Serving/400g	825	42.2	206	7.2	20.5	10.6	0.5
Steak & Guinness, Sainsbury's*	¼ Pie/137g	399	25.5	291	8.7	22.2	18.6	1.0
Steak & Kidney, Birds Eye*	1 Pie/146g	447	28.5	306	9.0	23.7	19.5	2.3
Steak & Kidney, Deep Fill, Sainsbury's*	½ Pie/125g	314	18.6	251	8.4	21.0	14.9	2.0
Steak & Kidney, Family, Iceland*	1/3 Pie/225g	502	29.2	223	10.2	16.3	13.0	2.1
Steak & Kidney, Individual	1 Pie/200g	646	42.4	323	9.1	25.6	21.2	0.9
Steak & Kidney, Premium, Tesco*	1 Serving/170g	428	26.4	252	9.9	18.3	15.5	1.2
Steak & Kidney, Princes*	½ Pack/212g	379	19.9	179	8.8	14.8	9.4	0.0
Steak & Kidney, Puff Pastry, Sainsbury's*	1 Pie/150g	423	23.6	282	8.2	26.9	15.7	0.9
Steak & Kidney, Pukka Pies Ltd*	1 Pie/238g	488	25.9	205	9.1	17.7	10.9	3.6
Steak & Kidney, Tesco*	1 Pie/150g	420	27.3	280	7.3	21.9	18.2	3.7
Steak & Kidney, Tinned, Fray Bentos*	½ Pie/212g	346	18.7	163	8.2	12.9	8.8	0.0

	Measure INFO/WEIGHT	per Measure KCAL	FAT	Nutrition Values per 100g / 100ml KCAL	PROT	CARB	FAT	FIBRE
PIE								
Steak & Mushroom, Asda*	1 Pie/130g	350	18.1	270	9.0	27.0	14.0	1.4
Steak & Mushroom, Deep Fill, Asda*	1/3 Pie/175g	476	28.0	272	11.0	21.0	16.0	1.1
Steak & Mushroom, Deep Fill, Puff Pastry, Tesco*	1 Slice/150g	339	20.7	226	9.1	16.3	13.8	1.9
Steak & Mushroom, Family, Iceland*	¼ Pie/164g	366	21.8	223	10.5	15.4	13.3	2.9
Steak & Mushroom, Finest, Tesco*	1 Pie/250g	640	36.5	256	9.2	21.9	14.6	1.1
Steak & Mushroom, HE, Tesco*	1 Serving/200g	380	11.4	190	10.5	24.2	5.7	1.9
Steak & Mushroom, Home Comforts, Weight Watchers*	1 Pie/136g	322	15.9	237	5.8	26.9	11.7	1.4
Steak & Mushroom, Individual, Birds Eye*	1 Pie/142g	389	24.1	274	7.5	22.7	17.0	2.0
Steak & Mushroom, McDougalls*	1 Pack/340g	779	57.8	229	9.0	10.0	17.0	1.0
Steak & Mushroom, Sainsbury's*	¼ Pie/130g	372	21.3	286	8.6	26.0	16.4	1.0
Steak & Onion, Farmfoods*	1 Pie/127g	382	24.3	301	6.0	26.4	19.1	1.0
Steak & Onion, Ginsters*	1 Pie/180g	481	30.8	267	8.0	20.3	17.1	1.3
Steak & Onion, Minced, Aberdeen Angus, Tesco*	½ Pie/300g	897	57.6	299	9.4	22.1	19.2	0.7
Steak & Potato, Asda*	1/3 Pie/173g	442	26.0	255	6.9	23.1	15.0	0.9
Steak & Red Wine, Puff Pastry, Pub, Sainsbury's*	1 Pie/240g	497	29.5	207	7.2	16.8	12.3	2.1
Summer Fruits, Orchard Tree*	1/8 Pie/75g	242	10.4	323	3.0	46.6	13.8	1.2
Teviot, Minced Beef, Morrisons*	½ Pie/250g	382	17.2	153	8.0	14.5	6.9	1.6
Tuna & Sweetcorn, HL, Tesco*	1 Pack/450g	392	12.2	87	7.1	8.6	2.7	2.0
Turkey & Ham, Farmfoods*	1 Pie/147g	404	21.9	275	8.6	26.5	14.9	1.4
Turkey & Ham, Shortcrust, M & S*	1/3 Pie/183g	494	29.1	270	11.9	19.5	15.9	1.0
Vegetable	1oz/28g	42	2.1	151	3.0	18.9	7.6	1.5
Vegetable, Mediterranean, Cheesy, COU, M & S*	1 Pack/400g	280	8.4	70	2.1	10.6	2.1	2.1
Vegetable, Retail, Average	1 Serving/200g	348	19.0	174	3.7	18.6	9.5	1.1
Vegetable & Cheddar Cheese, Waitrose*	1 Pie/210g	475	31.5	226	4.9	17.8	15.0	1.2
Vegetable & Cheese, Asda*	1 Pie/141g	330	16.2	234	5.8	26.9	11.5	1.0
Vegetable & Feta, Moroccan, Little, Higgidy*	1 Pie/180g	418	22.5	232	5.1	24.7	12.5	0.6
Vegetarian, Cottage, Mealpak, All About Weight*	1 Sachet/32g	120	2.8	375	28.6	36.0	8.6	10.0
Vegetarian, Deep Country, Linda McCartney*	1 Pie/166g	413	23.6	249	5.2	24.9	14.2	2.6
Vegetarian, Mushroom & Ale, Linda McCartney*	1 Pie/200g	439	23.5	219	4.1	25.0	11.7	1.2
Vegetarian, Shepherd's, Linda McCartney*	1 Pack/340g	286	7.5	84	3.7	12.3	2.2	2.3
Vegetarian, Vegetable Cumberland, M & S*	½ Pack/211g	190	5.5	90	2.8	13.4	2.6	1.6
PIE FILLING								
Apple, Sainsbury's*	1 Serving/75g	67	0.1	89	0.1	22.1	0.1	1.0
Black Cherry, Fruit, Sainsbury's*	1 Serving/100g	73	0.1	73	0.3	17.7	0.1	0.3
Blackcurrant, Fruit, Sainsbury's*	1 Serving/100g	82	0.1	82	0.4	20.0	0.1	1.6
Cherry	1oz/28g	23	0.0	82	0.4	21.5	0.0	0.4
Fruit	1oz/28g	22	0.0	77	0.4	20.1	0.0	1.0
Summer Fruits, Fruit, Tesco*	1 Can/385g	377	0.0	98	0.4	24.1	0.0	0.9
PIGEON								
Meat Only, Roasted, Average	***1 Pigeon/115g***	***215***	***9.1***	***187***	***29.0***	***0.0***	***7.9***	***0.0***
Meat Only, Roasted, Weighed with Bone, Average	***1oz/28g***	***25***	***1.0***	***88***	***13.6***	***0.0***	***3.7***	***0.0***
PIKELETS								
Classics, M & S*	1 Pikelet/35g	70	0.5	200	7.3	39.1	1.3	1.6
Free From, Tesco*	1 Pikelet/30g	58	1.3	194	2.8	36.2	4.3	1.4
Tesco*	1 Pikelet/35g	68	0.2	193	5.8	40.9	0.7	1.7
PILAF								
Bulgar Wheat, Sainsbury's*	1 Pack/381g	347	11.1	91	3.9	12.3	2.9	6.3
Forest Mushroom & Pine Nut, Bistro, Waitrose*	1 Serving/225g	338	14.6	150	7.0	15.8	6.5	1.5
with Tomato, Average	1oz/28g	40	0.9	144	2.5	28.0	3.3	0.4
PILCHARDS								
Fillets in Tomato Sauce, Average	1 Can/120g	158	7.8	132	16.2	2.2	6.5	0.1
Fillets in Virgin Olive Oil, Glenryck*	1 Serving/92g	223	14.4	242	23.3	2.0	15.7	0.0
in Brine, Average	***½ Can/77g***	***114***	***5.6***	***148***	***20.8***	***0.0***	***7.3***	***0.0***

	Measure INFO/WEIGHT	per Measure KCAL	FAT	Nutrition Values per 100g / 100ml KCAL	PROT	CARB	FAT	FIBRE
PIMMS*								
& Lemonade, Premixed, Canned, Pimms*	1 Can/250ml	160	0.0	64	0.0	8.4	0.0	0.0
25% Volume, Pimms*	***1 Serving/50ml***	***80***	***0.0***	***160***	***0.0***	***5.0***	***0.0***	***0.0***
PINE NUTS								
Average	***1oz/28g***	***195***	***19.2***	***695***	***15.7***	***3.9***	***68.6***	***1.9***
PINEAPPLE								
& Papaya, Dried, Garden Gang, Asda*	1 Pack/50g	142	0.8	283	2.8	64.0	1.7	8.0
Chunks, Average	1 Serving/100g	66	0.1	66	0.5	15.5	0.1	0.3
Deliciously Refreshing & Sweet, Love Life, Waitrose*	8 Chunks/80g	47	0.1	59	0.5	13.1	0.1	1.4
Dried, Soft, Love Life, Waitrose*	1 Serving/30g	93	0.1	309	3.0	73.7	0.2	3.1
Dried, Sweetened, Ready to Eat, Tesco*	1/5 Pack/50g	118	1.0	235	0.4	52.9	1.9	1.7
Dried, Tropical Wholefoods*	1 Slice/10g	30	0.0	305	2.9	73.9	0.2	5.2
Dried, Unsweetened, Sainsbury's*	1 Bag/75g	255	1.5	340	1.7	84.7	2.0	6.0
Fingers, Good to Go, Waitrose*	1 Pack/160g	90	0.2	56	0.5	13.1	0.1	1.4
in Juice, Canned, Average	***1 Can/106g***	***57***	***0.0***	***53***	***0.3***	***12.9***	***0.0***	***0.6***
in Own Juice, Del Monte*	1 Can/432g	298	0.4	69	0.4	15.5	0.1	0.0
in Syrup, Average	***1 Can/240g***	***158***	***0.0***	***66***	***0.3***	***16.1***	***0.0***	***0.8***
Lolly, Fresh, Great Stuff, Asda*	1 Pack/80g	36	0.2	45	0.4	9.8	0.2	1.2
Raw, Diced, Medley, Lozzas	1 Fruit/400g	200	0.9	42	0.4	10.0	0.2	1.0
Raw, Flesh Only, Average	***1 Pineapple/472g***	***200***	***0.9***	***42***	***0.4***	***10.0***	***0.2***	***1.0***
Sliced, Snack, Shapers, Boots*	1 Pack/80g	35	0.2	44	0.4	10.0	0.2	1.2
Tidbits, Dried, Graze*	1 Pack/30g	79	0.2	263	0.6	72.0	0.6	1.0
Yoghurt Coated, Pieces, Holland & Barrett*	1 Pack/100g	344	19.3	344	2.1	46.8	19.3	0.6
PISTACHIO NUTS								
Black Pepper, Graze*	1 Punnet/31g	104	9.7	331	10.0	5.0	31.0	3.0
Lightly Toasted, Graze*	1 Punnet/31g	104	9.7	331	10.0	5.0	31.0	3.0
Raw, Average, without Shells	1 Serving/20g	111	8.9	557	20.6	28.0	44.4	10.3
Roasted, Graze*	1 Pack/50g	166	15.5	333	9.9	4.6	31.0	0.0
Roasted & Salted, without Shells, Average	***1 Serving/25g***	***152***	***13.6***	***608***	***19.6***	***9.9***	***54.5***	***6.1***
Salted, Lemon, Graze*	1 Box/26g	148	12.0	568	21.4	26.8	46.0	0.0
Salted, Roasted, Weighed with Shell	1 Serving/100g	601	55.4	601	17.9	8.2	55.4	6.1
Shelled, Kernels, Wholesome, Love Life, Waitrose*	1 Serving/30g	181	16.6	603	17.9	8.2	55.4	10.3
PIZZA								
American Hot, 12 Inch, Supermarket, Pizza Express*	½ Pizza/264g	562	19.8	213	10.5	25.9	7.5	2.6
American Hot, 8 Inch, Supermarket, Pizza Express*	1 Pizza/295g	652	22.4	221	11.0	27.3	7.6	3.5
American Hot, Chicago Town*	1 Pizza/170g	445	20.1	262	8.2	30.8	11.8	0.9
Bacon, Mushroom & Tomato, HL, Tesco*	1 Pizza/231g	395	6.2	171	10.6	25.9	2.7	1.5
Bacon & Mushroom, Stone Bake, M & S*	1 Pizza/375g	750	24.0	200	9.9	27.2	6.4	1.6
Bacon & Mushroom, Stonebaked, Tesco*	1 Serving/157g	352	14.8	224	10.5	24.3	9.4	3.3
Bacon & Mushroom, Thin & Crispy, Sainsbury's*	½ Pizza/150g	396	15.9	264	12.9	29.2	10.6	1.7
Bacon & Mushroom, with Capers, Lozzas	1 Slice/157g	352	14.8	224	10.5	24.3	9.4	3.3
Bacon & Mushroom Pizzeria, Sainsbury's*	1 Pizza/355g	880	24.8	248	11.7	34.5	7.0	3.7
BBQ Chicken, M & S*	½ Pizza/210g	430	11.8	205	11.6	27.5	5.6	1.8
BBQ Chicken, Stonebaked, Tesco*	½ Pizza/158g	285	9.5	180	10.5	20.9	6.0	3.9
BBQ Chicken, Thin & Crispy, Sainsbury's*	½ Pizza/167g	399	12.4	238	11.4	30.4	7.4	2.2
BBQ Chicken, Weight Watchers*	1 Pizza/224g	412	7.8	184	11.5	26.5	3.5	2.7
BBQ Chicken Stuffed Crust, Asda*	½ Pizza/245g	612	24.5	250	13.0	27.0	10.0	2.7
Beef, Spicy, Goodfella's*	½ Pizza/148g	391	17.8	265	12.4	26.5	12.1	2.2
Bianca, Bistro, Waitrose*	½ Pizza/207g	618	32.6	298	12.9	26.2	15.7	2.3
Calzone Speciale, Ristorante, Dr Oetker*	½ Pizza/145g	378	23.2	261	11.5	22.1	16.0	0.0
Capricciosa, Pizza Express*	1 Serving/300g	753	29.3	251	13.6	29.0	9.8	0.0
Caprina, Pizza Express*	1 Pizza/300g	635	22.0	212	8.0	31.0	7.3	0.0
Cheese, Deep Pan, Tesco*	½ Pizza/455g	990	26.4	218	11.4	29.8	5.8	3.1
Cheese, Onion & Garlic, Pizzeria, Waitrose*	½ Pizza/245g	684	28.9	279	10.8	29.8	11.8	2.5

P

	Measure INFO/WEIGHT	per Measure KCAL	FAT	Nutrition Values per 100g / 100ml KCAL	PROT	CARB	FAT	FIBRE
PIZZA								
Cheese, Simply, Goodfella's*	¼ Pizza/82g	226	11.0	276	16.3	22.5	13.4	1.9
Cheese, Stuffed, Crust, Sainsbury's*	1 Pizza/525g	1428	52.5	272	14.0	31.5	10.0	2.0
Cheese, Thin & Crispy, Goodfella's*	1 Serving/275g	729	27.8	265	15.7	27.6	10.1	1.8
Cheese, Three, Slice, Microwaveable, Tesco*	1 Slice/160g	486	18.7	304	13.3	36.7	11.7	1.6
Cheese & Ham, Italian, The Little Big Food Company*	1 Pizza/95g	236	6.2	248	11.0	36.2	6.6	1.0
Cheese & Onion, Tesco*	1 Serving/22g	56	2.0	255	10.5	32.7	9.1	2.7
Cheese & Tomato, 12 inch, Fresh, Tesco*	1/3 Pizza/160g	413	13.8	258	9.6	36.3	8.6	1.4
Cheese & Tomato, Average	1 Serving/300g	711	35.4	237	9.1	25.2	11.8	1.4
Cheese & Tomato, Deep Pan, Goodfella's*	¼ Pizza/102g	259	10.8	253	11.5	29.6	10.5	3.7
Cheese & Tomato, Deep Pan, Sainsbury's*	1 Pizza/182g	470	15.8	258	11.7	33.1	8.7	1.9
Cheese & Tomato, French Bread, Co-Op*	1 Pizza/135g	270	8.1	200	9.0	27.0	6.0	2.0
Cheese & Tomato, French Bread, Findus*	1 Serving/143g	322	11.6	225	9.4	29.0	8.1	0.0
Cheese & Tomato, HE, Tesco*	1 Serving/100g	211	2.4	211	11.9	35.5	2.4	1.6
Cheese & Tomato, Italiano, Tesco*	1 Pizza/380g	969	35.0	255	11.4	31.7	9.2	3.3
Cheese & Tomato, Kids, Tesco*	1 Pizza/95g	219	5.2	231	11.5	33.9	5.5	1.9
Cheese & Tomato, Micro, McCain*	1 Pizza/122g	319	12.2	262	13.4	29.7	10.0	2.4
Cheese & Tomato, Mini, Bruschetta, Iceland*	1 Pizza/34g	63	2.3	188	8.0	23.0	7.0	2.1
Cheese & Tomato, Retail, Frozen	1oz/28g	70	3.0	250	7.5	32.9	10.7	1.4
Cheese & Tomato, Slice, Ross*	1 Slice/77g	148	6.6	192	6.5	22.2	8.6	2.0
Cheese & Tomato, Square, Sainsbury's*	1 Square/160g	435	11.7	272	14.0	37.6	7.3	2.1
Cheese & Tomato, Stonebaked, Thin & Crispy, Tesco*	½ Pizza/161g	388	13.8	241	11.6	29.4	8.6	2.1
Cheese & Tomato, Thin & Crispy, Carlos*	1 Pizza/155g	405	13.0	261	11.4	35.0	8.4	1.2
Cheese & Tomato, Thin & Crispy, Organic, Tesco*	½ Pizza/147g	369	14.4	251	10.6	30.1	9.8	1.3
Cheese & Tomato, Thin & Crispy, Waitrose*	1 Pizza/280g	658	28.3	235	12.3	23.6	10.1	2.3
Cheese Feast, Deep Pan, Asda*	½ Pizza/210g	422	18.9	201	13.0	17.0	9.0	2.3
Cheese Feast, Thin Crust, Chilled, Tesco*	½ Pizza/175g	467	22.4	267	14.7	23.4	12.8	2.5
Cheese Supreme, New Recipe, Goodfella's*	¼ Pizza/102g	269	10.2	264	12.3	31.2	10.0	2.2
Cheesefeast, Deep & Crispy 12", Takeaway, Iceland*	1 Slice/132g	342	11.1	259	13.1	32.8	8.4	1.5
Chicken, Chargrilled, & Vegetable, GFY, Asda*	½ Pizza/166g	355	3.3	214	13.0	36.0	2.0	2.0
Chicken, Chargrilled, & Vegetable, Low Fat, Bertorelli*	1 Pizza/180g	439	7.9	244	14.2	39.3	4.4	2.3
Chicken, Chargrilled, Iceland*	1 Pizza/381g	804	25.5	211	12.3	25.4	6.7	2.0
Chicken, Hot & Spicy, Deep Pan, Tesco*	½ Pizza/222g	423	7.3	191	10.5	30.0	3.3	2.1
Chicken, Spicy, Anytime, McCain*	1 Pizza/150g	382	11.7	255	15.1	32.2	7.8	2.0
Chicken, Spicy, Foccacia, Sainsbury's*	½ Pizza/245g	581	18.6	237	12.0	30.3	7.6	2.5
Chicken, Spicy, HL, Tesco*	1 Serving/252g	418	4.0	166	10.9	27.1	1.6	2.7
Chicken, Spicy, Iceland*	1 Pizza/345g	797	22.8	231	13.4	29.9	6.6	1.5
Chicken, Spicy, Micro, McCain*	1 Pizza/133g	388	20.0	292	12.4	26.9	15.0	0.0
Chicken & Bacon, Loaded, Tesco*	1 Serving/258g	622	25.3	241	12.8	25.4	9.8	1.9
Chicken & Bacon, Pizzeria, Italian, Sainsbury's*	½ Pizza/170g	508	24.1	300	13.6	29.4	14.2	2.7
Chicken & Chorizo, 12", TTD, Sainsbury's*	½ Pizza/290g	702	20.9	242	12.2	32.1	7.2	2.6
Chicken & Pesto, Californian Style, Asda*	½ Pizza/235g	533	16.4	227	10.0	31.0	7.0	2.0
Chicken & Red Pepper, HE, Tesco*	1 Pizza/260g	608	6.5	234	12.7	40.1	2.5	0.7
Chicken & Sweetcorn, Stonebaked, Tesco*	1 Serving/177g	354	9.6	200	11.9	26.0	5.4	2.0
Chicken & Vegetable, Chargrill, Italiano, Tesco*	½ Pizza/184g	383	14.7	208	10.6	23.3	8.0	2.4
Chicken & Vegetable, Stone Baked, GFY, Asda*	½ Pizza/161g	349	3.7	217	13.0	36.0	2.3	1.7
Chicken & Vegetables, Flamed, BGTY, Sainsbury's*	1 Pizza/260g	660	11.4	254	14.2	39.3	4.4	2.3
Chicken Alfredo, Chicago Town*	1 Pizza/265g	583	24.9	220	11.9	21.9	9.4	1.8
Chicken Arrabbiata, Italian Style, M & S*	½ Pizza/225g	495	15.8	220	12.3	26.3	7.0	2.0
Chicken Arrabbiata, Sainsbury's*	½ Pizza/191g	444	12.2	232	12.1	31.4	6.4	1.7
Chicken Provencal, Goodfella's*	½ Pizza/143g	388	18.0	272	13.7	25.9	12.6	2.1
Chicken Salsa, HE, Tesco*	½ Pizza/169g	313	2.2	185	13.0	30.3	1.3	1.5
Chicken Salsa, Thin Crust, Healthy Selection, Budgens*	½ Pizza/163g	295	3.1	181	10.5	30.5	1.9	1.4
Chicken Tikka, Stonebaked, Tesco*	1 Serving/153g	326	10.4	213	10.7	27.3	6.8	1.3

	Measure	per Measure		Nutrition Values per 100g / 100ml				
	INFO/WEIGHT	KCAL	FAT	KCAL	PROT	CARB	FAT	FIBRE
PIZZA								
Chilli Beef, Charged Up, Goodfella's*	½ Pizza/357g	857	32.8	240	12.8	26.4	9.2	1.6
Chilli Beef, Stone Bake, M & S*	1 Pizza/395g	790	22.9	200	9.6	26.7	5.8	1.9
Chorizo, Red Pepper & Chilli, Spicy, Classico, Tesco*	1 Serving/218g	474	17.4	218	10.3	26.4	8.0	2.5
Classic Italian, Stonebaked, Spinach & Ricotta, Tesco*	½ Pizza/190g	460	16.3	240	10.3	29.0	8.5	1.2
Cream Cheese & Pepperonata, Calzone, Waitrose*	½ Pizza/165g	383	15.8	232	7.0	29.4	9.6	1.5
Deep South, Chicago Town*	1 Pizza/171g	363	12.1	212	6.9	30.0	7.1	0.0
Diavolo, Pizza Express*	½ Pizza/164g	322	11.0	197	9.4	24.6	6.7	2.1
Four Cheese, Finest, Tesco*	½ Pizza/230g	575	21.2	250	12.1	29.8	9.2	1.3
Four Cheese, M & S*	1oz/28g	67	2.1	240	13.2	30.3	7.5	1.2
Four Cheese, Stuffed Crust, Takeaway, Chicago Town*	¼ Pizza/158g	433	17.0	275	10.8	33.0	10.8	1.9
Four Cheese, Thin & Crispy, Sainsbury's*	1 Pizza/265g	729	32.6	275	11.8	29.3	12.3	3.5
Four Cheese, Thin Crust, Tesco*	½ Pizza/142g	386	13.6	272	14.5	31.8	9.6	1.8
Four Cheese, Weight Watchers*	1 Pizza/186g	400	7.0	215	10.8	34.9	3.8	1.6
Four Cheese & Tomato, Pizzatilla, M & S*	1 Serving/69g	225	13.8	324	10.5	26.0	19.9	1.5
Four Seasons, Stonebaked, Truly Irresistible, Co-Op*	½ Pizza/245g	502	16.2	205	9.5	26.6	6.6	2.6
Four Seasons, Waitrose*	1/3 Pizza/174g	382	14.6	220	9.9	26.2	8.4	2.6
Garlic & Mushroom, Asda*	½ Pizza/241g	696	41.0	289	10.0	24.0	17.0	1.6
Garlic & Mushroom, Thin & Crispy, Sainsbury's*	1 Pizza/260g	829	43.2	319	11.1	31.2	16.6	1.7
Garlic Bread, Stonebaked, Italiono, Tesco*	1 Serving/117g	403	18.2	346	7.8	43.6	15.6	1.5
Garlic Chicken, Deep Pan, Sainsbury's*	½ Pizza/214g	464	13.9	217	11.2	28.3	6.5	3.3
Garlic Chicken, Thin & Crispy, Stonebake, Sainsbury's*	½ Pizza/160g	386	17.3	241	10.7	25.2	10.8	3.5
Garlic Mushroom, BGTY, Sainsbury's*	½ Pizza/123g	262	2.5	213	11.6	37.2	2.0	2.7
Garlic Mushroom, Classico, Tesco*	½ Pizza/208g	415	13.9	200	10.0	24.9	6.7	2.6
Garlic Mushroom, Tesco*	1 Pizza/425g	829	34.0	195	9.3	21.6	8.0	5.3
Garlic Mushroom, Thin & Crispy, Chicago Town*	1 Pizza/115g	283	13.3	246	9.0	26.4	11.6	1.9
Garlic Mushroom, Thin & Crispy, Weight Watchers*	1 Pizza/240g	410	3.1	171	11.2	28.8	1.3	3.0
Garlic Mushroom, Thin Crust, Tesco*	½ Pizza/163g	340	14.6	209	11.0	21.1	9.0	3.6
Giardiniera from Supermarket, Pizza Express*	½ Pizza/144g	291	10.5	202	8.6	25.5	7.3	2.1
Ham, Mushroom & Gruyere, Sainsbury's*	¼ Pizza/169g	404	13.7	239	10.2	31.3	8.1	3.7
Ham, Mushroom & Mascarpone, Italian Style, M & S*	1 Pizza/224g	515	21.7	230	10.0	25.5	9.7	2.9
Ham, Mushroom & Tomato, BGTY, Sainsbury's*	½ Pizza/150g	309	6.2	206	11.8	30.4	4.1	1.2
Ham, Pepperoni & Milano, M & S*	1 Pizza/290g	696	28.4	240	14.0	23.3	9.8	1.1
Ham, Smoked, & Mushroom, Thin & Crispy, Co-Op*	1 Pizza/400g	792	18.0	198	9.0	30.3	4.5	1.7
Ham, Smoked, & Peppers, HL, Tesco*	1 Serving/282g	386	5.6	137	8.7	21.1	2.0	1.8
Ham, Smoked, & Pineapple, Deep Pan, Co-Op*	1 Pizza/395g	1142	41.9	289	11.6	36.7	10.6	1.7
Ham, Smoked, & Pineapple, Weight Watchers*	1 Pizza/241g	429	7.0	178	10.3	27.6	2.9	1.5
Ham & Cheese, Chunky, Asda*	1 Serving/90g	211	3.0	234	12.0	39.0	3.3	4.7
Ham & Cheese, Ultra Thin, Sodebo*	1 Pizza/200g	400	8.6	200	11.3	29.1	4.3	0.0
Ham & Mushroom, Average	1 Serving/250g	533	16.0	213	10.5	28.4	6.4	2.1
Ham & Mushroom, BGTY, Sainsbury's*	1 Pizza/248g	526	3.5	212	12.1	37.8	1.4	2.9
Ham & Mushroom, Deep & Crispy, Tesco*	1 Serving/210g	420	10.3	200	9.7	29.2	4.9	1.1
Ham & Mushroom, Deep Pan, Waitrose*	½ Pizza/220g	453	13.6	206	10.9	26.6	6.2	1.0
Ham & Mushroom, HE, Tesco*	1 Pizza/252g	491	3.0	195	10.4	35.6	1.2	2.0
Ham & Mushroom, Stone Baked, Goodfella's*	½ Pizza/175g	439	20.0	251	9.6	27.6	11.4	1.2
Ham & Mushroom, Stonebaked, Stateside Foods*	¼ Pizza/101g	225	6.3	223	9.9	31.9	6.2	1.4
Ham & Mushroom, Thin & Crispy, Asda*	1 Pizza/360g	760	25.2	211	11.0	26.0	7.0	2.4
Ham & Mushroom Calzone, Waitrose*	½ Pizza/145g	362	13.5	250	10.0	31.6	9.3	1.6
Ham & Mushroom Slices, Farmfoods*	1 Slice/89g	170	2.3	191	8.0	34.0	2.6	0.9
Ham & Onion, Tesco*	1 Serving/181g	452	17.4	250	11.8	29.0	9.6	2.2
Ham & Pineapple, American Deep Pan, Sainsbury's*	1 Pizza/412g	1001	32.1	243	10.5	32.6	7.8	1.7
Ham & Pineapple, Average	1 Serving/250g	555	16.8	222	11.0	29.2	6.7	2.1
Ham & Pineapple, Chicago Town*	1 Pizza/435g	866	19.6	199	10.0	29.7	4.5	0.0
Ham & Pineapple, Deep & Loaded, Sainsbury's*	1 Pizza/515g	1102	26.8	214	10.2	31.7	5.2	3.5

	Measure INFO/WEIGHT	per Measure KCAL	FAT	Nutrition Values per 100g / 100ml KCAL	PROT	CARB	FAT	FIBRE
PIZZA								
Ham & Pineapple, Deep Pan, Ciabatta, Iceland*	½ Pizza/185g	440	14.4	238	11.6	30.3	7.8	0.8
Ham & Pineapple, Deep Pan, Tesco*	1 Pizza/237g	437	6.9	184	9.8	29.8	2.9	1.9
Ham & Pineapple, HL, Tesco*	¼ Pizza/105g	170	2.2	162	10.0	25.9	2.1	2.4
Ham & Pineapple, Thin & Crispy, 2 Pack, Sainsbury's*	1 Pizza/163g	417	13.2	256	13.8	32.0	8.1	1.7
Ham & Pineapple, Thin & Crispy, Goodfella's*	1 Serving/163g	333	12.7	204	10.6	22.8	7.8	2.4
Ham & Pineapple, Thin & Crispy, Iceland*	1 Serving/110g	301	13.1	274	9.9	31.9	11.9	3.0
Ham & Pineapple, Thin & Crispy, Waitrose*	1 Pizza/220g	616	21.1	280	12.8	33.3	9.6	2.2
Ham & Pineapple, Thin Crust, Tesco*	½ Pizza/175g	385	10.0	220	12.3	29.6	5.7	2.5
Ham & Pineapple Deep, Asda*	1 Pizza/486g	1055	22.4	217	11.3	32.5	4.6	3.0
Hawaiian, San Marco*	¼ Pizza/90g	208	8.3	231	8.9	29.7	9.2	1.5
Hawaiian, Stonebaked, Cucina, Aldi*	½ Pizza/165g	326	5.6	198	9.5	32.0	3.4	1.6
Hawaiian, Thin Crust, Tesco*	½ Pizza/192g	365	9.4	190	10.3	25.6	4.9	1.8
Hot & Spicy, Deep Dish, Chicago Town*	1 Pizza/177g	434	17.5	245	8.6	30.4	9.9	0.9
Hot & Spicy, Pizzeria Style, Sainsbury's*	1 Pizza/376g	986	46.3	262	12.5	25.5	12.3	2.4
Hot & Spicy, Thin & Crispy, Morrisons*	½ Pizza/170g	393	15.8	231	10.5	26.5	9.3	3.2
Leggera, Dr Oetker*	½ Pizza/175g	317	10.2	181	8.8	23.1	5.8	2.7
Margherita, 12 Inch, Supermarket, Pizza Express*	½ Pizza/230g	494	13.8	215	10.1	28.3	6.0	3.6
Margherita, Average	1 Slice/108g	239	8.6	239	11.0	30.5	8.6	1.2
Margherita, Cheese & Tomato, San Marco*	½ Pizza/200g	454	14.4	227	10.7	29.8	7.2	1.2
Margherita, HL, Tesco*	½ Pizza/125g	222	2.5	178	10.8	29.3	2.0	2.5
Margherita, Italian Stonebaked, Asda*	¼ Pizza/135g	323	10.8	240	11.0	31.0	8.0	1.8
Margherita, Italiano, Tesco*	1 Serving/173g	414	20.9	240	11.4	21.0	12.1	2.0
Margherita, LC, Tesco*	1 Pizza/200g	410	5.0	205	11.0	33.8	2.5	1.7
Margherita, Primafresco, Tesco*	½ Pizza/204g	500	20.4	245	10.7	27.4	10.0	2.4
Margherita, Stone Baked, GFY, Asda*	¼ Pizza/73g	158	1.4	217	11.0	39.0	1.9	1.8
Margherita, Stonebaked Ciabatta, Goodfella's*	½ Pizza/150g	404	17.2	270	11.3	32.8	11.5	2.6
Margherita, Thin & Crispy, Iceland*	½ Pizza/170g	391	14.4	230	12.7	25.9	8.5	2.8
Margherita, Tuscan, Finest, Tesco*	½ Pack/248g	557	22.0	225	8.2	27.7	8.9	1.3
Meat Feast, American Style, Sainsbury's*	½ Pizza/263g	642	26.0	244	12.6	26.2	9.9	2.9
Meat Feast, Deep & Crispy, Iceland*	1/6 Pizza/136g	345	11.3	254	11.2	33.7	8.3	2.0
Meat Feast, Deep & Loaded, Sainsbury's*	½ Pizza/298g	818	30.0	275	13.2	32.7	10.1	2.6
Meat Feast, Deep Pan, Co-Op*	1 Pizza/450g	1102	45.0	245	11.0	28.0	10.0	2.0
Meat Feast, Hot & Spicy, Thin & Crispy, Sainsbury's*	½ Pizza/170g	462	21.6	272	13.0	26.5	12.7	3.2
Meat Feast, Italian, Thin & Crispy, Waitrose*	1 Pizza/182g	477	22.9	262	10.7	26.5	12.6	1.8
Meat Feast, Stuffed Crust, Asda*	½ Pizza/238g	597	24.0	251	14.6	25.5	10.1	3.1
Meat Feast, Thin & Crispy, Asda*	½ Pizza/183g	410	14.6	224	11.0	27.0	8.0	1.4
Meat Feast, Thin Crust, Tesco*	½ Pizza/178g	430	20.2	242	13.6	21.3	11.4	2.3
Meat Feast, Ultimate, Sainsbury's*	1 Pizza/465g	1302	47.9	280	13.5	35.1	10.3	1.7
Mozzarella, Ristorante, Dr Oetker*	1 Pizza/335g	874	44.6	261	10.4	23.9	13.3	1.7
Mozzarella & Black Forest Ham, Italian, Asda*	¼ Pizza/110g	227	6.6	206	10.0	28.0	6.0	2.7
Mozzarella & Sunblush Tomato, 12", TTD, Sainsbury's*	½ Pizza/251g	638	17.8	254	12.4	35.0	7.1	2.6
Mozzarella & Tomato, Asda*	1 Pizza/360g	824	32.4	229	12.0	25.0	9.0	2.4
Mozzarella E Provolone, La Bottega, Goodfella's*	½ Pizza/156g	372	15.0	238	10.1	27.9	9.6	2.4
Napoletana, Sainsbury's*	½ Pizza/186g	424	14.3	228	9.7	29.9	7.7	3.1
Napoli, Tesco*	½ Pizza/184g	431	11.6	235	11.9	32.6	6.3	1.4
Napoli Ham & Mushroom, San Marco*	½ Pizza/219g	449	13.4	205	10.0	27.5	6.1	2.8
Pepper, Fire Roasted, Sainsbury's*	1 Pizza/344g	605	5.2	176	5.3	35.3	1.5	1.6
Pepper, Grilled, Weight Watchers*	1 Pizza/220g	392	5.1	178	10.0	29.3	2.3	1.8
Pepperonata, Delicata, Sainsbury's*	1 Pizza/330g	917	47.5	278	12.9	24.3	14.4	2.6
Pepperoni, Average	1 Serving/250g	671	28.4	269	11.8	29.6	11.4	2.1
Pepperoni, Deep & Crispy, Iceland*	1 Serving/175g	490	21.0	280	11.9	31.1	12.0	1.8
Pepperoni, Deep Pan, Goodfella's*	¼ Pizza/109g	294	12.6	270	12.7	28.9	11.6	1.6
Pepperoni, Deluxe, American Deep Pan, Sainsbury's*	1 Pizza/424g	1077	40.3	254	13.3	28.7	9.5	2.7

	Measure INFO/WEIGHT	per Measure KCAL	FAT	Nutrition Values per 100g / 100ml KCAL	PROT	CARB	FAT	FIBRE
PIZZA								
Pepperoni, Double, Italian, Chilled, Tesco*	½ Pizza/160g	455	23.3	285	12.4	25.6	14.6	2.4
Pepperoni, Extra, Chicago Town*	1 Pizza/460g	994	34.0	216	9.6	27.7	7.4	0.0
Pepperoni, Feast, Deep Dish, Schwan's*	1 Pizza/435g	1188	61.8	273	9.9	26.3	14.2	0.0
Pepperoni, Goodfella's*	1 Pizza/337g	900	43.5	267	13.2	26.3	12.9	1.7
Pepperoni, Hot & Spicy, Stuffed Crust, Asda*	1 Pizza/245g	666	30.0	272	13.9	26.5	12.2	2.4
Pepperoni, Hot & Spicy, Thin Crust, Chilled, Tesco*	½ Pizza/174g	486	25.5	280	12.4	24.0	14.7	2.2
Pepperoni, Italian Stonebaked, Asda*	¼ Pizza/132g	329	13.2	250	12.0	28.0	10.0	2.8
Pepperoni, Italian Style, Stonebaked, Stateside Foods*	½ Pizza/168g	436	17.9	260	11.8	29.0	10.7	2.1
Pepperoni, Mini, Tesco*	1 Serving/22g	71	3.7	323	11.8	30.5	16.8	2.7
Pepperoni, Pizzeria Style, Sainsbury's*	½ Pizza/183g	515	23.3	281	13.5	28.0	12.7	2.2
Pepperoni, Speciale, Sainsbury's*	½ Pizza/179g	448	19.5	250	11.9	26.6	10.9	2.3
Pepperoni, Stone Baked, Carlos*	1 Pizza/330g	832	39.6	252	13.0	23.0	12.0	0.0
Pepperoni, Stonebake, 10", Asda*	½ Pizza/170g	435	19.0	256	12.9	25.9	11.2	2.5
Pepperoni, Stonebaked, American Hot, Sainsbury's*	½ Pizza/276g	674	30.9	244	11.6	24.1	11.2	2.9
Pepperoni, Stonebaked Ciabatta, Goodfella's*	½ Pizza/181g	503	26.1	278	11.9	27.4	14.4	2.4
Pepperoni, Thin & Crispy, Essential, Waitrose*	½ Pizza/133g	380	18.0	286	12.3	28.8	13.5	1.0
Pepperoni, Thin & Crispy, Goodfella's*	1 Pizza/593g	1595	70.0	269	13.8	26.9	11.8	2.3
Pepperoni, Weight Watchers*	1 Pizza/300g	501	9.3	167	8.0	25.4	3.1	2.8
Pepperoni, Xxx Hot, Deep & Crispy, Chilled, Tesco*	½ Pizza/262g	656	27.0	250	9.1	30.1	10.3	2.0
Pepperoni, Zingy, Asda*	1 Serving/90g	255	6.3	283	12.0	43.0	7.0	4.0
Pepperoni & Cheese, Asda*	½ Pizza/150g	386	13.5	257	10.0	34.0	9.0	2.7
Pepperoni & Jalapeno Chill, Asda*	1 Pizza/277g	742	22.2	268	10.0	39.0	8.0	1.8
Pepperoni & Onion, 9", Sainsbury's*	½ Pizza/207g	615	26.9	297	13.4	31.7	13.0	1.9
Prosciutto, Ristorante, Dr Oetker*	1 Pizza/330g	752	32.3	228	10.3	24.6	9.8	0.0
Quattro Formaggi, 8 Inch, Supermarket, Pizza Express*	1 Pizza/266g	646	26.1	243	12.1	26.5	9.8	2.3
Quattro Formaggi, Ristorante, Dr Oetker*	½ Pizza/170g	457	23.8	269	10.8	24.1	14.0	1.6
Quattro Formaggi Pizzeria, Sainsbury's*	½ Pizza/175g	490	21.2	280	12.8	30.8	12.1	2.5
Quattro Formaggio, Tesco*	½ Pizza/219g	583	27.4	266	13.3	25.1	12.5	1.8
Salame, Ristorante, Dr Oetker*	½ Pizza/160g	455	24.5	285	10.4	26.3	15.3	0.0
Salami, Lidl*	1 Pizza/350g	854	32.2	244	8.1	29.4	9.2	0.0
Salami, Ultra Thin Italian, Tesco*	1 Serving/263g	692	25.5	263	12.0	31.9	9.7	1.0
Salami & Ham, Pizzeria, Waitrose*	½ Pizza/205g	443	13.7	216	10.1	28.7	6.7	1.8
Salami & Pepperoni, Waitrose*	½ Pizza/190g	578	30.8	304	13.4	23.9	16.2	2.1
Salami Con Mozarella, Lidl*	½ Pizza/200g	534	22.4	267	9.9	31.5	11.2	0.0
Salmon, Honey Roast, & Broccoli, BGTY, Sainsbury's*	1 Serving/280g	613	12.6	219	10.2	34.4	4.5	3.5
Sicilian, Premium, Co-Op*	1 Pizza/600g	1320	48.0	220	9.0	27.0	8.0	2.0
Slice Selection, M & S*	1 Serving/52g	120	4.1	230	9.4	30.3	7.8	1.9
Sloppy Joe, Take Away, Chicago Town*	¼ Pizza/158g	374	12.6	237	8.2	26.1	8.0	2.1
Spinach, with Bacon & Mushroom, GFY, Asda*	1 Serving/270g	618	12.2	229	13.0	34.0	4.5	2.6
Spinach & Bacon, Thin & Crispy, M & S*	1 Pizza/290g	740	35.1	255	10.6	26.8	12.1	1.0
Spinach & Ricotta, BGTY, Sainsbury's*	1 Pizza/265g	535	6.6	202	10.4	34.4	2.5	2.6
Spinach & Ricotta, Extra Special, Asda*	1 Pizza/400g	940	28.0	235	9.0	34.0	7.0	1.9
Spinach & Ricotta, Italian, Chilled, Sainsbury's*	1 Pizza/361g	859	34.7	238	9.3	28.7	9.6	2.3
Spinach & Ricotta, Perfectly Balanced, Waitrose*	½ Pizza/165g	272	2.8	165	9.7	27.7	1.7	2.6
Spinach & Ricotta, Pizzaria, Waitrose*	½ Pizza/238g	501	21.1	211	10.7	21.9	8.9	2.6
Spinach & Ricotta, Thin Crust, Italian, Tesco*	½ Pizza/190g	365	16.7	192	9.6	18.7	8.8	1.9
Super Supreme, Family, Chicago Town*	¼ Pizza/225g	526	24.3	234	9.6	24.5	10.8	0.0
Supreme, Deep Dish, Individual, Chicago Town*	1 Pizza/170g	456	20.4	268	9.2	30.8	12.0	1.0
Supreme, McCain*	1 Serving/125g	267	8.6	214	10.9	27.0	6.9	0.0
Supreme, Square to Share, Farmfoods*	1 Serving/93g	196	8.0	211	10.7	22.9	8.6	1.1
Sweet & Sour Chicken, Thin Crust, Tesco*	½ Pizza/186g	366	12.8	197	11.9	21.9	6.9	2.3
The Big Cheese, Deep Pan, Goodfella's*	1/6 Pizza/118g	295	12.7	250	12.2	25.9	10.8	1.1
The Big Eat Meat X-Treme, Deep Pan, Goodfella's*	½ Pizza/352g	806	28.9	229	11.6	27.1	8.2	3.6

	Measure INFO/WEIGHT	per Measure KCAL	FAT	Nutrition Values per 100g / 100ml KCAL	PROT	CARB	FAT	FIBRE
PIZZA								
Three Cheese, Ultra Thin, Sodebo*	1 Pizza/180g	450	18.4	250	10.9	28.5	10.2	1.8
Three Cheese & Cherry Tomato, Weight Watchers*	1 Pizza/256g	399	4.1	156	9.8	25.6	1.6	2.3
Three Cheese Calzone, Waitrose*	1 Pizza/265g	747	31.8	282	10.4	33.0	12.0	1.4
Three Cheeses & Tomato, Stonebaked, Co-Op*	1 Pizza/415g	888	33.6	214	10.0	25.2	8.1	1.5
Three Meat, Thin & Crispy, Sainsbury's*	½ Pizza/147g	344	15.7	234	12.5	23.4	10.7	1.3
Tomato	1oz/28g	54	3.0	193	3.3	22.6	10.6	1.4
Tomato, Aubergine & Spinach, Pizzeria, Waitrose*	½ Pizza/193g	403	7.7	209	7.8	35.4	4.0	3.6
Tomato, Basil & Garlic, Weight Watchers*	1 Serving/85g	169	2.9	199	12.3	29.8	3.4	1.6
Tomato, Mushroom & Bacon, Deep Pan, Co-Op*	1 Pizza/420g	882	33.6	210	9.0	25.0	8.0	2.0
Tomato, Roasted, & Mozzarella, BGTY, Sainsbury's*	1 Pizza/204g	526	16.4	258	17.8	28.6	8.0	6.0
Tomato & Cheese, Stone Bake, M & S*	1 Pizza/340g	782	28.6	230	10.8	30.1	8.4	1.6
Tomato & Cheese, Thin & Crispy, M & S*	1 Pizza/300g	705	28.2	235	11.0	27.7	9.4	1.2
Tomato & Pesto, Tesco*	1 Serving/176g	449	23.2	256	8.4	25.9	13.2	1.1
Tomato & Red Pepper, Perfectly Balanced, Waitrose*	½ Pizza/163g	313	2.4	192	6.6	38.1	1.5	1.9
Tomato & Ricotta, Waitrose*	½ Pizza/208g	444	18.5	214	7.8	25.7	8.9	2.2
Triple Cheese, Deep Dish, Chicago Town*	1 Serving/170g	418	18.2	246	9.9	27.6	10.7	0.0
Tuna & Caramelised Red Onion, COU, M & S*	1 Pizza/245g	429	5.6	175	9.6	26.7	2.3	1.2
Tuna Sweetcorn, BGTY, Sainsbury's*	1 Pizza/304g	602	5.8	198	13.5	31.7	1.9	2.7
Tuscana, Finest, Tesco*	1 Serving/255g	643	35.7	252	13.2	18.4	14.0	5.9
Vegetable, Average	1 Serving/250g	475	13.1	190	8.2	27.5	5.2	2.4
Vegetable, Chargrilled, Frozen, BGTY, Sainsbury's*	1 Pizza/290g	548	13.3	189	10.2	26.7	4.6	3.0
Vegetable, Chargrilled, HE, Tesco*	½ Pizza/143g	320	3.9	224	10.4	39.6	2.7	1.1
Vegetable, Chargrilled, Thin & Crispy, GFY, Asda*	1 Serving/188g	290	3.8	154	6.0	28.0	2.0	3.1
Vegetable, COU, M & S*	1 Pizza/294g	397	7.1	135	6.4	23.2	2.4	1.9
Vegetable, Deep Pan, Co-Op*	1 Pizza/425g	829	29.8	195	8.0	25.0	7.0	2.0
Vegetable, Frozen, HL, Tesco*	1 Pizza/400g	604	10.8	151	8.1	23.5	2.7	4.4
Vegetable, Mediterranean, Pizzeria, Sainsbury's*	1 Serving/211g	397	13.5	188	8.0	24.7	6.4	3.2
Vegetable, Mediterranean, Stonebaked, Sainsbury's*	½ Pizza/260g	622	16.4	239	9.8	35.7	6.3	3.1
Vegetable, Ristorante, Dr Oetker*	½ Pizza/185g	386	16.6	209	8.1	23.9	9.0	0.0
Vegetable, Roasted, for One, GFY, Asda*	1 Pizza/96g	190	3.6	198	9.0	32.0	3.8	1.5
Vegetable, Spicy, Low Fat, Bertorelli*	1 Pizza/180g	243	4.3	135	6.0	23.4	2.4	1.9
Vegetable, Stone Bake, M & S*	1 Serving/465g	837	26.0	180	7.8	25.0	5.6	1.5
Vegetable, Thin & Crispy, Iceland*	½ Pizza/200g	442	21.2	221	8.3	23.2	10.6	1.7
Vegetable Feast, Thin & Crispy, Iceland*	1 Slice/63g	148	6.9	237	7.8	26.5	11.1	1.8
Verona, Frozen, Finest, Tesco*	1 Serving/238g	542	23.3	228	11.6	23.2	9.8	2.7
PIZZA BASE								
Deep Pan, Napolina*	1 Base/260g	757	7.8	291	7.9	58.0	3.0	0.2
Garlic Bread, Sainsbury's*	¼ Base/59g	109	4.2	186	5.1	25.4	7.1	1.8
GF, Glutafin*	1 Base/110g	278	5.5	253	3.0	49.0	5.0	4.5
Gluten, Wheat & Dairy Free, Free From, Livwell*	1 Base/100g	237	2.6	237	5.2	48.3	2.6	4.7
Gluten & Wheat Free, Glutafin*	1 Base/110g	309	5.5	281	3.0	56.0	5.0	6.0
Italian, Classic, Sainsbury's*	1 Base/150g	452	7.2	301	7.6	57.0	4.8	1.5
Italian, Deep Pan, Sainsbury's*	1 Base/220g	684	11.0	311	7.0	59.5	5.0	1.4
Italian, The Pizza Company*	1 Base/260g	624	6.8	240	7.6	46.5	2.6	0.0
Italiana, Parmalat*	1 Base/150g	450	7.4	300	9.0	55.0	4.9	0.0
Light & Crispy, Napolina*	1 Base/150g	436	4.5	291	7.9	58.0	3.0	0.2
Mini, Napolina*	1 Base/75g	218	2.2	291	7.9	58.0	3.0	0.2
Pre Rolled, As Sold, Greenvale, Aldi*	1 Pack/400g	1048	16.4	262	9.3	46.0	4.1	2.6
Thin & Crispy, Sainsbury's*	1 Base/150g	504	7.8	336	9.9	62.3	5.2	4.3
Trufree*	1 Base/110g	345	6.6	314	3.0	63.0	6.0	4.0
PIZZA BASE MIX								
Morrisons*	1 Serving/77g	313	3.8	407	12.7	77.9	5.0	3.6
Sainsbury's*	1 Pack/145g	486	5.5	335	12.8	62.3	3.8	2.9

	Measure INFO/WEIGHT	per Measure KCAL	FAT	Nutrition Values per 100g / 100ml KCAL	PROT	CARB	FAT	FIBRE
PLAICE								
Fillets, Lightly Dusted, Average	1 Fillet/113g	188	9.2	166	12.9	10.4	8.2	0.6
Fillets, Raw, Average	***1oz/28g***	***24***	***0.4***	***87***	***18.2***	***0.0***	***1.5***	***0.0***
Fillets in Breadcrumbs, Average	1 Serving/150g	331	17.9	221	12.8	15.5	11.9	0.8
Goujons, Baked	1oz/28g	85	5.1	304	8.8	27.7	18.3	0.0
Goujons, Fried in Blended Oil	1oz/28g	119	9.0	426	8.5	27.0	32.3	0.0
Grilled	***1oz/28g***	***27***	***0.5***	***96***	***20.1***	***0.0***	***1.7***	***0.0***
Steamed	***1oz/28g***	***26***	***0.5***	***93***	***18.9***	***0.0***	***1.9***	***0.0***
PLAICE WITH								
Mushrooms & Prawns, Sainsbury's*	1 Serving/170g	354	18.2	208	12.0	15.9	10.7	1.7
Prawns, Fillets, Asda*	1oz/28g	24	1.3	86	11.0	0.4	4.5	0.7
Prawns, in Breadcrumbs, Aldi*	1 Serving/100g	212	8.4	212	8.6	25.4	8.4	0.0
Spinach & Cheddar Cheese, Fillets, Sainsbury's*	1 Serving/154g	222	13.3	144	13.6	3.1	8.6	0.8
Spinach & Ricotta Cheese, Whole, Sainsbury's*	1 Serving/159g	334	16.7	210	11.6	17.2	10.5	0.8
PLANTAIN								
Boiled in Unsalted Water	***1oz/28g***	***31***	***0.1***	***112***	***0.8***	***28.5***	***0.2***	***1.2***
Raw, Average	***1 Med/179g***	***218***	***0.7***	***122***	***1.3***	***31.9***	***0.4***	***2.3***
Ripe, Fried in Vegetable Oil	***1oz/28g***	***75***	***2.6***	***267***	***1.5***	***47.5***	***9.2***	***2.3***
PLUMS								
Average, Stewed without Sugar	***1oz/28g***	***8***	***0.0***	***30***	***0.5***	***7.3***	***0.1***	***1.3***
Fresh, Raw, Weighed without Stone, Average	1 Plum/66g	24	0.1	36	0.6	8.6	0.1	1.9
Weighed with Stone, Average	***1 Plum/90g***	***33***	***0.1***	***36***	***0.6***	***8.6***	***0.1***	***1.9***
Whole, Dried, Graze*	1 Pack/60g	143	0.3	239	2.6	56.0	0.5	0.0
Whole, Imperial, Graze*	1 Punnet/45g	124	0.0	275	2.6	56.0	0.1	7.1
POLENTA								
Dry, Merchant Gourmet*	1 Serving/65g	232	0.9	357	7.4	78.8	1.4	1.3
Organic, Dry, Kallo*	1 Serving/150g	543	2.7	362	8.5	78.0	1.8	0.0
POLLOCK								
Breaded, Asda*	1 Serving/97g	200	9.7	206	12.0	17.0	10.0	1.0
Fillets, Alaskan, Simply Bake to Perfection, Birds Eye*	1oz/28g	34	1.9	120	13.9	0.6	6.9	0.0
POLO								
Citrus Sharp, Nestle*	1 Tube/34g	134	0.3	393	0.0	96.6	1.0	0.0
Fruits, Nestle*	1 Tube/37g	142	0.0	383	0.0	96.0	0.0	0.0
Mints, Clear Ice, Nestle*	1 Sweet/4g	16	0.0	390	0.0	97.5	0.0	0.0
Mints, Original, Nestle*	1 Sweet/2g	8	0.0	402	0.0	98.2	1.0	0.0
Spearmint, Nestle*	1 Tube/35g	141	0.4	402	0.0	98.2	1.1	0.0
POMEGRANATE								
Raw, Fresh, Flesh Only, Average	***1 Sm Fruit/86g***	***59***	***0.3***	***68***	***1.0***	***17.2***	***0.3***	***0.6***
Raw, Weighed with Rind & Skin, Average	***1 Sm Fruit/154g***	***105***	***0.5***	***68***	***1.0***	***17.2***	***0.3***	***0.1***
Snack Pot, Morrisons*	1 Pot/100g	38	0.1	38	0.9	7.3	0.1	2.2
POMELO								
Fresh, Raw, Weighed with Skin & Seeds	***1 Serving/100g***	***18***	***0.1***	***18***	***0.4***	***4.1***	***0.1***	***0.0***
Raw, Flesh Only, Average	1 Fruit/340g	129	0.1	38	0.8	9.6	0.0	1.0
POP TARTS								
Blueberry, Unfrosted, Kellogg's*	1 Tart/52g	200	5.0	385	3.8	71.2	9.6	1.9
Bustin' Berry, Kellogg's*	1 Tart/50g	200	6.0	400	4.0	69.0	12.0	2.0
Chocolate, Kellogg's*	1 Tart/50g	198	8.5	396	5.0	136.0	17.0	2.0
Chocolate Chip, Kellogg's*	1 Tart/52g	210	6.0	404	5.8	69.2	11.5	1.9
Chocolate Chip Cookie Dough, Kellogg's*	1 Tart/50g	190	5.0	380	4.0	70.0	10.0	2.0
Chocomallow, Kellogg's*	1 Tart/50g	198	6.0	396	6.0	66.0	12.0	2.5
Cinnamon Roll, Kelloggs*	1 Tart/50g	210	7.0	420	4.0	68.0	14.0	2.0
Cookies 'n' Creme, Kellogg's*	1 Tart/50g	190	5.0	380	4.0	70.0	10.0	2.0
Cream Cheese & Cherry Swirl, Kellogg's*	1 Tart/62g	250	11.0	403	3.2	59.7	17.7	1.0
Frosted Blueberry, Kellogg's*	1 Tart/52g	200	5.0	385	3.8	73.1	9.6	1.9

P

	Measure INFO/WEIGHT	per Measure KCAL	FAT	Nutrition Values per 100g / 100ml KCAL	PROT	CARB	FAT	FIBRE
POP TARTS								
Frosted Confetti Cupcake, Kellogg's*	1 Tart/50g	190	4.0	380	4.0	72.0	8.0	2.0
Frosted S'mores, Kellogg's*	1 Tart/52g	200	5.0	385	5.8	69.2	9.6	1.9
Frosted Strawberry, Low Fat, Kellogg's*	1 Tart/50g	1800	25.0	360	4.0	74.0	5.0	6.0
Frosted Strawberry, Oatmeal Delights, Kellogg's*	1 Tart/50g	200	5.0	400	4.0	72.0	10.0	6.0
Strawberry Sensation, Kellogg's*	1 Tart/50g	198	5.5	395	4.0	70.0	11.0	2.0
POPCORN								
Air Popped, Plain, Average	1oz/28g	110	1.3	387	12.9	77.9	4.5	14.5
Butter, 6% Fat, Orville Redenbacher's*	1 Portion/21g	86	1.2	410	11.9	77.6	5.7	14.3
Butter, Microwave, 94% Fat Free, Act II*	½ Bag/41g	130	2.5	317	9.8	68.3	6.1	12.2
Butter, Microwave, Act II*	1 Bag/90g	425	16.2	472	9.0	69.0	18.0	9.0
Butter, Microwave, Butterkist*	1 Bag/100g	395	18.5	395	8.3	49.5	18.5	8.5
Butter Flavour, Microwave, Popz*	1 Serving/100g	480	27.5	480	7.5	51.1	27.5	9.2
Butter Toffee, Asda*	1 Serving/100g	364	8.0	364	2.1	71.0	8.0	4.1
Butter Toffee, Belgian Milk Chocolate Coated, M & S*	1 Pack/100g	505	25.0	505	6.5	60.4	25.0	4.1
Butter Toffee, Snack-A-Jacks, Quaker Oats*	1 Bag/35g	149	3.2	425	3.5	86.0	9.0	4.5
Butter Toffee, Yummies*	1 Serving/50g	228	6.4	455	2.5	82.4	12.8	3.1
Choc Full Of, Cadbury*	¼ Bag/32g	160	7.6	495	4.5	64.5	23.5	2.9
Chocolate & Pecan, M & S*	1 Packet/27g	130	5.2	480	3.3	72.9	19.3	3.6
Maize, Unpopped, Love Life, Waitrose*	1 Serving/33g	200	14.1	605	6.2	48.7	42.8	12.7
Microwave, Salted, Sunsnacks*	1 Pack/100g	498	22.9	498	10.7	51.3	22.9	10.8
Plain, Oil Popped, Average	1 Bag/74g	439	31.7	593	6.2	48.7	42.8	0.0
Popping Corn, Lightly Salted, Graze*	1 Punnet/28g	127	7.0	454	8.0	44.0	25.0	13.0
Popping Corn, Slightly Sweet, Graze*	1 Punnet/23g	95	3.6	415	8.1	55.9	15.5	13.3
Salt & Sweet, Pure*	1 Serving/25g	119	5.5	476	6.0	61.1	22.1	7.8
Salt & Vinegar, Diet Chef Ltd*	1 Serving/23g	106	3.6	461	10.4	69.8	15.8	13.0
Salt & Vinegar, Snack-A-Jacks, Quaker Oats*	1 Pack/13g	47	1.3	360	12.0	55.0	9.9	14.0
Salted, Blockbuster*	1 Bowl/25g	99	2.9	397	10.6	62.2	11.7	8.6
Salted, Bop, Microwave, Zanuy*	1 Serving/25g	119	5.8	477	10.7	56.9	23.0	0.0
Salted, Diet Chef Ltd*	1 Pack/23g	107	3.8	465	10.5	68.6	16.6	14.0
Salted, Light, Microwave, Act II*	1 Pack/85g	336	6.5	395	10.6	71.0	7.6	15.8
Salted, Manhatten Peanuts Limited*	1 Bag/30g	135	4.3	450	10.0	70.0	14.3	13.7
Salted, Microwave, 93% Fat Free, Act II*	1 Pack/85g	345	6.0	406	10.0	76.0	7.0	13.0
Salted, Sold At Cinema, Playtime Popcorn*	1 Sm/74g	384	24.9	519	8.3	45.9	33.6	0.0
Sea Salt Flavour, Skinny, Topcorn, Metcalfe's Food Co*	1 Pack/23g	108	5.6	471	6.6	63.7	24.4	15.2
Sweet, Best-In*	1 Serving/34g	161	5.8	473	7.3	72.6	17.0	0.0
Sweet, Butterkist, Butterkist*	1 Pack/120g	612	29.8	510	2.8	68.5	24.8	5.6
Sweet, Cinema Style, Butterkist*	1 Bag/120g	612	29.8	510	2.8	68.5	24.8	5.6
Sweet, Microwave, Butterkist*	½ Pack/50g	235	10.0	470	9.8	60.5	20.1	4.4
Sweet, Microwave, Cinema, Popz*	1 Bag/85g	420	21.7	494	6.0	60.0	25.5	8.2
Sweet, Vanilla & Sugar, Microwave, Act II*	1 Pack75g	369	18.1	492	7.9	60.8	24.1	10.4
Sweet & Salty, Propercorn*	1 Pack/30g	128	4.2	428	5.9	63.5	13.9	12.7
Sweet & Salty, Shapers, Boots*	1 Bag/20g	89	3.2	443	5.8	65.0	16.0	10.0
Sweet Maple, Diet Chef Ltd*	1 Pack/23g	111	3.6	483	9.7	75.2	15.7	13.0
Toffee, 90% Fat Free, Butterkist*	1 Pack/35g	142	3.3	406	2.8	77.7	9.3	0.0
Toffee, Best-In*	1 Bag/90g	356	3.2	396	5.0	85.9	3.6	0.0
Toffee, Butterkist*	1 Bag/30g	124	3.0	415	2.3	79.3	10.0	4.4
Toffee, Chicago Joes*	1 Serving/10g	31	0.5	314	3.1	84.6	4.8	0.0
Toffee, Milk Chocolate Coated, Butterkist*	1 Bag/50g	252	12.5	505	6.5	61.9	25.0	4.1
Toffee, Milk Chocolate Coated, Morrisons*	1 Serving/25g	119	5.0	479	4.1	68.9	20.0	3.3
Toffee, Milk Chocolate Coated, Sainsbury's*	¼ Bag/25g	130	6.6	520	6.5	64.1	26.4	1.3
Toffee, Sainsbury's*	1 Serving/50g	208	6.4	415	1.8	73.8	12.7	3.3
Toffee, Snack Pack, Butterkist*	1 Bag/25g	105	2.2	420	2.1	81.3	9.0	3.5
Vanilla, Cinema Sweet Microwave, Act II*	½ Pack/50g	234	8.0	468	9.0	71.0	16.0	12.0

	Measure INFO/WEIGHT	per Measure KCAL	per Measure FAT	KCAL	PROT	CARB	FAT	FIBRE
				Nutrition Values per 100g / 100ml				
POPCORN								
Wasabi, Pret a Manger*	1 Pack/29g	137	6.4	472	7.2	55.2	22.1	10.7
Wasabi Flavour, Skinny, Topcorn, Metcalfe's Food Co*	1 Bag/25g	121	6.6	484	8.4	54.1	26.2	9.7
POPPADOMS								
Fried in Vegetable Oil, Takeaway, Average	1 Poppadom/13g	65	5.0	501	11.5	28.3	38.8	5.8
Indian, Asda*	1 Pack/45g	232	15.7	516	14.5	36.2	34.8	7.8
Mini, Sainsbury's*	½ Pack/50g	249	16.2	498	14.9	36.9	32.3	7.6
Plain, Asda*	1 Poppadom/9g	44	2.5	484	18.0	40.0	28.0	0.0
Plain, Bilash, Aldi*	1 Poppadom/10g	46	2.2	463	15.2	48.7	22.3	0.0
Plain, Indian to Go, Sainsbury's*	1 Poppadom/8g	34	1.5	405	18.4	43.4	17.5	9.0
Plain, Tesco*	1 Serving/9g	41	2.0	439	17.8	44.4	21.1	4.6
Plain, Waitrose*	1 Serving/9g	37	1.7	408	21.0	39.3	18.6	9.1
Spicy, COU, M & S*	1 Pack/26g	84	0.6	325	23.5	51.9	2.4	8.1
Tesco*	1 Poppadum/9g	39	1.9	440	17.8	44.4	21.1	4.6
POPPETS*								
Chocolate Raisins, Poppets*	1 Pack/35g	140	4.7	401	4.9	65.4	13.3	0.0
Mint Cream, Poppets*	1oz/28g	119	3.6	424	2.0	75.0	13.0	0.0
Peanut, Poppets*	1 Box/100g	544	37.0	544	16.4	37.0	37.0	0.0
Toffee, Milk Chocolate, Poppets*	1 Box/100g	491	23.0	491	5.3	68.0	23.0	0.0
PORK								
Belly, Fresh, Raw, Weighed with Skin, Average	1 Serving/100g	518	53.0	518	9.3	0.0	53.0	0.0
Belly, Roasted, Lean & Fat	1oz/28g	82	6.0	293	25.1	0.0	21.4	0.0
Chitterlings, Raw, Average	1 Serving/100g	182	16.6	182	7.6	0.0	16.6	0.0
Chop, Lean & Fat, Boneless, Raw, Average	***1oz/28g***	***67***	***3.8***	***240***	***29.2***	***0.0***	***13.7***	***0.0***
Diced, Lean, Average	***1oz/28g***	***31***	***0.5***	***109***	***22.0***	***0.0***	***1.8***	***0.0***
Escalope, Average	***1 Escalope/75g***	***108***	***1.7***	***144***	***31.0***	***0.0***	***2.2***	***0.0***
Escalope, Lean, Healthy Range, Average	***1 Escalope/75g***	***80***	***1.5***	***106***	***22.0***	***0.0***	***2.0***	***0.0***
Ham, Hock, Raw, Weighed with Bone, Fat & Skin	1 Serving/100g	139	5.6	139	20.6	0.0	5.6	0.0
Joint, Ready to Roast, Average	***½ Joint/254g***	***375***	***18.0***	***148***	***19.2***	***2.3***	***7.1***	***0.2***
Joint with Crackling, Ready to Roast, Average	***1 Joint/567g***	***1283***	***80.1***	***226***	***24.2***	***0.8***	***14.1***	***0.0***
Leg, Joint, Healthy Range, Average	***1 Serving/200g***	***206***	***4.4***	***103***	***20.0***	***0.6***	***2.2***	***0.0***
Loin, Chops, Boneless, Grilled, Average	***1oz/28g***	***90***	***4.4***	***320***	***29.0***	***0.0***	***15.7***	***0.0***
Loin, Chops, Grilled, Lean	***1oz/28g***	***52***	***1.8***	***184***	***31.6***	***0.0***	***6.4***	***0.0***
Loin, Chops, Raw, Lean & Fat, Weighed with Bone	1 Chop/130g	295	23.7	227	15.7	0.0	18.2	0.0
Loin, Joint, Roast, Lean	***1oz/28g***	***51***	***1.9***	***182***	***30.1***	***0.0***	***6.8***	***0.0***
Loin, Joint, Roast, Lean & Fat	***1oz/28g***	***71***	***4.3***	***253***	***26.3***	***0.0***	***15.3***	***0.0***
Loin, Steak, Fried, Lean	***1oz/28g***	***53***	***2.0***	***191***	***31.5***	***0.0***	***7.2***	***0.0***
Loin, Steak, Fried, Lean & Fat	***1oz/28g***	***77***	***5.2***	***276***	***27.5***	***0.0***	***18.4***	***0.0***
Loin, Steak, Lean, Raw, Average	***1 Serving/175g***	***345***	***19.6***	***197***	***22.7***	***1.8***	***11.2***	***0.4***
Loin, Stuffed, Roast, M & S*	1 Slice/12g	22	0.9	180	24.4	2.4	7.9	0.0
Medallions, Average	***1 Medallion/125g***	***140***	***2.6***	***112***	***22.6***	***0.0***	***2.0***	***0.0***
Mince, Lean, Healthy Range, Average	***1 Pack/400g***	***504***	***20.2***	***126***	***19.8***	***0.4***	***5.0***	***0.3***
Mince, Raw	***1oz/28g***	***46***	***2.7***	***164***	***19.2***	***0.0***	***9.7***	***0.0***
Mince, Stewed	***1oz/28g***	***53***	***2.9***	***191***	***24.4***	***0.0***	***10.4***	***0.0***
Raw, Lean, Average	***1oz/28g***	***42***	***1.2***	***151***	***28.6***	***0.0***	***4.1***	***0.0***
Rib, Chops, Raw, Lean & Fat, Weighed with Bone	1 Chop/130g	287	19.2	221	22.0	0.0	14.8	0.0
Roast, Lean Only, Average	***1oz/28g***	***34***	***0.9***	***121***	***22.7***	***0.3***	***3.3***	***0.0***
Roast, Slices, Average	***1 Slice/30g***	***40***	***1.4***	***134***	***22.7***	***0.4***	***4.5***	***0.0***
Shoulder, Slices, Cured	***1oz/28g***	***29***	***1.0***	***103***	***16.9***	***0.9***	***3.6***	***0.0***
Shoulder, Whole, Lean & Fat, Raw, Average	***1 Serving/100g***	***236***	***18.0***	***236***	***17.2***	***0.0***	***18.0***	***0.0***
Shoulder, Whole, Lean Only, Roasted	1 Serving/150g	345	20.3	230	25.3	0.0	13.5	0.0
Steak, Lean, Stewed	***1oz/28g***	***49***	***1.3***	***176***	***33.6***	***0.0***	***4.6***	***0.0***
Steak, Lean & Fat, Average	***1oz/28g***	***61***	***3.8***	***219***	***23.8***	***0.0***	***13.7***	***0.1***
Stir Fry Strips, Lean, Healthy Range, Average	***¼ Pack/113g***	***118***	***2.3***	***104***	***21.3***	***0.0***	***2.0***	***0.0***

P

	Measure INFO/WEIGHT	per Measure KCAL	FAT	Nutrition Values per 100g / 100ml KCAL	PROT	CARB	FAT	FIBRE
PORK								
Streaky, Boneless, Slices, British, Tesco*	1 Pack/460g	1477	106.7	321	0.0	0.0	23.2	0.0
Tenderloin, Lean, Boneless, Raw, Average	1 Serving/100g	109	2.2	109	21.0	0.0	2.2	0.0
Tenderloin, Roulade, Waitrose*	1 Pack/171g	282	12.8	165	18.4	5.9	7.5	1.8
Tenderloin, Separable Lean & Fat, Raw, Average	1 Loin/265g	318	9.4	120	20.6	0.0	3.5	0.0
PORK CHAR SUI								
Chinese, Tesco*	1 Pack/400g	520	17.2	130	7.2	15.7	4.3	0.6
in Cantonese Sauce, Asda*	1 Pack/360g	623	7.9	173	9.8	28.4	2.2	0.5
Oriental, Finest, Tesco*	1 Pack/350g	245	5.2	70	6.8	6.2	1.5	2.1
Takeaway, Iceland*	1 Pack/400g	412	9.6	103	7.9	12.5	2.4	1.2
with Chicken & Egg Fried Rice, Tesco*	1 Serving/450g	602	16.2	134	7.1	18.3	3.6	0.9
PORK CHINESE								
Sliced, M & S*	1 Serving/140g	224	4.3	160	26.4	6.1	3.1	0.0
Style, GFY, Asda*	1 Serving/170g	286	6.0	168	18.8	15.3	3.5	0.4
with Noodles, Tesco*	1 Serving/450g	612	25.6	136	7.0	14.2	5.7	1.1
PORK DINNER								
Roast, Birds Eye*	1 Pack/340g	410	12.0	121	7.6	14.7	3.5	1.6
Roast Dinner, 103, Oakhouse Foods Ltd*	1 Dinner/400g	376	14.8	94	6.7	8.3	3.7	1.4
PORK IN								
Light Mustard Sauce, Fillet, COU, M & S*	1 Pack/390g	312	9.4	80	10.9	3.5	2.4	0.7
Mustard & Cream, Chops	1oz/28g	73	6.0	261	14.5	2.4	21.6	0.3
Rich Sage & Onion Gravy, Steaks, Tesco*	1 Serving/160g	218	10.4	136	16.0	3.2	6.5	1.5
PORK SCRATCHINGS								
Crunch, Mr Porky*	1 Pack/30g	159	9.6	531	60.4	0.5	31.9	4.6
KP Snacks*	1 Pack/20g	125	9.6	624	47.3	0.5	48.1	0.5
Tavern Snacks*	1 Pack/30g	187	14.4	624	47.3	0.5	48.1	0.5
PORK WITH								
Cheese & Pineapple, Loin Steaks, M & S*	1 Steak/141g	240	14.0	170	14.0	6.3	9.9	0.0
Herbes De Provence, Joint, Sainsbury's*	¼ Joint/200g	302	16.4	151	19.2	0.1	8.2	0.6
Honey & Mustard Sauce, Steaks, Tesco*	½ Pack/160g	258	11.8	161	16.3	8.7	7.4	1.4
Honey & Soy, Sainsbury's*	1 Serving/260g	260	7.5	100	12.3	6.2	2.9	0.3
Leek & Bacon Stuffing, Roast, Shoulder, Sainsbury's*	1 Serving/150g	237	12.4	158	18.8	2.4	8.3	0.5
Leek & Cheese Stuffing, Joint, Sainsbury's*	1 Serving/100g	231	10.5	231	31.0	3.0	10.5	1.1
Medallions with Bramley Apple, M & S*	1 Serving/380g	418	12.9	110	17.7	2.5	3.4	0.5
Noodles, Chinese, Tesco*	1 Serving/450g	464	13.5	103	5.3	13.7	3.0	1.4
Peppers, Marinated, Tapas, Waitrose*	1 Serving/105g	181	6.7	172	26.3	2.2	6.4	0.3
Rice & Beans, Jerk, Love Life, Waitrose*	1 Pack/380g	384	12.2	101	4.9	13.0	3.2	2.1
Roasted Rosemary Potatoes, Porchetta, Finest, Tesco*	½ Pack/370g	455	31.8	123	6.9	4.6	8.6	0.5
Sage, Onion & Lemon Stuffing, Joint, Sainsbury's*	1 Serving/260g	699	43.4	269	27.4	2.2	16.7	1.4
Sage & Onion Stuffing, Joint, BGTY, Sainsbury's*	1 Serving/150g	246	5.4	164	29.5	3.3	3.6	1.3
PORT								
Average	***1 Serving/50ml***	***78***	***0.0***	***157***	***0.1***	***12.0***	***0.0***	***0.0***
POT NOODLE*								
Beef & Tomato, Made Up, Pot Noodle*	1 Pot/320g	426	14.7	133	3.4	19.4	4.6	1.3
Bombay Bad Boy, Made Up, Pot Noodle*	1 Pot/320g	415	15.3	130	3.3	18.4	4.8	1.1
Chicken & Mushroom, Made Up, Pot Noodle*	1 Pot/305g	430	18.0	141	3.0	19.0	5.9	1.0
Chilli Beef, Made Up, Pot Noodle*	1 Pot/305g	384	14.6	126	3.0	17.7	4.8	0.8
Chow Mein Chinese, Made Up, Pot Noodle*	1 Pot/320g	416	14.7	130	3.2	19.0	4.6	1.3
Curry, Balti, Made Up, Pot Noodle*	1 Pot/301g	268	1.5	89	3.1	17.8	0.5	0.5
Curry, Chicken, Hot, Made Up, Pot Noodle*	1 Pot/300g	384	14.1	128	2.8	18.7	4.7	1.1
Curry, Korma, Made Up, Pot Noodle*	1 Pot/300g	273	3.3	91	2.9	17.4	1.1	0.4
Curry, Original, Made Up, Pot Noodle*	1 Pot/320g	431	15.0	135	3.1	20.0	4.7	1.2
Curry, Spicy, Made Up, Pot Noodle*	1 Pot/300g	393	14.4	131	2.9	19.1	4.8	1.1
Hot, Made Up, Pot Noodle*	1 Pot/300g	378	15.6	126	3.0	16.9	5.2	1.1

	Measure INFO/WEIGHT	per Measure KCAL	FAT	Nutrition Values per 100g / 100ml KCAL	PROT	CARB	FAT	FIBRE
POT NOODLE*								
Jamaican Jerk, Made Up, Pot Noodle*	1 Pot/310g	430	15.4	140	3.0	21.0	5.0	1.5
Nice & Spicy, Made Up, Pot Noodle*	1 Pot/300g	381	14.1	127	2.8	18.3	4.7	1.1
Piri Piri Chicken, Made Up, Pot Noodle*	1 Pot/307g	430	15.4	140	3.0	20.0	5.0	0.0
Seedy Sanchez, Made Up, Pot Noodle*	1 Pot/300g	396	14.4	132	3.1	19.1	4.8	1.1
Southern Fried Chicken, Made Up, Pot Noodle*	1 Pot/318g	427	15.0	134	3.1	19.8	4.7	1.2
Sweet & Sour, Oriental, Posh, Made Up, Pot Noodle*	1 Pot/300g	375	13.8	125	1.7	19.2	4.6	0.5
POTATO BOMBAY								
Aloo, M & S*	½ Pack/114g	108	5.2	95	1.8	10.3	4.6	2.3
Average	½ Pack/150g	176	10.2	117	2.0	13.7	6.8	1.2
Canned, Tesco*	1 Can/400g	380	11.6	95	2.5	13.5	2.9	2.3
Indian Takeaway for 1, Sainsbury's*	1 Serving/200g	202	10.4	101	1.8	11.8	5.2	1.7
Meal Solutions, Co-Op*	1 Pack/300g	210	12.0	70	1.0	8.0	4.0	2.0
POTATO CAKES								
Average	1 Cake/70g	127	1.2	180	3.8	37.5	1.7	2.4
Fried, Average	1oz/28g	66	2.5	237	4.9	35.0	9.0	0.8
POTATO FRITTERS								
Crispy, Oven Baked, Birds Eye*	1 Fritter/20g	29	1.6	145	2.0	16.3	8.0	1.2
with Sweetcorn, M & S*	1 Pack/135g	304	17.0	225	4.4	24.1	12.6	2.3
POTATO MASH								
Bacon & Cheese, Tesco*	1 Serving/200g	252	12.8	126	3.1	13.9	6.4	1.3
Bacon & Spring Onion, Finest, Tesco*	½ Pack/200g	214	10.4	107	4.3	10.8	5.2	1.6
Cheddar, Irish, Finest, Tesco*	½ Pack/250g	350	19.8	140	6.3	10.2	7.9	1.4
Cheese & Chive, Snack in a Pot, Tesco*	1 Pot/230g	304	21.6	132	2.2	9.6	9.4	0.9
Cheese & Onion, Tesco*	1 Serving/200g	210	9.4	105	3.2	12.6	4.7	1.0
Leek & Bacon, Tesco*	1 Serving/400g	356	14.4	89	3.0	11.1	3.6	1.9
Leek & Cheese, COU, M & S*	½ Pack/225g	180	4.7	80	3.0	12.0	2.1	1.3
Roast Onion, Snack in a Pot, Tesco*	1 Pot/218g	257	12.9	118	1.6	14.7	5.9	0.6
Sun Dried Tomato & Basil, COU, M & S*	1 Serving/170g	128	2.6	75	1.0	14.4	1.5	1.2
with Cracked Pepper & Sea Salt, Luxury, Sainsbury's*	½ Pack/225g	389	28.4	173	1.6	13.2	12.6	1.0
with Sweetcorn & Flaked Tuna, Quick, Sainsbury's*	1 Pot/224g	240	9.2	107	2.4	15.0	4.1	2.1
with Vegetables, GFY, Asda*	1 Pack/290g	186	3.2	64	1.6	12.0	1.1	2.3
POTATO RINGS								
Mature Cheddar & Red Onion, GFY, Asda*	1 Pack/10g	36	0.2	360	5.2	81.6	1.5	2.9
Ready Salted, M & S*	1 Serving/75g	375	21.1	500	3.5	58.9	28.1	2.6
Salt Vinegar, Sainsbury's*	1 Pack/25g	114	4.9	456	3.6	65.6	19.6	2.8
POTATO SKINS								
¼ Cut, Deep Fried, McCain*	1oz/28g	52	1.7	186	3.0	30.1	6.0	0.0
¼ Cut, Oven Baked, McCain*	1oz/28g	53	1.3	190	3.6	33.1	4.8	0.0
American Style, Loaded, Asda*	1 Serving/78g	294	18.0	375	15.0	27.0	23.0	2.4
Cheese & Bacon, Loaded, Tesco*	1 Skin/59g	150	9.1	255	9.2	19.5	15.5	3.0
Cheese & Bacon, Waitrose*	1 Serving/75g	146	9.4	195	7.3	13.1	12.6	3.5
Cheese & Chive, Sainsbury's*	2 Skins/150g	286	17.8	191	7.7	13.3	11.9	2.8
Cheese & Ham, Iceland*	2 Skins/108g	155	4.9	143	6.3	19.3	4.5	2.0
Cheese & Onion, Loaded, Tesco*	1 Skin/60g	114	6.5	190	5.8	17.6	10.8	1.4
Loaded, HE, Tesco*	1 Serving/340g	425	8.5	125	7.7	17.8	2.5	0.6
with Sour Cream	1 Serving/275g	541	34.6	197	7.2	13.8	12.6	2.2
POTATO SMILES								
Weighed Baked, McCain*	1 Serving/100g	237	10.1	237	3.4	33.4	10.1	3.1
Weighed Frozen, McCain*	1 Serving/100g	191	8.0	191	2.6	27.0	8.0	2.7
POTATO WAFFLES								
Frozen, Cooked	1oz/28g	56	2.3	200	3.2	30.3	8.2	2.3
Frozen, Grilled, Asda*	1 Waffle/57g	104	5.8	183	2.0	21.0	10.1	1.7
Mini, Sainsbury's*	1 Waffle/11g	27	1.8	242	2.8	20.1	16.7	1.0

	Measure	per Measure		Nutrition Values per 100g / 100ml				
	INFO/WEIGHT	KCAL	FAT	KCAL	PROT	CARB	FAT	FIBRE
POTATO WAFFLES								
Oven Baked, Mini, McCain*	1oz/28g	62	2.4	221	3.9	32.0	8.6	0.0
Southern Fried, Asda*	1 Waffle/51g	107	5.1	209	2.8	27.0	10.0	2.1
Uncooked, Average	1 Waffle/62g	113	5.1	182	2.4	24.4	8.3	1.8
POTATO WEDGES								
& Dip, M & S*	1 Pack/450g	698	33.3	155	2.5	20.4	7.4	1.8
Baked, GFY, Asda*	1 Pack/450g	616	11.7	137	3.4	25.0	2.6	3.4
BBQ Flavour, Asda*	1 Serving/100g	185	9.0	185	2.9	23.0	9.0	1.7
BGTY, Sainsbury's*	½ Pack/190g	179	3.4	94	3.0	16.4	1.8	3.4
Crispy, M & S*	1 Serving/200g	340	14.2	170	1.3	25.3	7.1	1.7
Four Cheese & Red Onion, Chicago Town*	1 Serving/150g	210	8.0	140	2.1	21.0	5.3	2.4
Frozen, Average	1 Serving/120g	145	4.1	121	2.0	20.5	3.4	2.2
Garlic & Herb, COU, M & S*	1 Pack/300g	300	7.8	100	2.3	16.4	2.6	3.2
Garlic & Herb Crusted, Chicago Town*	1 Serving/150g	216	6.4	144	1.9	24.4	4.3	2.2
Jacket, Spicy, American Style, Frozen, Sainsbury's*	1 Serving/125g	156	5.0	125	1.9	20.3	4.0	1.1
Jumbo, Finest, Tesco*	1 Serving/126g	145	2.6	115	1.4	22.7	2.1	1.7
Mexican, Inspire, Asda*	1 Pack/500g	525	17.0	105	2.2	16.5	3.4	1.8
Micro, Tesco*	1 Pack/100g	170	6.8	170	2.6	24.5	6.8	2.3
New York Style, HL, Tesco*	1 Serving/125g	129	3.0	103	2.0	18.3	2.4	2.3
Onion & Garlic, Spicy, Cooked, Champion, Aldi*	1 Serving/100g	135	4.7	135	2.5	19.4	4.7	2.7
Only 5% Fat, Weighed Baked, McCain*	1 Serving/100g	173	4.3	173	3.3	30.2	4.3	2.8
Only 5% Fat, Weighed Frozen, McCain*	1 Serving/100g	123	3.0	123	2.2	21.8	3.0	1.9
Perfectly Balanced, Waitrose*	1 Serving/275g	278	4.7	101	2.5	19.0	1.7	3.5
Savoury, Waitrose*	1/3 Bag/250g	350	10.8	140	2.3	22.9	4.3	1.9
Sea Salt & Black Pepper, Finest, Tesco*	½ Pack/200g	200	3.2	100	1.8	18.0	1.6	3.4
Slightly Spiced, Weighed Baked, Winners, McCain*	1 Serving/100g	187	5.2	187	2.7	26.9	5.2	1.8
Slightly Spiced, Weighed Frozen, Winners, McCain*	1 Serving/100g	144	5.9	144	2.0	20.8	5.9	1.7
Sour Cream & Chives, McCain*	1 Serving/100g	132	4.1	132	2.4	24.0	4.1	0.0
Southern Fried, Asda*	1 Serving/100g	157	4.5	157	3.0	26.0	4.5	3.5
Southern Fried Style, Tesco*	1 Serving/155g	232	14.1	150	3.0	14.1	9.1	2.0
Spicy, Asda*	1 Serving/100g	145	5.7	145	1.8	21.8	5.7	2.1
Spicy, M & S*	½ Pack/225g	349	14.6	155	2.4	21.8	6.5	1.3
Spicy, Occasions, Sainsbury's*	1 Serving/100g	144	4.3	144	2.5	23.7	4.3	0.4
Spicy, Simple Solutions, Tesco*	1 Serving/150g	141	4.5	94	4.6	12.2	3.0	1.4
Spicy & Garlic Dip, Linda McCartney*	1 Pack/300g	366	16.8	122	2.6	15.3	5.6	3.1
with a Parsley & Oil Dressing, Tesco*	½ Pack/280g	168	2.8	60	1.0	11.5	1.0	1.8
with Broccoli & Mozzarella Cheese, Weight Watchers*	1 Pack/320g	294	9.6	92	3.1	13.3	3.0	1.0
with Chilli, COU, M & S*	1 Pack/400g	380	10.8	95	5.2	13.7	2.7	2.3
with Chilli Beef, You Count, Love Life, Waitrose*	1 Pack/380g	379	8.7	100	5.4	13.2	2.3	2.4
with Olive Oil & Parsley Dressing, Inspire, Asda*	½ Pack/300g	219	7.2	73	0.1	12.7	2.4	2.1
POTATOES								
Anya, Raw, TTD, Sainsbury's*	1 Serving/100g	75	0.3	75	1.5	17.8	0.3	1.1
Baby, Dressed with Garlic & Rosemary, M & S*	1 Serving/185g	130	5.2	70	2.0	9.0	2.8	2.4
Baby, Garlic & Sea Salt Roasted, Finest, Tesco*	1 Serving/200g	192	6.6	96	3.1	13.5	3.3	1.0
Baby, New, with Butter, Mint & Parsley, Organic, Asda*	1 Pack/360g	414	10.4	115	1.7	20.4	2.9	2.5
Baby, Oven Bake, Aunt Bessie's*	1 Serving/120g	103	1.7	86	2.2	16.3	1.4	3.0
Baby, with Butter & Herbs, Sainsbury's*	¼ Pack/148g	103	0.9	70	1.9	14.2	0.6	2.0
Baby, with Herbs & Butter, Morrisons*	1 Serving/100g	94	2.3	94	1.9	14.6	2.3	1.9
Baby, with Paprika & Chilli Dressing, Morrisons*	1 Serving/120g	124	5.3	103	1.7	13.6	4.4	1.3
Baked, Flesh & Skin, Average	***1 Med/200g***	***218***	***0.2***	***109***	***2.3***	***25.2***	***0.1***	***2.4***
Baked, Flesh Only, Weighed with Skin, Average	***1oz/28g***	***26***	***0.0***	***93***	***2.0***	***21.6***	***0.1***	***1.5***
Baked, in Microwave, Flesh & Skin, Average	***1oz/28g***	***29***	***0.0***	***105***	***2.4***	***24.1***	***0.1***	***2.3***
Baked, in Microwave, Flesh Only, Average	***1oz/28g***	***28***	***0.0***	***100***	***2.1***	***23.3***	***0.1***	***1.6***
Baked, in Microwave, Skin Only, Average	***1oz/28g***	***37***	***0.0***	***132***	***4.4***	***29.6***	***0.1***	***5.5***

POTATOES	Measure INFO/WEIGHT	per Measure KCAL	FAT	Nutrition Values per 100g / 100ml KCAL	PROT	CARB	FAT	FIBRE
Baked, Jacket, Baby, Veg, COOK!, M & S*	1 Pack/675g	776	37.8	115	2.1	14.3	5.6	2.3
Baked, Jacket, Beef Chilli Filled, GFY, Asda*	1 Serving/300g	261	1.5	87	4.6	16.0	0.5	3.2
Baked, Jacket, Beef Chilli Filled, Mini, Classic, Asda*	1 Pack/300g	233	2.4	78	3.9	13.7	0.8	1.5
Baked, Jacket, Cheddar Cheese, COU, M & S*	1 Potato/164g	164	3.1	100	2.9	17.3	1.9	2.0
Baked, Jacket, Cheese, M & S*	1oz/28g	24	0.7	85	4.5	11.1	2.5	1.6
Baked, Jacket, Chicken Tikka, COU, M & S*	1 Serving/300g	240	4.8	80	5.4	10.9	1.6	1.3
Baked, Jacket, Chilli, BGTY, Sainsbury's*	1 Pack/350g	318	4.9	91	5.3	14.3	1.4	1.2
Baked, Jacket, Chilli Con Carne, COU, M & S*	1 Pack/300g	270	6.3	90	6.0	11.1	2.1	1.2
Baked, Jacket, Chilli Con Carne, Pro Cuisine*	1 Pack/340g	347	3.4	102	4.6	18.7	1.0	0.0
Baked, Jacket, Creamy Mushroom, Asda*	1 Serving/100g	124	2.4	124	3.5	22.0	2.4	1.7
Baked, Jacket, Garlic, Mini, Asda*	1 Serving/65g	59	2.1	91	2.2	13.0	3.3	0.0
Baked, Jacket, Garlic Butter Filling, Morrisons*	1 Potato/210g	239	12.4	114	1.7	13.6	5.9	0.9
Baked, Jacket, Garlic Mushrooms, BGTY, Sainsbury's*	1 Pack/350g	262	3.2	75	2.3	14.4	0.9	1.2
Baked, Jacket, Halves, M & S*	1 Serving/250g	188	2.8	75	2.0	14.2	1.1	1.7
Baked, Jacket, Ham & Cheddar Cheese, Asda*	1 Pack/300g	435	11.1	145	7.0	21.0	3.7	1.6
Baked, Jacket, Leek & Cheese, M & S*	1 Serving/206g	206	6.4	100	3.8	13.4	3.1	3.2
Baked, Jacket, Mature Cheddar Cheese, M & S*	½ Pack/206g	225	6.6	109	3.6	16.9	3.2	1.0
Baked, Jacket, Mature Cheddar Cheese, Morrisons*	1 Serving/400g	520	20.4	130	4.4	16.6	5.1	1.5
Baked, Jacket, Tuna & Sweetcorn, Average	1 Serving/300g	273	6.8	91	5.0	12.6	2.2	0.9
Baked, Jacket, Tuna & Sweetcorn, BGTY, Sainsbury's*	1 Pack/350g	360	9.5	103	6.5	13.2	2.7	1.3
Baked, Jacket, Tuna & Sweetcorn, COU, M & S*	1 Pack/300g	270	5.4	90	5.1	12.8	1.8	1.4
Baked, Jacket, with Baked Bean & Sausage, Asda*	1 Pack/300g	447	9.6	149	5.0	25.0	3.2	2.7
Baked, Jacket, with Baked Beans, Pro Cuisine*	1 Pack/340g	374	1.4	110	4.3	22.3	0.4	0.0
Baked, Jacket, with Beef Chilli, Asda*	1 Pack/300g	381	7.8	127	5.0	21.0	2.6	2.0
Baked, Jacket, with Beef Chilli, M & S*	1 Pack/360g	288	7.2	80	5.9	9.6	2.0	0.9
Baked, Jacket, with Cheese, Freshly Prepared, Tesco*	½ Pack/215g	150	3.0	70	3.9	9.7	1.4	2.8
Baked, Jacket, with Cheese, HL, Tesco*	1 Potato/225g	202	5.0	90	4.5	13.0	2.2	1.8
Baked, Jacket, with Cheese & Bacon, Finest, Tesco*	1 Potato/245g	360	19.6	147	6.0	12.6	8.0	2.5
Baked, Jacket, with Cheese & Butter, Tesco*	1 Potato/225g	263	11.2	117	3.1	14.9	5.0	2.3
Baked, Jacket, with Cheese Mash, GFY, Asda*	1 Potato/200g	192	5.6	96	4.8	13.0	2.8	2.2
Baked, Skin Only, Average	***1oz/28g***	***55***	***0.0***	***198***	***4.3***	***46.1***	***0.1***	***7.9***
Baking, Raw, Average	***1 Med/250g***	***198***	***0.2***	***79***	***2.1***	***18.0***	***0.1***	***1.6***
Boiled, Average	***1 Serving/120g***	***86***	***0.1***	***72***	***1.8***	***17.0***	***0.1***	***1.2***
Boiled, Organics, Asda*	1 Serving/200g	152	0.2	76	1.8	16.0	0.1	1.2
Boiled, with Skin	***1 Potato/125g***	***98***	***0.1***	***78***	***2.9***	***17.2***	***0.1***	***3.3***
Boulangere, M & S*	½ Pack/225g	180	2.0	80	2.8	15.9	0.9	0.9
Charlotte, Average	***1 Serving/184g***	***139***	***0.5***	***76***	***1.6***	***17.4***	***0.2***	***3.3***
Crispy Bites, Weighed Frozen, McCain*	1 Serving/100g	141	4.4	141	2.5	20.4	4.4	1.5
Crispy Slices, M & S*	1/3 Pack/159g	231	8.3	145	2.9	22.2	5.2	1.9
Crispy Slices, Weighed Baked, McCain*	1 Serving/100g	240	11.0	240	3.2	32.1	11.0	2.1
Crispy Slices, Weighed Frozen, McCain*	1 Portion/100g	163	7.4	163	2.1	21.9	7.4	1.4
Dauphinoise, Average	***1 Serving/200g***	***335***	***23.9***	***168***	***2.2***	***12.8***	***12.0***	***1.5***
Desiree, Average	***1 Serving/200g***	***152***	***0.4***	***76***	***2.2***	***16.4***	***0.2***	***0.6***
Exquisa, Finest, Tesco*	¼ Pack/247g	185	0.7	75	1.7	16.1	0.3	1.0
Frites, Fries, Golden, Crunchy, M & S*	½ Pack/100g	158	6.2	158	2.2	23.4	6.2	1.0
Garlic, Tapas Selection, Sainsbury's*	1 Serving/22g	49	4.2	224	2.6	10.4	19.1	0.7
Hasselback, Average	***1 Serving/175g***	***182***	***1.6***	***104***	***1.9***	***22.0***	***0.9***	***2.9***
Jersey Royal, Canned, Average	***1 Can/186g***	***116***	***0.2***	***62***	***1.4***	***14.0***	***0.1***	***1.2***
Jersey Royal, New, Raw, Average	***1oz/28g***	***21***	***0.1***	***75***	***1.6***	***17.2***	***0.2***	***1.5***
Jersey Royal, with Mint Butter, Extra Special, Asda*	½ Pack/172g	148	5.3	86	1.6	13.0	3.1	1.5
King Edward, Tesco*	1 Serving/100g	77	0.2	77	2.1	16.8	0.2	1.3
Lemon & Rosemary, Finest, Tesco*	½ Pack/200g	200	7.4	100	2.1	14.7	3.7	2.0
Maris Piper, Mashed, Eat Fresh, Tesco*	½ Pack/213g	191	4.0	90	1.9	14.7	1.9	1.6

	Measure INFO/WEIGHT	per Measure KCAL	FAT	Nutrition Values per 100g / 100ml KCAL	PROT	CARB	FAT	FIBRE
POTATOES								
Maris Piper, Raw, Average	***1 Serving/200g***	***151***	***0.4***	***75***	***2.0***	***16.5***	***0.2***	***1.4***
Mashed, Chosen By You, Asda*	½ Pack/250g	177	5.5	71	1.0	10.3	2.2	2.8
Mashed, Colcannon, Sainsbury's*	½ Pack/300g	192	12.0	64	0.4	6.7	4.0	1.4
Mashed, Colcannon, Waitrose*	½ Pack/225g	207	8.6	92	1.7	12.8	3.8	1.4
Mashed, Fresh, LC, Tesco*	1 Pack/400g	280	8.8	70	2.0	9.3	2.2	1.6
Mashed, from Supermarket, Average	½ Pack/200g	197	8.1	98	1.8	13.3	4.1	1.5
Mashed, from Supermarket, Healthy Range, Average	1 Serving/200g	160	3.1	80	1.8	14.6	1.6	1.3
Mashed, from Supermarket, Premium, Average	1 Serving/225g	305	17.8	136	1.7	14.4	7.9	1.1
Mashed, Home Prepared with Whole Milk	1 Cup/210g	162	1.2	77	1.9	17.6	0.6	2.0
Mashed, Mash Direct*	½ Pack/200g	190	3.8	95	1.7	17.7	1.9	1.3
Mashed, Olive Oil, HE, Tesco*	1 Serving/100g	90	2.2	90	2.1	15.5	2.2	0.9
Mashed, Vintage Cheddar Cheese, M & S*	½ Pack/225g	248	11.9	110	4.6	12.6	5.3	1.0
Mashed, with Cabbage & Spring Onion, COU, M & S*	½ Pack/225g	158	4.0	70	1.7	11.4	1.8	2.1
Mashed, with Carrot & Swede, COU, M & S*	1oz/28g	20	0.6	70	1.1	12.1	2.1	2.9
Mashed, with Carrot & Swede, M & S*	1 Serving/225g	214	14.4	95	1.6	8.3	6.4	1.4
Mashed, with Creme Fraiche & Seasoning, Waitrose*	½ Pack/225g	189	6.3	84	2.0	12.7	2.8	1.4
Mashed, with Leeks, Creamy, Birds Eye*	1 Pack/300g	300	21.0	100	2.0	7.3	7.0	0.8
Mashed, with Spring Onion, Weight Watchers*	1 Serving/100g	77	2.2	77	1.9	10.9	2.2	1.4
New, Average	***1 Serving/100g***	***75***	***0.3***	***75***	***1.5***	***17.8***	***0.3***	***1.1***
New, Baby, Average	***1 Serving/180g***	***135***	***0.5***	***75***	***1.7***	***17.1***	***0.3***	***1.6***
New, Baby, Canned, Average	***1 Can/120g***	***70***	***0.2***	***59***	***1.4***	***13.2***	***0.2***	***1.4***
New, Easy Steam with Herbs & Butter, Tesco*	1 Serving/125g	94	3.5	75	1.8	9.6	2.8	1.7
New, Garlic, Herb & Parsley Butter, Co-Op*	1 Serving/100g	115	5.0	115	1.0	15.0	5.0	2.0
New, in a Herb Marinade, Tesco*	¼ Pack/150g	152	7.4	101	1.3	13.0	4.9	1.5
New, with Butter, Chives & Mint, M & S*	¼ Pack/145g	116	2.0	80	1.1	16.2	1.4	2.3
New, with English Churned Butter, M & S*	1 Pack/180g	261	4.0	145	1.3	29.5	2.2	2.1
New, with Herbs & Butter, Asda*	½ Pack/170g	146	2.9	86	1.7	16.0	1.7	1.5
New, with Sunblush Tomato, M & S*	1 Pack/385g	346	6.9	90	1.6	17.2	1.8	1.3
Pan Fried, Aldi*	1 Serving/250g	182	2.0	73	2.7	13.7	0.8	0.0
Patatas Bravas, Bistro, M Kitchen, Morrisons*	½ Pack/126g	113	4.0	90	1.1	13.6	3.2	1.3
Raw, Peeled, Flesh Only	***1 Serving/100g***	***75***	***0.2***	***75***	***2.0***	***17.3***	***0.2***	***1.4***
Red, Flesh Only, Average	***1 Serving/300g***	***218***	***0.4***	***72***	***2.0***	***16.4***	***0.2***	***1.2***
Redskin, Roasted, Frozen, Lamb Weston*	½ Packet/200g	202	4.0	101	2.4	18.0	2.0	1.9
Roast, Dry, No Oil, No fat	1 Serving/100g	79	0.1	79	2.7	18.0	0.1	1.6
Roast, Extra Crispy, Oven Baked, Aunt Bessie's*	1 Serving/100g	223	11.8	223	2.9	26.1	11.8	3.6
Roast, Frozen, Average	1 Potato/70g	105	3.5	149	2.6	23.5	5.0	1.4
Roast, Frozen, Healthy Range, Average	1 Potato/70g	70	1.7	100	2.6	18.2	2.4	2.1
Roast, Garlic, Sainsbury's*	½ Pack/225g	358	21.8	159	3.2	14.6	9.7	1.4
Roast, in Lard, Average	***1oz/28g***	***42***	***1.3***	***149***	***2.9***	***25.9***	***4.5***	***1.8***
Roast, in Oil, Average	***1oz/28g***	***42***	***1.3***	***149***	***2.9***	***25.9***	***4.5***	***1.8***
Roast, New, Rosemary, Ainsley Harriott*	1 Serving/150g	133	4.0	89	2.0	16.0	2.7	1.3
Roast, Oven Baked, Aunt Bessie's*	1 Serving/165g	305	15.3	185	2.3	22.9	9.3	1.8
Roast, with Caramelised Onions, Finest, Tesco*	½ Pack/200g	500	16.4	250	5.5	38.6	8.2	2.9
Roasted with Goose Fat, TTD, Sainsbury's*	½ Pack/185g	216	4.4	117	2.7	21.1	2.4	3.0
Roasting, Average	***1 Serving/150g***	***202***	***5.2***	***135***	***2.5***	***23.4***	***3.5***	***1.6***
Rooster, Boiled, Albert Bartlett & Sons Ltd*	1 Potato/175g	126	0.2	72	1.8	17.0	0.1	1.2
Salad, Value, Tesco*	1 Serving/150g	111	0.4	74	1.7	16.1	0.3	1.0
Saute, Deep Fried, McCain*	1oz/28g	47	2.0	167	2.6	23.3	7.0	0.0
Saute, Oven Baked, McCain*	1oz/28g	56	1.1	199	4.4	36.9	3.8	0.0
Saute, with Onion & Bacon, Country Supper, Waitrose*	¼ Pack/100g	112	4.3	112	1.9	16.4	4.3	1.3
Slices, Garlic & Herb, Heinz*	1oz/28g	23	1.1	82	1.7	10.2	3.9	0.7
Slices, in Rich Crispy Batter, Crispy, Sainsbury's*	½ Pack/238g	591	37.0	249	2.4	24.8	15.6	2.8
Vivaldi, Boiled in Unsalted Water, Sainsbury's*	1 Serving/200g	144	0.2	72	1.8	17.0	0.1	1.2

P

	Measure INFO/WEIGHT	per Measure KCAL	FAT	Nutrition Values per 100g / 100ml KCAL	PROT	CARB	FAT	FIBRE
POTATOES								
Waves, Frozen, Lamb Weston*	1 Serving/100g	125	3.9	125	2.8	19.6	3.9	2.6
White, Raw, Flesh & Skin	1 Large/369g	284	0.3	77	2.0	17.5	0.1	2.2
White, Raw, Weighed with Skin, Flesh Only, Average	***1 Med/213g***	***160***	***0.3***	***75***	***2.0***	***16.8***	***0.2***	***1.3***
White, Vivaldi, TTD, Sainsbury's*	1 Serving/100g	76	0.1	76	1.8	17.0	0.1	1.2
POTATOES INSTANT								
Mashed, Butter Flavour, Premier Foods*	1 Serving/180g	288	4.1	160	1.4	9.1	2.3	0.8
Mashed, Dry, Tesco*	1 Serving/70g	225	0.1	321	7.7	72.0	0.2	7.1
Mashed, Dry, Value, Tesco*	1/6 Pack/42g	157	0.4	373	7.0	84.0	1.0	6.9
Mashed, Made Up with Water, Average	1 Serving/180g	118	0.3	66	1.7	14.5	0.2	1.3
Mashed, Original, Dry Weight, Smash*	1 Serving/30g	101	0.3	343	8.3	71.8	1.0	6.7
Mashed with Fried Onion, Smash*	½ Pack/269g	191	3.5	71	1.6	13.4	1.3	0.7
Mashed with Smoked Bacon, Smash*	1 Serving/169g	137	3.7	81	1.7	13.6	2.2	0.6
POUSSIN								
Meat & Skin, Raw, Average	***1oz/28g***	***57***	***3.9***	***202***	***19.1***	***0.0***	***13.9***	***0.0***
Spatchcock, British, Waitrose*	½ Poussin/225g	364	20.2	162	19.0	1.2	9.0	0.0
Spatchcock with Garlic & Herbs, Finest, Tesco*	½ Poussin/235g	348	17.2	148	19.7	1.0	7.3	0.5
POWERADE								
Berry & Tropical Fruit, Coca-Cola*	1 Bottle/500ml	120	0.0	24	0.0	5.6	0.0	0.0
Citrus Charge, Coca-Cola*	1 Bottle/500ml	120	0.0	24	0.0	6.0	0.0	0.0
Gold Rush, Coca-Cola*	1 Bottle/500ml	120	0.0	24	0.0	6.0	0.0	0.0
Ice Storm, Coca-Cola*	1 Bottle/500ml	120	0.0	24	0.0	6.0	0.0	0.0
Isotonic, Sports Drink, Coca-Cola*	1 Bottle/500ml	120	0.0	24	0.0	5.6	0.0	0.0
Zero, Coca-Cola*	1 Bottle/500ml	5	0.0	1	0.0	0.0	0.0	0.0
PRAWN COCKTAIL								
& Orkney Crab, M & S*	1 Serving/90g	180	13.8	200	14.2	1.8	15.3	0.6
20% More Prawns, M & S*	½ Pack/100g	330	31.6	330	8.9	2.2	31.6	0.2
Asda*	1oz/28g	124	12.2	443	8.6	3.3	43.6	0.0
BGTY, Sainsbury's*	1 Pack/200g	330	24.2	165	9.3	4.5	12.1	0.5
Delicious, Boots*	1 Pack/250g	285	6.5	114	5.5	17.0	2.6	1.2
King, Sainsbury's*	1 Pack/260g	328	15.1	126	5.8	12.7	5.8	2.3
LC, Tesco*	1 Pot/140g	210	16.0	150	7.5	4.3	11.4	1.3
Light, Asda*	1oz/28g	45	3.1	160	9.9	4.8	11.2	0.0
Reduced Fat, M & S*	1 Pack/200g	260	15.0	130	11.9	3.2	7.5	0.7
Sainsbury's*	1 Pot/200g	604	55.8	302	9.4	3.2	27.9	0.8
Tesco*	1 Tub/170g	476	39.1	280	6.6	10.2	23.0	1.0
TTD, Sainsbury's*	1 Serving/100g	333	30.6	333	11.5	2.9	30.6	0.5
PRAWN CRACKERS								
Asda*	1 Serving/25g	134	8.8	535	2.0	53.0	35.0	0.0
Cooked in Sunflower Oil, Sharwood's*	1 Cracker/2g	10	0.5	479	0.7	68.3	22.6	0.8
Food to Go, Sainsbury's*	1 Bag/40g	214	12.5	534	2.9	60.2	31.3	0.4
Green Thai Curry, M & S*	1 Pack/50g	250	12.9	500	3.2	62.2	25.8	1.6
M & S*	1 Bag/50g	262	15.6	525	2.8	57.4	31.3	0.8
Ready to Eat, Sharwood's*	1 Bag/60g	316	18.5	527	0.5	62.0	30.8	1.2
Red Mill*	1 Bag/50g	282	18.8	563	2.8	53.1	37.7	0.7
Sainsbury's*	1 Cracker/3g	16	1.0	537	2.4	60.4	31.7	0.8
Tesco*	1/3 Pack/20g	114	7.4	570	2.5	56.5	37.1	0.9
Uncooked, Sharwood's*	1oz/28g	136	8.3	487	0.7	52.7	29.7	1.7
Waitrose*	1 Pack/50g	266	16.0	533	2.4	58.6	32.1	1.6
PRAWN TOAST								
Baguette from Selection, Modern Asian, M & S*	1 Toast/23g	60	3.3	270	11.0	21.3	14.9	2.1
Chinese Snack Selection, Morrisons*	1 Toast/13g	41	2.6	328	11.3	23.1	21.2	6.6
Dim Sum Selection, Sainsbury's*	1 Toast/8g	23	1.5	283	9.9	19.2	18.5	2.0
from Chinese Selection, Ken Hom, Tesco*	1 Toast/12g	48	3.8	385	13.3	11.5	30.5	4.0

	Measure INFO/WEIGHT	per Measure KCAL	FAT	Nutrition Values per 100g / 100ml KCAL	PROT	CARB	FAT	FIBRE
PRAWN TOAST								
Mini, Oriental Selection, Party, Iceland*	1 Toast/15g	52	3.6	345	10.5	22.0	23.9	2.1
Oriental Selection, Waitrose*	1 Toast/14g	38	2.4	272	11.1	18.3	17.2	2.1
Sesame, Occasions, Sainsbury's*	1 Toast/12g	34	2.2	283	9.9	19.2	18.5	2.0
Sesame, Oriental Snack Selection, Sainsbury's*	1 Toast/12g	40	2.7	335	9.3	23.0	22.9	5.1
Sesame Prawn, Toasted Triangles, M & S*	1 Pack/220g	616	39.6	280	12.4	17.3	18.0	2.0
Waitrose*	1 Toast/21g	47	3.6	223	9.7	7.4	17.2	5.8
PRAWNS								
Batter Crisp, Lyons*	1 Pack/160g	350	20.3	219	8.0	18.2	12.7	1.1
Boiled	***1 Prawn/3g***	***3***	***0.0***	***99***	***22.6***	***0.0***	***0.9***	***0.0***
Cooked & Peeled, Average	***1oz/28g***	***21***	***0.2***	***77***	***17.6***	***0.2***	***0.6***	***0.0***
Dried, Average	***1 Prawn/3g***	***8***	***0.1***	***281***	***62.4***	***0.0***	***3.5***	***0.0***
Filo Wrapped & Breaded, M & S*	1 Serving/19g	45	2.5	235	9.5	20.4	13.0	1.4
Honduran, & Cocktail Sauce Dipper, M & S*	1 Pack/120g	258	21.6	215	13.6	0.0	18.0	1.1
Hot & Spicy, Average	1 Serving/170g	461	26.9	271	9.4	22.8	15.8	2.2
Icelandic, Raw, Average	***1oz/28g***	***30***	***0.4***	***106***	***22.7***	***0.0***	***1.6***	***0.0***
King, Raw, Average	***1 Bag/200g***	***145***	***1.9***	***72***	***15.8***	***0.2***	***1.0***	***0.1***
King, Tandoori, Average	1 Prawn/59g	33	0.6	55	5.7	5.9	1.1	0.7
Large, Wrapped, Party Food, M & S*	1 Wrap/26g	49	1.5	190	14.8	18.8	5.7	1.3
North Atlantic, Peeled, Cooked, Average	***1oz/28g***	***22***	***0.3***	***80***	***17.5***	***0.0***	***1.1***	***0.0***
North Atlantic, Raw, Average	***1oz/28g***	***17***	***0.1***	***62***	***14.4***	***0.0***	***0.4***	***0.0***
Raw, Average	***1oz/28g***	***22***	***0.2***	***79***	***17.8***	***0.2***	***0.7***	***0.0***
Tiger, Cooked & Peeled, Average	***1 Pack/180g***	***151***	***2.0***	***84***	***18.4***	***0.1***	***1.1***	***0.0***
Tiger, Jumbo, Average	***1 Serving/50g***	***39***	***0.2***	***78***	***18.2***	***0.3***	***0.5***	***0.0***
Tiger, Raw, Average	***1 Prawn/30g***	***19***	***0.2***	***64***	***14.2***	***0.0***	***0.7***	***0.0***
Tiger, Vegetarian, Crispy, Tkc*	½ Pack/150g	225	6.0	150	12.0	17.0	4.0	5.0
Tiger, Wrapped, M & S*	1 Pack/190g	477	25.8	251	11.3	20.7	13.6	1.3
PRAWNS CHILLI								
& Coriander, King, Honduran, M & S*	½ Pack/70g	70	2.2	100	17.2	0.1	3.2	0.4
& Coriander, King, Sainsbury's*	1 Pack/140g	112	1.8	80	16.6	0.4	1.3	0.5
Battered, M & S*	1oz/28g	63	3.2	225	7.2	23.8	11.5	0.5
Sweet, Crispy, Dipping Sauce, M & S*	1 Pack/240g	515	27.8	215	7.5	19.9	11.6	2.3
Sweet, Thai, King, Sainsbury's*	1 Serving/150g	177	6.2	118	6.4	13.9	4.1	1.9
with Spicy Chilli Dip, King, Sainsbury's*	½ Pack/150g	282	10.8	188	8.6	22.2	7.2	1.0
PRAWNS WITH								
a Spicy Cajun Dip, King, Sainsbury's*	1 Pack/240g	254	4.3	106	14.8	9.1	1.8	1.4
Chilli, Coriander & Lime, King, Waitrose*	1 Pack/140g	143	3.2	102	19.9	0.5	2.3	0.6
Creamy Lime Dip, King, Waitrose*	1 Pot/230g	518	40.7	225	15.8	0.8	17.7	0.2
Garlic & Herb Butter, King, Fresh, M & S*	1 Serving/200g	330	18.0	165	12.5	9.1	9.0	0.5
Ginger & Spring Onion, Sainsbury's*	1 Pack/300g	198	9.3	66	4.7	4.7	3.1	0.3
Green Thai Sauce, Tiger, Waitrose*	½ Pack/117g	108	2.7	92	16.1	0.8	2.3	0.1
Lemon & Pepper, Honduran, King, M & S*	1 Pack/140g	133	3.6	95	17.4	0.4	2.6	0.7
Rice, Sweet Chilli, Tesco*	1 Pack/460g	488	10.1	106	2.4	19.2	2.2	0.5
PRETZELS								
American Style, Salted, Sainsbury's*	1 Serving/50g	202	2.2	403	10.8	79.7	4.5	1.8
Cheddar Cheese, Penn State Pretzels*	1 Sm Bag/30g	124	2.8	412	10.0	71.6	9.3	3.8
Giant, Penn State Pretzels*	1 Pretzel/18g	66	0.7	374	10.5	74.7	3.7	4.1
Giant, Salted, Tesco*	1 Serving/25g	99	1.1	395	12.2	75.8	4.3	3.4
Jumbo, Tesco*	1 Serving/50g	194	3.4	388	9.7	71.9	6.8	5.4
Lightly Salted, Tesco*	1 Serving/25g	99	1.8	395	9.3	73.4	7.1	5.5
Mini, 99% Fat Free, Free Natural*	1 Serving/50g	188	0.5	376	10.1	81.7	1.0	0.0
Mini, M & S*	1 Pack/45g	194	6.0	430	10.4	66.6	13.4	4.9
New York Style, Salted, Mini, Shapers, Boots*	1 Bag/25g	94	0.5	375	10.0	79.0	2.1	4.2
Salt & Cracked Black Pepper, COU, M & S*	1 Pack/25g	100	0.6	390	11.4	79.1	2.4	2.6

	Measure INFO/WEIGHT	per Measure KCAL	FAT	Nutrition Values per 100g / 100ml KCAL	PROT	CARB	FAT	FIBRE
PRETZELS								
Salted, Average	1 Serving/30g	114	0.8	380	10.3	79.8	2.6	3.0
Salted, Mini, M & S*	1 Pack/25g	94	0.5	375	10.0	79.0	2.1	4.2
Salted, Stars, Tesco*	1oz/28g	104	1.3	371	8.2	73.7	4.8	3.1
Sea Salt & Black Pepper, Penn State Pretzels*	1 Serving/25g	94	1.0	375	10.4	73.7	4.2	4.7
Sea Salt & Black Pepper, Tesco*	1 Serving/50g	190	1.3	379	10.0	79.0	2.6	4.1
Selection Tray, M & S*	1oz/28g	112	1.9	401	9.7	75.5	6.7	3.4
Snacks, Fabulous Bakin' Boys*	1 Pack/24g	96	1.2	401	9.0	79.5	4.9	2.5
Soft, Cinnamon Sugar, Auntie Anne's*	1 Pretzel/112g	380	1.0	339	7.1	75.0	0.9	1.8
Soft, Salted, Original, Auntie Anne's*	1 Pretzel/112g	310	1.0	277	7.1	58.0	0.9	1.8
Soft, Sesame, Auntie Anne's*	1 Pretzel/112g	360	6.0	321	8.9	59.8	5.4	2.7
Sour Cream & Chive, Hoops, BGTY, Sainsbury's*	1 Bag/25g	98	0.6	391	10.4	80.9	2.3	1.6
Sour Cream & Chive, Mini, HL, Tesco*	1 Pack/25g	92	0.6	369	10.9	76.3	2.2	4.6
Sour Cream & Chive, Penn State Pretzels*	1 Serving/25g	111	3.2	443	8.9	71.8	12.9	2.0
Sour Cream & Chive Flavour, Mini, Shapers, Boots*	1 Packet/25g	93	0.7	371	11.0	74.0	2.7	7.3
Sour Cream & Onion, M & S*	1 Serving/30g	136	4.4	455	11.0	70.9	14.5	0.7
Sour Cream & Onion, Tesco*	1 Serving/25g	114	4.2	457	8.4	67.7	17.0	2.3
Wheat, GF, Trufree*	1 Bag/60g	282	12.0	470	0.5	72.0	20.0	0.7
PRINGLES*								
Barbecue, Pringles*	1 Serving/50g	266	18.0	533	4.9	48.0	36.0	5.1
BBQ Spare Rib, Rice Infusions, Pringles*	1 Pack/23g	108	5.3	469	5.1	60.0	23.0	2.6
Burger, Take Aways, Pringles*	1 Serving/25g	129	8.0	516	4.2	52.0	32.0	2.5
Cheese & Onion, Pringles*	1 Serving/25g	132	8.5	528	4.1	50.0	34.0	3.4
Chip n Ketchup, Pringles*	1 Serving/25g	129	8.0	516	3.9	52.0	32.0	2.5
Curry, Masala, Take Aways, Pringles*	1 Serving/25g	128	8.8	514	4.3	52.0	35.0	2.6
Hot & Spicy, Pringles*	1 Serving/25g	132	8.5	530	4.6	49.0	34.0	3.7
Light, Aromas, Greek Cheese & Avocado Oil, Pringles*	1 Serving/25g	122	6.2	488	4.6	57.0	25.0	3.6
Light, Original, Pringles*	1 Serving/25g	121	6.2	484	4.3	59.0	25.0	3.6
Light, Sour Cream & Onion, Pringles*	1 Serving/25g	122	6.2	487	4.7	57.0	25.0	3.6
Margarita Pizza, Classic Takeaways, Pringles*	1 Serving/25g	134	8.0	538	3.9	53.0	32.0	2.6
Minis, Original, Pringles*	1 Pack/23g	118	6.9	514	5.1	55.0	30.0	3.7
Minis, Salt & Vinegar, Pringles*	1 Pack/23g	115	6.4	502	4.5	55.0	28.0	3.6
Minis, Sour Cream & Onion, Pringles*	1 Pack/23g	118	6.7	511	5.2	56.0	29.0	3.5
Minis, Texas BBQ Sauce, Pringles*	1 Pack/23g	116	6.4	504	5.0	56.0	28.0	3.8
Original, Pringles*	1 Serving/25g	130	8.5	522	3.8	51.0	34.0	2.6
Paprika, Pringles*	1 Serving/25g	132	8.5	529	4.9	49.0	34.0	6.5
Prawn Cocktail, Pringles*	1 Serving/25g	130	8.0	518	4.1	53.0	32.0	2.5
Salt & Vinegar, Pringles*	1 Serving/25g	128	8.0	512	3.9	52.0	32.0	2.4
Sour Cream & Onion, Pringles*	1 Serving/25g	133	8.8	531	4.5	49.0	35.0	3.6
Texas BBQ Sauce, Pringles*	1 Serving/25g	132	8.5	527	4.2	50.0	34.0	3.5
PROFITEROLES								
Asda*	1 Serving/64g	218	17.2	343	5.0	20.0	27.0	0.0
Chocolate, Co-Op*	1 Pot/91g	260	13.7	285	6.0	33.0	15.0	3.0
Chocolate, Sainsbury's*	1/6 Pot/95g	192	8.5	202	5.4	25.1	8.9	0.8
Chocolate Covered, Tesco*	1 Serving/72g	295	21.2	410	5.7	29.3	29.5	2.0
Choux & Chocolate Sauce, Tesco*	1 Serving/77g	295	22.0	386	5.1	26.9	28.7	0.5
Classic French, Sainsbury's*	1 Serving/90g	284	15.5	316	6.6	33.7	17.2	0.1
Dairy Cream, Co-Op*	¼ Pack/70g	242	17.5	345	6.0	24.0	25.0	0.5
Filled with Cream, Stack, Fresh, M & S*	1 Serving/75g	281	21.4	375	5.3	23.6	28.5	1.9
in a Pot, Waitrose*	1 Pot/80g	207	11.3	259	6.3	25.6	14.1	2.9
Savoury, with Cheese & Chive, Chosen By You, Asda*	¼ Pack/15g	95	7.7	634	9.1	32.1	51.3	3.5
Waitrose*	4 Profiteroles/75g	269	17.9	359	4.8	31.1	23.9	0.7
PRUNES								
& Apricots, in Grape Juice, Asda*	1 Serving/100g	91	0.0	91	1.1	21.2	0.0	0.7

P

	Measure INFO/WEIGHT	per Measure KCAL	FAT	Nutrition Values per 100g / 100ml KCAL	PROT	CARB	FAT	FIBRE
PRUNES								
Dried, Average	***1 Serving/50g***	***79***	***0.2***	***158***	***2.5***	***36.4***	***0.4***	***5.8***
in Apple Juice, Average	***1 Serving/90g***	***76***	***0.1***	***84***	***0.8***	***19.8***	***0.1***	***1.4***
in Fruit Juice, Average	***1oz/28g***	***25***	***0.0***	***88***	***0.9***	***21.4***	***0.2***	***3.0***
in Syrup, Average	***1oz/28g***	***26***	***0.0***	***92***	***1.0***	***22.1***	***0.2***	***2.6***
Pitted, Californian, Ready to Eat, Sweetvine, Aldi*	4 Prunes/30g	48	0.1	161	2.5	34.0	0.4	5.7
Pitted, in Juice, 825g Jar, Tesco*	1 Serving/206g	165	1.0	80	0.8	17.0	0.5	3.3
Stewed with Sugar	***1oz/28g***	***29***	***0.1***	***103***	***1.3***	***25.5***	***0.2***	***3.1***
Stewed without Sugar	***1oz/28g***	***23***	***0.1***	***81***	***1.4***	***19.5***	***0.3***	***3.3***
PUDDING								
Bread, Retail Average	1 Slice/120g	301	8.0	251	8.4	41.8	6.7	0.5
Cherry Cobbler, GFY, Asda*	1 Pudding/100g	158	2.0	158	2.1	33.0	2.0	0.9
Chocolate, Gu*	1 Pack/240g	780	27.4	325	3.9	51.8	11.4	1.6
Chocolate, M & S*	¼ Pudding/76g	265	12.0	350	4.1	48.0	15.8	2.1
Chocolate, Melting Middle, M & S*	1 Pudding/155g	510	27.8	330	5.8	36.2	18.0	3.1
Chocolate, Perfectly Balanced, Waitrose*	1 Pot/105g	196	3.3	187	3.8	36.0	3.1	0.8
Chocolate, Raspberry & Chilli, Puds	1 Pot/85g	212	12.8	249	3.2	25.0	15.1	1.3
Chocolate & Vanilla Swirls, Sugar Free, Jell-O*	1 Pot/106g	60	1.5	57	0.9	12.3	1.4	0.0
Chocolate Bombe, Cooked, Fox's*	½ Pudding/114g	435	16.9	383	4.3	57.0	14.9	1.7
Chocolate Ganache, Mini Pot, Gu*	1 Pot/45g	199	16.6	442	3.3	26.4	36.8	2.3
Eve's, with Custard, Less Than 5% Fat, M & S*	1 Pudding/205g	318	9.4	155	3.4	24.7	4.6	0.7
Jam, Roly Poly, Aunt Bessie's*	1 Serving/75g	290	10.4	387	3.4	62.2	13.8	0.9
Jam, Roly Poly, Sainsbury's*	¼ Pack/81g	291	11.5	359	4.4	53.3	14.2	0.5
Jam Roly Poly, Custard, Diabetic, 928, Wiltshire Foods*	1 Serving/150g	234	10.4	156	2.5	21.9	6.9	0.8
Jam Roly Poly & Custard, Co-Op*	1 Serving/105g	262	7.4	250	3.0	44.0	7.0	0.8
Lemon, BGTY, Sainsbury's*	1 Serving/100g	151	1.9	151	2.9	31.0	1.9	0.5
Lemon, M & S*	1 Pudding/105g	328	16.0	312	4.3	39.4	15.2	2.3
Lemon Crunch, Bird's*	1oz/28g	125	3.9	445	5.5	74.0	14.0	0.7
Panettone, Finest, Tesco*	1oz/28g	94	4.2	335	3.8	45.7	14.9	5.3
Pineapple, Upside Down, Waitrose*	¼ Pudding/113g	303	12.7	269	3.3	38.0	11.3	1.2
Queen of Puddings	1oz/28g	60	2.2	213	4.8	33.1	7.8	0.2
Rhubarb & Custard, BGTY, Sainsbury's*	1 Pudding/140g	137	2.8	98	2.0	18.4	2.0	1.4
Souffle, Hot Chocolate, Gu*	1 Pot/65g	298	23.5	458	6.0	24.1	36.2	2.5
Sticky Toffee, Bistro, M Kitchen, Morrisons*	¼ Pack/100g	361	15.6	361	2.7	51.4	15.6	2.0
Sticky Toffee, Co-Op*	¼ Pudding/100g	355	20.0	355	3.0	40.0	20.0	0.7
Sticky Toffee, HL, Tesco*	1 Pack/125g	245	5.6	196	4.0	34.9	4.5	0.6
Sticky Toffee, Individual, Mr Kipling*	1 Pudding/85g	266	7.2	312	2.7	56.1	8.4	0.9
Sticky Toffee, Tesco*	1 Serving/110g	287	14.7	261	3.3	31.8	13.4	0.7
Sticky Toffee, Tryton Foods*	1oz/28g	88	1.5	314	3.7	62.7	5.4	1.0
Sticky Toffee, Weight Watchers*	1 Pudding/100g	172	1.1	172	3.0	27.2	1.1	20.5
Strawberry, Jelly Pud with Devon Custard, Ambrosia*	1 Pot/150g	129	1.2	86	0.7	19.4	0.8	0.0
Strawberry Jam, with Custard, Farmfoods*	1 Serving/145g	525	34.7	362	3.2	35.5	23.9	0.9
Summer, HE, Tesco*	1 Serving/100g	89	0.6	89	1.9	19.1	0.6	2.2
Summer Fruits, Eat Well, M & S*	1 Pudding/135g	128	0.7	95	1.7	20.8	0.5	3.0
Summer Pudding, BGTY, Sainsbury's*	1 Pot/110g	223	5.1	203	3.2	40.9	4.6	2.4
Summer Pudding, Waitrose*	1 Pot/120g	125	0.5	104	2.0	23.1	0.4	1.4
Syrup, Individual, Co-Op*	1 Pudding/170g	604	35.7	355	3.0	38.0	21.0	1.0
Syrup, M & S*	1 Serving/105g	370	10.5	352	3.9	61.7	10.0	0.8
PUMPKIN								
Boiled in Salted Water	***1oz/28g***	***4***	***0.1***	***13***	***0.6***	***2.1***	***0.3***	***1.1***
Kabocha, Tesco*	1 Serving 50g	20	0.0	39	1.1	8.3	0.1	1.6
Potimarron, Raw, Average	1 Serving/80g	21	0.1	26	1.0	6.5	0.1	1.9

	Measure INFO/WEIGHT	per Measure KCAL	FAT	Nutrition Values per 100g / 100ml KCAL	PROT	CARB	FAT	FIBRE
QUAVERS								
Cheese, Walkers*	1 Std Bag/20g	109	6.1	534	2.7	62.5	30.1	1.1
Prawn Cocktail, Walkers*	1 Bag/16g	88	5.1	537	2.1	62.0	31.0	1.2
Salt & Vinegar, Walkers*	1 Bag/16g	86	4.9	527	1.9	62.0	30.0	1.2
QUICHE								
Asparagus & Feta, Little, Higgidy*	1 Portion/155g	369	23.4	238	8.1	17.3	15.1	1.4
Asparagus & Mushroom, Tesco*	½ Quiche/200g	474	32.8	237	5.1	17.2	16.4	1.2
Asparagus & Vegetable, Herby Summer, Higgidy*	1 Quiche/400g	848	50.0	212	5.9	18.9	12.5	2.7
Bacon, Leek & Cheese, Weight Watchers*	1 Quiche/165g	327	15.7	198	8.2	18.0	9.5	1.8
Bacon, Leek & Mushroom, M & S*	¼ Quiche/100g	245	16.4	245	6.9	17.2	16.4	1.3
Bacon, Smoked, & Mature Cheddar, Higgidy*	1 Quiche/400g	1096	74.0	274	8.4	18.6	18.5	1.5
Bacon & Cheese, Pork Farms*	1 Pack/120g	378	24.0	315	11.1	20.8	20.0	0.0
Bacon & Cheese, Sainsbury's*	¼ Quiche/100g	237	15.0	237	7.0	18.6	15.0	0.7
Bacon & Leek, Asda*	¼ Quiche/100g	252	15.9	252	8.4	18.9	15.9	1.5
Bacon & Leek, Individual, Tesco*	1 Quiche/175g	485	32.4	277	8.3	19.4	18.5	0.9
Bacon & Leek, Tesco*	¼ Quiche/100g	260	18.0	260	6.9	17.5	18.0	1.2
Bacon & Tomato, Asda*	1 Serving/107g	201	8.6	188	8.0	21.0	8.0	1.1
Brie & Smoked Bacon, Asda*	¼ Quiche/90g	249	17.0	277	8.9	17.8	18.9	1.0
Broccoli, Budgens*	1 Serving/88g	213	15.5	243	6.3	14.8	17.7	1.0
Broccoli, Extra, Value, Tesco*	1 Serving/125g	341	24.0	273	10.0	15.1	19.2	0.8
Broccoli, HE, Tesco*	1 Quiche/175g	308	12.2	176	6.7	21.5	7.0	1.4
Broccoli, Tesco*	1 Serving/100g	249	17.2	249	6.0	17.6	17.2	1.4
Broccoli, Tomato & Cheese, BGTY, Sainsbury's*	1 Quiche/390g	632	32.0	162	6.4	15.7	8.2	1.3
Broccoli, Tomato & Cheese, Deep Filled, Sainsbury's*	¼ Quiche/100g	203	12.9	203	5.2	16.9	12.9	2.3
Broccoli & Stilton, Mini, Sainsbury's*	1 Quiche/14g	52	3.0	369	8.8	35.2	21.4	3.3
Broccoli & Stilton, with Cheddar Crumb, Higgidy*	½ Quiche/200g	558	38.6	279	9.2	17.2	19.3	1.4
Cheese, Broccoli & Tomato, Nisa Heritage*	1 Serving/85g	234	16.6	275	7.3	17.5	19.5	1.4
Cheese, Onion & Chive, HE, Tesco*	1 Serving/100g	202	8.2	202	10.9	21.2	8.2	1.3
Cheese, Onion & Chive, Tesco*	1oz/28g	90	6.7	320	10.6	15.5	24.0	0.6
Cheese & Bacon, Crustless, Tesco*	1 Serving/85g	199	12.8	234	10.0	14.4	15.0	0.6
Cheese & Bacon, Smart Price, Asda*	¼ Quiche/82g	211	13.9	257	6.0	20.0	17.0	0.7
Cheese & Broccoli, Morrisons*	1/3 Quiche/134g	338	22.4	253	7.1	18.4	16.8	1.7
Cheese & Chive, HE, Tesco*	1 Serving/86g	169	6.4	197	10.4	22.1	7.4	1.2
Cheese & Egg	1oz/28g	88	6.2	314	12.5	17.3	22.2	0.6
Cheese & Ham, Ready to Eat, Iceland*	¼ Quiche/95g	292	20.2	307	10.0	19.2	21.2	0.0
Cheese & Ham, Sainsbury's*	1 Serving/100g	266	19.0	266	9.3	14.4	19.0	1.2
Cheese & Mushroom, Budgens*	½ Quiche/170g	474	32.8	279	7.8	18.4	19.3	1.4
Cheese & Onion, 25% Reduced Fat, Asda*	½ Quiche/78g	163	7.0	209	11.0	21.0	9.0	2.4
Cheese & Onion, Crustless, Asda*	1 Quiche/160g	277	15.2	173	7.6	14.3	9.5	1.3
Cheese & Onion, Crustless, Weight Watchers*	1 Quiche/160g	267	12.3	167	11.3	11.1	7.7	4.3
Cheese & Onion, Deep Filled, Sainsbury's*	¼ Quiche/100g	254	17.2	254	7.3	17.2	17.2	2.2
Cheese & Onion, HL, Tesco*	¼ Quiche/100g	180	7.8	180	9.4	17.6	7.8	1.8
Cheese & Onion, Individual, Sainsbury's*	1 Quiche/180g	542	34.9	301	9.9	21.6	19.4	1.5
Cheese & Onion, Reduced Fat, Eat Smart, Morrisons*	1 Quiche/400g	824	36.8	206	7.7	16.9	9.2	0.7
Cheese & Onion, Retail, Average	¼ Quiche/100g	262	17.8	262	8.4	17.1	17.8	1.3
Cheese & Onion, Snack, Tasty Pastry*	1 Quiche/50g	137	8.6	274	4.9	24.9	17.2	1.2
Cheese & Onion, VLH Kitchens	1 Serving/80g	134	7.5	167	9.6	18.1	6.0	1.8
Cheese & Onion, Weight Watchers*	1 Quiche/165g	325	15.3	197	7.0	21.2	9.3	1.6
Cheese & Tomato, Retail, Average	¼ Quiche/100g	268	17.1	268	8.0	20.2	17.1	1.1
Chicken, Garlic & Herb, Asda*	1/8 Quiche/52g	137	8.3	264	10.0	20.0	16.0	1.2
Chicken & Basil, Finest, Tesco*	1 Serving/134g	381	24.9	284	9.3	19.8	18.6	1.3
Cumberland Sausage & Onion, Sainsbury's*	1 Serving/180g	486	33.3	270	7.0	18.8	18.5	1.3
Gammon, Leek & Mustard, Weight Watchers*	1 Quiche/165g	305	14.5	185	5.7	20.7	8.8	3.4
Garlic Mushroom, Asda*	¼ Quiche/105g	273	16.8	260	7.0	22.0	16.0	0.7

Q

	Measure INFO/WEIGHT	per Measure KCAL	FAT	Nutrition Values per 100g / 100ml KCAL	PROT	CARB	FAT	FIBRE
QUICHE								
Ham, Cheese & Chive, GFY, Asda*	1 Serving/78g	173	7.8	222	9.0	24.0	10.0	1.5
Ham & Mustard, GFY, Asda*	1 Quiche/155g	327	17.0	211	9.0	19.0	11.0	3.9
Ham & Soft Cheese, Tesco*	¼ Quiche/100g	280	20.1	280	7.4	17.5	20.1	1.9
Ham & Tomato, M & S*	½ Pack/200g	440	31.0	220	8.1	12.4	15.5	2.9
Leek, Cheese & Chive, Sainsbury's*	1/3 Quiche/125g	292	20.2	234	7.1	14.9	16.2	1.3
Leek & Sweet Potato, Waitrose*	½ Quiche/200g	440	29.0	220	5.3	17.0	14.5	2.3
Lorraine, Bacon, Smoked, & Cheese, M & S*	¼ Quiche/100g	270	18.4	270	9.7	16.4	18.4	1.6
Lorraine, BGTY, Sainsbury's*	1 Serving/128g	273	14.0	213	10.9	17.7	10.9	0.7
Lorraine, Crustless, Asda*	1 Quiche/160g	259	12.6	162	9.3	13.5	7.9	1.1
Lorraine, Crustless, LC, Tesco*	1 Pack/160g	280	13.4	175	12.6	11.8	8.4	2.5
Lorraine, Crustless, You Count, Love Life, Waitrose*	1 Quiche/160g	295	15.4	185	8.9	15.2	9.6	0.9
Lorraine, Finest, Tesco*	1 Serving/100g	330	25.1	330	8.4	17.5	25.1	1.5
Lorraine, Half Fat, Waitrose*	¼ Quiche/100g	189	8.9	189	8.1	19.0	8.9	1.4
Lorraine, Meat Free, Tesco*	1 Quiche/140g	335	19.3	240	9.4	19.1	13.8	2.8
Lorraine, Mini, M & S*	1oz/28g	95	6.6	340	11.6	21.0	23.6	1.6
Lorraine, Quiche Selection, M & S*	1 Slice/56g	160	11.5	285	12.8	12.3	20.6	2.1
Lorraine, Retail, Average	¼ Quiche/100g	280	19.5	280	9.0	16.8	19.5	2.0
Lorraine, Small, Waitrose*	1 Pack/170g	507	35.0	298	9.8	18.4	20.6	2.3
Lorraine, Snack, Morrisons*	1 Serving/50g	142	9.4	285	10.2	19.0	18.7	2.0
Lorraine, TTD, Sainsbury's*	1/3 Quiche/158g	402	28.3	254	10.9	12.3	17.9	2.5
Lorraine, Weight Watchers*	1 Quiche/165g	292	13.2	177	8.7	17.5	8.0	3.2
Mediterranean, GFY, Asda*	1 Serving/25g	54	2.2	217	9.0	25.0	9.0	2.4
Mediterranean, M & S*	1oz/28g	64	4.3	230	6.6	16.6	15.3	0.9
Mushroom	1oz/28g	80	5.5	284	10.0	18.3	19.5	0.9
Mushroom Medley, Waitrose*	¼ Quiche/100g	222	15.2	222	6.4	15.0	15.2	2.9
Onion, Caramelised, & Roquefort, Finest, Tesco*	1 Quiche/150g	401	26.7	267	7.2	17.0	17.8	5.1
Pepper, Sweetfire, Feta & Olive, Waitrose*	¼ Quiche/100g	238	16.9	238	5.7	15.7	16.9	1.4
Salmon & Asparagus, HE, Tesco*	1 Quiche/345g	621	26.6	180	7.5	20.2	7.7	1.2
Salmon & Broccoli, Asda*	¼ Quiche/106g	289	18.0	273	10.0	20.0	17.0	2.6
Salmon & Broccoli, Tesco*	1 Serving/133g	311	20.1	234	7.9	16.6	15.1	0.9
Salmon & Spinach, Sainsbury's*	1/3 Quiche/125g	318	21.9	254	8.2	15.9	17.5	1.0
Sausage & Onion, Sainsbury's*	1 Serving/100g	287	20.0	287	7.1	19.7	20.0	1.2
Spinach, Baby, & Gruyere, Sainsbury's*	¼ Quiche/93g	228	16.0	245	7.4	15.1	17.2	1.0
Spinach, Feta & Roasted Red Pepper, Higgidy*	1 Quiche/400g	888	53.2	222	5.8	19.9	13.3	2.2
Spinach & Gruyere, Sainsbury's*	¼ Quiche/100g	258	19.1	258	7.7	13.9	19.1	1.0
Spinach & Ricotta, M & S*	1oz/28g	73	5.3	260	8.0	14.9	18.8	1.7
Spinach & Ricotta, Tesco*	¼ Quiche/100g	237	14.9	237	5.8	19.9	14.9	1.0
Tomato, GFY, Asda*	¼ Quiche/50g	94	4.0	188	8.0	21.0	8.0	0.8
Tomato, Mozzarella, & Basil, Weight Watchers*	1 Quiche/165g	300	12.2	182	6.1	22.8	7.4	1.3
Tomato, Mushroom & Bacon, Sainsbury's*	1 Serving/187g	447	30.9	239	7.5	15.2	16.5	1.1
Tomato, Pesto & Mozzarella, TTD, Sainsbury's*	1/3 Quiche/158g	370	25.6	234	5.5	16.5	16.2	2.1
Tuna, Tomato & Basil, Asda*	1 Serving/125g	305	20.0	244	9.0	16.0	16.0	1.5
Vegetable, Garden, Crustless, Tesco*	½ Quiche/170g	270	13.8	160	6.5	12.2	8.2	3.5
Vegetable, Mediterranean, BGTY, Sainsbury's*	½ Quiche/90g	160	7.2	178	7.3	19.2	8.0	1.7
Vegetable, Mediterranean, Mini, M & S*	1oz/28g	78	4.9	280	6.8	23.9	17.5	1.6
Vegetable, Mediterranean, Weight Watchers*	1 Quiche/165g	285	13.5	173	3.8	21.1	8.2	4.0
Vegetable, Tesco*	1 Serving/100g	257	17.7	257	6.9	17.5	17.7	1.5
QUINCE								
Average	***1 Fruit/209g***	***54***	***0.2***	***26***	***0.3***	***6.3***	***0.1***	***1.9***
QUINOA								
Dry Weight, Average	***1 Serving/70g***	***258***	***4.2***	***368***	***14.1***	***64.2***	***6.1***	***7.0***
Flakes, Biofair*	1 Serving/40g	155	2.3	387	11.7	72.2	5.7	8.9
Organic, Dry Weight, Love Life, Waitrose*	1 Serving/40g	154	2.3	384	13.1	68.9	5.8	5.9

Q

	Measure INFO/WEIGHT	per Measure KCAL	FAT	Nutrition Values per 100g / 100ml KCAL	PROT	CARB	FAT	FIBRE
QUINOA								
Red	1 Serving/100g	358	6.0	358	12.9	62.2	6.0	9.7
QUORN*								
Balls, Swedish Style, Frozen, Quorn*	¼ Pack/75g	88	1.9	117	12.0	9.0	2.5	5.2
Biryani, Chicken Style, Lunch Pot, Quorn*	1 Pot/300g	300	13.0	100	3.5	10.9	4.4	1.7
Burger, Frozen, Quorn*	1 Burger/50g	75	3.0	150	14.4	7.7	6.0	4.0
Burger, Smoked Chilli & Lime, Chef's Selection, Quorn*	1 Burger/90g	147	6.3	163	17.0	6.6	7.0	3.0
Burgers, Chicken Style, Quorn*	1 Burger/67g	149	8.1	222	10.5	16.0	12.0	4.0
Burgers, Quarter Pounder, Quorn*	1 Burger/114g	170	6.8	150	14.4	7.7	6.0	4.0
Chicken Style Dippers, Quorn*	4 Dippers/92g	195	8.0	212	11.1	21.2	8.7	2.4
Chicken Style Pieces, Frozen or Chilled, Quorn*	1 Serving/87g	77	1.2	89	14.0	1.0	1.4	8.3
Chicken Style Tikka Pieces, Quorn*	1 Pack/175g	201	5.2	115	12.5	7.0	3.0	6.0
Cottage Pie, Quorn*	1 Lge Pack/500g	365	10.0	73	2.5	10.0	2.0	2.5
Curry, Red Thai, Quorn*	1 Serving/250g	240	12.0	96	5.6	6.1	4.8	3.6
Escalope, Mozzarella & Pesto, Quorn*	1 Escalope/120g	271	15.6	226	10.0	15.0	13.0	4.5
Escalope, Turkey Style, Sage & Onion, Quorn*	1 Escalope/100g	188	9.8	188	10.0	15.0	9.8	4.5
Escalopes, Cheese & Leek, Quorn*	1 Escalope/120g	256	13.2	213	9.0	17.0	11.0	5.0
Escalopes, Creamy Garlic & Mushroom, Quorn*	1 Escalope/120g	291	15.0	243	10.5	20.5	12.5	3.0
Escalopes, Goats Cheese & Cranberry, Quorn*	1 Escalope/120g	290	16.8	242	10.0	17.0	14.0	4.0
Escalopes, Gruyere Cheese, Quorn*	1 Escalope/110g	267	15.4	243	10.0	18.0	14.0	2.6
Escalopes, Lemon & Black Pepper, Quorn*	1 Escalope/110g	256	12.9	233	9.6	20.5	11.7	2.1
Fajita, Strips, Quorn*	½ Pack/70g	76	1.1	108	14.0	7.0	1.5	5.0
Fillets, Breaded, Mini, Quorn*	1 Fillet/30g	59	2.9	196	10.2	15.0	9.6	4.5
Goujons, Quorn*	1 Goujon/30g	59	2.9	196	10.2	15.0	9.6	4.5
Grills, Lamb Style, Quorn*	1 Grill/90g	126	4.0	140	16.0	5.6	4.4	5.5
Lasagne, Frozen or Chilled, Quorn*	1 Pack/300g	303	8.1	101	4.8	12.5	2.7	1.6
Mince, Frozen & Chilled, Quorn*	1 Serving/87g	91	1.7	105	14.5	4.5	2.0	5.5
Mini Savoury Eggs, Quorn*	1 Egg/20g	51	2.3	257	15.0	21.0	11.5	4.6
Nuggets, Crispy, Chicken Style, Quorn*	1 Nugget/17g	33	2.0	198	12.0	8.0	12.0	4.8
Pasty, Cornish Style, Quorn*	1 Pasty/150g	320	15.0	213	6.9	22.5	10.0	3.0
Pie, Chicken Style & Mushroom, Quorn*	1 Pie/235g	515	26.6	219	6.7	21.2	11.3	2.8
Pie, Mince & Potato, Quorn*	1 Pie/200g	388	16.0	194	6.5	22.5	8.0	3.0
Pork Steaks, Quorn*	1 Steak/83g	132	7.1	159	16.6	1.4	8.5	5.3
Sausage, Best of British, Chef's Selection, Quorn*	1 Sausage/60g	111	5.7	185	11.0	12.0	9.5	3.5
Sausage Roll, Chilled, Quorn*	1 Roll/130g	293	12.1	225	12.3	21.2	9.3	3.8
Sausages, Cumberland, Quorn*	1 Sausage/50g	86	3.5	172	13.5	12.0	7.0	3.5
Sausages, Frankfurter, Quorn*	1 Frankfurter/45g	92	6.3	205	13.5	4.5	14.0	3.5
Sausages, Leek & Pork Style, Quorn*	1 Sausage/44g	56	2.2	127	15.1	5.5	4.9	4.3
Sausages, Quorn*	1 Sausage/40g	71	3.1	177	10.2	13.4	7.8	6.2
Seasoned Steak, Strips, Quorn*	½ Pack/70g	76	0.9	109	14.0	7.5	1.3	5.5
Slices, Chicken Style, Deli, Quorn*	1 Slice/13g	13	0.3	107	16.3	4.5	2.6	6.0
Slices, Ham Style, Quorn*	¼ Pack/25g	30	0.5	122	16.0	6.5	2.2	5.8
Slices, Ham Style, Smoky, Quorn*	¼ Pack/25g	34	0.5	136	15.5	9.0	2.0	5.0
Slices, Peppered Beef Style, Quorn*	¼ Pack/25g	29	0.5	115	14.5	7.6	2.1	4.0
Slices, Pepperoni Style, Quorn*	1 Slice/5g	11	0.8	217	12.0	6.5	15.0	4.0
Spaghetti Bolognese, Quorn*	1 Pack/300g	255	1.8	85	4.4	14.8	0.6	1.5
Steak Strips, Frozen, Quorn*	¼ Pack/75g	75	1.8	100	14.3	4.3	2.4	6.0
Steaks, Peppered, Quorn*	1 Steak/98g	123	3.9	126	13.6	5.7	4.0	6.9

	Measure INFO/WEIGHT	per Measure KCAL	FAT	Nutrition Values per 100g / 100ml KCAL	PROT	CARB	FAT	FIBRE
RABBIT								
Meat Only, Raw	***1oz/28g***	***38***	***1.5***	***137***	***21.9***	***0.0***	***5.5***	***0.0***
Meat Only, Raw, Weighed with Bone	1 Serving/200g	274	11.0	137	21.9	0.0	5.5	0.0
Meat Only, Stewed	***1oz/28g***	***32***	***0.9***	***114***	***21.2***	***0.0***	***3.2***	***0.0***
Meat Only, Stewed, Weighed with Bone	***1oz/28g***	***19***	***0.5***	***68***	***12.7***	***0.0***	***1.9***	***0.0***
RADDICCIO								
Raw	***1oz/28g***	***4***	***0.1***	***14***	***1.4***	***1.7***	***0.2***	***1.8***
RADISH								
Red, Unprepared, Average	***1 Radish/8g***	***1***	***0.0***	***12***	***0.7***	***1.9***	***0.2***	***0.9***
White, Mooli, Raw	***1oz/28g***	***4***	***0.0***	***15***	***0.8***	***2.9***	***0.1***	***0.0***
RAISINS								
Cherry, Naturally Infused, Graze*	1 Pack/30g	90	0.0	299	3.0	79.0	0.0	0.0
Cherry Infused, Nak'd*	1 Pack/25g	68	0.0	272	2.1	79.0	0.0	2.0
Crazy Cola Infused, Nak'd*	1 Pack/25g	68	0.1	272	2.1	69.3	0.4	2.0
Lemon Infused, Nak'd*	1 Serving/25g	68	0.1	272	2.1	69.3	0.4	2.0
Lime Infused, Tangy, Nak'd*	1 Pack/25g	68	0.0	272	2.1	69.3	0.0	0.0
Orange, Naturally Infused, Graze*	1 Pack/30g	90	0.0	299	3.0	79.0	0.0	0.0
Pineapple Infused, Nak'd*	1 Packet/25g	68	0.0	272	3.0	79.0	0.0	4.0
Seedless, Average	***1 Serving/75g***	***215***	***0.4***	***287***	***2.2***	***68.5***	***0.5***	***3.2***
Sunny, Whitworths*	1 Box/43g	123	0.2	294	2.6	70.0	0.4	5.3
Very Cherry, Graze*	1 Punnet/40g	110	0.4	275	2.1	69.0	0.9	0.0
White Chocolate Coated, Graze*	1 Pack/30g	135	6.6	451	4.7	59.7	21.9	0.0
Yoghurt Coated, Graze*	1 Pack/40g	182	8.5	456	2.9	64.1	21.3	0.0
RAITA								
Cucumber & Mint, Patak's*	1oz/28g	18	0.5	64	3.4	8.4	1.8	0.0
Plain, Average	1oz/28g	16	0.6	57	4.2	5.8	2.2	0.0
RASPBERRIES								
Dried, Graze*	1 Pack/30g	85	0.8	284	3.2	62.0	2.6	0.0
Freeze Dried, Simply*	1 Serving/10g	37	0.0	370	10.0	80.0	0.0	20.0
Fresh, Raw, Average	***1 Serving/80g***	***20***	***0.2***	***25***	***1.3***	***4.7***	***0.3***	***6.5***
Frozen, Average	***1 Serving/100g***	***27***	***0.3***	***27***	***1.3***	***4.7***	***0.3***	***5.2***
in Fruit Juice, Average	***1oz/28g***	***9***	***0.0***	***32***	***0.8***	***6.7***	***0.2***	***1.7***
in Fruit Juice, Canned, John West*	1 Can/290g	93	0.6	32	0.9	6.7	0.2	1.5
in Syrup, Canned	***1oz/28g***	***25***	***0.0***	***88***	***0.6***	***22.5***	***0.1***	***1.5***
RATATOUILLE								
Average	1oz/28g	23	2.0	82	1.3	3.8	7.0	1.8
Princes*	1 Can/360g	86	1.4	24	1.0	4.2	0.4	0.0
Provencale, French Style Mixed Vegetables, Tesco*	½ Can/195g	76	3.9	39	1.1	4.2	2.0	1.9
RAVIOLI								
Asparagus, Waitrose*	1 Serving/150g	303	9.0	202	10.5	26.4	6.0	2.0
Basil & Parmesan, Organic, Sainsbury's*	½ Pack/192g	290	10.0	151	7.4	21.1	5.2	2.1
Beef	1 Serving/300g	501	13.7	167	6.4	25.0	4.6	1.4
Beef, Chef Boyardee*	1 Can/100g	190	5.0	190	6.0	31.0	5.0	2.0
Beef, GFY, Asda*	½ Pack/150g	288	4.8	192	7.0	33.9	3.2	1.9
Beef, in Rich Tomato Sauce, Corale, Aldi*	½ Can/200g	172	2.0	86	2.8	16.4	1.0	0.5
Beef, in Tomato Sauce, Canned, Asda*	1 Can/400g	352	8.0	88	3.6	14.0	2.0	3.0
Beef, Tesco*	1 Serving/194g	175	5.0	90	4.3	12.3	2.6	1.5
Beef, Weight Watchers*	1 Pack/300g	258	6.3	86	4.3	12.1	2.1	0.8
Beef & Shiraz, Finest, Tesco*	½ Pack/200g	358	9.0	179	8.4	26.1	4.5	1.8
Cheese, Garlic & Herb, Fresh, Organic, Tesco*	1 Serving/125g	382	19.5	306	11.3	30.1	15.6	0.9
Cheese, Tomato & Basil, Italiano, Tesco*	½ Pack/125g	309	11.0	247	13.1	28.5	8.8	2.1
Cheese & Asparagus, Waitrose*	1 Serving/100g	242	7.2	242	12.6	31.7	7.2	2.4
Cheese & Tomato, Fresh, Organic, Tesco*	1 Serving/125g	342	14.0	274	12.5	30.8	11.2	1.1
Cheese & Tomato, Heinz*	1 Can/400g	340	8.4	85	2.4	13.9	2.1	0.9

	Measure INFO/WEIGHT	per Measure KCAL	FAT	Nutrition Values per 100g / 100ml KCAL	PROT	CARB	FAT	FIBRE
RAVIOLI								
Chicken, Tomato & Basil, Finest, Tesco*	1 Serving/200g	358	12.0	179	9.6	21.7	6.0	1.0
Chicken & Bacon, Sainsbury's*	½ Pack/211g	335	11.4	159	5.5	22.2	5.4	2.0
Chicken & Mushroom, Finest, Tesco*	½ Pack/125g	268	8.9	214	11.6	25.8	7.1	1.1
Chicken & Rosemary, Perfectly Balanced, Waitrose*	½ Pack/125g	266	4.4	213	14.9	30.4	3.5	2.1
Chicken & Tomato, Perfectly Balanced, Waitrose*	1 Serving/125g	265	3.4	212	13.5	33.4	2.7	2.8
Feta Cheese, M & S*	1 Serving/100g	195	8.5	195	9.1	20.5	8.5	1.3
Five Cheese, Weight Watchers*	1 Pack/330g	271	9.2	82	3.2	11.1	2.8	0.8
Florentine, Weight Watchers*	1 Serving/241g	220	5.0	91	3.7	14.1	2.1	1.2
Four Cheese, Italian Choice, Asda*	1 Pack/449g	467	26.9	104	3.4	9.0	6.0	2.1
Fresh, Pasta Reale*	1 Serving/150g	459	8.8	306	13.1	53.3	5.9	0.0
Garlic & Herb, Italiano, Tesco*	1 Serving/100g	318	13.0	318	11.1	39.1	13.0	2.6
Goat's Cheese & Pesto, Asda*	½ Pack/150g	204	5.4	136	6.0	20.0	3.6	0.0
Goats Cheese & Roasted Red Pepper, Finest, Tesco*	½ Pack/125g	308	9.6	246	11.4	32.8	7.7	1.8
Grana Padano & Rocket, Finest, Tesco*	½ Pack/150g	270	7.5	180	7.5	26.0	5.0	1.8
Ham, Smoked, Bacon & Tomato, Italiano, Tesco*	1 Can/125g	302	9.6	242	10.8	32.3	7.7	2.9
in Tomato Sauce, Canned, Oaktree Estate*	½ Can/200g	175	2.1	90	3.0	15.9	1.1	1.1
in Tomato Sauce, Canned, Sainsbury's*	½ Can/200g	166	2.0	83	3.1	15.5	1.0	0.5
in Tomato Sauce, Heinz*	1 Can/400g	308	6.8	77	2.4	13.2	1.7	0.9
in Tomato Sauce, Meat Free, Heinz*	1 Can/410g	308	3.3	75	2.4	14.4	0.8	0.5
Meat, Italian, Fresh, Asda*	½ Pack/150g	261	6.3	174	8.0	26.0	4.2	0.0
Mozzarella, Tomato & Basil, Tesco*	1 Serving/125g	304	12.8	243	13.6	24.1	10.2	0.5
Mushroom, Fresh, Sainsbury's*	½ Pack/125g	196	5.1	157	7.4	22.6	4.1	1.9
Mushroom, Italiano, Tesco*	1 Serving/125g	332	16.1	266	10.4	27.0	12.9	3.0
Mushroom, Ready Meals, M & S*	1oz/28g	38	0.5	135	8.1	22.0	1.9	2.2
Mushroom, Wild, Finest, Tesco*	1 Serving/200g	472	12.2	236	10.8	34.4	6.1	1.9
Mushroomi, Tesco*	½ Pack/125g	332	16.1	266	10.4	27.0	12.9	3.0
Pancetta & Mozzarella, Finest, Tesco*	1 Serving/125g	344	13.2	275	12.2	32.8	10.6	1.8
Pepper, Sweet, & Chilli, Tesco*	½ Pack/125g	324	14.0	259	12.5	27.1	11.2	2.7
Pork, in Tomato Sauce, Low Fat, Morrisons*	1oz/28g	23	0.3	81	2.7	15.5	0.9	1.3
Prosciuttoi, Ready Meal, M & S*	1 Pack/100g	195	8.1	195	13.3	17.0	8.1	1.0
Red Pepper, Basil & Chilli, Waitrose*	½ Pack/125g	312	10.5	250	11.6	32.0	8.4	1.7
Salmon, Smoked, & Dill, Sainsbury's*	1 Serving/125g	256	8.9	205	8.7	26.5	7.1	0.7
Salmon & Dill, Sainsbury's*	1 Pack/300g	615	21.3	205	8.7	26.5	7.1	3.0
Smart Price, Asda*	1 Can/400g	272	0.4	68	2.7	14.0	0.1	1.3
Spinach & Ricotta, Waitrose*	1 Serving/125g	309	9.0	247	10.5	35.0	7.2	1.9
Tomato, Cheese & Meat, Sainsbury's*	1 Serving/125g	314	16.1	251	12.4	21.4	12.9	2.2
Vegetable, Canned, Sainsbury's*	1 Can/400g	328	2.8	82	2.6	16.3	0.7	0.7
Vegetable, in Tomato Sauce, Italiana, Weight Watchers*	1 Can/385g	266	8.1	69	1.7	11.0	2.1	0.5
Vegetable, Tesco*	½ Can/200g	164	1.4	82	2.6	16.3	0.7	0.7
Vegetable, with Omega 3, Heinz*	1 Can/200g	144	3.2	72	2.2	12.2	1.6	0.6
RED BULL*								
Energy Shot, Red Bull*	1 Can/60ml	27	0.0	45	0.0	10.7	0.0	0.0
Regular, Red Bull*	1 Can/250ml	112	0.0	45	0.0	11.3	0.0	0.0
REDCURRANTS								
Raw, Average	***1oz/28g***	***6***	***0.0***	***21***	***1.1***	***4.4***	***0.0***	***3.4***
Raw, Stalks Removed	1 Serving/100g	21	0.0	21	1.1	4.4	0.0	0.0
REEF*								
Orange & Passionfruit, Reef*	1 Bottle/275ml	179	0.0	65	0.0	9.5	0.0	0.0
REFRESHERS*								
Bassett's*	1oz/28g	106	0.0	377	4.3	78.1	0.0	0.0
RELISH								
Barbeque, Sainsbury's*	1 Serving/50g	50	1.0	100	1.0	19.3	2.1	1.1
Branston, Sweet Chilli & Ginger, Crosse & Blackwell*	1 Serving/20g	33	0.1	163	1.5	38.2	0.4	0.5

R

	Measure INFO/WEIGHT	per Measure KCAL	FAT	Nutrition Values per 100g / 100ml KCAL	PROT	CARB	FAT	FIBRE
RELISH								
Branston, Sweet Onion, Crosse & Blackwell*	1 Serving/10g	15	0.0	153	1.0	36.3	0.4	0.7
Branston, Tomato & Red Pepper, Crosse & Blackwell*	1 Serving/15g	24	0.1	160	1.3	37.4	0.4	0.7
Burger, Juicy, Asda*	1 Tbsp/15g	17	0.1	113	1.2	25.4	0.7	0.7
Caramelised Onion & Chilli, M & S*	1 Serving/20g	47	0.2	235	1.4	55.1	1.1	1.0
Caramelised Red Onion, Tesco*	1 Serving/10g	28	0.0	280	0.6	69.1	0.1	0.7
Hamburger, Bick's*	1oz/28g	27	0.1	96	1.3	22.3	0.2	0.0
Mango & Chilli, Levi Roots*	1 Serving/100g	110	0.2	110	0.7	25.0	0.2	1.1
Onion, M & S*	1oz/28g	46	0.8	165	1.0	32.1	3.0	1.1
Onion, Sainsbury's*	1 Serving/15g	23	0.1	151	0.9	36.0	0.4	0.7
Onion, Sweet, Heinz*	1 Tbsp/38g	38	0.2	102	1.0	23.5	0.4	0.6
Onion & Garlic, Spicy, Waitrose*	1 Tbsp/15g	35	0.2	232	0.8	54.2	1.1	1.7
Sweetcorn, American Style, Maryland, Tesco*	1 Serving/15g	15	0.0	101	1.1	23.9	0.1	0.9
Sweetcorn, Bick's*	1 Tbsp/22g	23	0.0	103	1.3	24.3	0.2	0.0
Tomato, M & S*	1oz/28g	36	0.1	130	1.8	30.2	0.3	1.5
Tomato, Sweet, Heinz*	1 Serving/25g	34	0.0	136	0.9	32.6	0.2	0.9
Tomato & Chilli Texan Style, Tesco*	1 Tbsp/14g	20	0.0	140	1.7	32.0	0.1	1.1
Tomato Spicy, Bick's*	1 Serving/28g	28	0.1	99	1.3	23.2	0.2	0.0
REVELS*								
Mars*	1 Packet/35g	168	7.3	480	5.1	68.0	20.9	0.0
RHUBARB								
in Juice, Canned, Drained, Average	1 Serving/100g	46	0.0	46	0.5	10.8	0.0	0.8
Raw, Average	***1 Stalk/51g***	***11***	***0.1***	***21***	***0.9***	***4.5***	***0.2***	***1.8***
Sliced, Frozen, Asda*	1 Serving/100g	11	0.1	11	0.9	0.8	0.1	1.4
Stewed with Sugar, Average	***1oz/28g***	***32***	***0.0***	***116***	***0.4***	***31.2***	***0.0***	***2.0***
RIBENA*								
Blackcurrant, Diluted with Water, Ribena*	1 Serving/100ml	46	0.0	46	0.0	11.4	0.0	0.0
Blackcurrant, No Added Sugar, Diluted, Ribena*	1 Serving/250ml	11	0.0	4	0.0	0.6	0.0	0.0
Blackcurrant, Original, Undiluted, Ribena*	1 Serving/50ml	108	0.0	216	0.0	53.0	0.0	0.0
Blackcurrant, Really Light, No Added Sugar, Ribena*	1 Carton/250ml	8	0.0	3	0.0	0.8	0.0	0.0
Blackcurrant & Cranberry, Ribena*	1 Bottle/500ml	205	0.0	41	0.0	9.9	0.0	0.0
Blackcurrant Juice Drink, Ready Made, Ribena*	1 Carton/200ml	82	0.0	41	0.0	10.6	0.0	0.0
Light, Ribena*	1 Carton/288ml	26	0.0	9	0.1	2.1	0.0	0.0
Orange, Juice Drink, Ribena*	1 Serving/288ml	98	0.0	34	0.1	8.1	0.0	0.0
Pineapple & Passion Fruit, Juice Drink, Ribena*	½ Bottle/250ml	103	0.0	41	0.0	9.9	0.0	0.0
Plus, Apple & Peach, Immunity Support, Ribena*	1 Carton/200ml	2	0.0	1	0.0	0.2	0.0	0.0
Plus, Blackcurrant, Carton, Ribena*	1 Carton/200ml	6	0.0	3	0.0	0.6	0.0	0.0
Really Light, Undiluted, Ribena*	1 Serving/25ml	20	0.0	80	0.0	2.5	0.0	0.0
Strawberry Juice Drink, Ribena*	1 Carton/288ml	130	0.0	45	0.0	10.9	0.0	0.0
RIBS								
Loin, BBQ, Sainsbury's*	1 Rib/42g	104	5.5	247	24.7	7.3	13.2	0.9
Loin, Chinese, Sainsbury's*	1 Rib/42g	103	5.0	246	27.2	7.2	12.0	0.9
Pork, Barbecue, Meat Only, Cooked, Average	1 Serving/100g	275	17.9	275	21.4	7.2	17.9	0.3
Pork, Barbeque, Weighed with Bone, Cooked, Average	1 Serving/100g	275	17.9	275	21.4	7.2	17.9	0.3
Pork, Chinese Style, Average	1 Serving/300g	736	44.7	245	17.9	10.0	14.9	0.7
Spare, Barbecue, Chinese Style, Farmfoods*	1 Pack/400g	464	25.2	116	9.3	5.6	6.3	0.1
Spare, Cantonese, Mini, Sainsbury's*	1 Rib/38g	97	5.0	259	17.2	17.3	13.4	1.0
Spare, Sweet, Sticky, Mini, M & S*	1 Pack/300g	615	34.5	205	16.6	8.6	11.5	0.2
RICE								
Arborio, Dry, Average	***1 Serving/80g***	***279***	***0.6***	***348***	***7.1***	***78.3***	***0.8***	***0.8***
Balti Style, Quick, Sainsbury's*	1 Serving/228g	192	1.1	84	4.3	15.7	0.5	2.0
Basmati, Boil in the Bag, Dry, Average	1 Serving/50g	176	0.4	352	8.4	77.8	0.8	0.4
Basmati, Brown, Butternut Squash, Tilda*	½ Pack/125g	164	5.1	131	3.3	20.3	4.1	1.2
Basmati, Brown, Dry, Average	***1 Serving/50g***	***177***	***1.5***	***353***	***9.5***	***71.8***	***3.0***	***2.2***

R

	Measure INFO/WEIGHT	per Measure KCAL	FAT	Nutrition Values per 100g / 100ml KCAL	PROT	CARB	FAT	FIBRE
RICE								
Basmati, Cooked, Average	***1 Serving/140g***	***189***	***1.0***	***135***	***3.1***	***29.0***	***0.7***	***0.4***
Basmati, Cooked, Tilda*	1 Serving/200g	214	0.2	107	2.4	24.0	0.1	1.2
Basmati, Dry Weight, Average	***1 Serving/60g***	***212***	***0.6***	***353***	***8.1***	***77.9***	***1.0***	***0.6***
Basmati, Indian, Dry, Average	***1 Serving/75g***	***260***	***0.7***	***346***	***8.4***	***76.1***	***0.9***	***0.1***
Basmati, Microwave, Cooked, Average	1 Serving/125g	182	2.3	146	2.7	30.0	1.8	0.0
Basmati, White, Dry, Average	***1 Serving/75g***	***262***	***0.4***	***349***	***8.1***	***77.1***	***0.6***	***2.2***
Basmati, Wholegrain, Cooked, Tilda*	1 Portion/180g	203	1.6	113	3.3	23.0	0.9	3.2
Basmati, with Mushroom, Dine In, Veetee*	1 Pack/280g	372	6.4	133	3.3	24.4	2.3	1.2
Basmati & Wild, Dry Weight, Tilda*	1 Serving/70g	244	0.3	349	9.4	77.0	0.5	1.0
Beef, Savoury, Batchelors*	1 Pack/120g	431	2.8	359	8.9	75.7	2.3	2.5
Black, Artemide, Eat Well, M & S*	1 Serving/75g	251	2.0	335	8.5	73.3	2.6	4.0
Brown, Cooked, Average	***1 Serving/140g***	***173***	***1.5***	***123***	***2.6***	***26.6***	***1.1***	***0.9***
Brown, Dry, Average	***1 Serving/75g***	***266***	***2.3***	***355***	***7.5***	***76.2***	***3.0***	***1.4***
Brown, Long Grain, Dry, Average	***1 Serving/50g***	***182***	***1.4***	***364***	***7.6***	***76.8***	***2.8***	***2.0***
Brown, Short Grain, Dry, Average	***1 Serving/50g***	***176***	***1.4***	***351***	***6.8***	***77.6***	***2.8***	***1.0***
Brown, Whole Grain, Cooked, Average	***1 Serving/170g***	***223***	***1.9***	***132***	***2.6***	***27.8***	***1.1***	***1.2***
Brown, Whole Grain, Dry, Average	***1 Serving/40g***	***138***	***1.2***	***344***	***7.4***	***71.6***	***2.9***	***3.0***
Chicken, Savoury, Batchelors*	1 Pack/124g	455	1.9	367	8.9	79.4	1.5	2.6
Chicken & Sweetcorn, Savoury, Asda*	½ Pack/60g	195	1.7	325	10.0	65.0	2.8	10.0
Chinese Savoury, Batchelors*	1 Serving/50g	177	1.2	354	9.9	73.1	2.4	2.8
Chinese Style, Express, Uncle Ben's*	1 Pack/250g	392	5.5	157	3.4	30.9	2.2	0.4
Coconut, M & S*	½ Pack/124g	217	5.0	175	3.1	31.8	4.0	0.3
Coconut, Thai, Sainsbury's*	½ Pack/100g	178	9.1	178	2.6	21.3	9.1	1.9
Coconut & Lime, Asda*	1 Pack/360g	695	17.6	193	4.5	32.7	4.9	0.9
Coriander & Herb, Packet, Cooked, Sainsbury's*	¼ Pack/150g	204	0.8	136	2.5	30.4	0.5	1.5
Coriander & Herbs, Batchelors*	1/3 Pack/76g	280	2.7	369	7.9	79.6	3.5	5.0
Egg, Chinese Style, Morrisons*	1 Serving/250g	285	11.9	114	2.1	16.8	4.8	0.7
Egg Fried, Average	1 Serving/300g	624	31.8	208	4.2	25.7	10.6	0.4
Egg Fried, Express, Uncle Ben's*	½ Pack/125g	216	5.2	173	4.0	29.9	4.2	0.3
Egg Fried, HL, Tesco*	1 Serving/250g	285	3.2	114	3.5	22.2	1.3	1.8
Egg Fried, Micro, Tesco*	1 Pack/250g	312	9.2	125	4.6	18.3	3.7	6.4
Fried, Chicken, Chinese Takeaway, Iceland*	1 Pack/340g	510	15.6	150	6.5	20.7	4.6	0.6
Fried, Duck, Chicken & Pork Celebration, Sainsbury's*	1 Pack/450g	544	16.2	121	7.9	14.2	3.6	1.5
Fried, Special, Cantonese, Sainsbury's*	½ Pack/250g	442	10.0	177	4.9	30.4	4.0	1.2
Fried, Special, Chinese, Tesco*	1 Serving/300g	618	33.3	206	6.5	19.9	11.1	0.8
Fried, Special, Chinese Takeaway, Iceland*	1 Pack/350g	630	17.5	180	5.5	28.2	5.0	1.2
Fried, Special, Waitrose*	1 Serving/350g	532	22.4	152	6.1	17.6	6.4	3.2
Garlic & Butter Flavoured, Batchelors*	1 Serving/50g	175	1.4	350	8.0	79.8	2.8	5.0
Garlic & Coriander Flavoured, Patak's*	1 Serving/125g	186	2.8	149	2.6	28.9	2.2	0.0
Ground, Whitworths*	1 Serving/28g	98	0.2	349	7.7	77.7	0.8	0.7
Long Grain, & Wild, Dry, Average	***1 Serving/75g***	***254***	***1.5***	***338***	***7.6***	***72.6***	***2.0***	***1.7***
Long Grain, American, Cooked, Average	***1 Serving/160g***	***229***	***2.8***	***143***	***3.0***	***28.8***	***1.8***	***0.2***
Long Grain, American, Dry, Average	***1 Serving/50g***	***175***	***0.5***	***350***	***7.2***	***77.8***	***1.1***	***0.6***
Long Grain, Brown, Micro Rice, Asda*	1 Portion/100g	153	1.4	153	3.8	30.2	1.4	2.4
Long Grain, Cooked, Value, Tesco*	1 Portion/50g	175	0.4	350	7.7	78.0	0.8	0.4
Long Grain, Dry, Average	***1 Serving/50g***	***169***	***0.5***	***337***	***7.4***	***75.5***	***1.0***	***1.7***
Long Grain, Microwavable, Cooked, Average	1 Serving/150g	180	0.9	120	2.7	25.8	0.6	0.7
Mexican Style, Ainsley Harriott*	1 Pack/170g	206	1.5	121	1.7	26.5	0.9	2.3
Mexican Style, Cooked, Express, Uncle Ben's*	1 Pack/250g	385	4.8	154	3.2	31.1	1.9	0.7
Mexican Style, Old El Paso*	1 Serving/75g	268	0.8	357	9.0	78.0	1.0	0.0
Mild Curry, Savoury, Batchelors*	1 Pack/120g	426	2.5	355	8.0	76.1	2.1	1.6
Mushroom & Coconut, Organic, Waitrose*	1 Pack/300g	474	15.0	158	3.7	24.5	5.0	1.4
Mushroom & Pepper, Savoury, Cooked, Morrisons*	1 Serving/200g	204	1.6	102	2.3	21.5	0.8	0.0

R

	Measure INFO/WEIGHT	per Measure KCAL	FAT	Nutrition Values per 100g / 100ml KCAL	PROT	CARB	FAT	FIBRE
RICE								
Mushroom Savoury, Batchelors*	½ Pack/61g	217	1.3	356	10.7	73.6	2.1	2.8
Peshwari, Special, Uncle Ben's*	½ Pack/125g	226	4.2	181	3.0	33.6	3.4	0.0
Pilau, Cooked, Average	***1 Serving/200g***	***349***	***8.8***	***174***	***3.5***	***30.3***	***4.4***	***0.8***
Pilau, Dry, Average	***1oz/28g***	***101***	***0.7***	***362***	***8.4***	***78.2***	***2.4***	***3.4***
Pilau, Indian Mushroom, Sainsbury's*	1 Serving/100g	119	2.4	119	3.0	21.3	2.4	1.9
Pilau, Mushroom, Bombay Brasserie, Sainsbury's*	1 Pack/400g	672	17.2	168	3.7	28.6	4.3	0.7
Pilau, Spinach, Bombay Brasserie, Sainsbury's*	1 Pack/401g	642	17.3	160	3.5	26.9	4.3	0.8
Pilau, Spinach & Carrot, Waitrose*	1 Pack/350g	466	8.4	133	3.1	24.8	2.4	1.2
Pilau, Waitrose*	½ Pack/175g	308	7.4	176	4.2	30.4	4.2	1.2
Pudding, Dry Weight, Average	1 Serving/100g	356	1.1	356	6.9	82.0	1.1	0.4
Risotto, Dry, Average	***1 Serving/50g***	***174***	***0.6***	***348***	***7.8***	***76.2***	***1.3***	***2.4***
Saffron, Cooked, Average	***1 Serving/150g***	***208***	***4.7***	***139***	***2.6***	***25.3***	***3.2***	***0.5***
Savoury, Golden, Dry Weight, Batchelors*	1 Pack/120g	437	3.4	364	10.1	74.7	2.8	2.4
Savoury, Golden, Nirvana*	1 Pack/120g	142	0.8	118	2.5	25.4	0.7	2.9
Stir Fry, Oriental Style, Oriental Express*	1 Serving/150g	216	5.1	144	4.2	24.1	3.4	1.9
Stir Fry, Thai Green, Tilda*	½ Pack/120g	155	4.8	129	2.9	20.3	4.0	4.0
Sweet & Sour, Savoury, Batchelors*	1 Serving/135g	418	2.8	310	9.4	75.6	2.1	3.1
Sweet & Sour, Savoury, Cooked, Asda*	½ Pack/126g	154	1.1	122	2.5	26.0	0.9	3.0
Sweet & Sour, Savoury, Sainsbury's*	1 Serving/145g	198	0.7	137	2.4	30.8	0.5	1.0
Sweet & Spicy, Express, Uncle Ben's*	1 Pack/250g	418	10.0	167	2.7	30.1	4.0	0.0
Tandoori, Savoury, Batchelors*	1 Serving/120g	430	3.0	358	10.3	73.5	2.5	3.0
Thai, Cooked, Average	***1 Serving/100g***	***136***	***1.8***	***136***	***2.5***	***27.4***	***1.8***	***0.3***
Thai, Dry, Average	***1 Serving/50g***	***174***	***0.2***	***348***	***7.1***	***78.9***	***0.4***	***0.9***
Thai, Fragrant, Dry, Average	***1 Serving/75g***	***272***	***0.5***	***363***	***7.2***	***82.0***	***0.7***	***0.3***
Thai, Glutinous, Sticky, White, Dry, Raw	1 Serving/100g	370	0.6	370	6.8	81.7	0.6	2.8
Vegetable, Golden, Freshly Frozen, Asda*	1 Sachet/200g	238	2.6	119	3.2	23.6	1.3	1.3
Vegetable, Golden, Savoury, Sainsbury's*	¼ Pack/100g	122	1.0	122	2.9	25.4	1.0	0.3
Vegetable, Original, Birds Eye*	1oz/28g	29	0.2	105	4.0	20.8	0.6	1.1
Vegetable, Savoury, Co-Op*	½ Pack/60g	210	0.6	350	9.0	76.0	1.0	3.0
White, Cooked, Average	***1 Serving/140g***	***182***	***1.1***	***130***	***2.6***	***28.7***	***0.8***	***0.2***
White, Cooked, Frozen, Average	***1 Serving/150g***	***168***	***0.8***	***112***	***2.9***	***23.8***	***0.6***	***1.2***
White, Flaked, Dry Weight, Average	***1oz/28g***	***97***	***0.3***	***346***	***6.6***	***77.5***	***1.2***	***0.0***
White, Fried	1oz/28g	37	0.9	131	2.2	25.0	3.2	0.6
White, Long Grain, Dry Weight, Average	***1 Serving/50g***	***181***	***1.0***	***362***	***7.1***	***79.1***	***1.9***	***0.4***
White, Microwave, Cooked, Average	½ Pack/125g	185	2.4	148	3.3	29.4	1.9	1.4
Wholegrain, Dry, Average	***1 Serving/50g***	***171***	***1.2***	***342***	***8.2***	***72.0***	***2.3***	***4.0***
Wholegrain, Microwave, Eat Well, M & S*	½ Pack/125g	181	1.5	145	2.5	31.0	1.2	2.2
Wild, Coronation, Sainsbury's*	¼ Pot/75g	140	4.8	186	3.1	29.1	6.4	0.9
Wild, Giant Canadian, Dry Weight, Tilda*	1 Serving/75g	262	0.6	350	11.5	74.2	0.8	1.9
Yellow, Ready Cooked, Tesco*	1oz/28g	32	0.4	113	2.7	27.1	1.3	0.1
RICE CAKES								
Caramel, Large, Tesco*	1 Cake/10g	34	0.2	344	6.5	73.9	2.5	5.1
Caramel, Less Than 3% Fat, Sainsbury's*	1 Pack/35g	134	0.6	382	5.6	86.4	1.6	1.8
Caramel Flavour, Kallo*	1 Cake/10g	38	0.5	383	6.2	78.9	4.8	3.9
Cheese, Jumbo, Free From, Tesco*	1 Serving/10g	44	1.8	439	8.1	62.1	17.6	3.8
Cheese & Onion, Namchow*	1 Serving/38g	141	1.2	377	7.2	79.5	3.3	0.0
Chilli, Mini, M & S*	1 Pack/22g	88	1.7	400	6.9	74.9	7.9	3.5
Chocolate, Dark, Organic, Kallo*	1 Cake/12g	57	2.9	471	6.8	57.2	24.1	7.4
Chocolate, Fabulous Bakin' Boys*	1 Biscuit/17g	83	3.7	490	6.4	66.7	22.0	1.6
Lightly Salted, Perfectly Balanced, Waitrose*	1 Cake/8g	31	0.2	387	8.3	82.4	2.7	2.1
Lightly Salted, Thick Slice, Low Fat, Kallo*	1 Cake/8g	28	0.2	372	8.0	78.7	2.8	5.1
Low Fat, Kallo*	1 Cake/10g	38	0.2	375	6.2	83.1	2.2	3.9
Multigrain, Ryvita*	3 Cakes/11g	43	0.5	384	9.1	76.2	4.7	5.3

	Measure INFO/WEIGHT	per Measure KCAL	FAT	Nutrition Values per 100g / 100ml KCAL	PROT	CARB	FAT	FIBRE
RICE CAKES								
Organic, Tesco*	1 Cake/8g	29	0.2	380	7.2	80.7	2.9	3.4
Paprika, Good Food*	1 Cake/12g	50	1.1	414	7.9	73.0	9.3	3.1
Salt & Vinegar, Jumbo, Tesco*	1 Cake/9g	31	0.2	347	8.4	72.7	2.5	6.0
Salt & Vinegar, Sainsbury's*	1 Pack/30g	121	2.5	403	8.3	73.3	8.3	2.7
Salt & Vinegar, Snack, Tesco*	1 Pack/35g	116	0.6	332	7.5	71.5	1.8	1.1
Savoury, Jumbo, HL, Tesco*	1 Cake/8g	31	0.2	369	11.9	75.0	2.4	3.6
Sea Salt & Balsamic Vinegar, Kallo*	1 Cake/9g	32	0.2	361	6.5	78.1	2.5	3.0
Sesame, No Added Salt, Thick Sliced, Organic, Kallo*	1 Cake/10g	37	0.3	373	8.0	78.0	3.2	5.4
Sesame, Slightly Salted, Thin Slice, Organic, Kallo*	1 Cake/5g	17	0.1	373	8.0	78.0	3.2	5.4
Sesame Garlic, Clearspring*	1 Serving/8g	29	0.2	382	7.8	82.3	2.4	0.0
Sesame Teriyaki, Clearspring*	1 Cake/7g	28	0.2	377	6.5	82.8	2.2	0.0
Slightly Salted, Mrs Crimble's*	1 Slice/6g	21	0.2	380	7.6	80.4	3.1	3.2
Slightly Salted, Organic, Thin Slice, Kallo*	1 Cake/5g	17	0.1	372	8.0	78.7	2.8	5.1
Slightly Salted, Thick Slice, Organic, Kallo*	1 Cake/8g	28	0.2	372	8.0	78.7	2.8	5.1
Sour Cream & Chive Flavour, Sainsbury's*	1 Pack/30g	119	2.6	396	7.9	72.0	8.5	2.9
Thin Slice, No Added Salt, Organic, Kallo*	1 Cake/5g	19	0.1	372	8.0	78.7	2.8	5.1
Thin Slice, Organic, Hawkwood*	1 Cake/6g	21	0.2	378	7.6	79.1	3.5	3.4
Thin Slice, Organic, Waitrose*	1 Serving/5g	17	0.1	340	8.0	70.0	2.0	4.0
Toasted Sesame, Ryvita*	1 Pack/11g	43	0.5	391	8.4	78.4	4.9	3.5
Wholegrain, Mild Chilli, Tesco*	1 Cake/10g	38	1.4	400	7.2	59.8	14.4	5.8
Wholegrain, No Added Salt, Thick Slice, Organic, Kallo*	1 Cake/9g	33	0.3	365	7.6	80.0	3.1	3.4
Wholegrain, Salt & Vinegar, Tesco*	1 Cake/9g	28	0.2	314	8.4	61.9	2.6	6.0
RICE CRACKERS								
Barbecue, Sakata*	½ Pack/50g	204	1.3	407	7.3	85.2	2.6	1.6
Barbecue Flavour, Tesco*	1 Pack/25g	102	1.8	409	6.7	78.8	7.4	1.7
Brown, Wakama*	1 Cracker/5g	19	0.0	375	8.0	84.8	0.4	0.0
Cheddar Gorge, Graze*	1 Punnet/26g	139	9.0	534	10.6	48.3	34.7	2.3
Cheese, Tesco*	1 Serving/25g	104	2.0	416	7.9	78.1	8.0	1.8
Chilli, Temptations, Tesco*	1 Serving/25g	128	7.2	512	4.4	58.0	28.8	0.0
Chilli, Whitworths*	½ Pack/50g	254	12.8	507	5.1	63.9	25.7	0.5
Cracked Pepper, Sakata*	½ Pack/50g	200	1.5	400	7.3	84.4	3.0	2.0
Japanese, Apollo*	1 Pack/75g	297	3.5	396	9.6	78.8	4.7	0.9
Japanese, Hider*	1 Pack/70g	303	12.1	433	11.3	61.7	17.3	0.0
Japanese, Julian Graves*	1 Serving/25g	92	0.4	369	8.8	79.5	1.7	3.8
Japanese, Mini, Sunrise*	1 Serving/50g	180	0.0	360	7.0	83.0	0.0	7.0
Japanese Seaweed, Very Nori-sh, Graze*	1 Punnet/14g	64	1.8	454	5.9	78.8	12.7	1.0
Korean Chilli, Graze*	1 Pack/19g	98	5.1	519	5.0	64.0	27.0	0.5
Mix, M & S*	½ Pack/63g	225	0.1	360	6.5	82.9	0.1	1.6
Paprika Flavour, Namchow*	1 Serving/38g	141	1.2	375	7.5	78.9	3.3	0.0
Sainsbury's*	1 Serving/20g	87	1.9	433	11.2	74.3	9.4	1.0
Salt & Pepper, Asda*	1 Cracker/5g	19	0.0	385	7.0	87.0	1.0	2.2
Salt & Vinegar, Namchow*	1 Serving/38g	139	1.4	370	6.7	77.5	3.7	0.0
Sour Cream & Chive, Sakata*	1 Serving/25g	107	2.0	430	7.8	80.6	7.9	0.0
Spicy Mix, Asda*	1 Serving/25g	115	4.2	461	6.4	71.2	16.7	0.2
Thai, M & S*	1 Serving/55g	209	1.8	380	7.0	80.2	3.3	1.2
Thai, Sesame & Soy Sauce, M & S*	1 Pack/55g	210	2.6	385	7.6	77.8	4.8	1.4
Thai, Wakama*	1 Cracker/2g	8	0.1	400	6.9	86.9	2.7	0.5
Thai Chilli, Nature's Harvest*	1 Pack/75g	401	22.3	535	4.6	61.5	29.7	4.2
Thin, Blue Dragon*	3 Crackers/5g	20	0.2	395	6.1	84.4	3.7	0.0
Veggie Sushi Plate, Graze*	1 Punnet/24g	107	3.1	444	11.1	68.4	12.8	3.9
RICE MILK								
Organic, Provamel*	1 Serving/250ml	122	3.8	49	0.1	9.5	1.5	0.0
Original, Rice Dream*	1 Serving/150ml	70	1.5	47	0.1	9.4	1.0	0.1

	Measure INFO/WEIGHT	per Measure KCAL	FAT	Nutrition Values per 100g / 100ml KCAL	PROT	CARB	FAT	FIBRE
RICE PUDDING								
50% Less Fat, Asda*	½ Can/212g	180	1.7	85	3.3	16.2	0.8	0.2
Apple, Mini Pot, Muller Rice, Muller*	1 Pot/95g	103	2.2	108	3.2	18.6	2.3	0.0
Apple, Muller Rice, Muller*	1 Pot/190g	205	4.4	108	3.2	18.6	2.3	0.4
Apple & Blackberry, Muller Rice, Muller*	1 Pot/190g	207	4.2	109	3.2	19.0	2.2	0.4
Apple Strudel Flavour Sauce, Muller Rice, Muller*	1 Pot/190g	205	4.4	108	3.2	18.6	2.3	0.4
Banana, Ambrosia*	1 Pot/150g	153	3.8	102	3.2	16.6	2.5	0.0
Banana & Toffee (Limited Edition), Muller Rice, Muller*	1 Pot/190g	207	4.2	109	3.1	19.3	2.2	0.4
Canned, Average	1oz/28g	25	0.7	89	3.4	14.0	2.5	0.2
Canned, BGTY, Sainsbury's*	1 Can/425g	344	2.6	81	3.3	15.5	0.6	0.4
Caramel, Ambrosia*	1 Pot/150g	149	3.8	99	3.1	16.1	2.5	0.0
Clotted Cream, Cornish, Waitrose*	1 Serving/150g	304	20.1	203	3.0	17.6	13.4	0.5
Clotted Cream, M & S*	1 Pudding/185g	431	30.7	233	3.0	19.2	16.6	0.2
COU, M & S*	1 Pot/171g	145	2.9	85	2.4	15.5	1.7	0.5
Creamed, Asda*	1 Serving/215g	196	3.4	91	3.2	16.0	1.6	0.0
Creamed, Canned, Ambrosia*	1 Can/425g	382	8.1	90	3.1	15.2	1.9	0.0
Creamed, Morrisons*	1 Can/212g	189	3.4	89	3.1	15.7	1.6	0.0
Creamed, Pot, Ambrosia*	1 Pot/150g	156	3.8	104	3.3	17.0	2.5	0.1
Creamed, Weight Watchers*	1 Pot/130g	108	0.9	83	3.2	16.0	0.7	0.3
Creamy, Ambrosia*	½ Can/212g	197	4.0	93	3.2	15.7	1.9	0.0
Creamy, Delicious, Taste of Home, Heinz*	½ Can/212g	225	4.0	106	3.4	18.6	1.9	0.2
Creamy, Shape, Danone*	1 Serving/175g	149	1.8	85	3.5	15.4	1.0	0.4
Creamy, with Strawberry Crunch, Ambrosia*	1 Pack/205g	297	8.6	145	3.9	23.0	4.2	0.7
Creamy, with Tropical Crunch, Ambrosia*	1 Pack/210g	307	8.8	146	3.6	23.4	4.2	0.6
Low Fat, Devon, Creamed, Ambrosia*	½ Can/213g	193	2.8	91	3.2	16.5	1.3	0.0
Low Fat, No Added Sugar, Canned, Weight Watchers*	½ Can/212g	155	3.2	73	3.7	11.4	1.5	0.0
Low fat, Tesco*	1 Can/425g	404	5.5	95	3.2	16.9	1.3	0.1
Organic, Ambrosia*	1 Can/425g	455	15.7	107	3.4	15.1	3.7	0.0
Organic, Evernat*	1oz/28g	39	0.8	141	5.5	22.9	3.0	0.0
Original, Jan Jac*	1 Pot/200g	258	7.2	129	2.6	21.6	3.6	0.0
Original, Muller Rice, Muller*	1 Pot/190g	196	4.9	103	3.6	16.3	2.6	0.3
Perfectly Balanced, Waitrose*	1 Serving/154g	140	2.5	91	3.4	15.7	1.6	1.2
Raspberry, BGTY, Sainsbury's*	1 Pot/135g	126	1.6	93	3.2	17.2	1.2	1.3
Raspberry, Mullerice, Muller*	1 Pot/190g	201	4.4	106	3.2	18.2	2.3	0.5
Rhubarb, Muller*	1 Pot/200g	226	4.4	113	3.2	20.0	2.2	0.0
Strawberry, Mullerrice, Muller*	1 Pot/200g	220	4.4	110	3.2	19.3	2.2	0.4
Strawberry Flavour, Jan Jac*	1 Pot/200g	256	6.4	128	2.4	22.4	3.2	0.2
Thick & Creamy, Co-Op*	1 Can/425g	531	25.5	125	3.0	16.0	6.0	0.0
Thick & Creamy, Nestle*	1 Can/425g	527	23.8	124	3.1	15.4	5.6	0.2
Toffee, Smooth, Muller Rice, Muller*	1 Pot/190g	201	4.4	106	3.3	18.0	2.3	0.3
Toffee Apple, Muller Rice, Muller*	1 Pot/190g	205	4.2	108	3.1	19.0	2.2	0.4
Toffee Flavour, Jan Jac*	1 Pot/200g	270	7.8	135	2.4	22.5	3.9	0.1
Vanilla Custard, Mullerrice, Muller*	1 Pot/200g	230	5.0	115	3.4	19.8	2.5	0.3
Venetian, Cafe Culture, M & S*	1 Serving/120g	300	19.7	250	3.4	21.8	16.4	0.2
RICE WINE								
Sake, Average	***1 Tbsp/15ml***	***20***	***0.0***	***134***	***0.5***	***5.0***	***0.0***	***0.0***
RIGATONI								
Carbonara, Tesco*	1 Serving/205g	236	11.9	115	5.2	10.6	5.8	1.2
Dry, Average	***1 Serving/80g***	***272***	***1.2***	***340***	***11.4***	***68.4***	***1.5***	***2.7***
Tomato & Cheese, Perfectly Balanced, Waitrose*	1 Pack/400g	664	9.2	166	7.6	28.6	2.3	2.3
Tuna, Diet Chef Ltd*	1 Pack/300g	336	13.2	112	5.9	12.2	4.4	1.0
RISOTTO								
Beef, Vesta*	1 Serving/100g	346	5.9	346	15.3	57.8	5.9	5.6
Beetroot & Goats Cheese, Lovely Vegetables, M & S*	1 Pack/379g	530	17.0	140	4.4	20.7	4.5	3.6

	Measure INFO/WEIGHT	per Measure KCAL	FAT	Nutrition Values per 100g / 100ml KCAL	PROT	CARB	FAT	FIBRE
RISOTTO								
Butternut, Pearl Barely, Veg Pot, Innocent*	1 Pot/390g	285	5.1	73	2.9	12.6	1.3	3.8
Butternut Squash, Fresh Ideas, M Kitchen, Morrisons*	1 Pot/350g	371	11.9	106	1.8	16.8	3.4	0.7
Cheese, Onion & Wine, Rice & Simple, Ainsley Harriott*	1 Pack/140g	253	7.0	181	3.1	31.0	5.0	1.6
Cheese Flavour, Made Up, Ainsley Harriott*	1 Sachet/140g	565	14.6	404	7.8	69.6	10.4	9.1
Cherry Tomato, COU, M & S*	1 Pack/360g	324	8.3	90	2.0	15.4	2.3	1.8
Chicken	1 Serving/380g	494	17.4	130	7.2	15.2	4.6	1.3
Chicken, & Bacon, Italiano, Tesco*	1 Pack/450g	652	20.2	145	5.9	20.2	4.5	1.5
Chicken, & Lemon, Weight Watchers*	1 Pack/330g	327	6.9	99	6.3	13.7	2.1	0.5
Chicken, & Mushroom, Waitrose*	1 Pack/350g	364	16.1	104	6.0	9.7	4.6	0.8
Chicken, & Mushroom, Weight Watchers*	1 Pack/320g	310	4.5	97	6.5	14.5	1.4	0.3
Chicken, BGTY, Sainsbury's*	1 Pack/327g	356	6.2	109	7.5	15.5	1.9	1.0
Chicken, Chargrilled, Ready Meal, M & S*	1 Pack/365g	493	25.2	135	6.4	11.6	6.9	0.7
Chicken, Enjoy, Birds Eye*	1 Pack/500g	735	31.5	147	8.5	14.0	6.3	0.5
Chicken, Lemon & Wild Rocket, Sainsbury's*	1 Pack/360g	683	41.0	190	16.2	5.6	11.4	0.1
Chicken, Little Dish*	1 Pack/200g	209	9.2	104	7.1	9.1	4.6	0.6
Chicken, Tomato & Mozzarella, GFY, Asda*	1 Pack/400g	356	4.0	89	8.1	11.9	1.0	1.2
Green Bean, Asparagus & Pecorino, Finest, Tesco*	1 Pack/400g	460	15.6	115	4.4	15.0	3.9	1.5
Haddock, Smoked, Italian, Tesco*	½ Pack/350g	400	15.1	114	4.2	14.3	4.3	0.8
Haddock & Mushroom, COU, M & S*	1 Pack/400g	320	3.2	80	6.4	12.1	0.8	2.0
King Prawn, & Snow Crab, M & S*	1 Pack/365g	402	16.4	110	4.1	12.7	4.5	0.5
King Prawn, Pea & Mint, M & S*	½ Pack/300g	405	18.6	135	3.8	15.9	6.2	0.9
Lemon & Mint, Perfectly Balanced, Waitrose*	1 Pack/350g	462	13.0	132	3.9	20.7	3.7	1.0
Mushroom, & Chestnut, Waitrose*	1 Pack/400g	496	90.0	124	14.6	58.4	22.5	7.2
Mushroom, Asda*	1 Pack/340g	340	11.6	100	2.3	15.0	3.4	0.6
Mushroom, Balls, Occasions, Sainsbury's*	1 Ball/25g	76	3.4	304	3.8	41.2	13.8	1.7
Mushroom, COU, M & S*	1 Pack/375g	338	5.6	90	3.0	16.1	1.5	1.5
Mushroom, Diet Chef Ltd*	1 Pack/250g	215	7.2	86	3.2	12.0	2.9	0.2
Mushroom, Low Saturated Fat, Waitrose*	1 Pack/400g	440	9.6	110	4.6	15.1	2.4	1.5
Mushroom, Perfectly Balanced, Waitrose*	1 Pack/400g	384	6.4	96	4.3	16.1	1.6	2.1
Mushroom, Wild, & Garlic, Tesco*	1 Pack/320g	522	14.1	163	3.6	27.2	4.4	1.6
Mushroom, Wild, Made Up, Ainsley Harriott*	1 Sachet/140g	785	21.7	561	12.0	93.3	15.5	14.7
Mushroom, Wild, Weight-Away*	1 Pack/250g	320	9.8	128	3.1	18.0	3.9	1.0
Red Pepper, Roasted, & Italian Cheese, M & S*	1 Pack/400g	500	13.2	125	2.9	20.4	3.3	1.0
Red Wine, with Creamed Spinach, Italian, Sainsbury's*	1 Pack/400g	596	27.6	149	2.4	19.3	6.9	0.4
Salmon, Hot Smoked, & Spinach, M & S*	½ Pack/300g	420	24.0	140	6.4	11.0	8.0	0.6
Salmon, Weight Watchers*	1 Pack/320g	261	2.5	82	4.7	13.8	0.8	0.3
Salmon & Prawn, Eat Smart, Morrisons*	1 Pack/381g	339	5.3	89	4.9	14.1	1.4	0.8
Seafood, HL, Tesco*	1 Pack/365g	328	3.6	90	5.3	14.1	1.0	0.9
Seafood, Youngs*	1 Pack/350g	424	13.0	121	4.5	17.4	3.7	0.1
Sun Dried Tomato, Balls, Occasions, Sainsbury's*	1 Ball/25g	71	3.8	285	6.8	30.8	15.0	2.9
Tomato, & Cheese, GFY, Asda*	1 Pack/400g	428	12.0	107	3.1	17.0	3.0	0.7
Tomato, & Mascarpone, M & S*	1 Pack/360g	468	19.1	130	2.7	17.5	5.3	0.9
Vegetable, Average	1oz/28g	41	1.8	147	4.2	19.2	6.5	2.2
Vegetable, Brown Rice, Average	1oz/28g	40	1.8	143	4.1	18.6	6.4	2.4
Vegetable, Great Stuff, Asda*	1 Pack/300g	315	5.7	105	4.3	17.6	1.9	1.3
Vegetable, Roasted, & Sunblush Tomato, Finest, Tesco*	½ Pack/200g	306	18.0	153	3.7	14.5	9.0	1.4
Vegetable, Roasted, Made Up, Ainsley Harriott*	1 Sachet/140g	766	18.2	547	11.0	96.5	13.0	15.5
Vegetable, Roasted, Stir-In, Uncle Ben's*	½ Pack/75g	86	7.3	115	1.7	5.0	9.7	0.0
Vegetable, Spring, M & S*	1 Serving/330g	330	13.2	100	2.0	14.2	4.0	0.9
RISSOLES								
Lentil, Fried in Vegetable Oil, Average	1oz/28g	59	2.9	211	8.9	22.0	10.5	3.6
ROCK SALMON								
Raw, Flesh Only, Average	***1oz/28g***	***43***	***2.7***	***154***	***16.6***	***0.0***	***9.7***	***0.0***

R

	Measure INFO/WEIGHT	per Measure KCAL	FAT	Nutrition Values per 100g / 100ml KCAL	PROT	CARB	FAT	FIBRE
ROCKET								
Baby Leaf, M & S*	½ Bag/40g	10	0.2	25	2.7	1.4	0.5	2.1
Fresh, Raw, Average	***1 Serving/80g***	***12***	***0.4***	***16***	***0.8***	***1.7***	***0.5***	***1.2***
Super Hot, Steve's Leaves*	1 Bag/30g	6	0.1	20	3.4	0.6	0.4	3.1
Wild, Morrisons*	1 Serving/100g	17	0.6	17	0.9	1.7	0.6	1.4
ROE								
Cod, Average	***1 Can/100g***	***96***	***2.8***	***96***	***17.1***	***0.5***	***2.8***	***0.0***
Cod, Hard, Coated in Batter, Fried	1oz/28g	53	3.3	189	12.4	8.9	11.8	0.2
Cod, Hard, Fried in Blended Oil	1oz/28g	57	3.3	202	20.9	3.0	11.9	0.1
Herring, Soft, Fried in Blended Oil	1oz/28g	74	4.4	265	26.3	4.7	15.8	0.2
Herring, Soft, Raw	***1oz/28g***	***25***	***0.7***	***91***	***16.8***	***0.0***	***2.6***	***0.0***
ROGAN JOSH								
Chicken, & Rice, Sainsbury's*	1 Pack/500g	675	27.0	135	6.7	14.1	5.4	2.4
Chicken, Breast, Chunks, Hot, Sainsbury's*	½ Pack/114g	143	2.0	126	23.6	3.9	1.8	1.0
Chicken, with Pilau Rice, Farmfoods*	1 Pack/325g	354	6.8	109	5.3	17.1	2.1	0.4
King Prawn, with Rice, HL, Tesco*	1 Pack/400g	365	6.0	91	4.8	14.6	1.5	1.6
Lamb, & Pilau Rice, Indian Takeaway, Asda*	1 Pack/569g	888	27.9	156	7.0	21.0	4.9	1.7
Lamb, & Pilau Rice, Tesco*	1 Pack/550g	770	29.2	140	6.0	16.9	5.3	1.0
Lamb, Indian, Takeaway, Chosen By You, Asda*	½ Pack/200g	218	12.0	109	8.0	5.1	6.0	1.4
Lamb, Sainsbury's*	1 Pack/400g	660	44.4	165	11.3	4.9	11.1	1.9
Lamb, Waitrose*	½ Pack/175g	242	13.3	138	12.4	5.0	7.6	1.3
Lamb, with Pilau Rice, Eastern Classics*	1 Pack/400g	604	21.6	151	5.6	19.9	5.4	1.0
Prawn, & Pilau Rice, BGTY, Sainsbury's*	1 Pack/401g	353	3.2	88	4.8	15.3	0.8	1.9
Prawn, COU, M & S*	1 Pack/400g	360	2.4	90	4.9	16.2	0.6	0.8
ROLL								
Cheese, Chunky, & Mustard, Finest, Tesco*	1 Roll/88g	260	9.0	295	10.9	40.0	10.2	2.4
Cheese, Tomato & Onion, Sainsbury's*	1 Pack/100g	518	28.1	518	18.4	47.9	28.1	0.0
Cheese & Chutney, M & S*	1 Roll/165g	256	1.2	155	13.9	23.1	0.7	1.2
Cheese & Onion, Asda*	1 Serving/67g	199	12.0	298	7.0	27.0	18.0	2.0
Cheese & Onion, King Size, Pork Farms*	1 Serving/130g	443	28.6	341	7.4	28.4	22.0	0.0
Cheese & Onion, M & S*	1 Roll/25g	80	5.1	320	9.6	24.7	20.5	1.3
Cheese & Onion, Sainsbury's*	1 Roll/67g	205	13.6	306	8.0	22.9	20.3	1.9
Cheese & Pickle, Sainsbury's*	1 Roll/136g	359	13.6	264	10.6	35.1	10.0	0.0
Chicken, Roast, & Mayonnaise, Big, Sainsbury's*	1 Pack/185g	479	27.4	259	9.6	21.8	14.8	0.0
Chicken, Roast, & Sweetcure Bacon, Boots*	1 Pack/245g	690	34.3	282	13.0	26.0	14.0	1.6
Chicken, Roast, Salad, Improved, Shapers, Boots*	1 Pack/188g	302	3.6	161	11.0	25.0	1.9	1.6
Chicken, Spicy, Crusty, M & S*	1 Roll/150g	382	16.6	255	12.8	25.8	11.1	2.0
Chicken & Herb, Shapers, Boots*	1 Roll/168g	290	4.7	173	12.0	25.0	2.8	1.7
Chicken & Stuffing, Tesco*	1 Roll/323g	1043	58.8	323	10.4	29.4	18.2	1.0
Chicken & Sun Dried Tomato, Weight Watchers*	1 Pack/170g	272	3.2	160	12.9	22.7	1.9	1.2
Chicken & Sweetcorn, Sainsbury's*	1 Serving/170g	462	23.6	272	12.5	24.2	13.9	0.0
Chicken Salad, HL, Tesco*	1 Serving/100g	149	2.0	149	10.6	22.3	2.0	1.2
Egg & Bacon, Sub, Shapers, Boots*	1 Serving/169g	320	7.3	189	11.0	27.0	4.3	1.3
Egg & Cress, HL, Tesco*	1 Pack/175g	322	6.8	184	9.6	27.7	3.9	1.2
Egg & Tomato, Shapers, Boots*	1 Roll/166g	301	5.3	181	8.0	30.0	3.2	2.6
Egg Mayo & Cress, Fullfillers*	1 Roll/125g	266	11.8	213	10.0	25.7	9.4	0.0
Egg Mayonnaise & Cress, Sub, Delicious, Boots*	1 Pack/205g	399	14.1	195	10.0	23.0	6.9	2.4
Ham, Darwins Deli*	1 Serving/125g	298	7.5	238	11.0	37.4	6.0	0.0
Ham & Cheese in Pastry, Pork Farms*	1 Roll/70g	216	12.5	308	8.0	28.8	17.9	0.0
Ham & Tomato, Taste!*	1 Serving/112g	211	4.8	188	10.4	27.0	4.3	0.0
Ham Salad, BGTY, Sainsbury's*	1 Roll/178g	292	3.4	164	10.8	25.9	1.9	0.0
Ham Salad, HL, Tesco*	1 Roll/203g	284	5.3	140	9.8	19.3	2.6	0.0
Mushroom & Bacon, Crusty, M & S*	1 Roll/160g	424	20.2	265	8.7	29.0	12.6	2.3
Ploughmans 4 Pack, Ginsters*	1 Roll/60g	220	16.3	367	9.2	21.4	27.2	2.1

R

	Measure INFO/WEIGHT	per Measure KCAL	FAT	Nutrition Values per 100g / 100ml KCAL	PROT	CARB	FAT	FIBRE
ROLL								
Pork, Roast, Stuffing & Apple Sauce, Boots*	1 Roll/218g	602	26.2	276	10.0	32.0	12.0	1.8
Tuna & Sweetcorn, with Mayonnaise, Shell*	1 Pack/180g	536	26.3	298	13.1	28.6	14.6	0.0
Tuna Mayo & Cucumber, Taste!*	1 Serving/111g	274	12.5	247	9.0	27.3	11.3	0.0
Tuna Mayonnaise with Cucumber, Yummies*	1 Serving/132g	340	18.6	257	10.4	22.5	14.0	0.0
Turkey, Stuffed, GFY, Asda*	½ Pack/225g	320	9.4	142	14.0	12.0	4.2	0.8
Turkey Salad, Northern Bites*	1 Roll/231g	323	8.3	140	8.6	19.6	3.6	3.0
ROLO								
Chocolate, Nestle*	2 Pieces/20g	102	5.3	509	4.1	62.6	26.6	1.3
Giant, Nestle*	1 Sweet/9g	42	1.8	470	3.1	70.1	19.7	0.3
Little, Nestle*	1 Pack/40g	196	9.4	491	4.0	65.5	23.5	0.5
Nestle*	1 Sweet/5g	24	1.0	478	4.4	68.2	20.4	1.1
ROOT BEER								
Average	1 Can/330ml	135	0.0	41	0.0	10.6	0.0	0.0
ROSE WATER								
The English Provender Co.*	1 Tsp/5g	0	0.0	2	0.1	0.6	0.1	0.1
ROSEMARY								
Dried	***1 Tsp/1g***	***3***	***0.2***	***331***	***4.9***	***46.4***	***15.2***	***0.0***
Fresh	***1 Tsp/0.7g***	***1***	***0.0***	***99***	***1.4***	***13.5***	***4.4***	***0.0***
ROSTI								
Garlic & Mushroom, Finest, Tesco*	1 Serving/200g	346	19.6	173	5.7	15.4	9.8	1.7
Oven Baked, McCain*	1 Rosti/100g	194	9.3	194	2.6	25.0	9.3	2.3
Potato, Chicken & Sweetcorn Bake, Asda*	1 Serving/400g	440	18.8	110	7.0	10.0	4.7	0.6
Potato, McCain*	1 Rosti/95g	161	8.6	169	2.2	19.6	9.1	0.0
Potato, Mini, Party Bites, Sainsbury's*	1 Serving/100g	218	11.5	218	2.5	26.2	11.5	3.0
Potato, Onion & Gruyere, Finest, Tesco*	½ Pack/200g	206	10.6	103	3.2	10.5	5.3	2.0
Potato, Spinach & Mozzarella, Tesco*	1 Serving/140g	228	7.7	163	3.8	24.5	5.5	2.0
Potato & Leek, Sainsbury's*	½ Pack/190g	296	20.9	156	4.5	9.8	11.0	0.3
Potato & Root Vegetable, COU, M & S*	1 Rosti/100g	85	2.7	85	1.6	13.3	2.7	1.5
Potato Cakes, Baby, M & S*	1 Rosti/23g	40	1.5	175	3.5	25.1	6.7	1.6
Spinach & Mozzarella, Vegetarian, Tesco*	1 Rosti/140g	245	13.6	175	4.8	17.0	9.7	2.3
Vegetable, Waitrose*	1 Pack/400g	248	9.2	62	1.4	8.8	2.3	1.3
ROULADE								
Chocolate, Finest, Tesco*	1 Serving/80g	222	4.5	277	3.4	53.2	5.6	2.3
Chocolate, Sainsbury's*	1 Serving/72g	264	15.7	367	5.7	36.9	21.8	1.8
Lemon, Asda*	1 Serving/100g	343	12.0	343	2.7	56.0	12.0	0.0
Mini, M & S*	1 Serving/63g	201	19.1	321	8.5	3.0	30.5	0.0
Orange & Lemon Meringue, Co-Op*	1 Serving/82g	287	9.8	350	3.0	57.0	12.0	0.3
Passion Fruit, M & S*	1oz/28g	83	2.6	295	2.8	50.0	9.2	0.2
Raspberry, M & S*	1oz/28g	88	3.1	315	3.3	50.3	11.0	0.1
Salmon, Smoked, & Asparagus, Sainsbury's*	1 Serving/60g	122	9.6	204	13.0	2.2	16.0	0.3
Salmon, Smoked, & Spinach, Finest, Tesco*	1 Serving/60g	91	6.1	152	11.5	3.6	10.2	0.6
Toffee, M & S*	1oz/28g	104	4.1	371	4.1	56.0	14.5	0.3
Toffee Pecan, Finest, Tesco*	1 Serving/60g	218	8.9	363	3.6	53.8	14.8	0.5
RUM								
37.5% Volume	***1 Shot/35ml***	***72***	***0.0***	***207***	***0.0***	***0.0***	***0.0***	***0.0***
40% Volume	***1 Shot/35ml***	***78***	***0.0***	***222***	***0.0***	***0.0***	***0.0***	***0.0***
Malibu, 21% Volume, Pernod Ricard*	***1 Shot/35ml***	***70***	***0.0***	***200***	***0.0***	***29.0***	***0.0***	***0.0***
White	***1 Shot/35ml***	***72***	***0.0***	***207***	***0.0***	***0.0***	***0.0***	***0.0***
RUSKS								
Banana, Farleys*	1 Serving/17g	70	1.5	409	7.3	75.1	8.8	2.9
Mini, Farleys*	1 Serving/30g	122	2.2	405	7.0	77.7	7.3	2.1
Original, Farleys*	1 Rusk/17g	69	1.2	406	7.1	77.6	7.1	2.4

	Measure INFO/WEIGHT	per Measure KCAL	FAT	Nutrition Values per 100g / 100ml KCAL	PROT	CARB	FAT	FIBRE
SAAG								
Aloo, Canned, Tesco*	½ Can/200g	124	3.8	62	1.8	9.3	1.9	2.0
Aloo, Fresh, Sainsbury's*	1 Pack/400g	388	13.2	97	2.0	14.7	3.3	4.8
Aloo, Jar, Sainsbury's*	½ Jar/135g	122	5.8	90	1.6	11.0	4.3	1.7
Aloo, North Indian, Sainsbury's*	1 Pack/300g	354	24.0	118	2.4	9.0	8.0	1.6
Aloo, Packet, Sainsbury's*	½ Pack/150g	184	12.4	123	2.1	9.9	8.3	2.7
Aloo, Sainsbury's*	1 Pack/300g	441	31.8	147	2.1	10.7	10.6	3.5
Aloo Gobi, M Kitchen, Morrisons*	1 Pack/225g	130	6.1	58	2.0	4.6	2.7	3.8
Aloo Gobi, Waitrose*	½ Pack/150	147	7.5	98	2.1	9.0	5.0	3.9
Chicken, Masala, Sainsbury's*	1oz/28g	36	2.0	127	13.2	2.4	7.2	2.3
Chicken, Masala, Waitrose*	1 Pack/400g	452	20.9	113	11.7	3.8	5.2	1.8
Gobi Aloo, Indian Takeaway, Sainsbury's*	1 Pack/334g	164	3.7	49	1.7	8.0	1.1	1.5
Gobi Aloo, M & S*	1 Pack/225g	270	19.1	120	1.9	9.3	8.5	2.4
Gobi Aloo, Tesco*	1 Serving/175g	166	8.9	95	2.1	9.5	5.1	1.9
Paneer, Sainsbury's*	1 Pack/300g	441	32.7	147	7.1	3.9	10.9	2.5
SAFFRON								
Average	***1 Tsp/1g***	***2***	***0.0***	***310***	***11.4***	***61.5***	***5.9***	***0.0***
SAGE								
Dried, Ground	***1 Tsp/1g***	***3***	***0.1***	***315***	***10.6***	***42.7***	***12.7***	***0.0***
Fresh	***1oz/28g***	***33***	***1.3***	***119***	***3.9***	***15.6***	***4.6***	***0.0***
SAGO								
Raw	***1oz/28g***	***99***	***0.1***	***355***	***0.2***	***94.0***	***0.2***	***0.5***
SALAD								
3 Bean, Sainsbury's*	1 Tub/270g	281	6.2	104	7.1	13.6	2.3	5.9
5 Bean & Mint, Asda*	1 Pack/340g	408	12.9	120	6.2	12.7	3.8	5.3
Alfresco Style, Tesco*	1 Serving/200g	40	0.6	20	0.9	3.3	0.3	2.1
All Seasons, Sainsbury's*	1oz/28g	3	0.1	12	1.0	1.5	0.2	1.2
American Ranch, Asda*	1 Serving/220g	253	19.8	115	2.5	6.0	9.0	2.0
American Style, Sweet & Crispy, Morrisons*	1 Serving/25g	7	0.1	28	1.2	4.2	0.3	2.0
Aromatic Herb, Waitrose*	¼ Pack/27g	4	0.1	15	0.9	1.7	0.5	1.0
Assorted, Asda*	1 Serving/100g	22	0.6	22	2.4	1.7	0.6	0.0
Avocado & Feta, Gourmet To Go, M & S*	1 Pack/320g	512	32.0	160	5.4	12.1	10.0	3.1
Baby Leaf, & Beetroot, Bistro, M & S*	1 Pack/165g	41	0.0	25	2.0	3.6	0.0	2.0
Baby Leaf, & Herb, Asda*	1 Serving/50g	7	0.1	14	2.3	0.7	0.2	2.4
Baby Leaf, Florette*	1 Serving/40g	5	0.1	12	2.0	0.4	0.3	1.0
Baby Leaf, Italian Style, M & S*	1 Serving/55g	11	0.3	20	1.3	2.3	0.5	1.3
Baby Leaf, Mild, Seasonal, Tesco*	½ Pack/42g	9	0.3	21	1.5	1.6	0.6	1.8
Baby Leaf, Organic, Sainsbury's*	1 Serving/20g	3	0.1	14	1.5	1.4	0.3	1.1
Baby Leaf, with Purple Basil, Finest, Tesco*	½ Pack/43g	7	0.1	17	2.9	0.9	0.2	1.8
Baby Leaf, with Watercress, Tesco*	1 Serving/30g	6	0.2	19	1.8	1.3	0.7	1.8
Bean, Mexican, Sainsbury's*	1 Pot/260g	291	8.1	112	5.2	12.9	3.1	5.8
Bean, Retail	1oz/28g	41	2.6	147	4.2	12.8	9.3	3.0
Bean, Spicy, Tesco*	1 Serving/125g	111	2.9	89	4.9	12.1	2.3	2.5
Bean & Cheese, Mexican Style, M & S*	½ Pot/150g	150	5.2	100	6.1	11.2	3.5	4.8
Bean & Chorizo, Tapas Selection, Sainsbury's*	1 Serving/22g	29	1.4	132	8.1	10.7	6.3	1.9
Bean & Sweetcorn, Side, M & S*	1 Serving/125g	131	9.0	105	2.5	7.0	7.2	1.3
Beetroot	1oz/28g	28	1.9	100	2.0	8.4	6.8	1.7
Beetroot, 1% Fat, M & S*	1 Serving/225g	130	6.1	58	1.1	7.7	2.7	1.7
Beetroot, Cous Cous & Quinoa, Tesco*	1 Serving/100g	70	0.6	70	2.3	12.9	0.6	2.3
Beetroot, Freshly Prepared, Tesco*	1 Pack/240g	58	0.7	24	1.9	3.3	0.3	2.7
Beetroot, Roast with Quinoa & Feta, Tesco*	1 Pack/400g	452	19.6	113	4.8	12.4	4.9	2.3
Beetroot & Carrot, Continental, Iceland*	1 Serving/100g	24	0.2	24	1.2	4.3	0.2	2.1
Beetroot & Cherry Tomato, & Lemon Dressing, M & S*	1 Pack/215g	129	8.2	60	1.3	5.2	3.8	1.5
Beetroot & Lettuce, Asda*	1 Serving/30g	5	0.0	16	1.4	2.7	0.0	2.5

S

	Measure INFO/WEIGHT	per Measure KCAL	FAT	Nutrition Values per 100g / 100ml KCAL	PROT	CARB	FAT	FIBRE
SALAD								
Bistro, Sainsbury's*	1 Pack/150g	26	0.3	17	1.9	2.0	0.2	2.0
Black Bean Salsa, Salad Bar, Waitrose*	1 Serving/100g	118	5.8	118	0.0	0.0	5.8	0.0
Black Olive, Tomato & Red Onion, Shapers, Boots*	1 Pack/80g	68	5.0	85	0.0	0.0	6.2	0.0
Bulgar Wheat, Lentil & Edamame Shaker, Waitrose*	1 Pack/190g	217	10.6	114	4.7	11.1	5.6	4.4
Bulgar Wheat & Carrot, Sainsbury's*	½ Pot/125g	167	6.7	134	2.8	16.1	5.4	4.8
Butternut Squash, Roast, & Fennel, TTD, Sainsbury's*	1 Pack/165g	214	7.6	130	3.4	15.2	4.6	6.9
Cabbage, Beetroot & Carrot, Mix, Florette*	½ Pack/100g	30	0.2	30	1.3	4.4	0.2	0.0
Cabbage & Leek, Crunchy Mix, Sainsbury's*	½ Pack/126g	24	0.8	19	1.2	2.1	0.6	1.9
Caesar	1 Serving/200g	352	27.8	176	4.8	8.1	13.9	0.7
Caesar, & New Potatoes with Asparagus, M & S*	1 Pack/200g	270	15.2	135	3.1	13.8	7.6	1.7
Caesar, Bacon, M & S*	1oz/28g	48	3.9	170	5.5	5.7	14.0	1.2
Caesar, Bacon, Sainsbury's*	1 Pack/256g	415	32.5	162	4.7	12.0	12.7	1.4
Caesar, Chicken, Asda*	1 Pack/273g	535	43.7	196	10.0	3.0	16.0	1.9
Caesar, Chicken, Bistro, M & S*	½ Pack/135g	189	14.3	140	5.0	6.5	10.6	0.6
Caesar, Chicken, Eat Well, M & S*	1 Pack/397g	595	24.6	150	9.9	18.7	6.2	2.1
Caesar, Chicken, Fresh, Sainsbury's*	1 Serving/200g	278	20.0	139	6.0	6.2	10.0	1.2
Caesar, Chicken, M & S*	½ Pack/140g	266	20.0	190	6.7	8.7	14.3	0.8
Caesar, Chicken, Shapers, Boots*	1 Pack/200g	205	5.8	102	8.2	10.0	2.9	1.0
Caesar, Chicken & Bacon, Gourmet, M & S*	1 Salad/250g	550	43.5	220	9.0	7.3	17.4	0.7
Caesar, Chicken & Bacon, Tesco*	1 Pack/200g	506	40.2	253	6.6	11.4	20.1	1.0
Caesar, Classic, Reduced Fat, M & S*	1 Serving/115g	132	5.6	115	4.8	12.7	4.9	0.5
Caesar, Florette*	1 Serving/100g	163	12.4	163	2.7	10.2	12.4	1.8
Caesar, GFY, Asda*	½ Pack/87g	76	2.6	87	8.0	7.0	3.0	1.5
Caesar, with Dressing, Croutons & Parmesan, M & S*	1 Serving/115g	190	15.5	165	4.3	6.4	13.5	1.4
Caesar, with Parmigiano Reggiano, Tesco*	1 Bag/275g	552	49.0	201	4.1	5.8	17.8	1.3
Caesar, with Romaine Lettuce, Kit, BGTY, Sainsbury's*	½ Pack/130g	139	7.9	107	3.7	9.2	6.1	1.4
Cannellini Bean & Chicken, M & S*	1 Serving/225g	250	14.7	111	5.9	7.4	6.5	3.1
Cannellini Bean & Chorizo, Sainsbury's*	1 Pack/250g	228	8.0	91	5.3	10.2	3.2	1.6
Cannellini Bean & Tuna, M & S*	1 Serving/255g	215	11.6	84	5.3	5.4	4.5	2.1
Caponata, Organic, Florentin*	1 Serving/100g	111	12.3	111	1.5	3.7	12.3	0.0
Carrot, Courgette & Coriander, Salad Bar, Waitrose*	1 Serving/100g	92	7.9	92	0.0	0.0	7.9	0.0
Carrot, M & S*	1 Pack/215g	280	7.3	130	3.1	22.4	3.4	2.7
Carrot, Peanut & Sultana, Asda*	1 Serving/20g	54	4.0	272	8.0	15.0	20.0	4.5
Carrot, with Fresh Coriander Vinaigrette, M & S*	½ Pack/105g	126	3.6	120	3.7	19.1	3.4	6.5
Carrot & Beetroot, with a Balsamic Dressing, Asda*	1 Pack/160g	101	6.6	63	0.9	5.6	4.1	1.0
Carrot & Sultana, BGTY, Sainsbury's*	½ Pack/100g	55	0.3	55	0.6	12.4	0.3	0.0
Celery, Nut & Sultana, Waitrose*	1oz/28g	54	4.6	192	2.8	8.4	16.4	1.0
Celery & Apple, Salad Bar, Waitrose*	1 Serving/100g	136	12.9	136	0.0	0.0	12.9	0.0
Cheese, HL, Tesco*	1 Serving/30g	32	0.9	107	18.0	2.0	3.0	0.0
Cheese, Layered, M & S*	½ Pack/230g	300	20.5	130	4.6	9.3	8.9	1.2
Cheese, Layered, Tesco*	1 Serving/225g	437	32.0	194	5.8	10.8	14.2	0.8
Cheese & Coleslaw, Tesco*	1 Serving/125g	135	10.9	108	3.4	3.4	8.7	1.1
Cherry Tomato, All Good Things*	1 Pack/185g	31	0.6	17	0.8	2.8	0.3	1.4
Cherry Tomato, Salad bar, Waitrose*	1 Serving/100g	77	5.3	77	0.0	0.0	5.3	0.0
Cherry Tomato, Tesco*	1 Pack/210g	136	9.4	65	0.9	4.2	4.5	1.1
Chick Pea & Cous Cous, Tesco*	1 Serving/250g	245	6.5	98	3.2	15.5	2.6	0.0
Chick Pea & Spinach, M & S*	1 Serving/260g	299	10.7	115	7.3	12.5	4.1	2.7
Chick Pea & Sweet Potato, Salad Bar, Sainsbury's*	1 Serving/100g	99	1.9	99	0.0	9.6	1.9	0.0
Chicken, & Cous Cous, Moroccan, Tesco*	1 Pack/210g	252	4.2	120	7.8	16.9	2.0	3.5
Chicken, Avocado & Bacon, M & S*	1 Serving/235g	235	13.6	100	8.5	2.8	5.8	2.8
Chicken, Chargrilled, & Pesto, Sainsbury's*	1 Pack/250g	375	15.2	150	7.9	15.8	6.1	1.3
Chicken, Chargrilled, & Quinoa, Shapers, Boots*	1 Pack/185g	139	1.8	75	6.2	10.0	1.0	1.8
Chicken, Chargrilled, Tesco*	1 Serving/300g	384	14.4	128	6.1	15.0	4.8	2.4

S

	Measure INFO/WEIGHT	per Measure KCAL	FAT	Nutrition Values per 100g / 100ml KCAL	PROT	CARB	FAT	FIBRE
SALAD								
Chicken, Chargrilled, Weight Watchers*	1 Pack/182g	265	3.8	146	11.7	20.0	2.1	2.2
Chicken, Chargrilled, Wholefood, M & S*	1 Pot/219g	230	4.2	105	10.1	11.6	1.9	4.8
Chicken, Italian Style, Snack Pot, Carb Check, Heinz*	1 Pot/218g	131	4.4	60	5.9	4.3	2.0	1.0
Chicken, Layered, Roast, HL, Tesco*	1 Salad/400g	268	4.4	67	5.8	8.4	1.1	2.1
Chicken, Roast, & Coleslaw, Boots*	1 Serving/245g	392	34.3	160	4.5	3.9	14.0	1.3
Chicken, Roast, 93 Cals, Shapers, Boots*	1 Pack/233g	93	0.9	40	8.6	0.6	0.4	1.8
Chicken, Roast, Tesco*	1 Salad/300g	348	22.2	116	5.3	7.0	7.4	1.0
Chicken, Sweet Chilli, BGTY, Sainsbury's*	1 Serving/200g	206	0.8	103	6.0	18.7	0.4	0.0
Chicken, Tesco*	1 Serving/300g	348	22.2	116	5.3	7.0	7.4	1.0
Chicken, Tomato Chilli, & Rice, COU, M & S*	1 Pack/340g	357	5.1	105	6.8	16.0	1.5	0.9
Chicken, with Mayonnaise, Waitrose*	1 Pack/208g	406	19.8	195	10.3	17.1	9.5	2.5
Chicken, with Tomato & Basil Cous Cous, Tesco*	1 Pack/200g	270	4.2	135	8.3	19.7	2.1	1.5
Chicken & Bacon, Asda*	1 Pack/381g	480	22.9	126	7.0	11.0	6.0	0.0
Chicken & Bacon, Carb Control, Tesco*	1 Serving/188g	244	14.7	130	13.2	1.7	7.8	0.5
Chicken & Bacon, Chargrilled, Gourmet, Atkins*	1 Pack/245g	311	20.1	127	12.0	2.5	8.2	1.0
Chicken & Bacon, Layered, Waitrose*	1 Serving/200g	246	14.8	123	6.7	7.4	7.4	2.1
Chicken & Bacon, Ranch, Sainsbury's*	1 Pack/210g	315	15.8	150	8.4	12.1	7.5	0.9
Chicken & Feta, Mediterranean Style, Shapers, Boots*	1 Pack/240g	143	6.1	59	5.9	3.1	2.5	0.0
Classic, Co-Op*	½ Pack/80g	16	0.2	20	0.8	2.9	0.3	2.2
Classic, with Chive Dressing, M & S*	½ Pack/138g	76	5.8	55	0.9	3.3	4.2	1.6
Classic, with Green Herb Dressing, Co-Op*	1 Serving/90g	86	8.1	95	1.0	2.0	9.0	1.0
Coleslaw, Classics, M & S*	1 Pot/190g	124	4.4	65	1.9	8.8	2.3	1.3
Coleslaw, Layered, Fresh Tastes, Asda*	1oz/28g	17	1.3	59	1.1	3.4	4.5	1.6
Coleslaw & Potato, 3% Fat, M & S*	1oz/28g	20	1.0	72	2.7	7.7	3.4	1.5
Continental, Co-Op*	1 Serving/80g	12	0.3	15	1.0	2.0	0.4	1.0
Continental, Four Leaf, Sainsbury's*	½ Pack/100g	13	0.2	13	1.2	1.7	0.2	1.9
Coronation Chicken, Salad Bar, Asda*	1oz/28g	82	6.4	293	5.7	16.4	22.7	0.7
Coronation Chicken & Rice, Asda*	1oz/28g	67	4.8	241	6.7	15.2	17.0	0.4
Coronation Rice, Tesco*	1 Serving/50g	104	7.6	207	2.0	15.9	15.1	0.8
Cosmopolitan, Fresh, Sainsbury's*	1 Bag/135g	20	0.5	15	1.2	1.6	0.4	1.9
Cous Cous, & Roast Vegetable, GFY, Asda*	1 Serving/100g	120	1.6	120	3.5	23.0	1.6	2.7
Cous Cous, & Roasted Vegetable, Waitrose*	1 Pack/220g	396	13.4	180	5.1	26.1	6.1	1.2
Cous Cous, BGTY, Sainsbury's*	1 Pot/200g	236	4.4	118	4.7	19.7	2.2	2.8
Cous Cous, Lemon, & Roasted Pepper, COU, M & S*	1 Pack/340g	306	7.8	90	3.2	14.6	2.3	1.8
Cous Cous, Tesco*	1 Serving/25g	35	0.4	141	4.8	26.9	1.6	0.6
Cous Cous, Waitrose*	1 Pot/200g	344	10.0	172	4.9	26.9	5.0	1.4
Crisp, Mixed, Morrisons*	1 Pack/230g	39	0.7	17	1.0	2.8	0.3	0.0
Crisp & Crunchy, Asda*	1 Pack/250g	55	1.5	22	0.8	3.3	0.6	1.4
Crisp & Crunchy, with French Dressing, GFY, Asda*	1/3 Pack/116g	26	0.7	22	0.8	3.3	0.6	1.4
Crisp & Light, M & S*	1 Serving/170g	51	1.4	30	0.5	5.4	0.8	1.0
Crisp & Sweet, Lettuce Leaves, Florette*	¼ Pack/70g	10	0.4	14	0.8	1.7	0.5	0.9
Crispy, Florette*	1 Portion/100g	22	0.3	22	1.5	3.4	0.3	3.0
Crispy Crunch, Lasting Leaf*	1 Serving/75g	14	0.3	18	1.1	1.5	0.4	1.9
Crunchy, Layered, Tesco*	1 Serving/54g	15	0.2	27	1.1	4.9	0.3	1.7
Crunchy, Mix, Co-Op*	1 Bag/200g	20	0.4	10	0.9	1.7	0.2	1.5
Crunchy, Oriental Slaw, Salad bar, Waitrose*	1 Serving/100g	68	2.8	68	0.0	0.0	2.8	0.0
Crunchy, Simple, M & S*	1 Serving/50g	8	0.2	15	1.0	1.6	0.5	1.8
Crunchy, Spring, Side, M & S*	1 Serving/160g	32	0.3	20	0.9	4.1	0.2	1.3
Cucumber, & Cherry Tomato, Fresh Tastes, Asda*	1 Serving/100g	22	0.3	22	1.6	2.4	0.3	0.0
Eat Me Keep Me, Tesco*	1 Serving/80g	14	0.2	18	0.8	3.0	0.3	1.7
Edamame & Butterbean, TTD, Sainsbury's*	1/3 Pack/62g	70	2.5	113	6.6	9.9	4.1	4.9
Edamame Bean, Oriental Style, Asda*	1 Pack/220g	183	8.4	83	4.8	7.3	3.8	4.0
Edamame Beans, & Peppers, Delicious, Boots*	1 Pack/87g	121	2.3	139	0.0	4.1	2.6	0.0

S

	Measure INFO/WEIGHT	per Measure KCAL	FAT	Nutrition Values per 100g / 100ml KCAL	PROT	CARB	FAT	FIBRE
SALAD								
Egg, Fresh4you*	1 Pack/55g	139	12.2	252	8.3	4.6	22.2	0.0
Egg & Baby Spinach, Waitrose*	1 Pack/215g	167	13.5	78	3.5	1.8	6.3	1.0
Egg & Coleslaw, Boots*	1 Pot/233g	405	37.3	174	3.0	4.6	16.0	1.0
Egg & Ham, with Salad Cream Dressing, M & S*	1 Pack/240g	145	7.2	60	4.9	3.2	3.0	1.2
Egg & Potato, Fresh, M & S*	1 Serving/250g	150	7.2	60	3.0	4.6	2.9	0.9
English Garden, Tesco*	1 Serving/180g	22	0.4	12	0.7	1.8	0.2	0.7
Fajita, Chicken, Shapers, Boots*	1 Pack/258g	181	3.4	70	7.0	7.4	1.3	2.7
Feta Cheese & Sunblushed Tomato, M & S*	1 Serving/190g	361	21.1	190	5.5	17.2	11.1	2.1
Fine Cut, Asda*	1oz/28g	7	0.1	24	1.2	4.1	0.3	2.1
Florida, Retail, Average	1oz/28g	63	5.7	224	0.9	9.7	20.5	1.0
Four Bean, Finest, Tesco*	1 Pack/225g	259	9.4	115	5.0	14.2	4.2	4.6
Four Bean, Sainsbury's*	½ Pot/113g	114	2.5	101	6.7	6.2	2.2	15.0
Four Bean & Buckwheat, Waitrose*	1 Pack/220g	319	14.5	145	5.3	16.0	6.6	6.1
Four Leaf, M & S*	1 Serving/130g	20	0.4	15	0.9	2.0	0.3	1.4
French Goat's Cheese, Extra Fine, Asda*	1 Pack/185g	462	35.2	250	8.4	11.4	19.0	0.8
French Style, M & S*	1 Pack/140g	140	13.6	100	1.0	2.5	9.7	0.9
Fresh & Crispy, Tesco*	1 Serving/230g	30	0.7	13	0.7	1.9	0.3	1.3
Fruity Moroccan Cous Cous, Waitrose*	1 Pack/90g	139	3.2	154	5.0	25.6	3.6	4.6
Fruity Tabbouleh, Salad Bar, Waitrose*	1 Serving/100g	184	6.6	184	0.0	0.0	6.6	0.0
Fusion, Fully Prepared, Sainsbury's*	½ Pack/63g	15	0.5	24	3.7	0.3	0.8	3.4
Garden, Classic, Morrisons*	1 Tray/175g	33	0.5	19	0.8	3.2	0.3	2.8
Garden, Side, Asda*	1 Pack/175g	32	0.5	18	0.9	2.8	0.3	1.3
Garden, Sweet & Crispy, Tesco*	1 Bag/225g	54	0.9	24	1.0	4.2	0.4	1.4
Garden, Tray, Asda*	½ Pack/88g	16	0.3	18	0.7	3.1	0.3	1.6
Garden, with Watercress, M & S*	1 Salad/80g	10	0.1	12	1.5	1.4	0.1	1.4
Garden, with Yoghurt & Mint Dressing, GFY, Asda*	1 Serving/195g	51	2.0	26	1.1	3.2	1.0	0.0
Goat's Cheese, & Cous Cous, Waitrose*	1 Pack/300g	372	14.4	124	4.8	15.3	4.8	2.2
Goat's Cheese, Sainsbury's*	1 Pack/192g	242	12.9	126	5.0	10.6	6.7	1.7
Gourmet Continental, Waitrose*	1 Serving/150g	22	0.8	15	0.8	1.7	0.5	0.9
Greek	1oz/28g	36	3.5	130	2.7	1.9	12.5	0.8
Greek, BGTY, Sainsbury's*	1 Serving/199g	133	5.0	67	2.0	9.0	2.5	0.8
Greek, Classic, Tesco*	1 Pack/255g	293	23.7	115	2.6	5.2	9.3	1.2
Greek, Complete, Hot, Sainsbury's*	1 Pack/299g	287	22.4	96	4.3	2.9	7.5	1.7
Greek, Salad Bar, Waitrose*	1 Serving/100g	103	7.8	103	0.0	0.0	7.8	0.0
Greek, with Basil & Mint Oil Dressing, M & S*	1 Pack/200g	220	19.6	110	3.6	2.2	9.8	1.5
Greek Feta & Pepper, with Cous Cous, Asda*	1 Pack/316g	262	10.4	83	3.2	10.2	3.3	0.0
Greek Style, Delphi*	1 Serving/220g	306	27.1	139	3.7	3.5	12.3	0.9
Greek Style, Fresh, Food Counter, Sainsbury's*	1 Serving/166g	247	23.2	149	1.9	2.7	14.0	0.0
Greek Style, Layered, Perfectly Balanced, Waitrose*	1 Pack/280g	134	7.8	48	2.4	3.2	2.8	0.7
Greek Style, Waitrose*	½ Pack/125g	54	2.8	43	1.9	4.0	2.2	1.2
Greek Style, with Herb Dressing, Tesco*	1 Pack/240g	305	28.3	127	3.2	2.0	11.8	1.0
Greek Style, with Houmous Dip & Pitta, Sainsbury's*	1 Bowl/195g	296	17.4	152	5.4	12.5	8.9	2.6
Greek Style, with White Wine Vinaigrette, Tesco*	1 Pack/235g	256	22.3	109	3.5	2.3	9.5	1.5
Greek Style Feta, Tip & Mix, M & S*	1 Pack/195g	214	18.3	110	4.0	2.5	9.4	1.6
Green, Average	1oz/28g	4	0.1	13	0.8	1.8	0.3	0.9
Green, Mixed, Average	1 Serving/100g	12	0.3	12	0.7	1.8	0.3	1.0
Green, with Chives, Tesco*	½ Pack/90g	13	0.4	14	1.0	1.6	0.4	1.7
Green, with Honey & Mustard Dressing, M & S*	1 Pack/200g	120	9.6	60	0.9	2.7	4.8	0.8
Green Butterhead & Peppercress, Duo, Florette*	1 Portion/30g	7	0.1	23	2.3	1.3	0.3	2.0
Green Lentil, Red Pepper & Spinach, Waitrose*	1 Pack/250g	485	20.0	194	8.6	22.0	8.0	2.9
Green Side, M & S*	1 Serving/200g	30	0.4	15	0.9	2.5	0.2	0.0
Ham & Egg, Free Range, British, M & S*	1 Pack/280g	182	6.4	65	6.1	5.3	2.3	1.0
Ham & Egg, Free Range, Fresh Tastes, Asda*	1 Bowl/265g	167	9.3	63	5.7	2.2	3.5	0.8

S

	Measure INFO/WEIGHT	per Measure KCAL	FAT	Nutrition Values per 100g / 100ml KCAL	PROT	CARB	FAT	FIBRE
SALAD								
Ham Hock, Waitrose*	1 Pack/350g	245	9.5	70	6.6	4.8	2.7	2.0
Herb, Asda*	1 Serving/20g	2	0.1	12	1.8	0.6	0.3	2.0
Herb, M & S*	1 Pack/100g	20	0.4	20	2.9	1.4	0.4	1.9
Herb, Sainsbury's*	1 Pack/120g	22	0.6	18	2.7	0.8	0.5	2.2
Herb, Tesco*	1oz/28g	4	0.1	16	1.1	1.8	0.5	0.9
Houmous, Delicious, Boots*	1 Pack/230g	154	4.4	67	5.3	7.4	1.9	3.1
Iceberg & Cabbage, Asda*	½ Pack/125g	24	0.4	19	1.0	3.1	0.3	1.5
Italian, Complete, Sainsbury's*	1 Pack/160g	237	14.4	148	5.4	11.4	9.0	1.6
Italian Style, Asda*	1 Serving/20g	3	0.1	15	1.1	1.6	0.5	1.2
Italian Style, Organic, Waitrose*	½ Pack/45g	7	0.2	15	0.8	1.7	0.5	0.9
Italian Style, with Rocket & Lambs Lettuce, M & S*	½ Bag/60g	12	0.3	20	1.3	2.3	0.5	1.3
Jardin, Tesco*	1 Serving/50g	7	0.3	14	0.8	1.8	0.6	1.4
King Prawn, & New Potato, COU, M & S*	1 Pack/300g	180	6.9	60	3.0	6.9	2.3	0.8
King Prawn, & Pasta, COU, M & S*	1 Pack/270g	284	6.5	105	5.9	15.1	2.4	2.7
King Prawn, GFY, Asda*	1 Serving/175g	112	2.6	64	4.7	8.0	1.5	1.3
King Prawn, Thai Style, M & S*	1 Pack/295g	266	7.4	90	4.4	12.6	2.5	1.3
Lambs Lettuce & Ruby Chard, Duo, Florette*	1 Serving/35g	7	0.1	21	2.0	1.0	0.4	2.9
Leaf, Crispy, Asda*	1 Serving/80g	11	0.4	14	0.8	1.6	0.5	0.9
Leafy, Organic, Sainsbury's*	½ Pack/50g	8	0.2	15	1.7	1.3	0.3	1.8
Leafy, Tesco*	1oz/28g	4	0.1	14	1.2	1.5	0.4	1.9
Leafy, with Tatsoi, Sainsbury's*	1 Bag/115g	17	0.4	15	1.0	1.6	0.3	1.7
Leaves, Oriental Mix, Waitrose*	1 Bag/100g	18	0.6	18	1.5	1.7	0.6	1.9
Lovely Summer, Jamie Oliver*	½ Bag/60g	48	4.0	80	1.7	4.0	6.6	1.2
Mediterranean, Side, Sainsbury's*	1 Pack/170g	44	2.2	26	0.9	2.7	1.3	1.3
Mediterranean Style, Asda*	½ Pack/135g	22	0.0	16	1.0	3.0	0.0	0.0
Mediterranean Style, Tray, Morrisons*	1 Tray/100g	26	0.3	26	1.2	3.6	0.3	1.8
Mixed, Crisp, Mild, Tesco*	½ Pack/145g	29	0.4	20	1.2	3.0	0.3	2.1
Mixed, Florette*	1 Serving/100g	20	0.2	20	1.3	3.4	0.2	3.0
Mixed, Green Leaf, Lasting Leaf*	1 Serving/69g	12	0.3	17	0.8	1.8	0.4	1.5
Mixed, Iceland*	1 Serving/50g	12	0.1	24	1.2	4.3	0.2	2.1
Mixed, Sainsbury's*	1 Serving/100g	21	0.2	21	1.4	3.4	0.2	2.1
Mixed, Sweet & Crispy, Tesco*	1 Serving/200g	48	0.6	24	1.0	4.2	0.3	2.0
Mixed, Sweet & Crunchy, Lasting Leaf*	1 Serving/62g	15	0.2	24	0.8	3.6	0.3	1.9
Mixed Bean, Asda*	½ Can/145g	126	3.6	87	5.0	11.0	2.5	6.0
Mixed Bean, Canned, Sainsbury's*	1 Can/270g	227	2.4	84	5.4	13.5	0.9	3.8
Mixed Bean, Tesco*	1 Serving/70g	49	0.4	70	3.2	13.1	0.5	1.9
Mixed Leaf, Asda*	1 Serving/100g	21	0.2	21	1.5	3.2	0.2	2.1
Mixed Leaf, Medley, Waitrose*	1 Serving/25g	4	0.1	15	0.8	1.7	0.5	1.4
Mixed Leaf, Tomato, Feta, Boots*	1 Pack/179g	218	17.0	122	3.7	5.4	9.5	1.0
Mixed Leaf, Tomato & Olive, Tesco*	1 Serving/170g	150	13.3	88	1.0	3.4	7.8	2.0
Mixed Leaves, Bondelle*	1 Serving/50g	10	0.1	21	1.4	3.3	0.2	0.0
Mixed Leaves, Tesco*	1 Serving/20g	3	0.1	14	0.9	1.6	0.4	0.9
Mixed Leaves, with Beetroot, Earthy, Waitrose*	1 Bag/140g	34	0.6	24	1.5	3.6	0.4	2.1
Mixed Pepper, Asda*	½ Pack/100g	24	0.3	24	1.0	4.3	0.3	1.7
Mixed Vegetable, Aldi*	1 Serving/200g	120	4.0	60	0.6	10.0	2.0	0.0
Mozzarella & Cherry Tomato, Shapers, Boots*	1 Bowl/194g	184	14.2	95	4.1	3.3	7.3	0.9
Mozzarella & Rocket, Asda*	1 Serving/265g	435	31.8	164	7.0	7.0	12.0	1.5
Mozzarella & Sunkissed Tomato, Tesco*	1 Bag/160g	270	22.9	169	4.6	4.3	14.3	2.1
Mozzarella & Tomato, M & S*	1 Serving/310g	400	14.8	129	5.5	15.5	4.8	0.9
Mozzarella & Tomato, no Dressing	1 Serving/105g	190	14.5	182	8.0	5.9	13.8	3.3
New Potato, Co-Op*	1 Serving/50g	98	8.0	195	1.0	10.0	16.0	2.0
New Potato, Less Than 5% Fat, M & S*	1 Serving/110g	88	3.4	80	1.3	12.1	3.1	1.5
New Potato, M & S*	1 Serving/60g	114	9.8	190	0.9	9.9	16.3	1.3

	Measure INFO/WEIGHT	per Measure KCAL	per Measure FAT	Nutrition Values per 100g / 100ml KCAL	PROT	CARB	FAT	FIBRE
SALAD								
New Potato, Tomato & Egg with Salad Cream, M & S*	1 Pack/300g	165	7.2	55	2.9	5.4	2.4	1.3
New Potato, Tuna & Egg, M & S*	1 Pack/340g	255	12.9	75	3.8	6.7	3.8	0.7
New Potato & Free Range Egg, M & S*	1 Pack/305g	214	11.6	70	2.5	7.0	3.8	0.8
New Potato & Free Range Egg, Side, Sainsbury's*	1 Pack/290g	174	12.2	60	2.5	3.1	4.2	1.4
New Potato & King Prawn, M & S*	1 Pack/210g	220	9.4	105	5.6	10.2	4.5	1.7
New Potato & Sweet Chilli Prawn, M & S*	1 Pack/210g	147	1.0	70	2.8	14.0	0.5	0.7
New Potato & Tuna Sweetcorn, Eat Well, M & S*	1 Pack/190g	133	3.4	70	5.4	8.4	1.8	1.9
Nicoise, Tesco*	1 Pack/260g	286	21.8	110	3.2	5.3	8.4	1.4
Nicoise Style, Layered, Waitrose*	1 Bowl/275g	129	3.8	47	2.7	5.8	1.4	1.0
Pancetta, Express, Pizza Express*	1 Salad/90g	200	17.9	223	7.4	3.3	20.0	0.0
Pea & Ham, M & S*	1 Pack/335g	420	13.8	125	7.1	12.6	4.1	4.7
Pea Shoots & Baby Leaves, Steve's Leaves*	1 Pack/60g	14	0.4	24	2.7	2.0	0.6	2.0
Pepper, Chargrilled, with Cous Cous, Asda*	1 Pack/325g	426	10.7	131	4.3	21.0	3.3	0.0
Pepper, Roast, Cous Cous, HL, Tesco*	1 Pot/220g	308	4.6	140	5.6	24.3	2.1	1.7
Pepper, Sweetcorn & Cucumber, Salad Bar, Waitrose*	1 Serving/100g	71	3.1	71	0.0	0.0	3.1	0.0
Ploughmans, Cheese, Asda*	1 Bowl/300g	246	10.8	82	3.6	8.9	3.6	1.0
Potato, 30% Less Fat, BGTY, Sainsbury's*	1 Serving/60g	64	3.7	106	1.7	11.1	6.1	1.1
Potato, Asda*	¼ Pot/57g	67	4.0	117	0.9	12.5	7.0	1.1
Potato, Creamy, Waitrose*	1 Serving/100g	163	11.9	163	1.3	12.7	11.9	1.1
Potato, Finest, Tesco*	1 Tub/250g	588	51.5	235	2.4	9.7	20.6	1.2
Potato, Heinz*	½ Can/97g	137	8.2	141	1.4	14.8	8.5	0.8
Potato, Iceland*	1 Serving/75g	162	14.7	216	1.1	8.9	19.6	0.6
Potato, Luxury, Asda*	1 Serving/50g	118	10.5	237	1.0	11.0	21.0	0.0
Potato, Perfectly Balanced, Waitrose*	½ Pot/125g	99	3.8	79	2.4	10.5	3.0	1.0
Potato, Reduced Calorie, Pre Packed	1oz/28g	27	1.1	97	1.3	14.8	4.1	0.8
Potato, Salad Bar, Asda*	1oz/28g	52	4.3	187	0.6	11.6	15.4	1.1
Potato, Side, Waitrose*	1 Pack/250g	181	11.0	72	3.0	5.2	4.4	1.0
Potato, Spiced, Salad Bar, Waitrose*	1 Serving/100g	88	2.0	88	0.0	0.0	2.0	0.0
Potato, Tesco*	1 Serving/100g	165	13.5	165	1.3	9.5	13.5	1.3
Potato, with Mayonnaise, Pre Packed	1oz/28g	67	5.8	239	1.6	12.2	20.8	0.9
Potato, with Onions & Chives, Co-Op*	1 Serving/50g	80	6.0	160	1.0	12.0	12.0	1.0
Potato & Cheese, Pasta & Mixed Leaf, Waitrose*	1 Serving/205g	266	17.4	130	3.2	10.1	8.5	1.1
Potato & Cheese, Sainsbury's*	1 Serving/125g	200	16.4	160	2.7	7.9	13.1	3.4
Potato & Egg, with Mayonnaise, Tesco*	½ Tub/150g	115	8.5	77	2.9	3.1	5.7	1.2
Prawn, King & Rice Noodle, M & S*	1 Pack/320g	208	2.6	65	2.9	11.6	0.8	0.9
Prawn, Layered, Asda*	1 Tub/380g	403	15.6	106	5.0	11.5	4.1	0.0
Prawn, Layered, Single Size, Asda*	1 Serving/197g	217	9.8	110	4.3	12.0	5.0	1.0
Prawn, Layered, Tesco*	1 Pack/180g	243	13.0	135	4.2	13.1	7.2	2.0
Prawn, Tesco*	1 Pack/280g	314	14.0	112	4.7	12.0	5.0	0.9
Prawn & Avocado, M & S*	1 Serving/220g	176	15.0	80	3.0	2.0	6.8	3.1
Prawn & Egg, Leaf, Shapers, Boots*	1 Pack/182g	193	14.4	106	6.7	2.1	7.9	1.0
Prawn Cocktail, Shapers, Boots*	1 Pack/245g	120	5.9	49	4.7	2.2	2.4	0.7
Prawn Cocktail, Tesco*	1 Pack/300g	360	18.0	120	5.7	10.9	6.0	0.8
Prawn Satay & Noodle, Tesco*	1 Serving/250g	320	17.0	128	7.1	9.5	6.8	1.2
Primavera, Finest, Tesco*	1 Pack/100g	25	0.6	25	2.4	2.4	0.6	2.6
Rainbow, Sainsbury's*	1 Pack/215g	300	14.8	140	5.5	13.8	6.9	3.9
Rice, Brown, Tossed*	1 Pack/200g	335	1.8	168	13.3	19.9	0.9	0.0
Rice, Courgette & Pine Nut, BGTY, Sainsbury's*	1/3 Pot/65g	68	1.0	105	2.7	20.0	1.6	1.5
Rice, Lentil & Mushroom, Salad Bar, Waitrose*	1 Serving/100g	135	5.4	135	0.0	0.0	5.4	0.0
Rocket, Leafy, Asda*	1 Serving/75g	10	0.1	13	1.5	1.4	0.1	1.8
Rocket, Tesco*	1oz/28g	4	0.1	14	0.8	1.7	0.5	0.9
Salmon, Honey Smoked, & New Potato, M & S*	1 Pack/270g	270	14.3	100	5.5	7.5	5.3	1.5
Salmon, Hot Smoked, with Potato Salad, M & S*	1 Pack/338g	270	7.4	80	4.5	10.3	2.2	1.3

S

	Measure INFO/WEIGHT	per Measure KCAL	FAT	Nutrition Values per 100g / 100ml KCAL	PROT	CARB	FAT	FIBRE
SALAD								
Salmon, Moroccan Style, Light Lunch, John West*	1 Pack/220g	299	11.7	136	11.7	8.8	5.3	3.4
Salmon & Roquette, M & S*	1 Serving/255g	306	20.4	120	3.9	8.5	8.0	1.0
Santini, Side, M & S*	1 Pack/195g	127	11.1	65	1.0	3.0	5.7	2.0
Seafood, Marinated, M & S*	1 Serving/90g	108	5.8	120	13.4	2.3	6.4	0.8
Seafood, Marinated, Waitrose*	1 Tub/160g	235	10.6	147	16.3	5.5	6.6	0.0
Seafood, Prawn & Calamari, Deli, M & S*	1 Pack/120g	132	6.1	110	14.7	1.2	5.1	0.8
Seafood, Sunkis*	1 Tub/100g	83	3.9	83	4.6	7.4	3.9	0.0
Selection, Fresh, M & S*	1 Pack/230g	32	0.7	14	0.7	2.1	0.3	0.9
Selection, Side, M & S*	1 Serving/255g	153	12.8	60	1.1	2.5	5.0	1.3
Spinach, Baby, & Red Mustard, M & S*	1 Pack/170g	264	26.7	155	1.7	1.1	15.7	0.1
Spinach, Rocket & Watercress, Asda*	1 Serving/100g	21	0.6	21	2.8	1.2	0.6	1.9
Spinach, Waitrose*	1 Pack/100g	25	0.8	25	2.8	1.6	0.8	2.1
Spring, American Style, M & S*	1 Serving/60g	9	0.1	15	1.9	1.4	0.2	1.3
Summer, M & S*	1oz/28g	6	0.1	20	0.8	3.6	0.4	1.2
Sweet, Layered, Tesco*	1 Serving/285g	80	1.1	28	1.1	5.0	0.4	1.6
Sweet, Shredded, Tesco*	1 Serving/100g	20	0.4	20	1.1	2.9	0.4	1.9
Sweet & Crispy, M & S*	1 Serving/140g	49	1.4	35	1.7	4.7	1.0	1.6
Sweet & Crispy, Side, Sainsbury's*	¼ Bag/93g	23	0.2	25	1.3	4.4	0.2	2.2
Sweet & Crunchy, Morrisons*	1 Serving/100g	23	0.3	23	0.8	3.4	0.3	1.8
Sweet & Crunchy, Sainsbury's*	1 Pack/150g	22	0.2	15	0.9	2.6	0.1	1.8
Sweet Green, M & S*	1 Serving/150g	22	0.4	15	1.5	1.3	0.3	2.0
Sweet Leaf, M & S*	1 Pack/110g	38	0.9	35	1.5	5.3	0.8	2.1
Sweet Leaf, Sainsbury's*	1 Serving/80g	19	0.2	24	0.8	3.6	0.3	1.9
Sweet Leaf & Carrot, Asda*	½ Pack/164g	34	0.5	21	0.9	3.6	0.3	1.4
Sweet Leaf & Carrot, Lasting Leaf*	1 Serving/70g	16	0.3	23	1.0	2.8	0.4	2.2
Sweet Leafy, Organic, Tesco*	1 Serving/250g	45	1.0	18	0.8	2.7	0.4	1.9
Tabbouleh, HL, Tesco*	1 Serving/200g	194	3.6	97	3.5	16.8	1.8	1.3
Tabbouleh, Salad Bar, Waitrose*	1 Serving/100g	94	1.7	94	0.0	0.0	1.7	0.0
Tabbouleh & Feta, Tesco*	1 Pack/225g	302	11.2	134	5.4	16.7	5.0	0.6
Tabbouleh Feta, Finest, Tesco*	1 Pack/225g	266	11.7	118	4.2	13.7	5.2	0.6
Three Bean, & Mint, Finest, Tesco*	½ Pack/115g	155	6.9	135	6.8	7.7	6.0	11.5
Three Bean, Pot, Tesco*	1 Pot/210g	204	9.2	97	4.1	10.2	4.4	2.3
Three Bean, Sainsbury's*	1 Serving/125g	108	6.3	86	4.2	6.0	5.0	0.0
Three Bean, Tinned, Tesco*	1 Tin/160g	176	1.6	110	7.7	17.6	1.0	5.3
Three Bean, with Mint Vinaigrette, M & S*	1 Pack/250g	250	6.0	100	5.9	8.2	2.4	11.1
Tomato, Avocado & Rocket, M & S*	1 Pack/350g	508	46.9	145	1.7	4.1	13.4	0.2
Tomato, Lettuce & Cucumber, Classics, M & S*	1 Serving/275g	151	11.6	55	0.9	3.3	4.2	1.6
Tomato & Cucumber, Ready To eat, Morrisons*	¼ Pack/81g	17	0.2	21	0.9	3.7	0.3	2.0
Tomato & Mozzarella, Finest, Tesco*	1 Pack/175g	254	21.4	145	5.6	3.3	12.2	0.7
Tomato & Mozzarella, M & S*	1 Pack/220g	264	16.5	120	9.8	2.8	7.5	1.1
Tomato & Onion	1oz/28g	20	1.7	72	0.8	4.0	6.1	1.0
Tuna, American, Lidl*	1oz/28g	25	0.8	91	7.4	8.5	3.0	0.0
Tuna, Breton Style, Snack Pot, Carb Check, Heinz*	1 Pot/219g	239	13.8	109	8.4	4.6	6.3	1.5
Tuna, French Style, Light Lunch, John West*	1 Pack/220g	218	6.2	99	7.5	9.8	2.8	2.5
Tuna, HE, Tesco*	1 Serving/300g	399	21.9	133	6.2	10.5	7.3	0.9
Tuna, Italian Style, Light Lunch, John West*	1 Pack/220g	205	5.7	93	7.3	9.8	2.6	0.5
Tuna, Layer, COU, M & S*	1 Pack/340g	272	8.8	80	6.2	7.5	2.6	1.5
Tuna, Layered, Waitrose*	1 Bowl/300g	636	58.8	212	4.0	4.8	19.6	1.0
Tuna, Mediterranean Style, Light Lunch, John West*	1 Pack/220g	211	4.2	96	8.5	10.0	1.9	2.4
Tuna, Mexican, Lidl*	1oz/28g	30	0.9	108	9.3	10.5	3.2	0.0
Tuna, Skipjack, John West*	1 Can/192g	190	11.7	99	7.3	3.7	6.1	0.0
Tuna, Tomato Salsa Style, Light Lunch, John West*	1 Pack/220g	187	2.9	85	7.6	10.8	1.3	0.8
Tuna, with Lemon Dressing, Tesco*	1 Serving/300g	282	24.0	94	4.2	1.4	8.0	1.0

	Measure INFO/WEIGHT	per Measure KCAL	per Measure FAT	Nutrition Values per 100g / 100ml KCAL	PROT	CARB	FAT	FIBRE
SALAD								
Tuna & Mixed Bean	1 Serving/220g	287	14.4	131	9.5	11.2	6.6	3.7
Tuna & Three Bean, Healthily Balanced, M & S*	1 Serving/350g	332	10.2	95	8.7	8.8	2.9	4.6
Tuna & Tomato, Boots*	1 Pack/171g	150	10.3	88	6.5	2.0	6.0	1.0
Tuna & Vegetable, Tesco*	½ Can/140g	189	10.1	135	9.0	8.5	7.2	3.3
Tuna Nicoise, BGTY, Sainsbury's*	1 Pack/300g	315	6.0	105	6.3	15.5	2.0	2.5
Tuna Nicoise, Finest, Tesco*	1 Serving/250g	430	23.5	172	8.5	13.3	9.4	0.8
Vegetable, Canned	1oz/28g	40	2.7	143	1.6	13.0	9.8	1.2
Vegetable, Chargrilled, M & S*	1 Tub/165g	91	5.4	55	1.4	5.3	3.3	2.6
Vegetable, Heinz*	1 Can/195g	259	16.6	133	1.5	12.6	8.5	1.3
Waldorf, Average	1 Serving/100g	193	17.7	193	1.4	7.5	17.7	1.3
Watercress, Morrisons*	1 Bag/100g	17	0.7	17	1.7	1.2	0.7	0.0
Watercress, Mustard Leaf & Mizuna, M & S*	½ Pack/60g	9	0.2	15	2.4	0.4	0.3	3.0
Watercress, Spinach & Rocket, Tesco*	1 Serving/30g	7	0.2	22	3.0	0.8	0.8	1.9
Watercress, Spinach & Rocket, Waitrose*	1 Bag/145g	30	1.2	21	2.2	1.2	0.8	1.5
Watercress & Spinach, Asda*	1 Serving/50g	10	0.3	21	2.8	1.2	0.6	1.9
SALAD BOWL								
Coleslaw, M & S*	1 Pack/325g	292	24.0	90	1.3	4.9	7.4	1.3
Coleslaw, Tesco*	1 Bowl/300g	327	30.3	109	1.0	3.4	10.1	1.3
Crispy, M & S*	1 Serving/250g	88	1.2	35	1.3	6.6	0.5	1.2
Egg Layered, Tesco*	1 Pack/410g	726	57.8	177	4.2	8.4	14.1	1.3
French Style, Sainsbury's*	1oz/28g	15	1.0	55	1.0	4.8	3.5	1.5
Frisee, Radicchio & Green Oak Leaf Lettuce, M & S*	1 Bowl/150g	30	0.6	20	1.1	2.6	0.4	1.1
Goats Cheese, Sainsbury's*	1 Serving/100g	161	11.9	161	5.8	7.6	11.9	1.3
Greek Style, M & S*	1 Bowl/223g	212	18.3	95	2.5	2.4	8.2	0.7
Large, Sainsbury's*	1/6 Pack/52g	12	0.2	23	0.9	4.3	0.3	1.1
Mixed, Medley, Waitrose*	¼ Pack/60g	9	0.3	15	0.9	1.7	0.5	1.0
Mixed, Waitrose*	¼ Pack/64g	9	0.3	14	0.8	1.6	0.5	1.4
Prawn, Sainsbury's*	1 Bowl/400g	632	46.8	158	3.7	9.4	11.7	1.2
Tomato, Sainsbury's*	½ Bowl/150g	93	6.8	62	0.9	4.4	4.5	1.6
Tomato & Basil, M & S*	1 Serving/225g	225	22.7	100	0.8	3.7	10.1	1.1
Tuna, BGTY, Sainsbury's*	½ Pack/175g	180	2.6	103	7.0	15.4	1.5	1.7
Tuna, Fresh, Asda*	1 Serving/160g	184	11.2	115	8.0	5.0	7.0	0.0
Tuna, Sainsbury's*	1 Serving/200g	336	21.4	168	6.1	11.7	10.7	1.5
SALAD CREAM								
Average	***1 Tsp/5g***	***17***	***1.4***	***335***	***1.7***	***18.6***	***27.8***	***0.1***
Heinz*	1 Tbsp/15g	50	4.0	332	1.4	20.0	26.8	0.0
Reduced Calorie, Average	***1 Tsp/5g***	***6***	***0.4***	***130***	***1.0***	***12.9***	***7.9***	***0.2***
Weight Watchers*	1 Serving/14g	16	0.6	115	1.5	16.2	4.4	0.0
SALAMI								
Ardennes Pepper, Waitrose*	1 Serving/7g	30	2.7	429	18.6	1.9	38.5	1.1
Average	***1 Slice/5g***	***18***	***1.3***	***360***	***28.4***	***1.8***	***26.2***	***0.0***
Danish, Average	***1 Serving/17g***	***89***	***8.8***	***524***	***13.2***	***1.3***	***51.7***	***0.0***
Emiliano, Sainsbury's*	1 Serving/70g	209	14.2	298	28.8	0.1	20.3	0.0
German, Average	***1 Serving/60g***	***200***	***16.4***	***333***	***20.3***	***1.6***	***27.3***	***0.1***
German, Peppered, Average	***3 Slices/25g***	***86***	***6.8***	***342***	***22.2***	***2.5***	***27.1***	***0.2***
Giganti, Sliced, TTD, Sainsbury's*	1 Slice/5g	21	1.8	411	25.0	0.1	34.4	0.6
Healthy Range, Average	***4 Slices/25g***	***55***	***3.6***	***220***	***22.4***	***0.6***	***14.3***	***0.0***
Meatster, Alpenmark, Aldi*	1 Serving/25g	124	11.0	497	24.0	1.0	44.0	0.5
Milano, Average	***1 Serving/70g***	***278***	***22.6***	***397***	***25.9***	***0.9***	***32.2***	***0.0***
Napoli, Average	***1 Slice/5g***	***17***	***1.3***	***342***	***27.1***	***0.8***	***25.5***	***0.0***
Pepperoni, Italian, Morrisons*	1 Slice/6g	23	1.9	406	24.0	0.9	34.0	0.0
Spanish, Wafer Thin, Tesco*	1 Pack/80g	273	18.8	341	25.5	6.8	23.5	0.0
Ungherese, Tesco*	1 Serving/35g	136	11.2	388	24.5	0.5	32.0	0.0

S

	Measure INFO/WEIGHT	per Measure KCAL	FAT	Nutrition Values per 100g / 100ml KCAL	PROT	CARB	FAT	FIBRE
SALMON								
Alaskan, Wild, TTD, Sainsbury's*	1 Fillet/115g	173	8.3	150	21.2	0.1	7.2	0.1
Cooked, Prepacked, Average	1 Fillet/93g	180	11.1	194	21.8	0.0	11.9	0.0
Fillets, Cajun, Waitrose*	1 Serving/150g	214	9.8	143	20.6	0.4	6.5	0.0
Fillets, Chargrilled, Sainsbury's*	1 Serving/270g	270	19.5	243	20.9	0.2	17.6	0.0
Fillets, Chilli & Lemon Pink, Aldi*	1 Fillet/140g	260	10.4	186	16.9	12.9	7.4	0.7
Fillets, Fresh, Value, Tesco*	1 Slice/85g	153	9.4	180	21.6	0.0	11.0	0.0
Fillets, Honey Roast, Co-Op*	1 Fillet/100g	250	13.8	250	26.7	4.7	13.8	0.1
Fillets, Lightly Smoked, TTD, Sainsbury's*	1 Serving/100g	201	13.2	201	20.2	0.3	13.2	0.6
Fillets, Lime & Coriander, Tesco*	1 Pack/250g	282	5.2	113	18.2	5.4	2.1	0.0
Fillets, Raw, Average	***1 Sm Fillet/120g***	***227***	***14.0***	***189***	***20.9***	***0.1***	***11.7***	***0.1***
Flakes, Honey Roast, Average	***1oz/28g***	***56***	***3.0***	***198***	***24.0***	***1.9***	***10.7***	***0.2***
Flakes, Honey Roast, Sainsbury's*	½ Pack/68g	166	9.5	244	25.9	3.6	14.0	0.0
Goujons, Average	1 Pack/150g	321	16.4	214	16.4	12.4	11.0	1.1
Gravadlax, Finest, Tesco*	1 Serving/70g	125	6.9	178	22.1	0.2	9.9	0.0
Gravadlax, M & S*	1 Serving/140g	294	16.0	210	18.4	5.3	11.4	0.5
Gravadlax, Scottish, M & S*	1 Serving/70g	147	8.0	210	18.4	5.3	11.4	0.5
Gravadlax, with Mustard Sauce, Waitrose*	1 Pack/200g	382	22.2	191	21.8	1.0	11.1	0.4
Grilled	***1oz/28g***	***60***	***3.7***	***215***	***24.2***	***0.0***	***13.1***	***0.0***
Hot Smoked, Average	***1 Serving/62g***	***103***	***4.4***	***166***	***24.0***	***0.9***	***7.2***	***0.1***
Juniper & Birch Smoked, TTD, Sainsbury's*	½ Pack/60g	132	8.4	220	23.3	0.3	14.0	0.1
Lemon & Rosemary, Easy Steam, BGTY, Sainsbury's*	1 Pack/350g	329	12.6	94	6.4	9.0	3.6	1.3
Lime & Coriander, Tesco*	1 Serving/120g	176	4.4	147	21.4	7.0	3.7	0.7
Mousse, Tesco*	1 Mousse/57g	100	7.0	177	13.5	2.9	12.4	0.2
Pink, Alaskan, Canned, Crown Prince*	¼ Cup/55g	90	4.0	164	20.0	0.0	7.3	0.0
Pink, Canned, Average	***1 Serving/125g***	***162***	***7.2***	***130***	***19.5***	***0.1***	***5.8***	***0.1***
Pink, in Brine, Average	***1 Sm Can/105g***	***161***	***6.9***	***153***	***23.5***	***0.0***	***6.6***	***0.0***
Poached, Average	***1 Serving/90g***	***176***	***10.5***	***195***	***22.5***	***0.2***	***11.7***	***0.3***
Potted, M & S*	1 Serving/75g	184	14.6	245	17.1	0.5	19.4	1.2
Red, Average	***½ Can/90g***	***141***	***7.4***	***156***	***20.4***	***0.1***	***8.2***	***0.1***
Red, in Brine, Average	***1oz/28g***	***47***	***2.5***	***169***	***22.4***	***0.0***	***8.9***	***0.0***
Rillettes, John West*	½ Can/62g	169	14.6	272	14.9	0.1	23.5	0.0
Roasted, Slices, Tesco*	1 Slice/33g	71	3.5	215	26.7	2.7	10.5	1.9
Smoked, Appetisers, Tesco*	1/3 Pack/33g	80	6.2	240	16.3	1.1	18.5	0.0
Smoked, Average	***1 Serving/70g***	***126***	***7.0***	***179***	***21.9***	***0.5***	***10.0***	***0.1***
Smoked, Parcels, TTD, Sainsbury's*	1 Serving/58g	144	11.1	250	13.4	5.7	19.3	1.0
Smoked, Pieces, Waitrose*	½ Pack/50g	87	4.3	174	23.9	0.3	8.6	0.1
Smoked, Sockeye, Wild, TTD, Sainsbury's*	½ Pack/60g	82	1.9	137	26.3	0.7	3.2	0.6
Smoked, Trimmings, Average	***1 Serving/55g***	***101***	***5.7***	***184***	***22.8***	***0.2***	***10.3***	***0.0***
Steaks	***1 Serving/100g***	***180***	***11.0***	***180***	***20.2***	***0.0***	***11.0***	***0.0***
Steamed	***1oz/28g***	***55***	***3.6***	***197***	***20.1***	***0.0***	***13.0***	***0.0***
Tail Joint, Lemon & Herb Butter, M & S*	1 Pack/480g	864	54.7	180	18.8	0.8	11.4	0.2
Whole, Raw, Average	1 Serving/100g	228	13.9	228	25.6	0.0	13.9	0.0
SALMON &								
Asparagus, Oakhouse Foods Ltd*	1 Meal/400g	396	17.2	99	6.1	9.0	4.3	0.7
Spinach, Roulade, Tesco*	1 Serving/60g	155	14.2	258	9.5	1.7	23.7	0.2
Thai Noodles, HE, Tesco*	1 Pack/350g	231	4.2	66	6.7	7.1	1.2	1.5
Vegetables, M & S*	1 Serving/200g	220	13.8	110	6.0	5.2	6.9	0.8
SALMON EN CROUTE								
Chilled, Youngs*	1 Pastry/200g	531	37.3	266	9.6	14.8	18.6	2.3
Frozen, Tesco*	1 Serving/166g	365	18.4	220	10.1	19.1	11.1	1.1
Frozen, Youngs*	1 Pastry/185g	542	38.3	293	10.2	16.5	20.7	1.0
Loved by Us, Co-Op*	1 Serving/135g	364	21.5	270	11.7	19.3	15.9	1.8
Luxury, M & S*	1oz/28g	59	3.8	210	11.9	9.4	13.7	2.2

S

	Measure INFO/WEIGHT	per Measure KCAL	per Measure FAT	KCAL	PROT	CARB	FAT	FIBRE
				Nutrition Values per 100g / 100ml				
SALMON EN CROUTE								
Retail, Average	1oz/28g	81	5.3	288	11.8	18.0	19.1	0.0
SALMON IN								
Chilli Lime & Ginger Dressing, The Saucy Fish Co.*	1 Fillet/140g	273	15.8	195	16.7	5.5	11.3	0.0
Dill Sauce, Youngs*	1 Pack/435g	265	10.0	61	6.1	4.2	2.3	0.1
Horseradish Sauce, Creamy, Fillets, Wonnemeyer*	1 Serving/300g	459	31.5	153	9.4	5.3	10.5	0.0
Lime & Coriander, Fillets, Good Choice, Iceland*	½ Pack/150g	189	4.4	126	19.8	5.1	2.9	0.8
Pancetta, Wrapped, Finest, Tesco*	1 Serving/150g	328	25.8	219	14.9	1.0	17.2	0.1
Tomato & Mascarpone Sauce, Fillets, Asda*	½ Pack/181g	279	19.9	154	13.0	0.8	11.0	0.6
Watercress Sauce, Creamy, Fillets, Scottish, Seafresh*	1 Pack 300g	528	38.7	176	13.7	1.2	12.9	0.1
Watercress Sauce, Pink, Wild Alaskan, Sainsbury's*	½ Pack/180g	194	9.7	108	13.9	0.9	5.4	0.8
Watercress Sauce, Waitrose*	½ Pack/150g	264	19.4	176	13.7	1.2	12.9	0.1
White Wine & Cream Sauce, Tesco*	1 Serving/170g	279	19.2	164	13.5	2.0	11.3	1.2
White Wine & Parsley Dressing, Fillets, Tesco*	1 Fillet/150g	291	20.4	194	17.5	0.3	13.6	0.6
White Wine Sauce, Creamy, 146, Oakhouse Foods Ltd*	1 Meal/400g	448	19.6	112	5.7	11.7	4.9	1.6
SALMON WITH								
Coriander & Lime, Pacific, Asda*	1 Serving/113g	154	3.4	137	27.0	0.5	3.0	0.0
Garlic & Herb Butter, Tesco*	1 Fillet/112g	291	23.1	260	17.6	0.0	20.6	0.0
Mozzarella & Tomato Crust, Just Cook, Sainsbury's*	½ Pack/171g	220	9.2	129	15.0	5.2	5.4	0.4
Pasta, Frozen, Youngs*	½ Bag/175g	234	7.7	134	7.4	16.3	4.4	1.2
Penne Pasta & Dill Sauce, SteamFresh, Birds Eye*	1 Pack/424g	335	6.4	79	6.4	9.9	1.5	1.1
Potatoes, Honey Roast, LC, Tesco*	1 Pack/350g	332	12.2	95	6.6	8.5	3.5	2.4
Prawns & Fusilli Pasta, Frozen, Youngs*	1 Pack/375g	439	27.8	117	5.6	7.0	7.4	1.1
Rice, Oriental Style, M & S*	1 Pot/210g	252	6.9	120	5.9	16.5	3.3	3.3
Spinach & Pasta, Smoked, Milson's Kitchen (Aldi)*	1 Pack/400g	472	16.0	118	5.6	15.0	4.0	1.7
Sweet Chilli, Fillets, Kiln Roasted, Tesco*	1 Fillet/93g	241	15.4	259	23.3	3.4	16.6	1.4
Sweet Chilli, Hot Smoked, Scottish, Tesco*	1 Fillet/120g	252	12.7	210	26.1	1.7	10.6	0.6
Sweet Chilli Lime & Ginger, Simply Fish, Tesco*	½ Pack/98g	235	17.2	240	17.4	3.2	17.5	0.0
SALSA								
Bottled, M & S*	½ Jar/136g	95	3.3	70	1.2	12.0	2.4	1.5
Chunky, Sainsbury's*	½ Pot/84g	43	1.4	51	1.1	7.8	1.7	1.2
Cool, Sainsbury's*	1 Serving/100g	31	0.3	31	1.0	6.1	0.3	1.2
Fresh, Asda*	1oz/28g	10	0.2	35	1.2	6.2	0.6	2.0
Fresh, Sainsbury's*	1oz/28g	15	0.6	54	1.7	7.0	2.1	0.9
GFY, Asda*	½ Pot/236g	85	0.9	36	1.1	7.0	0.4	0.7
Hot, Fresh, Chilled, Tesco*	1 Tub/200g	120	4.8	60	1.4	7.5	2.4	1.2
Hot, Primula*	1oz/28g	10	0.1	35	1.8	6.6	0.2	0.0
Medium Hot, Discovery*	1 Serving/30g	17	0.1	56	1.4	11.7	0.4	0.8
Mild, Heinz*	1 Serving/20g	16	0.0	79	1.2	17.9	0.1	0.8
Mild, Original, Old El Paso*	1 Sachet/144g	60	0.7	42	1.6	9.0	0.5	0.0
Original, from Dinner Kit, Old El Paso*	1 Jar/226g	71	0.7	32	1.2	6.0	0.3	0.0
Prawn & Tomato, Fresh, Anti Pasti, Asda*	1 Pot/150g	100	3.8	67	8.0	3.1	2.5	1.3
Red Onion & Tomato, Tapas Selection, Sainsbury's*	1 Serving/22g	17	1.0	77	3.0	6.0	4.5	0.9
Red Pepper, Sainsbury's*	1 Serving/85g	31	1.4	37	1.7	3.8	1.7	1.5
Smokey BBQ, Weight Watchers*	1 Serving/56g	20	0.1	36	1.1	7.6	0.1	2.3
Spiced Mango, Ginger & Chilli, Weight Watchers*	½ Pot/50g	42	0.1	85	1.0	19.9	0.2	2.6
Spicy, Less Than 3% Fat, M & S*	½ Pot/85g	30	0.7	35	1.3	5.6	0.8	0.8
Sweetcorn, Fresh, Sainsbury's*	¼ Pot/51g	32	0.9	63	1.1	10.5	1.8	1.3
Tomato, Chunky, Tesco*	1 Pot/170g	68	2.2	40	1.1	5.9	1.3	1.1
Tomato, Mexican Style, Dip, Morrisons*	½ Pack/50g	26	0.9	51	1.2	7.6	1.8	0.8
Tomato, Onion, Coriander & Chilli, Fresh, Waitrose*	1 Tub/170g	110	5.3	65	1.3	8.0	3.1	1.2
Tomato, Reduced Fat, Waitrose*	1 Serving/1g	0	0.0	27	1.5	4.7	0.2	1.4
Tomato, Spicy, Worldwide Sauces*	1 Serving/25g	8	0.0	30	1.2	5.9	0.2	1.2
Tomato, Sun Ripened, Tesco*	1 Serving/40g	46	1.7	115	5.0	14.2	4.2	4.6

	Measure INFO/WEIGHT	per Measure KCAL	FAT	Nutrition Values per 100g / 100ml KCAL	PROT	CARB	FAT	FIBRE
SALSA								
Tomato, Vine Ripened, Tesco*	½ Tub/100g	47	1.8	47	1.0	6.7	1.8	1.1
Tomato & Avocado, Chunky, COU, M & S*	½ Pack/86g	30	1.2	35	0.8	5.4	1.4	1.4
SALT								
Alternative, Reduced Sodium, Losalt*	1 Tsp/5g	0	0.0	0	0.0	0.0	0.0	0.0
Rock, Average	¼ Tsp/1g	0	0.0	0	0.0	0.0	0.0	0.0
Rock, Natural, Tidmans*	1 Serving/100g	0	0.0	0	0.0	0.0	0.0	0.0
Rock for Grinding, Saxa*	1 Serving/100g	0	0.0	0	0.0	0.0	0.0	0.0
Table, Average	***1 Tsp/5g***	***0***	***0.0***	***0***	***0.0***	***0.0***	***0.0***	***0.0***
SAMBUCA								
Average	***1 Shot/35ml***	***122***	***0.0***	***348***	***0.0***	***37.2***	***0.0***	***0.0***
SAMOSAS								
Chicken, Mumtaz*	1 Serving/105g	177	8.3	169	19.6	4.9	7.9	0.0
Chicken Tikka, Sainsbury's*	1 Samosa/50g	120	6.4	239	8.3	22.5	12.9	3.1
Dim Sum, Selection, Sainsbury's*	1 Samosa/12g	24	0.9	196	3.4	28.6	7.6	2.8
Indian Style, Selection, Co-Op*	1 Samosa/21g	50	2.7	240	5.0	27.0	13.0	3.0
Lamb, Morrisons*	1 Samosa/50g	144	7.8	288	9.8	27.0	15.7	1.5
Vegetable, Indian, Takeaway, Chosen By You, Asda*	1 Samosa/50g	126	5.2	250	5.2	32.5	10.3	3.3
Vegetable, Indian Starter Selection, M & S*	1 Samosa/21g	60	3.5	290	5.0	29.0	16.9	3.3
Vegetable, Large, Individual, Sainsbury's*	1 Samosa/110g	254	16.5	231	3.3	20.7	15.0	2.1
Vegetable, M & S*	1 Samosa/45g	115	6.9	255	5.1	24.8	15.3	2.8
Vegetable, Mini, Asda*	1 Samosa/23g	52	2.0	233	6.0	32.0	9.0	2.6
Vegetable, Mini, Indian, Party Selection, Tesco*	1 Samosa/30g	58	1.5	195	3.6	33.9	5.0	2.2
Vegetable, Mini, Indian Snack Selection, Sainsbury's*	1 Samosa/25g	70	4.0	280	4.7	29.8	15.8	3.2
Vegetable, Mini, Waitrose*	1 Samosa/29g	70	3.8	242	3.6	27.1	13.2	3.1
Vegetable, Morrisons*	1 Samosa/60g	101	3.5	169	4.9	24.1	5.8	2.0
Vegetable, Northern Indian, Sainsbury's*	1 Samosa/50g	126	5.9	252	5.8	30.6	11.8	2.6
Vegetable, Waitrose*	1 Samosa/50g	118	7.2	236	3.7	23.1	14.3	2.7
SANDWICH								
All Day Breakfast, Aramark*	1 Serving/206g	441	19.0	214	9.6	23.3	9.2	0.0
All Day Breakfast, BGTY, Sainsbury's*	1 Pack/188g	294	4.5	156	9.6	22.7	2.4	0.0
All Day Breakfast, Deep Fill, Ginsters*	1 Sandwich/215g	514	19.8	239	11.4	27.6	9.2	1.5
All Day Breakfast, Finest, Tesco*	1 Pack/275g	660	41.5	240	9.7	16.4	15.1	1.6
All Day Breakfast, Shapers, Boots*	1 Pack/207g	323	5.2	156	11.0	23.0	2.5	2.2
All Day Breakfast, Wall's*	1 Pack/225g	610	34.7	271	9.2	24.3	15.4	1.4
All Day Breakfast, Weight Watchers*	1 Pack/158g	298	4.3	189	11.0	30.2	2.7	1.9
Bacon, Brie & Mango Chutney, Daily Bread*	1 Serving/213g	555	22.7	261	12.7	28.6	10.7	0.0
Bacon, Cheese & Chicken, Triple, BGTY, Sainsbury's*	1 Serving/266g	506	16.8	190	12.7	20.7	6.3	2.6
Bacon & Brie, Asda*	1 Pack/181g	603	38.2	333	13.3	22.9	21.1	1.3
Bacon & Brie, Finest, Tesco*	1 Pack/201g	571	33.6	284	14.1	19.4	16.7	2.1
Bacon & Brown Sauce, Ashberry*	1 Pack/419g	1207	53.6	288	12.0	31.0	12.8	0.0
Bacon & Egg, Boots*	1 Pack/179g	480	28.6	268	12.0	19.0	16.0	1.4
Bacon & Egg, Co-Op*	1 Pack/188g	536	32.0	285	13.0	20.0	17.0	2.0
Bacon & Egg, Deep Fill, Spar*	1 Pack/191g	579	38.0	303	12.2	18.7	19.9	0.0
Bacon & Egg, Free Range, Daily Bread*	1 Serving/175g	425	22.9	243	10.1	21.5	13.1	0.0
Bacon & Egg, HL, Tesco*	1 Serving/178g	328	9.3	184	11.5	22.7	5.2	1.7
Bacon & Egg, on Malted Whole Grain Bread, Budgens*	1 Pack/175g	593	37.4	339	12.3	21.4	21.4	1.6
Bacon & Egg, Sainsbury's*	1 Pack/160g	384	17.8	240	13.0	22.0	11.1	1.8
Bacon & Egg, Scottish Slimmers, Tesco*	1 Pack/139g	279	6.4	201	13.6	26.3	4.6	1.2
Bacon & Egg, Shell*	1 Pack/191g	579	38.0	303	12.2	18.7	19.9	0.0
Bacon & Tomato, COU, M & S*	1 Pack/169g	270	4.6	160	9.5	25.6	2.7	2.5
Beef, Peppered, Shell*	1 Pack/181g	400	15.2	221	7.3	29.0	8.4	1.3
Beef, Roast, Daily Bread*	1 Pack/199g	281	5.4	141	8.7	20.0	2.7	0.0
Beef, Roast, Feel Good, Shell*	1 Pack/153g	390	14.8	255	17.6	24.2	9.7	0.0

S

	Measure INFO/WEIGHT	per Measure KCAL	FAT	Nutrition Values per 100g / 100ml KCAL	PROT	CARB	FAT	FIBRE
SANDWICH								
Beef, Roast, Finest, Tesco*	1 Sandwich/222g	455	15.1	205	13.2	22.3	6.8	2.5
Beef, Roast, Handmade, Tesco*	1 Pack/223g	439	15.8	197	12.5	20.7	7.1	1.6
Beef, Roast, Plain, From Restaurant, Average	1 Sandwich/139g	346	13.8	249	15.5	24.1	9.9	0.0
Beef, Roast, Sainsbury's*	1 Pack/174g	426	17.4	245	9.4	29.3	10.0	0.0
Beef & Horseradish, Deep Filled, BGTY, Sainsbury's*	1 Pack/202g	313	4.8	155	11.4	22.0	2.4	2.4
Beef & Horseradish, Sainsbury's*	1 Pack/187g	389	13.3	208	12.0	24.1	7.1	0.0
Beef & Horseradish, Shapers, Boots*	1 Pack/156g	276	2.7	177	12.0	28.0	1.7	1.8
Beef & Horseradish Mayonnaise, Shapers, Boots*	1 Pack/159g	266	3.3	167	12.0	25.0	2.1	2.6
Beef & Onion, Co-Op*	1 Pack/221g	530	24.3	240	11.0	24.0	11.0	1.0
Beef & Onion, Roast, Deep Filled, Asda*	1 Pack/258g	550	27.9	213	11.3	22.6	10.8	1.1
Beef & Onion, Roast, HL, Tesco*	1 Pack/185g	278	3.5	150	13.3	20.0	1.9	2.7
Beef & Pate, M & S*	1 Pack/188g	310	7.3	165	11.2	21.6	3.9	2.4
Beef & Salad, Deep Fill, Iceland*	1 Pack/188g	317	9.2	169	11.1	20.1	4.9	2.7
Beef & Salad, Gibsons*	1 Pack/185g	348	10.6	188	10.6	23.5	5.7	0.0
Beef & Salad, Roast, Daily Bread*	1 Pack/202g	319	8.3	158	9.0	21.4	4.1	0.0
BLT, & Chicken Salad, Co-Op*	1 Pack/230g	472	20.7	205	10.0	21.0	9.0	2.0
BLT, Bacon, Lettuce & Tomato, LC, Tesco*	1 Pack/155g	310	7.9	200	9.9	26.5	5.1	2.2
BLT, BGTY, Sainsbury's*	1 Pack/196g	331	4.4	169	10.4	27.0	2.2	0.0
BLT, COU, M & S*	1 Pack/174g	278	4.7	160	9.5	25.6	2.7	2.5
BLT, Daily Bread*	1 Pack/171g	344	18.8	201	9.1	21.6	11.0	0.0
BLT, Deep Fill, Tesco*	1 Pack/231g	635	38.1	275	11.8	19.8	16.5	1.2
BLT, Deep Filled, Asda*	1 Pack/206g	606	35.0	294	13.3	21.8	17.0	3.0
BLT, GFY, Asda*	1 Pack/171g	294	6.0	172	9.0	26.0	3.5	1.6
BLT, HL, Tesco*	1 Pack/190g	287	2.7	151	10.1	24.5	1.4	1.6
BLT, Impress*	1 Pack/189g	381	13.4	202	11.5	22.8	7.1	0.0
BLT, Max, Shell*	1 Pack/249g	665	35.1	267	10.8	24.1	14.1	0.0
BLT, Salt Controlled, Shapers, Boots*	1 Pack/180g	290	6.1	161	9.3	23.0	3.4	3.0
BLT, Shapers, Boots*	1 Pack/169g	254	6.3	150	10.7	18.9	3.7	5.9
BLT, Sutherland*	1 Pack/216g	624	37.9	289	9.1	23.8	17.5	0.0
BLT, Taste!*	1 Pack/169g	353	16.0	209	8.5	22.4	9.5	0.0
BLT, with Mayo, Malted Bread, Just Tasty, Aldi*	1 Pack/186g	437	17.9	235	14.0	22.0	9.6	2.4
Brie, with Apple & Grapes, Sainsbury's*	1 Pack/220g	473	24.2	215	8.2	20.8	11.0	0.0
Brie & Grape, Finest, Tesco*	1 Pack/209g	527	31.6	252	8.5	20.6	15.1	1.5
Cheddar & Bacon, Deep Fill, Ginsters*	1 Serving/170g	550	28.2	324	14.1	28.3	16.6	2.3
Cheddar & Celery, M & S*	1 Pack/200g	540	31.8	270	9.7	22.4	15.9	1.5
Cheddar & Coleslaw, Simply, Boots*	1 Pack/185g	538	33.3	291	9.2	23.0	18.0	1.8
Cheddar & Ham, British, M & S*	1 Serving/165g	395	18.6	240	15.1	20.0	11.3	1.7
Cheddar & Ham, M & S*	1 Pack/165g	396	18.6	240	15.1	20.0	11.3	1.7
Cheddar & Ham, Oldfields*	1 Pack/246g	674	39.6	274	11.7	20.5	16.1	2.0
Cheddar & Ham, Smoked, Deep Filled, Tesco*	1 Serving/203g	573	33.1	282	14.3	19.5	16.3	1.2
Cheddar & Ham, with Pickle, Smoked, Finest, Tesco*	1 Pack/217g	532	24.7	245	11.9	23.7	11.4	3.9
Cheddar & Pickle, Mature, Sainsbury's*	1 Pack/171g	588	27.0	344	14.3	38.7	15.8	7.0
Cheddar & Salad, Mature, Upper Crust*	1 Pack/225g	466	22.1	207	9.5	20.3	9.8	0.0
Cheddar & Tomato, Mature, Big, Sainsbury's*	1 Pack/233g	596	25.6	256	12.9	26.3	11.0	0.0
Cheddar & Tomato, Red, Tesco*	1 Pack/182g	526	31.7	289	9.2	24.0	17.4	1.1
Cheddar Gorge, Cranks*	1 Pack/190g	454	23.2	239	11.5	19.4	12.2	3.0
Cheese, Apple & Celery, Asda*	1 Pack/173g	244	4.8	141	8.0	21.0	2.8	2.7
Cheese, Apple & Grape, COU, M & S*	1 Pack/186g	270	2.2	145	8.5	24.9	1.2	2.0
Cheese, Asda*	1 Pack/262g	618	31.4	236	12.2	20.3	12.0	3.0
Cheese, Ham, & Pickle, Healthy Range, Average	1 Pack/185g	299	5.1	162	13.6	20.6	2.8	2.5
Cheese, Ham & Pickle, Shapers, Boots*	1 Pack/184g	318	8.5	173	13.0	20.0	4.6	2.5
Cheese, Ham & Pickle, Simply, Boots*	1 Pack/225g	551	29.2	245	11.0	21.0	13.0	2.4
Cheese, Three & Onion, Boots*	1 Pack/169g	566	33.8	335	11.0	28.0	20.0	1.9

S

	Measure INFO/WEIGHT	per Measure KCAL	FAT	Nutrition Values per 100g / 100ml KCAL	PROT	CARB	FAT	FIBRE
SANDWICH								
Cheese, Three & Spring Onion, Shell*	1 Pack/168g	672	50.9	400	11.1	20.8	30.3	0.0
Cheese & Celery, Shapers, Boots*	1 Pack/181g	288	4.2	159	11.0	24.0	2.3	3.0
Cheese & Coleslaw, Asda*	1 Pack/262g	799	51.4	305	10.1	22.1	19.6	3.3
Cheese & Coleslaw, M & S*	1 Pack/186g	498	32.4	268	10.2	17.6	17.4	3.2
Cheese & Coleslaw, Shapers, Boots*	1 Pack/224g	338	4.7	151	11.0	22.0	2.1	3.2
Cheese & Coleslaw, Sutherland*	1 Pack/185g	376	8.3	203	10.7	29.9	4.5	0.0
Cheese & Ham, Baxter & Platts*	1 Pack/168g	408	21.8	243	11.3	20.5	13.0	1.7
Cheese & Ham, Smoked, Co-Op*	1 Pack/167g	334	8.4	200	15.0	24.0	5.0	2.0
Cheese & Marmite, No Mayonnaise, Boots*	1 Pack/156g	420	20.0	269	12.2	26.3	12.8	1.7
Cheese & Onion, Deep Fill, Tesco*	1 Pack/212g	742	51.9	350	12.3	20.2	24.5	1.3
Cheese & Onion, GFY, Asda*	1 Pack/156g	317	4.1	203	14.0	31.0	2.6	2.7
Cheese & Onion, Ginsters*	1 Pack/172g	491	26.8	286	11.1	25.4	15.6	1.8
Cheese & Onion, HL, Tesco*	1 Pack/168g	314	9.9	187	10.3	23.2	5.9	1.7
Cheese & Onion, LC, Tesco*	1 Pack/144g	310	9.4	215	12.7	26.5	6.5	3.6
Cheese & Onion, Morrisons*	1 Pack/142g	260	2.4	183	14.1	27.8	1.7	2.9
Cheese & Onion, Reduced Fat, NUME, Morrisons*	1 Pack/142g	348	13.6	245	11.8	26.1	9.6	3.5
Cheese & Onion, Tesco*	1 Pack/178g	573	37.9	322	11.6	21.0	21.3	3.5
Cheese & Onion, Waitrose*	1 Pack/176g	579	38.7	329	12.5	20.2	22.0	2.8
Cheese & Pickle, Heinz*	1 Pack/178g	543	26.9	305	13.8	28.4	15.1	3.8
Cheese & Pickle, Shapers, Boots*	1 Pack/165g	342	8.1	207	9.8	31.0	4.9	2.3
Cheese & Pickle, Tesco*	1 Pack/140g	400	19.3	286	12.7	27.8	13.8	1.4
Cheese & Pickle, Virgin Trains*	1 Pack/158g	444	19.6	281	11.5	31.1	12.4	0.0
Cheese & Salad, Budgens*	1 Pack/169g	250	3.0	148	10.9	21.9	1.8	1.6
Cheese & Salad, COU, M & S*	1 Pack/188g	244	3.0	130	12.1	17.0	1.6	2.4
Cheese & Salad, Shapers, Boots*	1 Pack/205g	308	5.1	150	9.7	22.0	2.5	2.2
Cheese & Spring Onion, Asda*	1 Pack/160g	576	39.9	361	13.0	21.0	25.0	1.9
Cheese & Spring Onion, Mixed, Scottish Slimmers*	1 Pack/139g	298	9.1	214	12.4	26.5	6.5	2.1
Cheese & Spring Onion, Sainsbury's*	1 Serving/177g	605	39.5	342	11.4	24.0	22.3	1.1
Cheese & Tomato, Asda*	1 Pack/154g	388	19.7	252	11.0	23.2	12.8	3.7
Cheese & Tomato, Co-Op*	1 Pack/155g	365	18.5	235	10.6	21.8	11.9	1.9
Cheese & Tomato, Freshmans*	1 Pack/111g	248	18.6	223	11.0	8.0	16.8	0.0
Cheese & Tomato, Organic, M & S*	1 Pack/165g	559	35.3	339	11.8	24.8	21.4	1.9
Cheese & Tomato, Sainsbury's*	1 Pack/216g	542	26.3	251	12.9	22.8	12.2	0.0
Cheese Hamwich, Iceland*	1 Hamwich/54g	165	11.9	306	11.0	16.0	22.0	3.0
Cheesy Coleslaw, Ginsters*	1 Pack/164g	481	27.7	293	9.9	25.4	16.9	2.4
Chicken, Bacon, & Avocado, M & S*	1 Pack/242g	508	28.3	210	10.7	15.8	11.7	3.2
Chicken, Bacon, & Cheese, Club, M & S*	1 Pack/383g	805	37.2	210	11.9	18.5	9.7	1.9
Chicken, Bacon & Guacamole, Darwins Deli*	1 Pack/198g	340	16.4	172	3.6	15.9	8.3	1.7
Chicken, Bacon & Salad, Big, Sainsbury's*	1 Pack/249g	610	31.6	245	11.1	21.7	12.7	0.0
Chicken, Bacon & Sweet Chilli, Feel Good, Shell*	1 Pack/174g	366	8.7	211	14.1	29.2	5.0	0.0
Chicken, Bacon & Tomato, BGTY, Sainsbury's*	1 Pack/190g	270	4.4	142	11.4	19.0	2.3	0.0
Chicken, Basil & Sunblush Tomato, Harry Mason*	1 Pack/164g	272	5.2	166	13.0	21.8	3.2	0.6
Chicken, Bechamel & Leek, Daily Bread*	1 Pack/210g	383	7.2	182	11.0	26.8	3.4	0.0
Chicken, BLT, Daily Bread*	1 Pack/187g	322	13.1	172	9.0	19.5	7.0	0.0
Chicken, BLT, Deli Continental*	1 Pack/224g	509	26.9	227	12.4	17.3	12.0	0.0
Chicken, BLT, Taste!*	1 Pack/239g	458	19.8	192	10.3	19.0	8.3	0.0
Chicken, Breast, BGTY, Sainsbury's*	1 Pack/165g	251	0.8	152	12.2	24.7	0.5	0.0
Chicken, Breast, Millers*	1 Pack/162g	343	14.4	212	13.8	19.3	8.9	0.0
Chicken, Breast, Oldfields*	1 Pack/193g	311	8.1	161	11.7	19.8	4.2	3.0
Chicken, British, & Chorizo, Finest, Tesco*	1 Pack/186g	391	12.6	210	15.7	21.2	6.8	2.7
Chicken, Caesar, & Salad, GFY, Asda*	1 Pack/163g	289	4.6	177	11.0	27.0	2.8	2.1
Chicken, Caesar, & Salad, Sainsbury's*	1 Pack/186g	299	7.1	161	11.2	20.4	3.8	0.0
Chicken, Caesar, Boots*	1 Pack/226g	531	27.1	235	9.8	22.0	12.0	1.7

S

	Measure INFO/WEIGHT	per Measure KCAL	FAT	Nutrition Values per 100g / 100ml KCAL	PROT	CARB	FAT	FIBRE
SANDWICH								
Chicken, Caesar, Chargrilled, Big, Sainsbury's*	1 Pack/216g	657	36.9	304	12.2	25.3	17.1	0.0
Chicken, Caesar, Deli Continental*	1 Pack/169g	455	25.4	269	13.0	20.4	15.0	0.0
Chicken, Caesar, Finest, Tesco*	1 Pack/199g	454	19.9	228	15.4	19.2	10.0	1.4
Chicken, Chargrilled, Ginsters*	1 Pack/209g	431	17.3	206	11.3	21.6	8.3	0.0
Chicken, Chargrilled, No Mayo, Rustlers*	1 Pack/150g	228	1.2	152	16.0	20.1	0.8	0.0
Chicken, Chargrilled, Pitta Pocket, M & S*	1 Pack/208g	279	7.3	134	11.2	14.5	3.5	1.6
Chicken, Chargrilled, with Salad, Weight Watchers*	1 Pack/181g	264	3.8	146	11.7	20.0	2.1	2.2
Chicken, Cheese, Bacon, Big, Sainsbury's*	1 Pack/254g	734	45.5	289	11.7	18.0	17.9	0.0
Chicken, Chilli, Fresh, Taste!*	1 Pack/155g	224	4.9	145	5.6	23.4	3.2	0.0
Chicken, Chinese, Low Calorie, Tesco*	1 Pack/169g	270	4.2	160	11.8	22.6	2.5	2.0
Chicken, Chinese, Malted Brown Bread, Waitrose*	1 Pack/164g	333	11.2	203	13.5	21.9	6.8	3.3
Chicken, Chinese, Snack & Shop, Esso*	1 Pack/178g	409	16.0	230	13.0	22.8	9.0	4.0
Chicken, Chinese, Treat Yourself, Shell*	1 Pack/178g	409	17.1	230	13.0	22.8	9.6	0.0
Chicken, Chorizo & Chipotle Mayonaise, Tesco*	1 Pack/174g	365	13.4	210	12.1	22.7	7.7	2.3
Chicken, Coronation, in Pitta Bread, COU, M & S*	1 Serving/207g	269	2.5	130	9.2	20.4	1.2	2.0
Chicken, Coronation, Indulgence, Taste!*	1 Pack/159g	396	18.8	249	9.1	26.5	11.8	0.0
Chicken, Coronation, M & S*	1 Pack/210g	420	20.4	200	11.2	20.2	9.7	3.1
Chicken, Coronation, on Onion Bread, M & S*	1 Pack/260g	520	21.3	200	10.7	20.0	8.2	1.9
Chicken, Coronation, Sainsbury's*	1 Pack/212g	411	14.4	194	9.7	21.5	6.8	4.1
Chicken, Coronation, Taste!*	1 Pack/178g	367	13.4	206	10.6	24.0	7.5	0.0
Chicken, Creole & Italian Leaves, Northern Bites*	1 Pack/190g	298	4.6	157	13.1	22.1	2.4	2.4
Chicken, Curry, Lifestyle*	1 Serving/160g	211	9.6	132	13.0	6.0	6.0	0.0
Chicken, Flame Grilled, Rustlers*	1 Pack/150g	346	14.2	231	16.3	20.1	9.5	0.0
Chicken, Ham, & Prawn, Triple, Weight Watchers*	1 Pack/250g	337	3.7	135	9.8	20.5	1.5	2.6
Chicken, Ham, Prawn, Triple Pack, HL, Tesco*	1 Pack/247g	350	5.2	142	10.7	20.2	2.1	2.2
Chicken, Ham & Pepperoni, Meat Feast, Tesco*	1 Pack/196g	470	22.5	240	14.7	19.4	11.5	1.5
Chicken, Harvester, Taste!*	1 Pack/200g	295	8.0	148	7.6	20.3	4.0	0.0
Chicken, Healthier Choice, Ginsters*	1 Pack/183g	247	2.6	135	10.2	20.5	1.4	0.0
Chicken, Honey & Mustard, BGTY, Sainsbury's*	1 Pack/171g	296	4.6	173	13.1	24.0	2.7	0.0
Chicken, Jalfrezi, Naan, Ready to Go, M & S*	1 Pack/288g	576	18.1	200	9.8	26.3	6.3	2.9
Chicken, Kashmir, French Cuisiniers*	1 Pack/145g	204	2.3	141	12.9	20.3	1.6	2.9
Chicken, Mexican, Healthy Choices, Shell*	1 Serving/168g	376	11.8	224	12.2	28.1	7.0	0.0
Chicken, No Mayo, Cafe Revive, M & S*	1 Pack/153g	230	3.7	150	14.1	17.9	2.4	3.1
Chicken, No Mayo, Daily Bread*	1 Pack/160g	279	7.1	174	8.6	23.8	4.4	0.0
Chicken, No Mayo, M & S*	1 Pack/142g	248	3.3	175	16.6	20.6	2.3	3.2
Chicken, No Mayonnaise, Waitrose*	1 Pack/173g	332	9.5	192	11.6	24.0	5.5	2.1
Chicken, Red Thai, BGTY, Sainsbury's*	1 Pack/195g	326	3.7	167	11.3	26.4	1.9	0.0
Chicken, Red Thai, Foo-Go*	1 Pack/188g	358	14.9	190	10.2	19.4	7.9	4.4
Chicken, Red Thai, Taste!*	1 Pack/164g	335	9.8	204	11.5	26.1	6.0	0.0
Chicken, Roast, & Salad, Shapers, Boots*	1 Pack/183g	274	4.4	150	12.0	20.0	2.4	3.4
Chicken, Roast, Breast, BGTY, Sainsbury's*	1 Pack/174g	275	4.4	158	14.8	20.9	2.5	1.8
Chicken, Roast, HL, Tesco*	1 Pack/155g	288	5.3	186	13.5	25.4	3.4	1.4
Chicken, Roast, Salad, BGTY, Sainsbury's*	1 Pack/182g	268	4.0	147	11.9	19.9	2.2	2.7
Chicken, Roast, Shapers, Boots*	1 Pack/163g	259	2.1	159	16.0	21.0	1.3	2.5
Chicken, Roast, Tesco*	1 Pack/158g	412	19.8	261	13.1	23.9	12.5	1.5
Chicken, Rustlers*	1 Pack/150g	346	14.2	231	16.3	20.1	9.5	0.0
Chicken, Salad, Aldi*	1 Pack/195g	338	4.5	173	11.5	23.8	2.3	2.0
Chicken, Salad, M & S*	1 Pack/226g	350	9.3	155	10.6	18.8	4.1	3.0
Chicken, Salad on Malted Bread, BGTY, Sainsbury's*	1 Pack/216g	346	7.3	160	12.7	19.7	3.4	2.7
Chicken, Shell*	1 Pack/121g	334	15.7	276	13.9	25.9	13.0	0.0
Chicken, Simply, Healthy Selection, Budgens*	1 Pack/148g	286	3.7	193	14.3	28.4	2.5	2.1
Chicken, Smokey, BGTY, Sainsbury's*	1 Pack/178g	276	1.8	155	11.1	25.6	1.0	0.0
Chicken, Southern Spiced, M & S*	1 Pack/179g	421	23.3	235	11.2	21.7	13.0	3.1

	Measure INFO/WEIGHT	per Measure KCAL	FAT	Nutrition Values per 100g / 100ml KCAL	PROT	CARB	FAT	FIBRE
SANDWICH								
Chicken, Spicy, Deep Filled, Co-Op*	1 Pack/216g	421	15.1	195	10.0	24.0	7.0	3.0
Chicken, Stuffing & Red Onion, Co-Op*	1 Pack/180g	360	10.6	200	13.0	22.4	5.9	2.7
Chicken, Sun Dried Tomato & Herb, Bells*	1 Pack/198g	400	18.8	202	10.2	18.9	9.5	0.0
Chicken, Tandoori, Finest, Tesco*	1 Pack/224g	421	16.8	188	10.8	19.2	7.5	1.4
Chicken, Tandoori, Waitrose*	1 Pack/181g	302	5.6	167	11.6	23.0	3.1	4.1
Chicken, Thai, BGTY, Sainsbury's*	1 Pack/196g	280	5.1	143	10.2	19.6	2.6	0.6
Chicken, Thai, Deep Fill, Spar*	1 Pack/143g	291	6.6	204	13.9	26.8	4.6	0.0
Chicken, Tomato & Basil, HE, Tesco*	1 Pack/176g	266	4.0	151	11.5	21.1	2.3	2.0
Chicken, Tomato & Rocket, LC, Tesco*	1 Pack/184g	285	3.9	155	10.3	23.4	2.1	2.6
Chicken, Triple, GFY, Asda*	1 Pack/230g	453	11.5	197	13.0	25.0	5.0	1.6
Chicken, Triple, Shapers, Boots*	1 Serving/228g	440	12.3	193	13.0	23.0	5.4	2.3
Chicken & Bacon, Antony Worrall Thompson's*	1 Pack/191g	577	27.3	302	16.0	25.9	14.3	2.1
Chicken & Bacon, Baton, Tesco*	1 Pack/201g	511	26.3	254	9.4	24.7	13.1	1.7
Chicken & Bacon, COU, M & S*	1 Pack/179g	250	3.6	140	13.5	15.8	2.0	3.8
Chicken & Bacon, Deep Fill, Ginsters*	1 Pack/200g	435	15.7	224	12.4	25.3	8.1	2.4
Chicken & Bacon, HE, Tesco*	1 Pack/155g	240	2.6	155	10.4	24.6	1.7	1.7
Chicken & Bacon, Healthy Living, Co-Op*	1 Pack/179g	277	3.4	155	12.3	21.8	1.9	3.4
Chicken & Bacon, HL, Tesco*	1 Pack/193g	318	6.2	165	13.5	19.5	3.2	2.7
Chicken & Bacon, M & S*	1 Pack/185g	509	27.2	275	15.9	20.2	14.7	2.1
Chicken & Bacon, on Pepper Bread, M & S*	1 Serving/177g	265	1.6	150	13.2	22.7	0.9	2.1
Chicken & Bacon, Roast, Boots*	1 Pack/175g	413	14.0	236	15.4	26.3	8.0	2.2
Chicken & Bacon, Shapers, Boots*	1 Pack/179g	317	9.0	177	14.0	19.0	5.0	3.1
Chicken & Bacon, Sutherland Deli*	1 Pack/169g	453	20.1	268	14.6	25.7	11.9	2.7
Chicken & Bacon, Waitrose*	1 Serving/191g	495	23.5	259	11.8	25.3	12.3	2.2
Chicken & Coleslaw, Tesco*	1 Pack/160g	305	7.1	191	12.0	25.7	4.4	2.4
Chicken & Coriander, Taste!*	1 Serving/159g	228	4.6	143	5.6	23.3	2.9	0.0
Chicken & Coriander, with Lime, BGTY, Sainsbury's*	1 Pack/168g	282	5.9	168	10.6	23.5	3.5	0.0
Chicken & Ham, Healthy Living, Co-Op*	1 Pack/150g	285	6.0	190	12.0	28.0	4.0	3.0
Chicken & Ham, HL, Tesco*	1 Serving/244g	327	2.7	134	13.2	17.9	1.1	1.3
Chicken & Ham, Oak Smoked, Big, Sainsbury's*	1 Pack/244g	461	17.6	189	12.3	18.8	7.2	0.0
Chicken & Ham, Roast, Ginsters*	1 Pack/180g	425	24.5	236	11.2	18.5	13.6	0.0
Chicken & Ham, Roast, Tesco*	1 Pack/228g	561	31.9	246	13.3	16.6	14.0	1.2
Chicken & Mayo, The Sandwich Company*	1 Pack/72g	251	10.7	348	17.8	35.9	14.8	0.0
Chicken & Mayo, Wholemeal, Sodhexo*	1 Pack/128g	346	17.4	270	13.1	24.0	13.6	3.6
Chicken & Mayonnaise, Country Harvest*	1 Pack/120g	268	9.0	223	13.1	27.6	7.5	0.0
Chicken & Mayonnaise, Simply, Oldfields*	1 Pack/128g	357	16.4	279	12.8	30.2	12.8	2.1
Chicken & Pepperonata, COU, M & S*	1 Pack/171g	240	2.9	140	10.4	20.9	1.7	1.3
Chicken & Pesto, Shapers, Boots*	1 Pack/181g	311	4.2	172	12.0	26.0	2.3	1.7
Chicken & Pesto Salad, Bells*	1 Pack/196g	430	22.9	220	12.0	16.6	11.7	0.0
Chicken & Salad, Bernard Matthews*	1 Pack/162g	269	8.4	166	7.0	22.7	5.2	0.0
Chicken & Salad, Best for You, BHS*	1 Pack/315g	992	16.7	315	23.2	43.1	5.3	3.3
Chicken & Salad, Co-Op*	1 Pack/195g	448	21.4	230	10.0	24.0	11.0	2.0
Chicken & Salad, COU, M & S*	1 Pack/194g	262	3.7	135	9.8	19.0	1.9	1.6
Chicken & Salad, Deep Filled, Tesco*	1 Pack/238g	440	19.5	185	13.1	14.6	8.2	2.8
Chicken & Salad, Deli-Lite, Brambles*	1 Pack/175g	268	2.3	153	11.7	23.7	1.3	2.0
Chicken & Salad, GFY, Asda*	1 Pack/194g	252	2.9	130	12.0	17.0	1.5	2.6
Chicken & Salad, Ham & Cheese, Twin, Tesco*	1 Pack/189g	434	21.5	230	10.8	21.1	11.4	2.3
Chicken & Salad, Healthy Living, Co-Op*	1 Pack/196g	265	3.5	135	10.4	19.1	1.8	3.9
Chicken & Salad, Heinz*	1 Pack/166g	331	15.9	200	8.6	19.9	9.6	2.0
Chicken & Salad, Low Fat, Heinz*	1 Pack/166g	246	2.2	148	11.8	22.3	1.3	5.3
Chicken & Salad, Low Fat, Waitrose*	1 Pack/188g	291	8.1	155	10.4	18.6	4.3	2.1
Chicken & Salad, Roast, COU, M & S*	1 Pack/196g	265	4.5	135	8.9	19.6	2.3	2.2
Chicken & Salad, Roast, Feel Good, Shell*	1 Pack/191g	326	9.0	171	9.8	22.4	4.7	0.0

S

	Measure INFO/WEIGHT	per Measure KCAL	FAT	Nutrition Values per 100g / 100ml KCAL	PROT	CARB	FAT	FIBRE
SANDWICH								
Chicken & Salad, Roast, Weight Watchers*	1 Pack/186g	266	8.0	143	10.3	15.8	4.3	2.8
Chicken & Salad, Sainsbury's*	1 Pack/240g	425	14.2	177	12.1	18.8	5.9	0.0
Chicken & Salad, Scottish Slimmers*	1 Pack/169g	275	6.4	163	9.5	22.8	3.8	1.8
Chicken & Salad, Shell*	1 Pack/201g	404	19.7	201	8.7	19.4	9.8	0.0
Chicken & Salad, Tesco*	1 Pack/193g	386	17.6	200	11.9	17.6	9.1	1.5
Chicken & Salad, Waitrose*	1 Pack/208g	406	19.8	195	10.3	17.1	9.5	2.5
Chicken & Salad, Wild Bean Cafe*	1 Pack/210g	273	1.0	130	12.4	18.9	0.5	2.8
Chicken & Salad, with Mayo, BGTY, Sainsbury's*	1 Serving/200g	314	4.8	157	12.0	21.9	2.4	0.0
Chicken & Salad, with Mayo, Roast, Big, Sainsbury's*	1 Pack/269g	559	23.9	208	11.0	20.9	8.9	9.0
Chicken & Stuffing, Antony Worrall Thompson's*	1 Pack/198g	485	28.3	245	16.0	13.1	14.3	2.8
Chicken & Stuffing, LC, Tesco*	1 Pack/172g	275	4.8	160	14.4	18.7	2.8	6.9
Chicken & Stuffing, M & S*	1 Pack/182g	400	12.6	220	13.9	24.5	6.9	2.5
Chicken & Stuffing, Roast, Deep Fill, Tesco*	1 Serving/220g	532	26.8	242	14.0	19.0	12.2	1.3
Chicken & Stuffing, Roast, Shapers, Boots*	1 Pack/186g	324	3.9	174	14.0	25.0	2.1	3.1
Chicken & Stuffing, Roast, Weight Watchers*	1 Pack/159g	283	4.5	178	14.1	24.2	2.8	3.1
Chicken & Stuffing, Shapers, Boots*	1 Serving/185g	327	5.2	177	13.0	25.0	2.8	2.2
Chicken & Stuffing, Sutherland*	1 Pack/201g	505	25.8	251	11.9	22.1	12.8	3.0
Chicken & Stuffing, Waitrose*	1 Pack/183g	450	18.8	246	12.8	25.6	10.3	1.5
Chicken & Sweet Chilli, Flora Light, Flora*	1 Pack/154g	296	5.7	192	13.1	27.0	3.7	1.9
Chicken & Sweetcorn, Scottish Slimmers*	1 Pack/147g	289	7.2	197	11.1	27.4	4.9	2.2
Chicken & Sweetcorn, Shapers, Boots*	1 Pack/180g	324	6.3	180	12.0	25.0	3.5	2.0
Chicken & Sweetcorn with Mayo, Benedicts*	1 Pack/185g	437	19.8	236	12.2	20.6	10.7	0.0
Chicken & Watercress, Chargrilled, M & S*	1 Pack/173g	285	2.9	165	12.8	23.9	1.7	2.1
Chicken & Watercress, COU, M & S*	1 Pack/164g	266	2.8	162	12.8	23.9	1.7	2.1
Chicken Jalfrezi, Deep Fill, Ginsters*	1 Pack/171g	389	14.6	227	8.4	29.3	8.5	1.7
Chicken Tikka, Asda*	1 Pack/186g	316	8.7	170	11.0	21.0	4.7	1.5
Chicken Tikka, COU, M & S*	1 Pack/185g	268	3.3	145	12.1	20.5	1.8	3.2
Chicken Tikka, HE, Tesco*	1 Pack/159g	270	4.3	170	14.5	21.9	2.7	1.8
Chicken Tikka, M & S*	1 Pack/180g	391	19.6	217	10.4	19.5	10.9	2.0
Chicken Tikka, on Pepper Chilli Bread, Shapers, Boots*	1 Pack/172g	296	4.5	172	13.0	25.0	2.6	2.5
Chicken Tikka, Taste!*	1 Pack/196g	368	11.7	188	11.7	21.7	6.0	0.0
Chicken Tikka, Thai Style, Korma, Big, Sainsbury's*	1 Pack/268g	581	26.0	217	11.9	20.5	9.7	0.0
Chicken Tikka, Weight Watchers*	1 Pack/158g	250	2.2	158	13.1	23.2	1.4	2.9
Chicken Tikka & Yoghurt, Taste!*	1 Pack/215g	437	21.1	203	8.2	20.4	9.8	0.0
Chicken Tikka Masala, Go Foods Wonderfill*	1 Pack/136g	343	17.4	252	11.4	23.5	12.8	0.0
Corned Beef, on White, Simply, Brambles*	1 Pack/126g	325	10.8	258	14.2	30.8	8.6	1.4
Corned Beef, Tomato & Onion, Salad Garden*	1 Pack/137g	338	14.8	247	14.2	23.0	10.8	0.0
Crayfish & Lemon Mayonnaise, Daily Bread*	1 Pack/173g	391	11.4	226	9.5	31.0	6.6	0.0
Crayfish & Rocket, Bells*	1 Pack/144g	276	11.8	192	11.2	18.4	8.2	2.0
Crayfish & Rocket, Bistro, Waitrose*	1 Pack/193g	422	19.5	219	11.5	20.4	10.1	2.4
Crayfish & Rocket, Shapers, Boots*	1 Pack/172g	291	3.8	169	11.0	26.0	2.2	2.5
Cream Cheese, Red Pepper & Spinach, Daily Bread*	1 Pack/156g	273	8.1	175	7.4	24.0	5.2	0.0
Cream Cheese & Ham, Tesco*	1 Pack/212g	655	36.7	309	11.0	27.2	17.3	1.2
Cream Cheese & Peppers, Taste!*	1 Pack/154g	296	10.5	192	7.3	25.5	6.8	0.0
Cream Cheese & Salad, Sandwich Box*	1 Pack/138g	250	8.0	181	5.6	26.3	5.8	0.0
Cumberland Sausage, Ginsters*	1 Pack/210g	564	29.5	268	9.3	26.0	14.0	2.4
Duck, Peking, No Mayo, Boots*	1 Pack/222g	399	10.2	180	7.7	27.0	4.6	1.7
Edam, Oldfields*	1 Pack/175g	326	9.9	186	9.8	23.9	5.7	0.0
Edam & Tomato, Low Fat, Oldfields*	1 Pack/173g	306	6.4	177	9.6	26.3	3.7	2.7
Egg, Co-Op*	1 Pack/190g	285	7.0	150	6.8	22.1	3.7	3.7
Egg & Bacon, & Lincolnshire Sausage, Waitrose*	1 Pack/249g	655	32.9	263	11.3	24.7	13.2	0.9
Egg & Bacon, Deep Fill, Ginsters*	1 Pack/216g	503	21.8	233	14.5	21.0	10.1	2.3
Egg & Bacon, Handmade, Tesco*	1 Pack/217g	489	20.4	225	13.4	20.8	9.4	2.0

	Measure INFO/WEIGHT	per Measure KCAL	FAT	Nutrition Values per 100g / 100ml KCAL	PROT	CARB	FAT	FIBRE
SANDWICH								
Egg & Bacon, Weight Watchers*	1 Pack/139g	246	5.0	177	10.1	26.1	3.6	1.9
Egg & Bacon Mayo, Delifresh*	1 Pack/129g	310	12.6	240	10.1	29.7	9.8	2.1
Egg & Cress, BGTY, Sainsbury's*	1 Pack/145g	268	7.5	185	9.1	25.4	5.2	2.7
Egg & Cress, Co-Op*	1 Pack/159g	398	23.8	250	9.0	21.0	15.0	2.0
Egg & Cress, COU, M & S*	1 Pack/192g	240	5.2	125	9.8	15.5	2.7	2.8
Egg & Cress, Free Range, M & S*	1 Pack/192g	307	9.0	160	10.7	17.8	4.7	3.0
Egg & Cress, Free Range, Sainsbury's*	1 Pack/204g	404	16.9	198	10.5	20.3	8.3	3.3
Egg & Cress, Heinz*	1 Pack/200g	610	21.6	305	14.4	37.5	10.8	4.0
Egg & Cress, M & S*	1 Pack/182g	331	17.7	182	10.1	13.6	9.7	3.2
Egg & Cress, No Mayo, LC, Tesco*	1 Pack/160g	280	7.2	175	9.4	23.7	4.5	3.0
Egg & Cress, on Wheat Germ Bread, Tesco*	1 Pack/150g	255	6.9	169	9.5	21.7	4.6	1.4
Egg & Cress, Organic, M & S*	1 Pack/185g	444	26.3	240	9.6	18.0	14.2	3.6
Egg & Cress, Reduced Fat, Asda*	1 Pack/164g	290	8.7	177	9.8	22.4	5.3	0.0
Egg & Cress, Reduced Fat, Waitrose*	1 Pack/162g	262	10.4	162	9.7	16.5	6.4	6.4
Egg & Ham, Asda*	1 Pack/262g	590	33.5	225	10.4	16.8	12.8	2.1
Egg & Salad, Co-Op*	1 Pack/190g	285	7.6	150	7.0	22.0	4.0	4.0
Egg & Salad, Deep Filled, Asda*	1 Pack/231g	395	16.2	171	8.0	19.0	7.0	1.0
Egg & Salad, Free Range, Sainsbury's*	1 Pack/225g	449	16.8	200	8.5	24.5	7.5	0.0
Egg & Salad, GFY, Asda*	1 Pack/157g	229	4.5	146	8.0	22.0	2.9	2.9
Egg & Salad, Shapers, Boots*	1 Pack/184g	304	8.5	165	6.9	24.0	4.6	1.1
Egg & Salad, Weight Watchers*	1 Pack/172g	237	4.6	138	7.1	21.3	2.7	2.2
Egg & Salad, with Mayonnaise, Wholemeal, Waitrose*	1 Pack/180g	257	8.8	143	8.3	16.5	4.9	3.6
Egg & Tomato, Delicious, Boots*	1 Pack/218g	362	10.0	166	8.2	22.0	4.6	2.0
Egg & Tomato, on Softgrain Bread, Daily Bread*	1 Pack/160g	279	7.1	174	8.6	23.8	4.4	0.0
Egg & Tomato, Organic, Waitrose*	1 Pack/192g	359	18.6	187	9.7	15.3	9.7	4.0
Egg & Tomato, Tesco*	1 Pack/172g	311	10.8	181	8.5	22.6	6.3	2.3
Egg & Tomato, with Salad Cream, Big, Sainsbury's*	1 Pack/266g	463	15.4	174	9.1	21.3	5.8	0.0
Egg Mayo, Free Range, Asda*	1 Sandwich/178g	311	10.1	175	9.3	21.5	5.7	2.1
Egg Mayo, Free Range, on Oatmeal Bread, M & S*	1 Pack/180g	315	12.2	175	9.4	18.2	6.8	2.8
Egg Mayonnaise, & Bacon, Boots*	1 Serving/200g	426	14.0	213	13.5	23.5	7.0	2.8
Egg Mayonnaise, & Cress, Co-Op*	1 Pack/159g	405	24.0	255	8.8	20.8	15.1	1.9
Egg Mayonnaise, & Cress, Go Simple, Asda*	1 Pack/169g	370	18.6	219	10.0	20.0	11.0	1.7
Egg Mayonnaise, & Cress, Millers*	1 Pack/166g	369	20.3	222	9.4	18.8	12.2	0.0
Egg Mayonnaise, & Cress, Reduced Fat, Waitrose*	1 Pack/162g	300	12.8	185	10.4	18.1	7.9	3.4
Egg Mayonnaise, & Cress, Shapers, Boots*	1 Pack/156g	292	7.6	187	11.0	25.0	4.9	2.6
Egg Mayonnaise, & Cress, Weight Watchers*	1 Pack/126g	238	4.2	189	8.8	31.1	3.3	3.3
Egg Mayonnaise, & Gammon Ham, Strollers*	1 Pack/170g	400	19.3	236	13.0	20.5	11.4	0.0
Egg Mayonnaise, & Iceburg Lettuce, Northern Bites*	1 Serving/152g	333	17.2	219	7.7	20.9	11.3	0.0
Egg Mayonnaise, & Salad, Superdrug*	1 Pack/169g	286	12.3	169	7.6	18.3	7.3	2.4
Egg Mayonnaise, Boots*	1 Pack/184g	448	23.9	244	9.7	22.0	13.0	2.3
Egg Mayonnaise, Deep Fill, Benedicts*	1 Pack/195g	560	21.6	287	9.6	36.3	11.1	0.0
Egg Mayonnaise, Free Range, Finest, Tesco*	1 Pack/217g	412	19.1	190	10.9	16.8	8.8	2.3
Egg Mayonnaise, on Hi Bran Bread, Ginsters*	1 Pack/143g	343	21.7	240	10.7	17.6	15.2	0.0
Egg Mayonnaise, on Malted Wheatgrain, Taste!*	1 Serving/169g	394	20.8	233	10.6	20.0	12.3	0.0
Egg Mayonnaise, Shell*	1 Pack/189g	522	29.1	276	9.8	24.7	15.4	0.0
Egg Mayonnaise, Simply, Ginsters*	1 Serving/163g	365	15.9	224	10.1	24.0	9.8	3.1
Egg Mayonnaise, Snack & Shop, Esso*	1 Pack/240g	624	32.2	260	9.4	25.5	13.4	0.0
Egg Mayonnaise, Waitrose*	1 Pack/180g	396	20.5	220	10.1	19.1	11.4	3.4
Feta Cheese, & Salad, Tastte*	1 Pack/178g	367	13.4	206	10.6	24.0	7.5	0.0
Feta Cheese, Bells*	1 Pack/223g	468	26.3	210	7.1	18.8	11.8	0.0
Fish, Triple, Co-Op*	1 Serving/233g	420	9.3	180	10.0	26.0	4.0	3.0
Goats Cheese, & Chargrilled Vegetables, Finest, Tesco*	1 Pack/214g	482	19.7	225	7.7	27.8	9.2	1.4
Goat's Cheese, & Cranberry, Shapers, Boots*	1 Pack/150g	323	6.3	216	8.4	36.0	4.2	2.6

S

	Measure INFO/WEIGHT	per Measure KCAL	FAT	Nutrition Values per 100g / 100ml KCAL	PROT	CARB	FAT	FIBRE
SANDWICH								
Goat's Cheese, Sunblush Tomato, Deli Continental*	1 Pack/179g	480	29.4	268	9.5	20.5	16.4	0.0
Greek Salad, Classic, Cafe, Primo*	1 Serving/216g	513	26.9	238	8.6	23.1	12.5	1.8
Ham, Just Ham, Shoprite*	1 Pack/148g	286	7.1	193	12.4	25.0	4.8	0.0
Ham, M & S*	1 Pack/200g	220	5.2	110	17.2	3.2	2.6	0.0
Ham, Smoked, Fresh, Taste!*	1 Pack/187g	286	9.0	153	9.1	18.4	4.8	0.0
Ham & Cheese, & Mayo, Brown Bread, Mattessons*	1 Pack/172g	439	18.1	255	13.8	27.0	10.5	2.2
Ham & Cheese, & Pickle, Average	1 Pack/220g	524	25.1	238	12.2	21.6	11.4	2.5
Ham & Cheese, & Pickle, BGTY, Sainsbury's*	1 Sandwich/198g	325	5.0	164	14.0	21.3	2.5	2.1
Ham & Cheese, & Pickle, Deep Fill, Tesco*	1 Pack/225g	495	20.7	220	14.6	19.4	9.2	2.4
Ham & Cheese, & Pickle, Healthy Living, Co-Op*	1 Pack/185g	370	7.4	200	13.0	27.0	4.0	3.0
Ham & Cheese, & Pickle, Heinz*	1 Pack/188g	466	24.2	248	11.3	21.7	12.9	4.8
Ham & Cheese, & Pickle, in a Soft Wrap, Sainsbury's*	1 Pack/195g	503	23.2	258	10.9	26.8	11.9	0.9
Ham & Cheese, & Pickle, Taste!*	1 Pack/174g	414	21.7	238	11.1	20.3	12.5	0.0
Ham & Cheese, Ginsters*	1 Sandwich/170g	434	20.9	256	14.1	22.1	12.3	2.5
Ham & Cheese, LC, Tesco*	1 Pack/158g	284	5.1	180	14.5	22.8	3.2	5.0
Ham & Cheese, Morrisons*	1 Serving/183g	273	4.6	149	12.5	19.2	2.5	4.1
Ham & Coleslaw, Smoked, Brambles*	1 Pack/166g	283	4.1	171	8.2	28.8	2.5	1.8
Ham & Dijon Mustard, Healthy Selection, Budgens*	1 Pack/120g	190	3.0	158	9.7	21.9	2.5	2.0
Ham & Edam, Smoked, Shapers, Boots*	1 Pack/183g	315	11.9	172	9.3	19.0	6.5	2.7
Ham & Emmental, Tesco*	1 Pack/179g	305	6.8	170	10.7	22.1	3.8	1.3
Ham & Mustard, Ginsters*	1 Pack/140g	307	9.4	219	11.8	28.0	6.7	2.5
Ham & Mustard, Heinz*	1 Pack/180g	460	20.7	255	11.8	25.6	11.5	5.0
Ham & Mustard, Smoked, Tesco*	1 Pack/131g	315	11.4	240	11.5	28.0	8.7	1.4
Ham & Mustard, Tesco*	1 Pack/147g	437	27.9	297	10.6	20.8	19.0	1.2
Ham & Mustard Mayo, on White, Urban Eat*	1 Pack/130g	299	11.2	230	11.0	27.2	8.6	1.4
Ham & Philadelphia Light, Dry Cured, Boots*	1 Pack/172g	339	9.3	197	12.8	24.4	5.4	2.5
Ham & Pineapple Salsa, Maple Flavoured, Waitrose*	1 Pack/194g	329	8.9	170	8.4	23.8	4.6	3.1
Ham & Salad, Foo-Go*	1 Pack/178g	297	7.1	167	9.8	22.9	4.0	0.0
Ham & Salad, Ginsters*	1 Pack/179g	287	6.2	160	8.8	23.6	3.4	0.0
Ham & Salad, Healthy, Spar*	1 Serving/181g	286	6.7	158	8.4	22.7	3.7	0.0
Ham & Salad, Shapers, Boots*	1 Pack/195g	269	2.7	138	9.4	22.0	1.4	1.8
Ham & Salad, Smoked, Ainsley Harriott*	1 Pack/218g	307	6.3	141	8.9	19.9	2.9	0.0
Ham & Salad, Smoked, Taste!*	1 Serving/188g	309	9.7	164	9.8	19.8	5.2	0.0
Ham & Salad, Snack & Shop, Esso*	1 Pack/191g	304	6.5	159	9.2	22.9	3.4	5.0
Ham & Salad, Wild Bean Cafe*	1 Pack/212g	301	5.5	142	10.7	18.8	2.6	2.0
Ham & Salad, with Mustard, Finest, Tesco*	1 Pack/200g	466	21.0	233	15.3	19.3	10.5	1.3
Ham & Soft Cheese, Tesco*	1 Serving/164g	333	12.1	203	11.6	22.5	7.4	2.2
Ham & Swiss Cheese, Big, Sainsbury's*	1 Pack/218g	652	36.4	299	11.6	25.4	16.7	0.5
Ham & Swiss Cheese, M & S*	1 Pack/159g	393	20.0	247	14.7	18.9	12.6	3.3
Ham & Tomato, GFY, Asda*	1 Pack/173g	254	2.9	147	10.0	23.0	1.7	1.4
Ham & Tomato, Honey Roast, Feel Good, Shell*	1 Pack/171g	388	18.8	227	9.8	22.1	11.0	0.0
Ham & Turkey, & Salad, Sutherland*	1 Pack/185g	303	4.8	164	9.8	25.2	2.6	0.0
Ham & Turkey, Healthy, Felix Van Den Berghe*	1 Pack/149g	263	5.9	177	9.4	26.2	4.0	0.0
Ham & Turkey with Salad, Co-Op*	1 Pack/188g	263	5.6	140	9.0	21.0	3.0	2.0
Hey Pesto, Cranks*	1 Pack/155g	427	22.5	275	10.0	24.9	14.5	2.5
Houmous & Carrot, Shapers, Boots*	1 Pack/204g	323	10.2	158	7.5	21.0	5.0	5.2
Houmous & Grilled Vegetable, Deep Filled, Dd's*	1 Pack/200g	314	6.0	157	6.4	26.2	3.0	1.5
Houmous & Olive Bread, Flora Light, Flora*	1 Pack/160g	258	9.2	161	5.0	22.4	5.8	1.9
Houmous Tomato, & Red Onion, Daily Bread*	1 Serving/184g	367	17.7	199	6.9	22.7	9.6	0.0
It's The Slaw, Cranks*	1 Pack/155g	465	26.2	300	8.6	27.4	16.9	1.9
King Prawn, Sainsbury's*	1 Pack/204g	424	16.3	208	11.6	22.3	8.0	0.0
King Prawn & Avocado, Finest, Tesco*	1 Pack/185g	370	16.6	200	9.1	19.6	9.0	2.5
King Prawn & Harissa, Foo-Go*	1 Pack/180g	282	6.8	157	9.1	21.6	3.8	3.4

	Measure INFO/WEIGHT	per Measure KCAL	FAT	Nutrition Values per 100g / 100ml KCAL	PROT	CARB	FAT	FIBRE
SANDWICH								
Mozzarella, Pesto & Pine Nuts, Sainsbury's*	1 Pack/180g	423	17.5	235	10.2	26.8	9.7	2.8
Mozzarella, Tomato, & Basil, Healthy Options, Oldfields*	1 Pack/175g	285	8.4	163	8.1	22.1	4.8	3.3
Mozzarella & Pepperoni, Sainsbury's*	1 Pack/171g	380	12.2	222	10.5	29.0	7.1	0.0
Mozzarella & Roast Vegetables, Felix Van Den Berghe*	1 Pack/158g	330	13.3	209	9.5	23.8	8.4	0.0
Mozzarella & Tomato, Waitrose*	1 Pack/193g	359	18.1	186	9.7	15.7	9.4	2.3
Mozzarella & Tomato Calzone, Waitrose*	1 Pack/175g	410	19.4	234	10.8	22.7	11.1	2.2
Mozzarella Italian Style, Taste!*	1 Pack/183g	390	19.4	213	9.2	20.1	10.6	2.0
New York Deli, Boots*	1 Pack/245g	397	12.5	162	10.0	19.0	5.1	1.7
New York Deli, Chosen By You, Asda*	1 Pack/200g	320	7.3	160	9.8	20.1	3.6	0.0
New York Deli, Extra Special, Asda*	1 Pack/201g	403	15.4	201	12.4	20.6	7.7	3.8
Ploughman's, Cheddar, Heinz*	1 Pack/208g	552	27.7	265	9.3	27.1	13.3	2.4
Ploughman's, Cheddar, Mature Vintage, Sainsbury's*	1 Pack/204g	439	20.2	215	9.3	22.3	9.9	0.0
Ploughman's, Cheddar Cheese, Deep Fill, Asda*	1 Pack/229g	471	22.9	206	9.0	20.0	10.0	4.3
Ploughman's, Cheddar Cheese, Gibsons*	1 Pack/198g	469	22.8	237	9.8	23.7	11.5	0.0
Ploughman's, Cheese, BGTY, Sainsbury's*	1 Pack/193g	326	8.1	169	9.8	22.8	4.2	3.6
Ploughman's, Cheese, Deep Fill, Sutherland*	1 Pack/220g	558	32.3	254	9.2	21.4	14.7	0.0
Ploughman's, Deep Fill, Ginsters*	1 Pack/232g	636	40.8	274	9.6	20.8	17.6	0.0
Ploughman's, Deep Fill, Tesco*	1 Pack/245g	551	27.4	225	10.9	20.2	11.2	1.4
Pork & Apple Sauce, Bells*	1 Pack/180g	341	8.1	190	11.5	26.1	4.5	0.0
Prawn, Crayfish & Rocket, Tesco*	1 Pack/193g	425	17.4	220	11.4	22.3	9.0	2.0
Prawn, Creme Fraiche, on Oatmeal Bread, Choice*	1 Pack/153g	265	5.2	173	11.7	23.8	3.4	1.9
Prawn, Egg & Chicken, Triple, Weight Watchers*	1 Pack/224g	367	6.0	164	10.2	24.8	2.7	2.9
Prawn, Marie Rose, Felix Van Den Berghe*	1 Pack/163g	372	16.3	228	12.8	21.9	10.0	0.0
Prawn, Marie Rose, Fulfilled*	1 Pack/149g	292	6.1	196	13.4	26.3	4.1	0.0
Prawn, Marie Rose, Waitrose*	1 Pack/164g	226	5.6	138	8.8	18.0	3.4	1.9
Prawn, Mayo, Tomato & Lettuce, Deep Fill, Benedicts*	1 Pack/200g	330	7.8	165	10.2	21.9	3.9	0.0
Prawn, Salad, COU, M & S*	1 Pack/200g	230	3.6	115	8.0	16.6	1.8	3.8
Prawn, Shell*	1 Pack/209g	523	27.4	250	9.4	23.7	13.1	0.0
Prawn, Thai Style, Ginsters*	1 Pack/183g	313	9.0	171	9.2	22.5	4.9	0.0
Prawn & Egg, Deep Filled, Asda*	1 Pack/250g	570	30.0	228	12.0	17.0	12.0	2.3
Prawn & Salmon, Waitrose*	1 Pack/154g	345	14.6	224	12.5	22.0	9.5	2.8
Prawn & Thai Dressing, Tiger, Waitrose*	1 Pack/200g	342	8.6	171	9.6	23.6	4.3	2.2
Prawn Cocktail, Classic, Heinz*	1 Pack/193g	409	16.8	212	8.4	25.0	8.7	2.5
Prawn Cocktail, Jumbo Tiger, Benedicts*	1 Serving/225g	349	10.8	155	7.4	20.4	4.8	0.0
Prawn Cocktail, Platter, M & S*	1 Sandwich/200g	460	25.6	230	8.1	22.3	12.8	2.2
Prawn Cocktail, Waitrose*	1 Pack/196g	300	8.0	153	8.3	20.7	4.1	2.5
Prawn Cocktail, Weight Watchers*	1 Pack/168g	252	7.7	150	8.9	18.1	4.6	2.8
Prawn Mayonnaise, Cafe Collection*	1 Pack/165g	454	27.7	275	11.6	20.7	16.8	1.7
Prawn Mayonnaise, Co-Op*	1 Pack/154g	285	6.0	185	9.7	27.3	3.9	3.2
Prawn Mayonnaise, COU, M & S*	1 Pack/155g	240	3.6	155	10.2	22.9	2.3	2.8
Prawn Mayonnaise, Daily Bread*	1 Pack/157g	374	17.2	239	11.9	23.0	11.0	0.0
Prawn Mayonnaise, GFY, Asda*	1 Pack/160g	251	4.5	157	10.0	23.0	2.8	2.8
Prawn Mayonnaise, Ginsters*	1 Pack/160g	397	21.1	248	9.1	23.3	13.2	2.4
Prawn Mayonnaise, Heinz*	1 Pack/180g	493	28.4	274	8.9	24.0	15.8	2.5
Prawn Mayonnaise, M & S*	1 Pack/156g	328	12.0	210	10.0	24.7	7.7	2.2
Prawn Mayonnaise, Nutritionally Balanced, M & S*	1 Pack/162g	300	10.7	185	10.2	21.2	6.6	1.9
Prawn Mayonnaise, Oatmeal Bread, Co-Op*	1 Pack/159g	445	22.3	280	11.0	28.0	14.0	2.0
Prawn Mayonnaise, Oatmeal Bread, Waitrose*	1 Pack/180g	463	27.0	257	10.2	20.4	15.0	3.2
Prawn Mayonnaise, Origin Foods*	1 Pack/149g	355	18.5	238	9.3	22.4	12.4	2.0
Prawn Mayonnaise, Sainsbury's*	1 Pack/151g	323	14.0	214	11.6	20.9	9.3	0.0
Prawn Mayonnaise, Sayers Bakery*	1 Pack/155g	449	27.7	290	9.7	22.5	17.9	2.1
Prawn Mayonnaise, Shapers, Boots*	1 Pack/160g	293	7.5	183	9.4	25.6	4.7	2.5
Prawn Mayonnaise, Triple, Asda*	1 Pack/248g	635	39.7	256	9.0	19.0	16.0	3.4

	Measure INFO/WEIGHT	per Measure KCAL	FAT	Nutrition Values per 100g / 100ml KCAL	PROT	CARB	FAT	FIBRE
SANDWICH								
Prawn Mayonnaise, Upper Crust*	1 Pack/208g	343	10.4	165	9.2	20.9	5.0	0.0
Salad, Falafel & Houmous, Spicy, Delifresh*	1 Pack/209g	429	19.7	205	6.1	24.0	9.4	2.6
Salad, Healthy, Cambridge University Catering*	1 Pack/156g	246	4.4	158	5.9	27.4	2.8	0.0
Salad, Northern Bites*	1 Pack/210g	193	4.2	92	4.1	15.3	2.0	3.0
Salad, Serious About Sandwiches*	1 Pack/237g	322	11.6	136	5.8	17.1	4.9	0.8
Salad, Simply, Shapers, Boots*	1 Pack/216g	300	6.3	139	5.2	23.0	2.9	1.8
Salad, Taste!*	1 Serving/200g	246	6.5	123	4.4	18.9	3.2	0.0
Salad & Salad Cream, Fulfilled*	1 Pack/172g	244	7.1	142	4.9	21.5	4.1	0.0
Salmon & Black Pepper, Smoked, Fulfilled*	1 Pack/120g	293	10.3	244	13.8	29.0	8.6	0.0
Salmon & Cucumber, Brown Bread, Waitrose*	1 Pack/150g	296	10.6	197	10.5	22.7	7.1	1.4
Salmon & Cucumber, Healthly Choice, Sutherland*	1 Pack/164g	321	9.2	196	9.8	26.6	5.6	0.0
Salmon & Cucumber, M & S*	1 Pack/168g	329	13.9	196	11.0	19.5	8.3	2.6
Salmon & Cucumber, Red, Healthy Choice, Asda*	1 Pack/149g	285	11.5	191	10.6	19.9	7.7	2.1
Salmon & Cucumber, Red, Tesco*	1 Pack/144g	284	9.2	197	11.1	23.8	6.4	1.9
Salmon & Cucumber, White Bread, Waitrose*	1 Pack/161g	305	8.6	189	9.8	25.5	5.3	1.7
Salmon & Rocket, Poached, M & S*	1 Pack/180g	495	26.8	275	13.5	21.2	14.9	2.1
Salmon & Soft Cheese, Feel Good, Shell*	1 Pack/174g	404	12.9	232	13.5	28.0	7.4	1.0
Salmon & Soft Cheese, Smoked, Waitrose*	1 Pack/154g	300	10.0	195	14.8	19.2	6.5	4.2
Salmon & Spinach, Poached, Shapers, Boots*	1 Pack/168g	284	7.6	169	9.2	23.0	4.5	3.1
Salmon Poached, Prawn & Rocket, Waitrose*	1 Pack/166g	308	8.6	186	11.2	23.5	5.2	2.1
Salsa Chicken, HL, Tesco*	1 Pack/182g	300	3.3	165	13.4	23.6	1.8	1.9
Sausage, Egg & Bacon, Boots*	1 Pack/325g	887	52.0	273	9.3	23.0	16.0	2.2
Sausage, Speedy Snacks*	1 Serving/93g	258	9.4	279	11.6	35.2	10.2	0.0
Sausage, Triple Pack, GFY, Asda*	1 Pack/215g	424	9.7	197	9.0	30.0	4.5	2.3
Seafood, Mixed, Tesco*	1 Pack/184g	502	30.9	273	7.3	23.2	16.8	0.8
Seafood Cocktail, Asda*	1 Pack/190g	486	30.0	256	6.7	21.3	15.8	1.6
Seafood Cocktail, Daily Bread*	1 Pack/147g	292	6.9	199	8.3	31.0	4.7	0.0
Seafood Cocktail, Waitrose*	1 Pack/210g	267	6.3	127	7.3	17.6	3.0	8.1
Seafood Medley, M & S*	1 Pack/227g	468	28.1	206	7.2	16.3	12.4	3.5
Soft Cheese & Roasted Pepper, Weight Watchers*	1 Pack/158g	289	6.0	183	9.4	27.7	3.8	1.5
Sub, Beef & Onion, M & S*	1 Pack/207g	611	31.7	295	13.3	25.6	15.3	1.5
Sub, Beef & Onion, Roast, Sainsbury's*	1 Serving/174g	426	17.4	245	9.4	29.3	10.0	0.0
Sub, Chicken & Bacon, Compass Foods*	1 Pack/165g	450	20.1	273	12.2	28.7	12.2	0.0
Sub, Chicken & Bacon, Sainsbury's*	1 Pack/190g	554	27.0	291	13.4	27.4	14.2	0.8
Sub, Chicken & Salad, Asda*	1 Sub/200g	460	27.2	230	9.4	17.4	13.6	0.9
Sub, Chicken & Stuffing, Shell*	1 Serving/183g	437	11.7	239	13.3	32.0	6.4	0.0
Sub, Chicken Caesar, Sainsbury's*	1 Roll/210g	590	34.4	281	11.3	22.1	16.4	1.9
Sub, Egg Mayonnaise, Daily Bread*	1 Pack/165g	441	22.3	267	9.6	29.6	13.5	0.0
Sub, Ham, & Tomato Salad, Shapers, Boots*	1 Pack/170g	286	3.9	168	9.2	28.0	2.3	1.4
Sub, Turkey, Stuffing, & Cranberry, Sainsbury's*	1 Sub/265g	603	19.1	227	10.6	29.2	7.2	1.9
Sweet Chilli Chicken, in Pitta Bread, Shapers, Boots*	1 Pack/178g	245	5.0	138	9.2	19.0	2.8	2.2
Sweet Chilli Chicken, Special Edition, Ginsters*	1 Pack/172g	351	9.5	204	12.5	26.3	5.5	2.3
Tuna, Heinz*	1 Serving/183g	277	2.9	151	12.3	21.6	1.6	6.8
Tuna, Mediterranean, COU, M & S*	1 Pack/260g	364	5.7	140	10.3	19.6	2.2	1.6
Tuna, Melt, Swedish Bread, Shapers, Boots*	1 Pack/163g	254	3.6	156	14.0	20.0	2.2	2.1
Tuna, Nicoise, Taste!*	1 Pack/218g	404	14.4	185	11.3	20.1	6.6	0.0
Tuna & Celery, Waitrose*	1 Pack/168g	254	6.1	151	10.2	19.5	3.6	3.0
Tuna & Chargrilled Vegetables, BGTY, Sainsbury's*	1 Pack/196g	329	8.6	168	10.7	21.5	4.4	0.0
Tuna & Cucumber, & Red Onion, Brambles*	1 Pack/161g	264	3.9	164	11.3	24.3	2.4	1.6
Tuna & Cucumber, Antony Worrall Thompson's*	1 Pack/188g	284	4.3	151	11.6	21.0	2.3	2.9
Tuna & Cucumber, BGTY, Sainsbury's*	1 Pack/178g	268	3.2	151	11.3	22.3	1.8	3.1
Tuna & Cucumber, BHS*	1 Pack/210g	479	24.2	228	10.8	24.2	11.5	1.2
Tuna & Cucumber, Feel Good, Shell*	1 Pack/214g	518	16.0	242	12.6	31.2	7.5	0.0

S

	Measure INFO/WEIGHT	per Measure KCAL	FAT	Nutrition Values per 100g / 100ml KCAL	PROT	CARB	FAT	FIBRE
SANDWICH								
Tuna & Cucumber, Finest, Tesco*	1 Pack/169g	380	16.7	225	10.2	23.4	9.9	2.7
Tuna & Cucumber, Healthy Living, Co-Op*	1 Pack/192g	250	3.5	130	10.9	17.9	1.8	3.0
Tuna & Cucumber, Less Than 350 Cals, Ginsters*	1 Serving/193g	298	7.5	154	10.8	19.0	3.9	3.1
Tuna & Cucumber, on Oatmeal Bread, Ginsters*	1 Pack/175g	290	7.2	166	11.7	20.7	4.1	2.4
Tuna & Cucumber, Perfectly Balanced, Waitrose*	1 Pack/178g	240	3.6	135	11.0	18.3	2.0	3.6
Tuna & Cucumber, Shell*	1 Pack/188g	431	19.2	229	12.3	21.9	10.2	0.0
Tuna & Cucumber, Weight Watchers*	1 Pack/173g	279	2.9	161	11.4	25.1	1.7	1.4
Tuna & Cucumber, You Count, Love Life, Waitrose*	1 Pack/195g	321	5.3	165	13.0	21.4	2.7	1.4
Tuna & Green Pesto, BGTY, Sainsbury's*	1 Pack/211g	279	4.7	132	11.0	17.0	2.2	0.0
Tuna & Lemon Mayo, Shapers, Boots*	1 Pack/206g	318	9.7	154	10.0	18.0	4.7	1.7
Tuna & Salad, Bloomer, M & S*	1 Pack/231g	600	36.9	260	11.8	17.8	16.0	2.6
Tuna & Salad, Classic*	1 Pack/230g	449	15.9	195	8.7	27.3	6.9	2.1
Tuna & Salad, M & S*	1 Pack/250g	575	31.5	230	12.5	16.8	12.6	2.1
Tuna & Salad, Tesco*	1 Pack/197g	339	14.6	172	9.9	16.5	7.4	2.8
Tuna & Sweetcorn, & Red Onion, Co-Op*	1 Pack/256g	614	28.2	240	11.0	23.0	11.0	4.0
Tuna & Sweetcorn, BGTY, Sainsbury's*	1 Pack/187g	309	5.1	165	10.8	24.7	2.7	2.8
Tuna & Sweetcorn, COU, M & S*	1 Pack/180g	270	4.3	150	12.6	19.0	2.4	3.8
Tuna & Sweetcorn, Felix Van Den Berghe*	1 Pack/129g	372	16.0	289	10.4	29.3	12.4	0.0
Tuna & Sweetcorn, Ginsters*	1 Pack/169g	348	11.4	205	9.6	26.4	6.7	2.4
Tuna & Sweetcorn, Heinz*	1 Pack/208g	528	27.5	254	10.4	23.5	13.2	1.6
Tuna & Sweetcorn, on Malt Bread, Tesco*	1 Pack/175g	350	8.2	200	11.6	27.5	4.7	2.2
Tuna & Sweetcorn, Sainsbury's*	1 Pack/183g	392	15.6	214	12.1	22.3	8.5	0.0
Tuna & Sweetcorn, Shapers, Boots*	1 Pack/170g	295	4.4	174	12.4	25.3	2.6	2.0
Tuna & Tomato, & Onion, COU, M & S*	1 Pack/177g	250	4.2	141	11.1	18.8	2.4	2.2
Tuna Crunch, HL, Tesco*	1 Pack/180g	261	4.3	145	11.0	19.9	2.4	0.5
Tuna Crunch, Shapers, Boots*	1 Pack/200g	290	6.4	145	9.1	20.0	3.2	3.2
Tuna Mayonnaise, & Cucumber, Daily Bread*	1 Pack/190g	392	16.6	206	12.1	19.8	8.7	0.0
Tuna Mayonnaise, & Cucumber, Darwins Deli*	1 Pack/155g	370	14.6	239	9.6	21.9	9.4	0.0
Tuna Mayonnaise, & Cucumber, Simply, Boots*	1 Pack/200g	498	26.0	249	12.0	21.0	13.0	2.4
Tuna Mayonnaise, & Sweetcorn, Whistlestop*	1 Pack/140g	378	17.7	271	13.6	25.5	12.7	0.0
Tuna Mayonnaise, Menu, Boots*	1 Pack/182g	451	20.0	248	13.0	23.0	11.0	1.1
Tuna Mayonnaise, on White Bread, Oldfields*	1 Pack/142g	394	18.1	278	15.2	27.4	12.8	2.0
Tuna Mayonnaise, White Bread, Open Choice Foods*	1 Pack/120g	298	10.1	248	12.0	29.6	8.4	0.0
Turkey, Gibsons*	1 Pack/138g	260	5.3	188	12.5	26.0	3.8	0.0
Turkey, Northern Bites*	1 Pack/200g	354	8.6	177	11.9	22.8	4.3	0.0
Turkey, Smoked on Wholemeal, Sodhexo*	1 Pack/128g	259	6.1	202	16.1	23.8	4.8	3.6
Turkey, Stuffing & Cranberry, Boots*	1 Pack/192g	328	2.1	171	12.0	28.0	1.1	2.5
Turkey & Bacon, COU, M & S*	1 Pack/165g	256	4.0	155	12.0	21.0	2.4	1.7
Turkey & Cheese, & Bacon, Bernard Matthews*	1 Serving/192g	482	21.5	251	9.2	28.3	11.2	0.0
Turkey & Cranberry, COU, M & S*	1 Pack/180g	279	3.1	155	12.1	22.8	1.7	2.9
Turkey & Cranberry Salad, Fullfillers*	1 Serving/180g	319	5.8	177	13.0	23.3	3.2	0.0
Turkey & Lettuce & Tomato, Shapers, Boots*	1 Pack/217g	310	4.8	143	9.8	21.0	2.2	2.9
Turkey & Sage, & Mayonnaise, Bells*	1 Pack/164g	414	22.1	253	11.6	21.2	13.5	0.0
Turkey & Salad, Brambles*	1 Pack/170g	248	2.0	146	9.3	24.5	1.2	2.0
Turkey & Salad, Fullfillers*	1 Serving/218g	320	7.0	147	10.3	18.6	3.2	0.0
Turkey & Salad, Healthy Eating, Wild Bean Cafe*	1 Serving/230g	315	2.5	137	10.0	21.5	1.1	1.8
Turkey & Stuffing, & Bacon, Bernard Matthews*	1 Pack/127g	250	8.7	196	12.0	21.6	6.8	2.0
Turkey & Stuffing, M & S*	1 Pack/190g	352	9.3	185	12.3	23.1	4.9	1.9
Turkey & Sun Dried Tomato, Festive Feast, Taste!*	1 Pack/159g	401	22.1	252	8.8	23.0	13.9	0.0
Turkey with All the Christmas Trimmings, Tesco*	1 Pack/189g	425	14.2	225	10.8	28.0	7.5	1.9
Vegetable, M & S*	1 Serving/180g	252	4.1	140	6.1	23.5	2.3	2.1
Vegetable, Roasted, Open, COU, M & S*	1 Pack/150g	260	2.2	173	8.4	31.3	1.5	4.4
Vegetable & Chilli Bean, Roasted, M & S*	1 Pack/200g	340	11.4	170	5.2	24.5	5.7	2.1

	Measure INFO/WEIGHT	per Measure KCAL	FAT	Nutrition Values per 100g / 100ml KCAL	PROT	CARB	FAT	FIBRE
SANDWICH FILLER								
Beef & Onion, Deli, Asda*	1 Serving/50g	78	6.5	157	10.0	0.1	13.0	1.1
Big Breakfast, Asda*	1 Serving/125g	314	26.2	251	12.0	3.5	21.0	0.5
Cajun Chicken, Sainsbury's*	1 Serving/60g	109	8.1	182	13.4	1.8	13.5	1.8
Chargrilled Vegetable, Sainsbury's*	½ Pot/85g	192	19.3	226	3.4	2.2	22.7	0.6
Cheese & Bacon, Tesco*	1 Serving/50g	199	18.8	398	12.2	2.6	37.6	1.2
Cheese & Ham, Sainsbury's*	1 Serving/25g	124	12.3	497	12.4	0.8	49.3	0.3
Cheese & Onion, Reduced Fat, Supermarket, Average	1 Serving/100g	227	18.1	227	11.8	4.4	18.1	1.7
Cheese & Onion, Supermarket, Average	1 Serving/100g	405	38.6	405	10.2	4.1	38.6	1.3
Cheese & Onion, Tesco*	1 Pack/170g	721	72.4	424	10.0	0.2	42.6	1.5
Cheese & Spring Onion, M & S*	1 Serving/56g	199	18.8	355	8.5	5.0	33.6	0.2
Chicken, Bacon & Sweetcorn, BGTY, Sainsbury's*	1 Tub/300g	399	18.3	133	14.0	5.5	6.1	0.5
Chicken, Stuffing & Bacon, COU, M & S*	1 Pack/170g	170	3.7	100	13.1	6.2	2.2	1.3
Chicken, Sweetcorn & Bacon, Tesco*	1 Serving/50g	167	14.8	334	12.3	4.3	29.7	1.6
Chicken, Sweetcorn & Sage, HE, Tesco*	1 Serving/125g	105	1.6	84	9.4	8.8	1.3	1.3
Chicken, Tomato & Sweetcure Bacon, M & S*	1 Pot/170g	502	44.9	295	11.4	2.8	26.4	0.7
Chicken, with Salad Vegetables, Heinz*	1 Serving/56g	114	8.5	203	5.1	11.7	15.1	0.5
Chicken & Bacon with Sweetcorn, Sainsbury's*	1 Serving/60g	123	9.4	205	12.0	4.0	15.7	0.9
Chicken & Stuffing, Sainsbury's*	½ Tub/120g	397	37.8	331	6.5	5.3	31.5	1.7
Chicken & Sweetcorn, Sainsbury's*	1 Tub/170g	396	33.7	233	11.0	2.7	19.8	1.9
Chicken Caesar, BGTY, Sainsbury's*	½ Jar/85g	117	6.1	137	15.6	2.5	7.2	2.2
Chicken Fajita, Tesco*	1 Serving/50g	78	4.2	155	13.8	5.9	8.5	1.4
Chicken Tikka, BGTY, Sainsbury's*	½ Pot/85g	99	2.6	117	16.5	6.0	3.0	1.0
Chicken Tikka, HE, Tesco*	1 Serving/100g	110	3.6	110	7.1	12.4	3.6	1.0
Chicken Tikka, Mild, Heinz*	1 Serving/52g	102	7.3	196	5.2	12.3	14.0	0.7
Chicken Tikka & Citrus Raita, COU, M & S*	½ Pot/85g	76	1.7	90	12.6	4.9	2.0	0.9
Chickpea, Moroccan Style, Sainsbury's*	½ Tub/120g	160	9.4	133	4.1	11.7	7.8	4.2
Corned Beef & Onion, Deli, Asda*	1 Serving/50g	170	15.5	340	12.0	3.3	31.0	0.7
Coronation Chicken, 50 % Less Fat, Tesco*	1 Serving/50g	102	6.3	205	11.5	9.7	12.6	2.7
Coronation Chicken, BGTY, Sainsbury's*	1 Portion/50g	73	3.5	146	11.9	8.9	7.0	1.4
Coronation Chicken, Sainsbury's*	¼ Tub/60g	183	14.8	305	12.1	8.9	24.6	1.2
Coronation Chicken, Tesco*	1 Tbsp/30g	88	7.0	293	11.4	9.2	23.2	0.7
Coronation Tuna, BGTY, Sainsbury's*	1 Can/80g	90	2.1	112	16.5	5.7	2.6	1.0
Egg & Bacon, Free Range, Deli, Essential, Waitrose*	½ Pot/85g	267	23.6	314	12.7	3.3	27.8	0.5
Egg & Bacon, Fresh, Tesco*	1 Serving/45g	112	9.0	248	12.7	4.2	20.1	0.6
Egg & Salad Cream, Chosen By You, Asda*	1 Serving/100g	165	10.4	165	10.3	7.2	10.4	0.5
Egg Mayonnaise, 50% Less Fat, Chosen By You, Asda*	1 Serving/50g	67	4.2	134	10.3	4.2	8.3	0.5
Egg Mayonnaise, BGTY, Sainsbury's*	1 Serving/63g	71	4.1	113	10.2	3.4	6.5	0.1
Egg Mayonnaise, Chunky Free Range, Tesco*	1 Serving/50g	104	8.9	209	11.3	0.9	17.8	1.6
Egg Mayonnaise, Country Fresh, Aldi*	¼ Pack/50g	106	8.9	211	9.8	2.9	17.8	0.0
Egg Mayonnaise, Deli, Asda*	1 Serving/50g	114	10.0	227	11.0	0.8	20.0	0.3
Egg Mayonnaise, M & S*	1oz/28g	62	5.5	220	10.1	0.8	19.7	1.1
Egg Mayonnaise, Morrisons*	1 Serving/50g	71	5.3	142	10.0	1.7	10.6	0.0
Egg Mayonnaise & Bacon, Free Range, Co-Op*	1 Pot/200g	500	44.0	250	13.0	0.9	22.0	0.6
Egg Mayonnaise 50% Less Fat, Tesco*	1 Serving/50g	65	3.8	130	10.2	3.8	7.6	0.5
Egg Mayonniase, Reduced Fat, Tesco*	1 Serving/50g	50	2.6	100	11.0	1.0	5.3	3.5
Ham & Salad Vegetables, Heinz*	1oz/28g	57	4.5	204	5.3	10.0	15.9	0.4
Peppered Mackerel, Creamy, Shippam*	1 Serving/15g	27	2.8	177	7.8	6.5	18.6	0.0
Poached Salmon & Cucumber, Deli, M & S*	1 Pot/170g	348	27.7	205	14.0	1.0	16.3	0.5
Prawn Marie Rose, Sainsbury's*	1 Serving/60g	121	10.6	201	8.1	2.5	17.6	0.9
Prawn Mayonnaise, Deli, Asda*	1 Serving/50g	170	16.5	339	9.0	1.6	33.0	0.4
Prawn Mayonnaise, GFY, Asda*	1 Serving/57g	101	7.4	177	12.0	3.0	13.0	0.1
Prawn Mayonnaise, Waitrose*	1 Pot/170g	537	52.9	316	8.9	0.2	31.1	0.0
Seafood, BGTY, Sainsbury's*	1oz/28g	36	2.0	128	8.7	7.6	7.0	0.5

	Measure INFO/WEIGHT	per Measure KCAL	FAT	Nutrition Values per 100g / 100ml KCAL	PROT	CARB	FAT	FIBRE
SANDWICH FILLER								
Seafood Cocktail, M & S*	1oz/28g	76	6.7	272	6.4	8.2	23.8	0.2
Seafood Cocktail, Sainsbury's*	½ Tub/120g	314	27.6	262	5.7	8.1	23.0	1.0
Tuna, Carb Check, Heinz*	1 Serving/52g	84	6.2	161	6.6	6.3	12.0	0.7
Tuna, Tomato & Black Olive, BGTY, Sainsbury's*	1 Pack/100g	88	1.6	88	12.6	5.9	1.6	1.2
Tuna & Sweetcorn, Reduced Fat, Supermarket, Average	1 Serving/100g	119	5.4	119	11.5	5.8	5.4	1.2
Tuna & Sweetcorn, Supermarket, Average	1 Serving/100g	228	17.8	228	11.6	5.7	17.8	1.4
Tuna Mayonnaise, BGTY, Sainsbury's*	1 Serving/100g	114	3.4	114	17.6	3.5	3.4	0.1
Tuna Mayonnaise & Cucumber, Choice, Tesco*	1 Serving/200g	463	22.8	232	12.8	23.2	11.4	1.6
SANDWICH FILLING								
Baked Beans, Paste, British Classics, Princes*	1 Jar/75g	82	0.3	110	5.0	21.6	0.4	0.0
Cheese & Onion, Asda*	1 Serving/56g	288	28.5	515	9.8	4.4	50.9	0.3
Cheese & Onion, Co-Op*	1 Serving/56g	269	26.3	480	10.0	4.0	47.0	0.5
Cheese & Onion, GFY, Asda*	1 Serving/80g	206	16.8	257	11.0	6.0	21.0	0.8
Chicken & Bacon, Asda*	1 Serving/100g	341	29.0	341	17.0	3.0	29.0	0.5
Chicken & Sweetcorn, Asda*	1 Serving/60g	187	16.8	312	11.0	4.0	28.0	2.0
Chicken Tikka, Asda*	1 Serving/28g	80	5.6	284	13.0	13.0	20.0	0.7
Chicken Tikka, Less Than 5% Fat, Asda*	1 Serving/56g	65	2.6	116	11.0	7.3	4.7	1.2
Crab, BGTY, Sainsbury's*	1oz/28g	36	2.0	128	8.7	7.6	7.0	0.5
Egg Mayonnaise, Asda*	1oz/28g	72	6.5	258	10.3	1.9	23.3	0.7
Egg Mayonnaise, Co-Op*	1oz/28g	66	5.9	235	10.0	1.0	21.0	1.0
Egg Mayonnaise, with Chives, Asda*	1oz/28g	92	8.9	327	9.1	1.1	31.8	0.0
Houmous & Vegetable, Asda*	1/3 Tub/57g	133	9.7	233	8.0	12.0	17.0	3.5
Prawns, with Seafood Sauce, Asda*	1oz/28g	107	10.3	382	11.7	1.4	36.8	0.0
Sausage & Tomato, Paste, British Classics, Princes*	1 Jar/75g	163	11.1	217	14.6	6.3	14.8	0.0
Smokey Bacon, Paste, Princes*	1 Jar/75g	136	8.2	181	14.1	6.3	11.0	0.0
Tuna & Sweetcorn, Asda*	1oz/28g	83	7.4	295	8.2	6.0	26.5	0.6
Tuna & Sweetcorn, Reduced Fat, Co-Op*	1 Serving/50g	102	7.0	205	13.0	7.0	14.0	0.9
Tuna & Sweetcorn, Reduced Fat, Morrisons*	1oz/28g	48	2.9	172	13.2	6.9	10.2	0.0
SANDWICH SPREAD								
Beef, Classic, Shippam*	1 Pot/75g	133	8.8	177	15.5	2.2	11.8	0.0
Chicken, Classic, Shippam*	1 Serving/35g	64	4.4	182	15.5	1.8	12.5	0.0
Chicken & Bacon, Asda*	¼ Jar/43g	153	13.2	359	18.0	2.0	31.0	1.0
Chicken Tikka, Asda*	1 Serving/50g	77	5.0	154	7.0	9.0	10.0	0.2
Crab, Classic, Shippam*	1 Jar/35g	60	3.8	170	13.1	4.6	10.9	0.0
Heinz*	1 Tbsp/10ml	22	1.3	220	1.0	24.0	13.0	1.0
Light, Heinz*	1 Tbsp/10g	16	0.9	161	1.1	18.2	9.2	0.9
Salmon, Classic, Shippam*	1 Serving/35g	70	4.9	200	14.7	4.2	14.1	0.0
Tuna & Mayonnaise, Shippam*	1 Pot/75g	189	13.9	252	18.3	3.1	18.5	0.0
SARDINES								
Boneless, in Tomato Sauce, John West*	1 Can/120g	197	12.0	164	17.0	1.5	10.0	0.0
Grilled	***1oz/28g***	***55***	***2.9***	***195***	***25.3***	***0.0***	***10.4***	***0.0***
in BBQ Sauce, John West*	1 Tin/121g	177	7.7	146	16.1	6.2	6.4	0.0
in Brine, Canned, Drained	***1oz/28g***	***48***	***2.7***	***172***	***21.5***	***0.0***	***9.6***	***0.0***
in Oil, Canned, Drained	***1oz/28g***	***62***	***3.9***	***220***	***23.3***	***0.0***	***14.1***	***0.0***
in Olive Oil, Canned, Ambrosia*	1 Can/100g	320	13.7	320	22.3	0.7	13.7	0.0
in Peri Peri Sauce, John West*	1 Can/120g	181	12.3	150	12.3	2.3	10.2	0.3
in Tomato Sauce, Canned	1oz/28g	45	2.8	162	17.0	1.4	9.9	0.0
Raw, Whole, with Head	***1oz/28g***	***46***	***2.6***	***165***	***20.6***	***0.0***	***9.2***	***0.0***
SATAY								
Chicken, Breast, Iceland*	1 Satay/10g	15	0.1	155	34.1	2.7	0.9	0.1
Chicken, Breast, Party Bites, Sainsbury's*	1 Stick/10g	16	0.1	157	34.1	2.7	0.9	0.1
Chicken, GFY, Asda*	1 Serving/168g	242	6.1	144	22.0	6.0	3.6	0.8
Chicken, Indonesian, Charlie Bigham's*	½ Pack/300g	555	36.6	185	14.2	4.9	12.2	1.5

S

	Measure INFO/WEIGHT	per Measure KCAL	FAT	Nutrition Values per 100g / 100ml KCAL	PROT	CARB	FAT	FIBRE
SATAY								
Chicken, Indonesian, Mini, Sainsbury's*	1 Stick/10g	17	0.7	171	23.0	4.0	7.0	0.7
Chicken, Kebab, Waitrose*	½ Pack/125g	246	13.5	197	18.9	6.0	10.8	0.5
Chicken, M & S*	1 Satay/43g	90	5.5	210	19.1	4.4	12.7	0.7
Chicken, Mini, Iceland*	1 Satay/8g	19	1.1	236	23.0	4.5	14.0	0.7
Chicken, Occasions, Sainsbury's*	1 Satay/10g	15	0.6	150	22.0	2.0	6.0	0.7
Chicken, Oriental, Tesco*	1 Serving/100g	160	5.0	160	23.6	5.1	5.0	0.4
Chicken, Taste Original*	1 Stick/20g	33	1.3	164	23.0	2.5	6.5	0.7
Chicken, with Peanut Sauce, Waitrose*	1 Pack/250g	492	27.0	197	18.9	6.0	10.8	0.5
Chicken & Turkey, Sainsbury's*	1 Stick/20g	44	2.8	222	20.0	4.0	14.0	1.9
SATSUMAS								
Fresh, Raw, Flesh Only, Average	***1 Sm/56g***	***21***	***0.0***	***37***	***0.9***	***8.6***	***0.1***	***1.3***
Weighed with Peel, Average	***1 Sm/60g***	***22***	***0.1***	***37***	***0.9***	***8.6***	***0.1***	***0.9***
SAUCE								
Apple, Baxters*	1 Tsp/15g	7	0.1	49	0.1	11.1	0.4	0.7
Apple, Bramley, M & S*	1 Tbsp/15g	21	0.0	140	0.2	32.6	0.3	0.4
Apple, Bramley, Sainsbury's*	1 Tsp/15g	17	0.0	111	0.2	27.2	0.1	1.8
Apple, Heinz*	1 Tsp/15g	8	0.0	56	0.3	13.4	0.2	1.5
Apple & Brandy, Asda*	1 Serving/125g	56	0.0	45	0.2	11.0	0.0	0.0
Apricot & Almond Tagine, Sainsbury's*	1/3 Jar/120g	98	1.9	82	2.0	17.9	1.6	2.5
Arrabbiata, Don Pomodoro*	½ Pot/185g	231	20.4	125	0.5	6.0	11.0	0.0
Arrabbiata, Fresh, Waitrose*	1 Serving/100g	52	2.5	52	1.4	5.9	2.5	2.0
Arrabbiata, Italian, Tesco*	½ Pot/175g	72	0.5	41	1.3	8.3	0.3	1.1
Arrabbiata, Lazio, Sainsbury's*	1/3 Jar/113g	154	12.3	136	2.2	7.2	10.9	0.0
Arrabbiata, Weight Watchers*	½ Pot/150g	44	0.8	29	1.1	5.0	0.5	1.7
Balti, 97% Fat Free, Homepride*	1 Serving/230g	133	4.4	58	1.1	9.1	1.9	1.8
Balti, Cooking, BGTY, Sainsbury's*	¼ Jar/129g	98	4.0	76	1.1	10.9	3.1	0.6
Balti, Cooking, Indian Inspired, Asda*	1 Jar/320g	243	10.9	76	0.9	10.5	3.4	1.8
Balti, Cooking, Organic, Perfectly Balanced, Waitrose*	1 Jar/450g	302	5.8	67	1.6	12.1	1.3	3.1
Balti, Cooking, Sharwood's*	¼ Jar/140g	120	8.3	86	1.2	7.1	5.9	1.4
Balti, Ready Made, Average	1 Serving/100g	98	6.1	98	2.0	8.3	6.1	1.8
Balti, Tomato & Coriander, Canned, Patak's*	1 Can/283g	235	17.0	83	0.8	6.5	6.0	1.2
Balti Curry, Tesco*	1 Serving/200g	126	9.2	63	1.7	4.3	4.6	1.7
Barbecue, Asda*	1 Serving/135g	128	0.3	95	1.2	22.0	0.2	0.6
Barbecue, Chicken Tonight, Knorr*	¼ Jar/125g	76	0.5	61	2.0	12.4	0.4	0.9
Barbeque, Cook in, Homepride*	1 Can/500g	375	7.5	75	0.7	14.6	1.5	0.6
Barbeque, Simply Sausages Ranch, Colman's*	1 Serving/130g	96	0.1	74	1.8	16.6	0.1	1.1
Basil & Onion, Italian, Slow Cooked, Dolmio*	1 Jar/350g	322	24.5	92	1.8	5.6	7.0	1.3
BBQ, Heinz*	1 Serving/20g	28	0.1	139	1.1	31.7	0.3	0.5
BBQ, HP*	1 Serving/20ml	29	0.0	143	0.8	33.1	0.2	0.0
Bearnaise, Mary Berry*	1 Serving/100g	435	39.8	435	1.7	17.3	39.8	0.4
Bearnaise, Sainsbury's*	1 Tbsp/15g	59	6.2	393	0.6	5.0	41.0	0.0
Bechamel, for Lasagne, Loyd Grossman*	1 Jar/400g	396	33.2	99	0.6	5.4	8.3	0.1
Beef in Ale, Cooking, Asda*	1 Jar/500g	160	1.0	32	1.6	6.0	0.2	0.0
Bhuna, Cooking, Sharwood's*	1/3 Jar/140g	116	7.6	83	1.2	7.6	5.4	1.6
Black Bean, Asda*	1 Serving/55g	55	0.8	100	2.9	19.0	1.4	0.0
Black Bean, Canton, Stir Fry, Blue Dragon*	½ Pack/60g	53	1.2	88	2.8	14.8	2.0	1.5
Black Bean, Cantonese, Sharwood's*	½ Jar/212g	131	3.0	62	1.9	10.5	1.4	1.2
Black Bean, Cooking, Tesco*	1 Tbsp/15g	14	0.3	90	2.5	14.9	2.0	0.6
Black Bean, Finest, Tesco*	1 Jar/350g	252	1.8	72	0.8	16.1	0.5	0.8
Black Bean, Fresh, Sainsbury's*	1 Sachet/50ml	78	1.3	156	6.7	27.5	2.6	1.7
Black Bean, Iceland*	¼ Jar/125g	131	5.2	105	1.3	15.3	4.2	0.7
Black Bean, Loyd Grossman*	1 Serving/175g	177	7.9	101	2.4	12.6	4.5	0.7
Black Bean, Ready to Stir Fry, M & S*	1 Sachet/120g	78	1.1	65	2.5	11.5	0.9	1.4

S

SAUCE	Measure INFO/WEIGHT	per Measure KCAL	FAT	Nutrition Values per 100g / 100ml KCAL	PROT	CARB	FAT	FIBRE
Black Bean, Stir Fry, Fresh, M & S*	1 Pot/120g	120	0.7	100	2.6	20.3	0.6	1.4
Black Bean, Stir Fry, Sainsbury's*	½ Pack/75ml	91	3.2	121	3.3	17.6	4.3	1.7
Black Bean, Stir Fry, Sharwood's*	1 Jar/195g	127	0.6	65	2.3	12.9	0.3	0.0
Black Bean, Stir Fry Additions, Tesco*	1 Sachet/50g	69	1.5	138	4.1	23.6	3.0	0.0
Black Bean, Uncle Ben's*	1 Serving/125g	89	1.6	71	2.0	12.8	1.3	0.0
Black Pepper, Lee Kum Kee*	1 Serving/90g	107	3.0	119	3.2	19.0	3.3	1.3
Black Pepper, Stir Fry, Blue Dragon*	½ Sachet/60g	47	2.6	79	1.6	8.4	4.4	0.1
Bolognese, Italiano, Tesco*	1 Serving/175g	194	13.1	111	5.9	4.8	7.5	0.8
Bolognese, Loyd Grossman*	¼ Jar/106g	80	3.1	75	2.0	10.2	2.9	1.4
Bolognese, Original, Deliciously Good, Homepride*	¼ Jar/112g	39	0.2	35	1.3	7.1	0.2	0.8
Bolognese, Smooth, Dolmio*	1 Serving/125g	61	1.0	49	1.5	8.0	0.8	0.0
Bolognese, Tinned, Sainsbury's*	1/3 Can/141g	86	3.1	61	4.5	5.7	2.2	1.0
Bolognese, Waitrose*	1 Serving/175g	150	8.6	86	5.4	5.3	4.9	2.0
Bourguignon, Beef Tonight, Knorr*	¼ Jar/125g	71	3.2	57	0.6	7.6	2.6	0.4
Branston, Brown, Crosse & Blackwell*	1 Serving/15g	18	0.0	121	0.7	29.0	0.2	0.7
Branston, Rich & Fruity, Crosse & Blackwell*	1 Serving/15g	20	0.0	130	0.0	31.5	0.0	1.6
Branston, Smooth, Crosse & Blackwell*	1 Serving/25g	35	0.0	139	0.6	34.0	0.1	1.4
Bread, Christmas, Tesco*	1 Serving/60g	64	3.2	107	3.3	11.8	5.3	0.5
Bread, Luxury, M & S*	1 Serving/115g	196	16.2	170	3.2	8.1	14.1	2.2
Bread, M & S*	1 Serving/85g	153	12.4	180	3.1	8.7	14.6	0.2
Bread, Made with Semi-Skimmed Milk	1 Serving/45g	42	1.4	93	4.3	12.8	3.1	0.3
Brown, Bottled	1 Tsp/6g	6	0.0	99	1.1	25.2	0.0	0.7
Brown, Chop, Hammonds of Yorkshire*	1 Tbsp/15g	10	0.0	66	0.3	16.1	0.1	0.3
Brown, Original, HP*	1 Tbsp/15g	18	0.0	122	0.9	28.3	0.1	0.4
Brown, Reduced Salt & Sugar, HP*	1 Tbsp/15g	13	0.0	87	0.7	20.0	0.1	0.3
Brown, Tiptree, Wilkin & Sons*	1 Serving/100g	104	0.0	104	1.1	42.0	0.0	0.0
Butter & Tarragon, Chicken Tonight, Knorr*	¼ Jar/125g	132	13.0	106	1.0	2.1	10.4	0.7
Butter Chicken, Patak's*	1 Jar/500g	725	60.0	145	1.2	7.6	12.0	1.4
Butter Chicken, Simmer, Passage To India*	½ Pack/100g	188	11.7	188	2.2	18.9	11.7	3.2
Butter Chicken, TTD, Sainsbury's*	½ Pack/174g	272	23.5	156	1.8	6.7	13.5	0.9
Cantonese, Sizzling, Uncle Ben's*	½ Jar/270g	416	16.5	154	0.7	24.0	6.1	0.0
Caramelised Onion & Red Wine, M & S*	1 Serving/52g	31	1.6	60	1.9	6.7	3.1	0.6
Carbonara, TTD, Sainsbury's*	½ pot/175g	347	31.0	198	5.2	4.5	17.7	0.5
Caribbean Curry, Levi Roots*	½ Jar/175g	182	14.2	104	0.4	7.2	8.1	0.3
Chasseur, Classic, Chicken Tonight, Knorr*	¼ Jar/125g	61	3.6	49	0.6	5.3	2.9	0.7
Chasseur, Cook in, Homepride*	1 Can/390g	160	0.4	41	0.7	9.2	0.1	0.4
Cheese, Basics, Sainsbury's*	¼ Pot/124g	71	3.1	57	2.5	6.1	2.5	0.5
Cheese, Dry, Asda*	1 Serving/27g	101	3.0	373	4.4	64.0	11.0	7.0
Cheese, Fresh, Italiano, Tesco*	½ Tub/175g	236	16.1	135	6.8	6.2	9.2	0.0
Cheese, Fresh, Waitrose*	1 Pot/350g	458	34.3	131	5.1	5.7	9.8	0.0
Cheese, Instant, Morrisons*	1 Serving/14g	38	2.8	272	7.9	14.3	20.3	0.0
Cheese, Italian, Tesco*	½ Carton/175g	238	15.6	136	5.8	8.3	8.9	0.0
Cheese, Made with Semi-Skimmed Milk	1 Serving/60g	107	7.6	179	8.1	9.1	12.6	0.2
Cheese, Made with Whole Milk	1 Serving/60g	118	8.8	197	8.0	9.0	14.6	0.2
Cheese, Sainsbury's*	1 Serving/125g	140	9.4	112	5.0	6.1	7.5	1.2
Chickpea & Spinach, Asda*	1 Jar/500g	365	14.0	73	3.5	8.4	2.8	2.0
Chilli, Amoy*	1 Tsp/6g	2	0.0	25	1.0	5.2	0.0	1.0
Chilli, Barbeque, Encona*	1 Tbsp/15ml	19	0.0	129	1.3	30.7	0.1	0.0
Chilli, Cooking, Casa Mexico*	1 Jar/500g	275	2.5	55	1.5	10.0	0.5	2.7
Chilli, Hot, Asda*	1 Jar/570g	319	2.3	56	2.1	11.0	0.4	1.9
Chilli, Hot, Blue Dragon*	1 Tbsp/15ml	14	0.0	96	0.5	23.0	0.2	0.0
Chilli, Hot, Heinz*	1 Portion/10g	8	0.0	80	1.4	18.0	0.0	0.0
Chilli, HP*	1 Tsp/6g	8	0.0	134	1.2	32.3	0.0	0.0

S

	Measure INFO/WEIGHT	per Measure KCAL	FAT	Nutrition Values per 100g / 100ml KCAL	PROT	CARB	FAT	FIBRE
SAUCE								
Chilli, Iceland*	1 Serving/115g	75	0.8	65	2.7	12.0	0.7	1.6
Chilli, Medium, Deliciously Good, Homepride*	1 Jar/460g	258	2.3	56	2.3	10.4	0.5	1.2
Chilli, Mild, Healthy Eating, Asda*	½ Jar/250g	172	5.8	69	2.1	10.0	2.3	1.7
Chilli, Seeds of Change*	1 Jar/400g	408	6.0	102	4.0	18.2	1.5	2.2
Chilli, Sweet, Thai, Dipping, Original, Blue Dragon*	1 Serving/30ml	69	0.2	229	0.6	55.1	0.7	1.6
Chilli, Tesco*	1 Tsp/5ml	4	0.2	90	1.3	14.0	3.2	1.1
Chilli, Tomato Based, Bottled, Average	***1 Tbsp/15g***	***16***	***0.0***	***104***	***2.5***	***19.8***	***0.3***	***5.9***
Chilli & Garlic, Blue Dragon*	1 Serving/30ml	26	0.1	85	1.1	19.7	0.2	0.0
Chilli & Garlic, Lea & Perrins*	1 Tsp/6g	4	0.0	60	1.0	14.9	0.0	0.0
Chilli & Garlic, Lee Kum Kee*	1 Tsp/15g	16	0.0	110	2.1	24.7	0.3	4.3
Chilli & Garlic, Stir Fry, M & S*	1 Serving/83g	120	1.0	145	0.7	32.4	1.2	1.1
Chilli Con Carne, Asda*	1 Lge Jar/570g	370	4.0	65	2.6	12.0	0.7	0.0
Chilli Con Carne, Classic, Loyd Grossman*	1 Jar/350g	242	10.5	69	2.2	7.6	3.0	1.3
Chilli Con Carne, Cook in, BGTY, Sainsbury's*	¼ Jar/125g	69	0.6	55	1.7	11.0	0.5	2.5
Chilli Con Carne, Cook in, Homepride*	1 Can/390g	234	2.3	60	2.5	11.2	0.6	0.0
Chilli Con Carne, Hot, Sainsbury's*	1 Serving/116g	66	0.2	57	2.4	11.3	0.2	1.6
Chilli Con Carne, Hot, Uncle Ben's*	1 Jar/500g	295	3.0	59	2.3	10.9	0.6	1.7
Chilli Con Carne, Sizzle & Stir, Knorr*	1 Jar/455g	505	32.3	111	2.7	9.1	7.1	2.7
Chilli Soy, Amoy*	1 Tbsp/15g	8	0.0	55	4.6	9.1	0.0	0.0
Chinese, Curry, Farmfoods*	1 Sachet/200g	220	17.6	110	0.6	7.1	8.8	0.7
Chinese, Stir Fry, Sainsbury's*	½ Sachet/75g	61	1.9	81	0.4	14.1	2.5	1.0
Chinese Style, Stir Fry, Fresh, Asda*	½ Sachet/50ml	93	6.0	186	1.5	18.0	12.0	0.0
Chocolate, Dry, Sainsbury's*	1 Serving/30g	108	3.5	360	1.3	62.8	11.6	0.9
Chocolate, Sainsbury's*	1 Serving/25g	81	1.6	323	1.8	64.7	6.3	2.7
Chocolate Flavour, Dry, Lyle's*	1 Serving/10g	30	0.0	305	1.0	74.0	0.5	0.0
Cholula Hot Sauce*	1 Tbsp/12g	3	0.1	22	1.0	2.5	1.0	0.0
Chop Suey, Blue Dragon*	½ Sachet/60g	34	1.4	57	0.5	8.3	2.4	0.5
Chop Suey, Cantonese, Sharwood's*	1 Serving/200g	146	2.8	73	0.6	14.4	1.4	0.4
Chop Suey, Stir Fry, Sharwood's*	1 Jar/160g	120	2.4	75	0.7	14.6	1.5	0.2
Chow Mein, Sainsbury's*	1 Serving/50g	36	1.2	71	1.8	10.5	2.4	0.0
Chow Mein, Stir Fry, Asda*	½ Jar/98g	97	1.0	99	1.6	21.0	1.0	0.1
Chow Mein, Stir Fry, Blue Dragon*	1 Sachet/120g	110	3.5	92	1.1	15.4	2.9	0.4
Chow Mein, Stir Fry, Straight to Wok, Amoy*	1 Packet/120g	172	7.0	143	0.9	21.9	5.8	0.5
Coconut, Chilli & Lime, Cook-In, Homepride*	1 Serving/115g	110	8.6	96	1.1	5.9	7.5	0.0
Coconut, Ginger & Lemon Grass, Stir Fry, Wagamama*	½ Jar/125g	144	7.1	115	1.2	14.7	5.7	0.4
Coconut, Lime & Coriander, Cooking, Nando's*	1 Serving/65g	88	6.5	135	1.5	12.2	10.0	1.2
Coconut, Thai Style, Stir Fry, Waitrose*	½ Pack/50ml	52	4.3	105	1.5	5.5	8.6	1.8
Coronation, Heinz*	1 Tbsp/10g	33	3.1	334	0.8	13.1	31.0	0.9
Coronation Chicken, Cook in, Homepride*	1 Serving/250g	232	10.5	93	0.8	13.2	4.2	0.0
Coronation Chicken, Schwartz*	1 Pack/35g	124	5.1	354	14.9	29.1	14.5	23.8
Country French, Chicken Tonight, Knorr*	¼ Jar/125g	110	8.8	89	0.4	5.3	7.1	0.8
Country French, Low Fat, Chicken Tonight, Knorr*	¼ Jar/125g	56	3.6	45	0.4	4.4	2.9	0.7
Cranberry, Sainsbury's*	1 Tsp/15g	23	0.0	154	0.8	37.1	0.3	1.3
Cranberry, with Brandy & Orange Zest, Finest, Tesco*	1 Serving/10g	24	0.1	235	0.3	57.2	0.6	1.3
Cranberry & Port, M & S*	1 Serving/75g	71	0.3	95	2.3	20.2	0.4	2.1
Cranberry Jelly, Baxters*	1 Tsp/15g	40	0.0	268	0.0	67.0	0.0	0.0
Curry, 98% Fat Free, Homepride*	1oz/28g	16	0.5	56	1.1	8.6	1.9	0.5
Curry, Bettabuy, Morrisons*	1 Jar/440g	295	10.1	67	0.7	10.8	2.3	1.0
Curry, Chinese Style, Cooking, Chosen By You, Asda*	1 Serving/140g	89	4.3	64	1.5	7.4	3.1	3.5
Curry, Cook in, Homepride*	½ Can/250g	140	4.8	56	1.1	8.6	1.9	0.5
Curry, Creamy, Chicken Tonight, Knorr*	½ Jar/250g	208	18.5	83	0.6	3.6	7.4	0.8
Curry, Creamy, Cooking, BGTY, Sainsbury's*	¼ Jar/125g	94	3.8	75	1.8	10.1	3.0	1.0
Curry, Deliciously Good, Homepride*	1/3 Jar/149g	91	2.7	61	1.1	10.0	1.8	0.5

SAUCE	Measure INFO/WEIGHT	per Measure KCAL	FAT	Nutrition Values per 100g / 100ml KCAL	PROT	CARB	FAT	FIBRE
Curry, Green Thai, BGTY, Sainsbury's*	¼ Jar/125g	61	3.2	49	0.6	5.7	2.6	1.4
Curry, Green Thai, Cooking, TTD, Sainsbury's*	½ Pack/175g	152	11.9	87	0.9	5.5	6.8	1.0
Curry, Kashmiri, Bibijis*	¼ Packet/119g	51	1.7	43	2.1	7.1	1.4	1.5
Curry, Mild, Tesco*	1 Jar/500g	420	14.0	84	1.1	13.4	2.8	0.8
Curry, Red Thai, BGTY, Sainsbury's*	1 Serving/124g	77	4.8	62	0.6	6.0	3.9	1.4
Curry, Red Thai, Sainsbury's*	½ Pouch/250g	390	35.8	156	1.7	5.0	14.3	1.5
Curry, Red Thai, Sharwood's*	1 Serving/138g	150	11.0	109	1.2	7.9	8.0	0.2
Curry, Sri Lanken, Seasoned Pioneers*	½ Pack/200g	194	16.8	97	1.8	3.4	8.4	0.8
Curry, Sweet	1 Serving/115g	105	6.4	91	1.2	9.6	5.6	1.4
Curry, Thai Coconut, Uncle Ben's*	1 Serving/125g	128	6.0	102	1.4	13.2	4.8	0.0
Dhansak, Medium, Sharwood's*	1 Jar/420g	370	13.4	88	3.6	11.1	3.2	1.0
Dhansak, Sharwood's*	1 Jar/445g	668	34.7	150	4.7	15.2	7.8	1.4
Dill & Lemon, Delicate for Fish, Schwartz*	1 Pack/300g	387	34.2	129	1.1	5.6	11.4	0.5
Dill & Mustard for Gravadlax, Dry, Waitrose*	1 Sachet/35g	123	9.0	352	2.5	27.8	25.7	0.6
Dipping, for Dim Sum, Amoy*	1 Tbsp/15ml	28	0.0	190	0.0	48.0	0.0	0.0
Dopiaza, Cooking, Tesco*	1 Serving/166g	176	11.0	106	2.2	9.4	6.6	1.9
Dopiaza, Tomato & Onion, Original, Glass Jar, Patak's*	1 Jar/540g	605	39.4	112	1.6	9.8	7.3	1.2
Enchilada, Medium, Old El Paso*	1 Can/270g	92	4.6	34	0.0	5.0	1.7	0.0
Fajita, M & S*	1oz/28g	24	1.7	85	1.3	6.4	6.1	2.2
Fish Pie, Fresh, The Saucy Fish Co.*	1 Pack/230g	179	12.9	78	2.4	4.6	5.6	0.0
Four Cheese, for Pasta, Waitrose*	1 Pot/300g	392	24.8	112	6.6	5.5	7.1	0.5
Four Cheese, Reduced Fat, Morrisons*	½ Tub/175g	161	9.5	92	6.1	4.8	5.4	0.5
Fruity, HP*	1 Tsp/6g	8	0.0	141	1.2	35.1	0.1	0.0
Garlic, Heinz*	1 Serving/10ml	32	3.0	323	1.0	12.1	29.9	1.2
Garlic, Lea & Perrins*	1 Tsp/6g	20	1.7	337	1.8	17.8	29.0	0.0
Garlic & Chive, Heinz*	1 Serving/10ml	35	3.3	350	1.0	11.3	33.2	0.1
Garlic & Chive, Table & Dip, Heinz*	1 Serving/10ml	32	3.0	323	1.0	12.1	29.9	0.2
Garlic & Herb, Cooking, Simply Stir, Philadelphia*	1 Serving/60g	81	7.2	135	2.5	4.6	12.0	0.4
Green Peppercorn, Dry, Sainsbury's*	1 Tbsp/15ml	68	7.3	455	0.4	3.8	48.5	0.1
Green Thai, Cooking, Perfectly Balanced, Waitrose*	½ Jar/215g	112	6.9	52	0.8	4.9	3.2	1.5
Green Thai, Loyd Grossman*	½ Jar/175g	182	11.2	104	1.6	10.0	6.4	0.8
Green Thai, Stir Fry, Sainsbury's*	½ Pack/75g	112	8.0	149	1.2	11.9	10.7	1.0
Hoi Sin, Chosen By You, Asda*	1 Jar/210g	309	2.3	147	0.8	31.3	1.1	1.4
Hoi Sin, M & S*	½ Pot/50ml	80	1.0	160	3.2	31.8	2.0	2.2
Hoi Sin, Sharwood's*	1 Tbsp/15g	32	0.0	211	2.7	49.5	0.3	0.1
Hoi Sin, Stir Fry, Tesco*	½ Sachet/60g	87	2.9	145	1.1	23.9	4.9	0.5
Hoi Sin & Garlic, Blue Dragon*	1 Serving/60g	80	1.6	133	1.2	26.1	2.6	0.0
Hoi Sin & Plum, Chinatown, Knorr*	¼ Jar/131g	96	0.9	73	0.8	15.8	0.7	1.2
Hoi Sin & Plum, Sweet & Fruity, Stir Fry, Sharwood's*	1 Serving/136g	128	1.8	94	0.7	19.9	1.3	0.9
Hoi Sin & Spring Onion, Stir Fry, Sharwood's*	1 Jar/165g	196	1.5	119	1.3	26.5	0.9	0.8
Hollandaise, Classic, for Fish, Schwartz*	1 Sachet/300g	456	49.2	152	0.7	0.4	16.4	2.0
Hollandaise, Classic, Knorr*	1 Serving/100ml	202	20.5	202	0.6	3.9	20.5	0.4
Hollandaise, Dry, M & S*	1oz/28g	115	12.2	410	0.9	3.6	43.6	0.5
Hollandaise, Dry, Maille*	1 Serving/30g	148	15.2	495	1.0	10.8	50.6	0.0
Hollandaise, Fresh, Average	1 Pack/150g	342	32.4	228	2.4	6.1	21.6	0.0
Hollandaise, Homemade, Average	1oz/28g	198	21.3	707	4.8	0.0	76.2	0.0
Hollandaise, Mary Berry*	1 Serving/100g	472	43.8	472	1.4	17.8	43.8	0.3
Hollandaise, Sainsbury's*	1 Tbsp/15g	72	7.6	478	0.2	5.9	50.4	0.4
Honey & Coriander, Stir Fry, Blue Dragon*	1 Pack/120g	115	0.7	96	0.5	22.1	0.6	0.3
Honey & Mustard, Chicken Tonight, Knorr*	¼ Jar/125g	132	6.6	106	1.0	12.6	5.3	1.8
Honey & Mustard, COU, M & S*	½ Jar/160g	112	4.6	70	2.3	9.2	2.9	0.7
Honey & Mustard, for Cooking, Asda*	1 Serving/200g	234	14.0	117	0.6	13.0	7.0	0.0
Honey & Mustard, Low Fat, Chicken Tonight, Knorr*	¼ Jar/131g	105	3.0	80	1.0	13.8	2.3	0.8

	Measure INFO/WEIGHT	per Measure KCAL	FAT	Nutrition Values per 100g / 100ml KCAL	PROT	CARB	FAT	FIBRE
SAUCE								
Horseradish, Asda*	1oz/28g	38	2.0	135	2.2	14.0	7.0	2.0
Horseradish, Colman's*	1 Tbsp/15ml	17	0.9	112	1.9	9.8	6.2	2.6
Horseradish, Creamy, Sainsbury's*	1 Tsp/5g	11	0.6	223	2.8	28.9	11.8	1.6
Horseradish, Hot, Morrisons*	1 Serving/20g	22	1.1	110	1.6	10.9	5.6	1.1
Horseradish, Mustard, Sainsbury's*	1 Tsp/5g	8	0.3	163	7.9	18.2	6.6	3.5
Horseradish, Sainsbury's*	1 Dtsp/10g	14	0.7	145	1.5	17.8	6.6	2.4
Jalfrezi, Cooking, Chosen By You, Asda*	1 Jar/570g	445	27.4	78	1.1	7.2	4.8	0.9
Jalfrezi, Cooking, Sainsbury's*	1 Serving/250g	160	6.0	64	1.0	9.6	2.4	1.7
Jalfrezi, Cooking, Shere Khan*	1 Jar/425g	202	13.6	48	0.8	3.9	3.2	0.0
Jalfrezi, Spice & Stir, Geeta's*	½ Jar/175g	156	11.2	89	1.4	6.5	6.4	1.4
Jalfrezi, Stir Fry, Patak's*	1 Jar/250g	260	18.8	104	1.4	7.6	7.5	1.4
Jambalaya, Cajun, Seasoned Pioneers*	1 Pack/400g	248	20.4	62	0.8	3.2	5.1	1.0
Jerk/BBQ, Levi Roots*	¼ Bottle/78g	94	0.1	121	1.1	28.8	0.1	0.5
Korma, Asda*	1 Serving/225g	434	33.8	193	2.5	12.0	15.0	2.2
Korma, Authentic, VLH Kitchens	1 Serving/118g	180	11.0	153	1.9	6.7	13.0	0.8
Korma, Cooking, BGTY, Sainsbury's*	¼ Jar/125g	100	3.4	80	1.1	12.9	2.7	1.2
Korma, Cooking, Patak's*	¼ Jar/125g	211	17.5	169	1.3	9.3	14.0	2.4
Korma, Cooking, Sharwood's*	1 Jar/420g	680	42.8	162	1.7	15.9	10.2	2.2
Korma, Free From, Sainsbury's*	½ Jar/175g	191	13.8	109	1.9	7.6	7.9	1.2
Korma, GFY, Asda*	1 Serving/240g	336	21.6	140	1.7	13.0	9.0	1.5
Korma, Homepride*	1 Serving/160g	110	3.2	69	1.3	11.6	2.0	0.0
Korma, Indian Style, Iceland*	¼ Jar/112g	150	10.2	134	1.5	11.4	9.1	1.0
Korma, Organic, Patak's*	¼ Jar/106g	148	12.7	140	1.9	5.9	12.0	0.9
Korma, Royal, TTD, Sainsbury's*	½ Pack/175g	207	12.3	118	2.4	11.4	7.0	3.9
Korma, Sizzle & Stir, Knorr*	1 Jar/455g	1092	96.5	240	1.2	11.2	21.2	2.7
Korma, with Flaked Almonds, Weight Watchers*	1 Serving/175g	107	3.7	61	2.0	8.5	2.1	1.6
Laksa, Finest, Tesco*	1/3 Jar/111g	105	8.2	95	1.3	5.5	7.4	1.8
Lemon, Amoy*	1 Tsp/5ml	5	0.0	104	0.0	26.0	0.0	0.0
Lemon, Stir Fry, Straight to Wok, Amoy*	½ Sachet/50g	81	0.1	162	0.3	40.0	0.2	0.0
Lemon & Ginger, Stir Fry, Finest, Tesco*	¼ Jar/85g	144	0.2	169	0.2	41.7	0.2	0.2
Lemon & Sesame, Stir Fry, Sharwood's*	1 Serving/100g	125	0.1	125	0.1	30.9	0.1	0.1
Lime & Coriander, Tangy for Fish, Schwartz*	1 Pack/300g	381	37.2	127	1.1	2.7	12.4	1.3
Lime Honey & Ginger, Stir Fry, Sharwood's*	1 Serving/50g	34	0.0	69	0.3	16.6	0.1	0.2
Madras, Cooking, HL, Tesco*	1 Serving/128g	55	2.6	43	1.6	4.8	2.0	2.3
Mango, Kashmiri Style, Finest, Tesco*	½ Jar/175g	285	23.8	163	2.4	7.7	13.6	0.9
Marie Rose, Fresh, The Saucy Fish Co.*	1 Pack/150g	590	59.7	393	1.6	7.0	39.8	0.0
Mint, Baxters*	1oz/28g	17	0.1	62	1.7	13.2	0.3	0.0
Mint, Sainsbury's*	1 Dtsp/10g	13	0.0	126	2.5	28.7	0.1	4.0
Moglai, Tomato & Fennel, Cooking, Patak's*	1 Jar/283g	374	25.2	132	3.1	9.7	8.9	1.8
Mornay, Cheese, Asda*	¼ Pot/71g	114	9.0	161	6.8	6.6	12.7	0.4
Moroccan, Spread & Bake, Heinz*	¼ Jar/70g	64	1.6	91	1.7	15.8	2.3	2.1
Mushroom, Creamy, Asda*	1 Serving/125g	76	4.6	61	0.8	6.0	3.7	0.5
Mushroom, Creamy, Chicken Tonight, Knorr*	¼ Jar/125g	99	7.1	79	0.5	6.0	5.7	1.0
Mushroom, Creamy, Cooking, M & S*	1 Jar/510g	663	57.6	130	1.3	5.4	11.3	0.5
Mushroom, Creamy, Homepride*	1 Portion/100g	76	5.6	76	1.1	5.2	5.6	0.3
Mushroom, Creamy, Knorr*	1 Serving/125g	111	9.6	89	0.4	4.5	7.7	0.4
Mushroom, Creamy, Low Fat, Chicken Tonight, Knorr*	¼ Jar/125g	59	3.6	47	0.8	7.3	2.9	0.4
Napoletana, Fresh, Sainsbury's*	½ Pot/150g	94	4.5	63	1.7	7.3	3.0	2.3
Napoletana, Italian, Tesco*	1 Pot/350g	178	4.2	51	1.5	8.5	1.2	1.0
Napoletana, Waitrose*	1 Pot/600g	252	8.4	42	1.8	5.5	1.4	1.7
Onion, Made with Semi-Skimmed Milk	1 Serving/60g	52	3.0	86	2.9	8.4	5.0	0.4
Onion, Made with Skimmed Milk	1 Serving/60g	46	2.4	77	2.9	8.4	4.0	0.4
Oyster, Blue Dragon*	1 Tsp/5ml	6	0.0	121	3.4	26.9	0.0	0.0

S

	Measure INFO/WEIGHT	per Measure KCAL	FAT	Nutrition Values per 100g / 100ml KCAL	PROT	CARB	FAT	FIBRE
SAUCE								
Oyster, Stir Fry, Sainsbury's*	1 Tbsp/15g	9	0.0	61	1.6	13.3	0.1	0.2
Oyster & Garlic, Stir Fry, Straight to Wok, Amoy*	½ Pack/50g	98	1.5	195	4.9	37.0	3.0	0.0
Parsley, Fresh, Sainsbury's*	½ Pot/150g	117	7.6	78	2.0	5.9	5.1	0.5
Parsley, Instant, Dry, Asda*	1 Serving/23g	82	1.6	355	7.0	66.0	7.0	4.4
Parsley, Instant, Made Up, Semi Skim Milk, Sainsbury's*	¼ Sachet/51ml	34	1.1	67	3.5	8.6	2.1	0.1
Parsley, Made Up, Bisto*	1 Serving/50ml	41	2.4	82	0.6	9.2	4.8	0.0
Peanut, Sainsbury's*	1 Sachet/70g	185	9.2	264	1.9	34.7	13.1	1.6
Peking Lemon, Stir Fry, Blue Dragon*	1 Serving/35g	47	0.2	134	0.0	31.6	0.7	0.5
Pepper, Creamy, Schwartz*	1 Pack/170g	116	9.2	68	1.5	3.4	5.4	1.0
Pepper, Creamy, Tesco*	1 Serving/85ml	128	11.4	151	1.2	6.4	13.4	0.5
Peppercorn, Creamy, Asda*	¼ Jar/137g	137	11.0	100	1.1	6.0	8.0	0.2
Peppercorn, Creamy, Chicken Tonight, Knorr*	¼ Jar/125g	110	9.8	88	0.3	3.8	7.8	0.4
Peppercorn & Whisky, Creamy, Baxters*	1 Pack/320g	422	34.6	132	1.9	6.7	10.8	0.2
Peri-Peri, Extra Hot, Nando's*	1 Serving/5g	4	0.2	71	0.7	8.8	3.7	1.4
Peri-Peri, Garlic, Nando's*	1 Serving/15g	9	0.5	59	0.5	6.6	3.4	0.8
Peri-Peri, Hot, Nando's*	1 Serving/5g	4	0.2	75	0.6	9.6	3.8	1.3
Peri-Peri, Sweet, Nando's*	1 Tbsp/25g	36	0.5	142	0.5	30.7	2.1	0.0
Plum, Spiced, Heinz*	1 Serving/25g	32	0.0	128	0.5	31.1	0.1	1.0
Plum & Ginger, Stir Fry, Asda*	½ Jar/97g	94	0.7	97	0.7	22.0	0.7	0.3
Plum & Sesame, Stir Fry, M & S*	½ Jar/115g	138	0.1	120	0.9	29.0	0.1	1.8
Prawn Cocktail, Morrisons*	1 Portion/15ml	81	8.5	540	1.4	5.5	56.9	1.1
Puttanesca, Fresh, Waitrose*	½ Pot/176g	118	7.7	67	1.8	6.2	4.4	1.2
Red & Yellow Pepper, Roasted, Sacla*	1 Serving/290g	232	17.1	80	1.1	5.5	5.9	0.0
Red Pepper, Fresh, Asda*	¼ Pot/82g	35	1.0	43	1.4	6.8	1.2	1.1
Red Pepper, GFY, Asda*	1 Serving/100g	43	1.1	43	1.2	7.0	1.1	0.0
Red Pepper, Sainsbury's*	1 Serving/37g	118	11.6	320	4.3	5.0	31.4	0.0
Red Thai, Cooking, Asda*	½ Jar/160g	136	9.1	85	0.9	6.8	5.7	1.5
Red Thai, Loyd Grossman*	1Jar/350g	438	22.8	125	2.8	13.7	6.5	1.5
Red Wine, Cook in, Homepride*	¼ Can/98g	47	0.6	48	0.5	10.1	0.6	0.0
Red Wine, Cooking, BGTY, Sainsbury's*	1 Serving/125g	52	0.6	42	0.5	8.8	0.5	0.8
Red Wine, Cooking, Homepride*	1 Serving/250ml	115	1.5	46	0.4	9.8	0.6	0.0
Red Wine & Onion, Rich, Simply Sausages, Colman's*	¼ Jar/125g	49	0.2	39	0.9	8.5	0.2	1.3
Redcurrant, Colman's*	1 Tsp/12g	44	0.0	368	0.7	90.0	0.0	0.0
Reggae Reggae, Cooking, Levi Roots*	½ Jar/175g	215	0.9	123	1.3	28.5	0.5	0.7
Reggae Reggae, Jerk BBQ, Levi Roots*	1 Jar/310g	375	0.3	121	1.1	28.8	0.1	0.5
Risotto, Mushroom & White Wine, Sacla*	1 Serving/95g	151	12.4	159	3.7	6.9	13.0	0.0
Rogan Josh, 99% Fat Free, Homepride*	1/3 Jar/153g	92	1.1	60	1.8	11.6	0.7	2.0
Rogan Josh, Asda*	¼ Jar/125g	135	10.0	108	0.9	8.0	8.0	0.6
Rogan Josh, Cooking, LC, Tesco*	¼ Jar/125g	58	3.0	46	1.4	4.8	2.4	2.5
Rogan Josh, Curry, The Curry Sauce Company*	1 Serving/235g	310	23.7	132	1.9	8.4	10.1	1.5
Rogan Josh, Medium, Sharwood's*	½ Jar/210g	151	7.6	72	1.4	8.6	3.6	0.5
Rogan Josh, Sharwood's*	½ Jar/210g	220	16.8	105	1.2	7.0	8.0	1.5
Rogan Josh, VLH Kitchens	1 Serving/460g	374	1.2	82	1.4	6.1	5.3	1.4
Satay, Indonesian, Sharwood's*	1oz/28g	45	3.0	159	5.4	10.0	10.8	5.1
Satay, Stir Fry & Dipping, Finest, Tesco*	1 Tsp/5g	22	1.7	432	9.0	20.7	34.8	2.7
Satay, with Peanuts & Chillies, Cooking, Blue Dragon*	1 Serving/110g	198	10.7	180	4.3	18.0	9.7	1.5
Sausage Casserole, Cook in, Homepride*	½ Jar/250g	92	0.5	37	0.7	8.0	0.2	0.6
Seafood, 25% Less Fat, Tesco*	1 Tsp/5g	17	1.4	344	2.7	18.2	28.5	0.3
Seafood, Atkins & Potts*	1 Serving/30g	195	20.8	650	2.1	4.1	69.5	0.2
Seafood, Average	1 Tsp/5g	20	1.9	410	1.4	15.4	38.0	0.2
Seafood, Baxters*	1oz/28g	149	15.2	533	1.5	9.9	54.2	0.7
Seafood, Colman's*	1 Tbsp/15g	44	3.4	296	0.9	21.5	22.9	0.4
Seafood, GFY, Asda*	1 Dstp/10ml	31	2.7	313	0.6	17.0	27.0	0.0

	Measure INFO/WEIGHT	per Measure KCAL	FAT	Nutrition Values per 100g / 100ml KCAL	PROT	CARB	FAT	FIBRE
SAUCE								
Seafood, Organic, Simply Delicious*	1 Serving/35g	192	18.9	549	2.3	13.6	53.9	0.3
Sloppy Joe, Manwich, Original, Hunt's*	¼ Cup/64g	40	0.0	62	1.6	14.1	0.0	3.1
Soy, Average	1 Tsp/5ml	3	0.0	64	8.7	8.3	0.0	0.0
Soy, Dark, Average	1 Tsp/5g	4	0.0	84	4.0	16.7	0.1	0.2
Soy, Light, Amoy*	1 Tsp/5ml	3	0.0	52	2.5	10.5	0.0	0.0
Soy, Light, Sharwood's*	1 Tsp/5ml	2	0.0	37	2.7	6.4	0.2	0.0
Soy, Naturally Brewed, Kikkoman*	1 Tbsp/15g	11	0.0	74	10.3	8.1	0.0	0.0
Soy, Premium, Light, Heinz*	1 Serving/15g	11	0.1	71	7.4	9.1	0.5	0.0
Soy, Reduced Salt, Amoy*	1 Tsp/5ml	3	0.0	56	4.0	10.0	0.0	0.0
Soy, Rich, Sharwood's*	1 Tsp/5ml	4	0.0	79	3.1	16.6	0.4	0.0
Stir Fry, Chinese, Tesco*	1 Serving/90g	86	3.2	95	1.3	14.3	3.5	0.6
Stroganoff, Asda*	1 Serving/285g	305	25.6	107	1.5	5.0	9.0	0.3
Stroganoff, M & S*	1oz/28g	30	2.2	107	3.8	4.9	8.0	0.6
Stroganoff, Mushroom, Creamy, M & S*	1 Serving/75g	86	6.9	115	3.3	4.8	9.2	0.6
Stroganoff, Tesco*	1 Serving/100g	89	7.3	89	0.7	5.3	7.3	0.4
Sweet & Sour, Aromatic, Stir Fry Sensations, Amoy*	1 Pack/160g	312	0.5	195	0.4	46.8	0.3	0.8
Sweet & Sour, Basics, Sainsbury's*	¼ Jar/110g	59	0.3	54	0.3	12.4	0.3	0.4
Sweet & Sour, Cantonese, Loyd Grossman*	1 Serving/225g	306	4.7	136	1.2	28.0	2.1	0.5
Sweet & Sour, Chinese, Sainsbury's*	½ Jar/150g	222	0.2	148	0.2	36.6	0.1	0.1
Sweet & Sour, Classic, Canned, Homepride*	1 Can/500g	510	0.5	102	0.4	24.9	0.1	0.5
Sweet & Sour, Cook In, Glass Jar, Homepride*	1 Jar/500g	335	0.5	67	0.3	16.2	0.1	0.5
Sweet & Sour, Cooking, Chinese, Sainsbury's*	¼ Jar/125g	155	0.1	124	0.6	30.1	0.1	0.7
Sweet & Sour, Cooking, LC, Tesco*	1 Jar/510g	357	0.5	70	0.3	16.1	0.1	0.5
Sweet & Sour, Cooking, Organic, Sainsbury's*	1/3 Jar/150g	150	1.4	100	0.8	22.1	0.9	0.5
Sweet & Sour, Extra Pineapple, Uncle Ben's*	1 Serving/165g	147	0.3	89	0.3	21.2	0.2	0.7
Sweet & Sour, Fresh, Sainsbury's*	1 Sachet/50ml	102	4.3	205	0.8	31.2	8.6	0.3
Sweet & Sour, Fresh Ideas, Tesco*	1 Serving/50ml	77	0.7	154	1.1	34.3	1.4	0.5
Sweet & Sour, GFY, Asda*	½ Jar/164g	77	0.3	47	0.4	11.0	0.2	0.3
Sweet & Sour, HL, Tesco*	1 Jar/510g	326	0.5	64	0.4	15.4	0.1	0.5
Sweet & Sour, Light, Uncle Ben's*	¼ Jar/125g	71	0.1	57	0.4	12.6	0.1	0.9
Sweet & Sour, Organic, Seeds of Change*	1 Jar/350g	350	0.4	100	0.4	24.4	0.1	0.6
Sweet & Sour, Oriental, Chicken Tonight, Knorr*	½ Jar/262g	217	2.6	83	0.4	20.8	1.0	0.5
Sweet & Sour, Original, Uncle Ben's*	1 Pack/300g	264	0.6	88	0.4	21.9	0.2	0.8
Sweet & Sour, Peking Style, Finest, Tesco*	1 Serving/175g	147	0.2	84	0.6	20.1	0.1	0.5
Sweet & Sour, Perfectly Balanced, Waitrose*	1 Serving/175g	140	0.4	80	0.6	18.9	0.2	1.1
Sweet & Sour, Seeds of Change*	1 Serving/200g	174	0.0	87	0.3	21.3	0.0	0.7
Sweet & Sour, Sizzling, Uncle Ben's*	½ Jar/270g	375	18.1	139	0.6	19.2	6.7	0.0
Sweet & Sour, Stir Fry, GFY, Asda*	½ Pack/51ml	43	2.1	85	0.9	11.0	4.1	3.4
Sweet & Sour, Stir Fry, M & S*	1 Pack/120g	150	0.5	125	0.7	29.8	0.4	1.3
Sweet & Sour, Stir Fry, Pouch, Average	1 Serving/100g	124	1.9	124	0.8	25.7	1.9	1.0
Sweet & Sour, Stir Fry, Sachet, Blue Dragon*	1 Sachet/120g	145	0.1	122	0.2	29.7	0.1	0.3
Sweet & Sour, Stir Fry, Sharwood's*	1 Jar 160g	168	0.8	105	0.6	24.5	0.5	0.8
Sweet & Sour, Stir Fry, Tesco*	½ Jar/222g	164	0.4	74	0.6	17.0	0.2	0.4
Sweet & Sour, Stir Fry, Waitrose*	1 Serving/50ml	94	2.2	187	1.2	35.6	4.4	1.8
Sweet & Sour, Stir Fry Additions, Tesco*	1 Sachet/50g	84	0.5	167	0.8	38.7	1.0	0.5
Sweet & Sour, Take-Away	1oz/28g	44	1.0	157	0.2	32.8	3.4	0.0
Sweet & Sour, Two Stage, Uncle Ben's*	½ Jar/200g	314	18.2	157	1.0	18.1	9.1	0.0
Sweet Chilli, Dipping, M & S*	1 Tbsp/15g	34	0.1	225	0.9	53.2	0.7	0.6
Sweet Chilli, Dipping, Sharwood's*	1 Bottle/150ml	339	3.9	226	0.6	51.5	2.6	1.6
Sweet Chilli, Dipping, Thai, Amoy*	1 Serving/10g	14	0.3	142	0.5	34.2	2.8	0.3
Sweet Chilli, Heinz*	1 Serving/25g	38	0.1	150	0.3	36.5	0.4	6.4
Sweet Chilli, Lee Kum Kee*	1 Jar/215g	518	0.4	241	0.4	59.4	0.2	0.6
Sweet Chilli & Coriander, Sizzling, Homepride*	1 Serving/100g	51	0.2	51	0.7	11.5	0.2	0.0

	Measure INFO/WEIGHT	per Measure KCAL	FAT	Nutrition Values per 100g / 100ml KCAL	PROT	CARB	FAT	FIBRE
SAUCE								
Sweet Chilli & Garlic, Stir Fry & Dipping, Tesco*	½ Jar/95ml	78	0.0	82	0.3	20.1	0.0	0.1
Sweet Chilli & Lemon Grass, Stir Fry, Sharwood's*	1 Serving/155g	127	0.2	82	0.3	19.7	0.1	0.3
Sweet Chilli & Lime, Chinatown, Knorr*	1 Jar/525g	635	17.3	121	0.6	22.0	3.3	0.5
Sweet Pepper, Stir in, Dolmio*	½ Pot/75g	77	4.6	103	1.4	9.6	6.2	1.6
Sweet Soy & Roasted Red Chilli, Stir Fry, Blue Dragon*	½ Pack/60g	49	0.0	81	0.4	19.5	0.0	0.2
Sweet Soy & Sesame, Uncle Ben's*	1 Serving/100g	110	1.7	110	0.7	23.0	1.7	0.0
Sweet Soy & Spring Onion, Stir Fry Sensations, Amoy*	1 Pouch/160g	312	10.4	195	2.0	31.5	6.5	0.6
Sweet Thai Chilli, Uncle Ben's*	¼ Jar/125g	131	0.4	105	0.8	23.6	0.3	1.1
Szechuan, Spicy Tomato, Stir Fry, Blue Dragon*	½ Sachet/60g	59	1.8	98	1.3	15.8	3.0	0.9
Szechuan, Stir Fry, Sharwood's*	1 Jar/150g	126	1.6	84	3.0	15.5	1.1	0.4
Szechuan Style, Stir Fry, Fresh Ideas, Tesco*	1 Sachet/50g	114	4.8	228	1.9	33.4	9.7	0.1
Tabasco, Tabasco*	1 Tsp/5ml	1	0.0	12	1.3	0.8	0.8	0.6
Tartare	1oz/28g	84	6.9	299	1.3	17.9	24.6	0.0
Tartare, Atkins & Potts*	1 Tbsp/15g	73	7.7	487	2.5	3.4	51.5	0.9
Tartare, Baxters*	1oz/28g	144	14.9	515	1.0	8.0	53.3	0.3
Tartare, Colman's*	1 Tbsp/15g	45	3.7	290	1.5	17.0	24.0	0.6
Tartare, Iceland*	1 Serving/100g	290	21.4	290	1.3	21.5	21.4	0.2
Tartare, Mild & Creamy, Heinz*	1 Tbsp/15g	47	4.2	312	0.9	13.4	28.3	0.1
Tartare, Rich, Colman's*	1 Tsp/5ml	14	1.2	284	1.2	17.0	23.0	0.6
Tartare, Sainsbury's*	1 Serving/20ml	94	9.8	469	0.4	5.8	49.0	1.0
Tartare, with Olives, The English Provender Co.*	1 Tbsp/15g	64	6.6	425	2.2	5.7	43.7	0.7
Teriyaki, Asda*	1 Serving/98g	99	0.1	101	2.1	23.0	0.1	0.0
Teriyaki, Fresh, The Saucy Fish Co.*	1 Pack/150g	318	2.8	212	2.8	45.8	1.9	0.0
Teriyaki, Japanese Grill, Kikkoman*	1 Serving/15ml	24	0.0	158	4.5	30.8	0.1	0.0
Teriyaki, Lee Kum Kee*	1 Serving/15g	27	0.0	178	2.2	42.4	0.0	0.5
Teriyaki, Sticky, Oven Cook, Blue Dragon*	1 Jar/310g	391	0.3	126	0.7	30.4	0.1	0.0
Teriyaki, Stir Fry, Blue Dragon*	1 Sachet/120g	124	0.0	103	0.5	25.0	0.0	0.0
Teriyaki, Stir Fry, Fresh Ideas, Tesco*	1 Serving/25g	33	0.6	133	1.1	26.9	2.3	0.0
Teriyaki, Stir Fry, Sharwood's*	1 Jar/150g	144	0.4	96	0.9	22.5	0.3	0.3
Thai, Lemon Grass, Lime, & Chilli, Stir Fry, Sainsbury's*	1 Serving/50ml	145	13.2	290	4.0	10.2	26.5	3.5
Thai, Sweet Chilli, Blue Dragon*	1 Serving/15g	28	0.1	188	0.5	45.5	0.6	0.0
Thai Green, Barts*	½ Pack/150ml	210	18.0	140	2.0	6.0	12.0	0.0
Thai Green, Sainsbury's*	¼ Pack/125g	170	11.9	136	1.8	10.8	9.5	2.1
Tikka, Cooking, BGTY, Sainsbury's*	1 Jar/500g	370	9.5	74	1.2	12.9	1.9	0.3
Tikka, Creamy, Chicken Tonight, Knorr*	1oz/28g	36	2.3	129	1.7	12.1	8.2	0.7
Tikka Bhuna, Sizzle & Stir, Chicken Tonight, Knorr*	½ Jar/230g	267	21.6	116	1.2	6.7	9.4	1.1
Tikka Masala, 98% Fat Free, Homepride*	1oz/28g	14	0.5	49	1.4	7.9	1.7	0.8
Tikka Masala, Deliciously Good, Homepride*	¼ Jar/149g	121	5.4	81	2.1	10.0	3.6	1.5
Tikka Masala, GFY, Asda*	½ Jar/250g	190	8.0	76	2.9	9.0	3.2	0.5
Tikka Masala, Hot & Spicy in Glass Jar, Patak's*	1 Jar/350g	332	23.8	95	1.7	6.5	6.8	1.7
Tikka Masala, LC, Tesco*	¼ Jar/125g	100	3.4	80	2.0	11.1	2.7	1.2
Tikka Masala, Lemon & Coriander, Canned, Patak's*	1 Can/283g	487	36.8	172	2.5	11.0	13.0	1.1
Tikka Masala, Medium, Cooking, Sharwood's*	1/3 Jar/140g	150	9.7	107	1.3	9.7	6.9	0.5
Tikka Masala, Perfectly Balanced, Waitrose*	½ Jar/175g	107	1.4	61	2.7	10.7	0.8	1.5
Tikka Masala, Shere Khan*	1 Serving/213ml	176	14.7	83	1.3	3.9	6.9	0.0
Tikka Masala, TTD, Sainsbury's*	½ Pack/175g	247	18.0	141	1.6	10.5	10.3	3.0
Tikka Masala for One, Express, Uncle Ben's*	1 Sachet/170g	168	10.7	99	1.5	9.0	6.3	0.0
Tikka Masala with Coriander, Weight Watchers*	½ Jar/175g	130	3.7	74	2.6	11.2	2.1	0.7
Toffee, GFY, Asda*	1 Serving/5g	15	0.1	306	2.2	68.0	2.8	0.0
Toffee, Luxury, Rowse*	1 Serving/20g	67	0.7	336	1.9	73.9	3.7	0.4
Toffee Fudge, Sainsbury's*	1 Serving/40g	134	1.5	336	1.9	73.9	3.7	0.4
Tomato, Heinz*	1 Tbsp/17g	18	0.0	103	0.9	24.1	0.1	0.7
Tomato & Basil, Cooking, BGTY, Sainsbury's*	1 Jar/500g	335	6.5	67	2.6	11.3	1.3	0.7

	Measure INFO/WEIGHT	per Measure KCAL	FAT	Nutrition Values per 100g / 100ml KCAL	PROT	CARB	FAT	FIBRE
SAUCE								
Tomato & Basil, Cooking, M & S*	1 Serving/130g	78	4.4	60	1.4	5.7	3.4	1.2
Tomato & Basil, for Meatballs, Dolmio*	¼ Jar/125g	48	0.2	38	1.5	6.9	0.2	1.3
Tomato & Basil, Fresh, Asda*	½ Tub/175g	100	3.7	57	1.5	7.9	2.1	0.5
Tomato & Basil, Fresh, Organic, Waitrose*	¼ Pot/175g	77	3.0	44	1.0	6.2	1.7	0.8
Tomato & Basil, Italian, Sainsbury's*	½ Pot/175g	80	3.7	46	1.6	5.1	2.1	2.5
Tomato & Basil, Sun-Ripened, Microwaveable, Dolmio*	1 Sachet/170g	95	3.6	56	1.4	7.9	2.1	0.0
Tomato & Basil for Pasta Stir & Serve, Homepride*	1 Jar/480g	278	13.9	58	1.2	6.7	2.9	0.0
Tomato & Basil Sauce, Fresh, Tesco*	1 Pot/500g	245	9.0	49	1.5	6.8	1.8	0.8
Tomato & Chilli, Table & Dip, Heinz*	1 Tsp/10ml	8	0.0	76	1.4	16.6	0.2	0.8
Tomato & Chilli, Waitrose*	1 Pot/350g	182	9.1	52	10.0	6.2	2.6	3.2
Tomato & Herb, Italian, Sainsbury's*	¼ Jar/126g	88	2.5	70	2.0	11.1	2.0	1.4
Tomato & Marscapone, Finest, Tesco*	1 Serving/350g	270	17.5	77	2.7	5.4	5.0	0.8
Tomato & Marscapone, Italiano, Tesco*	1 Serving/175g	194	15.2	111	2.8	5.4	8.7	0.6
Tomato & Mascarpone, Asda*	½ Tub/175g	152	10.2	87	1.8	7.0	5.8	0.5
Tomato & Mascarpone, Fresh, Sainsbury's*	1/3 Pot/100g	91	6.6	91	2.1	5.9	6.6	1.2
Tomato & Mascarpone, Italian, Sainsbury's*	½ Tub/175g	158	10.2	90	2.6	6.8	5.8	1.2
Tomato & Mascarpone, LC, Tesco*	½ Pot/175g	77	3.5	44	1.6	4.9	2.0	0.8
Tomato & Mozzarella, Finest, Tesco*	1 Serving/175g	89	5.6	51	1.6	4.1	3.2	0.6
Tomato & Onion, Cook in, Homepride*	1 Can/390g	183	2.0	47	0.9	9.8	0.5	0.0
White, for Lasagne, Dolmio*	1 Jar/470g	451	34.3	96	0.6	7.0	7.3	0.0
White, Savoury, Made with Semi-Skimmed Milk	1oz/28g	36	2.2	128	4.2	11.1	7.8	0.2
White, Savoury, Made with Whole Milk	1oz/28g	42	2.9	150	4.1	10.9	10.3	0.2
White Wine, Chardonnay, M & S*	1 Serving/160ml	184	16.0	115	1.4	4.6	10.0	0.9
White Wine, Cooking, Iceland*	1 Serving/220g	198	12.8	90	1.1	8.3	5.8	0.2
White Wine & Cream, Cook in, Classic, Homepride*	¼ Can/125g	101	5.1	81	1.0	8.0	4.1	0.4
White Wine & Mushroom, BGTY, Sainsbury's*	¼ Jar/125g	81	2.5	65	2.8	9.0	2.0	0.3
White Wine & Tarragon, French for Fish, Schwartz*	1 Pack/300g	372	33.3	124	1.1	5.0	11.1	0.8
Worcestershire, Average	***1 Tsp/5g***	***3***	***0.0***	***65***	***1.4***	***15.5***	***0.1***	***0.0***
Worcestershire, Lea & Perrins*	1 Tsp/5ml	4	0.0	88	1.1	22.0	0.0	0.0
Worcestershire, Special Edition, Lea & Perrins*	1 Serving/10ml	13	0.0	130	1.3	28.8	0.2	0.1
Yellow Bean, Stir Fry, Sainsbury's*	½ Jar/100g	126	1.3	126	1.8	26.7	1.3	0.8
Yellow Bean, Stir Fry, Straight to Wok, Amoy*	1oz/28g	44	0.1	158	1.6	36.9	0.5	0.0
Yellow Bean & Cashew, Tesco*	½ Jar/210g	170	6.1	81	1.6	11.9	2.9	0.3
Yellow Bean & Ginger, Stir Fry, Finest, Tesco*	1 Jar/350g	318	3.5	91	2.1	18.3	1.0	1.1
SAUCE MIX								
Beef Bourguignon, Colman's*	1 Pack/40g	136	0.8	340	7.0	72.0	2.0	3.0
Beef Stroganoff, Colman's*	1 Pack/40g	140	3.6	350	11.6	56.1	8.9	2.7
Bread, As Sold, Knorr*	1 Pack/46g	179	5.1	390	12.0	59.0	11.0	4.0
Bread, Colman's*	1 Pack/40g	131	0.4	327	11.4	67.9	1.1	3.2
Bread, Luxury as Sold, Schwartz*	1 Pack/40g	148	1.5	369	11.5	70.3	3.8	3.7
Bread, Made Up, Colman's*	1 Serving/75ml	70	1.5	95	5.0	14.0	2.0	0.6
Cheddar Cheese, Colman's*	1 Pack/40g	164	6.0	410	19.0	51.0	15.0	2.0
Cheddar Cheese, Dry Mix, Schwartz*	1 Pack/40g	144	3.0	361	18.4	55.1	7.4	2.3
Cheddar Cheese, Lidl*	1 Pack/40g	140	4.6	350	18.6	43.0	11.5	0.0
Cheese, Instant, Made Up, Mrs Carters*	1 Serving/100ml	59	1.4	59	1.0	10.7	1.4	0.1
Cheese, Knorr*	1 Pack/58g	132	2.8	227	7.8	38.0	4.9	1.8
Cheese, Made Up, Crosse & Blackwell*	1 Pack/30g	26	1.0	86	5.1	9.2	3.2	0.7
Cheese, Made Up with Skimmed Milk	1 Serving/60g	47	1.4	78	5.4	9.5	2.3	0.0
Cheese & Bacon, for Pasta, Colman's*	1 Pack/50g	180	3.4	359	15.6	58.7	6.8	2.7
Chicken Chasseur, Colman's*	1 Pack/45g	128	0.7	284	8.0	59.2	1.6	3.8
Chicken Chasseur, Schwartz*	1 Pack/40g	126	1.8	316	9.6	59.1	4.6	6.8
Chicken Korma, Colman's*	½ Pack/50g	230	15.4	459	6.6	38.8	30.8	13.2
Chicken Supreme, Colman's*	1 Pack/40g	143	3.7	358	12.1	56.7	9.2	2.4

S

	Measure INFO/WEIGHT	per Measure KCAL	FAT	Nutrition Values per 100g / 100ml KCAL	PROT	CARB	FAT	FIBRE
SAUCE MIX								
Chilli Con Carne, Asda*	1 Sachet/50g	157	0.8	314	7.0	68.0	1.6	2.5
Chilli Con Carne, Hot, Colman's*	1 Pack/40g	127	1.2	317	10.4	62.4	2.9	7.0
Chilli Con Carne, Schwartz*	1 Pack/41g	120	1.5	293	7.9	57.2	3.6	9.5
Chip Shop Curry, Dry Weight, Bisto*	1 Dtsp/9g	38	1.6	427	3.4	63.5	17.7	1.3
Coq Au Vin, Colman's*	1 Pack/50g	150	0.9	301	5.6	65.6	1.8	3.3
Curry, Batchelors*	1 Serving/100g	359	8.3	359	7.1	63.9	8.3	3.9
Curry, Dinaclass, Kerry Group*	1 Bag/382g	1282	32.0	336	17.2	47.1	8.4	1.6
Dauphinoise Potato Bake, Schwartz*	1 Pack/40g	161	10.5	402	6.8	34.7	26.3	15.8
Four Cheese, Colman's*	1 Pack/35g	127	3.9	362	17.1	48.4	11.1	1.8
Hollandaise, Colman's*	1 Pack/28g	104	3.1	372	6.4	61.6	11.1	1.8
Hollandaise, Schwartz*	1 Pack/25g	98	3.2	394	10.6	59.2	12.8	3.7
Lamb Hotpot, Colman's*	1 Pack/40g	119	0.7	297	6.9	63.3	1.7	2.1
Lasagne, Mediterranean Vegetable, Schwartz*	1 Pack/30g	79	1.3	263	9.3	46.0	4.4	15.2
Lasagne, Schwartz*	1 Pack/36g	106	0.5	294	7.0	63.4	1.4	7.0
Mixed Herbs for Chicken, So Juicy, Maggi*	1 Pack/34g	97	1.0	285	8.3	53.8	2.8	5.5
Onion, Creamy, Schwartz*	1 Pack/25g	90	2.3	362	10.1	59.6	9.2	5.3
Onion as Sold, Colman's*	1 Pack/35g	116	0.5	330	12.0	68.0	1.5	7.0
Paprika, for Chicken, So Juicy, Maggi*	1 Pack/34g	91	1.4	267	8.8	45.5	4.0	7.1
Paprika Chicken, Creamy, Schwartz*	1 Pack/34g	116	3.3	342	9.7	53.9	9.8	9.5
Parsley, Creamy, Made Up, Schwartz*	1 Serving/79g	59	2.0	75	4.2	8.7	2.5	0.3
Parsley, Dry, Colman's*	1 Pack/20g	63	0.3	313	7.2	67.9	1.4	3.8
Parsley, Knorr*	1 Sachet/48g	210	11.6	437	4.2	50.6	24.2	0.8
Parsley & Chive for Fish, Schwartz*	1 Pack/38g	132	3.2	348	9.0	58.9	8.5	7.7
Pepper, Creamy, Colman's*	1 Pack/25g	88	2.8	352	13.0	50.0	11.0	0.0
Savoury Mince, Schwartz*	1 Pack/35g	108	0.7	310	14.6	58.3	2.0	1.8
Shepherds Pie, Bramwells*	1 Pack/50g	168	3.0	336	8.6	62.0	6.0	6.9
Shepherd's Pie, Schwartz*	1 Pack/38g	104	1.0	273	7.9	54.4	2.6	11.1
Spaghetti Bolognese, Colman's*	1 Pack/40g	120	0.4	300	8.9	64.1	0.9	5.2
Spaghetti Bolognese, Schwartz*	1 Pack/40g	114	0.6	285	9.2	59.0	1.6	7.0
Spaghetti Carbonara, Schwartz*	1 Pack/32g	135	6.4	421	10.4	49.4	20.1	7.2
Stroganoff, Beef, Schwartz*	1 Pack/35g	125	3.6	358	15.6	50.8	10.3	4.4
Stroganoff, Mushroom, Schwartz*	1 Pack/35g	113	1.9	324	10.0	59.2	5.3	9.6
Sweet & Sour, Colman's*	1 Pack/40g	133	0.2	333	2.6	79.9	0.4	2.2
Sweet & Sour, for Chicken, So Juicy, Maggi*	½ Pack/15g	42	0.3	279	7.1	55.8	2.3	3.5
Thai Green Curry, Schwartz*	1 Pack/41g	137	3.3	333	7.6	57.6	8.1	13.0
Thai Red Curry, Schwartz*	1 Pack/35g	120	2.5	342	5.9	63.5	7.1	7.6
Tikka Masala, Creamy, Schwartz*	1 Pack/31g	100	3.5	324	11.9	43.5	11.4	18.1
Tuna & Pasta Bake, Colman's*	1 Pack/45g	144	2.4	319	10.4	57.1	5.4	5.2
Tuna Napolitana, Schwartz*	1 Pack/30g	107	3.9	357	10.3	49.6	13.1	0.5
Vegetable Pasta, Bake, Colman's*	1 Pack/50g	223	13.1	446	12.0	40.1	26.2	3.6
White, Dry Weight, Bisto*	1 Dtsp/9g	45	2.5	496	3.2	57.4	28.2	0.4
White, Instant, Made Up, Sainsbury's*	1 Serving/90ml	65	2.5	72	0.8	10.9	2.8	0.1
White, Made Up with Semi-Skimmed Milk	1oz/28g	20	0.7	73	4.0	9.6	2.4	0.0
White, Made Up with Skimmed Milk	1oz/28g	17	0.3	59	4.0	9.6	0.9	0.0
White, Savoury, Colman's*	1 Pack/25g	105	3.8	420	9.0	63.0	15.0	2.0
White, Savoury, Knorr*	½ Pack/16g	46	0.9	290	7.8	52.2	5.6	5.2
White, Savoury, Schwartz*	1 Pack/25g	108	5.7	434	11.5	45.6	22.9	5.9
White Wine, with Herbs, Creamy, Schwartz*	1 Pack/26g	86	1.7	330	8.0	60.0	6.5	9.1
SAUERKRAUT								
Average	***1oz/28g***	***4***	***0.0***	***13***	***1.3***	***1.9***	***0.0***	***1.1***
SAUSAGE								
Beef, Average	***1 Sausage/60g***	***151***	***11.1***	***252***	***14.5***	***7.0***	***18.5***	***0.6***
Billy Bear, Kids, Tesco*	1 Slice/20g	37	2.2	185	13.7	7.5	11.2	0.4

S

	Measure INFO/WEIGHT	per Measure KCAL	FAT	Nutrition Values per 100g / 100ml KCAL	PROT	CARB	FAT	FIBRE
SAUSAGE								
Bockwurst, Average	***1 Sausage/45g***	***114***	***10.4***	***253***	***10.8***	***0.8***	***23.0***	***0.0***
Bratwurst, Frozen, Lidl*	1 Sausage/80g	235	21.4	294	12.8	0.5	26.8	0.0
Cheese & Leek, Tesco*	1 Sausage/55g	135	7.9	245	6.6	21.3	14.4	3.9
Chicken, Manor Farm*	1 Sausage/65g	126	8.1	194	13.7	6.6	12.5	1.2
Chicken & Tarragon, Butchers Choice, Sainsbury's*	1 Sausage/47g	106	6.8	225	18.1	5.8	14.4	0.2
Chicken & Turkey, Morrisons*	1 Sausage/57g	86	4.1	152	16.0	5.8	7.2	1.1
Chilli & Coriander, TTD, Sainsbury's*	1 Sausage/44g	136	10.7	310	18.5	4.2	24.4	1.2
Chilli Beef, Boston Style, Waitrose*	1 Sausage/67g	135	9.7	203	14.7	3.4	14.6	0.9
Chipolata, Average	***1 Sausage/28g***	***81***	***6.5***	***291***	***12.1***	***8.7***	***23.1***	***0.7***
Chipolata, Lamb & Rosemary, Tesco*	1 Sausage/32g	69	4.9	218	11.3	8.3	15.5	0.0
Chipolata, Pork, Extra Lean, BGTY, Sainsbury's*	1 Sausage/24g	46	2.1	189	16.9	10.9	8.6	0.5
Chipolata, Pork & Tomato, Organic, Tesco*	1 Sausage/28g	79	6.7	283	12.2	4.3	24.1	0.9
Chipolata, Premium, Average	***1 Serving/80g***	***187***	***13.8***	***234***	***14.8***	***4.7***	***17.3***	***1.2***
Chorizo, Average	***1 Serving/80g***	***250***	***19.4***	***313***	***21.1***	***2.6***	***24.2***	***0.2***
Chorizo, Lean, Average	***1 Sausage/67g***	***131***	***9.2***	***195***	***15.7***	***2.3***	***13.7***	***0.8***
Cocktail, Average	***1 Sausage/7g***	***23***	***1.9***	***323***	***12.1***	***8.6***	***26.7***	***0.9***
Cumberland, Average	***1 Sausage/57g***	***167***	***13.0***	***293***	***13.8***	***8.6***	***22.8***	***0.8***
Cumberland, Healthy Range, Average	***1 Sausage/53g***	***75***	***2.1***	***142***	***17.4***	***9.0***	***4.0***	***0.9***
Cumberland, Weight Watchers*	1 Sausage/39g	55	1.3	140	18.6	8.3	3.4	1.1
Debrecziner, Spicy Smoked, Gebirgsjager*	1 Sausage/37g	118	10.4	320	16.0	1.0	28.0	0.0
Extrawurst, German, Waitrose*	1 Slice/28g	80	7.1	281	13.0	1.0	25.0	0.0
Free From, Wheat & Gulten, Sainsbury's*	1 Serving/23g	61	4.8	268	15.2	4.5	21.0	1.8
Garlic, Average	***1 Slice/11g***	***25***	***2.0***	***227***	***15.7***	***0.8***	***18.2***	***0.0***
Irish, Average	***1 Sausage/40g***	***119***	***8.3***	***298***	***10.7***	***17.2***	***20.7***	***0.7***
Lamb & Mint, M & S*	1oz/28g	63	4.6	225	13.3	6.6	16.3	1.7
Lincolnshire, Average	***1 Sausage/42g***	***122***	***9.1***	***291***	***14.6***	***9.2***	***21.8***	***0.6***
Lincolnshire, Healthy Range, Average	***1 Sausage/50g***	***89***	***4.3***	***177***	***15.8***	***9.0***	***8.6***	***0.8***
Lorne, Average	***1 Sausage/25g***	***78***	***5.8***	***312***	***10.8***	***16.0***	***23.1***	***0.6***
Merguez	1 Merguez/55g	165	14.3	300	16.0	0.6	26.0	0.0
Mortadella, Sainsbury's*	1 Slice/13g	34	2.8	261	17.3	0.1	21.2	0.1
Polish Kabanos, Sainsbury's*	1 Sausage/25g	92	7.6	366	23.0	0.1	30.4	0.1
Polony Slicing, Asda*	1oz/28g	60	3.9	214	11.0	11.0	14.0	0.0
Pork, Apricot & Herb, Waitrose*	1 Sausage/67g	165	11.1	246	11.2	12.9	16.6	1.3
Pork, Average	***1 Sausage/45g***	***139***	***11.2***	***309***	***11.9***	***9.8***	***25.0***	***0.8***
Pork, Bacon & Cheese, Asda*	¼ Pack/114g	329	23.9	289	18.0	7.0	21.0	0.4
Pork, Battered, Thick, Average	1oz/28g	126	10.2	448	17.3	21.7	36.3	2.0
Pork, Casserole, Diet Chef Ltd*	1 Portion/300g	303	18.3	101	6.6	4.9	6.1	1.4
Pork, Cumberland, TTD, Sainsbury's*	1 Sausage/46g	132	9.7	288	21.4	3.1	21.1	0.6
Pork, Extra Lean, Average	***1 Sausage/54g***	***84***	***3.7***	***155***	***17.3***	***6.1***	***6.8***	***0.8***
Pork, Free From, Tesco*	1 Sausage/57g	124	8.6	218	12.1	8.5	15.0	2.2
Pork, Frozen, Fried	***1oz/28g***	***88***	***6.9***	***316***	***13.8***	***10.0***	***24.8***	***0.0***
Pork, Frozen, Grilled	***1oz/28g***	***81***	***5.9***	***289***	***14.8***	***10.5***	***21.2***	***0.0***
Pork, Garlic & Herb, Average	***1 Sausage/76g***	***203***	***16.5***	***268***	***12.0***	***6.0***	***21.8***	***1.2***
Pork, Gourmet, Waitrose*	2 Sausages/133g	285	20.1	214	14.1	5.6	15.1	0.4
Pork, Low Fat, Skinny Lizzie*	1 Sausage/66g	87	0.9	132	16.9	13.1	1.3	1.6
Pork, Premium, Average	***1 Sausage/74g***	***191***	***13.6***	***258***	***14.9***	***8.3***	***18.4***	***1.0***
Pork, Reduced Fat, Chilled, Grilled	***1 Sausage/45g***	***104***	***6.2***	***230***	***16.2***	***10.8***	***13.8***	***1.5***
Pork, Reduced Fat, Chilled, Raw	***1oz/28g***	***50***	***3.0***	***180***	***13.0***	***8.7***	***10.6***	***1.2***
Pork, Reduced Fat, Healthy Range, Average	***1 Sausage/57g***	***86***	***3.4***	***151***	***15.6***	***9.0***	***6.0***	***0.9***
Pork, Skinless, Average	***1oz/28g***	***81***	***6.6***	***291***	***11.7***	***8.2***	***23.6***	***0.6***
Pork, Smoked, Reduced Fat, Mattessons*	½ Pack/113g	288	21.5	255	14.0	7.0	19.0	0.9
Pork, Thick, Average	***1 Sausage/39g***	***115***	***8.7***	***296***	***13.3***	***10.0***	***22.4***	***1.0***
Pork, Thick, Reduced Fat, Healthy Range, Average	***1 Sausage/52g***	***90***	***3.8***	***172***	***14.0***	***12.3***	***7.4***	***0.8***

S

	Measure INFO/WEIGHT	per Measure KCAL	FAT	Nutrition Values per 100g / 100ml KCAL	PROT	CARB	FAT	FIBRE
SAUSAGE								
Pork & Apple, Average	***1 Sausage/57g***	***146***	***10.7***	***256***	***14.5***	***7.5***	***18.8***	***1.9***
Pork & Beef, Average	***1 Sausage/45g***	***133***	***10.2***	***295***	***8.7***	***13.6***	***22.7***	***0.5***
Pork & Herb, Average	***1 Sausage/75g***	***231***	***19.5***	***308***	***13.2***	***5.4***	***26.0***	***0.4***
Pork & Herb, Healthy Range, Average	***1 Sausage/59g***	***75***	***1.4***	***126***	***16.0***	***10.8***	***2.4***	***1.1***
Pork & Leek, Average	***1oz/28g***	***73***	***5.6***	***262***	***14.6***	***6.0***	***20.0***	***1.1***
Pork & Onion, GF, Asda*	1 Sausage/41g	105	7.0	257	20.0	6.0	17.0	1.8
Pork & Red Onion, TTD, Sainsbury's*	1 Sausage/48g	138	8.8	288	18.5	12.4	18.3	1.4
Pork & Stilton, Average	***1 Sausage/57g***	***180***	***15.2***	***316***	***13.2***	***5.8***	***26.7***	***0.3***
Pork & Sweet Chilli, Waitrose*	1 Sausage/67g	151	10.1	226	15.5	6.9	15.1	2.7
Pork & Tomato, Grilled, Average	***1 Sausage/47g***	***127***	***9.7***	***273***	***13.9***	***7.5***	***20.8***	***0.4***
Premium, Chilled, Fried	***1oz/28g***	***77***	***5.8***	***275***	***15.8***	***6.7***	***20.7***	***0.0***
Premium, Chilled, Grilled	***1oz/28g***	***82***	***6.3***	***292***	***16.8***	***6.3***	***22.4***	***0.0***
Premium, Pork, (8 Pack), Weight Watchers*	1 Sausage/39g	60	1.6	155	20.0	7.8	4.2	1.7
Round, Breakfast Pack, Healthy Choice, Asda*	1 Sausage/53g	85	2.6	160	23.0	6.0	4.9	0.0
Saucisson Montagne, Waitrose*	1 Slice/5g	21	1.8	421	20.7	1.9	36.7	0.0
Saveloy, The Delicatessen, Tesco*	1 Saveloy/65g	185	14.9	285	9.5	8.3	23.0	2.3
Schinkenwurst, German, Waitrose*	1 Slice/13g	28	2.2	224	16.0	0.8	17.6	0.0
Sicilian Style, TTD, Sainsbury's*	1 Sausage/50g	146	12.2	293	17.6	0.7	24.4	0.9
Smoked, Average	***1 Sausage/174g***	***588***	***52.2***	***338***	***13.0***	***4.0***	***30.0***	***0.0***
Spanish, Wafer Thin, Asda*	1 Slice/4g	12	0.8	298	25.4	4.1	20.0	0.0
Thick, Irish, Fresh, Grilled, Richmond*	2 Sausages/80g	203	12.7	254	11.7	16.0	15.9	2.6
Toulouse, M & S*	1 Sausage/57g	123	8.9	215	12.4	5.8	15.6	1.3
Turkey, Average	***1 Sausage/57g***	***90***	***4.6***	***157***	***15.7***	***6.3***	***8.0***	***0.0***
Turkey & Chicken, Average	***1 Sausage/57g***	***126***	***8.2***	***222***	***14.4***	***8.2***	***14.6***	***1.8***
Tuscan, M & S*	1 Sausage/66g	145	10.6	220	14.9	4.6	16.0	0.6
Venison, Grilled, Finest, Tesco*	1 Sausage/41g	86	5.5	215	16.6	6.3	13.7	0.6
Venison, Oisin, M & S*	1 Serving/25g	41	2.3	165	16.8	3.8	9.3	0.7
Venison & Pork, Waitrose*	1 Sausage/64g	93	4.0	146	16.5	5.3	6.3	1.1
Venison & Red Wine, TTD, Sainsbury's*	1 Sausage/39g	88	5.2	228	20.7	5.8	13.6	1.7
Wiejska, Polish, Sainsbury's*	1/8 Pack/50g	78	4.5	157	18.7	0.4	9.0	0.5
Wild Boar	1 Sausage/85g	220	17.0	259	16.5	1.2	20.0	0.0
SAUSAGE & MASH								
	1 Serving/231g	285	16.1	123	4.5	10.4	7.0	1.0
221, Oakhouse Foods Ltd*	1 Meal/400g	504	27.2	126	5.5	11.0	6.8	1.4
GFY, Asda*	1 Pack/400g	330	10.0	82	4.2	10.8	2.5	1.8
Vegetarian, GFY, Asda*	1 Pack/400g	292	8.8	73	4.2	9.0	2.2	2.1
Vegetarian, Tesco*	1 Pack/410g	398	15.6	97	4.6	11.1	3.8	2.0
SAUSAGE MEAT								
Pork, Average	***1oz/28g***	***96***	***8.2***	***344***	***9.9***	***10.2***	***29.4***	***0.6***
SAUSAGE ROLL								
BGTY, Sainsbury's*	1 Roll/65g	200	11.4	308	9.6	27.9	17.6	1.4
Cocktail, Average	1 Roll/15g	57	3.7	378	8.9	29.4	24.9	1.9
Cumberland, Chosen By You, Asda*	1 Roll/66g	201	10.9	304	8.3	28.9	16.5	3.1
Frozen, Greggs Iceland Exclusive*	1 Roll/103g	371	26.3	360	8.0	22.0	25.5	1.5
Go Large, Asda*	1 Roll/170g	660	47.6	388	9.0	25.0	28.0	0.9
Jumbo, Sainsbury's*	1 Roll/145g	492	34.4	339	8.2	23.2	23.7	1.5
Kingsize, Pork Farms*	½ Roll/50g	241	15.9	483	10.5	39.9	31.8	0.0
Large, Freshbake*	1 Roll/52g	153	9.5	294	6.6	25.9	18.3	4.6
Large, Frozen, Tesco*	1 Roll/50g	182	11.9	365	6.0	31.0	23.8	0.9
Lincolnshire, Geo Adams*	1 Roll/130g	474	31.6	365	8.3	28.2	24.3	1.1
Mini, Tesco*	1 Roll/15g	53	3.7	356	9.0	23.9	24.9	1.5
Party, Sainsbury's*	1 Roll/13g	54	4.0	422	8.7	26.7	31.1	1.2
Pork, 30% Less Fat, Chosen By You, Asda*	1 Roll/66g	207	12.3	313	9.8	26.4	18.7	1.2

	Measure INFO/WEIGHT	per Measure KCAL	FAT	Nutrition Values per 100g / 100ml KCAL	PROT	CARB	FAT	FIBRE
SAUSAGE ROLL								
Pork, Morrisons*	1 Roll/70g	195	9.0	278	9.6	31.2	12.8	1.5
Pork, Spicy, 5 Pack, Chosen By You, Asda*	1 Roll/66g	201	10.9	304	8.3	28.9	16.5	3.1
Pork Farms*	1 Roll/54g	196	12.9	363	7.9	30.0	23.9	0.0
Puff Pastry	1 Med/60g	230	16.6	383	9.9	25.4	27.6	1.0
Puff Pastry, Sainsbury's*	1 Roll/65g	250	18.1	384	8.3	25.0	27.9	0.9
Reduced Fat, Sainsbury's*	1 Roll/66g	191	9.4	289	10.5	29.8	14.2	1.8
Snack, GFY, Asda*	1 Roll/34g	112	7.0	329	9.4	26.5	20.6	0.9
Snack, Sainsbury's*	1 Roll/34g	130	8.5	383	9.7	29.9	25.0	2.1
Snack Size, Tesco*	1 Roll/32g	118	8.8	369	9.1	21.7	27.4	2.3
TTD, Sainsbury's*	1 Roll/115g	440	31.9	383	11.9	21.3	27.8	2.0
SAUSAGE ROLL VEGETARIAN								
Linda McCartney*	1 Roll/52g	145	7.1	278	13.1	26.0	13.7	1.6
Mini, Linda McCartney*	1 Roll/14g	41	2.2	293	11.3	23.7	15.8	5.2
SAUSAGE VEGETARIAN								
Asda*	1 Sausage/43g	81	3.9	189	20.0	7.0	9.0	2.9
Braai Flavour, Fry's Special Vegetarian*	1 Sausage/63g	86	4.4	138	16.5	10.0	7.0	4.0
Cumberland, Cauldron Foods*	1 Sausage/46g	75	4.0	163	14.0	6.5	8.6	2.0
Glamorgan, Cooked, Asda*	1 Sausage/50g	113	6.2	226	5.3	21.8	12.4	2.8
Glamorgan, Leek & Cheese, Goodlife*	1 Sausage/50g	94	4.9	188	4.9	20.0	9.8	2.3
Glamorgan, Organic, Cauldron Foods*	1 Sausage/41g	67	3.8	162	12.5	7.3	9.2	1.7
Glamorgan Leek & Cheese, Sainsbury's*	1 Sausage/50g	98	5.2	197	4.3	21.3	10.5	2.7
Granose*	1oz/28g	63	3.8	226	8.5	17.5	13.5	0.0
Italian, Linda McCartney*	1 Sausage/50g	76	2.8	152	16.8	6.9	5.6	3.4
Leek & Cheese, Organic, Cauldron Foods*	1 Sausage/41g	80	4.1	194	14.4	11.3	10.1	1.7
Lincolnshire, Asda*	1 Sausage/56g	96	4.5	172	17.0	8.0	8.0	1.4
Lincolnshire, Chilled, Cauldron Foods*	1 Sausage/46g	76	4.1	165	14.0	6.5	8.8	2.0
Lincolnshire, Frozen, Tesco*	1 Sausage/50g	78	2.5	155	15.5	10.8	5.0	3.0
Linda McCartney*	1 Sausage/50g	101	4.4	202	22.5	8.3	8.8	1.6
Realeat*	1 Sausage/40g	66	3.9	165	17.2	2.0	9.8	8.1
Red Onion & Rosemary, Linda McCartney*	2 Sausages/100g	128	3.7	128	14.2	9.7	3.7	5.8
Roasted Garlic & Oregano, Cauldron Foods*	1 Sausage/50g	90	5.0	179	13.1	9.0	10.1	2.1
Smoked Paprika & Chilli, Cauldron Foods*	1 Sausage/50g	76	4.1	152	7.8	11.8	8.2	2.6
Spinach, Leek & Cheese, Gourmet, Wicken Fen*	1 Sausage/46g	92	4.7	201	10.3	17.0	10.2	1.9
Sun Dried Tomato & Black Olive, Cauldron Foods*	1 Sausage/50g	71	3.8	142	8.7	9.4	7.7	2.6
Sun Dried Tomato & Herb, Linda McCartney*	1 Sausage/35g	93	5.4	266	21.8	10.1	15.4	1.7
SAVOURY EGGS								
Bites, Mini, Sainsbury's*	1 Egg/12g	35	2.2	288	9.4	21.7	17.8	1.6
Mini, Iceland*	1 Egg/20g	66	4.8	327	11.0	17.5	23.7	1.1
Mini, Tesco*	1 Egg/20g	55	3.5	274	9.2	20.2	17.4	2.3
SCALLOPS								
Asda*	1oz/28g	33	0.4	118	23.2	1.4	1.4	0.0
Breaded, Thai Style with Plum Sauce, Finest, Tesco*	1 Serving/210g	401	14.7	191	11.5	20.6	7.0	0.8
Canadian, Finest, Tesco*	½ Pack/100g	80	0.2	80	16.4	2.6	0.2	0.1
Hotbake Shells, Sainsbury's*	1 Serving/140g	241	15.7	172	9.5	8.4	11.2	0.8
Lemon Grass & Ginger, Tesco*	½ Pack/112g	90	1.1	80	15.2	2.5	1.0	0.6
Raw, Bay or Sea with Roe, Average	***1 Scallop/15g***	***13***	***0.1***	***88***	***16.8***	***2.4***	***0.8***	***0.0***
Steamed, Average	1oz/28g	33	0.4	118	23.2	3.4	1.4	0.0
SCAMPI								
Bites, Everyday, Value, Tesco*	½ pack/125g	262	10.0	210	9.4	23.4	8.0	1.2
Breaded, Baked, Average	½ Pack/255g	565	27.4	222	10.7	20.5	10.7	1.0
Breaded, Fried in Oil, Average	1 Serving/100g	237	13.6	237	9.4	20.5	13.6	0.0
Breaded & Chips, Oakhouse Foods Ltd*	1 Meal/300g	456	16.5	152	4.6	21.5	5.5	2.3
Provencale	1 Serving/100g	500	49.0	500	7.0	4.0	49.0	1.0

	Measure INFO/WEIGHT	per Measure KCAL	FAT	Nutrition Values per 100g / 100ml KCAL	PROT	CARB	FAT	FIBRE
SCAMPI								
Wholetail, Breaded, Frozen, Chosen By You, Asda*	1 Serving/93g	197	8.7	212	9.7	21.4	9.4	1.3
Wholetail, in Crunchy Crumb, Morrisons*	1 Pack/250g	508	21.8	203	9.6	19.9	8.7	1.7
Wholetail, Premium, Youngs*	1 Serving/125g	256	11.4	205	29.5	21.6	9.1	2.1
Wholetail, with a Hint of Lemon, Youngs*	1 Pack/228g	505	20.5	202	9.6	22.4	8.2	1.2
SCAMPI & CHIPS								
Chunky, Finest, Tesco*	1 Pack/280g	420	15.4	150	5.9	18.3	5.5	1.4
with Peas	1 Serving/490g	822	43.6	168	10.1	11.3	8.9	1.2
with Peas, 531, Wiltshire Farm Foods*	1oz/28g	42	1.3	149	6.3	20.0	4.8	2.9
Youngs*	1oz/28g	42	1.5	150	5.0	20.3	5.4	1.7
SCHNAPPS								
Vodkat, Intercontinental Brands Ltd*	1 Serving/25ml	31	0.0	124	0.0	0.8	0.0	0.0
SCHNITZEL VEGETARIAN								
Breaded, Tivall*	1 Schnitzel/100g	172	8.0	172	16.0	9.0	8.0	5.0
SCONE								
3% Fat, M & S*	1 Scone/65g	179	1.6	275	7.2	55.1	2.5	2.3
Cheese, Average	1 Scone/40g	145	7.1	363	10.1	43.2	17.8	1.6
Cheese, Cornish, TTD, Sainsbury's*	1 Scone/74g	267	13.8	361	12.3	36.1	18.6	2.3
Cheese & Black Pepper, Mini, M & S*	1 Scone/18g	67	3.3	370	10.2	41.1	18.3	1.7
Cherry, Double Butter, Genesis Crafty*	1 Scone/63g	198	4.8	314	6.8	54.5	7.6	1.4
Cherry, Genesis Crafty*	1 Scone/81g	226	5.8	279	4.9	50.5	7.1	0.0
Cherry, M & S*	1 Scone/60g	202	7.3	337	6.9	49.7	12.2	1.9
Clotted Cream, Cornish, TTD, Sainsbury's*	1 Scone/70g	269	12.7	384	8.4	46.6	18.2	2.1
Cream, Sainsbury's*	1 Scone/50g	172	8.7	345	4.6	42.5	17.4	3.1
Derby, Asda*	1 Scone/59g	202	5.9	342	7.0	56.0	10.0	0.0
Derby, Mother's Pride*	1 Scone/60g	208	8.4	347	5.2	49.8	14.0	1.5
Devon, M & S*	1 Scone/59g	225	9.6	380	7.1	50.8	16.2	1.5
Devon, Sainsbury's*	1 Scone/54g	201	8.4	372	7.1	51.1	15.5	1.6
Fresh Cream, Finest, Tesco*	1 Serving/133g	469	23.2	354	4.6	44.5	17.5	1.7
Fresh Cream, with Strawberry Jam, Tesco*	1 Scone/83g	290	15.6	352	4.7	40.7	18.9	1.1
Fruit, Average	1 Scone/40g	126	3.9	316	7.3	52.9	9.8	0.0
Fruit, Breakfast Griddle, Genesis Crafty*	1 Scone/65g	192	5.5	296	6.2	50.7	8.5	1.9
Fruit, Economy, Sainsbury's*	1 Scone/34g	111	3.2	326	7.9	52.5	9.4	1.7
Fruit, Genesis Crafty*	1 Scone/78g	231	6.6	296	6.2	50.7	8.5	0.0
Fruit, Waitrose*	1 Scone/59g	190	4.8	325	6.3	56.5	8.2	2.2
Luxury, Hovis*	1 Scone/85g	267	7.9	314	5.6	51.8	9.3	2.2
Plain, Average	1 Scone/40g	145	5.8	362	7.2	53.8	14.6	1.9
Plain, Genesis Crafty*	1 Scone/74g	227	7.4	307	6.8	49.1	10.0	0.0
Potato, Average	1 Scone/40g	118	5.7	296	5.1	39.1	14.3	1.6
Potato, Mother's Pride*	1 Scone/37g	77	0.8	207	4.7	42.0	2.2	4.3
Strawberry, Fresh Cream, BGTY, Sainsbury's*	1 Scone/50g	154	5.6	309	5.1	47.0	11.2	1.1
Strawberry, Fresh Cream, Sainsbury's*	1 Scone/60g	218	11.2	363	6.5	42.5	18.6	1.4
Sultana, BGTY, Sainsbury's*	1 Scone/63g	178	1.8	283	7.7	56.7	2.8	2.4
Sultana, Finest, Tesco*	1 Scone/70g	238	7.6	340	8.9	50.9	10.9	2.1
Sultana, M & S*	1 Scone/66g	231	8.2	350	6.5	53.0	12.5	2.0
Sultana, Reduced Fat, Waitrose*	1 Scone/65g	187	3.4	287	6.6	53.2	5.3	2.6
Sultana, Sainsbury's*	1 Scone/54g	176	5.9	327	6.9	50.2	11.0	6.5
Sultana, TTD, Sainsbury's*	1 Scone/70g	239	8.1	341	6.5	52.9	11.5	2.6
Tattie, Scottish, Nick Nairn's*	1 Scone/21g	42	0.3	199	4.0	34.7	1.6	0.7
Wholemeal	1 Scone/40g	130	5.8	326	8.7	43.1	14.4	5.2
Wholemeal, Fruit	1 Scone/40g	130	5.1	324	8.1	47.2	12.8	4.9
SCOTCH EGGS								
Cumberland, Waitrose*	1 Egg/114g	243	14.3	214	13.0	12.1	12.6	1.6
Free Range, Sainsbury's*	1 Egg/113g	284	19.0	252	12.4	12.5	16.9	2.5

	Measure INFO/WEIGHT	per Measure KCAL	FAT	Nutrition Values per 100g / 100ml KCAL	PROT	CARB	FAT	FIBRE
SCOTCH EGGS								
Ginsters*	1 Egg/95g	228	15.1	240	15.3	9.7	15.9	0.6
Retail	1 Egg/120g	301	20.5	251	12.0	13.1	17.1	0.0
Super Mini, Asda*	1 Egg/13g	38	2.6	305	10.0	19.0	21.0	2.1
SEA BASS								
Cooked, Dry Heat, Average	***1 Fillet/101g***	***125***	***2.6***	***124***	***23.6***	***0.0***	***2.6***	***0.0***
Fillet, in Beurre Blanc & Dill Sauce, The Saucy Fish Co.*	2 Fillets/210g	357	23.5	170	16.8	0.7	11.2	0.0
Fillet, with Lemon & Parsley Butter, Iceland*	½ Pack/110g	197	13.2	179	17.6	0.1	12.0	0.1
Raw, Fillet, Average	***1 Fillet/95g***	***108***	***3.4***	***113***	***20.3***	***0.0***	***3.5***	***0.1***
SEA BREAM								
Fillets, Raw, Average	***1oz/28g***	***27***	***0.8***	***96***	***17.5***	***0.0***	***2.9***	***0.0***
SEAFOOD COCKTAIL								
Average	1oz/28g	24	0.4	87	15.6	2.9	1.5	0.0
Frozen, Chosen By You, Asda*	1 Bag/300g	213	1.5	71	15.3	1.0	0.5	0.6
Premium Quality, Lyons Seafood Co*	1 Serving/100g	76	0.9	76	13.2	3.7	0.9	1.1
SEAFOOD SELECTION								
Asda*	1 Pack/240g	173	1.9	72	13.4	2.9	0.8	0.0
Fresh, Tesco*	1 Pack/234g	187	2.3	80	17.7	0.1	1.0	0.0
M & S*	1 Serving/200g	170	2.0	85	17.4	1.6	1.0	0.5
SEAFOOD STICKS								
Average	1 Stick/15g	16	0.0	106	8.0	18.4	0.2	0.2
Chilled or Frozen, Youngs*	1 Stick/14g	15	0.2	108	9.0	15.4	1.2	0.6
SEASONING MIX								
Beef Taco, Colman's*	1 Pack/30g	76	3.6	252	9.1	26.9	12.0	14.0
Chicken, Piri Piri, Tray Bake, Maggi*	1 Pack/40g	120	2.0	300	9.6	49.5	4.9	9.6
Chicken, Simply Shake, Schwartz*	1 Serving/100g	273	8.1	273	12.3	67.9	8.1	29.1
Chicken & Chorizo Gratin, Schwartz*	1 Pack/35g	108	0.5	310	5.8	63.4	1.4	10.4
Chicken Provencal, Schwartz*	1 Packet/35g	104	0.7	296	9.3	55.3	2.0	9.9
Chilli, Old El Paso*	1 Pack/39g	117	2.0	301	7.0	57.0	5.0	0.0
Fajita, Chicken, Colman's*	1 Pack/40g	138	2.5	344	9.4	62.5	6.3	4.8
Fish, Schwartz*	1 Tsp/4g	9	0.1	222	6.5	55.5	2.3	11.6
Garlic, for Chicken, Cook in Bag, Average	1 Bag/36g	108	0.7	300	9.6	58.3	2.0	5.9
Garlic, Papyrus Sheets, SoTender, Maggi*	1 Sheet/6g	25	1.9	438	6.3	24.4	32.5	11.4
Garlic & Herb Mash, Perfect Shake, Schwartz*	1 Serving/10g	29	2.2	290	7.6	43.0	21.9	20.2
Italian Herb, Schwartz*	1 Tsp/1g	3	0.0	338	11.0	64.5	4.0	0.0
Italian Herbs, Papyrus Sheets, SoTender, Maggi*	1 Sheet/6g	26	2.0	440	7.3	22.1	34.1	7.7
Jamaican Jerk Chicken, Recipe, Schwartz*	1 Pack/27g	75	0.8	276	9.8	69.8	3.0	17.2
Lemon & Herb, Cous Cous, Asda*	1 Tbsp/15g	46	1.0	305	10.6	52.0	6.5	10.2
Lemon & Herb, for Chicken, Cook in Bag, Average	1 Bag/34g	121	1.9	356	10.8	63.7	5.5	4.1
Mediterranean, for Chicken, Cook in Bag, Average	1 Bag/33g	99	0.7	302	10.6	56.6	2.0	7.0
Mediterranean Roasted Vegetable, Schwartz*	1 Pack/30g	86	1.2	288	6.9	56.1	4.0	10.3
Paprika, for Chicken, Cook in Bag, Average	1 Bag/34g	96	1.3	283	12.3	45.8	4.0	8.1
Paprika, Papyrus Sheets, SoTender, Maggi*	1 Sheet/6g	25	2.0	431	9.1	12.2	35.2	14.5
Potato Roasties, Rosemary & Garlic, Crispy, Schwartz*	1 Pack/33g	88	2.6	267	13.0	36.1	7.8	21.1
Potato Roasties, Southern Fried, Crispy, Schwartz*	1 Pack/35g	78	1.5	222	9.2	36.2	4.4	25.1
Potato Wedges, Cajun, Schwartz*	1 Pack/38g	112	2.9	295	9.1	47.6	7.6	14.3
Potato Wedges, Garlic & Herb, Schwartz*	1 Pack/38g	106	1.9	278	11.4	47.1	4.9	11.7
Potato Wedges, Nacho Cheese, Schwartz*	1 Pack/38g	114	3.7	299	13.6	39.3	9.7	7.7
Potato Wedges, Onion & Chive, Schwartz*	1 Pack/38g	113	0.7	297	10.9	59.4	1.8	6.5
Season-All, Schwartz*	1 Tsp/6g	4	0.1	72	2.3	11.6	1.8	0.0
Shepherd's Pie, Colman's*	1 Pack/50g	141	0.7	282	12.5	54.7	1.4	4.3
Shotz, Cajun Chicken Seasoning, Schwartz*	1 Pack/3g	8	0.2	268	9.9	45.6	5.2	0.0
Shotz, Garlic Pepper Steak Seasoning, Schwartz*	1 Pack/3g	11	0.2	370	14.0	67.0	5.0	0.0
Shotz, Moroccan Chicken Seasoning, Schwartz*	1 Pack/3g	9	0.2	312	9.7	56.7	5.2	0.0

	Measure INFO/WEIGHT	per Measure KCAL	FAT	Nutrition Values per 100g / 100ml KCAL	PROT	CARB	FAT	FIBRE
SEASONING MIX								
Shotz, Seven Pepper Steak Seasoning, Schwartz*	1 Pack/3g	7	0.1	246	8.2	47.8	2.4	0.0
Spanish Roasted Vegetables, Schwartz*	1 Pack/15g	22	0.9	147	9.1	14.1	6.0	22.6
Sticky Spare Ribs, Season & Shake, Colman's*	1 Pack/52g	179	1.5	344	5.1	72.7	2.8	4.0
Taco, Old El Paso*	¼ Pack/9g	30	0.4	334	5.5	69.0	4.0	0.0
Thai Seven Spice, Schwartz*	1 Serving/10g	24	0.4	243	7.5	44.1	4.1	0.0
SEAWEED								
Chuka Wakame, Daiwa*	1 Serving/100g	70	3.3	70	1.3	8.8	3.3	1.4
Crispy, Average	***1oz/28g***	***182***	***17.3***	***651***	***7.5***	***15.6***	***61.9***	***7.0***
Irish Moss, Raw	***1oz/28g***	***2***	***0.1***	***8***	***1.5***	***0.0***	***0.2***	***12.3***
Kombu, Dried, Raw	***1oz/28g***	***12***	***0.4***	***43***	***7.1***	***0.0***	***1.6***	***58.7***
Nori, Dried, Raw	***1oz/28g***	***38***	***0.4***	***136***	***30.7***	***0.0***	***1.5***	***44.4***
Wakame, Dried, Raw	***1oz/28g***	***20***	***0.7***	***71***	***12.4***	***0.0***	***2.4***	***47.1***
SEEDS								
Chia, Black, The Chia Company*	1 Tbsp/15g	69	4.6	458	20.4	37.0	30.4	36.0
Chia, White, The Chia Company*	1 Tbsp/15g	69	5.1	458	20.4	37.0	34.0	36.0
Chocolate Covered, Munchy Seeds*	1 Pack/50g	275	14.2	550	15.2	37.2	28.4	14.2
Fenugreek, Average	***1 Tsp/4g***	***12***	***0.2***	***323***	***23.0***	***58.4***	***6.4***	***24.6***
Fiery, Graze*	1 Pack/34g	173	14.8	510	21.8	17.3	43.5	7.9
Hemp, Raw, Organic, Navitas Naturals*	1 Serving/15g	80	7.0	533	33.3	20.0	46.7	6.7
Hemp, Shelled, Linwoods*	2 Tbsps/30g	178	14.8	593	35.1	7.6	49.5	5.9
Melon, Average	***1 Tbsp/15g***	***87***	***7.2***	***583***	***28.5***	***9.9***	***47.7***	***0.0***
Mixed, Snacking, Chosen By You, Asda*	1 Serving/25g	145	10.9	581	33.1	10.9	43.5	6.7
Mixed, Wholesome, Love Life, Waitrose*	1 Serving/30g	166	13.6	554	21.3	15.5	45.2	8.0
Mustard, Average	***1 Tsp/3g***	***15***	***0.9***	***469***	***34.9***	***34.9***	***28.8***	***14.7***
Nigella, Average	***1 Tsp/5g***	***20***	***1.7***	***392***	***21.3***	***1.9***	***33.3***	***8.4***
Poppy, Average	***1 Tbsp/9g***	***47***	***3.9***	***533***	***18.0***	***23.7***	***44.7***	***10.0***
Pumpkin, Average	***1 Tbsp/10g***	***57***	***4.6***	***568***	***27.9***	***13.0***	***45.9***	***3.8***
Pumpkin, Whole, Roasted, Salted, Average	***1 Serving/50g***	***261***	***21.1***	***522***	***33.0***	***13.4***	***42.1***	***3.9***
Sesame, Average	1oz/28g	171	15.8	610	22.3	3.6	56.4	7.8
Soy, Roasted, Graze*	1 Punnet/34g	202	16.0	593	21.0	21.0	47.0	9.0
Sunflower, Average	***1 Tbsp/10g***	***59***	***4.9***	***585***	***23.4***	***15.0***	***48.7***	***5.7***
SEMOLINA								
Average	***1oz/28g***	***98***	***0.5***	***348***	***11.0***	***75.2***	***1.8***	***2.1***
Pudding, Creamed, Ambrosia*	1 Can/425g	344	7.2	81	3.3	13.1	1.7	0.2
Pudding, Creamed, Co-Op*	1 Can/425g	382	8.5	90	4.0	15.0	2.0	0.0
SHALLOTS								
Pickled in Hot & Spicy Vinegar, Tesco*	1 Onion/18g	14	0.0	77	1.0	18.0	0.1	1.9
Raw, Average	***1 Serving/80g***	***16***	***0.2***	***20***	***1.5***	***3.3***	***0.2***	***1.4***
SHANDY								
Bavaria*	1 Can/300ml	109	0.0	36	0.0	0.0	0.0	0.0
Bitter, Original, Ben Shaws*	1 Can/330ml	89	0.0	27	0.0	6.0	0.0	0.0
Canned, Morrisons*	1 Can/330ml	36	0.0	11	0.0	1.8	0.0	0.0
Homemade, Average	1 Pint/568ml	148	0.0	26	0.2	2.9	0.0	0.0
Lemonade, Schweppes*	1 Can/330ml	76	0.0	23	0.0	5.1	0.0	0.0
Lemonade, Traditional Style, Tesco*	1 Can/330ml	63	0.0	19	0.0	4.7	0.0	0.0
Traditional, Fentiman's*	1 Bottle/275ml	102	0.0	37	0.4	8.7	0.0	0.0
SHARK								
Raw	***1oz/28g***	***29***	***0.3***	***102***	***23.0***	***0.0***	***1.1***	***0.0***
SHARON FRUIT								
Average	***1oz/28g***	***20***	***0.0***	***73***	***0.8***	***18.6***	***0.0***	***1.6***
SHERRY								
Dry, Average	***1 Glass/120ml***	***139***	***0.0***	***116***	***0.2***	***1.4***	***0.0***	***0.0***
Medium	***1 Serving/50ml***	***58***	***0.0***	***116***	***0.1***	***5.9***	***0.0***	***0.0***

	Measure INFO/WEIGHT	per Measure KCAL	FAT	Nutrition Values per 100g / 100ml KCAL	PROT	CARB	FAT	FIBRE
SHERRY								
Sweet	***1 Serving/50ml***	***68***	***0.0***	***136***	***0.3***	***6.9***	***0.0***	***0.0***
SHORTBREAD								
All Butter, Assorted, Aldi*	1oz/28g	143	7.5	511	6.5	61.0	26.8	2.0
All Butter, Deans*	1 Biscuit/15g	77	3.8	511	4.9	65.7	25.4	1.2
All Butter, Fingers, Highland, Sainsbury's*	2 Biscuits/40g	208	11.5	521	4.8	59.4	28.8	2.7
All Butter, Fingers, McVitie's*	1 Finger/20g	106	5.4	530	6.5	64.7	27.2	0.0
All Butter, Fingers, Royal Edinburgh Bakery*	1 Biscuit/17g	88	4.8	519	5.8	60.3	28.3	1.8
All Butter, Fingers, Scottish, M & S*	1 Finger/18g	90	4.9	510	5.7	58.9	27.8	4.7
All Butter, Petticoat Tails, Co-Op*	1 Biscuit/13g	68	3.8	520	5.0	60.0	29.0	2.0
All Butter, Petticoat Tails, Gardiners of Scotland*	1 Biscuit/12g	64	3.4	514	5.2	62.1	27.2	0.0
All Butter, Round, Luxury, M & S*	1 Biscuit/20g	105	5.8	525	6.2	60.0	29.0	2.0
All Butter, Royal Edinburgh, Asda*	1 Biscuit/18g	93	5.1	519	5.8	60.3	28.3	1.8
All Butter, Scottish, M & S*	1 Biscuit/34g	173	9.5	510	5.7	58.9	27.8	2.3
All Butter, Thins, M & S*	1 Biscuit/10g	50	2.2	485	5.8	68.4	21.1	3.5
All Butter, Trufree*	1 Biscuit/11g	58	3.1	524	2.0	66.0	28.0	0.9
Assortment, Parkside*	1 Serving/30g	155	8.6	517	5.4	59.8	28.5	2.0
Average	1oz/28g	139	7.3	498	5.9	63.9	26.1	1.9
Bites, Murray*	1 Bar/21g	80	3.5	381	4.8	76.2	16.7	14.3
Caramel, Millionaires, Fox's*	1 Serving/16g	75	3.9	483	6.1	57.9	25.3	0.1
Choc Chip, Fair Trade, Co-Op*	1 Biscuit/19g	100	6.0	526	5.3	57.9	31.6	2.6
Chocolate Chip, Jacob's*	1 Biscuit/17g	87	4.7	513	5.2	61.2	27.5	1.8
Chocolate Chip, Tesco*	1 Serving/20g	105	6.1	525	7.5	55.0	30.6	3.0
Chocolate Chunk, Belgian, TTD, Sainsbury's*	1 Biscuit/19g	101	5.7	521	5.1	59.1	29.4	2.0
Clotted Cream, Finest, Tesco*	1 Biscuit/20g	109	6.4	543	5.2	58.0	32.2	1.7
Crawfords*	1 Biscuit/13g	67	3.4	533	6.6	65.0	27.4	2.0
Demerara, Rounds, TTD, Sainsbury's*	1 Biscuit/22g	113	5.9	508	5.1	62.2	26.5	1.8
Dutch, M & S*	1 Biscuit/17g	90	5.1	540	5.4	59.0	30.8	2.5
Fingers, Asda*	1 Finger/18g	93	5.1	519	5.8	60.3	28.3	18.0
Fingers, Cornish Cookie*	1 Finger/25g	124	6.4	498	6.4	61.0	25.5	0.0
Fingers, Deans*	1 Finger/24g	115	5.9	488	5.1	60.1	24.8	1.4
Fingers, Highland, Organic, Sainsbury's*	1 Serving/16g	84	4.8	527	5.8	58.7	29.9	1.9
Fingers, Scottish, Finest, Tesco*	1 Biscuit/21g	104	5.0	498	5.1	65.5	23.9	2.0
Free From, Sainsbury's*	1 Biscuit/20g	98	5.2	490	6.0	58.0	26.0	6.0
Highland, Organic, Duchy Originals*	1 Biscuit/16g	80	4.2	515	5.2	61.8	27.4	1.7
Honey & Oatmeal, Walkers*	1 Biscuit/34g	158	7.6	465	6.7	64.1	22.4	3.8
Mini Bites, Co-Op*	1 Biscuit/10g	53	3.0	530	7.0	59.0	30.0	2.0
Mini Bites, Country Table*	1 Biscuit/10g	52	3.0	525	7.1	59.3	29.5	1.5
Reduced Sugar, Tesco*	1 Biscuit/17g	86	4.9	519	6.7	57.1	29.4	2.1
Rings, Handbaked, Border*	1 Biscuit/17g	86	4.9	520	6.2	61.2	29.5	0.0
Royal Edinburgh*	1 Biscuit/11g	56	2.9	507	6.1	61.1	26.5	4.5
Shrewsbury, M & S*	1oz/28g	128	6.5	458	7.5	63.9	23.3	4.5
Stem Ginger, Waitrose*	1 Biscuit/15g	71	3.3	487	4.7	66.0	22.7	1.6
Wheat & GF, Free From Range, Tesco*	1 Biscuit/20g	98	5.2	490	6.0	58.0	26.0	6.0
SHRIMP								
Boiled, Average	***1 Serving/60g***	***70***	***1.4***	***117***	***23.8***	***0.0***	***2.4***	***0.0***
Dried, Average	***1oz/28g***	***69***	***0.7***	***245***	***55.8***	***0.0***	***2.4***	***0.0***
Frozen, Average	***1oz/28g***	***20***	***0.2***	***73***	***16.5***	***0.0***	***0.8***	***0.0***
in Brine, Canned, Drained, Average	***1oz/28g***	***26***	***0.3***	***94***	***20.8***	***0.0***	***1.2***	***0.0***
SKATE								
Grilled	***1oz/28g***	***22***	***0.1***	***79***	***18.9***	***0.0***	***0.5***	***0.0***
in Batter, Fried in Blended Oil	1oz/28g	47	2.8	168	14.7	4.9	10.1	0.2
Raw, Edible Portion	***1oz/28g***	***18***	***0.1***	***64***	***15.1***	***0.0***	***0.4***	***0.0***

	Measure INFO/WEIGHT	per Measure KCAL	per Measure FAT	Nutrition Values per 100g / 100ml KCAL	PROT	CARB	FAT	FIBRE
SKIPS								
Bacon, KP Snacks*	1 Bag/17g	81	3.8	474	6.5	62.1	22.2	2.3
Cheesy, KP Snacks*	1 Bag/17g	89	5.0	524	6.2	58.5	29.5	1.0
Pickled Onion, KP Snacks*	1 Bag/13g	67	4.0	512	3.4	56.4	30.3	1.4
SKITTLES								
Mars*	1 Pack/55g	223	2.4	406	0.0	90.6	4.4	0.0
SLICES								
Apple & Raisin, Asda*	3 Slices/43g	173	3.3	400	6.5	74.7	7.7	2.8
Bacon & Cheese, Pastry, Tesco*	1 Slice/165g	480	32.0	291	7.4	21.7	19.4	1.0
Beef, Minced, Morrisons*	1 Slice/143g	457	29.6	320	8.8	24.6	20.7	1.0
Beef, Minced Steak & Onion, Tesco*	1 Slice/150g	424	27.2	283	8.7	21.3	18.1	1.6
Broccoli, Leek & Cheese, En Croute, M & S*	½ Pack/220g	550	30.6	250	5.6	25.2	13.9	1.5
Cheddar Cheese & Onion, Ginsters*	1 Slice/180g	583	40.9	324	7.1	22.8	22.7	1.0
Cheese, Leek & Red Onion Plait, Linda McCartney*	1 Plait/170g	473	28.1	278	6.7	25.9	16.5	2.4
Cheese, Potato & Onion, Pastry, Taste!*	1 Slice/155g	501	30.4	323	8.6	28.1	19.6	0.0
Cheese & Ham, Pastry, Sainsbury's*	1 Slice/118g	352	23.2	298	7.8	22.5	19.7	1.8
Cheese & Onion, Pastry, Tesco*	1 Slice/150g	502	37.0	335	8.0	20.1	24.7	1.4
Chicken, Spicy, Deep Fill, Ginsters*	1 Slice/180g	499	30.6	277	9.2	21.8	17.0	1.4
Chicken & Ham, Taste!*	1 Slice/155g	356	15.3	230	10.8	24.2	9.9	0.0
Chicken & Leek, Taste!*	1 Slice/155g	406	19.1	262	10.1	27.6	12.3	0.0
Chicken & Mushroom, Asda*	1 Slice/128g	354	21.7	277	7.0	24.0	17.0	2.1
Chicken & Mushroom, Ginsters*	1 Slice/180g	439	26.8	244	8.3	19.1	14.9	1.8
Chicken & Mushroom, Sainsbury's*	1 Slice/164g	427	26.5	259	7.3	21.3	16.1	1.0
Chicken Lattice, Ginsters*	1 Lattice/400g	1060	66.8	265	10.6	18.0	16.7	1.5
Chocolate, Belgian, Weight Watchers*	1 Slice/30g	99	2.0	329	5.9	61.3	6.7	2.3
Custard, Pastry, Tesco*	1 Slice/108g	275	11.1	255	2.8	37.2	10.3	1.3
Fresh Cream, Tesco*	1 Slice/75g	311	21.0	414	3.5	37.4	27.9	1.0
Goats Cheese & Spinach, Crisp & Creamy, Waitrose*	1 Slice/100g	351	22.7	351	7.6	28.3	22.7	1.8
Ham & Cheese, Ginsters*	1 Pack/180g	511	33.7	284	8.5	20.4	18.7	2.5
Ham & Cheese, Pastry, Ginsters*	1 Slice/155g	625	43.7	403	9.8	31.9	28.2	4.2
Minced Steak & Onion, Sainsbury's*	1 Slice/165g	475	29.9	288	15.2	16.0	18.1	2.5
Mushroom, Creamy, Quorn*	1 Slice/164g	653	29.5	398	9.8	49.2	18.0	1.6
Pork & Egg, Gala, Tesco*	1 Slice/105g	333	24.2	317	10.3	17.2	23.0	3.4
Prawn & Avocado, Plait, Extra Special, Asda*	1 Serving/198g	331	6.7	167	11.0	23.0	3.4	1.3
Raisin, Crispy, LC, Tesco*	1 Biscuit/15g	56	0.6	370	6.0	76.6	3.9	5.5
Spicy Chicken, Ginsters*	1 Slice/180g	448	27.4	249	6.7	21.4	15.2	1.9
Spinach & Ricotta, Sainsbury's*	1 Slice/165g	500	35.3	303	6.5	21.1	21.4	2.9
Steak, Peppered, Deep Fill, Ginsters*	1 Slice/180g	513	36.2	285	9.4	16.1	20.1	3.1
Steak, Peppered, Ginsters*	1 Slice/180g	457	27.0	254	8.4	21.3	15.0	1.6
Steak & Onion, Aberdeen Angus, Tesco*	1 Slice/165g	444	27.7	269	8.7	20.7	16.8	1.3
Steak (4-pack), Ginsters*	1 Slice/105g	274	14.5	261	9.3	25.0	13.8	1.6
SLIMFAST*								
Cafe Latte, Ready To Drink, Slim Fast*	1 Bottle/325ml	230	6.5	71	4.5	7.0	2.0	1.0
Caramel Temptation Shake Powder, Slim Fast*	2 Scoops/60g	230	3.6	380	14.0	62.0	6.0	11.0
Meal Bar, Fruits of the Forest, Slim Fast*	1 Bar/60g	211	6.1	351	23.7	42.1	10.1	7.3
Meal Bar, Yoghurt & Muesli, Slim Fast*	1 Bar/60g	208	6.5	347	23.9	42.2	10.8	7.4
Milk Shake, Banana, Canned, Slim Fast*	1 Can/325ml	214	8.4	66	4.2	10.6	2.6	4.9
Milk Shake, Chocolate, Ready to Drink, Slim Fast*	1 Bottle/325ml	211	5.2	65	4.6	8.0	1.6	1.5
Milk Shake, Peach, Canned, Slim Fast*	1 Can/325ml	214	2.6	66	4.2	10.6	0.8	1.5
Shake, Blissful Banana, Ready To Drink, Slim Fast*	1 Bottle/325ml	230	6.6	70	4.5	7.0	2.0	1.5
Shake, Chocolate, Powder, Dry, Slim Fast*	2 Scoops/38g	136	2.8	363	13.9	59.0	7.5	10.9
Shake, Summer Strawberry, Ready to Drink, Slim Fast*	1 Bottle/325ml	230	6.6	70	4.5	7.0	2.0	1.0
Shake, Vanilla, Powder, Dry, Slim Fast*	2 Scoops/37g	131	2.4	360	13.4	60.9	6.5	11.0
Snacks, Chocolate Caramel Bar, Slim Fast*	1 Bar/26g	99	3.2	382	3.4	69.6	12.4	1.2

	Measure INFO/WEIGHT	per Measure KCAL	FAT	Nutrition Values per 100g / 100ml KCAL	PROT	CARB	FAT	FIBRE
SLIMFAST*								
Snacks, Sour Cream & Chive Pretzels, Slim Fast*	1 Pack/23g	96	2.0	416	9.5	75.2	8.6	3.4
Soup, Chicken & Vegetable Pasta, Hearty's*	1 Pack/295ml	212	5.6	72	6.6	7.0	1.9	0.7
SMARTIES								
Giants, Nestle*	1 Pack/186g	882	35.9	474	4.6	70.4	19.3	0.7
Mini Cones, Nestle*	1 Serving/44g	145	5.8	330	4.5	45.0	13.1	0.0
Mini Eggs, Nestle*	1 Lge Bag/100g	496	20.4	496	3.9	72.9	20.4	2.8
Nestle*	1 Tube/40g	188	7.1	469	3.9	72.5	17.7	2.4
Tree Decoration, Nestle*	1 Chocolate/18g	95	5.4	529	5.6	58.9	30.1	0.8
SMIRNOFF*								
Ice, Smirnoff*	1 Bottle/275ml	188	0.0	68	1.8	12.0	0.0	0.0
SMOOTHIE								
Apple, Grapes & Blackcurrant, PJ Smoothies*	1 Bottle/250ml	125	0.8	50	0.8	11.1	0.3	0.7
Apple, Kiwi & Lime, SunJuice*	1 Bottle/250ml	132	0.2	53	0.5	13.4	0.1	0.8
Apple, Strawberry, Cherry & Banana, M & S*	1 Bottle/250ml	125	0.8	50	0.5	11.2	0.3	0.6
Apples & Blackcurrant, for Kids, Innocent*	1 Carton/180ml	104	0.2	58	0.3	14.1	0.1	0.1
Apricot & Peach, COU, M & S*	1 Bottle/250ml	100	0.9	40	0.9	8.3	0.4	0.4
Banana, Dairy, Probiotic, Boots*	1 Bottle/250ml	148	1.2	59	1.6	12.0	0.5	1.0
Banana, Dairy, Tesco*	1 Bottle/250ml	165	1.0	66	1.6	14.0	0.4	0.4
Banana, M & S*	1 Bottle/500ml	400	2.0	80	1.8	16.8	0.4	1.2
Banana, Shapers, Boots*	1 Bottle/251ml	176	0.8	70	2.8	14.0	0.3	0.8
Banana & Mango, Juice, Calypso*	1 Carton/200ml	106	0.0	53	0.0	12.8	0.0	1.0
Berry, Prepacked, Average	1 Serving/250ml	133	0.5	53	0.7	11.6	0.2	0.9
Blackberries, Strawberries & Blackcurrants, Innocent*	1 Serving/200ml	108	0.0	54	0.6	11.9	0.0	1.5
Blackberries, Strawberries & Boysenberries, Innocent*	1 Serving/250ml	130	0.0	52	0.6	11.8	0.0	1.3
Blackberries & Blueberries, Innocent*	1 Bottle/250ml	120	0.2	48	0.5	12.0	0.1	2.1
Blackberry, Strawberry, Raspberry, Prepacked, Average	1 Serving/250ml	122	1.0	49	1.2	9.6	0.4	1.1
Blackberry & Blueberry, Wild Orchard*	1 Bottle/250ml	110	0.0	44	0.6	10.8	0.0	1.9
Blackcurrant & Apple, Sweetbird*	1 Serving/330ml	191	0.0	58	0.5	13.8	0.0	0.0
Blackcurrants & Gooseberries for Autumn, Innocent*	1 Bottle/250ml	118	0.2	47	0.5	12.5	0.1	1.0
Blueberry, Blackberry & Strawberry, COU, M & S*	1 Bottle/250ml	150	0.8	60	0.8	13.1	0.3	0.3
Blueberry, Blackcurrant & Beetroot, Love Life, Waitrose*	1 Serving/250ml	90	0.2	36	0.2	8.5	0.1	0.8
Blueberry & Pear, COU, M & S*	1 Bottle/250ml	112	0.8	45	0.3	10.4	0.3	0.3
Cappuccino, with Yoghurt, Island Oasis*	1 Carton/473ml	300	3.5	63	1.7	12.5	0.7	0.0
Cherries & Strawberries, Innocent*	1 Bottle/250ml	122	0.2	49	0.6	12.6	0.1	0.0
Cherry, Grape & Raspberry, Juiceburst*	1 Bottle/250ml	170	0.5	68	0.7	14.9	0.2	1.2
Cranberries, Blueberries, Cherries, Innocent*	1 Serving/250ml	138	0.0	55	0.3	12.8	0.0	1.3
Cranberries, Yumberries & Blackcurrants, Innocent*	1 Bottle/250ml	130	0.2	52	0.5	14.2	0.1	1.5
Cranberries & Raspberries, Innocent*	1 Bottle/250ml	112	0.0	45	0.5	12.0	0.0	2.3
Cranberries & Strawberries, Innocent*	1 Bottle/250ml	102	0.5	41	0.5	9.5	0.2	0.0
Fruit, Cranberry & Raspberry, Juice Republic*	1 Bottle/250ml	182	1.0	73	0.5	16.0	0.4	0.0
Fruit, The Green One, Ella's Kitchen*	1 Pack/90g	52	0.0	58	0.4	13.4	0.0	1.8
Fruit, The Purple One, Ella's Kitchen*	1 Pack/90g	57	0.0	63	0.7	13.8	0.0	3.3
Fruit, The Red One, Ella's Kitchen*	1 Pack/90g	48	0.1	53	0.6	11.6	0.1	1.9
Fruit, The Yellow One, Ella's Kitchen*	1 Pack/90g	63	0.2	70	0.7	15.3	0.2	2.1
Fruit, Tropical, Free From, Tesco*	1 Pouch/90g	72	1.8	80	0.7	13.4	2.0	1.1
Guavas, Mangoes & Goji Berries, Innocent*	1 Bottle/250ml	112	0.2	45	0.6	12.0	0.1	2.1
Kiwi, Apples & Limes, Innocent*	1 Bottle/250ml	125	0.2	50	0.5	11.0	0.1	1.8
Mango, Mini-me, Skinny, Boost*	1 Sm/480ml	178	1.4	37	0.5	7.7	0.3	0.4
Mango & Orange, Smoothie Smile*	1 Bottle/250ml	130	1.0	52	0.4	11.7	0.4	0.0
Mango & Orange, Sweetbird*	1 Serving/330ml	182	0.7	55	0.7	11.9	0.2	0.0
Mango & Passionfrruit, Weight Watchers*	1 Serving/90ml	90	0.1	100	0.3	23.9	0.1	0.5
Mango & Passionfruit, Prepacked, Average	1 Serving/250ml	145	0.3	58	0.6	12.7	0.1	1.5
Mango & Passionfruit, Tesco*	1 Glass/250ml	150	0.2	60	0.5	12.7	0.1	1.8

	Measure INFO/WEIGHT	per Measure KCAL	FAT	Nutrition Values per 100g / 100ml KCAL	PROT	CARB	FAT	FIBRE
SMOOTHIE								
Mangoes, Coconuts & Lemon Grass, Innocent*	1 Bottle/250ml	172	3.5	69	0.6	12.9	1.4	1.2
Mangoes & Passion Fruits, Pure Fruit, Innocent*	1 Bottle/250ml	142	0.5	57	0.6	12.5	0.2	1.6
Mixed Berry, Chosen By You, Asda*	1 Glass/250ml	143	0.0	57	0.6	12.6	0.0	1.6
Orange, Banana & Pineapple, Innocent*	1 Bottle/250ml	120	1.0	48	0.6	10.8	0.4	0.0
Orange, Mandarin & Guava, PJ Smoothies*	1 Bottle/250ml	122	0.0	49	0.7	10.9	0.0	1.6
Orange, Mango, Banana & Passion Fruit, Asda*	1 Serving/100ml	55	0.2	55	0.8	12.0	0.2	1.1
Orange, Mango & Pineapple, Prepacked, Average	1 Serving/250ml	131	0.2	52	0.6	11.9	0.1	0.7
Orange, Mango & Pumpkin, Love Life, Waitrose*	1 Bottle/250ml	98	0.5	39	0.6	8.8	0.2	1.1
Orange, Strawberry & Guava, Sainsbury's*	1 Serving/300ml	159	0.6	53	0.3	12.0	0.2	0.8
Orange & Mango, Prepacked, Average	1 Serving/250ml	138	0.4	55	0.6	12.4	0.2	0.4
Oranges, Bananas & Pineapples, Innocent*	1 Bottle/250ml	142	0.2	57	0.6	14.1	0.1	0.0
Oranges, Mangoes & Pineapples For Kids, Innocent*	1 Carton/180ml	94	0.2	52	0.7	11.7	0.1	0.9
Peaches, Bananas & Passionfruit, PJ Smoothies*	1 Bottle/250g	128	0.2	51	0.4	12.1	0.1	0.0
Peaches & Passion Fruits, Innocent*	1 Bottle/250ml	120	0.2	48	0.5	10.7	0.1	1.7
Pineapple, Banana & Coconut, Prepacked, Average	1 Serving/250ml	163	3.0	65	0.6	12.8	1.2	0.9
Pineapple, Banana & Pear, Asda*	1 Bottle/250ml	147	0.3	59	0.5	13.6	0.1	0.3
Pineapple, Mango & Lime, WTF, Sainsbury's*	1 Bottle/250g	120	0.2	48	0.4	11.3	0.1	0.3
Pineapple, Mango & Passion Fruit, Extra Special, Asda*	½ Bottle/250ml	100	0.5	40	0.5	9.0	0.2	1.3
Pineapple, Strawberries & Passion Fruit, PJ Smoothies*	1 Bottle/330ml	152	0.3	46	0.6	10.8	0.1	1.3
Pineapple & Passion Fruit, Sweetbird*	1 Serving/330ml	175	0.3	53	0.8	12.3	0.1	0.0
Pineapples, Bananas & Coconuts, Innocent*	1 Bottle/250ml	172	2.8	69	0.7	13.6	1.1	1.0
Pomegranate, Raspberry & Cranberry, PJ Smoothies*	1 Bottle/250ml	132	0.5	53	1.1	11.6	0.2	0.0
Raspberry, Banana & Peach, Sainsbury's*	1 Bottle/251ml	138	0.3	55	0.8	12.8	0.1	1.5
Raspberry, M & S*	1 Bottle/250ml	138	1.5	55	1.7	12.2	0.6	1.9
Raspberry & Bio Yoghurt, M & S*	1 Bottle/500ml	275	1.5	55	2.0	10.8	0.3	0.9
Raspberry & Blueberry, Plus, Tesco*	1 Serving/100ml	59	0.3	59	2.6	11.6	0.3	0.5
Raspberry & Boysenberry, Shapers, Boots*	1 Bottle/248ml	109	0.0	44	0.7	10.0	0.0	1.6
Raspberry & Cranberry, Smoothie Plus, Tesco*	1 Bottle/250ml	140	0.4	56	0.6	13.0	0.2	3.0
Raspberry & Red Pepper, Love Life, Waitrose*	1 Bottle/250ml	90	0.2	36	0.3	8.5	0.1	0.7
Strawberries, Blackberries, Raspberries, Kids, Innocent*	1 Carton/180ml	81	0.2	45	0.5	9.9	0.1	1.3
Strawberries & Bananas, PJ Smoothies*	1 Bottle/250ml	118	0.2	47	0.4	11.0	0.1	0.0
Strawberries & Bananas, Pure Fruit, Innocent*	1 Bottle/250ml	132	0.2	53	0.7	13.1	0.1	1.3
Strawberries & Raspberries, Squeezie, Innocent*	1 Squeezie/40g	16	0.0	39	0.3	8.5	0.0	2.1
Strawberry, Dairy, Finest, Tesco*	1 Bottle/250ml	162	0.2	65	2.9	13.2	0.1	0.1
Strawberry, Raspberry, Apple & Banana, PJ Smoothies*	1 Bottle/250ml	132	0.8	53	0.8	11.9	0.3	0.7
Strawberry, Raspberry & Banana, Waitrose*	1 Bottle/250ml	122	0.2	49	0.7	10.8	0.1	0.8
Strawberry, with Yoghurt, Finest, Tesco*	1 Serving/100ml	62	1.2	62	2.1	10.5	1.2	0.6
Strawberry & Banana, Don Simon, Don Simon*	1 Carton/250ml	132	0.0	53	0.6	12.2	0.0	0.3
Strawberry & Banana, Fruit, Serious Food Company*	1 Bottle/250ml	135	0.0	54	0.5	12.7	0.0	1.3
Strawberry & Banana, Juice, Calypso*	1 Carton/200ml	100	0.0	50	0.0	11.9	0.0	0.0
Strawberry & Banana, Prepacked, Average	1 Serving/250ml	131	0.2	53	0.6	11.9	0.1	0.9
Strawberry & Cherry, Organic, M & S*	1 Bottle/250ml	138	0.8	55	0.8	12.3	0.3	0.4
Strawberry & Raspberry, Fruity, Sainsbury's*	1 Glass/200ml	106	0.0	53	0.6	11.9	0.0	2.4
Strawberry & Raspberry, Rhapsody, M & S*	1 Glass/200ml	90	0.2	45	0.6	9.4	0.1	0.9
Strawberry & Raspberry, Shapers, Boots*	1 Bottle/250ml	122	0.5	49	0.3	12.0	0.2	0.6
Summer Fruits, Tesco*	1 Bottle/250ml	140	0.0	56	0.2	13.8	0.0	0.5
Super Berry, M & S*	1 Bottle/250ml	150	1.0	60	0.9	13.0	0.4	1.2
Vanilla & Honey, Sainsbury's*	1 Bottle/250ml	238	6.0	95	3.2	14.8	2.4	0.3
Vanilla Bean, M & S*	1 Bottle/500ml	450	13.0	90	3.3	13.9	2.6	0.0
Yoghurt, Vanilla Bean & Honey, Thickie, Innocent*	1 Bottle/250g	242	4.5	97	4.1	16.2	1.8	0.1
Zumo Berry, Zumo*	1 Regular/375ml	158	2.2	42	1.4	7.8	0.6	0.0
SNACK-A-JACKS								
Apple Danish, Jumbo, Quaker Oats*	1 Cake/10g	39	0.2	390	5.0	87.0	2.5	1.0

S

	Measure INFO/WEIGHT	per Measure KCAL	FAT	Nutrition Values per 100g / 100ml KCAL	PROT	CARB	FAT	FIBRE
SNACK-A-JACKS								
Barbecue, Jumbo, Quaker Oats*	1 Cake/10g	38	0.2	380	8.0	83.0	2.0	1.7
Barbecue, Snack, Quaker Oats*	1 Bag/30g	123	1.8	410	7.5	81.0	6.0	1.0
Barbeque, Snack-A-Jacks, Quaker Oats*	1 Pack/26g	106	1.6	408	7.3	81.1	6.1	0.9
Caramel, Jumbo, Snack-A-Jacks, Quaker Oats*	1 Cake/13g	51	0.3	390	5.5	87.0	2.1	1.4
Caramel, Snack, Snack-A-Jacks, Quaker Oats*	1 Bag/30g	122	0.9	405	6.0	88.0	3.0	0.8
Cheese, Jumbo, Quaker Oats*	1 Cake/10g	38	0.2	380	8.5	81.0	2.5	1.7
Cheese, Snack, Quaker Oats*	1 Bag/26g	108	2.1	415	8.5	77.0	8.0	0.9
Cheese & Onion, Snack, Quaker Oats*	1 Bag/30g	120	2.2	400	6.7	77.0	7.5	1.5
Chocolate & Caramel, Delights, Quaker Oats*	1 Cake/15g	62	0.9	415	6.0	83.0	6.0	1.6
Chocolate & Orange, Delights, Quaker Oats*	1 Cake/15g	59	0.7	394	5.5	83.0	4.5	1.0
Chocolate Chip, Jumbo, Snack-A-Jacks, Quaker Oats*	1 Cake/15g	62	1.0	410	6.0	81.0	7.0	1.7
Prawn Cocktail, Snack, Quaker Oats*	1 Bag/30g	123	2.2	410	7.0	78.0	7.5	0.8
Prawn Cocktail, Snack-A-Jacks, Quaker Oats*	1 Bag/26g	106	2.0	408	6.9	78.3	7.5	0.9
Roast Chicken, Snack, Quaker Oats*	1 Bag/30g	124	2.4	415	7.0	77.5	8.0	1.0
Salt & Vinegar, Jumbo, Snack-A-Jacks, Quaker Oats*	1 Cake/10g	41	0.6	391	7.4	75.4	5.7	1.6
Sweet Chilli Flavour, Snack-A-Jacks, Quaker Oats*	1 Packet/26g	108	2.0	414	7.3	78.9	7.5	1.1
SNAILS								
in Garlic Butter, Average	6 Snails/50g	219	20.8	438	9.7	8.0	41.5	1.0
Raw, Average	1 Snail/5g	4	0.1	90	16.1	2.0	1.4	0.0
SNAPPER								
Red, Fried in Blended Oil	***1oz/28g***	***35***	***0.9***	***126***	***24.5***	***0.0***	***3.1***	***0.0***
Red, Weighed with Bone, Raw	***1oz/28g***	***25***	***0.4***	***90***	***19.6***	***0.0***	***1.3***	***0.0***
SNICKERS								
Cruncher, Mars*	1 Bar/40g	209	12.0	523	9.0	57.0	30.0	2.3
Mars*	1 Snacksize/41g	208	11.5	511	9.4	54.3	28.2	1.3
SOPOCKA								
Sliced, Cured, Pork Loin	1 Serving/100g	101	2.9	101	17.8	0.8	2.9	0.0
SORBET								
Blackcurrant, Del Monte*	1oz/28g	30	0.0	106	0.4	27.1	0.1	0.0
Blackcurrant, Iceland*	¼ Pot/100g	100	0.0	100	0.0	25.0	0.0	0.0
Elderflower, Bottle Green*	1 Serving/100g	104	0.0	104	0.1	25.6	0.0	0.0
Lemon	1 Scoop/60g	79	0.0	131	0.9	34.2	0.0	0.0
Lemon, Del Monte*	1 Sorbet/500g	570	0.5	114	0.1	29.2	0.1	0.0
Lemon, Organic, Evernat*	1oz/28g	27	0.1	96	0.1	22.8	0.5	0.0
Lemon, Sticks, Haagen-Dazs*	1oz/28g	67	3.2	238	1.5	32.5	11.3	0.0
Lemon, The Real Ice Company*	1 Serving/100g	117	0.1	117	0.1	29.1	0.1	0.4
Lemon, Zesty, Haagen-Dazs*	1 Serving/125ml	120	0.0	96	0.0	24.8	0.0	1.0
Lemon Harmony, Haagen-Dazs*	1 Serving/90ml	214	10.2	238	1.5	32.5	11.3	0.0
Mango, Del Monte*	1 Sorbet/500g	575	0.5	115	0.2	29.6	0.1	0.0
Mango, Organic, M & S*	1 Serving/100g	99	0.1	99	0.3	24.1	0.1	0.9
Mango, Tesco*	1 Serving/100g	107	0.0	107	0.1	26.5	0.0	0.3
Mango, Tropicale, Haagen-Dazs*	1oz/28g	32	0.0	116	0.2	28.6	0.1	0.0
Mango, Waitrose*	1 Pot/100g	90	0.0	90	0.1	22.1	0.0	0.6
Mango Berry Swirl, Ben & Jerry's*	1 Serving/100g	100	0.0	100	0.2	25.0	0.0	1.5
Orange, Del Monte*	1 Sorbet/500g	625	0.5	125	0.2	32.1	0.1	0.0
Pineapple, Del Monte*	1 Sorbet/500g	600	0.5	120	0.3	30.6	0.1	0.0
Raspberry, Haagen-Dazs*	½ Cup/105g	120	0.0	114	0.0	28.6	0.0	1.9
Raspberry, Sticks, Haagen-Dazs*	1oz/28g	28	0.0	99	0.2	24.2	0.1	0.0
Raspberry, Tesco*	1 Serving/70ml	97	0.0	138	0.5	34.0	0.0	0.0
Raspberry, Waitrose*	1 Pot/750ml	690	0.8	92	0.5	22.2	0.1	1.1
Raspberry & Blackberry, Fat Free, M & S*	1 Sorbet/125g	140	0.0	112	0.4	27.5	0.0	0.6
Sicilian Lemon, Seriously Fruity, Waitrose*	1/5 Pot/100ml	77	0.1	77	18.8	13.5	0.1	0.2
Strawberry, Fruit Ice, Starburst, Mars*	1 Stick/93ml	99	0.1	106	0.1	26.7	0.1	0.0

	Measure INFO/WEIGHT	per Measure KCAL	FAT	Nutrition Values per 100g / 100ml KCAL	PROT	CARB	FAT	FIBRE
SORBET								
Strawberry, M & S*	1oz/28g	27	0.0	95	0.3	23.4	0.1	0.5
Strawberry & Champagne, Sainsbury's*	¼ Pot/89g	95	0.0	107	0.2	25.5	0.0	0.6
Summer Berry, Swirl, Asda*	¼ Pack/89g	97	0.4	109	3.0	26.0	0.4	0.0
SOUFFLE								
Cheese	1oz/28g	71	5.4	253	11.4	9.3	19.2	0.3
Cheese, Alizonne*	1 Serving/33g	129	3.4	392	60.5	14.5	10.2	0.2
Cheese, Mini, Waitrose*	1 Souffle/14g	32	2.4	232	16.0	2.9	17.4	2.4
Chocolate, Gu*	1 Pot/70g	307	24.9	439	6.3	24.4	35.6	2.9
Chocolate & Toffee, Gu*	1 Pot/95g	353	15.8	372	4.6	46.4	16.6	2.5
Lemon, Finest, Tesco*	1 Pot/80g	270	20.5	338	2.9	24.1	25.6	0.2
Plain	1oz/28g	56	4.1	201	7.6	10.4	14.7	0.3
SOUP								
Asparagus, Fresh, M & S*	1 Serving/300g	135	10.8	45	1.1	2.5	3.6	0.9
Asparagus, M & S*	1 Serving/300g	180	13.5	60	1.1	3.3	4.5	0.7
Asparagus, New Covent Garden Food Co*	½ Carton/300g	132	7.2	44	1.5	4.1	2.4	0.9
Asparagus, Slimline, Cup, Waitrose*	1 Sachet/204ml	51	1.4	25	0.4	4.3	0.7	0.7
Bacon & Bean, Smoked, Diet Chef Ltd*	1 Pack/300g	162	3.3	54	2.8	8.2	1.1	2.1
Bacon & Lentil, Chosen By You, Asda*	1 Pot/600g	348	7.2	58	3.3	7.7	1.2	1.6
Bacon & Three Bean, Smoked, Chunky, Baxters*	1 Can/400g	232	4.8	58	2.9	8.8	1.2	1.8
Bean, Spicy Mixed, Big Soup, Heinz*	1 Serving/200g	78	0.6	39	2.3	6.8	0.3	2.0
Bean, Tuscan, Chunky, Love Life, Waitrose*	½ Can/200g	90	1.0	45	2.6	7.6	0.5	2.3
Bean, Tuscan, GFY, Asda*	1 Carton/400ml	224	3.6	56	2.9	9.0	0.9	0.8
Bean, Tuscan, New Covent Garden Food Co*	½ Carton/300g	84	2.4	28	1.6	3.7	0.8	1.0
Bean & Sausage, Tuscan Style, Chunky, M & S*	1 Can/415g	249	9.1	60	2.4	7.7	2.2	1.0
Bean & Vegetable, Chunky, Chosen By You, Asda*	1 Can/400g	224	1.2	56	2.6	9.7	0.3	1.9
Beef, Mushroom & Red Wine, Farmers Market, Heinz*	1 Can/515g	263	9.3	51	2.4	6.4	1.8	0.7
Beef, Spicy, & Tomato, Diet Chef Ltd*	1 Pack/300g	165	5.7	55	2.3	7.3	1.9	1.9
Beef & Ale, Canned, M & S*	1 Can/400g	150	4.0	38	1.0	5.4	1.0	1.4
Beef & Mushroom, Big Soup, Heinz*	1 Can/515g	216	2.6	42	2.3	7.0	0.5	0.7
Beef & Tomato, Cup a Soup, Made Up, Batchelors*	1 Serving/252g	83	1.6	33	0.6	6.3	0.6	0.4
Beef & Tomato, Spicy, Diet Chef Ltd*	1 Pouch/300g	165	5.7	55	2.3	7.3	1.9	1.9
Beef & Vegetable, Big Soup, Heinz*	1 Can/400g	212	4.0	53	3.5	7.5	1.0	0.9
Beef & Vegetable, Ten Calorie, Gourmet Cuisine*	1 Sachet/200g	10	0.1	5	0.3	1.0	0.0	0.1
Beef Broth, Big Soup, Heinz*	1 Can/400g	184	2.8	46	2.5	7.0	0.7	0.9
Beef Broth, Chosen By You, Asda*	1 Pot/300g	174	3.6	58	2.6	8.6	1.2	1.3
Beef Broth, Classic, Heinz*	1 Can/400g	180	2.0	45	1.9	7.6	0.5	0.8
Broccoli, Salmon & Watercress, Stay Full, Baxters*	1 Can/400g	244	8.8	61	3.3	5.8	2.2	2.4
Broccoli & Cauliflower, Cup, BFY, Morrisons*	1 Sachet/15g	56	2.1	376	4.9	57.2	14.2	4.9
Broccoli & Stilton, Classics, Fresh, Tesco*	½ Pot/300g	180	8.4	60	2.9	5.8	2.8	1.1
Broccoli & Stilton, Cup Soup, Ainsley Harriott*	1 Satchet/229ml	87	1.8	38	1.0	7.0	0.8	1.3
Broccoli & Stilton, English, Dry, Knorr*	1 Pack/65g	331	24.6	509	11.7	30.3	37.9	1.6
Broccoli & Stilton, Farmers Market, Heinz*	½ Can/200g	108	7.4	54	1.5	3.2	3.7	0.9
Broccoli & Stilton, Fresh, Sainsbury's*	½ Pot/300ml	141	9.9	47	2.7	1.8	3.3	1.5
Broccoli & Stilton, New Covent Garden Food Co*	1 Carton/600ml	240	14.4	40	2.2	1.9	2.4	1.1
Butternut Squash, & Ginger, Waitrose*	½ Pot/300g	210	17.4	70	0.9	3.5	5.8	1.0
Butternut Squash, Curried, & Lentil, Seeds of Change*	1 Pack/400g	164	1.2	41	2.3	7.2	0.3	1.9
Butternut Squash, Diet Chef Ltd*	1 Pack/300g	135	5.4	45	0.8	6.5	1.8	1.6
Butternut Squash & Red Pepper, Vegetarian, Baxters*	1 Can/415g	149	2.5	36	0.9	6.6	0.6	0.5
Carrot, Honey & Coriander, Cully And Sully*	1 Bowl/200g	56	3.2	28	0.5	3.3	1.6	1.0
Carrot, Onion & Chickpea, Healthy, Baxters*	1 Can/415ml	170	0.8	41	1.9	8.0	0.2	1.2
Carrot, Orange & Coriander, COU, M & S*	1 Pack/415g	145	2.5	35	0.6	6.9	0.6	1.2
Carrot, Orange & Ginger, Go Organic*	1 Jar/495g	119	4.0	24	0.5	3.6	0.8	1.4
Carrot & Butterbean, Diet Chef Ltd*	1 Pack/300g	174	2.1	58	2.7	10.3	0.7	2.8

S

	Measure	per Measure		Nutrition Values per 100g / 100ml				
	INFO/WEIGHT	KCAL	FAT	KCAL	PROT	CARB	FAT	FIBRE
SOUP								
Carrot & Butterbean, Vegetarian, Baxters*	1 Can/415g	237	7.9	57	1.5	7.2	1.9	2.2
Carrot & Coriander, Average	1 Serving/200g	83	4.3	42	0.6	4.8	2.2	1.0
Carrot & Coriander, Blended, Heinz*	½ Can/200g	104	5.4	52	0.7	6.2	2.7	0.6
Carrot & Coriander, Carton, Campbell's*	1 Serving/250ml	110	5.5	44	0.7	5.4	2.2	0.0
Carrot & Coriander, Classic, Classic, Heinz*	1 Can/400g	164	6.4	41	0.4	5.8	1.6	0.9
Carrot & Coriander, Fresh, Organic, Simply Organic*	1 Pot/600g	276	18.0	46	0.5	4.5	3.0	1.3
Carrot & Coriander, Low Calorie, Average	1 Serving/200g	45	1.3	22	0.6	3.5	0.6	1.1
Carrot & Coriander, Soup-A-Cup, Asda*	1 Serving/26g	102	3.6	392	4.6	62.0	14.0	4.5
Carrot & Coriander, Weight Watchers*	1 Pouch/300g	102	3.9	34	0.4	5.1	1.3	0.6
Carrot & Coriander, with Creme Fraiche, Heinz*	1 Can/515g	232	9.3	45	0.7	6.6	1.8	0.9
Carrot & Ginger, Fresh, Sainsbury's*	1 Pot/600g	150	5.4	25	0.4	3.9	0.9	1.0
Carrot & Ginger, Perfectly Balanced, Waitrose*	½ Pot/300g	66	2.7	22	0.4	3.1	0.9	1.0
Carrot & Lentil, Microwave, Heinz*	1 Can/303g	94	0.3	31	1.5	6.1	0.1	0.8
Carrot & Lentil, Weight Watchers*	1 Can/295g	87	0.3	29	1.3	5.5	0.1	0.7
Carrot & Orange	1oz/28g	6	0.1	20	0.4	3.7	0.5	1.0
Carrot & Orange, Pouch, Heinz*	½ Pack/300g	165	6.6	55	0.6	8.3	2.2	1.0
Chick Pea, Moroccan, M & S*	1oz/28g	20	0.6	70	3.6	8.8	2.1	2.0
Chick Pea & Chorizo, Truly Irresistible, Co-Op*	½ Pack/300g	170	5.3	55	2.7	7.0	1.7	1.2
Chicken, Barley & Vegetable, Fuller Longer, M & S*	1 Pack/400g	200	6.0	50	4.9	4.5	1.5	1.6
Chicken, Coconut & Lemon Grass, Fresh, Waitrose*	½ Pot/300g	303	24.9	101	2.6	4.1	8.3	0.8
Chicken, Condensed, 99% Fat Free, Campbell's*	1 Can/295g	77	2.1	26	1.0	3.8	0.7	0.1
Chicken, Cream of, in Seconds, Dry, Knorr*	1 Pack/58g	300	21.2	518	11.2	36.0	36.6	0.3
Chicken, Cream of, Mealpak, All About Weight*	1 Pack/40g	152	3.6	380	36.1	32.1	9.0	13.3
Chicken, Cream of, Reduced Salt, Heinz*	1 Can/400g	216	12.0	54	1.7	4.9	3.0	0.1
Chicken, Cream of, Soupreme, Aldi*	1 Can/400g	228	15.2	57	1.8	3.8	3.8	0.4
Chicken, Creamed, Basics, Sainsbury's*	1 Can/400ml	120	6.0	30	0.6	3.5	1.5	0.1
Chicken, Fresh, Sainsbury's*	½ Carton/300g	126	5.7	42	2.2	4.0	1.9	0.3
Chicken, Green Thai, Sainsbury's*	1 Pot/600g	366	19.8	61	1.9	5.8	3.3	0.3
Chicken, Green Thai, Spiced, M & S*	½ Pot/300g	195	11.4	65	2.0	6.3	3.8	0.6
Chicken, in a Cup, Dry, Symingtons*	1 Serving/22g	93	4.0	424	7.0	57.7	18.4	11.7
Chicken, Indian, Glorious!*	½ Pot/300g	201	7.5	67	3.4	7.6	2.5	0.7
Chicken, Leek & Potato, Weight Watchers*	1 Tin/295g	80	1.2	27	0.9	5.0	0.4	0.3
Chicken, Low Fat, Condensed, Batchelors*	1 Can/295g	148	4.1	50	1.9	7.5	1.4	0.2
Chicken, M & S*	1 Pack/213g	196	15.3	92	1.6	5.5	7.2	0.2
Chicken, Moroccan, Finest, Tesco*	½ Pot/300g	180	5.1	60	3.6	6.8	1.7	1.2
Chicken, Moroccan, New Covent Garden Food Co*	1 Serving/300g	108	5.7	36	2.1	2.7	1.9	0.4
Chicken, Mushroom & Rice, Chilled, M & S*	½ Pot/300g	225	10.2	75	3.2	7.3	3.4	1.8
Chicken, New Covent Garden Food Co*	1 Carton/600g	510	32.4	85	3.8	5.4	5.4	0.6
Chicken, Packet, Knorr*	1 Packet/85g	423	27.5	498	7.7	44.3	32.3	0.2
Chicken, Potato, & Lentil, Weight Watchers*	1 Can/400g	136	3.6	34	1.2	5.3	0.9	0.3
Chicken, Potato & Bacon, Big Soup, Heinz*	1 Can/515g	294	11.3	57	3.0	6.1	2.2	0.5
Chicken, Potato & Leek, Weight Watchers*	1 Can/295g	97	2.4	33	1.1	5.1	0.8	0.3
Chicken, Red Thai, Waitrose*	1 Pot/6400g	316	14.8	79	6.5	5.1	3.7	0.7
Chicken, Roasted, Canned, Tesco*	1 Can/400g	220	10.8	55	1.0	6.6	2.7	0.3
Chicken, Sweetcorn & Potato, Heinz*	1 Can/400g	204	11.2	51	1.2	5.4	2.8	0.3
Chicken, Ten Calorie, Gourmet Cuisine*	1 Serving/200g	10	0.1	5	0.2	1.1	0.0	0.0
Chicken, Thai, Diet Chef Ltd*	1 Sachet/300g	114	4.5	38	1.0	5.1	1.5	1.0
Chicken, Thai, Fresh, Finest, Tesco*	½ Tub/300g	255	16.2	85	4.1	4.2	5.4	1.1
Chicken, Thai, GFY, Asda*	1 Serving/200g	85	3.0	42	1.7	5.5	1.5	0.5
Chicken, Thai, New Covent Garden Food Co*	½ Carton/300g	174	10.5	58	2.6	4.1	3.5	0.8
Chicken, Thai Style, Canned, Soupreme, Aldi*	1 Can/400g	200	10.8	50	2.5	3.8	2.7	1.1
Chicken, Thick & Creamy, M & S*	1oz/28g	31	2.2	110	5.8	3.9	8.0	0.5
Chicken, Weight Watchers*	1 Can/295g	97	3.0	33	1.6	4.4	1.0	0.0

	Measure INFO/WEIGHT	per Measure KCAL	FAT	Nutrition Values per 100g / 100ml KCAL	PROT	CARB	FAT	FIBRE
SOUP								
Chicken, West Indian, Bowl Soups*	1 Bowl/400g	240	4.8	60	2.4	8.1	1.2	1.4
Chicken & Barley, Broth, Heinz*	1 Can/400g	128	1.2	32	1.3	5.9	0.3	0.8
Chicken & Broccoli, Soup a Cups, GFY, Asda*	1 Cup/226ml	52	1.4	23	0.5	4.0	0.6	0.4
Chicken & Broccoli, Soup-A-Slim, Asda*	1 Sachet/16g	55	1.4	341	7.0	58.0	9.0	6.0
Chicken & Country Vegetable, Big Soup, Heinz*	1 Can/400g	200	2.8	50	3.1	7.4	0.7	1.0
Chicken & Country Vegetable, Farmers Market, Heinz*	½ Can/200g	106	4.6	53	2.2	5.3	2.3	1.3
Chicken & Country Vegetable, Soupfulls, Batchelors*	1 Serving/400g	164	3.6	41	5.1	3.0	0.9	1.3
Chicken & Ham, Big, Heinz*	½ Can/200g	92	2.0	46	2.3	6.9	1.0	0.7
Chicken & King Prawn, Noodle, Fresh, Tesco*	1 Pot/400g	180	1.6	45	4.7	5.5	0.4	0.4
Chicken & Leek, Big Soup, Heinz*	½ Can/258g	162	5.2	63	3.0	8.2	2.0	0.6
Chicken & Leek, Cup a Soup, Made Up, Batchelors*	1 Serving/259g	96	4.7	37	0.5	4.7	1.8	0.7
Chicken & Leek, Instant, Cup, Average	1 Packet/19g	73	2.7	382	5.0	58.2	14.4	8.5
Chicken & Leek, Simmer & Serve, Dried, Sainsbury's*	1/3 Sachet/200ml	62	1.8	31	0.4	5.2	0.9	0.3
Chicken & Mushroom, BFY, Dry, Morrisons*	1 Serving/14g	47	0.9	337	16.0	54.8	6.1	2.5
Chicken & Mushroom, Creamy, Very Special, Heinz*	1 Serving/260g	130	6.2	50	1.9	5.3	2.4	0.0
Chicken & Mushroom, Extra, Slim a Soup, Batchelors*	1 Serving/257g	90	1.5	35	1.4	5.9	0.6	0.3
Chicken & Mushroom, in a Cup, Sainsbury's*	1 Sachet/223ml	107	4.2	48	0.7	7.1	1.9	0.1
Chicken & Mushroom, Soup-A-Slim, Asda*	1 Sachet/14g	51	1.4	362	10.0	58.0	10.0	4.2
Chicken & Noodle, Laksa, Fuller Longer, M & S*	1 Pot/385g	289	7.7	75	7.0	7.1	2.0	0.9
Chicken & Orzo, Tuscan, Glorious!*	½ Pot/300g	120	1.2	40	2.8	6.2	0.4	0.7
Chicken & Pasta, Big, Heinz*	½ Can/200g	68	0.8	34	1.8	5.9	0.4	0.8
Chicken & Sweetcorn, Asda*	1 Pot/600g	246	8.4	41	2.2	4.9	1.4	1.6
Chicken & Sweetcorn, Canned, BGTY, Sainsbury's*	½ Can/200g	56	0.8	28	1.5	4.5	0.4	0.2
Chicken & Sweetcorn, Canned, Tesco*	1 Can/400ml	240	6.0	60	1.6	8.2	1.5	0.7
Chicken & Sweetcorn, Cantonese, Fresh, Sainsbury's*	½ Pot/300ml	135	1.5	45	2.1	7.9	0.5	0.5
Chicken & Sweetcorn, Fresh, Average	1 Serving/300g	146	3.1	48	2.4	7.3	1.0	0.6
Chicken & Sweetcorn, GFY, Asda*	1 Can/400g	108	2.0	27	1.5	4.2	0.5	0.2
Chicken & Sweetcorn, in a Cup, BGTY, Sainsbury's*	1 Sachet/15g	57	1.3	379	7.6	68.3	9.0	1.4
Chicken & Sweetcorn, Instant, Cup, Average	1 Packet/13g	46	1.5	356	7.0	56.2	11.7	4.1
Chicken & Sweetcorn, New Covent Garden Food Co*	1 Carton/600g	282	5.4	47	1.0	8.7	0.9	0.5
Chicken & Sweetcorn, Soupreme, Aldi*	1 Serving/250g	90	0.8	36	2.7	5.6	0.3	1.7
Chicken & Tarragon, Thick & Creamy, Batchelors*	1 Sachet/281g	118	6.5	42	0.8	5.7	2.3	0.3
Chicken & Thyme, Diet Chef Ltd*	1 Pack/300g	147	9.0	49	2.2	3.4	3.0	0.7
Chicken & Vegetable, Big Soup, Heinz*	½ Can/200g	104	2.8	52	3.3	6.7	1.4	0.8
Chicken & Vegetable, Canned, Average	1 Can/400g	192	8.5	48	2.5	4.6	2.1	0.8
Chicken & Vegetable, Casserole, Chunky, Baxters*	1 Can/415g	195	2.9	47	2.4	7.8	0.7	1.1
Chicken & Vegetable, Casserole, Heinz*	1 Pot/430g	331	16.8	77	3.9	6.7	3.9	0.8
Chicken & Vegetable, Chunky, Eat Well, M & S*	½ Can/213g	138	4.0	65	4.6	6.9	1.9	1.0
Chicken & Vegetable, Classic, Heinz*	1 Can/400g	132	1.6	33	1.2	6.2	0.4	0.6
Chicken & Vegetable, Fresh, M & S*	½ Pot/300g	120	4.2	40	3.0	2.9	1.4	0.8
Chicken & Vegetable, Healthy, Baxters*	1 Can/415g	170	2.1	41	1.9	6.3	0.5	1.8
Chicken & Vegetable, Loyd Grossman*	1 Pack/400g	272	15.2	68	0.5	8.0	3.8	0.6
Chicken & Vegetable, Moroccan, Love Life, Waitrose*	½ Pot/300g	192	5.7	64	3.7	7.9	1.9	1.9
Chicken & Vegetable, with Croutons, Cup, Campbell's*	1 Sachet/222ml	100	4.0	45	0.7	5.9	1.8	0.9
Chicken & Vegetable, with Pasta, Select, Campbell's*	1 Can/480ml	220	1.0	46	2.9	7.9	0.2	0.8
Chicken & White Wine, Campbell's*	1 Serving/295g	145	9.7	49	1.0	4.0	3.3	0.0
Chicken Broth, Favourites, Baxters*	1 Can/400g	128	0.8	32	1.4	5.7	0.2	0.8
Chicken Curry, & Brown Rice, Sainsbury's*	1 Can/400g	208	4.4	52	3.1	6.3	1.1	2.1
Chicken Curry, Big Soup, Heinz*	1 Can/400g	196	2.8	49	2.8	7.3	0.7	1.0
Chicken Curry, Chosen By You, Asda*	½ Pot/300g	216	5.4	72	5.0	8.6	1.8	0.5
Chicken Curry, Mild, Indian, Soups of the World, Heinz*	1 Can/515g	381	21.1	74	3.6	5.9	4.1	0.3
Chicken Flavour, Tony Ferguson*	1 Pack/59g	203	1.9	344	25.6	49.8	3.2	5.1
Chicken Mix, Telma*	1 Serving/7g	20	0.5	286	14.3	42.9	7.1	0.0

	Measure INFO/WEIGHT	per Measure KCAL	FAT	Nutrition Values per 100g / 100ml KCAL	PROT	CARB	FAT	FIBRE
SOUP								
Chicken Noodle, & Vegetable, Slim a Soup, Batchelors*	1 Serving/203g	55	1.0	27	0.8	4.8	0.5	0.6
Chicken Noodle, Batchelors*	1 Pack/284g	71	0.6	25	1.6	4.2	0.2	0.3
Chicken Noodle, Canned, Sainsbury's*	½ Can/217g	78	0.7	36	1.7	7.4	0.3	0.7
Chicken Noodle, Chinese, Dry, Knorr*	1 Pack/45g	138	2.0	307	15.1	51.8	4.4	2.9
Chicken Noodle, Chunky, Campbell's*	½ Can/200g	86	1.2	43	2.8	6.5	0.6	0.0
Chicken Noodle, Classic, Heinz*	1 Can/400g	124	1.2	31	1.2	6.0	0.3	0.2
Chicken Noodle, Clear, Weight Watchers*	1 Can/295g	51	0.6	17	0.8	3.1	0.2	0.2
Chicken Noodle, Cup, Asda*	1 Sachet/13g	40	0.2	305	9.0	63.0	1.9	3.6
Chicken Noodle, Cup, GFY, Asda*	1 Sachet/215ml	43	0.2	20	0.6	4.2	0.1	0.1
Chicken Noodle, Cup Soup, Dry, Heinz*	1 Sachet/20g	48	0.5	240	8.0	46.0	2.5	1.5
Chicken Noodle, Cup Soup, Made Up, Heinz*	1 Serving/218ml	48	0.4	22	0.7	4.3	0.2	0.1
Chicken Noodle, Dry, Symingtons*	½ Pack/15g	48	0.4	318	8.6	65.4	2.4	2.4
Chilli, Meal, Chunky, Canned, Tesco*	½ Can/200g	120	2.4	60	5.0	6.3	1.2	1.6
Chilli Bean, Chosen By You, Asda*	1 Pot/600g	258	1.8	43	2.1	6.8	0.3	2.2
Chilli Bean, M & S*	½ Carton/300g	150	7.5	50	2.5	4.7	2.5	2.7
Chilli Bean, Mexican, Tesco*	1 Carton/600g	270	6.6	45	2.2	6.4	1.1	1.9
Chilli Beef, Mighty, Asda*	1 Can/400g	236	5.6	59	4.9	6.8	1.4	1.2
Chilli Con Carne, Chunky, Sainsbury's*	½ Can/200g	110	1.8	55	3.6	8.0	0.9	1.5
Chorizo & Bean, TTD, Sainsbury's*	1 Pack/298g	161	2.4	54	4.0	7.6	0.8	5.8
Chowder, Bacon & Corn, M & S*	½ Pot/300g	195	10.8	65	2.5	6.0	3.6	1.8
Chowder, Clam, New England, Select, Campbell's*	1 Cup/240ml	221	14.4	92	2.5	6.0	6.0	0.8
Chowder, Corn, Spicy, New Covent Garden Food Co*	½ Carton/300g	132	5.4	44	1.6	4.3	1.8	2.2
Chowder, Haddock, Smoked, Asda*	1 Serving/300g	462	12.0	154	1.6	28.0	4.0	0.5
Chowder, Ham & Sweetcorn, Diet Chef Ltd*	1 Pack/300g	165	3.6	55	1.9	9.2	1.2	0.9
Chowder, Prawn, Manhattan, Fresh, Sainsbury's*	1 Serving/300g	177	6.9	59	1.6	7.9	2.3	0.1
Chowder, Seafood, Waitrose*	1 Can/404g	226	11.3	56	2.2	5.6	2.8	0.6
Chowder, Sweetcorn & Chicken, Heinz*	1 Serving/200g	148	5.6	74	3.3	9.1	2.8	0.6
Chowder, Vegetable, New Covent Garden Food Co*	½ Carton/300g	159	5.1	53	2.9	6.6	1.7	1.1
Cock-A-Leekie, Favourites, Baxters*	1 Can/400g	116	2.4	29	1.1	4.7	0.6	0.3
Courgette & Parmesan, Fresh, Sainsbury's*	1 Pack/300ml	198	16.8	66	1.5	2.5	5.6	0.4
Cumberland Sausage & Vegetable, Big Soup, Heinz*	1 Can/515g	221	4.1	43	1.9	6.7	0.8	0.8
Dhansak, TTD, Sainsbury's*	½ Pot/300g	180	3.9	60	3.2	9.0	1.3	1.6
Egg, Drop, Average	1 Bowl/500g	470	30.0	94	6.0	4.0	6.0	0.0
Fish, Bouillabaise, Bistro, M & S*	1 Pack/820g	2665	18.0	325	10.0	4.3	2.2	1.3
Fish, Frozen, Findus*	1 Serving/85g	128	4.7	150	11.0	13.0	5.5	0.0
Fish, Mediterranean, Waitrose*	½ Pot/300g	108	2.7	36	3.4	3.5	0.9	0.7
French Onion	1oz/28g	11	0.6	40	0.2	5.7	2.1	1.0
French Onion, & Cider, Waitrose*	1 Can/425g	94	0.4	22	0.5	4.8	0.1	0.4
French Onion, & Croutons, Dry, Tesco*	1 Serving/30g	106	2.3	353	7.3	63.7	7.7	2.0
French Onion, & Gruyere Cheese, Fresh, Finest, Tesco*	½ Pot/300g	210	15.3	70	1.4	4.7	5.1	0.5
French Onion, Favourites, Baxters*	½ Can/200g	68	1.2	34	0.6	6.0	0.6	0.6
French Onion, GFY, Asda*	½ Pot/253g	91	1.3	36	1.9	6.0	0.5	0.4
French Onion, Knorr*	1 Pack/40g	118	1.0	296	6.0	62.5	2.5	6.6
French Onion, Simmer & Serve, Dried, Sainsbury's*	1/3 Sachet/204ml	37	0.2	18	0.3	3.8	0.1	0.2
French Onion, Tinned, M & S*	½ Can/200g	40	0.4	20	0.4	3.9	0.2	0.3
Game, Luxury, Baxters*	1 Can/415g	245	4.6	59	6.2	6.0	1.1	0.5
Game, Royal, Favourites, Baxters*	1 Can/400g	152	0.8	38	1.8	6.9	0.2	0.3
Gazpacho, Canned, Average	1 Can/400g	76	0.4	19	2.9	1.8	0.1	0.2
Gazpacho, New Covent Garden Food Co*	1 Carton/600g	276	17.4	46	1.0	3.3	2.9	1.2
Gumbo, Spicy, Fresh, Sainsbury's*	½ Pot/300g	120	5.4	40	1.5	4.5	1.8	0.9
Haddock, Smoked, Chowder, M & S*	½ Pot/300g	180	7.2	60	3.1	6.4	2.4	0.8
Haddock, Smoked, Fresh, Finest, Tesco*	1 Pot/550g	302	13.8	55	2.7	5.1	2.5	0.8
Haggis, Broth, Favourites, Baxters*	1 Can/400g	180	6.0	45	1.8	6.1	1.5	0.6

	Measure INFO/WEIGHT	per Measure KCAL	FAT	Nutrition Values per 100g / 100ml KCAL	PROT	CARB	FAT	FIBRE
SOUP								
Highlander's Broth, Favourites, Baxters*	1 Can/400g	192	5.6	48	1.7	6.3	1.4	0.9
Italian, Chunky, New Covent Garden Food Co*	½ Carton/300g	111	4.2	37	1.5	4.7	1.4	0.9
Italian Wedding, Deli Inspired, Baxters*	1 Can/400g	199	5.4	48	2.1	6.9	1.3	0.9
Jammin Jamaica, New Covent Garden Food Co*	1 Carton/600g	324	15.6	54	1.0	6.0	2.6	1.6
Lamb, Minted, Hot Pot, Big Soup, Heinz*	1 Can/400g	228	5.2	57	2.9	8.1	1.3	1.0
Lamb & Cous Cous, M & S*	½ Can/208g	100	3.7	48	2.1	6.2	1.8	0.9
Lamb & Vegetable, Big Soup, Heinz*	½ Can/200g	120	2.6	60	3.0	9.1	1.3	1.3
Lamb & Vegetable, Mega, Morrisons*	1 Pack/410g	172	4.1	42	1.9	6.3	1.0	0.8
Lamb Casserole, Chunky, Baxters*	1 Can/415g	232	3.3	56	2.4	9.0	0.8	1.6
Leek, Cream of, Favourites, Baxters*	1 Can/400g	228	16.8	57	1.1	3.8	4.2	0.7
Leek & Chicken, Knorr*	1 Serving/300ml	82	5.2	27	0.6	2.4	1.7	0.1
Leek & Ham, Philpotts*	1 Pot/100g	87	4.4	87	1.3	9.6	4.4	1.7
Leek & Potato, Chunky, Meal, Canned, Tesco*	½ Can/200g	60	2.6	30	1.0	3.5	1.3	1.0
Leek & Potato, Creamy, Fresh, Asda*	1 Serving/300g	106	2.4	35	1.0	5.4	0.8	1.2
Leek & Potato, Cup a Soup, Batchelors*	1 Sachet/28g	121	4.9	432	5.2	63.2	17.6	1.8
Leek & Potato, Cup Soup, GFY, Asda*	1 Sachet/219ml	57	0.9	26	0.4	5.3	0.4	0.2
Leek & Potato, Fresh, Chilled, Chosen By You, Asda*	½ Pot/300g	105	2.4	35	1.0	5.4	0.8	1.2
Leek & Potato, Fresh, Sainsbury's*	½ Pot/300ml	141	7.2	47	1.0	5.3	2.4	0.4
Leek & Potato, Fresh with Cream, Tesco*	½ Tub/300g	180	7.2	60	1.5	8.0	2.4	0.9
Leek & Potato, in a Cup, BGTY, Sainsbury's*	1 Serving/218ml	59	1.5	27	0.3	4.9	0.7	0.2
Leek & Potato, Maris Piper, Chilled, M & S*	1 Serving/300g	165	11.4	55	0.6	4.5	3.8	0.9
Leek & Potato, Slim a Soup, Batchelors*	1 Serving/204g	57	1.4	28	0.4	5.0	0.7	0.2
Leek & Potato, Smooth, Vie, Knorr*	1 Pack/500ml	155	4.5	31	0.9	4.8	0.9	1.0
Leek & Potato, Thick & Creamy, Soup in a Mug, Tesco*	1 Serving/25g	94	2.4	378	4.2	68.5	9.7	4.9
Leek & Potato, Weight Watchers*	1 Sachet/215ml	58	1.1	27	0.5	5.1	0.5	0.1
Lentil, Average	1 Carton/600g	594	22.8	99	4.4	12.7	3.8	1.1
Lentil, Bacon & Mixed Bean, Low Fat, Aldi*	1 Serving/400g	260	3.6	65	4.7	9.5	0.9	1.6
Lentil, Campbell's*	1 Can/295g	139	1.8	47	2.6	7.7	0.6	0.0
Lentil, Canned	1 Serving/220g	86	0.4	39	3.1	6.5	0.2	1.2
Lentil, Carrot & Cumin, Canned, BGTY, Sainsbury's*	1 Can/400g	204	3.6	51	2.3	8.4	0.9	0.1
Lentil, Chilled, Spicy, Morrisons*	1 Serving/300ml	271	8.6	90	3.9	12.3	2.9	4.0
Lentil, Classic, Heinz*	1 Can/400g	192	0.8	48	2.3	8.7	0.2	0.8
Lentil, Moroccan, Waitrose*	½ Pot/300g	153	1.5	51	3.5	8.2	0.5	3.4
Lentil, Puy, & Vine Ripened Tomato, Finest, Tesco*	1 Pot/600g	360	7.8	60	2.8	9.2	1.3	1.5
Lentil, Red, & Chilli, Fresh, Love Life, Waitrose*	½ Pot/300g	138	4.5	46	1.7	6.4	1.5	1.3
Lentil, Red, & Ham, Waitrose*	½ Pot/300g	147	3.3	49	3.9	5.8	1.1	2.0
Lentil, Red, & Smoked Bacon, M & S*	½ Pot/300g	225	9.6	75	4.3	6.6	3.2	1.9
Lentil, Red, & Tomato, Canned, Tesco*	½ Can/300g	189	3.9	63	4.0	8.9	1.3	1.1
Lentil, Red, & Vegetable, Favourites, Baxters*	1 Can/400g	192	2.0	48	2.6	8.3	0.5	1.2
Lentil, Redemption*	1 Pot/600g	138	1.2	23	1.6	3.2	0.2	0.0
Lentil, Spicy, COU, M & S*	1 Pack/415g	187	3.7	45	2.6	6.7	0.9	1.2
Lentil, Spicy, Cup, Made Up, Ainsley Harriott*	1 Sachet/226ml	86	1.1	38	1.1	7.3	0.5	0.4
Lentil, Spicy, in a Mug, LC, Tesco*	1 Sachet/221ml	62	0.0	28	1.1	5.9	0.0	0.0
Lentil, Spicy, Organic, Suma*	1 Can/400g	232	4.8	58	2.7	9.0	1.2	1.6
Lentil, Spicy, Seeds of Change*	1 Pack/422g	190	0.8	45	2.5	8.2	0.2	1.9
Lentil, Tomato & Vegetable, M & S*	1 Can/415g	170	3.4	41	2.0	6.3	0.8	1.4
Lentil & Bacon, Canned, Tesco*	1 Serving/200g	96	1.4	48	3.2	7.2	0.7	0.5
Lentil & Bacon, Classic, Heinz*	1 Can/400g	232	5.6	58	2.7	8.4	1.4	0.7
Lentil & Bacon, Favourites, Baxters*	1 Can/400g	216	4.4	54	3.3	7.4	1.1	0.8
Lentil & Bacon, M & S*	1oz/28g	18	0.4	63	4.1	8.6	1.6	0.7
Lentil & Bean, Spicy, Canned, Organic, Asda*	1 Can/400g	212	3.2	53	2.8	8.6	0.8	3.0
Lentil & Chick Pea, Fresh, Organic, Tesco*	1 Serving/300ml	117	2.4	39	1.9	6.1	0.8	0.5
Lentil & Pancetta, Tesco*	½ Can/192g	115	2.5	60	3.1	8.0	1.3	1.6

S

	Measure INFO/WEIGHT	per Measure KCAL	FAT	Nutrition Values per 100g / 100ml KCAL	PROT	CARB	FAT	FIBRE
SOUP								
Lentil & Parsley, Simply Organic*	1 Pot/600g	390	1.8	65	4.4	11.8	0.3	1.4
Lentil & Potato, Spiced, Heinz*	1 Can/295g	118	0.6	40	2.0	7.7	0.2	0.7
Lentil & Red Pepper, Sainsbury's*	½ Pot/300g	162	3.6	54	3.5	7.4	1.2	1.6
Lentil & Smoked Bacon, New Covent Garden Food Co*	½ Carton/300g	153	3.0	51	3.7	8.9	1.0	4.3
Lentil & Tomato, New Covent Garden Food Co*	½ Pack/284g	162	3.1	57	3.6	8.1	1.1	0.7
Lentil & Tomato, Spicy, Chunky, Fresh, Tesco*	½ Pot/300g	195	5.4	65	2.6	9.7	1.8	1.3
Lentil & Vegetable, Diet Chef Ltd*	1 Pack/300g	156	0.9	52	2.6	9.6	0.3	2.1
Lentil & Vegetable, Healthy, Baxters*	1 Can/415g	174	1.2	42	1.9	7.4	0.3	1.2
Lentil & Vegetable, LC, Tesco*	1 Can/400g	188	0.8	47	2.5	8.8	0.2	1.1
Lentil & Vegetable, Spicy, Chilled, M & S*	½ Serving/300g	150	2.4	50	2.7	8.0	0.8	1.1
Lentil & Vegetable, Spicy, Chosen By You, Asda*	1 Pot/330g	178	3.3	54	2.4	8.5	1.0	0.7
Lentil & Vegetable, Spicy, Micro, Tesco*	1 Serving/330g	214	6.3	65	2.2	9.4	1.9	0.9
Lentil & Vegetable, with Bacon, Organic, Baxters*	½ Can/211g	93	1.5	44	1.9	7.6	0.7	1.0
Lobster Bisque, Luxury, with Brandy & Cream, Baxters*	1 Can/400g	272	17.2	68	2.6	4.8	4.3	0.2
Lobster Bisque, New Covent Garden Food Co*	½ Carton/300g	108	1.8	36	3.2	4.4	0.6	0.4
Masala Dhal, Moreish, Tesco*	1 Pot/400g	276	10.8	69	3.2	7.9	2.7	1.7
Meatball, Marvellous, Tesco*	1 Pot/400g	240	8.8	60	2.3	7.6	2.2	0.8
Meatball & Tomato, Italian, Big Soup, Heinz*	1 Can/515g	319	14.9	62	2.5	6.4	2.9	1.8
Meatball & Tomato, Italian, Soups of the World, Heinz*	1 Can/515g	319	14.9	62	2.5	6.4	2.9	1.8
Minestrone, Calorie Counter, Low Calorie Cup, Co-Op*	1 Sachet/13g	40	0.3	310	7.0	66.0	2.0	3.0
Minestrone, Canned, Average	1 Can/400g	252	12.0	63	1.8	7.6	3.0	0.9
Minestrone, Chilled, M & S*	½ Pot/300g	135	3.9	45	2.0	5.8	1.3	1.9
Minestrone, Chosen By You, Asda*	½ Can/200g	70	1.0	35	0.4	6.4	0.5	1.6
Minestrone, Chunky, Big Soup, Heinz*	½ Can/200g	74	1.6	37	1.3	6.2	0.8	1.1
Minestrone, Chunky, Classic, Meal, Canned, Tesco*	½ Can/200g	92	1.2	46	2.0	8.3	0.6	1.2
Minestrone, Chunky, COU, M & S*	1 Bowl/400g	300	7.2	75	3.0	11.8	1.8	0.8
Minestrone, Chunky, Fresh, Baxters*	1 Serving/250g	95	1.8	38	1.5	6.5	0.7	1.1
Minestrone, Classic, Heinz*	1 Can/400g	128	0.8	32	1.0	6.2	0.2	0.8
Minestrone, Diet Chef Ltd*	1 Pack/300g	123	2.7	41	1.4	6.9	0.9	1.2
Minestrone, Favourites, Baxters*	1 Can/400g	156	2.4	39	1.5	5.5	0.6	1.3
Minestrone, for One, Heinz*	1 Can/300g	96	2.1	32	1.4	5.2	0.7	0.7
Minestrone, Fresh, Average	1 Carton/600g	244	4.9	41	1.7	6.8	0.8	1.2
Minestrone, Fresh, Baxters*	1 Box/568ml	233	5.7	41	1.8	6.2	1.0	0.6
Minestrone, Hearty, 99% Fat Free, Campbell's*	1 Can/295g	77	0.3	26	0.7	5.6	0.1	0.0
Minestrone, Hearty, Chilled, Farmers Market, Heinz*	½ Carton/300g	123	2.7	41	1.4	6.9	0.9	0.5
Minestrone, in a Cup, BGTY, Sainsbury's*	1 Serving/200ml	54	0.2	27	0.8	6.0	0.1	0.6
Minestrone, Instant, Cup, Average	1 Packet/23g	79	0.7	351	7.7	72.1	3.3	3.4
Minestrone, Instant, Under 60 Calories, Tesco*	1 Sachet/19g	58	0.5	307	7.3	63.6	2.6	2.3
Minestrone, Italian, Dry, Knorr*	1 Pack/62g	193	2.5	311	11.5	57.1	4.1	7.8
Minestrone, Mediterranean, Campbell's*	½ Carton/250ml	95	2.8	38	0.9	6.1	1.1	0.6
Minestrone, Mighty, Dry, Asda*	1 Serving/38g	131	0.5	343	9.0	74.0	1.2	2.4
Minestrone, Organic, M & S*	1 Pack/208g	83	1.0	40	1.4	8.9	0.5	1.1
Minestrone, Organic, Seeds of Change*	1 Pack/350g	228	11.6	65	1.4	7.4	3.3	0.9
Minestrone, Packet, Dry, Knorr*	1 Pack/61g	204	2.4	335	12.0	58.8	4.0	6.9
Minestrone, Verde, New Covent Garden Food Co*	½ Carton/300g	123	2.4	41	1.8	6.1	0.8	1.2
Minestrone, with Basil & Parmesan, Stay Full, Baxters*	1 Can/400g	276	5.2	69	3.5	9.2	1.3	2.6
Minestrone, with Borlotti Beans, Tuscan Style, Heinz*	½ Can/200g	90	1.5	45	1.4	8.0	0.8	1.1
Minestrone, with Croutons, Dry, Soupreme, Aldi*	1 Serving/27g	94	1.7	349	7.6	65.3	6.4	4.4
Minestrone, with Croutons, Slim a Soup, Batchelors*	1 Serving/203g	55	1.2	27	0.6	4.8	0.6	0.6
Minestrone, with Meatballs, Fuller Longer, M & S*	1 Pack/400g	260	10.0	65	5.2	5.8	2.5	1.2
Minestrone, with Pasta, Chunky, Co-Op*	1 Pack/400g	140	2.4	35	1.0	6.0	0.6	0.7
Minestrone, with Ribbon Noodles, Extra, Dry, Aldi*	1 Serving/34g	107	0.7	315	11.0	62.8	2.2	2.0
Miso, Chicken, Noodle, Waitrose*	1 Pot/400g	268	8.8	67	5.9	5.9	2.2	0.9

	Measure INFO/WEIGHT	per Measure KCAL	FAT	Nutrition Values per 100g / 100ml KCAL	PROT	CARB	FAT	FIBRE
SOUP								
Miso, Instant, Blue Dragon*	1 Sachet/18g	25	0.7	139	10.0	14.4	3.9	0.0
Miso, Japanese, Made Up, Yutaka*	1 Serving/250ml	24	0.7	10	0.6	1.1	0.3	0.0
Miso, Wakama*	1 Sachet/8g	27	0.6	336	18.7	48.6	7.6	0.0
Miso, with Sea Vegetables, Clearspring*	1 Sachet/10g	26	0.9	260	20.0	26.0	9.0	11.0
Miso, with Tofu, Instant, Kikkoman*	1 Sachet/10g	35	1.0	350	30.0	30.0	10.0	0.0
Mulligatawny	1 Serving/220g	213	15.0	97	1.4	8.2	6.8	0.9
Mulligatawny, Beef Curry, Heinz*	1oz/28g	15	0.5	54	2.0	7.2	1.9	0.6
Mulligatawny, Chicken, Chunky, Weight Watchers*	1 Pack/340g	163	4.4	48	2.2	6.8	1.3	1.5
Mulligatawny, Chicken, Finest, Tesco*	½ Pot/300g	240	12.0	80	4.0	7.0	4.0	0.8
Mulligatawny, Chicken, Perfectly Balanced, Waitrose*	1 Serving/300g	138	6.0	46	1.7	5.3	2.0	0.4
Mulligatawny, Classic, Heinz*	1 Can/400g	232	7.6	58	1.9	8.0	1.9	0.5
Mulligatawny, in a Cup, Symingtons*	1 Serving/232ml	95	1.4	41	0.7	8.3	0.6	0.5
Mulligatawny, Vegetable, Tesco*	½ Pack/300g	210	7.5	70	1.9	9.0	2.5	1.1
Mushroom, Canned, HL, Tesco*	1 Can/400g	132	5.6	33	0.5	4.4	1.4	0.2
Mushroom, Chosen By You, Asda*	½ Pot/300g	108	5.1	36	1.0	3.8	1.7	0.9
Mushroom, Country, Selection, Campbell's*	1 Serving/250ml	80	4.5	32	0.6	3.4	1.8	0.5
Mushroom, Cream of, Canned	1 Serving/220g	101	6.6	46	1.1	3.9	3.0	0.1
Mushroom, Cream of, Classics, Heinz*	1 Can/400g	208	11.2	52	1.5	5.2	2.8	0.1
Mushroom, Cream of, Crosse & Blackwell*	1 Can/400g	186	9.9	47	1.3	4.7	2.5	0.0
Mushroom, Cream of, Favourites, Baxters*	1 Can/400g	244	15.2	61	1.0	5.6	3.8	0.2
Mushroom, Cream of, Fresh, Tesco*	½ Tub/300g	96	2.4	32	1.4	4.8	0.8	0.5
Mushroom, Cream of, Jeremy's Soups Ltd*	1 Serving/300g	135	12.6	45	0.8	1.2	4.2	0.2
Mushroom, Creamy, Asda*	1 Pot/500g	228	14.0	46	1.1	4.0	2.8	1.3
Mushroom, Creamy, Farmers Market, Heinz*	1 Can/515g	237	15.4	46	1.0	3.5	3.0	0.3
Mushroom, Cully & Sully*	1 Carton/400g	192	17.6	48	0.8	1.3	4.4	1.0
Mushroom, Diet Chef Ltd*	1 Pack/300g	105	5.1	35	1.9	3.2	1.7	0.9
Mushroom, Dry, Symingtons*	1 Serving/23g	80	2.1	348	17.8	48.4	9.2	6.7
Mushroom, for One, Heinz*	1 Can/290g	148	7.8	51	1.4	5.1	2.7	0.1
Mushroom, Forest, Heinz*	1oz/28g	12	0.6	43	1.0	4.5	2.3	0.1
Mushroom, Four, Loyd Grossman*	1 Pack/420g	202	16.4	48	0.8	2.5	3.9	0.2
Mushroom, Fresh, Average	1 Serving/300g	146	9.3	49	1.3	4.0	3.1	0.8
Mushroom, in a Cup, Sainsbury's*	1 Serving/200ml	96	3.8	48	0.5	7.0	1.9	0.2
Mushroom, Low Fat, Fresh, Sainsbury's*	½ Pot/300g	132	8.7	44	0.7	3.7	2.9	0.6
Mushroom, Moreish, New Covent Garden Food Co*	1 Carton/300g	90	3.0	30	1.3	2.9	1.0	1.4
Mushroom, Morrisons*	1 Serving/500g	250	18.0	50	1.3	3.2	3.6	0.3
Mushroom, Simmer & Serve, Dried, Sainsbury's*	½ Pack/600ml	234	9.6	39	0.6	5.5	1.6	0.3
Mushroom, Weight Watchers*	1 Can/295g	83	2.1	28	1.1	4.5	0.7	0.1
Mushroom, Wild, & Maderia, Fresh, Finest, Tesco*	½ Tub/300g	250	16.8	85	2.1	5.2	5.7	0.7
Mushroom, Wild, Carton, Soupreme, Aldi*	1 Carton/500g	135	6.0	27	1.1	2.9	1.2	0.5
Mushroom, Wild, Farmers Market, Heinz*	½ Carton/300g	93	3.3	31	0.9	4.4	1.1	0.5
Mushroom, Wild, in a Cup, BGTY, Sainsbury's*	1 Serving/200ml	56	1.8	28	0.4	4.5	0.9	0.2
Mushroom, Wild, New Covent Garden Food Co*	1 Carton/600g	222	7.2	37	1.5	4.1	1.2	0.9
Mushroom, with Croutons, Soup in a Mug, Tesco*	1 Pack/26g	113	4.6	435	6.1	63.3	17.5	2.9
Mushroom, with Croutons in a Cup, Waitrose*	1 Sachet/212g	102	4.2	48	0.6	6.8	2.0	0.5
Mushroom, Woodland, Farmers Market, Heinz*	1 Can/515g	227	12.4	44	0.9	4.7	2.4	0.3
Onion, Ten Calorie, Gourmet Cuisine*	1 Serving/200g	10	0.2	5	0.3	0.8	0.1	0.1
Oxtail, Average	1 Can/400g	163	4.5	41	2.0	5.8	1.1	0.4
Oxtail, Canned	1 Serving/220g	97	3.7	44	2.4	5.1	1.7	0.1
Oxtail, Classic, Heinz*	1 Can/400g	168	2.0	42	1.9	7.3	0.5	0.3
Oxtail, Condensed, Classics, Diluted, Campbell's*	1 Can/590g	236	8.8	40	1.4	5.3	1.5	0.0
Oxtail, Cup Soup, Co-Op*	1 Sachet/19g	67	1.7	355	7.0	63.0	9.0	1.0
Oxtail, Diet Chef Ltd*	1 Pack/300g	144	3.6	48	1.8	7.5	1.2	0.5
Oxtail, Favourites, Baxters*	1 Can/400g	192	4.4	48	1.8	6.8	1.1	0.5

S

	Measure INFO/WEIGHT	per Measure KCAL	FAT	Nutrition Values per 100g / 100ml KCAL	PROT	CARB	FAT	FIBRE
SOUP								
Oxtail, For One, Heinz*	1 Can/300g	126	1.5	42	1.9	7.3	0.5	0.3
Oxtail, Hearty, Canned, Crosse & Blackwell*	1 Can/400g	180	7.6	45	2.1	4.6	1.9	0.3
Oxtail, New Covent Garden Food Co*	1 Carton/600g	198	3.0	33	2.5	4.5	0.5	0.5
Oxtail, Simmer & Serve, Dried, Sainsbury's*	1 Pack/600ml	180	5.4	30	0.6	4.9	0.9	0.2
Oxtail, Soup in a Cup, Sainsbury's*	1 Serving/223ml	69	1.1	31	1.0	5.7	0.5	0.2
Parsnip, Creamy, New Covent Garden Food Co*	½ Carton/300g	174	9.0	58	1.2	6.6	3.0	1.6
Parsnip, Fresh, Morrisons*	½ Pot/250g	100	3.8	40	0.9	5.8	1.5	1.4
Parsnip, Fresh, VLH Kitchens	1 Serving/400g	180	0.4	45	0.9	5.8	1.6	1.4
Parsnip, Honey & Ginger, COU, M & S*	1 Can/415g	124	2.5	30	0.7	5.3	0.6	0.7
Parsnip, Leek & Ginger, New Covent Garden Food Co*	1 Carton/600g	162	1.8	27	1.2	4.9	0.3	1.3
Parsnip, Mr Bean's*	1 Tin/400g	208	7.6	52	1.9	6.7	1.9	0.0
Parsnip, Spicy, Average	1 Serving/400g	212	11.2	53	0.9	6.0	2.8	1.6
Parsnip, Spicy, New Covent Garden Food Co*	½ Box/297g	116	3.9	39	0.9	5.8	1.3	1.8
Parsnip, Spicy, Vegetarian, Baxters*	1 Can/425g	212	10.6	50	0.7	5.3	2.5	1.7
Parsnip & Apple, COU, M & S*	1 Can/415g	187	10.4	45	0.7	5.4	2.5	1.2
Parsnip & Apple, Spicy, NUME, Morrisons*	½ Can/200g	98	1.6	49	1.6	8.4	0.8	1.0
Parsnip & Butternut Squash, The Best, Morrisons*	1 Can/400g	244	8.4	61	2.4	8.1	2.1	1.6
Parsnip & Chilli, Diet Chef Ltd*	1 Serving/300g	102	4.2	34	0.8	4.6	1.4	1.3
Parsnip & Honey, Diet Chef Ltd*	1 Pack/300g	153	7.5	51	0.9	6.3	2.5	1.8
Parsnip & Honey, Fresh, Sainsbury's*	½ Carton/300g	192	12.6	64	1.1	5.4	4.2	1.5
Pea, Cream of, Garden, Jeremy's Soups Ltd*	1 Serving/300g	138	9.3	46	1.6	2.9	3.1	1.2
Pea, in a Cup, Symingtons*	1 Sachet/31g	95	2.2	311	7.2	54.1	7.2	6.9
Pea, Organic, Suma*	1 Can/400g	272	8.8	68	2.7	9.4	2.2	0.7
Pea, Souper, New Covent Garden Food Co*	½ Carton/300g	153	6.0	51	4.3	4.1	2.0	1.1
Pea & Ham	1 Serving/220g	154	4.6	70	4.0	9.2	2.1	1.4
Pea & Ham, Campbell's*	1 Can/500g	310	4.5	62	4.6	7.4	0.9	2.8
Pea & Ham, Canned, Favourites, Baxters*	1 Can/400g	218	4.0	55	3.3	7.1	1.0	2.0
Pea & Ham, Classic, Heinz*	1 Can/400g	252	3.2	63	2.8	10.1	0.8	1.1
Pea & Ham, Creamy, Chunky, Meal, Weight Watchers*	1 Pack/340g	156	3.7	46	2.3	6.8	1.1	2.0
Pea & Ham, Diet Chef Ltd*	1 Portion/300g	138	3.3	46	3.2	5.8	1.1	2.6
Pea & Ham, Extra Thick, in a Cup, Sainsbury's*	1 Sachet/224ml	85	1.8	38	1.1	6.7	0.8	0.4
Pea & Ham, Fresh, Sainsbury's*	½ Pack/300ml	120	1.5	40	1.9	7.0	0.5	0.3
Pea & Ham, Fresh, Waitrose*	1 Serving/300g	196	10.0	65	2.9	6.2	3.3	1.6
Pea & Mint, Baxters*	1 Serving/300g	186	9.6	62	2.3	6.1	3.2	1.5
Pea & Mint, Canned, Sainsbury's*	½ Can/200g	94	1.2	47	2.2	7.3	0.6	1.6
Pea & Mint, Fresh, Chosen By You, Asda*	½ Pot/300g	111	0.6	37	2.1	6.0	0.2	1.3
Pea & Mint, Fresh, Finest, Tesco*	1 Serving/300g	165	7.2	55	1.3	6.0	2.4	1.5
Pea & Mint, Fresh, Sainsbury's*	½ Pot/300g	102	2.7	34	1.4	5.0	0.9	1.9
Pea & Mint, Green, Fresh, Waitrose*	1oz/28g	27	2.2	97	1.8	5.5	7.7	1.2
Pea & Mint, Tinned, Tesco*	1 Can/400g	180	2.8	45	2.0	7.8	0.7	1.3
Potato, Leek & Bacon, Fresh, Baxters*	½ Pot/300g	249	16.8	83	2.0	6.1	5.6	0.7
Potato, Leek & Chicken, Canned, BGTY, Sainsbury's*	½ Can/200g	62	0.8	31	1.6	5.3	0.4	0.4
Potato, Leek & Thyme, Farmers Market, Heinz*	1 Can/515g	294	15.4	57	0.9	6.7	3.0	0.6
Potato & Leek	1oz/28g	15	0.7	52	1.5	6.2	2.6	0.8
Potato & Leek, Classics, Canned, Heinz*	1 Can/400g	184	7.2	46	0.8	6.7	1.8	0.6
Potato & Leek, Favourites, Baxters*	1 Can/400g	192	7.2	48	1.0	6.6	1.8	0.9
Potato & Leek, Instant, Cup, Average	1 Packet/22g	83	1.9	379	5.0	70.0	8.7	4.0
Prawn Laksa, Waitrose*	1 Pot/400g	388	25.2	97	2.5	9.7	6.3	0.6
Pumpkin, Creamy, Very Special, Heinz*	1 Sm Can/290g	188	5.5	65	1.3	9.9	1.9	1.1
Pumpkin, Spicy, Fresh, Sainsbury's*	½ Pot/300g	87	3.0	29	0.9	4.2	1.0	1.3
Pumpkin, Sweet Potato & Red Pepper, SO, Sainsbury's*	½ Pot/300g	111	3.9	37	0.8	5.6	1.3	0.8
Pumpkin & Ginger, in a Cup, Symingtons*	1 Serving/200ml	66	2.8	33	0.4	4.7	1.4	0.4
Pumpkin Ghoulash, New Covent Garden Food Co*	1 Carton/600g	186	1.2	31	1.3	5.2	0.2	1.2

	Measure INFO/WEIGHT	per Measure KCAL	FAT	Nutrition Values per 100g / 100ml KCAL	PROT	CARB	FAT	FIBRE
SOUP								
Red Pepper, & Goats Cheese, Diet Chef Ltd*	1 Pack/300g	138	6.6	46	2.2	4.4	2.2	0.9
Red Pepper, & Rocket, New Covent Garden Food Co*	½ Carton/300g	129	2.7	43	1.7	6.9	0.9	1.0
Red Pepper, & Tomato, Canned, Sainsbury's*	1 Can/400g	120	4.4	30	0.9	4.1	1.1	1.6
Red Pepper, & Tomato, Canned, Weight Watchers*	1 Can/295g	35	0.2	12	0.4	2.4	0.1	0.4
Red Pepper, Roasted, & Tomato, M & S*	1 Serving/150g	105	7.4	70	1.4	5.0	4.9	0.6
Red Pepper, Roasted, & Tomato, Weight Watchers*	1 Can/400g	136	0.4	34	0.7	7.7	0.1	0.6
Red Pepper, Roasted, Finest, Tesco*	1 Pot/600g	290	12.6	48	1.4	5.4	2.1	1.1
Red Pepper, Roasted, Fresh, Waitrose*	1 Pack/600g	172	9.0	29	0.8	3.0	1.5	1.0
Red Pepper, Tomato & Basil, M & S*	1 Can/415g	83	1.2	20	1.3	2.7	0.3	0.8
Scotch Broth, British, Sainsbury's*	1 Can/415g	149	2.9	36	1.9	5.4	0.7	0.9
Scotch Broth, Canned, Tesco*	½ Can/200g	85	2.6	42	1.3	5.9	1.3	0.8
Scotch Broth, Classic, Heinz*	1 Can/400g	156	2.4	39	1.4	6.7	0.6	0.6
Scotch Broth, Favourites, Baxters*	1 Can/400g	196	6.0	49	1.8	6.2	1.5	1.5
Scotch Broth, Fresh, Baxters*	1 Serving/300g	108	2.1	36	1.6	5.9	0.7	0.6
Scotch Broth, Fresh, Tesco*	½ Pack/300g	129	5.4	43	1.7	5.0	1.8	1.4
Scotch Broth, M & S*	1 Serving/300g	150	7.2	50	2.1	5.1	2.4	1.1
Split Pea, Yellow, Simply Organic*	1 Pot/600g	354	3.0	59	4.3	10.4	0.5	2.6
Split Pea & Ham, Asda*	1 Serving/300g	129	0.6	43	3.5	6.9	0.2	0.7
Steak, Potato & Ale, Chunky, Sainsbury's*	1 Can/400g	152	2.4	38	2.2	5.9	0.6	0.8
Steak & Guiness Casserole, Taste of Home, Heinz*	1 Pot/410g	260	7.0	63	3.2	8.4	1.7	0.7
Steak & Onion, Angus, Big Soup, Heinz*	½ Can/250g	135	2.1	54	3.3	7.7	0.8	0.9
Steak & Potato, Angus, Big Soup, Heinz*	½ Can/250g	120	2.0	48	3.1	6.8	0.8	0.6
Stilton, Celery & Watercress, Morrisons*	1 Serving/250g	272	23.0	109	3.9	3.1	9.2	0.3
Stilton & White Port, Baxters*	1oz/28g	25	1.8	88	2.5	5.4	6.3	0.3
Sun Dried Tomato & Basil, Heinz*	1 Serving/275ml	124	5.2	45	0.6	6.5	1.9	0.1
Sun Dried Tomato & Basil, Microwaveable Cup, Heinz*	1 Cup/275ml	118	5.0	43	0.6	6.2	1.8	0.1
Sweetcorn, Cream of, Campbell's*	1 Serving/80g	41	2.2	51	0.6	6.2	2.7	0.5
Sweetcorn & Chicken, Cup, Calorie Counter, Co-Op*	1 Sachet/11g	35	1.2	315	5.0	49.0	11.0	11.0
Sweetcorn & Chilli, COU, M & S*	½ Can/275g	138	6.6	50	0.9	6.1	2.4	0.4
Sweetcorn & Chilli Chowder, Simply Organic*	½ Pot/300g	126	2.7	42	2.2	6.1	0.9	3.8
Three Bean, Chunky, M & S*	1 Can/415g	208	5.0	50	2.3	7.5	1.2	1.8
Three Bean, Spicy, Tesco*	½ Carton/300g	165	4.5	55	2.8	7.3	1.5	2.1
Three Bean & Chorizo, Diet Chef Ltd*	1 Pack/300g	162	2.4	54	4.0	7.6	0.8	5.8
Three Bean & Red Pepper, Farmers Market, Heinz*	½ Can/200g	124	3.0	62	2.2	9.1	1.5	2.0
Three Bean & Tomato, Autumn, Farmers Market, Heinz*	½ Carton/300g	132	1.5	44	2.3	7.5	0.5	0.5
Three Bean & Vegetable, LC, Tesco*	½ Can/200g	110	0.6	55	2.6	9.7	0.3	1.9
Tomato, 99% Fat Free, Wattie's*	1 Serving/105g	32	0.4	31	1.0	5.6	0.4	1.1
Tomato, Basil & Chilli, Microwave, Sainsbury's*	1 Pot/345g	100	2.1	29	1.0	5.0	0.6	1.2
Tomato, Canned, HL, Tesco*	½ Can/200g	110	4.0	55	0.7	7.4	2.0	0.5
Tomato, Canned, LC, Tesco*	½ Can/200g	90	3.8	45	0.9	5.9	1.9	0.4
Tomato, Cannellini & Borlotti Bean, M & S*	½ Pot/300g	195	9.9	65	2.1	6.7	3.3	2.5
Tomato, Chunky, Organic, Canned, Amy's Kitchen*	1 Can/400g	212	5.6	53	1.2	8.6	1.4	1.2
Tomato, Classic, Soup at Hand, Campbell's*	1 Serving/305g	427	1.5	140	3.0	30.0	0.5	0.0
Tomato, Co-Op*	½ Can/200g	80	2.6	40	0.7	6.9	1.3	0.2
Tomato, Cream of, Canned, Average	1 Can/400g	208	12.0	52	0.8	5.9	3.0	0.7
Tomato, Cream of, Canned, Crosse & Blackwell*	1 Can/400g	228	10.0	57	0.9	7.4	2.5	0.8
Tomato, Cream of, Classic, Heinz*	½ Can/200g	118	6.0	59	0.9	6.7	3.0	0.4
Tomato, Cream of, Condensed, Batchelors*	1 Can/295g	454	19.5	154	1.7	21.9	6.6	0.6
Tomato, Cream of, Condensed, Prepared, Heinz*	1oz/28g	15	0.7	55	0.9	7.1	2.6	0.4
Tomato, Cream of, Dry, Knorr*	1 Pack/90g	392	21.2	435	4.3	51.3	23.6	3.3
Tomato, Cream of, for One, Heinz*	1 Can/300g	189	10.8	63	0.8	6.9	3.6	0.4
Tomato, Cream of, in a Cup, Sainsbury's*	1 Sachet/233ml	112	2.1	48	0.7	9.3	0.9	0.1
Tomato, Cream of, Microwave, Heinz*	1 Pack/300g	204	11.4	68	0.9	7.5	3.8	0.4

	Measure INFO/WEIGHT	per Measure KCAL	FAT	Nutrition Values per 100g / 100ml KCAL	PROT	CARB	FAT	FIBRE
SOUP								
Tomato, Cream of, Microwaveable Cup, Heinz*	1 Cup/275ml	169	9.4	61	0.8	6.9	3.4	0.4
Tomato, Cream of, Organic, Heinz*	1 Can/400g	220	10.4	55	1.0	7.0	2.6	0.4
Tomato, Cream of, Prepared, Campbell's*	½ Can/295g	195	9.4	66	0.8	8.5	3.2	0.0
Tomato, Cream of, Soup & Go, Heinz*	1 Cup/293ml	161	8.5	55	0.9	6.4	2.9	0.4
Tomato, Creamy, Very Special, Heinz*	1 Serving/290g	148	6.4	51	0.7	6.5	2.2	0.0
Tomato, Cup a Soup, Made Up, Batchelors*	1 Sachet/256g	92	2.3	36	0.3	6.7	0.9	0.3
Tomato, Diet Chef Ltd*	1 Pack/300g	159	5.4	53	1.3	7.7	1.8	1.2
Tomato, Harissa & Mint, Vine, The Best, Morrisons*	1 Pot/600g	294	11.4	49	1.5	6.4	1.9	1.1
Tomato, Hi Taste Low Cal, Cup Soup, Ainsley Harriott*	1 Sachet/22g	70	0.5	318	8.6	65.9	2.3	3.6
Tomato, in a Cup, Mediterranean, Waitrose*	1 Sachet/18g	52	1.5	289	8.3	45.6	8.3	10.0
Tomato, in a Cup, Symingtons*	1 Sachet/32g	97	1.6	308	3.5	62.0	5.0	3.8
Tomato, in a Cup, Tesco*	1 Serving/23g	75	0.7	328	6.4	68.5	3.2	0.1
Tomato, Lighter Life*	1 Pack/36g	125	2.6	347	34.7	33.9	7.2	7.5
Tomato, Mealpak, All About Weight*	1 Pack/37g	152	7.5	416	35.0	22.4	20.6	5.0
Tomato, Mediterranean, Campbell's*	1 Can/295g	83	0.0	28	0.6	6.4	0.0	0.0
Tomato, Mediterranean, COU, M & S*	1 Pack/415g	104	2.1	25	0.7	4.8	0.5	0.6
Tomato, Mediterranean, Fresh, Organic, Sainsbury's*	1 Serving/250ml	78	3.5	31	1.3	3.3	1.4	1.0
Tomato, Mediterranean, Instant, Weight Watchers*	1 Serving/200ml	50	0.2	25	0.7	5.2	0.1	0.1
Tomato, Mediterranean, Slim a Soup, Cup, Batchelors*	1 Serving/208g	56	1.2	27	0.5	4.8	0.6	0.4
Tomato, Mediterranean, Vegetarian, Baxters*	1 Can/400g	126	0.4	32	0.9	5.6	0.1	0.8
Tomato, Mixed Bean & Vegetable, Tesco*	1oz/28g	18	0.1	64	2.4	9.8	0.3	1.6
Tomato, Onion & Basil, GFY, Asda*	1 Can/400g	96	2.8	24	1.0	3.4	0.7	1.7
Tomato, Original, Cup a Soup, Batchelors*	1 Sachet/24g	90	2.1	387	3.9	70.5	9.0	3.4
Tomato, Simmer & Serve, Dried, Sainsbury's*	1 Serving/200ml	70	2.2	35	0.3	6.0	1.1	0.4
Tomato, Slow Roasted, New Covent Garden Food Co*	½ Carton/300g	96	1.5	32	0.9	5.5	0.5	1.1
Tomato, Smoky, Atkins & Potts*	1 Pack/400g	336	23.2	84	1.1	6.1	5.8	0.6
Tomato, Ten Calorie, Gourmet Cuisine*	1 Sachet/200g	10	0.1	5	0.3	1.0	0.0	0.1
Tomato, Vegetable Garden, Campbell's*	1 Can/310g	240	2.7	77	1.6	16.1	0.9	0.0
Tomato, Vine Ripend, Green Giant*	1 Pouch/330g	129	3.0	39	0.6	7.7	0.9	1.6
Tomato, Weight Watchers*	1 Can/295g	76	1.5	26	0.7	4.6	0.5	0.3
Tomato & Basil, Campbell's*	1 Pack/500ml	205	6.5	41	0.7	6.7	1.3	1.1
Tomato & Basil, Canned, M & S*	1 Can/400g	140	2.8	35	0.7	5.8	0.7	0.5
Tomato & Basil, Diet Chef Ltd*	1 Pack/300g	159	5.4	53	1.3	7.7	1.8	1.2
Tomato & Basil, Fresh, Finest, Tesco*	½ Pot/300g	219	14.7	73	1.0	6.3	4.9	0.6
Tomato & Basil, Fresh, Low Fat, Sainsbury's*	½ Carton/300ml	75	1.8	25	1.1	4.1	0.6	0.7
Tomato & Basil, Fresh, M & S*	½ Pot/300g	120	5.1	40	1.0	5.0	1.7	1.3
Tomato & Basil, Fresh, Sainsbury's*	½ Pot/300g	114	3.0	38	1.1	5.9	1.0	0.7
Tomato & Basil, Fresh, So Organic, Sainsbury's*	½ Carton/200g	100	4.0	50	0.5	7.5	2.0	0.2
Tomato & Basil, Fresh, The Fresh Soup Company*	½ Pot/250g	85	2.2	34	1.3	5.1	0.9	0.6
Tomato & Basil, Instant, Cup, Average	1 Packet/22g	76	1.2	346	6.1	67.8	5.4	4.2
Tomato & Basil, Italian, 99% Fat Free, Baxters*	½ Can/208g	119	2.1	57	2.6	9.3	1.0	1.1
Tomato & Basil, Italian, Canned, Organic, Suma*	½ Can/200g	82	2.4	41	1.4	5.2	1.2	1.7
Tomato & Basil, Italian, Go Organic*	1 Jar/495g	183	10.4	37	1.2	3.3	2.1	0.8
Tomato & Basil, Italian Style, Co-Op*	1 Pack/500g	200	10.0	40	1.0	4.0	2.0	0.6
Tomato & Basil, Loyd Grossman*	½ Pack/210g	97	4.0	46	0.8	6.4	1.9	0.2
Tomato & Basil, Soup-A-Slim, Asda*	1 Sachet/16g	52	0.3	326	7.0	70.0	2.0	3.9
Tomato & Basil, Squeeze & Stir, Heinz*	1 Made Up/196g	114	5.7	58	0.9	6.8	2.9	0.4
Tomato & Basil, Vie, Knorr*	1 Pack/500ml	145	2.0	29	0.8	5.5	0.4	0.9
Tomato & Basil, Vine Ripened, Fresh, Avonmore*	1 Serving/300g	141	8.1	47	1.0	4.7	2.7	0.3
Tomato & Basil, Weight Watchers*	1 Serving/295g	77	1.8	26	0.6	4.4	0.6	0.5
Tomato & Brown Lentil, Healthy Choice, Heinz*	½ Can/208g	112	0.6	54	3.1	9.6	0.3	1.5
Tomato & Butterbean, Classic, Heinz*	½ Can/200g	92	1.4	46	1.3	8.1	0.7	0.8
Tomato & Butterbean, Vegetarian, Baxters*	1 Can/415g	166	5.0	40	1.2	6.1	1.2	1.0

	Measure INFO/WEIGHT	per Measure KCAL	FAT	Nutrition Values per 100g / 100ml KCAL	PROT	CARB	FAT	FIBRE
SOUP								
Tomato & Chorizo, Mediterranean, Tesco*	1 Serving/200g	130	6.8	65	2.0	6.1	3.4	0.3
Tomato & Herb, Campbell's*	1 Carton/500ml	180	6.5	36	1.0	5.0	1.3	0.0
Tomato & Lentil, M & S*	½ Can/211g	95	0.4	45	2.3	8.4	0.2	1.5
Tomato & Lentil, Mediterranean, Weight Watchers*	1 Can/400g	184	2.4	46	2.3	7.8	0.6	1.0
Tomato & Lentil, Spicy, Canned, Tesco*	1 Can/400g	180	0.8	45	2.1	8.7	0.2	0.8
Tomato & Lentil, Truly Irresistible, Co-Op*	½ Pot/300g	165	2.1	55	3.1	8.0	0.7	1.2
Tomato & Orange, HE, Tesco*	1 Pack/400g	132	0.8	33	0.6	7.1	0.2	0.4
Tomato & Pesto, Diet Chef Ltd*	1 Pack/300g	171	6.6	57	1.3	7.9	2.2	1.1
Tomato & Spinach, Organic, Waitrose*	1 Serving/300g	126	5.7	42	1.4	4.9	1.9	0.7
Tomato & Three Bean, Canned, BGTY, Sainsbury's*	½ Can/200g	118	1.8	59	3.7	9.1	0.9	1.7
Tomato & Three Bean, Co-Op*	½ Can/200g	130	1.8	65	3.7	10.2	0.9	2.0
Tomato & Vegetable, Cup a Soup, Batchelors*	1 Serving/218g	107	2.6	49	1.1	8.5	1.2	0.6
Tomato & Vegetable, Instant, Cup, Average	1 Packet/22g	80	1.5	364	6.2	69.9	6.6	3.0
Tomato & Vegetable, Mediterranean, Fresh, Tesco*	½ Pot/300g	105	2.1	35	1.0	6.2	0.7	0.7
Tomato & Vegetable, Mighty, Asda*	1 Sachet/38g	140	2.2	368	10.5	68.4	5.8	3.7
Tomato & Vegetable, Organic, Baxters*	1 Can/400g	200	3.2	50	1.6	9.2	0.8	0.8
Tomato & Vegetable, Spicy, Healthy Living, Co-Op*	1 Can/400g	180	3.2	45	2.0	8.0	0.8	2.0
Tomato & Vegetable, Spicy, Meal in a Mug, Tesco*	1 Sachet/20g	74	2.1	370	5.5	62.3	10.5	4.3
Tomato Flavoured, Tony Ferguson*	1 Pack/58g	205	2.1	354	26.2	49.2	3.6	5.2
Turkey Broth, Canned, Baxters*	½ Can/208g	79	1.5	38	1.3	6.5	0.7	0.7
Turkey Broth, Favourites, Baxters*	1 Can/400g	152	2.8	38	1.3	6.5	0.7	0.7
Vegetable, 99% Fat Free, Wattie's*	1 Serving/105g	30	0.2	28	0.8	5.9	0.2	0.8
Vegetable, Batchelors*	1 Can/400g	168	3.6	42	1.0	5.3	0.9	4.4
Vegetable, Broth, Canned, HL, Tesco*	½ Can/200g	74	0.4	37	1.2	7.4	0.2	1.0
Vegetable, Broth, Hearty, Weight Watchers*	1 Can/295g	135	0.6	46	2.0	8.2	0.2	1.4
Vegetable, Broth, M & S*	1 Pack/213g	85	3.0	40	1.0	6.3	1.4	0.8
Vegetable, Canned, Average	1 Can/400g	208	16.0	52	0.9	3.2	4.0	0.9
Vegetable, Canned, Country, Heinz, Weight Watchers*	1 Can/295g	97	0.6	33	1.2	5.9	0.2	1.0
Vegetable, Chunky, Diet Chef Ltd*	1 Pack/300g	105	1.8	35	1.9	5.5	0.6	3.0
Vegetable, Chunky, Fresh, Organic, Simply Organic*	½ Tub/300g	153	4.5	51	1.9	9.0	1.5	1.4
Vegetable, Chunky, Fresh, Waitrose*	½ Pot/300g	117	5.4	39	1.3	4.5	1.8	2.1
Vegetable, Chunky, Organic, Tesco*	½ Pot/300g	150	3.6	50	1.7	8.0	1.2	2.1
Vegetable, Classic, Heinz*	1 Can/400g	188	3.2	47	1.1	8.3	0.8	0.9
Vegetable, Condensed, Campbell's*	1 Can/295g	103	2.4	35	0.8	6.2	0.8	0.0
Vegetable, Condensed, Classic, Campbell's*	1 Can/295g	221	5.0	75	1.7	13.2	1.7	1.7
Vegetable, Country, Asda*	1 Serving/125g	59	3.6	47	0.6	4.5	2.9	0.8
Vegetable, Country, Chunky, Baxters*	1 Can/400g	188	2.4	47	1.6	7.2	0.6	2.0
Vegetable, Country, Erin*	1 Bowl/250ml	78	2.4	31	0.9	4.8	1.0	0.3
Vegetable, Country, Fresh, Chilled, Eat Well, M & S*	½ Pot/300g	135	6.0	45	1.0	5.2	2.0	1.4
Vegetable, Country, Fresh, Sainsbury's*	½ Pot/300g	123	2.7	41	1.6	6.6	0.9	2.5
Vegetable, Country, Knorr*	1 Pack/500ml	160	3.5	32	0.9	5.5	0.7	1.2
Vegetable, Country, Weight Watchers*	1 Can/295g	97	0.3	33	1.2	6.3	0.1	1.0
Vegetable, Country Garden, Green Giant*	1 Pack/330g	129	2.0	39	1.0	7.2	0.6	2.0
Vegetable, Cream of, Cup a Soup, Batchelors*	1 Sachet/33g	134	5.3	406	5.8	59.8	16.0	6.2
Vegetable, Cream of, Fresh, Sainsbury's*	1 Pot/600g	216	12.6	36	0.5	3.8	2.1	1.2
Vegetable, Cream of, Jeremy's Soups Ltd*	1 Serving/300g	99	8.1	33	0.6	1.6	2.7	0.7
Vegetable, Cully & Sully*	1 Pack/400g	204	14.4	51	0.6	4.2	3.6	0.9
Vegetable, Cup Soup, Dry, Heinz*	1 Sachet/16g	54	1.1	348	5.8	64.5	7.1	3.2
Vegetable, Cup Soup, Made Up, Heinz*	1 Cup/200g	50	1.0	25	0.4	4.7	0.5	0.2
Vegetable, Extra Thick, Canned, Sainsbury's*	1 Can/400g	184	2.4	46	1.5	8.6	0.6	1.4
Vegetable, Farmhouse, Canned, BGTY, Sainsbury's*	½ Can/200ml	52	1.6	26	0.5	4.4	0.8	0.9
Vegetable, Farmhouse, Fresh, Avonmore*	½ Carton/250g	138	5.0	55	1.9	7.4	2.0	0.8
Vegetable, Farmhouse, Thick, Co-Op*	1 Can/400g	140	1.6	35	1.0	7.0	0.4	0.3

	Measure INFO/WEIGHT	per Measure KCAL	FAT	Nutrition Values per 100g / 100ml KCAL	PROT	CARB	FAT	FIBRE
SOUP								
Vegetable, Florida Spring, Dry, Knorr*	1 Pack/36g	104	2.0	290	7.8	52.2	5.6	5.2
Vegetable, for One, Heinz*	1 Can/300g	129	2.1	43	1.1	8.1	0.7	0.9
Vegetable, Fresh, Average	1 Serving/300g	118	4.1	40	1.4	5.4	1.4	1.3
Vegetable, Garden, Dry, Slim Fast*	1 Serving/60g	224	6.2	373	23.8	45.0	10.3	7.0
Vegetable, Garden, Heinz*	1 Can/400g	160	3.2	40	0.9	7.2	0.8	0.9
Vegetable, Garden, with Barley, Co-Op*	1 Pot/600g	240	0.6	40	2.1	7.4	0.1	0.7
Vegetable, Golden, Asda*	1 Pack/300g	150	6.0	50	1.9	6.0	2.0	0.0
Vegetable, Golden, Cup, GFY, Asda*	1 Sachet/217ml	52	1.1	24	0.5	4.4	0.5	0.2
Vegetable, Golden, Dry, Knorr*	1 Pack/76g	299	14.4	394	10.4	45.4	19.0	3.3
Vegetable, Golden, in a Mug, Tesco*	1 Sachet/17g	60	1.3	351	8.2	62.0	7.8	3.7
Vegetable, Golden, Slim a Soup, Batchelors*	1 Sachet/207g	58	1.7	28	0.5	4.7	0.8	0.7
Vegetable, Golden, Soup-A-Slim, Asda*	1 Sachet/15g	50	1.2	336	6.0	60.0	8.0	1.9
Vegetable, Heinz, Canned, Weight Watchers*	1 Can/295g	86	0.9	29	0.9	5.6	0.3	0.8
Vegetable, in a Cup, HL, Tesco*	1 Sachet/18g	66	1.4	367	7.2	66.1	7.8	2.8
Vegetable, in a Cup, Weight Watchers*	1 Serving/100g	57	1.2	57	1.2	10.4	1.2	0.5
Vegetable, Instant, Cup, Average	1 Packet/19g	69	2.0	362	8.7	57.1	10.5	5.5
Vegetable, Mediterranean, Aldi*	1 Serving/250g	78	0.5	31	5.2	2.0	0.2	0.9
Vegetable, Mediterranean, Canned, Tesco*	½ Can/200g	76	1.8	38	0.6	6.8	0.9	0.5
Vegetable, Mediterranean, GFY, Asda*	½ Pot/250g	80	4.2	32	0.5	3.6	1.7	1.6
Vegetable, Mediterranean, Homepride*	1 Serving/250ml	82	3.2	33	0.9	4.3	1.3	0.0
Vegetable, Mediterranean, Tesco*	½ Pot/300g	105	2.1	35	1.0	6.2	0.7	0.7
Vegetable, Nupo*	1 Serving/32g	111	2.1	347	37.0	39.0	6.7	9.8
Vegetable, Provencal, M & S*	1 Serving/300g	150	7.5	50	1.0	6.0	2.5	1.1
Vegetable, Roasted, Chunky, M & S*	1 Can/400g	140	2.4	35	1.3	5.8	0.6	1.1
Vegetable, Roasted, Fresh, Sainsbury's*	½ Pot/300ml	78	1.5	26	0.5	4.8	0.5	1.2
Vegetable, Scotch, Baxters*	1 Can/425g	183	2.6	43	1.9	7.4	0.6	1.2
Vegetable, Soup in a Mug, As Consumed, HL, Tesco*	1 Serving/218ml	70	1.2	30	0.7	5.5	0.5	0.4
Vegetable, Soup-A-Cups, Asda*	1 Sachet/200ml	59	1.1	30	0.6	5.5	0.6	0.4
Vegetable, Soupreme, Aldi*	½ Can/200g	62	0.8	31	1.2	4.8	0.4	1.6
Vegetable, Spring, Classic, Heinz*	1 Can/400g	148	1.6	37	0.8	7.0	0.4	0.8
Vegetable, Spring, Sainsbury's*	½ Can/200g	72	0.8	36	0.8	7.4	0.4	0.6
Vegetable, Spring, Simmer & Serve, Dried, Sainsbury's*	½ Sachet/200ml	32	0.4	16	0.2	3.2	0.2	0.2
Vegetable, Spring,Condensed, Campbell's*	1 Can/295g	62	0.3	21	0.5	4.5	0.1	0.0
Vegetable, Summer, New Covent Garden Food Co*	1 Carton/600g	336	14.4	56	1.7	6.5	2.4	0.7
Vegetable, Tesco*	½ Carton/200g	78	2.6	39	0.9	5.8	1.3	1.0
Vegetable, Thick & Creamy, Soup in a Mug, Tesco*	1 Serving/26g	104	4.3	399	5.2	57.4	16.5	7.5
Vegetable, Tuscan, Organic, Tideford Organics*	1 Pack/300g	195	7.8	65	2.4	8.1	2.6	0.0
Vegetable, Tuscan, Organic, Tideford*	1 Carton/300g	144	3.3	48	2.2	6.2	1.1	2.4
Vegetable, White Winter, Cully Ans Sully*	1 Pot/400g	172	10.8	43	0.8	4.2	2.7	1.1
Vegetable, Winter, Broth, Classic, Heinz*	1 Serving/200g	56	0.2	28	0.8	5.3	0.1	0.8
Vegetable, Winter, Chosen By You, Asda*	1 Pot/600g	234	4.2	39	1.6	5.9	0.7	1.1
Vegetable, Winter, New Covent Garden Food Co*	½ Pack/300g	117	2.1	39	2.0	5.1	0.7	2.3
Vegetable, Winter, Organic, Sainsbury's*	½ Can/200g	100	2.0	50	2.3	7.9	1.0	1.3
Vegetable, with Croutons, Soup in a Mug, Tesco*	1 Pack/23g	90	3.7	392	6.2	55.2	16.3	8.0
Vegetable & Chilli, Chunky, Fresh, Sainsbury's*	½ Pot/300g	117	1.8	39	1.6	6.9	0.6	2.6
Vegetable & Herb, Country, Farmers Market, Heinz*	½ Carton/300g	114	3.6	38	1.2	5.7	1.2	0.9
Vegetable & Lentil, Waitrose*	½ Pot/300g	138	4.5	46	2.9	5.2	1.5	3.5
Vegetable & Rosemary, Fresh, Sainsbury's*	½ Pack/300g	96	3.0	32	0.9	4.9	1.0	1.3
Watercress, M & S*	½ Pot/300g	75	5.1	25	1.3	1.5	1.7	0.6
Watercress & Cream, Soup Chef*	1 Jar/780g	413	22.6	53	0.8	5.9	2.9	0.3
Wonton, Blue Dragon*	1 Can/410g	102	5.3	25	1.2	2.0	1.3	0.2
SOUTHERN COMFORT								
37.5% Volume	***1 Shot/35ml***	***72***	***0.0***	***207***	***0.0***	***0.0***	***0.0***	***0.0***

S

	Measure INFO/WEIGHT	per Measure KCAL	FAT	Nutrition Values per 100g / 100ml KCAL	PROT	CARB	FAT	FIBRE
SOYA								
Barbeque Chilli, Vegelicious, Tesco*	1 Portion/450g	450	15.8	100	3.1	12.9	3.5	2.7
Bolognese Style, Sainsbury's*	½ Pack/168g	113	1.2	67	3.1	13.9	0.7	2.7
Chunks, Dried, Cooked, Sainsbury's*	1oz/28g	27	0.1	98	14.0	9.8	0.3	1.1
Chunks, Protein, Natural, Nature's Harvest*	1 Serving/50g	172	0.5	345	50.0	35.0	1.0	4.0
Hot Pot, with Sweet Potato, Vegelicious, Tesco*	1 Pack/450g	518	21.6	115	3.3	14.5	4.8	2.2
Mince, Dry Weight, Sainsbury's*	1 Serving/50g	164	0.4	328	47.2	33.2	0.8	3.6
Mince, Granules	***1oz/28g***	***74***	***1.5***	***263***	***43.2***	***11.0***	***5.4***	***0.0***
Mince, with Onion, Cooked, Sainsbury's*	½ Pack/180g	122	2.9	68	5.4	8.0	1.6	1.8
SOYA MILK								
Banana Flavour, Provamel*	1 Serving/250ml	195	5.5	78	3.8	10.4	2.2	0.6
Choco Flavour, Provamel*	1 Serving/250ml	208	6.0	83	3.8	11.1	2.4	1.1
Chocolate, So Good Beverages*	1 Serving/250ml	160	2.5	64	3.6	10.8	1.0	0.0
Fat Free, Original, So Good Beverages*	1 Serving/250ml	100	0.2	40	3.6	6.4	0.1	0.0
Flavoured, Average	1 fl oz/30ml	12	0.5	40	2.8	3.6	1.7	0.0
No Added Sugar, Unsweetened, Average	***1 Serving/250ml***	***85***	***4.8***	***34***	***3.3***	***0.9***	***1.9***	***0.4***
Omega Original, (Best Taste Ever), So Good Beverages*	1 Serving/250ml	98	3.8	39	2.0	4.4	1.5	0.0
Omega Vanilla, So Good Beverages*	1 Serving/250ml	130	3.0	52	3.6	7.6	1.2	0.0
Original, No Added Sugar, So Good Beverages*	1 Serving/250ml	80	2.5	32	3.6	2.0	1.0	0.8
Plain, Organic, Kirkland*	1 Glass/250ml	118	5.5	47	4.0	3.7	2.2	0.5
Strawberry, So Good Beverages*	1 Serving/250ml	160	2.5	64	3.6	10.4	1.0	0.0
Strawberry Flavour, Provamel*	1 Serving/250ml	160	5.2	64	3.6	7.7	2.1	1.2
Sweetened, Average	***1 Glass/200ml***	***94***	***4.2***	***47***	***3.4***	***3.7***	***2.1***	***0.4***
Sweetened, Calcium Enriched, Average	1 Glass/200ml	91	3.9	46	3.4	3.7	2.0	0.3
Uht, Non Dairy, Alternative to Milk, Waitrose*	1 Serving/250ml	102	4.8	41	3.3	2.7	1.9	0.2
Unsweetened, Organic, Waitrose*	1 Serving/60ml	19	1.1	31	3.3	0.2	1.9	0.0
Vanilla, Fat Free, So Good Beverages*	1 Serving/250ml	140	0.2	56	3.6	10.4	0.1	0.0
Vanilla, Organic, Heinz*	1 Serving/200ml	106	3.2	53	2.6	6.9	1.6	0.2
Vanilla, So Good Beverages*	1 Serving/250ml	180	5.0	72	3.6	10.4	2.0	0.0
Vanilla Flavour, Organic, Provamel*	1 Serving/250ml	150	5.5	60	3.8	6.2	2.2	0.6
Vitasoy*	1 Serving/250ml	130	3.8	52	3.0	5.5	1.5	2.0
SPAGHETTI								
Cooked, Average	***1oz/28g***	***33***	***0.2***	***119***	***4.1***	***24.8***	***0.6***	***1.1***
Dried, Waitrose*	1 Serving/75g	256	1.0	341	11.5	70.7	1.3	3.7
Dry, Average	***1oz/28g***	***98***	***0.4***	***350***	***12.1***	***72.1***	***1.5***	***2.4***
Dry, Carb Check, Heinz*	1 Serving/75g	219	1.7	292	52.7	15.2	2.3	20.8
Durum Wheat, Dry, Average	***1oz/28g***	***97***	***0.1***	***348***	***12.4***	***71.8***	***0.4***	***1.4***
Fresh, Cooked, Average	***1 Serving/125g***	***182***	***2.2***	***146***	***6.1***	***26.9***	***1.7***	***1.8***
Fresh, Dry, Average	***1 Serving/100g***	***278***	***3.0***	***278***	***10.8***	***53.0***	***3.0***	***2.2***
in Tomato & Cheese, Sainsbury's*	1 Serving/300g	345	10.2	115	4.4	16.8	3.4	1.4
in Tomato Sauce, Canned	1oz/28g	18	0.1	64	1.9	14.1	0.4	0.7
in Tomato Sauce, Heinz*	½ Can/200g	120	0.6	60	1.7	12.7	0.3	2.4
in Tomato Sauce, HP*	1 Can/410g	247	0.8	60	1.5	13.1	0.2	0.4
In Tomato Sauce, Multigrain, Heinz*	½ Can/200g	120	0.6	60	1.7	12.7	0.3	2.4
in Tomato Sauce, with Parsley, Weight Watchers*	1 Sm Can/200g	100	0.4	50	1.8	9.9	0.2	0.6
Marinara	1 Serving/450g	675	18.9	150	8.0	19.0	4.2	0.9
TTD, Sainsbury's*	1 Serving/90g	321	1.5	357	12.3	73.1	1.7	2.5
Wheat Free, Tesco*	1 Serving/100g	340	2.0	340	8.0	72.5	2.0	2.5
Whole Wheat, Cooked, Average	***1oz/28g***	***32***	***0.3***	***113***	***4.7***	***23.2***	***0.9***	***3.5***
Whole Wheat, Dry, Average	***1 Serving/100g***	***324***	***2.6***	***324***	***13.5***	***62.2***	***2.6***	***8.0***
Wholewheat, Cooked, Cucina, Aldi*	1 Serving/100g	130	0.6	130	5.3	24.0	0.6	3.4
with Sausages, in Tomato Sauce, Heinz*	1 Can/400g	352	14.0	88	3.4	10.8	3.5	0.5
with Tomato & Cheese, Tesco*	½ Pack/250g	280	6.5	112	4.0	18.1	2.6	1.1

	Measure INFO/WEIGHT	per Measure KCAL	FAT	Nutrition Values per 100g / 100ml KCAL	PROT	CARB	FAT	FIBRE
SPAGHETTI & MEATBALLS								
American, Superbowl, Asda*	1 Pack/453g	594	17.7	131	11.0	13.0	3.9	1.1
Chicken, in Tomato Sauce, Heinz*	1 Can/400g	332	9.2	83	4.2	11.3	2.3	0.5
Healthy Range, Average	1 Serving/400g	375	8.3	94	5.7	12.9	2.1	1.7
Italian Cuisine, Tesco*	1 Pack/400g	500	17.6	125	5.9	14.6	4.4	1.7
Sainsbury's*	1 Pack/400g	497	18.4	124	6.5	14.2	4.6	2.8
Tesco*	1 Serving/475g	641	30.9	135	5.1	14.1	6.5	0.9
SPAGHETTI BOLOGNESE								
Al Forno, Sainsbury's*	1 Pack/400g	460	19.6	115	7.8	10.0	4.9	1.1
BGTY, Sainsbury's*	1 Pack/400g	416	9.2	104	6.3	14.4	2.3	1.1
Canned, Asda*	½ Can/205g	174	5.7	85	4.2	10.7	2.8	0.6
Chosen By You, Asda*	1 Pack/100g	108	2.0	108	6.0	15.6	2.0	2.0
Cook*	1 Portion/430g	636	24.9	148	7.6	16.2	5.8	1.0
Co-Op*	1 Pack/300g	285	12.0	95	4.0	11.0	4.0	1.0
Eat Smart, Morrisons*	1 Pack/399g	311	8.8	78	4.8	9.7	2.2	1.2
Frozen, Tesco*	1 Pack/450g	472	9.0	105	5.8	15.0	2.0	1.8
GFY, Asda*	1 Pack/400g	352	6.4	88	4.9	13.4	1.6	2.2
Healthy Choice, Iceland*	1 Pack/400g	428	4.0	107	6.8	17.8	1.0	1.1
Hidden Veg, Heinz*	1 Can/400g	312	6.4	78	3.4	12.6	1.6	0.9
HP*	1 Pack/410g	312	7.8	76	3.8	11.3	1.9	0.7
Italian, Chilled, Tesco*	1 Pack/400g	520	17.2	130	6.5	15.9	4.3	1.5
Lean Cuisine, Findus*	1 Pack/320g	275	7.4	86	4.5	11.5	2.3	1.1
M & S*	1 Pack/400g	380	8.4	95	7.5	11.7	2.1	1.7
Meat Free, Heinz*	1 Serving/200g	162	3.4	81	3.3	13.1	1.7	0.6
Perfectly Balanced, Waitrose*	1 Pack/400g	380	6.8	95	6.7	13.4	1.7	1.1
Ross*	1 Serving/320g	288	3.5	90	4.2	15.7	1.1	0.9
Vegetarian, Tesco*	1 Pack/340g	374	13.3	110	5.1	13.7	3.9	1.2
Weight Watchers*	1 Pack/320g	293	6.1	91	5.7	12.6	1.9	0.8
SPAGHETTI CARBONARA								
Chicken, Mushroom & Ham, Asda*	1 Pack/700g	686	14.0	98	10.0	10.0	2.0	1.5
Chicken & Asparagus, Sainsbury's*	1 Pack/450g	657	27.4	146	6.6	16.2	6.1	1.1
COU, M & S*	1 Pack/330g	346	7.2	105	6.1	15.7	2.2	0.8
Creamy, Mini Meals, Heinz*	1 Sm Can/200g	130	2.7	65	3.8	9.0	1.4	0.6
GFY, Asda*	1 Pack/400g	406	7.6	102	5.5	15.3	1.9	0.7
Italian, Fresh, Chilled, Tesco*	1 Pack/430g	606	26.2	141	7.6	13.9	6.1	1.3
Italian Express*	1 Pack/320g	310	11.8	97	4.3	11.6	3.7	1.1
LC, Tesco*	1 Pack/400g	460	9.6	115	6.9	15.7	2.4	1.2
Ready Meal, Average	1 Pack/400g	524	21.5	131	5.9	14.4	5.4	1.1
SPAGHETTI HOOPS								
& Sausages, Tesco*	1 Serving/205g	184	6.8	90	3.1	11.9	3.3	0.2
Canned, Smart Price, Asda*	½ Can/205g	127	0.6	62	1.7	13.0	0.3	0.4
in Tomato Sauce, Heinz*	½ Can/200g	106	0.4	53	1.7	11.1	0.2	0.5
in Tomato Sauce, Hidden Veg, Heinz*	1 Can/400g	244	2.0	61	1.7	12.4	0.5	1.1
in Tomato Sauce, Multigrain, Snap Pot, Heinz*	1 Pot/190g	112	0.6	59	1.6	12.7	0.3	1.5
in Tomato Sauce, Snap Pot, Heinz*	1 Pot/192g	113	0.6	59	1.6	12.7	0.3	1.5
Tesco*	½ Can/205g	123	0.4	60	1.6	12.9	0.2	0.5
SPAGHETTI RINGS								
in Tomato Sauce, Canned, Sainsbury's*	1 Serving/213g	136	0.8	64	1.9	13.3	0.4	0.5
SPAGHETTINI								
Wholewheat, Great Stuff, Asda*	1 Serving/100g	99	0.7	99	3.4	19.7	0.7	2.4
SPAM*								
Fritters, Hormel Foods*	1 Fritter/80g	221	14.5	276	10.2	18.1	18.1	2.2
Pork & Ham, Chopped, Spam*	1 Serving/100g	296	24.2	296	14.5	3.2	24.2	0.0

	Measure	per Measure		Nutrition Values per 100g / 100ml				
	INFO/WEIGHT	KCAL	FAT	KCAL	PROT	CARB	FAT	FIBRE
SPELT								
Organic, Easy Grain, The Food Doctor*	1 Pack/225g	326	4.0	145	5.2	26.6	1.8	5.9
Pearled, Sharpham Park*	1 Portion/100g	314	1.8	314	12.0	68.4	1.8	6.0
SPICE MIX								
Chilli Con Carne, Tex Mex, Recipe Mix, Schwartz*	1 Sachet/35g	97	2.3	277	12.9	66.6	6.6	24.6
for Burritos, Old El Paso*	½ Packet/23g	68	0.9	304	13.0	54.0	4.0	0.0
for Fajitas, Old El Paso*	1 Pack/35g	107	2.1	306	9.0	54.0	6.0	0.0
for Mexican Fajitas, Discovery*	½ Pack/15g	34	1.0	230	8.0	35.0	6.5	17.5
SPINACH								
Baby, Average	***1 Serving/90g***	***22***	***0.7***	***25***	***2.8***	***1.6***	***0.8***	***2.1***
Boiled or Steamed, Average	***1 Serving/80g***	***17***	***0.6***	***21***	***2.6***	***0.9***	***0.8***	***2.1***
Canned, Average	***1 Serving/80g***	***18***	***0.4***	***22***	***3.0***	***1.4***	***0.5***	***3.0***
Chopped, Frozen, Waitrose*	1 Serving/80g	20	0.6	25	2.8	1.6	0.8	2.7
Creamed, Frozen, Weight Watchers*	1 Portion/112g	48	1.1	43	2.5	5.0	1.0	1.5
Frozen, Leaf, GutBio*	1 Portion/50g	13	0.2	26	3.0	1.0	0.5	2.8
Leaf, Frozen, Organic, Waitrose*	1 Serving/80g	20	0.6	25	2.8	1.6	0.8	2.1
Raw, Average	***1 Serving/80g***	***19***	***0.6***	***24***	***2.9***	***1.4***	***0.7***	***2.2***
SPIRALI								
Dry, Average	***1 Serving/50g***	***176***	***0.8***	***352***	***12.2***	***72.6***	***1.6***	***2.8***
SPIRITS								
37.5% Volume	***1 Shot/35ml***	***72***	***0.0***	***207***	***0.0***	***0.0***	***0.0***	***0.0***
40% Volume	***1 Shot/35ml***	***78***	***0.0***	***222***	***0.0***	***0.0***	***0.0***	***0.0***
SPLIT PEAS								
Dried, Average	***1oz/28g***	***89***	***0.5***	***319***	***22.1***	***57.4***	***1.7***	***3.2***
Green, Dried, Boiled, Average	***1 Tbsp/35g***	***40***	***0.2***	***115***	***8.3***	***19.8***	***0.6***	***3.9***
Yellow, Morrisons*	1 Serving/120g	338	1.4	282	21.3	62.2	1.2	15.6
Yellow, Wholefoods, Tesco*	1 Serving/15g	52	0.4	345	22.1	58.2	2.4	6.3
SPONGE FINGERS								
Boudoir, Sainsbury's*	1 Finger/5g	20	0.2	396	8.1	82.8	3.6	0.4
Tesco*	1 Finger/5g	19	0.2	386	7.6	80.6	3.7	1.0
SPONGE PUDDING								
Average	1 Portion/170g	578	27.7	340	5.8	45.3	16.3	1.1
Blackcurrant, Low Fat, Iceland*	1 Pudding/90g	159	1.0	177	2.2	39.5	1.1	1.6
Canned, Average	1 Serving/75g	214	8.6	285	3.1	45.4	11.4	0.8
Chocolate, & Chocolate Sauce, HE, Tesco*	1 Pudding/90g	186	3.7	207	3.9	38.7	4.1	2.1
Chocolate, & Sauce, Co-Op*	1 Pack/225g	608	29.2	270	5.0	34.0	13.0	0.6
Chocolate, & Sauce, Iceland*	1 Serving/130g	407	22.6	313	3.8	35.4	17.4	1.9
Chocolate, BGTY, Sainsbury's*	1 Pudding/105g	137	2.5	131	4.4	23.1	2.4	2.7
Chocolate, Cadbury*	1 Pack/370g	1276	73.3	345	4.9	36.7	19.8	0.0
Chocolate, Free From, Sainsbury's*	1 Pudding/110g	388	10.2	353	5.2	62.0	9.3	0.3
Chocolate, Heinz*	¼ Pudding/77g	229	8.9	298	4.6	44.0	11.5	1.2
Chocolate, M & S*	¼ Pudding/131g	524	32.2	400	6.1	38.6	24.6	1.8
Chocolate, Sainsbury's*	¼ Pudding/110g	464	28.3	422	5.4	42.3	25.7	0.8
Chocolate, Tesco*	1 Pudding/110g	337	16.6	306	4.7	37.7	15.1	1.8
Fruit, Co-Op*	1 Can/300g	1110	48.0	370	3.0	53.0	16.0	2.0
Fruited, with Brandy Sauce, Sainsbury's*	1 Pudding/125g	261	8.4	209	3.6	33.6	6.7	0.8
Ginger, with Plum Sauce, Waitrose*	1 Pudding/120g	424	17.9	353	3.1	51.7	14.9	0.7
Jam, M & S*	1oz/28g	87	2.8	311	3.6	51.5	10.1	1.6
Jam, Tesco*	1 Pudding/110g	367	13.1	334	3.3	53.3	11.9	0.5
Lemon, COU, M & S*	1 Pudding/100g	157	2.3	157	2.0	32.1	2.3	1.9
Lemon, Waitrose*	1 Serving/105g	212	2.5	202	3.4	41.7	2.4	1.4
Lemon Curd, Heinz*	¼ Can/78g	236	9.1	302	2.6	46.7	11.7	0.6
Pear & Ginger, COU, M & S*	1 Pudding/100g	175	0.7	175	1.9	39.8	0.7	1.1
Raspberry Jam, Asda*	½ Pudding/147g	481	16.2	327	3.1	54.0	11.0	4.1

	Measure INFO/WEIGHT	per Measure KCAL	FAT	Nutrition Values per 100g / 100ml KCAL	PROT	CARB	FAT	FIBRE
SPONGE PUDDING								
Sticky Toffee, COU, M & S*	1 Pack/150g	278	2.6	185	2.5	39.3	1.7	1.8
Sticky Toffee, Microwavable, Heinz*	1 Serving/75g	233	9.0	311	3.3	47.4	12.0	0.7
Sticky Toffee, Smart Price, Asda*	½ Can/150g	452	19.5	301	2.0	44.0	13.0	0.0
Strawberry, Co-Op*	1 Can/300g	960	39.0	320	2.0	48.0	13.0	0.8
Strawberry Jam, Heinz*	¼ Can/82g	230	6.2	281	2.6	50.4	7.6	0.6
Sultana, with Toffee Sauce, HL, Tesco*	1 Serving/80g	280	2.2	350	3.2	60.2	2.8	1.0
Syrup, & Custard, Iceland*	1 Pudding/130g	410	21.1	315	3.6	38.8	16.2	0.4
Syrup, & Custard, M & S*	1oz/28g	76	2.4	271	3.3	44.9	8.7	1.1
Syrup, BGTY, Sainsbury's*	1 Pudding/110g	338	4.5	307	2.8	64.6	4.1	0.4
Syrup, Finest, Tesco*	1 Pudding/115g	330	9.0	287	3.1	51.2	7.8	0.6
Syrup, GFY, Asda*	1 Sponge/105g	207	4.3	197	2.0	38.0	4.1	2.6
Syrup, Individual, Tesco*	1 Pudding/110g	390	14.5	355	3.1	55.6	13.2	0.5
Syrup, Value, Tesco*	1 Serving/100g	307	10.2	307	2.1	51.7	10.2	0.6
Syrup & Custard, Morrisons*	1 Serving/125g	290	8.6	232	3.4	39.1	6.9	0.8
Treacle, Heinz*	1 Serving/160g	445	13.0	278	2.5	48.9	8.1	0.6
Treacle, Super Sticky, Heinz*	1 Pudding/110g	318	12.2	289	1.9	45.3	11.1	1.6
Treacle, Waitrose*	1 Pudding/105g	385	13.8	367	2.8	59.5	13.1	0.5
Treacle,with Custard, Farmfoods*	1 Serving/145g	539	33.1	372	3.2	38.4	22.8	0.8
with Custard	1 Serving/200g	521	24.9	261	4.8	34.1	12.4	0.9
with Dried Fruit	1oz/28g	93	4.0	331	5.4	48.1	14.3	1.2
with Jam or Treacle	1oz/28g	93	4.0	333	5.1	48.7	14.4	1.0
with Lyles Golden Syrup, Heinz*	½ Pudding/95g	368	14.4	386	3.1	53.3	15.1	0.5
SPOTTED DICK								
Average	1 Serving/105g	343	17.5	327	4.2	42.7	16.7	1.0
with Custard	1 Serving/210g	438	15.6	209	3.4	31.5	7.4	1.3
SPRATS								
Fried	***1oz/28g***	***116***	***9.8***	***415***	***24.9***	***0.0***	***35.0***	***0.0***
Raw	***1oz/28g***	***48***	***3.1***	***172***	***18.3***	***0.0***	***11.0***	***0.0***
SPREAD								
Baking, Cook's Range, Lurpak*	1 Serving/100g	635	70.0	635	0.5	0.6	70.0	0.0
Butter Me Up, Light, Tesco*	1 Thin Spread/7g	24	2.7	350	0.3	0.5	38.0	0.0
Butter Me Up, Tesco*	1 Thin Spread/7g	38	4.1	540	0.8	1.2	59.0	0.0
Butterlicious, Vegetable, Sainsbury's*	1 Thin Spread/7g	44	4.8	628	0.6	1.1	69.0	0.0
Buttersoft, Light, Reduced Fat, Sainsbury's*	1 Thin Spread/7g	38	4.2	544	0.4	0.5	60.0	0.0
Butterspread, British, Asda*	1 Serving/10g	70	7.7	699	0.4	0.5	77.3	0.0
Buttery Taste, Benecol*	1 Thin Spread/7g	40	4.4	575	0.0	0.8	63.3	0.0
Clover, Light, Dairy Crest Ltd*	1 Serving/7g	32	3.4	455	0.7	2.9	49.0	0.0
Dairy Free, Organic, Pure Spreads*	1 Thin Spread/7g	37	4.1	533	0.5	0.0	59.0	0.0
Diet, Delight*	1 Thin Spread/7g	16	1.6	228	3.6	1.6	23.0	0.0
Gold, Low Fat, Omega 3, St Ivel*	1 Thin Spread/7g	25	2.7	360	0.5	3.1	38.0	0.0
Gold, Low Fat, St Ivel*	1 Thin Spread/7g	23	2.4	330	0.5	3.1	35.0	0.0
Gold, Lowest Fat with Omega 3, St Ivel*	1 Thin Spread/7g	13	1.3	192	0.8	4.3	19.0	1.3
Light, Benecol*	1 Thin Spread/7g	23	2.4	333	2.5	0.0	35.0	0.0
Lighter Than Light, Flora*	1 Serving/10g	19	1.8	188	5.0	1.6	18.0	0.0
Low Fat, Average	1 Thin Spread/7g	27	2.8	390	5.8	0.5	40.5	0.0
Olive, Light, GFY, Asda*	1 Thin Spread/7g	24	2.7	345	0.8	0.0	38.0	0.0
Olive, Light, Sainsbury's*	1 Thin Spread/7g	24	2.7	348	1.5	0.0	38.0	0.0
Olive, Reduced Fat, Asda*	1 Thin Spread/7g	38	4.1	536	0.2	1.1	59.0	0.0
Olive, Reduced Fat, M & S*	1 Thin Spread/7g	38	4.1	536	0.2	1.1	59.0	0.0
Olive, Reduced Fat, So Organic, Sainsbury's*	1 Thin Spread/7g	38	4.2	537	0.1	0.4	59.5	0.0
Olive, Waitrose*	1 Thin Spread/7g	37	4.1	534	0.2	0.5	59.0	0.0
Olive Oil, 55% Reduced Fat, Benecol*	1 Thin Spread/7g	35	3.8	498	0.3	0.5	55.0	0.0
Olive Oil, Bertolli*	1 Thin Spread/7g	38	4.1	536	0.2	1.0	59.0	0.0

	Measure INFO/WEIGHT	per Measure KCAL	FAT	Nutrition Values per 100g / 100ml KCAL	PROT	CARB	FAT	FIBRE
SPREAD								
Olivite, Low Fat, Weight Watchers*	1 Thin Spread/7g	25	2.7	351	0.0	0.2	38.9	0.0
Organic, Dairy Free, M & S*	1 Thin Spread/7g	37	4.1	531	0.0	0.0	59.0	0.0
Soft, Economy, Sainsbury's*	1 Thin Spread/7g	32	3.5	450	0.2	1.0	50.0	0.0
Soft, Reduced Fat, Basics, Sainsbury's*	1 Thin Spread/7g	30	3.4	425	0.0	0.0	48.1	0.0
Soft, Sainsbury's*	1 Thin Spread/7g	44	4.9	630	0.1	0.1	70.0	0.0
Sunflower, Average	1 Thin Spread/7g	42	4.6	595	0.1	0.4	65.9	0.4
Sunflower, Enriched, Light, HL, Tesco*	1 Thin Spread/7g	24	2.7	350	0.3	1.0	38.0	0.0
Sunflower, Enriched, Tesco*	1 Thin Spread/7g	37	4.1	535	0.1	0.2	59.0	0.0
Sunflower, Light, BFY, Morrisons*	1 Thin Spread/7g	24	2.7	342	0.0	0.0	38.0	0.0
Sunflower, Light, BGTY, Sainsbury's*	1 Thin Spread/7g	19	2.0	265	0.1	0.8	29.0	0.0
Sunflower, Light, Reduced Fat, Asda*	1 Thin Spread/7g	24	2.7	347	0.3	1.0	38.0	0.1
Sunflower, Reduced Fat, Suma*	1 Thin Spread/7g	38	4.2	537	0.0	0.4	59.5	0.0
Vegetable, Dairy Free, Free From, Sainsbury's*	1 Thin Spread/7g	44	4.9	630	0.0	0.0	70.0	3.0
Vegetable, Soft, Tesco*	1 Thin Spread/7g	46	5.1	661	0.1	1.0	73.0	0.0
Vegetable, with Buttermilk, Beautifully Butterfully*	1 Serving/10g	49	5.4	488	0.4	0.0	54.0	0.0
Vitalite, St Ivel*	1 Thin Spread/7g	35	3.9	503	0.0	0.0	56.0	0.0
SPRING ROLLS								
Chicken, & Chilli, Sainsbury's*	1 Roll/50g	92	4.6	185	9.6	15.6	9.3	2.8
Chicken, Asda*	1 Roll/58g	115	5.2	199	4.6	25.0	9.0	3.4
Chicken, Oriental, Asda*	1 Roll/60g	106	4.2	178	3.7	25.0	7.0	0.4
Chicken, Tesco*	1 Roll/50g	116	5.6	231	8.1	24.5	11.2	1.5
Dim Sum, Sainsbury's*	1 Roll/12g	26	1.2	216	4.1	28.2	9.6	2.9
Duck, M & S*	1 Roll/30g	75	3.4	250	9.8	27.7	11.2	1.5
Duck, Mini, Asda*	1 Roll/18g	47	1.9	259	8.7	32.8	10.3	1.9
Duck, Party Bites, Sainsbury's*	1 Roll/20g	49	1.8	245	10.1	31.4	8.8	1.0
Duck, Roast, M & S*	1 Roll/31g	85	4.9	275	7.8	26.2	15.7	1.4
Duck, with Sweet Chilli Sauce, Waitrose*	1 Roll/72g	66	1.4	92	5.1	14.0	1.9	0.9
Mini, Sainsbury's*	1 Roll/12g	27	1.2	221	4.2	28.7	9.9	1.6
Prawn, Cantonese, Sainsbury's*	1 Roll/28g	46	1.7	162	6.8	20.3	6.0	2.5
Prawn, Crispy, M & S*	1 Roll/34g	75	3.4	220	10.0	22.2	9.9	1.3
Prawn, Tesco*	1 Roll/33g	70	3.1	211	8.7	22.8	9.4	1.4
Prawn, Thai, Waitrose*	1 Roll/50g	110	4.8	219	8.0	25.4	9.5	2.4
Thai, Sainsbury's*	1 Roll/30g	69	3.4	229	2.9	28.8	11.3	3.5
Vegetable, & Chicken, Tesco*	1 Roll/60g	110	4.6	183	6.1	22.2	7.7	2.5
Vegetable, Cantonese, Sainsbury's*	1 Roll/36g	84	4.2	233	3.6	28.1	11.7	1.4
Vegetable, Chilled, Tesco*	1 Roll/68g	149	7.6	221	4.0	25.9	11.3	1.6
Vegetable, Cocktail, Tiger Tiger*	1 Roll/15g	38	2.0	254	6.4	26.7	13.4	2.0
Vegetable, Frozen, Tesco*	1 Roll/60g	123	6.4	205	3.5	23.0	10.6	1.3
Vegetable, M & S*	1 Roll/37g	80	3.6	215	4.3	27.8	9.6	2.0
Vegetable, Mini, Nirvana*	1 Roll/26g	54	2.7	208	3.5	25.1	10.4	1.7
Vegetable, Mini, Occasions, Sainsbury's*	1 Roll/24g	52	2.3	216	4.1	28.2	9.6	2.9
Vegetable, Mini, Oriental Selection, Waitrose*	1 Roll/18g	35	1.2	192	4.2	28.6	6.8	1.7
Vegetable, Oriental, Sainsbury's*	1 Roll/61g	137	7.2	224	3.8	24.3	11.8	2.9
Vegetable, Oriental Selection, Party, Iceland*	1 Roll/15g	36	1.4	241	4.3	34.1	9.7	2.1
Vegetable, Waitrose*	1 Roll/57g	107	5.3	187	3.7	22.1	9.3	3.4
Vegetable Roll	1 Roll/85g	185	10.6	218	6.6	21.0	12.5	0.0
Waitrose*	1 Roll/33g	61	2.8	184	3.6	23.1	8.6	2.5
SPRITE*								
Sprite*	1 Bottle/500ml	215	0.0	43	0.0	10.5	0.0	0.0
Zero, Lemon & Lime, Sprite*	1 Bottle/500ml	6	0.0	1	0.0	0.0	0.0	0.0
Zero, Sprite*	1 Can/330ml	3	0.0	1	0.0	0.0	0.0	0.0
SPRITZER								
Rose & Grape, Non Alcoholic, Extra Special, Asda*	1 Bottle/750ml	90	0.0	12	0.0	3.0	0.0	0.0

	Measure INFO/WEIGHT	per Measure KCAL	FAT	Nutrition Values per 100g / 100ml KCAL	PROT	CARB	FAT	FIBRE
SPRITZER								
White Wine, Echo Falls*	1 Serving/125ml	78	0.0	39	0.0	0.0	0.0	0.0
with White Zinfadel, Echo Falls*	1 Serving/200ml	216	0.0	108	0.0	0.0	0.0	0.0
SQUASH								
Apple, Blackcurrant, Low Sugar, Diluted, Sainsbury's*	1 Glass/250ml	5	0.2	2	0.1	0.2	0.1	0.1
Apple, Cherry & Raspberry, High Juice, Robinson's*	1 Serving/25ml	49	0.0	196	0.2	47.6	0.1	0.0
Apple, Hi Juice, Tesco*	1 fl oz/30ml	52	0.0	173	0.0	42.5	0.0	0.0
Apple, No Added Sugar, Morrisons*	1 Serving/40ml	8	0.0	21	0.1	4.1	0.0	0.0
Apple & Blackcurrant, Fruit, Robinson's*	1 Glass/50ml	18	0.0	36	0.1	8.0	0.0	0.0
Apple & Blackcurrant, No Added Sugar, Tesco*	1 Serving/30ml	4	0.0	15	0.2	2.0	0.0	0.0
Apple & Blackcurrant, Special R, Diluted, Robinson's*	1 fl oz/30ml	2	0.0	8	0.1	1.1	0.1	0.0
Apple & Blackcurrant, Special R, Robinson's*	1 Serving/30ml	2	0.0	8	0.1	1.1	0.0	0.0
Blackcurrant, High Juice, M & S*	1 Glass/250ml	50	0.0	20	0.1	5.2	0.0	0.1
Blackcurrant, High Juice, Tesco*	1 Serving/75ml	215	0.0	287	0.3	70.0	0.0	0.0
Cranberry, Light, Classic, Undiluted, Ocean Spray*	1 Serving/50ml	32	0.0	63	0.2	14.1	0.0	0.0
Dandelion & Burdock, Morrisons*	1 Serving/50ml	2	0.0	3	0.0	0.0	0.0	0.0
Fruit & Barley, no Added Sugar, Robinson's*	1 fl oz/30ml	4	0.0	14	0.3	2.0	0.0	0.0
Grape & Passion Fruit, High Juice, Diluted, Sainsbury's*	1 Serving/250ml	100	0.2	40	0.1	9.8	0.1	0.1
Grapefruit, High Juice, No Added Sugar, Sainsbury's*	1 Serving/25ml	2	0.0	6	0.1	1.1	0.0	0.0
Lemon, High Juice, Diluted, Sainsbury's*	1 Glass/250ml	98	0.2	39	0.1	9.1	0.1	0.1
Lemon, High Juice, Tesco*	1 Serving/80ml	141	0.1	176	0.3	43.6	0.1	0.0
Lemon, No Added Sugar, Double Concentrate, Tesco*	1 Serving/25ml	4	0.0	16	0.3	0.7	0.0	0.0
Lemon, No Sugar, Asda*	1 Serving/200ml	5	0.2	2	0.1	0.3	0.1	0.1
Lemon Barley Water, Made Up, Robinson's*	1 Serving/250ml	48	0.0	19	0.1	4.4	0.0	0.0
Mixed Fruit, Diluted, Kia Ora*	1 Serving/250ml	5	0.0	2	0.0	0.3	0.0	0.0
Mixed Fruit, Low Sugar, Sainsbury's*	1 Glass/250ml	5	0.2	2	0.1	0.2	0.1	0.1
Mixed Fruit, Tesco*	1 Serving/75ml	13	0.0	17	0.0	3.5	0.0	0.0
Orange, Fruit & Barley, Chosen By You, Asda*	1 Serving/100ml	2	0.0	2	0.0	0.2	0.0	0.0
Orange, Fruit & Barley, Diluted, Robinson's*	1 Serving/50ml	6	0.0	12	0.2	1.7	0.0	0.1
Orange, High Juice, Undiluted, Robinson's*	1 Serving/200ml	364	0.2	182	0.3	44.0	0.1	0.0
Orange, No Added Sugar, High Juice, Sainsbury's*	1 Serving/100ml	6	0.1	6	0.1	1.1	0.1	0.1
Orange, Sainsbury's*	1 Glass/250ml	8	0.2	3	0.1	0.5	0.1	0.1
Orange, Special R, Diluted, Robinson's*	1 fl oz/30ml	2	0.0	8	0.2	0.7	0.1	0.0
Orange & Mango, Low Sugar, Sainsbury's*	1 Serving/250ml	5	0.2	2	0.1	0.2	0.1	0.1
Orange & Mango, No Added Sugar, Robinson's*	1 Serving/25ml	2	0.0	8	0.2	0.9	0.0	0.0
Orange & Pineapple, No Sugar Added, Robinson's*	1 Serving/25ml	2	0.0	8	0.2	0.7	0.0	0.2
Orange & Pineapple, Original, Undiluted, Robinson's*	1 Serving/250ml	138	0.0	55	1.0	13.0	0.0	0.0
Peach, High Juice, Undiluted, Robinson's*	1 fl oz/30ml	54	0.0	181	0.5	43.0	0.1	0.0
Pink Grapefruit, High Juice, Diluted, Sainsbury's*	1 Serving/250ml	85	0.0	34	0.0	8.1	0.0	0.0
Pink Grapefruit, High Juice, Low Sugar, Tesco*	1 Serving/75ml	12	0.1	16	0.2	3.7	0.1	0.0
Pink Grapefruit, High Juice, Tesco*	1 Serving/75ml	135	0.1	180	0.2	44.6	0.1	0.0
Pink Grapefruit, High Juice, Undiluted, Robinson's*	1 Glass/250ml	455	0.2	182	0.2	43.3	0.1	0.0
Red Apple, No Added Sugar, Diluted, Ribena*	1 Serving/250ml	12	0.0	5	0.0	0.9	0.0	0.0
Summer Fruit, No Added Sugar, Sainsbury's*	1 Serving/250ml	5	0.2	2	0.1	0.2	0.1	0.1
Summer Fruits, High Juice, Undiluted, Robinson's*	1 fl oz/30ml	61	0.0	203	0.1	49.0	0.1	0.0
Summer Fruits, High Juice, Waitrose*	1 Serving/250ml	102	0.0	41	0.0	10.0	0.0	0.0
Summer Fruits, Robinson's*	1 Measure/25ml	14	0.0	56	0.1	13.0	0.0	0.0
Summer Fruits & Barley, no Added Sugar, Tesco*	1 Serving/50ml	6	0.0	11	0.2	1.7	0.0	0.0
Tropical, Fruit & Barley, No Added Sugar, Robinson's*	1 Serving/60ml	7	0.0	12	0.2	1.6	0.0	0.0
Tropical, High Juice, Tesco*	1 Glass/75ml	141	0.1	188	0.2	46.6	0.1	0.1
Tropical Fruits, Sainsbury's*	1 Serving/250ml	95	0.2	38	0.1	9.3	0.1	0.1
Whole Orange, Spar*	1 Serving/250ml	10	0.1	4	0.0	0.8	0.0	0.0
Whole Orange, Tesco*	1 Serving/100ml	45	1.0	45	0.2	10.1	1.0	1.0
Winter, Acorn, Baked, Average	***1oz/28g***	***16***	***0.0***	***56***	***1.1***	***12.6***	***0.1***	***3.2***

S

	Measure INFO/WEIGHT	per Measure KCAL	FAT	Nutrition Values per 100g / 100ml KCAL	PROT	CARB	FAT	FIBRE
SQUASH								
Winter, Acorn, Raw, Average	***1oz/28g***	***11***	***0.0***	***40***	***0.8***	***9.0***	***0.1***	***2.3***
Winter, All Varieties, Flesh Only, Raw, Average	***1oz/28g***	***10***	***0.0***	***34***	***1.0***	***8.6***	***0.1***	***1.5***
Winter, Butternut, Baked, Average	***1oz/28g***	***9***	***0.0***	***32***	***0.9***	***7.4***	***0.1***	***1.4***
Winter, Butternut, Raw, Prepared, Average	1 Serving/80g	29	0.1	36	1.1	8.3	0.1	1.6
Winter, Butternut, Raw, Unprepared, Average	***1 Serving/80g***	***29***	***0.1***	***36***	***1.1***	***8.3***	***0.1***	***1.6***
Winter, Spaghetti, Baked	***1oz/28g***	***6***	***0.1***	***23***	***0.7***	***4.3***	***0.3***	***2.1***
SQUID								
Dried, Average	***1oz/28g***	***88***	***1.3***	***313***	***63.3***	***4.8***	***4.6***	***0.0***
in Batter, Fried in Blended Oil, Average	1oz/28g	55	2.8	195	11.5	15.7	10.0	0.5
Pieces in Squid Ink, Palacio De Oriente*	1 Can/120g	274	21.6	228	13.0	3.6	18.0	0.0
Raw, Average	***1oz/28g***	***23***	***0.5***	***81***	***15.4***	***1.2***	***1.7***	***0.0***
STAR FRUIT								
Average, Tesco*	***1oz/28g***	***9***	***0.1***	***32***	***0.5***	***7.3***	***0.3***	***1.3***
STARBAR								
Cadbury*	1 Bar/53g	260	14.8	491	10.7	49.0	27.9	0.0
STARBURST								
Fruit Chews, Tropical, Mars*	1 Tube/45g	168	3.3	373	0.0	76.9	7.3	0.0
Joosters, Mars*	1 Pack/45g	160	0.0	356	0.0	88.8	0.1	0.0
Juicy Gums, Mars*	1 Pack/45g	139	1.8	309	5.9	71.0	4.1	0.0
Mars*	1 Pack/45g	185	3.4	411	0.3	85.3	7.6	0.0
STEAK & KIDNEY PUDDING								
M & S*	1 Pudding/121g	260	13.4	215	9.2	19.4	11.1	3.2
Sainsbury's*	1 Pudding/435g	1135	62.6	261	10.5	22.3	14.4	0.8
Tesco*	1 Serving/190g	437	22.6	230	10.0	20.7	11.9	1.2
Waitrose*	1 Pudding/223g	497	26.1	223	8.9	20.4	11.7	1.2
STEW								
Bean, Tuscan, Tasty Veg Pot, Innocent*	1 Pot/400g	320	7.6	80	3.1	12.5	1.9	3.6
Beef, Asda*	½ Can/196g	178	4.9	91	10.0	7.0	2.5	1.5
Beef, Meal for One, M & S*	1 Pack/440g	350	8.4	80	7.0	8.7	1.9	2.0
Beef, Value, Tesco*	1 Serving/200g	170	9.8	85	4.0	6.2	4.9	1.0
Beef & Dumplings	1 Serving/652g	766	32.7	117	7.4	10.7	5.0	0.8
Beef & Dumplings, 216, Oakhouse Foods Ltd*	1 Meal/400g	424	15.2	106	5.1	14.0	3.8	2.0
Beef & Dumplings, Birds Eye*	1 Pack/400g	308	8.4	77	4.4	10.0	2.1	0.9
Beef & Dumplings, British Classics, Tesco*	1 Pack/450g	563	29.7	125	7.9	8.6	6.6	0.5
Beef & Dumplings, Countryside*	1 Pack/300g	246	6.9	82	8.1	7.3	2.3	0.5
Beef & Dumplings, Frozen, Asda*	1 Pack/400g	392	13.2	98	6.0	11.0	3.3	0.8
Beef & Dumplings, Iceland*	1 Serving/400g	468	20.0	117	4.5	13.5	5.0	0.5
Beef & Dumplings, Plumrose*	½ Can/196g	143	3.9	73	6.1	9.0	2.0	0.0
Beef & Dumplings, Weight Watchers*	1 Pack/327g	262	6.9	80	5.2	10.0	2.1	0.8
Chicken, Morrisons*	1 Pack/400g	492	7.6	123	17.6	8.9	1.9	0.5
Chicken & Chorizo, with Patatas Bravas, Co-Op*	1 Pack/400g	380	12.8	95	8.0	8.6	3.2	1.6
Chicken & Dumplings, Birds Eye*	1 Pack/320g	282	8.6	88	7.0	8.9	2.7	0.5
Chicken & Dumplings, Tesco*	1 Serving/450g	567	29.7	126	7.6	9.1	6.6	0.7
Chickpea, Roast Sweet Potato, & Feta, Stewed!*	½ Pot/250g	188	7.2	75	3.3	8.8	2.9	2.7
Gumbo, Pearl Barley, Chosen By You, Asda*	1 Pack/350g	336	6.6	96	3.0	14.5	1.9	4.4
Irish, Asda*	¼ Can/196g	172	7.8	88	6.0	7.0	4.0	1.0
Irish, Diet Chef Ltd*	1 Pack/300g	252	8.1	84	8.7	6.3	2.7	1.7
Irish, Morrisons*	1 Can/392g	243	4.7	62	3.8	8.9	1.2	0.0
Irish, Plumrose*	1 Can/392g	318	9.8	81	7.5	7.2	2.5	0.0
Irish, Sainsbury's*	1 Pack/450g	274	9.4	61	5.7	4.8	2.1	0.5
Irish, Smart Price, Asda*	1 Can/392g	298	14.1	76	3.0	8.0	3.6	0.9
Vegetable, Mixed, Topped with Herb Dumplings, Tesco*	1 Pack/420g	508	26.0	121	1.9	14.5	6.2	1.3

S

	Measure INFO/WEIGHT	per Measure KCAL	FAT	Nutrition Values per 100g / 100ml KCAL	PROT	CARB	FAT	FIBRE
STIR FRY								
Baby Leaf, Waitrose*	1 Pack/265g	50	0.3	19	1.7	2.9	0.1	2.0
Bean Sprout, Chinese, Sainsbury's*	1 Pack/300g	144	8.4	48	1.9	5.1	2.8	1.5
Bean Sprout, Ready to Eat, Washed, Sainsbury's*	1 Serving/150g	82	5.8	55	1.5	3.3	3.9	1.8
Beef, BGTY, Sainsbury's*	½ Pack/125g	156	5.1	125	22.0	0.1	4.1	0.0
Beef, Less Than 10% Fat, Asda*	1 Pack/227g	275	6.4	121	24.0	0.0	2.8	0.8
Chicken, Chinese, as Consumed, Iceland*	½ Pack/371g	353	2.6	95	6.5	15.2	0.7	1.0
Chicken, Chinese, Sizzling, Oriental Express*	1 Pack/400g	400	8.0	100	6.6	13.8	2.0	1.7
Chicken, Chinese Style, GFY, Asda*	1 Pack/338g	362	5.8	107	6.0	17.0	1.7	1.5
Chicken, Chow Mein, Orient Express, Oriental Express*	1 Pack/400g	384	10.8	96	7.3	10.7	2.7	2.2
Chicken, Noodle, GFY, Asda*	1 Pack/330g	403	10.9	122	7.0	16.0	3.3	2.4
Chinese Style, Tesco*	1oz/28g	8	0.1	30	2.2	4.4	0.4	2.1
Edamame Bean, Morrisons*	½ Pack/175g	220	8.4	126	10.9	7.7	4.8	5.2
Edamame Bean & Ginger, Tesco*	1 Pack/290g	145	4.6	50	4.1	4.9	1.6	2.5
Exotic, Asda*	1 Serving/250g	102	4.2	41	2.3	4.2	1.7	2.7
Exotic, Tesco*	1 Pack/191g	42	0.4	22	1.3	3.8	0.2	1.5
Mushroom, Chinese, Sainsbury's*	1 Serving/175g	66	4.2	38	1.7	2.4	2.4	1.7
Mushroom, Just Stir Fry, Sainsbury's*	1 Pack/350g	172	9.5	49	2.8	3.3	2.7	2.8
Mushroom, Tesco*	1 Portion/100g	34	0.5	34	2.6	3.9	0.5	2.0
Mushroom, Waitrose*	½ Pack/165g	43	0.7	26	2.3	3.3	0.4	1.6
Noodle, Spicy Thai Style, Tesco*	1 Pack/500g	335	13.0	67	2.6	8.4	2.6	1.3
Noodles, & Bean Sprouts, Tesco*	½ Pack/125g	131	2.6	105	4.2	16.1	2.1	0.7
Noodles, Chinese, Oriental Express*	1 Serving/100g	70	0.5	70	2.7	14.7	0.5	1.4
Oriental, Chinese, Waitrose*	1 Serving/150g	40	0.6	27	2.2	3.9	0.4	1.4
Oriental, Ready Prepared, M & S*	½ Pack/260g	65	1.6	25	2.3	2.1	0.6	1.9
Pak Choi, Oriental Style, M & S*	1 Pack/220g	165	12.5	75	2.2	3.5	5.7	2.4
Pepper, Mixed, & Sweet Chilli Sauce, Asda*	1 Pack/300g	180	6.0	60	1.6	9.0	2.0	2.6
Pepper, Mixed, HL, Tesco*	1 Pack/325g	62	0.3	19	1.9	2.6	0.1	1.5
Pepper, Mixed, Sainsbury's*	1 Pack/300g	188	12.9	70	1.5	4.6	4.8	1.2
Pepper, Mixed, Tesco*	1/3 Pack/100g	23	0.1	23	1.9	3.7	0.1	1.9
Pepper, Sweet, M & S*	1 Pack/400g	160	7.2	40	2.3	3.5	1.8	0.6
Pepper & Vegetable, Mixed, Asda*	½ Pack/150g	42	1.5	28	1.6	3.2	1.0	2.6
Prawn, Chinese, Asda*	1 Serving/375g	345	2.2	92	3.6	18.0	0.6	1.8
Prawn, Chinese, Iceland*	1 Pack/340g	235	4.4	69	3.1	11.1	1.3	2.1
Rainbow, Fresh Tastes, Asda*	1 Portion/225g	119	5.0	53	1.8	4.6	2.2	3.8
Singaporean Noodle, Sainsbury's*	½ Pack/160g	202	11.7	126	3.2	11.9	7.3	2.4
Sweet & Sour, Tesco*	1 Pack/350g	161	1.0	46	1.8	9.1	0.3	1.3
Tatsoi & Sugar Snap Pea, M & S*	½ Pack/125g	25	0.4	20	2.0	3.0	0.3	1.9
Tender Shoot, Sainsbury's*	½ Pack/126g	113	8.3	90	4.4	2.8	6.6	0.8
Thai Style, M & S*	1 Serving/150g	44	0.5	29	1.0	4.4	0.3	2.0
Turkey, Chinese Style, Asda*	½ Pack/210g	321	6.0	153	23.8	8.1	2.9	0.8
Vegetable, & Beansprout, Waitrose*	1 Pack/300g	78	0.9	26	1.4	4.5	0.3	2.1
Vegetable, & Broccoli, Fresh Tastes, Asda*	½ Bag/175g	88	3.5	50	2.5	3.7	2.0	3.7
Vegetable, & Mushroom, Asda*	½ Pack/160g	59	2.4	37	2.4	3.4	1.5	3.4
Vegetable, & Noodle, Asda*	1 Pack/330g	465	14.8	141	4.0	21.0	4.5	3.0
Vegetable, Asda*	1 Pack/300g	132	6.9	44	1.6	4.2	2.3	3.1
Vegetable, Cantonese, Sainsbury's*	1 Serving/150g	90	5.2	60	2.8	4.2	3.5	2.7
Vegetable, Chinese, Mixed, Amoy*	1 Serving/110g	27	0.3	25	1.8	3.7	0.3	0.0
Vegetable, Chinese, Oriental Express*	½ Pack/200g	44	0.4	22	1.4	3.7	0.2	2.2
Vegetable, Chinese, Tesco*	1 Serving/175g	93	0.7	53	1.6	10.8	0.4	1.3
Vegetable, Chop Suey, Chinese, Sharwood's*	1 Pack/310g	223	3.4	72	1.5	13.9	1.1	0.6
Vegetable, Crunchy, Waitrose*	1 Pack/300g	81	0.3	27	1.6	4.8	0.1	2.4
Vegetable, Green, M & S*	1 Pack/220g	165	13.0	75	3.1	2.5	5.9	2.2
Vegetable, Mexican, Lidl*	1 Serving/100g	97	5.7	97	3.4	8.1	5.7	0.0

S

	Measure INFO/WEIGHT	per Measure KCAL	FAT	Nutrition Values per 100g / 100ml KCAL	PROT	CARB	FAT	FIBRE
STIR FRY								
Vegetable, Mixed, Asda*	1 Serving/200g	96	5.0	48	1.7	4.7	2.5	3.0
Vegetable, Oriental, Frozen, Asda*	1 Serving/150g	116	6.8	77	2.1	7.0	4.5	1.7
Vegetable, Oriental Style, Sainsbury's*	1 Pack/300g	195	14.4	65	1.5	4.1	4.8	2.1
Vegetable, Premium, Sainsbury's*	½ Pack/150g	90	5.2	60	2.8	4.2	3.5	2.7
Vegetable, Ready Prepared, M & S*	½ Pack/150g	38	0.4	25	2.2	3.5	0.3	2.2
Vegetable, Sweet & Crunchy, Waitrose*	1 Pack/300g	69	0.3	23	1.8	3.6	0.1	1.4
Vegetable, Szechuan, Spicy, Oriental, Sainsbury's*	1 Pack/350g	224	15.4	64	1.3	4.9	4.4	1.7
Vegetable, Tesco*	¼ Bag/100g	35	0.4	35	1.8	4.7	0.4	2.5
Vegetable, with Chinese Style Sauce, Tesco*	1 Serving/350g	133	3.5	38	1.4	5.6	1.0	1.2
Vegetable, with Oyster Sauce, Chinese, Tesco*	1 Pack/350g	98	0.7	28	2.0	4.6	0.2	1.1
Vegetable & Bean Sprout, M & S*	1 Pack/350g	105	1.4	30	1.8	4.6	0.4	2.0
Vegetable & Beansprouts, Family Pack, Fresh, Tesco*	1 Pack/600g	108	0.6	18	2.0	2.2	0.1	2.1
Vegetable & Peashoot, Mixed, Tesco*	1 Serving/100g	36	0.5	36	2.1	4.7	0.5	2.0
Vegetables, Fresh, Asda*	½ Pack/150g	106	7.5	71	1.7	4.9	5.0	1.7
Vegetables, Frozen, Farm Foods*	1 Pack/650g	208	3.2	32	1.9	4.9	0.5	2.2
Vegetables, Mixed Pepper, M & S*	½ Pack/150g	52	0.6	35	1.9	4.9	0.4	1.9
STOCK								
Beef, Cooks' Ingredients, Waitrose*	1 Jar/500g	74	0.5	15	3.0	0.3	0.1	0.8
Beef, Fresh, Tesco*	1 Serving/300ml	54	0.9	18	2.1	1.6	0.3	0.5
Beef, Made Up, Stock Pot, Knorr*	1 Serving/100ml	10	0.4	10	0.2	1.0	0.4	0.0
Beef, Pots, Unprepared, Sainsbury's*	1 Pot/28g	31	1.7	112	4.1	8.5	6.2	2.9
Beef, Signature, Sainsbury's*	1 Pack/500g	65	1.0	13	2.7	0.0	0.2	0.0
Beef, Simply Stock, Knorr*	1 Serving/100ml	6	0.0	6	1.4	0.1	0.0	0.0
Beef, Slowly Prepared, Sainsbury's*	1 Serving/100g	7	0.3	7	0.7	0.3	0.3	0.5
Chicken, as Sold, Stock Pot, Knorr*	1 Serving/100ml	8	2.4	160	4.0	26.0	45.0	0.8
Chicken, Asda*	½ Pot/150g	26	1.4	17	1.8	0.7	0.9	0.2
Chicken, Concentrated, M & S*	1 Tsp/5g	16	0.9	315	25.6	12.2	18.1	0.8
Chicken, Cooks' Ingredients, Waitrose*	1 Pack/500ml	75	0.5	15	3.2	0.3	0.1	0.2
Chicken, Fresh, Sainsbury's*	½ Pot/142ml	23	0.1	16	3.7	0.1	0.1	0.3
Chicken, Fresh, Tesco*	1 Serving/300ml	27	0.3	9	1.6	0.5	0.1	0.5
Chicken, Granules, Knorr*	1 Tsp/5g	10	0.2	232	13.1	36.5	3.7	0.4
Chicken, Home Prepared, Average	***1 fl oz/30ml***	***7***	***0.3***	***24***	***3.8***	***0.7***	***0.9***	***0.3***
Chicken, Made Up, Stock Pot, Knorr*	1 Serving/125ml	15	0.3	12	0.2	1.6	0.2	0.0
Chicken, Prepared, Tesco*	1 Serving/300ml	54	0.3	18	2.4	1.8	0.1	0.5
Chicken, Simply Stock, Knorr*	1 Pack/450ml	27	0.0	6	1.5	0.1	0.0	0.1
Chicken, Slowly Prepared, Sainsbury's*	1 Pot/300g	27	0.3	9	0.6	1.3	0.1	0.5
Fish, Fresh, Finest, Tesco*	1 Serving/100g	10	0.0	10	0.6	1.8	0.0	0.5
Fish, Home Prepared, Average	***1 Serving/250ml***	***42***	***2.0***	***17***	***2.3***	***0.0***	***0.8***	***0.0***
Vegetable, As Sold, Stock Pot, Knorr*	1 Serving/100ml	9	0.5	180	6.0	19.0	9.0	1.5
Vegetable, Campbell's*	1 Serving/250ml	38	1.8	15	0.3	2.0	0.7	0.0
Vegetable, Concentrated, M & S*	1 Tsp/5g	19	1.0	380	3.3	43.0	19.0	1.2
Vegetable, Cooks Ingredients, Waitrose*	1 Pouch/500ml	15	0.5	3	0.2	0.4	0.1	0.5
Vegetable, Granules, Knorr*	2 Tsp/9g	18	0.1	199	8.5	39.9	0.6	0.9
Vegetable, Made Up, Stock Pot, Knorr*	1 Serving/100ml	10	0.5	10	0.4	1.0	0.5	0.1
Vegetable, Tablets, Sainsbury's*	1 Tablet/11g	1	0.1	7	0.4	0.2	0.5	0.1
STOCK CUBES								
Beef, Dry Weight, Bovril*	1 Cube/6g	12	0.2	197	10.8	29.3	4.1	0.0
Beef, Dry Weight, Oxo*	1 Cube/6g	15	0.3	265	17.3	38.4	4.7	1.5
Beef, Knorr*	1 Cube/10g	31	2.3	310	5.0	19.0	23.0	0.0
Beef, Organic, Kallo*	1 Cube/12g	25	1.0	208	16.7	16.7	8.3	0.0
Beef, Telma*	1 Serving/15g	20	1.0	133	0.0	0.0	6.7	0.0
Beef, Tesco*	1 Cube/7g	17	0.2	260	9.7	48.9	2.8	1.3
Beef Flavour, Made Up, Oxo*	1 Cube/189ml	17	0.4	9	0.6	1.3	0.2	0.1

	Measure INFO/WEIGHT	per Measure KCAL	FAT	Nutrition Values per 100g / 100ml KCAL	PROT	CARB	FAT	FIBRE
STOCK CUBES								
Chicken	1 Cube/6g	14	0.9	237	15.4	9.9	15.4	0.0
Chicken, Dry, Average	1 Cube/10g	29	1.8	293	7.3	25.5	18.0	0.4
Chicken, Dry, Oxo*	1 Cube/7g	17	0.2	249	10.9	44.0	3.3	0.9
Chicken, Just Bouillon, Kallo*	1 Cube/12g	30	1.3	247	11.8	26.1	10.6	1.0
Chicken, Knorr*	1 Cube/10g	31	2.0	310	4.0	29.0	20.0	0.0
Chicken, Made Up, Average	1 Pint/568ml	43	1.0	8	0.4	1.1	0.2	0.1
Chicken, Prepared, Oxo*	1 Cube/100ml	9	0.1	9	0.4	1.5	0.1	0.1
Chicken, Telma*	1 Cube/15g	25	0.2	167	0.0	0.0	1.0	0.0
Fish, Knorr*	1 Cube/10g	32	2.4	321	8.0	18.0	24.0	1.0
Fish, Sainsbury's*	1 Cube/11g	31	2.2	282	19.1	7.3	20.0	0.9
Garlic, Dry Weight, Oxo*	1 Cube/6g	18	0.3	298	13.4	48.5	5.5	3.6
Ham, Knorr*	1 Cube/10g	31	1.9	313	11.8	24.4	18.7	0.0
Indian, Dry Weight, Oxo*	1 Cube/6g	17	0.5	291	11.5	43.9	7.7	6.7
Italian, Dry Weight, Oxo*	1 Cube/6g	19	0.4	309	11.9	48.9	7.3	4.6
Lamb, Made Up, Knorr*	1 Cube/10g	32	2.5	320	11.0	14.0	25.0	0.0
Parsley & Garlic, Herb Cubes, Knorr*	1 Cube/10g	42	2.7	422	8.6	35.2	27.4	1.8
Vegetable, Average	1 Cube/7g	18	1.2	253	13.5	11.6	17.3	0.0
Vegetable, Dry, Oxo*	1 Cube/6g	17	0.3	251	10.4	41.4	4.9	1.4
Vegetable, Knorr*	1 Cube/10g	33	2.4	330	10.0	25.0	24.0	1.0
Vegetable, Low Salt, Organic, Made Up, Kallo*	1 Serving/500ml	50	3.5	10	0.3	0.7	0.7	0.2
Vegetable, Made Up, Organic, Kallo*	2 Cubes/100ml	7	0.4	7	0.1	0.5	0.4	0.1
Vegetable, Made Up, Oxo*	1 Cube/100ml	9	0.2	9	0.4	1.4	0.2	0.1
Vegetable, Organic, Evernat*	1oz/28g	2	0.1	6	0.3	0.0	0.5	0.0
Vegetable, Organic, Yeast Free, Dry, Kallo*	1 Cube/11g	37	3.1	334	11.4	8.2	27.8	2.3
Vegetable, Premium, Made Up, Kallo*	1 Serving/125ml	7	0.4	6	0.4	0.4	0.3	0.1
Vegetable, Telma*	1 Serving/14g	35	2.4	253	0.0	2.2	17.3	0.0
Vegetable, Yeast Free, Made Up, Kallo*	1 Cube/500ml	35	3.0	7	0.3	0.2	0.6	0.1
Vegetable Bouillon, Vegetarian, Amoy*	1 Cube/10g	30	2.0	300	0.0	20.0	20.0	0.0
Vegetable Bouillon, Yeast Free, Made Up, Marigold*	1 Serving/250ml	19	1.6	8	0.0	0.5	0.6	0.0
STOLLEN								
Slices, Average	1 Slice/42g	160	6.3	381	5.5	55.8	15.0	3.1
STRAWBERRIES								
Dried, Graze*	1 Pack/35g	131	0.2	374	1.0	91.0	0.7	0.0
Dried, Urban Fresh Fruit*	1 Pack/35g	111	0.1	318	1.6	77.0	0.4	5.9
Freeze Dried, Slices, Crunchy in Munchcup, Benjoy*	1 Pot/6g	21	0.2	350	6.6	65.1	2.9	18.6
Fresh, Raw, Average	***1 Strawberry/12g***	***3***	***0.0***	***28***	***0.8***	***6.0***	***0.1***	***1.4***
Frozen, Average	***1 Serving/100g***	***30***	***0.2***	***30***	***0.8***	***6.3***	***0.2***	***1.0***
in Fruit Juice, Canned, Average	***1/3 Can/127g***	***58***	***0.0***	***46***	***0.4***	***11.0***	***0.0***	***1.0***
in Light Syrup, Canned, Drained, Tesco*	1 Can/149g	100	0.1	67	0.5	16.0	0.1	0.7
in Raspberry Sauce, WT5, Sainsbury's*	1 Serving/170g	110	0.2	65	0.7	15.3	0.1	2.3
in Syrup, Canned, Average	1 Serving/100g	63	0.0	63	0.4	15.2	0.0	0.6
STROGANOFF								
Beef, & Rice, TTD, Sainsbury's*	1 Pack/410g	595	20.9	145	9.6	15.2	5.1	1.7
Beef, 115, Oakhouse Foods Ltd*	1 Meal/400g	428	19.6	107	5.0	10.8	4.9	0.6
Beef, Asda*	1 Serving/120g	276	20.4	230	16.0	3.3	17.0	0.6
Beef, BGTY, Sainsbury's*	1 Pack/400g	416	10.4	104	5.6	14.6	2.6	0.6
Beef, Finest, Tesco*	½ Pack/200g	330	13.4	165	9.4	16.2	6.7	0.7
Beef, Sainsbury's*	1 Can/200g	232	12.0	116	12.5	3.0	6.0	0.2
Beef, Weight Watchers*	1 Pack/330g	297	7.6	90	4.3	13.0	2.3	0.1
Beef, with Rice, 'n' Peppers, Tesco*	1 Pack/450g	562	19.8	125	7.5	13.1	4.4	0.4
Beef, with Rice, Naturally Good Food, Tesco*	1 Pack/400g	425	9.4	106	7.1	13.9	2.4	1.3
Beef, with White & Wild, Rice, Classic, Tesco*	1 Pack/500g	770	29.6	154	9.5	15.5	5.9	2.3
Beef, with White & Wild Rice, Low Fat, Waitrose*	1 Pack/401g	429	6.4	107	7.9	15.3	1.6	1.0

S

	Measure INFO/WEIGHT	per Measure KCAL	FAT	Nutrition Values per 100g / 100ml KCAL	PROT	CARB	FAT	FIBRE
STROGANOFF								
Chicken, with Rice, BGTY, Sainsbury's*	1 Pack/415g	448	5.4	108	7.0	17.1	1.3	1.1
Chicken & Mushroom, COU, M & S*	1 Serving/400g	400	8.0	100	3.2	16.7	2.0	0.1
Mushroom, Diet Chef Ltd*	1 Pouch/250g	202	14.8	81	2.6	4.5	5.9	1.7
Mushroom, Eat Smart, Morrisons*	1 Pack/400g	312	4.4	78	2.6	14.3	1.1	1.0
Mushroom, with Rice, BGTY, Sainsbury's*	1 Serving/450g	418	6.8	93	3.3	16.6	1.5	1.0
Pork, with Rice, HE, Tesco*	1 Pack/450g	482	8.1	107	7.0	15.8	1.8	0.5
STRUDEL								
Apple, Co-Op*	1 Slice/100g	225	12.0	225	3.0	28.0	12.0	3.0
Apple, Frozen, Sainsbury's*	1 Serving/100g	283	15.4	283	3.2	32.8	15.4	1.9
Apple, Sainsbury's*	1/6 Strudel/90g	255	13.9	283	3.2	32.8	15.4	1.9
Apple, Tesco*	1 Serving/150g	432	21.6	288	3.3	36.4	14.4	2.8
Apple & Mincemeat, Tesco*	1 Serving/100g	322	16.7	322	3.3	39.6	16.7	2.0
Fruit, Woodland, Sainsbury's*	1/6 Strudel/95g	276	14.8	290	3.7	34.0	15.5	2.0
STUFFING								
Chestnut, Olde English, Sainsbury's*	1 Serving/110g	216	12.8	196	9.4	13.5	11.6	2.1
Chestnut & Pork, M & S*	1oz/28g	67	4.7	240	6.6	16.3	16.7	2.9
Parsley & Thyme, Co-Op*	1 Serving/28g	95	0.8	340	10.0	67.0	3.0	6.0
Pork, Chestnut & Onion, Cooked, Finest, Tesco*	¼ Pack/98g	230	11.5	235	9.5	21.5	11.7	1.7
Sage & Onion, for Chicken, Paxo*	1 Serving/50g	62	0.9	123	3.6	23.0	1.8	1.7
Sage & Onion with Lemon, Paxo*	1 Serving/50g	61	0.6	122	3.4	24.2	1.2	1.9
Sausagemeat, Sainsbury's*	1 Serving/100g	175	4.2	175	7.0	27.0	4.2	2.3
Sausagemeat & Thyme, Made Up, Celebrations, Paxo*	1 Serving/50g	80	1.8	160	6.3	25.8	3.5	4.0
STUFFING BALLS								
Pork, Sage & Onion, Cooked, British, Finest, Tesco*	2 Balls/49g	110	5.0	224	13.9	17.4	10.2	2.2
Pork, Sausagemeat, Aunt Bessie's*	1 Ball/26g	55	2.1	212	7.2	27.3	8.2	3.0
Sage & Onion, Aunt Bessie's*	1 Ball/26g	63	2.3	243	6.4	34.4	8.9	3.1
Sage & Onion, Meat-Free, Aunt Bessie's*	1 Ball/28g	54	1.9	193	5.4	28.0	6.7	1.7
Sage & Onion, Tesco*	1 Serving/20g	64	4.4	322	10.0	21.1	22.0	1.9
Tesco*	1 Ball/21g	65	4.1	315	9.6	23.5	20.0	1.4
STUFFING MIX								
Apple, Mustard & Herb, Paxo*	1 Serving/50g	83	1.0	166	4.2	32.8	2.0	4.0
Apple & Herb, Special Recipe, Sainsbury's*	1 Serving/41g	68	0.9	165	3.8	32.4	2.2	2.2
Apricot & Walnut, Made Up, Celebrations, Paxo*	1 Serving/50g	80	1.8	161	4.3	28.0	3.5	2.8
Chestnut, Morrisons*	1 Serving/20g	33	0.7	165	4.6	29.1	3.4	3.7
Chestnut & Cranberry, Celebration, Paxo*	1 Serving/25g	35	0.5	141	4.0	26.7	2.0	2.4
Date, Walnut & Stilton, Special Recipe, Sainsbury's*	1 Serving/25g	49	2.1	196	5.2	25.0	8.4	2.0
Dry, Average	1 Serving/25g	84	1.0	338	9.6	70.1	3.8	5.3
Herb & Onion, GF, Allergycare*	1 Serving/12g	43	0.3	360	7.9	76.8	2.4	0.0
Parsley, Thyme & Lemon, Paxo*	1 Serving/45g	68	0.9	150	4.3	28.4	2.1	2.4
Sage & Onion, Asda*	1 Serving/27g	29	0.2	107	3.4	22.0	0.6	1.3
Sage & Onion, Dry Weight, Tesco*	1 Std Pack/170g	578	4.1	340	10.3	69.3	2.4	6.3
Sage & Onion, Made Up, Paxo*	1 Serving/60g	74	1.1	123	3.6	23.0	1.8	1.7
Sage & Onion, Prepared, Tesco*	1 Serving/100g	50	0.4	50	1.5	10.1	0.4	0.9
Sage & Onion, Value, Tesco*	1 Ball/38g	133	1.1	350	10.2	70.7	2.9	5.1
Sage & Onion, with Apple, Made Up, Paxo*	1 Serving/50g	69	0.8	138	3.8	26.0	1.6	2.2
Sausage Meat, Morrisons*	1 Serving/20g	35	0.5	174	6.8	30.8	2.6	2.9
SUET								
Beef, Shredded, Original, Atora*	1 Pack/200g	1592	163.0	796	1.1	14.6	81.5	0.5
Vegetable, Average	***1oz/28g***	***234***	***24.6***	***836***	***1.2***	***10.1***	***87.9***	***0.0***
SUET PUDDING								
Average	***1oz/28g***	***94***	***5.1***	***335***	***4.4***	***40.5***	***18.3***	***0.9***
SUGAR								
Brown, Soft, Average	***1 Tsp/4g***	***15***	***0.0***	***382***	***0.0***	***96.5***	***0.0***	***0.0***

S

	Measure INFO/WEIGHT	per Measure KCAL	FAT	Nutrition Values per 100g / 100ml KCAL	PROT	CARB	FAT	FIBRE
SUGAR								
Brown, Soft, Light, Average	***1 Tsp/5g***	***20***	***0.0***	***393***	***0.2***	***97.8***	***0.1***	***0.0***
Caster, Average	***1 Tsp/5g***	***20***	***0.0***	***399***	***0.0***	***99.8***	***0.0***	***0.0***
Dark Brown, Muscovado, Average	***1 Tsp/7g***	***27***	***0.0***	***380***	***0.2***	***94.8***	***0.0***	***0.0***
Dark Brown, Soft, Average	***1 Tsp/5g***	***18***	***0.0***	***369***	***0.1***	***92.0***	***0.0***	***0.0***
Demerara, Average	***1 Tsp/5g***	***18***	***0.0***	***368***	***0.2***	***99.2***	***0.0***	***0.0***
for Making Jam, Silver Spoon*	1oz/28g	111	0.0	398	0.0	99.5	0.0	0.0
Fructose, Fruit Sugar, Tate & Lyle*	1 Tsp/4g	16	0.0	400	0.0	100.0	0.0	0.0
Golden, Unrefined, Average	***1 Tsp/4g***	***16***	***0.0***	***399***	***0.0***	***99.8***	***0.0***	***0.0***
Granulated, Organic, Average	***1 Tsp/4g***	***16***	***0.0***	***398***	***0.2***	***99.7***	***0.0***	***0.0***
Icing, Average	***1 Tsp/4g***	***16***	***0.0***	***394***	***0.0***	***102.2***	***0.0***	***0.0***
Icing, Golden, Cane, Natural, Unrefined, Billingtons*	1oz/28g	111	0.0	397	0.5	98.7	0.0	0.0
Icing, Homegrown, Silver Spoon*	1 Serving/100g	400	70.0	400	0.0	99.4	70.0	0.0
Light Or Diet, Average	***1 Tsp/4g***	***16***	***0.0***	***394***	***0.0***	***98.5***	***0.0***	***0.0***
Maple, Average	1 Tsp/5g	18	0.0	354	0.1	90.9	0.2	0.0
Muscovado, Light, Average	1 Tsp/5g	19	0.0	384	0.0	96.0	0.0	0.0
Vanilla, Fairtrade, Cooks' Ingredients, Waitrose*	1 Serving/100g	399	0.0	399	0.0	99.7	0.0	0.0
Vanilla, Fiddes Payne*	1 Serving/100g	397	0.1	397	0.1	99.2	0.1	0.5
White, Granulated, Average	***1 Tsp/5g***	***20***	***0.0***	***398***	***0.0***	***100.0***	***0.0***	***0.0***
White, Plus Stevia Blend, Light at Heart, Tate & Lyle*	1 Serving/2g	8	0.0	398	0.0	99.6	0.0	0.0
SULTANAS								
Average	***1oz/28g***	***82***	***0.1***	***291***	***2.8***	***69.2***	***0.4***	***2.0***
SUNDAE								
Banoffee, Perfectly Balanced, Waitrose*	1 Pot/115g	143	2.2	124	3.1	23.6	1.9	0.8
Blackcurrant, M & S*	1 Sundae/53g	212	10.2	400	3.0	54.2	19.2	1.9
Chocolate, & Cookie, Weight Watchers*	1 Pot/82g	128	2.8	156	2.5	30.3	3.4	2.2
Chocolate, & Sticky Toffee, Asda*	1 Sundae/215g	755	51.6	351	2.8	31.0	24.0	0.5
Chocolate, & Vanilla, Tesco*	1 Sundae/70g	140	6.0	199	2.8	27.5	8.6	0.5
Chocolate, Individual, M & S*	1oz/28g	69	3.6	247	4.1	28.5	12.9	0.6
Chocolate, M & S*	1oz/28g	80	5.1	285	3.1	27.2	18.2	0.0
Chocolate, Mini, Asda*	1 Pot/86g	199	12.9	231	3.1	21.0	15.0	1.7
Chocolate, Sainsbury's*	1 Pot/140g	393	29.8	281	2.5	19.3	21.3	0.6
Chocolate Brownie, Finest, Tesco*	1 Serving/215g	778	56.5	362	2.7	28.7	26.3	2.3
Chocolate Mint, COU, M & S*	1 Pot/90g	108	2.3	120	5.4	17.8	2.6	0.5
Chocolate Nut	1 Serving/70g	195	10.7	278	3.0	34.2	15.3	0.1
Hot Fudge, Two Scoop, Baskin Robbins*	1 Serving/203g	530	29.0	261	3.9	30.5	14.3	0.0
Ice Cream	1 Serving/170g	482	15.4	284	5.9	45.3	9.1	0.3
Raspberry, Perfectly Balanced, Waitrose*	1 Pot/175ml	150	1.0	86	1.7	18.9	0.6	0.0
Strawberry, & Vanilla, Tesco*	1 Serving/68g	120	3.9	177	2.0	29.5	5.7	0.1
Strawberry, & Vanilla, Weight Watchers*	1 Pot/105g	148	2.2	141	1.2	29.1	2.1	0.3
Strawberry, M & S*	1 Sundae/45g	173	8.0	385	3.4	53.3	17.8	1.0
Toffee, Asda*	1 Serving/120g	322	19.2	268	2.1	29.0	16.0	0.0
Toffee & Vanilla, Tesco*	1 Serving/70g	133	4.5	189	2.1	30.7	6.4	0.1
SUNNY DELIGHT*								
Californian Style, No Added Sugar, Sunny Delight*	1 Serving/200ml	20	0.4	10	0.1	1.4	0.2	0.1
Florida Style, Sunny Delight*	1 Serving/200ml	70	0.2	35	0.4	7.4	0.1	0.2
Original, Sunny Delight*	1 Glass/200ml	88	0.4	44	0.1	10.0	0.2	0.0
SUSHI								
Aya Set, Waitrose*	1 Pack/110g	200	4.3	182	5.4	31.7	3.9	1.5
California Roll Box, M & S*	1 Pack/230g	391	12.0	170	7.0	22.0	5.2	1.1
California Roll Selection, Classics, M & S*	1 Pack/225g	326	6.1	145	7.0	23.2	2.7	1.1
California Rolls 8 Pack	1 Pack/206g	354	9.3	172	5.1	27.5	4.5	1.4
California Set, Waitrose*	1 Pack/120g	223	9.1	186	3.8	25.2	7.6	1.7
Californian, Yakatori, M & S*	1 Serving/200g	340	9.4	170	6.4	25.0	4.7	1.0

S

	Measure INFO/WEIGHT	per Measure KCAL	per Measure FAT	Nutrition Values per 100g / 100ml KCAL	PROT	CARB	FAT	FIBRE
SUSHI								
Californian Roll, Nigiri & Maki Selection, M & S*	1 Pack/210g	294	4.4	140	4.4	25.9	2.1	2.2
Californian Roll & Nigiri, Selection, M & S*	1 Pack/215g	355	5.8	165	7.1	28.0	2.7	1.1
Chicken, M & S*	1 Pack/186g	260	4.1	140	6.0	24.4	2.2	1.0
Chicken, Tesco*	1 Pack/147g	243	3.5	165	5.2	30.0	2.4	1.0
Deluxe, Shapers, Boots*	1 Serving/235g	355	3.5	151	5.3	29.0	1.5	2.7
Fish, & Veg Selection, Tesco*	1 Pack/150g	248	3.4	165	6.7	29.2	2.3	0.4
Fish, Japanese Style, Shapers, Boots*	1 Pack/144g	230	4.3	160	4.5	28.0	3.0	1.0
Fish, Large Pack, Tesco*	1 Pack/284g	469	11.1	165	5.5	27.0	3.9	1.5
Fish, Selection, M & S*	1 Pack/191g	295	4.6	155	5.6	26.8	2.4	0.9
Fish, Selection, Medium, Sainsbury's*	1 Pack/157g	256	3.9	163	5.6	28.6	2.5	1.9
Fish, Snack, Tesco*	1 Pack/104g	159	2.6	153	4.5	28.0	2.5	1.5
Hagi Set, Waitrose*	1 Pack/370g	688	9.6	186	7.1	33.6	2.6	1.1
Hana Set, Waitrose*	1 Serving/175g	324	4.0	185	5.4	35.7	2.3	1.4
Irodori Set, with Fish, Cucumber & Avocado, Waitrose*	1 Pack/281g	472	12.4	168	5.2	26.7	4.4	1.3
Japanese Style, Sampler, Shapers, Boots*	1 Pack/80g	124	2.0	155	3.0	30.0	2.5	1.4
Large, Boots*	1 Pack/324g	480	5.8	148	5.0	28.0	1.8	0.7
Maki Rolls, Box, Sainsbury's*	1 Pack/127g	197	2.2	155	4.5	30.5	1.7	0.8
Maki Selection, Shapers, Boots*	1 Pack/158g	225	2.1	142	3.5	29.0	1.3	1.1
Medium Pack, Tesco*	1 Pack/139g	211	3.2	152	6.3	26.6	2.3	2.3
Mini, Boots*	1 Pack/99g	153	1.9	155	5.5	29.0	1.9	0.8
Nigiri, M & S*	1 Serving/190g	303	5.9	159	7.3	25.3	3.1	0.6
Nigiri, Selection, Tesco*	1 Pack/152g	236	1.5	155	4.6	31.2	1.0	0.6
Nigiri Set, Taiko, Salmon & Tuna, Waitrose*	1 Pack/113g	174	2.3	154	6.3	26.0	2.0	0.6
Oriental Fish Box, M & S*	1 Pack/205g	318	8.4	155	6.1	23.3	4.1	0.9
Prawn & Salmon, Selection, M & S*	1 Serving/175g	255	2.9	146	5.5	27.4	1.7	0.6
Prawn Feast, M & S*	1 Pack/219g	350	8.1	160	5.7	25.8	3.7	1.1
Roll Selection, Sainsbury's*	1 Pack/217g	363	8.0	167	5.0	28.4	3.7	0.5
Salmon, Nigri Crayfish, Red Pepper, Sainsbury's*	1 Serving/150g	232	4.5	155	5.5	26.4	3.0	1.0
Salmon, Smoked, Snack Pack, Tesco*	1 Pack/69g	114	1.9	165	5.0	29.1	2.7	0.9
Salmon & Roll Set, Sainsbury's*	1 Serving/101g	167	2.6	165	4.9	30.4	2.6	0.8
Selection, Shapers, Boots*	1 Pack/162g	245	2.6	151	5.6	29.0	1.6	1.7
Taiko, Fuji Set, Waitrose*	1 Pack/332g	515	10.0	155	5.0	28.0	3.0	1.0
Tokyo Set, M & S*	1 Pack/150g	240	4.6	160	7.3	25.3	3.1	0.6
Trial Pack, Asda*	1 Pack/115g	186	2.8	162	4.1	31.0	2.4	0.0
Tuna, to Snack Selection, Food to Go, M & S*	1 Serving/150g	225	3.9	150	5.2	26.4	2.6	2.3
Veg Selection, Ichiban*	1 Pack/130g	198	1.7	152	2.7	32.3	1.3	1.2
Vegetable, Mixed, Pick & Mix, Snack Pack, Tesco*	1 Pack/85g	132	2.0	155	3.7	28.6	2.4	1.4
Vegetarian, Japanese Style, Shapers, Boots*	1 Pack/145g	218	3.2	150	2.9	29.0	2.2	1.3
Vegetarian, Medium, Taiko Foods*	1 Pack/267g	403	5.3	151	4.0	36.0	2.0	1.0
Vegetarian, Selection, M & S*	1 Pack/171g	248	2.4	145	3.0	28.5	1.4	2.4
Vegetarian, Snack Selection, Tesco*	1 Pack/85g	106	2.8	125	3.7	20.1	3.3	0.6
Vegetarian, with Pickled Vegetables, Waitrose*	1 Pack/135g	244	4.9	181	5.0	27.8	3.6	1.7
Yo!, Bento Box, Sainsbury's*	1 Pack/208g	530	6.2	255	8.4	48.7	3.0	0.9
Yo!, Salmon Lunch Set, Sainsbury's*	1 Pack/150g	242	4.2	161	5.9	28.1	2.8	0.8
SWEDE								
Boiled, Average	***1oz/28g***	***3***	***0.0***	***11***	***0.3***	***2.3***	***0.1***	***0.7***
Mash, COU, M & S*	1oz/28g	15	0.3	55	1.1	9.5	1.2	2.1
Raw, Flesh Only, Peeled	***1 Serving/100g***	***24***	***0.3***	***24***	***0.7***	***5.0***	***0.3***	***1.6***
Raw, Unprepared, Average	***1oz/28g***	***6***	***0.1***	***21***	***0.8***	***4.4***	***0.3***	***1.9***
SWEET & SOUR								
Beef, Feeling Great, New, Findus*	1 Pack/350g	420	8.8	120	4.5	20.0	2.5	1.3
Chicken, & Noodles, BGTY, Sainsbury's*	1 Pack/400g	356	2.4	89	7.5	13.3	0.6	0.7
Chicken, & Noodles, Chinese Takeaway, Tesco*	1 Pack/350g	350	0.7	100	5.7	18.8	0.2	0.2

	Measure INFO/WEIGHT	per Measure KCAL	per Measure FAT	KCAL	PROT	CARB	FAT	FIBRE
				Nutrition Values per 100g / 100ml				
SWEET & SOUR								
Chicken, & Rice, Chilled, Tesco*	1 Pack/450g	540	5.8	120	4.9	21.9	1.3	0.9
Chicken, Balls, Chinese Takeaway, Iceland*	1 Pack/255g	311	3.3	122	9.9	17.5	1.3	6.0
Chicken, Breasts, Tesco*	1 Serving/185g	172	1.8	93	14.6	6.5	1.0	0.1
Chicken, Canned, Tesco*	1 Can/400g	408	6.4	102	9.6	12.4	1.6	1.1
Chicken, Crispy, Fillets, Tesco*	1 Pack/350g	508	19.6	145	7.2	15.3	5.6	0.9
Chicken, Crispy, Iceland*	1 Serving/125g	221	6.5	177	18.3	14.2	5.2	1.2
Chicken, Diet Chef Ltd*	1 Pack/270g	270	4.9	100	8.9	12.1	1.8	1.1
Chicken, Healthy Options, Birds Eye*	1 Meal/348g	390	3.8	112	4.8	20.7	1.1	0.6
Chicken, in Batter, Cantonese, Chilled, Sainsbury's*	1 Pack/350g	560	21.0	160	8.9	22.4	6.0	0.9
Chicken, Low Fat, Iceland*	1 Pack/400g	444	6.8	111	8.1	15.7	1.7	1.1
Chicken, M & S*	1 Pack/300g	465	10.8	155	6.6	24.4	3.6	0.8
Chicken, Oriental, Tesco*	1 Pack/350g	340	4.0	97	9.3	12.2	1.1	0.8
Chicken, Tinned, M & S*	1 Serving/481g	553	20.2	115	11.4	7.8	4.2	1.9
Chicken, Waitrose*	1 Serving/400g	372	3.2	93	9.8	11.7	0.8	1.4
Chicken, with Egg Fried Rice, GFY, Asda*	1 Pack/400g	500	7.6	125	6.0	20.3	1.9	1.8
Chicken, with Egg Fried Rice, M Kitchen, Morrisons*	1 Pack/450g	706	16.2	157	8.1	22.2	3.6	1.9
Chicken, with Long Grain Rice, Weight Watchers*	1 Pack/330g	300	1.6	91	5.4	15.5	0.5	1.4
Chicken, with Noodles, Feeling Great, Findus*	1 Pack/350g	385	8.8	110	5.0	17.0	2.5	1.5
Chicken, with Rice, 233, Oakhouse Foods Ltd*	1 Meal/400g	488	10.4	122	6.1	18.5	2.6	0.7
Chicken, with Rice, Chilled, BGTY, Sainsbury's*	1 Pack/400g	344	3.6	86	6.0	13.5	0.9	1.0
Chicken, with Rice, Oriental Express*	1 Pack/340g	350	2.0	103	4.4	21.3	0.6	0.7
Chicken, with Vegetable Rice, COU, M & S*	1 Pack/400g	400	5.6	100	6.9	14.9	1.4	1.1
Pork	1oz/28g	48	2.5	172	12.7	11.3	8.8	0.6
Pork, Battered, Sainsbury's*	½ Pack/175g	306	8.8	175	7.3	25.1	5.0	0.6
Pork, Cantonese, & Egg Fried Rice, Farmfoods*	1 Pack/327g	520	19.0	159	4.8	22.0	5.8	0.1
Pork, with Rice, 229, Oakhouse Foods Ltd*	1 Meal/400g	484	12.0	121	5.1	18.4	3.0	0.7
Vegetables, Roasted, Cantonese, Sainsbury's*	1 Pack/348g	327	4.2	94	1.1	19.6	1.2	0.9
Vegetables, with Rice, Waitrose*	1 Pack/400g	384	4.4	96	1.9	19.5	1.1	1.1
SWEET POTATO								
Baked, Flesh Only, Average	***1 Med/130g***	***150***	***0.5***	***115***	***1.6***	***27.9***	***0.4***	***3.3***
Boiled in Salted Water, Average	***1 Med/200g***	***168***	***0.6***	***84***	***1.1***	***20.5***	***0.3***	***2.3***
Dried	1 Serving/100g	110	3.0	110	1.6	19.7	3.0	3.2
Organic, Tesco*	1 Serving/100g	93	0.3	93	1.2	21.3	0.3	2.4
Raw, Peeled, Average	1 Sm Potato/130g	112	0.1	86	1.6	20.1	0.0	3.0
Steamed, Average	***1 Med/200g***	***168***	***0.6***	***84***	***1.1***	***20.4***	***0.3***	***2.3***
with Rosemary & Garlic, Frozen, McCain*	1 Serving/150g	172	5.6	115	2.1	18.4	3.7	2.8
SWEETBREAD								
Lamb, Fried	***1oz/28g***	***61***	***3.2***	***217***	***28.7***	***0.0***	***11.4***	***0.0***
SWEETCORN								
& Petit Pois, M & S*	1oz/28g	20	0.4	73	4.6	10.8	1.3	3.6
Baby, Canned, Drained, Average	1 Serving/80g	18	0.3	23	2.9	2.0	0.4	1.5
Baby, Frozen, Average	***1oz/28g***	***7***	***0.1***	***24***	***2.5***	***2.7***	***0.4***	***1.7***
Boiled, Average	***1oz/28g***	***31***	***0.6***	***111***	***4.2***	***19.6***	***2.3***	***2.2***
Canned, No Sugar & Salt, Average	½ Can/125g	99	1.3	79	2.7	15.0	1.1	1.6
Canned, Weight Watchers*	1 Portion/143g	103	1.4	72	2.5	12.0	1.0	2.0
Canned, with Sugar & Salt, Average	***1 Lge Can/340g***	***376***	***4.0***	***111***	***3.2***	***21.9***	***1.2***	***1.9***
Frozen, Average	***1 Sachet/115g***	***121***	***2.4***	***105***	***3.8***	***17.9***	***2.1***	***1.8***
Original, Reduced Salt & Sugar, Canned, Bonduelle*	1 Can/165g	182	2.6	110	3.1	20.7	1.6	2.9
Supersweet, Field Fresh, Birds Eye*	1 Portion/80g	67	0.6	84	2.6	16.9	0.7	2.4
with Peppers, Canned, Average	***1 Serving/50g***	***40***	***0.2***	***79***	***2.6***	***16.4***	***0.3***	***0.6***
SWEETENER								
Aspartamo, Artificial Sugar, Zen*	1 Tbsp/2g	8	0.0	383	1.8	94.0	0.0	0.0
Calorie Free, Truvia*	1 Sachet/2g	0	0.0	0	0.0	99.0	0.0	0.0

	Measure INFO/WEIGHT	per Measure KCAL	FAT	Nutrition Values per 100g / 100ml KCAL	PROT	CARB	FAT	FIBRE
SWEETENER								
Canderel, Spoonful, Canderel*	1 Tsp/0.5g	2	0.0	384	2.9	93.0	0.0	0.0
Granulated, Low Calorie, Splenda*	1 Tsp/0.5g	2	0.0	391	0.0	97.7	0.0	0.0
Granulated, Silver Spoon*	1 Tsp/0.5g	2	0.0	387	1.0	96.8	0.0	0.0
Granulated, Tesco*	1 Tsp/1g	4	0.0	383	1.8	94.0	0.0	0.0
Lucuma Powder, Navitas*	1 Tbsp/15g	60	0.0	400	6.7	86.7	0.0	0.0
Natural, Pure Via*	1 Sachet/2g	3	0.0	149	0.0	95.7	0.0	0.0
Natural Syrup, Fruit, Dark, Sweet Freedom*	1 Tsp/5g	13	0.0	292	0.0	79.0	0.0	0.0
Silver Spoon*	1 Tablet/0.05g	0	0.0	325	10.0	71.0	0.0	0.0
Simply Sweet*	1 Tbsp/2g	8	0.0	375	1.4	92.3	0.0	0.0
Spoonfull, Low Calorie, SupaSweet*	1 Tsp/1g	4	0.0	392	3.0	95.0	0.0	0.0
Sweet' N Low*	1 Sachet/1g	3	0.0	368	0.0	92.0	0.0	0.0
Sweetex*	1oz/28g	0	0.0	0	0.0	0.0	0.0	0.0
Tablet, Average	1 Tablet/0.1g	0	0.0	355	8.7	73.0	0.0	0.8
Tablets, Low Calorie, Canderel*	1 Tablet/0.1g	0	0.0	342	13.0	72.4	0.0	0.0
Tablets, Splenda*	1 Tablet/0.1g	0	0.0	345	10.0	76.2	0.0	1.6
Tablets, Tesco*	1 Tablet/1g	0	0.0	20	2.0	2.0	0.5	0.0
Tagatesse (Granulated), Damhert*	1 Serving/5g	14	2.0	275	0.0	79.8	39.9	20.1
Tagatesse (Tablet), Damhert*	1 Tablet/0.075g	0	0.0	266	2.7	76.3	0.0	0.0
Xylosweet, Xylitol*	1 Serving/4g	10	0.0	240	0.0	100.0	0.0	0.0
SWEETS								
Almonds, Sugared, Dragee*	1 Sweet/4g	17	0.6	472	10.0	68.3	17.9	2.5
Alphabet Candies, Asda*	1 Pack/80g	306	0.0	382	0.5	95.0	0.0	0.0
Banana, Baby Foam, M & S*	1/3 Pack/34g	131	0.0	385	4.1	92.7	0.0	0.0
Big Purple One, Quality Street, Nestle*	1 Sweet/39g	191	9.9	490	4.7	60.5	25.5	0.7
Black Jacks & Fruit Salad, Bassett's*	1 Serving/190g	760	11.8	400	0.7	84.9	6.2	0.0
Blackcurrant & Liquorice, M & S*	1 Sweet/8g	32	0.3	400	0.6	89.0	4.3	0.0
Butter Candies, Original, Werther's*	1 Sweet/5g	21	0.4	424	0.1	85.7	8.9	0.1
Butterscotch Candies, Weight Watchers*	1 Box/42g	95	0.0	226	0.0	81.9	0.0	14.5
Campino, Oranges & Cream, Bendicks*	1oz/28g	116	2.3	416	0.1	85.8	8.1	0.0
Campino, Strawberries & Cream, Bendicks*	1oz/28g	117	2.3	418	0.1	86.2	8.1	0.0
Candy Cane, Average	1oz/28g	100	0.0	357	3.6	85.7	0.0	0.0
Candy Floss, Asda*	1 Tub/75g	292	0.0	390	0.0	100.0	0.0	0.0
Candy Foam Shapes, Fun Fruits, Value, Tesco*	1 Serving/25g	94	0.0	374	3.1	90.3	0.1	0.5
Cherry Drops, Bassett's*	1 Sweet/5g	18	0.0	390	0.0	98.1	0.0	0.0
Cherry Lips, Chewits*	1 Serving/100g	319	0.2	319	5.6	72.1	0.2	0.0
Chewits, Blackcurrant, Leaf*	1 Chew/3g	12	0.1	385	0.2	87.5	3.0	0.0
Chewits, Cola, Leaf*	1 Chew/3g	12	0.1	385	0.2	87.5	3.0	0.0
Chewits, Fruit Salad, Leaf*	1 Chew/3g	12	0.1	385	0.2	87.5	3.0	0.0
Chewits, Strawberry, Leaf*	1 Chew/3g	12	0.1	385	0.2	87.5	3.0	0.0
Chewitts, Blackcurrant	1 Pack/33g	125	0.9	378	0.3	86.9	2.7	0.0
Chews, Just Fruit, Fruit-tella*	1 Serving/43g	170	2.8	400	0.9	79.5	6.5	0.0
Chews, Spearmint, Victoria, Aldi*	1 Sweet/10g	40	0.8	405	0.3	83.8	7.6	0.0
Chews, Strawberry Mix, Starburst*	1 Sweet/4g	15	0.3	401	0.0	83.9	7.3	0.0
Choco Toffee, Sula*	1 Sweet/8g	21	1.2	267	3.3	31.7	15.8	0.0
Chocolate Caramels, Diabetic, Boots*	5 Sweets/40g	109	13.2	272	3.2	33.0	33.0	2.0
Chocolate Caramels, Milk, Tesco*	1 Sweet/3g	15	0.5	444	2.7	72.1	16.1	0.1
Chocolate Eclairs, Cadbury*	1 Sweet/8g	36	1.4	455	4.5	68.9	17.9	0.0
Chocolate Limes, Pascall*	1 Sweet/8g	27	0.2	333	0.3	77.2	2.5	0.0
Clear Fruits, Sainsbury's*	1 Sweet/7g	26	0.0	372	0.1	92.9	0.0	0.0
Cola Bottles, Asda*	1 Serving/100g	329	0.2	329	9.0	73.0	0.2	0.0
Cola Bottles, Fizzy, M & S*	1 Pack/200g	650	0.0	325	6.4	75.0	0.0	0.0
Cough, Herbs, Swiss, Orginal, Ricola*	1 Packet/37g	148	0.0	400	0.0	98.0	0.0	0.0
Crazy Crocs, Chewits*	1 Serving/100g	316	0.2	316	3.8	73.9	0.2	0.0

S

	Measure INFO/WEIGHT	per Measure KCAL	FAT	Nutrition Values per 100g / 100ml KCAL	PROT	CARB	FAT	FIBRE
SWEETS								
Cream Caramel, Sula*	1 Sweet/3g	10	0.0	297	0.4	86.1	0.0	0.0
Crunchies, Fruit, Fruit-tella*	1 Box/23g	90	1.2	390	0.7	86.0	5.0	0.0
Dolly Mix, Bassett's*	1 Bag/45g	171	1.4	380	3.0	85.1	3.1	0.4
Drops, Lemon & Orange, M & S*	1 Pack42g	97	0.0	230	0.0	61.0	0.0	0.0
Drumstick, Matlow's*	1 Pack/40g	164	2.2	409	0.4	88.3	5.5	0.0
Edinburgh Rock, Gardiners of Scotland*	1 Piece/2g	8	0.0	380	0.1	94.4	0.3	0.8
Fizzy Cola, Weight Watchers*	1 Sweet/2g	5	0.0	249	0.3	98.6	0.6	0.3
Fizzy Lemon Fish, Asda*	1 Sweet/4g	14	0.0	325	5.0	76.0	0.1	0.0
Fizzy Mix, Tesco*	½ Bag/50g	166	0.0	332	5.2	75.2	0.0	0.0
Flipsters, Starburst*	1 Pack/37g	145	0.0	392	0.0	98.1	0.0	0.0
Flumps, Bassett's*	1 Serving/5g	16	0.0	325	4.0	77.0	0.0	0.0
Flumps, Fluffy Mallow Twists, Fat Free, Bassett's*	1 Twist/13g	30	0.0	230	4.1	77.1	0.0	0.0
Flying Suacers, Asda*	1 Serving/23g	82	0.6	355	0.1	83.0	2.5	0.8
Foamy Mushrooms, Chewy, Asda*	1 Sweet/3g	9	0.0	347	4.2	82.0	0.2	0.0
Fruit, Mentos*	1 Sweet/3g	10	0.0	333	0.0	100.0	0.0	0.0
Fruit Drops, Co-Op*	1 Sweet/6g	24	0.0	395	0.2	98.0	0.0	0.0
Fruit Gums & Jellies	1 Tube/33g	107	0.0	324	6.5	79.5	0.0	0.0
Fruit Rocks, Assorted, M & S*	1oz/28g	107	0.0	381	0.0	95.2	0.0	0.0
Fruit Sherbets, Assorted, M & S*	1 Sweet/9g	35	0.4	405	0.3	91.6	4.3	0.1
Fruit Tingles, Wonka*	1 Sweet/8g	8	0.0	104	0.0	26.0	0.0	0.0
Fruities, Lemon & Lime, Weight Watchers*	1 Sweet/2g	3	0.0	134	0.0	54.0	0.0	33.0
Fruity Babies, Bassett's*	1 Sweet/3g	10	0.0	310	4.6	72.7	0.2	0.0
Fruity Chews, Starburst*	1 Sweet/8g	34	0.6	404	0.0	83.4	7.4	0.0
Fruity Flutterbies, Chewits*	1 Serving/100g	316	0.2	316	3.8	73.9	0.2	0.0
Fruity Frogs, Rowntree's*	1 Serving/40g	128	0.1	321	4.7	74.5	0.2	0.0
Fruity Mallows, Fizzy, Asda*	1 Pack/400g	1252	0.0	313	4.3	74.0	0.0	0.0
Gobstoppers, Everlasting, Wonka*	9 Pieces/15g	60	0.0	400	0.0	93.3	0.0	0.0
Gummy Bears	10 Bears/22g	85	0.0	386	0.0	98.9	0.0	98.9
Gummy Mix, Tesco*	1 Pack/100g	327	0.1	327	5.9	75.7	0.1	0.0
Gummy Worms	10 Worms/74g	286	0.0	386	0.0	98.9	0.0	98.9
Ice Cream Sundae, Asda*	1 Sweet/2g	8	0.0	343	4.1	81.0	0.2	0.1
Jellies, Very Berry, Rowntrees*	1 Sweet/4g	12	0.0	326	5.0	74.8	0.2	0.1
Jelly Babies, Morrisons*	1 Serving/227g	781	0.0	344	5.3	80.7	0.0	0.0
Jelly Beans, Lucozade*	1 Packet/30g	111	0.0	370	0.0	92.0	0.0	0.0
Jelly Beans, Tesco*	¼ Bag/63g	243	0.2	385	0.1	94.5	0.3	0.3
Kisses, Hershey*	1 Sweet/5g	28	1.6	561	7.0	59.0	32.0	0.0
Laces, Apple Flavour, Tesco*	5 Laces/15g	52	0.5	347	3.6	74.8	3.2	2.1
Laces, Strawberry, Sainsbury's*	1 Serving/25g	94	1.2	377	3.3	76.3	4.6	0.1
Lances, Strawberry & Cream Flavour, Tesco*	1 Bag/75g	276	0.9	368	3.2	86.1	1.2	2.1
Lances, Strawberry Flavour, Fizzy, Tesco*	½ Pack/50g	177	1.3	354	2.8	79.8	2.6	1.8
Lemon Mint Flavour, Herb Drops, Sugar Free, Ricola*	1 Sweet/3g	7	0.0	235	0.0	96.0	0.0	0.0
Liquorice & Fruit, Fruit-tella*	1 Sweet/4g	16	0.3	395	0.9	83.0	6.5	0.0
Liquorice Torpedoes, Sweets For Life*	1 Serving/100g	368	0.3	368	4.1	87.1	0.3	1.4
Lovehearts, Giant, Swizzels*	1 Pack/42g	165	0.0	393	0.0	100.0	0.0	0.0
Lovehearts, Swizzels*	1oz/28g	100	0.0	359	0.7	88.2	0.0	0.0
Maoam Sour, Haribo*	1 Pack/22g	85	1.4	386	1.2	80.0	6.5	0.1
Maynards Sours, Bassett's*	1 Pack/52g	169	0.0	325	6.1	75.0	0.0	0.0
Midget Gems, Maynards*	1 Sweet/1g	3	0.0	340	8.7	76.2	0.0	0.0
Parma Violets, Swizzlers*	1 Small Tube/10g	41	0.0	406	0.9	99.1	0.0	0.0
Pear Drops, Bassett's*	1 Sweet/4g	16	0.0	390	0.0	96.4	0.0	0.0
Percy Pig & Pals, Soft, M & S*	1 Sweet/8g	30	0.0	344	5.8	80.0	0.1	0.0
Randoms, Rowntree's*	1 Pack/50g	164	0.2	328	4.9	75.7	0.3	0.6
Rhubarb & Custards, Tesco*	1 Sweet/9g	36	0.0	396	0.3	97.6	0.5	0.1

	Measure INFO/WEIGHT	per Measure KCAL	FAT	Nutrition Values per 100g / 100ml KCAL	PROT	CARB	FAT	FIBRE
SWEETS								
Salzige Heringe, Katjes*	1 Serving/50g	172	0.0	345	5.8	80.0	0.1	0.0
Scary Mix, Tesco*	1 Bag/100g	327	0.5	327	9.5	71.1	0.5	0.3
Scary Sours, Rowntree's*	1 Serving/100g	321	0.0	321	3.5	74.7	0.0	0.0
Sherbert Cocktails, Sainsbury's*	1 Sweet/9g	36	0.7	400	0.0	83.1	7.5	0.0
Sherbert Dib Dab, with Strawberry Lolly, Barratt*	1 Pack/23g	90	0.0	385	0.1	95.6	0.1	0.0
Sherbert Lemons, Weight Watchers*	1 Box/35g	84	0.2	239	0.0	94.7	0.5	0.0
Sherbet Lemons, Bassett's*	1 Sweet/7g	25	0.0	375	0.0	93.9	0.0	0.0
Shrimps & Bananas, Sainsbury's*	½ Pack/50g	188	0.0	376	2.5	91.3	0.1	0.5
Snakes, Bassett's*	1 Sweet/9g	30	0.0	320	3.5	76.8	0.1	0.0
Soft Fruits, Trebor*	1 Roll/45g	165	0.0	367	0.0	90.9	0.0	0.0
Sour Squirms, Bassett's*	1 Serving/7g	21	0.0	325	3.1	78.1	0.0	0.0
Strawberry & Cream, Sugar Free, Sula*	1 Sweet/3g	9	0.2	267	0.2	90.5	5.4	0.0
Sugar Free, Sula*	1 Sweet/3g	7	0.0	231	0.0	96.1	0.0	0.0
Sweetshop Favourites, Bassett's*	1 Sweet/5g	17	0.0	340	0.0	84.3	0.0	0.0
Tic Tac, Cool Cherry, Ferrero*	1 Pack/18g	69	0.1	382	0.2	92.2	0.7	0.0
Toffees, Value, Tesco*	3 Toffees/23g	101	3.3	450	2.1	77.3	14.8	0.3
Toffo*	1 Tube/43g	194	9.5	451	2.2	69.8	22.0	0.0
Tootsie Roll, Small Midgees, Tootsie*	1 Sweet/7g	23	0.5	350	2.5	70.0	7.5	0.0
Tooty Frooties, Rowntree's*	1 Bag/28g	111	1.0	397	0.1	91.5	3.5	0.0
Wazzly Wobble Drops, Wonka*	1 Bag/42g	186	6.8	443	3.0	71.6	16.1	0.2
Wiggly Worms, Sainsbury's*	1 Serving/10g	32	0.0	317	5.6	72.7	0.4	0.2
Wine Gummies, Matlow, Swizzels*	1 Pack/16g	52	0.0	324	0.0	58.7	0.0	0.0
Xtra Sour Spiders, Rowntree's*	1 Pack/35g	112	0.0	321	3.5	74.8	0.0	0.0
SWORDFISH								
Grilled, Average	***1oz/28g***	***39***	***1.5***	***139***	***22.9***	***0.0***	***5.2***	***0.0***
Raw, Average	***1oz/28g***	***42***	***2.0***	***149***	***21.1***	***0.0***	***7.2***	***0.0***
SYRUP								
Amaretto, Fabbri*	1 Serving/20ml	70	0.0	349	0.0	86.0	0.0	0.0
Amaretto, Sugar Free, Monin*	1 Serving/30ml	0	0.0	0	0.0	13.3	0.0	0.0
Balsamic, Merchant Gourmet*	1 Tsp/5g	12	0.0	232	0.4	60.0	0.1	0.0
Butterscotch, Monin*	1 Serving/30ml	100	0.0	333	0.0	80.0	0.0	0.0
Caramel, for Coffee, Lyle's*	2 Tsps/10ml	33	0.0	329	0.0	83.0	0.0	0.0
Caramel, Sugar Free, Monin*	1 Serving/30ml	0	0.0	0	0.0	13.3	0.0	0.0
Chocolate Mint, Monin*	1 Serving/30ml	100	0.0	333	0.0	80.0	0.0	0.0
Cinnamon, Monin*	1 Serving/30ml	100	0.0	333	0.0	80.0	0.0	0.0
Corn, Dark, Average	***1 Tbsp/20g***	***56***	***0.0***	***282***	***0.0***	***76.6***	***0.0***	***0.0***
Gingerbread, Monin*	1 Serving/30ml	90	0.0	300	0.0	76.7	0.0	0.0
Golden, Average	***1 Tbsp/20g***	***61***	***0.0***	***304***	***0.4***	***78.2***	***0.0***	***0.0***
Hazelnut, Monin*	1 Serving/30ml	90	0.0	300	0.0	73.3	0.0	0.0
Maple, Average	***1 Tbsp/20g***	***52***	***0.0***	***262***	***0.0***	***67.2***	***0.2***	***0.0***
Organic Rice Malt, Clearspring*	2 Tbsp/42g	133	0.2	316	1.5	76.8	0.4	0.0
Peppermint, Monin*	1 Serving/30ml	96	0.0	320	0.0	80.0	0.0	0.0
Praline, Monin*	1 Serving/30ml	94	0.0	313	0.0	76.7	0.0	0.0
Strawberry, Aardbeien Siroop, Plein Sud, Lidl*	1 Serving/20ml	56	0.0	280	0.0	71.0	0.0	0.0
Sugar	1 Tbsp/20g	64	0.0	319	0.0	83.9	0.0	0.0
Toffee Nut, Monin*	1 Serving/30ml	90	0.0	300	0.0	70.0	0.0	0.0
Vanilla, Fabbri*	1 Serving/20ml	70	0.0	349	0.0	86.0	0.0	0.0
Vanilla, Monin*	1 Shot/35ml	119	0.0	340	0.0	84.4	0.0	0.0
Vanilla, Sugar Free, Monin*	1 Serving/30ml	0	0.0	0	0.0	13.3	0.0	0.0

	Measure INFO/WEIGHT	per Measure KCAL	FAT	Nutrition Values per 100g / 100ml KCAL	PROT	CARB	FAT	FIBRE
TABOO*								
Average, Taboo*	1 Shot/35ml	80	0.0	230	0.0	33.0	0.0	0.0
TABOULEH								
Average	***1oz/28g***	***33***	***1.3***	***119***	***2.6***	***17.2***	***4.6***	***0.0***
TACO SHELLS								
Corn, Crunchy, Old El Paso*	1 Taco/10g	51	2.6	506	7.0	61.0	26.0	0.0
Old El Paso*	1 Taco/12g	57	2.7	478	7.4	60.8	22.8	0.0
Taco, Crunchy, Taco Bell*	1 Serving/78g	133	7.8	170	8.0	13.0	10.0	1.0
Traditional, Discovery*	1 Taco/11g	55	3.2	489	5.7	53.4	28.1	6.0
TAGLIATELLE								
Basil, M & S*	1 Serving/100g	365	2.8	365	15.1	69.0	2.8	4.0
Bicolore, Asda*	¼ Pack/125g	202	3.0	162	7.0	28.0	2.4	1.4
Carbonara, Frozen, Tesco*	1 Pack/450g	428	8.6	95	5.2	14.1	1.9	0.9
Carbonara, Low Fat, Bertorelli*	1 Pack/350g	301	7.7	86	5.3	12.0	2.2	0.9
Carbonara, Naturally Less 5% Fat, Asda*	1 Pack/400g	440	9.6	110	4.2	18.0	2.4	0.8
Carbonara, Perfectly Balanced, Waitrose*	1 Pack/350g	357	12.6	102	5.3	12.1	3.6	0.7
Carbonara, Ready Meal, Average	1 Serving/400g	460	13.4	115	5.5	15.8	3.3	1.0
Carbonara, TTD, Sainsbury's*	1 Pack/405g	644	25.9	159	7.8	17.6	6.4	1.6
Chicken, Chargrilled, & Tomato, Asda*	1 Pack/400g	392	12.4	98	5.8	11.7	3.1	1.4
Chicken, Italia, M & S*	1 Pack/360g	342	6.5	95	8.1	12.1	1.8	1.2
Chicken, Italian, Sainsbury's*	1 Pack/450g	567	15.8	126	6.5	17.0	3.5	2.6
Chicken & Mushroom, GFY, Asda*	1 Pack/400g	359	7.0	90	7.2	11.2	1.8	0.7
Chicken & Tomato, Italiano, Tesco*	1 Pack/400g	416	8.4	104	6.6	14.8	2.1	0.8
Dry, Average	***1 Serving/100g***	***356***	***1.8***	***356***	***12.6***	***72.4***	***1.8***	***1.0***
Egg, Dry, Average	***1 Serving/75g***	***272***	***2.5***	***362***	***14.2***	***68.8***	***3.3***	***2.3***
Egg, Fresh, Chosen By You, Asda*	1 Serving/125g	179	1.4	143	5.6	26.9	1.1	1.7
Egg, Fresh, Dry, Average	***1 Serving/125g***	***345***	***3.5***	***276***	***10.6***	***53.0***	***2.8***	***2.1***
Egg & Spinach, M & S*	1 Serving/100g	365	2.7	365	15.5	69.6	2.7	3.0
Fresh, Dry, Average	***1 Serving/75g***	***211***	***2.0***	***281***	***11.4***	***53.3***	***2.6***	***2.6***
Garlic & Herb, Cooked, Sainsbury's*	1oz/28g	41	0.5	147	6.5	26.3	1.8	1.9
Garlic & Herb, Fresh, Tesco*	1 Serving/125g	361	4.6	289	12.0	51.8	3.7	1.5
Garlic & Herb, Fresh, Waitrose*	1 Serving/125g	328	3.1	262	11.8	48.1	2.5	2.1
Garlic & Herbs, Cooked, Pasta Reale*	1 Pack/250g	390	2.8	156	6.2	30.4	1.1	1.0
Garlic Mushroom, BGTY, Sainsbury's*	1 Pack/400g	416	9.2	104	4.7	16.2	2.3	2.0
Garlic Mushroom, Italiano, Tesco*	1 Pack/450g	738	41.0	164	5.2	15.2	9.1	0.6
Ham & Mushroom, Asda*	1 Pack/340g	469	12.9	138	6.0	20.0	3.8	0.2
Ham & Mushroom, BGTY, Sainsbury's*	1 Pack/400g	368	4.8	92	4.2	15.5	1.2	1.1
Ham & Mushroom, Italian, Sainsbury's*	1 Pack/400g	548	19.6	137	5.0	17.5	4.9	1.3
Ham & Mushroom, LC, Tesco*	1 Pack/400g	400	8.8	100	6.0	13.8	2.2	1.8
Multigrain, BGTY, Uncooked, Sainsbury's*	1 Serving/190g	294	4.8	155	7.0	26.0	2.5	3.0
Mushroom, Creamy, Chosen By You, Asda*	1 Pak/400g	428	10.8	107	3.7	16.3	2.7	1.4
Mushroom & Bacon, BGTY, Sainsbury's*	1 Pack/400g	368	9.6	92	4.0	13.5	2.4	1.0
Mushroom & Bacon, Sainsbury's*	1 Pack/450g	585	23.4	130	7.1	13.8	5.2	0.5
Nests, Dry Weight, Napolina*	1oz/28g	93	0.4	332	11.5	68.0	1.5	3.7
Prawn, Eat Smart, Morrisons*	1 Pack/380g	296	6.8	78	6.1	9.4	1.8	0.9
Prawn, Primavera, Sainsbury's*	1 Pack/400g	383	6.1	100	6.1	15.3	1.6	1.4
Salmon, Hot Smoked, HL, Tesco*	1 Packet/400g	420	11.6	105	6.0	12.8	2.9	1.4
Salmon, Perfectly Balanced, Waitrose*	1 Pack/400g	376	10.8	94	5.4	11.7	2.7	0.8
Salmon, Smoked, Ready Meals, M & S*	1 Pack/360g	612	40.3	170	6.2	10.6	11.2	0.9
Salmon & King Prawn, HL, Tesco*	1 Pack/400g	480	9.6	120	6.5	17.2	2.4	1.7
Salmon & Prawn, Perfectly Balanced, Waitrose*	1 Pack/401g	341	13.2	85	6.8	7.1	3.3	1.1
Sun Dried Tomato, Fresh, Morrisons*	1 Pack/250g	748	8.2	299	11.1	56.4	3.3	3.5
Sweet Chilli & Prawn, Tesco*	1 Pack/400g	440	12.4	110	5.5	14.9	3.1	1.3
Tricolore, Waitrose*	½ Pack/125g	351	3.6	281	12.0	51.6	2.9	1.6

	Measure INFO/WEIGHT	per Measure KCAL	FAT	Nutrition Values per 100g / 100ml KCAL	PROT	CARB	FAT	FIBRE
TAGLIATELLE								
Vegetables, Retail	1oz/28g	21	0.8	74	1.6	11.0	3.0	0.7
Verdi, Dry, Barilla*	1 Serving/150g	555	5.2	370	14.0	70.5	3.5	0.0
Verdi, Fresh, Average	***1 Serving/125g***	***171***	***1.8***	***137***	***5.5***	***25.5***	***1.5***	***1.8***
TAHINI PASTE								
Average	***1 Tsp/6g***	***36***	***3.5***	***607***	***18.5***	***0.9***	***58.9***	***8.0***
TAMARIND								
Pulp	***1oz/28g***	***76***	***0.1***	***273***	***3.2***	***64.5***	***0.3***	***0.0***
Whole, Raw, Weighed with Pod, Average	***1oz/28g***	***67***	***0.2***	***239***	***2.8***	***62.5***	***0.6***	***5.1***
TANGERINES								
Fresh, Raw	***1oz/28g***	***10***	***0.0***	***35***	***0.9***	***8.0***	***0.1***	***1.3***
Fresh, Raw, Weighed with Peel, Average	***1 Med/70g***	***18***	***0.1***	***25***	***0.7***	***5.8***	***0.1***	***0.9***
TANGO*								
Cherry, Britvic*	1 Bottle/500ml	55	0.0	11	0.0	2.4	0.0	0.0
Orange, Britvic*	1 Can/330ml	63	0.0	19	0.1	4.4	0.0	0.0
TAPIOCA								
Creamed, Ambrosia*	½ Can/213g	159	3.4	75	2.6	12.6	1.6	0.2
Raw	***1oz/28g***	***101***	***0.0***	***359***	***0.4***	***95.0***	***0.1***	***0.4***
TARAMASALATA								
Average	1 Tbsp/30g	143	14.4	478	4.2	7.9	47.9	1.1
BGTY, Sainsbury's*	1oz/28g	71	5.7	253	4.3	13.5	20.2	0.7
Reduced Fat, Tesco*	½ Pot/85g	256	23.0	301	3.8	10.5	27.1	1.5
Reduced Fat, Waitrose*	1 Pack/170g	522	48.3	307	4.0	8.9	28.4	1.5
Supreme, Waitrose*	1 Serving/20g	84	8.1	421	7.4	6.3	40.7	2.9
TARRAGON								
Dried, Ground	***1 Tsp/2g***	***5***	***0.1***	***295***	***22.8***	***42.8***	***7.2***	***0.0***
Fresh, Average	***1 Tbsp/4g***	***2***	***0.0***	***49***	***3.4***	***6.3***	***1.1***	***0.0***
TART								
Apple, & Custard, Asda*	1 Tart/84g	227	11.0	270	3.1	35.0	13.1	0.1
Apple, & Fresh Cream, Asda*	½ Tart/50g	134	8.0	267	3.4	33.0	16.0	0.8
Apricot, Lattice, Sainsbury's*	1 Slice/125g	321	14.2	257	3.4	35.3	11.4	2.6
Asparagus, Pea & Mint, Frozen, Meat Free, Morrisons*	1 Tart/141g	385	22.8	273	7.3	22.9	16.2	3.3
Aubergine, & Feta, Roast Marinated, Sainsbury's*	1 Serving/105g	227	15.2	216	4.8	16.6	14.5	1.7
Bakewell, Average	1 Tart/50g	228	14.8	456	6.3	43.5	29.7	1.9
Bakewell, Cherry, Morrisons*	1 Tart/46g	198	9.8	430	4.6	54.9	21.4	1.3
Bakewell, Free From, Tesco*	1 Tart/50g	170	4.6	340	1.6	63.0	9.2	4.8
Bakewell, Lemon, Average	1 Tart/46g	206	9.7	447	3.7	60.9	21.1	0.9
Bakewell, Lemon, Holmefield Bakery*	1 Tart/46g	207	11.3	449	4.8	52.9	24.6	0.0
Bakewell, Lyons*	1/6 Tart/52g	205	8.9	397	3.8	56.7	17.2	0.9
Bakewell, Toffee, Morrisons*	1 Tart/47g	201	7.4	422	3.0	67.2	15.5	0.9
Bakewell, Weight Watchers*	1 Tart/43g	156	5.0	363	3.6	65.2	11.7	3.2
Bannoffi, Finest, Tesco*	1/6 Tart/87g	291	16.8	334	3.0	37.2	19.3	0.5
Blackcurrant Sundae, Asda*	1 Tart/55g	227	10.4	413	3.5	57.0	19.0	2.3
Chocolate, Co-Op*	1 Tart/22g	102	6.8	465	4.0	42.0	31.0	0.7
Coconut, & Cherry, Asda*	1 Serving/50g	215	10.0	430	4.4	58.0	20.0	4.0
Coconut, & Raspberry, Waitrose*	1 Tart/48g	204	11.5	426	5.0	45.0	24.0	3.9
Coconut, M & S*	1 Tart/53g	220	9.6	415	5.8	57.8	18.1	3.6
Egg Custard, Individual, Average	1 Tart/94g	260	13.6	277	6.3	32.4	14.5	1.2
Feta Cheese & Spinach, Puff Pastry, Tesco*	1 Tart/108g	306	19.2	283	7.1	23.5	17.8	0.9
Frangipane, Chocolate & William Pear, Waitrose*	1/6 Pack/80g	219	12.4	274	3.5	29.9	15.5	2.5
Frangipane, Lutowska Cherry Amaretto, Sainsbury's*	1 Serving/66g	264	12.9	400	6.0	50.0	19.5	1.3
Frangipane, Spiced Winter Fruit, Rustic Bake, Waitrose*	1 Slice/87g	315	13.6	363	7.2	48.3	15.7	2.1
Gruyere, Pancetta & Balsamic Onion, Finest, Tesco*	¼ Tart/106g	320	21.9	301	7.7	21.3	20.6	3.3
Jam, Assorted, VLH Kitchens	1 Serving/34g	44	42.4	130	3.4	56.0	14.4	1.3

T

	Measure INFO/WEIGHT	per Measure KCAL	FAT	Nutrition Values per 100g / 100ml KCAL	PROT	CARB	FAT	FIBRE
TART								
Jam, Average	1 Slice/90g	342	13.4	380	3.3	62.0	14.9	1.6
Jam, Real Fruit, Mr Kipling*	1 Tart/35g	136	5.2	388	3.8	67.9	14.9	1.7
Leek & Stilton, Morrisons*	1 Serving/125g	392	26.9	314	6.9	23.1	21.5	0.3
Lemon, M & S*	1/6 Tart/50g	208	14.6	415	5.0	32.7	29.3	0.9
Lemon, Sainsbury's*	1/8 Tart/56g	258	15.8	459	4.4	47.0	28.1	0.6
Lemon, Zesty, Tesco*	1/6 Tart/64g	260	15.5	405	5.3	41.0	24.2	0.7
Lemon & Almond, Italian, Sainsbury's*	1 Slice/49g	182	11.6	371	7.4	31.9	23.7	4.1
Lemon & Raspberry, Finest, Tesco*	1 Tart/120g	360	16.8	300	5.2	38.4	14.0	2.9
Lemon Curd, Asda*	1 Tart/30g	121	4.5	402	2.8	64.0	15.0	2.2
Lemon Curd, Lyons*	1 Tart/30g	122	5.1	406	3.7	59.3	17.0	0.0
Manchester, M & S*	1oz/28g	104	6.6	370	4.1	36.0	23.5	1.1
Mince, Gluten & Wheat Free, Florentines, Lovemore*	1 Tart/45g	183	8.3	407	4.5	55.7	18.4	2.5
Mincemeat, Whisky, Glenfiddich, Glenfiddich*	1 Tart/62g	247	9.0	398	3.1	63.1	14.5	1.6
Raspberry & Blueberry, Tesco*	1 Serving/85g	168	7.5	198	2.7	27.0	8.8	2.8
Raspberry Flavoured, Value, Tesco*	1 Tart/29g	113	4.8	389	3.8	56.6	16.4	1.6
Red Pepper, Serrano Ham & Goats Cheese, Waitrose*	1 Serving/100g	293	19.2	293	8.7	21.3	19.2	3.2
Spinach & Ricotta, Individual, TTD, Sainsbury's*	1 Quiche/170g	466	33.7	274	7.5	16.5	19.8	1.4
Strawberry, & Fresh Cream, Finest, Tesco*	1 Tart/129g	350	19.1	271	3.3	31.1	14.8	1.2
Strawberry, Fresh, M & S*	1 Tart/120g	305	18.4	255	3.1	26.4	15.4	2.4
Strawberry, Reduced Sugar, Asda*	1 Tart/37g	141	3.7	380	4.6	67.5	10.1	1.2
Strawberry, Sainsbury's*	1 Serving/206g	521	26.2	253	2.6	32.0	12.7	0.7
Strawberry, Waitrose*	1 Serving/101g	241	12.0	239	3.8	29.2	11.9	1.2
Strawberry Custard, Asda*	1 Tart/100g	335	15.0	335	3.1	47.0	15.0	0.0
Strawberry Sundae, Asda*	1 Tart/46g	187	8.3	407	3.3	58.0	18.0	1.3
Toffee Apple, Co-Op*	1 Tart/20g	69	3.2	345	3.0	47.0	16.0	0.7
Toffee Bakewell, Sainsbury's*	1 Tart/45g	200	8.7	444	3.4	64.2	19.3	1.1
Toffee Pecan, M & S*	1 Tart/91g	414	24.1	455	6.0	48.5	26.5	2.0
Toffee Pecan, Waitrose*	¼ Tart/133g	564	19.1	423	4.3	69.3	14.3	1.6
Tomato, Cherry, & Mascarpone, Asda*	1 Tart/160g	290	18.0	181	4.4	15.6	11.2	1.1
Tomato, Mozzarella & Basil Puff, Sainsbury's*	1/3 Tart/120g	318	25.0	265	9.2	10.2	20.8	0.9
Treacle, & Custard, Apetito*	1 Pack/142g	330	10.2	232	2.0	39.2	7.2	0.8
Treacle, Average	1 Portion/125g	460	17.6	368	3.7	60.4	14.1	1.1
Treacle, Lattice, Lyons*	1/6 Tart/70g	255	8.4	364	4.4	59.3	12.0	1.1
Treacle, with Custard	1 Serving/251g	586	23.5	233	3.1	36.1	9.4	0.8
Treacle Lattice, Mr Kipling*	1/6 Tart/70g	256	8.5	365	4.4	59.8	12.1	1.1
Vegetable, & Feta, Deli, M & S*	½ Tart/115g	315	18.4	274	5.0	20.0	16.0	6.0
Vegetable, Roasted, Finest, Tesco*	¼ Tart/113g	226	13.2	200	3.1	20.6	11.7	2.3
TARTAR								
Cream of, Leavening Agent	***1 Tsp/3g***	***8***	***0.0***	***258***	***0.0***	***61.5***	***0.0***	***0.0***
TARTE								
Au Citron, Frozen, Tesco*	1/6 Tarte/81g	255	11.8	315	5.4	39.4	14.6	0.7
Au Citron, Frozen, TTD, Sainsbury's*	1/6 Tarte/80g	232	13.4	290	4.7	40.7	16.8	7.7
Au Citron, Seriously Lemony, Large, Waitrose*	1 Tarte/470g	1589	81.8	338	4.6	40.8	17.4	0.5
Au Citron, Waitrose*	1 Tarte/100g	325	18.1	325	4.9	35.7	18.1	1.0
Aux Cerises, Finest, Tesco*	1 Serving/98g	219	7.0	225	4.9	35.4	7.2	0.6
Bacon, Leek & Roquefort, Bistro, Waitrose*	¼ Tarte/100g	277	18.2	277	8.4	19.8	18.2	0.6
Normande, French Style, M & S*	1/6 Tarte/85g	245	16.1	290	3.3	26.8	19.0	0.7
Spinach & Goats Cheese, Flamme, TTD, Sainsbury's*	1/3 Quiche/77g	227	16.7	296	6.9	18.1	21.8	5.0
Tatin, Sainsbury's*	1 Serving/120g	244	8.0	203	2.9	32.8	6.7	1.9
TARTLETS								
Asparagus & Leek, Linda McCartney*	1 Tartlet/150g	375	21.8	250	8.4	19.8	14.5	3.4
Butternut Squash & Goats Cheese, Linda McCartney*	1 Tartlet/150g	405	25.0	270	6.3	24.2	16.7	1.2
Cheddar, Vintage, Potato & Leek, Waitrose*	1 Tartlet/130g	391	25.0	301	7.7	23.3	19.2	2.2

	Measure INFO/WEIGHT	per Measure KCAL	per Measure FAT	Nutrition Values per 100g / 100ml KCAL	PROT	CARB	FAT	FIBRE
TARTLETS								
Cheese & Roast Onion, Asda*	1 Tartlet/50g	135	7.5	270	6.0	28.0	15.0	1.9
Mandarin, Mini, M & S*	1 Tartlet/29g	80	4.7	280	3.4	30.4	16.3	0.6
Mushroom & Watercress, Waitrose*	1 Tartlet/120g	308	24.6	257	8.4	19.1	20.5	2.6
Mushroom Medley, BGTY, Sainsbury's*	1 Tartlet/80g	134	8.0	167	4.7	14.5	10.0	3.4
Onion, Caramelised, & Gruyere, Sainsbury's*	1 Tartlet/145g	381	27.6	263	5.8	17.3	19.0	1.3
Raspberry, Mini, M & S*	1 Tartlet/27g	90	5.4	330	4.3	34.4	19.6	0.5
Red Onion & Goats Cheese, Sainsbury's*	1 Tartlet/113g	335	21.8	297	7.0	23.7	19.3	1.5
Red Pepper, Roasted, BGTY, Sainsbury's*	1 Tartlet/80g	143	7.4	179	3.1	21.0	9.2	3.4
Redcurrant & Blackcurrant, Mini, M & S*	1 Tartlet/29g	85	4.9	290	3.9	30.5	16.8	1.1
Salmon & Watercress, Hot Smoked, Waitrose*	1 Tartlet/130g	315	19.9	242	8.1	18.0	15.3	3.0
Sausage & Tomato, Sainsbury's*	1 Tartlet/135g	323	21.3	239	4.8	19.5	15.8	1.6
Spinach, Ricotta & Sun Dried Tomato, Filo, Tesco*	1 Tartlet/135g	358	23.1	265	5.2	22.4	17.1	1.9
Tomato, Cherry, & Aubergine, M & S*	1 Tartlet/160g	320	20.2	200	3.1	17.8	12.6	1.7
Tomato & Goats Cheese, Waitrose*	1 Tartlet/130g	295	19.0	227	6.6	17.4	14.6	2.0
TEA								
Assam, Blended, TTD, Sainsbury's*	1 Serving/2g	0	0.0	0	0.0	0.0	0.0	0.0
Blackberry & Nettle, Twinings*	1 Cup/250ml	5	0.0	2	0.0	0.3	0.0	0.0
Blackcurrant, Fruit Creations, Typhoo*	1 Sm Cup/100ml	5	0.0	5	0.2	0.8	0.0	0.2
Camomile, Pure, Classic Herbal, Twinings*	1 Serving/200ml	4	0.0	2	0.0	0.3	0.0	0.0
Camomile, Smile, Tetley*	1oz/28g	1	0.0	2	0.0	0.5	0.0	0.0
Chai, Twinings*	1 Cup/200ml	2	0.0	1	0.1	0.0	0.0	0.0
Damask, Rose, Chinese, Choi Time*	1 Mug/500ml	0	0.3	0	0.0	0.0	0.1	0.0
Decaf, Tetley*	1 Cup/100ml	1	0.0	1	0.0	0.3	0.0	0.0
Earl Grey, Green, Twinings*	1 Cup/200ml	2	0.0	1	0.0	0.2	0.0	0.0
Earl Grey, Infusion with Water, Average	1 Mug/250ml	2	0.0	1	0.0	0.2	0.0	0.0
Fennel, Sweet, Twinings*	1 fl oz/30ml	1	0.0	2	0.0	0.3	0.0	0.0
Fruit, Twinings*	1 Mug/227ml	4	0.0	2	0.0	0.4	0.0	0.0
Fruit Or Herbal, Made with Water, Twinings*	1 Mug/200ml	8	0.0	4	0.0	1.0	0.0	0.0
Fruits of the Forest, Westminster Tea*	1 Bag/250ml	5	0.0	2	0.0	0.6	0.0	0.0
Ginger, Herbal, Brit & Tang*	1 Tea Bag/2g	5	0.0	278	0.0	55.6	0.0	0.0
Green, Powder, Matcha*	1 Serving/10g	30	0.0	300	0.0	50.0	0.0	30.0
Green, Pure, Twinings*	1 Serving/100g	1	0.0	1	0.0	0.2	0.0	0.0
Green, with Citrus, Twinings*	1 Serving/200ml	2	0.0	1	1.0	0.2	0.0	0.0
Green, with Jasmine, Twinings*	1 Serving/100ml	1	0.0	1	0.0	0.2	0.0	0.0
Green, with Lemon, Jackson's*	1 Serving/200ml	2	0.0	1	0.0	0.2	0.0	0.0
Green, with Mango, Brewed with Water, Twinings*	1 Cup/200ml	2	0.0	1	0.0	0.2	0.0	0.0
Green, with Mint, Whittards of Chelsea*	1 Cup/100ml	1	0.0	1	0.2	0.1	0.0	0.0
Herbal, Wellbeing Blends, Infusions, Twinings*	1 Serving/200ml	4	0.0	2	0.0	0.3	0.0	0.0
Ice, with Lemon, Lipton*	1 Bottle/325ml	91	0.0	28	0.0	6.9	0.0	0.0
Ice, with Mango, Lipton*	1 Bottle/500ml	165	0.0	33	0.0	8.1	0.0	0.0
Ice, with Peach, Lipton*	1 Bottle/500ml	140	0.0	28	0.0	6.8	0.0	0.0
Iced, Green, Orange, Lipton*	1 Bottle/500ml	100	0.0	20	0.0	5.0	0.0	0.0
Iced, Lemon, San Benedetto*	1 Bottle/500ml	170	0.0	34	0.1	8.3	0.0	0.0
Iced, Peach, Twinings*	1 Serving/200ml	60	0.2	30	0.1	7.3	0.1	0.0
Jasmine, Twinings*	1 fl oz/30ml	0	0.0	1	0.0	0.2	0.0	0.0
Lemon, Instant, Original, Lift*	1 Serving/15g	53	0.0	352	0.0	87.0	0.0	0.0
Lemon, Instant, Tesco*	1 Serving/7g	23	0.0	326	1.0	80.5	0.0	0.0
Lemon & Limeflower, Infused, M & S*	1 Bottle/330ml	99	0.0	30	0.0	7.8	0.0	0.0
Made with Water	1 Mug/227ml	0	0.0	0	0.1	0.0	0.0	0.0
Made with Water, with Semi-Skimmed Milk, Average	1 Cup/200ml	14	0.4	7	0.5	0.7	0.2	0.0
Made with Water, with Skimmed Milk, Average	1 Mug/270ml	16	0.5	6	0.5	0.7	0.2	0.0
Made with Water, with Whole Milk, Average	1 Cup/200ml	16	0.8	8	0.4	0.5	0.4	0.0
Morning Detox, Twinings*	1 Serving/200ml	5	0.0	2	0.0	0.3	0.0	0.0

T

	Measure INFO/WEIGHT	per Measure KCAL	per Measure FAT	KCAL	PROT	CARB	FAT	FIBRE
				Nutrition Values per 100g / 100ml				
TEA								
Nettle & Peppermint, Twinings*	1 Cup/200ml	2	0.0	1	0.0	0.2	0.0	0.0
Nettle & Sweet Fennel, Twinings*	1 Cup/200ml	4	0.0	2	0.0	0.3	0.0	0.0
Peach Flavour, Lift*	1 Cup/15g	58	0.0	384	0.3	95.6	0.0	0.0
Peppermint, Made with Water, Average	1 Serving/200ml	3	0.0	2	0.0	0.2	0.0	0.0
Raspberry & Cranberry, T of Life, Tetley*	1 Serving/100ml	36	0.0	36	0.0	9.0	0.0	0.0
Red Bush, Made with Water, Tetley*	1 Mug/250ml	2	0.0	1	0.0	0.1	0.0	0.0
TEACAKES								
Caramel, Highlights, Mallows, Cadbury*	1 Teacake/15g	61	1.9	408	6.2	69.1	12.4	3.6
Fruit, Average	1 Teacake/60g	178	4.5	296	8.0	52.5	7.5	0.0
Fruity, Warburton's*	1 Teacake/63g	160	2.2	256	8.7	48.0	3.5	2.7
G H Sheldon*	1 Teacake/95g	274	2.6	288	8.5	57.4	2.7	0.0
Hovis*	1 Teacake/60g	155	1.5	258	9.0	49.9	2.5	3.0
Jam, Castello*	1 Teacake/13g	60	2.4	470	5.3	70.1	18.4	1.3
Large, Sainsbury's*	1 Teacake/100g	291	6.8	291	8.3	49.1	6.8	3.4
Large, TTD, Sainsbury's*	1 Teacake/90g	264	3.5	293	7.5	57.0	3.9	2.6
Lees*	1 Teacake/19g	81	2.9	426	4.2	67.7	15.4	0.0
Mallow, Tesco*	1 Teacake/14g	63	2.7	450	4.1	65.4	19.1	1.0
Mallow, Value, Tesco*	1 Teacake/14g	60	2.3	425	3.6	65.8	16.2	1.4
Marshmallow, Milk Chocolate, Tunnock's*	1 Teacake/24g	106	4.6	440	4.9	61.9	19.2	2.4
Mini Bites, M & S*	1 Bite/6g	29	1.2	484	3.2	72.6	20.3	2.1
Toasted, Average	1 Teacake/60g	197	5.0	329	8.9	58.3	8.3	0.0
Value, Tesco*	1 Teacake/68g	180	2.4	265	9.6	47.8	3.6	4.9
with Orange Filling, M & S*	1 Teacake/20g	80	2.8	410	4.5	66.6	14.2	0.9
TEMPEH								
Average	***1oz/28g***	***46***	***1.8***	***166***	***20.7***	***6.4***	***6.4***	***4.3***
TEQUILA								
Average	***1 Shot/35ml***	***78***	***0.0***	***224***	***0.0***	***0.0***	***0.0***	***0.0***
THYME								
Dried, Ground, Average	***1 Tsp/1g***	***3***	***0.1***	***276***	***9.1***	***45.3***	***7.4***	***0.0***
Fresh, Average	***1 Tsp/1g***	***1***	***0.0***	***95***	***3.0***	***15.1***	***2.5***	***0.0***
TIA MARIA								
Original	***1 Shot/35ml***	***105***	***0.0***	***300***	***0.0***	***0.0***	***0.0***	***0.0***
TIC TAC								
Extra Strong Mint, Ferrero*	2 Tic Tacs/1g	4	0.0	381	0.0	95.2	0.0	0.0
Fresh Mint, Ferrero*	2 Tic Tacs/1g	4	0.0	390	0.0	97.5	0.0	0.0
Lime & Orange, Ferrero*	2 Tic Tacs/1g	4	0.0	386	0.0	95.5	0.0	0.0
Orange, Ferrero*	2 Tic Tacs/1g	4	0.0	385	0.0	95.5	0.0	0.0
Spearmint, Ferrero*	1 Box/16g	62	0.0	390	0.0	97.5	0.0	0.0
TIKKA MASALA								
Chicken, & Pilau Rice, Asda*	1 Pack/400g	608	19.6	152	7.0	20.0	4.9	1.5
Chicken, & Pilau Rice, BGTY, Sainsbury's*	1 Pack/400g	380	4.8	95	8.1	13.0	1.2	1.1
Chicken, & Pilau Rice, Takeaway, Asda*	1 Pack/561g	852	27.5	152	7.0	20.0	4.9	1.5
Chicken, & Pilau Rice, Waitrose*	1 Pack/500g	797	34.5	159	8.2	16.1	6.9	0.8
Chicken, & Rice, 231, Oakhouse Foods Ltd*	1 Meal/400g	528	18.0	132	5.5	17.2	4.5	0.6
Chicken, & Rice, LC, Tesco*	1 Pack/450g	472	7.2	105	7.9	14.6	1.6	1.3
Chicken, & Rice, M & S*	1 Pack/400g	700	35.2	175	7.4	17.0	8.8	1.0
Chicken, Asda*	1 Pack/340g	388	20.4	114	9.0	6.0	6.0	1.5
Chicken, Birds Eye*	1 Serving/400g	420	7.2	105	5.6	16.6	1.8	0.3
Chicken, Boiled Rice & Naan, Meal for One, GFY, Asda*	1 Pack/605g	823	18.8	136	6.0	21.0	3.1	0.0
Chicken, Breast, GFY, Asda*	1 Pack/380g	486	14.4	128	19.0	4.5	3.8	0.2
Chicken, Canned, Chosen By You, Asda*	½ Can/200g	222	10.6	111	10.9	4.0	5.3	1.7
Chicken, COU, M & S*	1 Pack/400g	400	6.8	100	7.6	14.1	1.7	1.3
Chicken, Healthy Choice, Iceland*	1 Pack/399g	431	4.4	108	6.5	18.0	1.1	0.9

T

	Measure INFO/WEIGHT	per Measure KCAL	FAT	Nutrition Values per 100g / 100ml KCAL	PROT	CARB	FAT	FIBRE
TIKKA MASALA								
Chicken, Hot, Sainsbury's*	1 Pack/400g	604	37.2	151	13.2	3.6	9.3	1.5
Chicken, Hot, Tesco*	1 Pack/400g	588	34.4	147	8.7	8.6	8.6	1.0
Chicken, Indian, Medium, Sainsbury's*	1 Pack/400g	848	61.2	212	13.2	5.3	15.3	0.1
Chicken, Indian, Takeaway, Chosen By You, Asda*	½ Pack/225g	256	11.0	114	8.6	8.3	4.9	1.2
Chicken, Indian, Tesco*	1 Pack/350g	560	32.6	160	11.6	7.2	9.3	0.6
Chicken, Indian Meal for One, BGTY, Sainsbury's*	1 Serving/241g	200	1.9	83	13.9	5.1	0.8	1.0
Chicken, Large, Sainsbury's*	1 Pack/650g	1105	68.9	170	11.7	7.0	10.6	0.3
Chicken, Low Fat, Iceland*	1 Pack/400g	360	4.0	90	7.8	12.5	1.0	0.5
Chicken, M & S*	½ Pack/175g	245	13.0	140	12.5	5.6	7.4	1.6
Chicken, Medium Spiced, without Rice, Tesco*	½ Pack/175g	231	13.1	132	10.2	5.9	7.5	0.9
Chicken, Microwave Meal, Good Choice, Iceland*	1 Pack/400g	488	6.0	122	6.6	20.4	1.5	0.6
Chicken, Mild, Diet Chef Ltd*	1 Pack/300g	291	6.6	97	10.4	9.0	2.2	0.6
Chicken, Rice Bowl, Uncle Ben's*	1 Pack/350g	382	8.4	109	5.9	15.9	2.4	0.0
Chicken, Sharwood's*	1 Pack/375g	562	25.1	150	7.2	15.1	6.7	0.8
Chicken, Smart Price, Asda*	1 Pack/300g	414	18.0	138	13.0	8.0	6.0	1.6
Chicken, The Authentic Food Company*	1 Serving/375g	510	31.5	136	10.6	5.5	8.4	0.9
Chicken, Tinned, M & S*	½ Can/213g	309	18.1	145	14.5	2.9	8.5	2.2
Chicken, Waitrose*	½ Pack/200g	298	19.4	149	12.8	2.6	9.7	1.6
Chicken, Weight Watchers*	1 Pack/331g	344	4.6	104	7.0	15.8	1.4	0.2
HE, Tesco*	1 Serving/220g	191	10.3	87	1.0	10.2	4.7	0.5
King Prawn & Rice, Finest, Tesco*	1 Pack/475g	618	30.4	130	6.0	16.6	6.4	1.2
Prawn, COU, M & S*	1 Pack/400g	400	6.4	100	6.9	14.7	1.6	1.9
Prawn, King, Perfectly Balanced, Waitrose*	1 Pack/400g	372	3.6	93	5.2	16.0	0.9	1.7
Spicy, with Long Grain Rice, Rice Time, Uncle Ben's*	1 Tub/300g	399	11.7	133	2.3	21.7	3.9	0.9
Vegetable, Aldi*	1 Can/400g	496	33.6	124	1.9	10.3	8.4	1.4
Vegetable, Asda*	1 Pack/340g	316	20.7	93	2.0	7.4	6.1	1.1
Vegetable, Canned, Waitrose*	1 Can/200g	152	4.4	76	3.6	10.5	2.2	0.0
Vegetable, Indian, Tesco*	1 Pack/225g	234	13.5	104	2.4	10.4	6.0	2.4
Vegetable, Waitrose*	1 Serving/196g	149	4.3	76	3.6	10.5	2.2	3.8
Vegetable, with Rice, Tesco*	1 Pack/450g	500	19.4	111	2.6	15.5	4.3	0.9
Vegetarian, with Pilau Rice, Tesco*	1 Serving/440g	519	17.2	118	5.0	15.6	3.9	1.5
TILAPIA								
Raw, Average	***1 Serving/100g***	***95***	***1.0***	***95***	***20.0***	***0.0***	***1.0***	***0.0***
TIME OUT								
Break Pack, Cadbury*	1 Serving/20g	108	6.3	530	6.2	58.3	30.7	0.0
Chocolate Fingers, Cadbury*	2 Fingers/35g	186	10.6	530	7.1	57.3	30.3	1.1
Orange, Snack Size, Cadbury*	1 Finger/11g	61	3.6	555	5.0	59.4	32.9	0.0
TIRAMISU								
Asda*	1 Pot/100g	252	11.0	252	4.3	34.0	11.0	0.5
BGTY, Sainsbury's*	1 Pot/90g	140	2.4	156	4.5	28.3	2.7	0.3
Choc & Mascarpone, Tiramigu, Gu*	1 Pud/90g	316	23.3	351	3.3	26.1	25.9	1.0
COU, M & S*	1 Tub/95g	138	2.6	145	3.7	26.9	2.7	0.6
Dine in Dessert, M & S*	½ Dessert/145g	515	36.7	355	2.6	28.8	25.3	0.7
Family Size, Tesco*	1 Serving/125g	356	18.1	285	4.3	34.5	14.5	4.3
Italian, Co-Op*	1 Pack/90g	230	9.0	255	5.0	37.0	10.0	0.4
LC, Tesco*	1 Pot/90g	162	3.5	180	7.7	27.6	3.9	2.4
Morrisons*	1 Pot/90g	248	9.9	276	4.0	38.0	11.0	0.0
Raspberry, M & S*	1 Serving/84g	197	12.1	235	3.8	22.9	14.4	0.2
Sainsbury's*	1 Serving/100g	263	10.0	263	4.4	40.2	10.0	0.1
Single Size, Tesco*	1 Pot/100g	290	12.9	290	3.8	35.1	12.9	4.5
Trifle, Sainsbury's*	1 Serving/100g	243	15.7	243	2.3	23.2	15.7	0.6
Waitrose*	1 Pot/90g	221	11.2	246	6.4	27.2	12.4	0.0

T

	Measure INFO/WEIGHT	per Measure KCAL	FAT	Nutrition Values per 100g / 100ml KCAL	PROT	CARB	FAT	FIBRE
TOAD IN THE HOLE								
& Potatoes, M & S*	1 Serving/100g	200	12.9	200	6.4	14.6	12.9	0.9
Average	1 Serving/231g	640	40.2	277	11.9	19.5	17.4	1.1
Frozen, Cooked, Chosen By You, Asda*	1 Slice/72g	168	7.5	232	9.2	24.2	10.4	2.6
Large, Great Value, Asda*	¼ Pack/81g	238	13.8	293	10.0	25.0	17.0	2.3
Vegetarian, Aunt Bessie's*	1 Pack/190g	502	19.4	264	15.6	27.5	10.2	2.7
Vegetarian, Linda McCartney*	1 Pack/190g	359	16.7	189	13.6	13.9	8.8	1.1
Vegetarian, Meat Free, Asda*	1 Serving/173g	407	19.0	235	9.0	25.0	11.0	3.1
Vegetarian, Tesco*	1 Pack/190g	471	19.0	248	13.1	26.5	10.0	2.8
Vegetarian, Tryton Foods*	1oz/28g	73	4.0	262	14.8	18.6	14.2	1.6
TOASTIE								
All Day Breakfast, M & S*	1 Serving/174g	375	13.8	215	11.2	25.0	7.9	1.7
Cheese & Ham, Tayto*	1 Serving/50g	260	14.8	519	6.8	58.0	29.7	0.0
Cheese & Onion, Ginsters*	1 Toastie/122g	330	12.3	269	10.9	33.1	10.0	1.5
Cheese & Pickle, M & S*	1 Toastie/136g	320	9.1	235	10.4	33.5	6.7	2.6
Ham & Cheddar, British, M & S*	1 Pack/128g	269	8.6	210	15.5	22.3	6.7	1.3
Ham & Cheese, Ginsters*	1 Toastie/129g	308	11.9	239	12.4	26.0	9.2	1.3
Ham & Cheese, Tesco*	1 Serving/138g	388	18.2	281	11.5	29.1	13.2	1.0
Ham & Cheese, White Bread	1 Toastie/150g	409	14.9	273	14.5	31.3	9.9	0.9
TOFFEE APPLE								
Average	1 Apple/141g	188	3.0	133	1.2	29.2	2.1	2.3
TOFFEE CRISP								
Biscuit, Nestle*	1 Original/44g	228	12.1	519	3.7	62.8	27.6	1.4
Bitesize, Nestle*	1 Serving/20g	101	5.4	518	3.8	63.0	27.6	1.3
TOFFEES								
Assorted, Bassett's*	1 Toffee/8g	35	1.1	434	3.8	73.1	14.0	0.0
Assorted, Sainsbury's*	1 Sweet/8g	37	1.3	457	2.2	76.5	15.8	0.2
Brazil Nut, Diabetic, Thorntons*	1 Serving/20g	93	7.0	467	3.2	49.0	35.1	0.5
Butter, Smart Price, Asda*	1 Toffee/8g	37	1.3	440	1.3	75.0	15.0	0.0
Butter Candies, Sugar Free, Hard, Original, Werther's*	1 Pack/80g	231	7.0	289	0.2	86.8	8.8	0.1
Chewy, Werther's*	1 Toffee/5g	22	0.8	436	3.5	71.3	15.2	0.1
Chocolate, Milk, Covered, Thorntons*	1 Bag/215g	1120	66.0	521	4.1	57.2	30.7	0.9
Chocolate, Milk, Smothered, Thorntons*	1 Pack/125g	655	38.5	524	4.3	57.5	30.8	1.1
Dairy, Smart Price, Asda*	1 Sweet/9g	37	1.3	407	1.3	68.4	14.2	0.0
Dairy, Waitrose*	1 Toffee/8g	37	1.1	458	2.0	80.2	14.3	0.5
Devon Butter, Thorntons*	1 Sweet/9g	40	1.5	444	1.7	72.2	16.7	0.0
English Butter, Co-Op*	1 Toffee/8g	38	1.6	470	2.0	71.0	20.0	0.0
Liquorice, Thorntons*	1 Bag/100g	506	29.4	506	1.9	58.8	29.4	0.0
Mixed, Average	1oz/28g	119	5.2	426	2.2	66.7	18.6	0.0
No Added Sugar, Boots*	1 Serving/7g	23	1.0	324	1.3	52.0	14.0	0.0
Original, Thorntons*	1 Bag/100g	514	30.1	514	1.8	59.3	30.1	0.0
Squares, No Added Sugar, Russell Stover*	1 Piece/15g	57	3.9	380	6.0	49.3	26.0	1.3
TOFU								
Average	***1 Pack/250g***	***297***	***16.5***	***119***	***13.4***	***1.4***	***6.6***	***0.1***
Beech Smoked, Organic, Cauldron Foods*	½ Pack/110g	124	7.8	113	10.9	1.0	7.1	0.5
Firm, Silken Style, Blue Dragon*	1 Pack/216g	134	5.8	62	6.9	2.4	2.7	0.0
Fresh, Drained, Kong Nam*	1 Tub/575g	397	21.3	69	7.7	1.3	3.7	0.5
Fried, Average	***1oz/28g***	***75***	***4.0***	***268***	***28.6***	***9.3***	***14.1***	***0.0***
Marinated, Pieces, Organic, Cauldron Foods*	1 Pack/160g	363	27.2	227	17.5	1.0	17.0	2.7
Original, Organic, Cauldron Foods*	¼ Pack/99g	84	4.2	85	10.0	1.9	4.2	0.9
Smoked, Organic, Evernat*	1oz/28g	36	1.8	127	16.3	0.8	6.6	0.0
Traditional Luncheon, Bean Supreme*	1 Serving/100g	210	13.1	210	23.4	7.8	13.1	0.0
TOMATILLOS								
Raw	***1 Med/34g***	***11***	***0.3***	***32***	***1.0***	***5.8***	***1.0***	***1.9***

	Measure INFO/WEIGHT	per Measure KCAL	FAT	Nutrition Values per 100g / 100ml KCAL	PROT	CARB	FAT	FIBRE
TOMATO PASTE								
Average	***1 Tbsp/20g***	***19***	***0.0***	***96***	***5.0***	***19.2***	***0.2***	***1.5***
Sun Dried, Average	***1 Heap Tsp/10g***	***38***	***3.5***	***385***	***3.2***	***13.8***	***35.2***	***0.0***
TOMATO PUREE								
Average	***1 Tsp/5g***	***4***	***0.0***	***76***	***4.5***	***14.1***	***0.2***	***2.3***
Double Concentrate, Average	1 Tbsp/15g	13	0.0	85	4.9	14.9	0.2	3.6
Sun Dried, & Olive Oil & Herbs, GIA*	1 Serving/20g	41	4.3	204	2.6	0.5	21.6	0.0
TOMATOES								
Cherry, Average	***1 Tomato/15g***	***3***	***0.0***	***18***	***0.7***	***3.0***	***0.3***	***0.5***
Cherry, Canned, TTD, Sainsbury's*	½ Can/204g	47	0.4	23	1.4	4.0	0.2	0.9
Cherry, on the Vine, Average	***1 Serving/80g***	***15***	***0.3***	***18***	***0.7***	***3.1***	***0.3***	***1.2***
Cherry, Tinned, Napolina*	1 Can/400g	92	2.4	23	1.2	3.3	0.6	0.0
Chopped, Canned, Average	1 Serving/100g	19	0.2	19	1.1	3.3	0.2	0.9
Chopped, Canned, Branded Average	***1 Serving/130g***	***27***	***0.2***	***21***	***1.1***	***3.8***	***0.1***	***0.8***
Chopped, Italian, Average	***½ Can/200g***	***47***	***0.2***	***23***	***1.3***	***4.4***	***0.1***	***0.9***
Chopped, Italian, with Olive Oil & Garlic, Waitrose*	1 Serving/100g	33	1.6	33	1.1	3.6	1.6	0.0
Chopped, Italian, with Olives, Waitrose*	1 Can/400g	184	7.2	46	1.4	6.0	1.8	0.8
Chopped, with Chilli, Sainsbury's*	½ Can/200g	44	1.0	22	1.0	3.5	0.5	0.9
Chopped, with Garlic, Average	***½ Can/200g***	***43***	***0.3***	***21***	***1.2***	***3.8***	***0.1***	***0.8***
Chopped, with Herbs, Average	***½ Can/200g***	***42***	***0.3***	***21***	***1.1***	***3.8***	***0.1***	***0.8***
Chopped, with Olive Oil & Roasted Garlic, Sainsbury's*	1 Pack/390g	187	8.2	48	1.3	5.9	2.1	1.0
Chopped, with Onion & Herbs, Napolina*	1 Can/400g	84	0.4	21	1.0	4.0	0.1	0.4
Chopped, with Onions, Italian, Tesco*	½ Can/200g	46	0.4	23	1.4	4.0	0.2	0.9
Chopped, with Peppers & Onions, Sainsbury's*	½ Can/200g	40	0.2	20	1.2	3.5	0.1	0.9
Creamed, Sainsbury's*	1oz/28g	6	0.0	22	1.5	5.0	0.1	1.6
Diced, Freshly Frozen, Tesco*	1 Serving/80g	14	0.2	18	0.7	3.1	0.3	1.0
Fresh, Raw, Average	***1 Medium/123g***	***22***	***0.2***	***18***	***0.9***	***3.9***	***0.2***	***1.2***
Fried in Blended Oil	1 Med/85g	77	6.5	91	0.7	5.0	7.7	1.3
Green Tiger, Raw, M & S*	1 Serving/80g	16	0.2	20	0.7	3.1	0.3	1.0
Grilled, Average	1oz/28g	6	0.1	20	0.8	3.5	0.3	1.5
Plum, Baby, Average	***1 Serving/50g***	***9***	***0.2***	***18***	***1.5***	***2.3***	***0.3***	***1.0***
Plum, in Tomato Juice, Average	***1 Can/400g***	***71***	***0.4***	***18***	***1.0***	***3.3***	***0.1***	***0.7***
Plum, in Tomato Juice, Premium, Average	***1 Can/400g***	***93***	***1.2***	***23***	***1.3***	***3.8***	***0.3***	***0.7***
Pomodorino, TTD, Sainsbury's*	1 Tomato/8g	1	0.0	17	0.7	3.1	0.4	1.3
Puglian, Sun Drenched, Waitrose*	½ Pack/100g	190	16.2	190	2.2	8.8	16.2	3.8
Ripened on the Vine, Average	***1 Medium/123g***	***22***	***0.4***	***18***	***0.7***	***3.1***	***0.3***	***0.7***
San Marzano, TTD, Sainsbury's*	½ Can/200g	34	0.2	17	0.9	3.1	0.1	2.9
Santini, M & S*	1 Serving/80g	16	0.2	20	0.7	3.1	0.3	1.0
Stuffed, with Rice Based Filling, Average	1oz/28g	59	3.8	212	2.1	22.2	13.4	1.1
Sun Dried, Average	***3 Pieces/20g***	***43***	***3.2***	***214***	***4.7***	***13.0***	***15.9***	***3.3***
Sun Dried, Cooks Ingredients, Waitrose*	4 Pieces/15g	26	0.1	175	7.3	35.2	0.4	13.9
Sun Dried, in Oil, GIA*	1 Serving/10g	15	1.4	153	1.9	7.5	13.9	0.0
Sun Dried, in Olive Oil, M & S*	1 Jar/280g	644	57.1	230	3.9	7.9	20.4	6.7
Sun Dried, in Sunflower Oil, Deli Express, Asda*	1 Serving/50g	76	3.0	153	5.8	15.9	6.0	9.0
Sun Dried, in Vegetable Oil, Aldi*	1 Serving/50g	76	3.0	153	5.8	15.9	6.0	9.0
Sun Dried, Italian, Merchant Gourmet*	1 Serving/50g	56	0.4	111	5.7	20.4	0.7	1.3
Sun Dried, Moist, Waitrose*	1 Serving/25g	44	0.5	175	11.8	27.4	2.0	7.2
Sun Dried, with Herbs & Extra Virgin Olive Oil, Waitrose*	1 Serving/50g	72	5.2	145	3.4	9.1	10.5	7.1
Sun Dried in Oil	1 serving/10g	30.1	2.5	301	5.8	13.5	24.8	7.0
Sunblush, TTD, Sainsbury's*	¼ Pack/30g	42	3.2	140	2.4	8.8	10.6	5.8
Sweet, Aromatico, Extra Special, Extra Special, Asda*	1 Serving/100g	21	0.5	21	0.7	3.1	0.5	1.3
TONGUE								
Lunch, Average	***1oz/28g***	***51***	***3.0***	***181***	***20.1***	***1.8***	***10.6***	***0.0***
Ox from Deli Counter, Sainsbury's*	1 Serving/100g	195	13.3	195	18.3	0.5	13.3	0.1

T

	Measure INFO/WEIGHT	per Measure KCAL	FAT	Nutrition Values per 100g / 100ml KCAL	PROT	CARB	FAT	FIBRE
TONGUE								
Slices, Average	***1oz/28g***	***56***	***3.9***	***201***	***18.7***	***0.0***	***14.0***	***0.0***
TONIC WATER								
Average	1 Glass/250ml	82	0.0	33	0.0	8.8	0.0	0.0
Diet, Asda*	1 Glass/200ml	2	0.0	1	0.0	0.0	0.0	0.0
Indian, Britvic*	1 Mini Can/150ml	39	0.2	26	0.1	6.2	0.1	0.1
Indian, Diet, Schweppes*	1 Glass/100ml	1	0.0	1	0.0	0.0	0.0	0.0
Indian, Fever Tree*	1 Bottle/200ml	76	0.0	38	0.0	9.0	0.0	0.0
Indian, Schweppes*	1 Serving/500ml	110	0.0	22	0.0	5.1	0.0	0.0
Indian, Slimline, Schweppes*	1 Serving/188ml	3	0.0	2	0.4	0.0	0.0	0.0
Indian, Sugar Free, Essential, Waitrose*	1 Serving/50ml	1	0.0	2	0.0	0.0	0.0	0.0
Indian, with a Hint of Lemon, Low Calorie, Asda*	1 Serving/300ml	3	0.3	1	0.0	0.0	0.1	0.0
Indian with Lime, Low Calorie, Tesco*	1 Glass/250ml	5	0.0	2	0.0	0.0	0.0	0.0
Light, Royal Club*	1 Glass/250ml	2	0.0	1	0.0	0.0	0.0	0.0
Low Calorie, Indian, Co-Op*	1 Serving/100ml	2	0.0	2	0.0	0.0	0.0	0.0
Low Calorie, Tesco*	1 Serving/200ml	4	0.0	2	0.0	0.5	0.0	0.0
Quinine, Schweppes*	1 Glass/125ml	46	0.0	37	0.0	9.0	0.0	0.0
Soda Stream*	1 Glass/100ml	15	0.0	15	0.0	3.2	0.0	0.0
TONIC WINE								
Original, Sanatogen*	1 Bottle/700ml	889	0.0	127	0.0	124.4	0.0	0.0
TOPIC								
Mars*	1 Bar/47g	234	12.3	498	6.2	59.6	26.2	1.7
TORTE								
Chocolate, & Pecan Brownie, Gu*	1/6 Torte/67g	292	17.7	436	5.3	45.1	26.4	3.1
Chocolate, Half Fat, Waitrose*	1/6 Torte/70g	135	4.1	193	5.4	29.7	5.8	2.2
Chocolate, Mint, Weight Watchers*	1 Pot/88g	174	4.1	198	4.7	34.3	4.7	5.2
Chocolate, Orange & Almond, Gu*	1 Serving/65g	273	19.8	420	5.0	28.2	30.5	2.7
Chocolate, Tesco*	1 Serving/50g	126	6.0	251	3.6	32.3	11.9	1.0
Chocolate Fondant, Gu*	1/8 Torte/63g	264	18.9	423	5.7	32.0	30.2	1.8
Chocolate Truffle, Waitrose*	1 Serving/116g	359	20.1	309	4.6	30.1	17.3	1.4
Lemon, Farmfoods*	1/6 Torte/70g	136	7.0	195	4.3	21.9	10.0	0.5
Lemon, Tesco*	1 Serving/62g	142	6.1	230	2.3	32.9	9.9	0.5
Lemon & Mango, Waitrose*	1 Serving/80g	142	2.4	177	3.9	33.6	3.0	0.6
Raspberry, BGTY, Sainsbury's*	1 Serving/100g	154	3.9	154	2.6	27.0	3.9	1.2
TORTELLINI								
3 Cheese, Sainsbury's*	1 Serving/50g	196	4.4	391	14.4	63.8	8.7	3.0
Aubergine & Pecorino, Sainsbury's*	½ Pack/150g	354	6.4	236	8.9	40.3	4.3	3.2
Beef & Red Wine, Italian, Asda*	½ Pack/150g	242	4.2	161	9.0	25.0	2.8	0.0
Beef Bolognese, Rich, Italian, Giovanni Rana*	½ Pack/125g	222	9.0	178	7.6	20.6	7.2	4.1
Cheese, Fresh, Sainsbury's*	½ Pack/180g	329	9.0	183	7.6	26.8	5.0	1.7
Cheese, Tomato & Basil, Cooked, Tesco*	1 Serving/270g	551	15.1	204	6.7	30.5	5.6	2.5
Cheese, Weight Watchers*	1 Can/395g	245	6.3	62	2.3	9.7	1.6	0.4
Cheese & Ham, Italiano, Tesco*	½ Pack/150g	396	12.3	264	12.8	34.8	8.2	3.0
Chicken, Spicy, Big Eat, Heinz*	1 Pot/350g	404	23.1	115	2.9	11.2	6.6	0.4
Four Cheese, Tesco*	½ Pack/150g	405	11.8	270	12.3	37.3	7.9	3.4
Four Cheese, with Tomato & Basil Sauce, Tesco*	1 Pack/400g	500	14.8	125	6.1	16.9	3.7	0.6
Four Cheese & Tomato, Italian, Asda*	1 Serving/150g	249	5.7	166	8.0	25.0	3.8	0.0
Garlic, Basil & Ricotta, Asda*	½ Pack/175g	318	10.5	182	6.0	26.0	6.0	2.6
Garlic & Herb, Fresh, Sainsbury's*	½ Pack/150g	364	11.7	243	11.1	32.2	7.8	1.8
Ham & Cheese, Fresh, Asda*	½ Pack/150g	255	9.0	170	6.0	23.0	6.0	1.7
Ham & Cheese, Tesco*	1 Serving/225g	578	12.6	257	13.5	38.1	5.6	1.8
Italian, Diet Chef Ltd*	1 Pack/300g	234	1.5	78	2.3	16.0	0.5	0.2
Meat, Italian, Tesco*	1 Serving/125g	332	9.5	266	10.6	38.9	7.6	2.3
Mozzarella & Tomato, Fresh, Asda*	1oz/28g	46	1.1	166	8.0	25.0	3.8	0.0

T

	Measure INFO/WEIGHT	per Measure KCAL	FAT	Nutrition Values per 100g / 100ml KCAL	PROT	CARB	FAT	FIBRE
TORTELLINI								
Mushroom, Asda*	1 Serving/125g	218	5.2	174	6.0	28.0	4.2	2.3
Mushroom, BGTY, Sainsbury's*	½ Can/200g	180	6.2	90	2.2	13.2	3.1	0.7
Pepperoni, Italian, Asda*	½ Pack/150g	250	6.0	167	6.7	26.0	4.0	0.0
Pepperoni, Spicy, Asda*	½ Pack/150g	252	6.0	168	7.0	26.0	4.0	0.0
Pepperoni, Spicy, Fresh, Asda*	½ Pack/150g	249	6.0	166	7.0	26.0	4.0	0.0
Pesto & Goats Cheese, Fresh, Sainsbury's*	½ Pack/150g	310	12.2	207	8.9	24.6	8.1	2.6
Pork & Beef, BGTY, Sainsbury's*	½ Can/200g	148	3.0	74	3.7	11.2	1.5	0.6
Ricotta & Spinach, Giovanni Rana*	½ Pack/125g	319	10.0	255	9.0	35.5	8.0	10.0
Sausage & Ham, Italiano, Tesco*	1 Pack/300g	816	27.9	272	13.1	34.0	9.3	3.7
Spinach & Ricotta, Italian, Asda*	½ Pack/150g	189	3.6	126	5.0	21.0	2.4	0.6
Spinach & Ricotta, Pasta Reale*	½ Pack/125g	319	5.2	255	11.2	45.5	4.2	2.6
Spinach & Ricotta, Verdi, Asda*	1 Serving/125g	186	5.6	149	6.0	21.0	4.5	2.4
Tomato & Mozzarella, Fresh, Asda*	½ Pack/150g	236	4.2	157	8.0	25.0	2.8	0.0
Tomato & Mozzarella, Fresh, Sainsbury's*	½ Pack/150g	291	12.0	194	7.5	23.0	8.0	3.4
TORTELLONI								
Arrabbiata, Sainsbury's*	½ Pack/210g	407	11.8	194	7.1	28.8	5.6	2.6
Basil, Mozzarella & Tomato, Weight Watchers*	½ Pack/125g	278	3.4	222	9.0	40.5	2.7	4.8
Beef & Chianti, TTD, Sainsbury's*	½ Pack/125g	300	8.0	240	11.3	34.3	6.4	1.9
Beef & Pancetta, Aberdeen Angus, Grandi, Budgens*	½ Pack/125g	314	5.4	251	12.4	40.5	4.3	2.9
Cheese, Garlic & Herb, Co-Op*	1 Serving/125g	331	7.5	265	10.0	43.0	6.0	0.0
Cheese, Garlic & Herb, Fresh, Budgens*	½ Pack/125g	334	7.5	267	10.3	46.1	6.0	3.3
Cheese, Tomato, & Basil, Sainsbury's*	½ Pack/150g	272	9.8	181	8.0	22.7	6.5	1.7
Cheese & Ham, Fresh, Budgens*	1 Serving/100g	268	6.5	268	12.6	42.0	6.5	2.2
Cheese & Smoked Ham, Waitrose*	1 Serving/250g	625	17.0	250	11.5	35.8	6.8	1.8
Chicken & Bacon, As Consumed, Italiano, Tesco*	½ Pack/280g	567	14.0	202	6.8	30.7	5.0	3.7
Chicken & Ham, Morrisons*	1 Serving/150g	366	5.8	244	12.3	38.6	3.9	2.4
Chorizo & Tomato, Morrisons*	1 Serving/150g	447	12.9	298	12.8	45.1	8.6	2.6
Five Cheese, Sainsbury's*	1 Serving/125g	285	11.6	228	10.8	25.2	9.3	2.9
Four Cheese, Asda*	½ Pack/150g	312	13.0	208	7.6	24.9	8.7	1.6
Four Cheese, Express, Dolmio*	1 Pack/220g	411	16.7	187	7.6	22.1	7.6	0.0
Four Cheese, Waitrose*	½ Pack/125g	298	8.4	238	10.3	34.2	6.7	1.6
Fresh, Ham & Cheese, Asda*	½ Pack/150g	315	11.4	210	8.8	26.7	7.6	1.4
Fresh, Morrisons*	1 Serving/150g	430	14.6	287	11.2	41.0	9.7	2.4
Garlic & Herb, Cooked, Pasta Reale*	1 Pack/300g	546	11.7	182	6.7	30.1	3.9	0.9
Goats Cheese & Red Pepper, Morrisons*	1 Pack/150g	450	16.6	300	11.5	38.4	11.1	3.8
Ham & Cheese, M Kitchen, Morrisons*	½ Pack/150g	279	7.0	186	9.6	25.5	4.7	1.4
Meat, Italian, Asda*	½ Pack/150g	266	6.8	177	7.0	27.0	4.5	2.4
Meat & Cheese, Fresh, Sainsbury's*	½ Pack/125g	304	10.5	243	13.5	28.3	8.4	2.6
Mushroom, Basics, Sainsbury's*	¼ Pack/125g	196	6.2	157	6.1	21.8	5.0	3.0
Mushroom, Perfectly Balanced, Waitrose*	½ Pack/125g	300	4.0	240	10.9	41.8	3.2	2.2
Mushroom, Wild, Italian, Sainsbury's*	½ Pack/150g	309	12.3	206	7.7	25.4	8.2	2.3
Olive & Ricotta, Sainsbury's*	½ Pack/175g	403	18.4	230	8.8	25.1	10.5	2.3
Pasta, Fresh, Cream Cheese, Garlic & Herb, Morrisons*	1 Serving/150g	400	9.0	267	10.3	46.1	6.0	3.2
Pesto, Italian, Tesco*	1 Pack/300g	885	33.9	295	10.7	36.7	11.3	3.0
Pesto, LC, Tesco*	½ Pack/150g	278	8.7	185	6.5	26.5	5.8	2.0
Ricotta & Basil, Asda*	½ Pack/150g	322	12.9	215	9.2	25.1	8.6	1.6
Sausage & Red Wine, Italian Style, Morrisons*	½ Pack/150g	420	10.8	280	11.1	45.5	7.2	2.7
Sicilian Style & Tuna, Morrisons*	½ Pack/150g	398	8.8	265	12.1	43.0	5.9	2.3
Smoked Ham, Bacon & Tomato, Tesco*	½ Packet/150g	450	17.6	300	12.0	35.7	11.7	2.5
Spicy Red Pepper & Tomato, Pasta Reale*	½ Pack/125g	310	5.5	248	10.0	42.0	4.4	3.3
Spinach & Ricotta, Chilled, Italiano, Tesco*	½ Pack/150g	412	12.8	275	10.4	38.1	8.5	3.3
Spinach & Ricotta, Emma Giordani*	1 Pack/250g	685	15.0	274	10.0	45.0	6.0	0.0
Spinach & Ricotta, Fresh, Waitrose*	½ Pack/150g	239	5.3	159	6.3	24.4	3.5	2.5

T

	Measure INFO/WEIGHT	per Measure KCAL	FAT	Nutrition Values per 100g / 100ml KCAL	PROT	CARB	FAT	FIBRE
TORTELLONI								
Spinach & Ricotta, Sainsbury's*	½ Pack/150g	326	10.8	217	7.8	30.2	7.2	2.4
Spinach & Ricotta Cheese, Co-Op*	½ Pack/126g	315	6.3	250	10.0	41.0	5.0	4.0
Tomato & Mozzarella, Sainsbury's*	1 Serving/175g	340	14.0	194	7.5	23.0	8.0	3.4
Walnut & Gorgonzola, Fresh, Sainsbury's*	½ Pack/210g	414	12.2	197	8.4	27.8	5.8	2.4
TORTIGLIONI								
Dry, Average	***1 Serving/75g***	***266***	***1.4***	***355***	***12.5***	***72.2***	***1.9***	***2.1***
TORTILLA CHIPS								
Black Pepper & Jalapeno, Love Life, Waitrose*	1 Bag/22g	92	1.9	420	6.7	76.0	8.8	3.2
Blazing BBQ, Sainsbury's*	1 Serving/50g	237	11.8	474	6.8	58.9	23.5	4.6
Chilli, Organic, Evernat*	1oz/28g	137	6.2	490	8.0	65.0	22.0	0.0
Cool, Salted, Sainsbury's*	1 Serving/50g	253	13.6	506	6.5	58.6	27.3	4.3
Cool, Tesco*	1 Serving/40g	190	9.9	474	6.3	56.7	24.7	7.8
Cool Flavour, BGTY, Sainsbury's*	1 Packet/22g	94	2.7	425	7.1	71.4	12.3	4.5
Cool Flavour, Sainsbury's*	1 Serving/50g	232	9.4	463	5.7	68.1	18.7	3.7
Cool Sour Cream, Love Life, Waitrose*	1 Bag/22g	95	2.7	434	7.1	7.1	12.3	4.5
Easy Cheesy!, Sainsbury's*	1 Serving/50g	249	13.0	498	7.1	58.7	26.1	4.5
Honey BBQ, Love Life, Waitrose*	1 Bag/22g	94	2.2	425	6.6	76.0	9.8	3.3
Hot Chilli Flavour, Weight Watchers*	1 Bag/18g	83	3.3	461	4.6	67.7	18.2	4.2
Lightly Salted, M & S*	1 Serving/20g	98	4.8	490	7.2	61.5	24.1	4.5
Lightly Salted, Tesco*	1 Serving/50g	248	13.8	495	4.8	56.8	27.6	7.5
Lightly Salted, Waitrose*	1 Serving/40g	187	8.6	468	7.1	61.2	21.6	6.5
Mexican, Classic, Phileas Fogg*	1 Serving/35g	162	6.7	464	5.9	67.2	19.1	3.8
Mexicana Cheddar, Kettle Chips*	1 Serving/50g	249	13.3	498	7.9	56.7	26.6	5.1
Nacho Cheese Flavour, M & S*	1 Serving/30g	144	6.7	480	7.5	62.0	22.4	4.2
Nacho Cheese Flavour, Mexican Style, Co-Op*	1 Serving/50g	248	13.5	495	7.0	58.0	27.0	4.0
Nacho Cheese Flavour, Morrisons*	1 Serving/25g	126	6.6	504	7.2	59.4	26.4	3.6
Nacho Cheese Flavour, Weight Watchers*	1 Pack/18g	83	3.3	459	5.2	66.6	18.2	4.1
Nachos Kit, Asda*	1 Serving/100g	448	24.0	448	7.0	51.0	24.0	0.7
Pita, Multigrain, Stacy's*	9 Chips/28g	140	5.0	500	10.7	67.9	17.9	0.0
Plain	1 Serving/100g	486	21.1	486	6.8	62.0	21.1	4.2
Salsa, Asda*	1 Serving/25g	122	6.0	488	6.0	62.0	24.0	6.0
Salsa, M & S*	½ Bag/75g	364	18.8	485	5.7	59.1	25.1	6.1
Slightly Salted, Organic, Sainsbury's*	1 Serving/50g	226	6.6	453	10.0	73.3	13.3	13.3
Taco, Tesco*	1 Serving/50g	248	12.7	495	7.4	59.3	25.4	4.4
TORTILLAS								
Corn, GF, Discovery*	1 Tortilla/22g	53	0.5	243	5.4	53.8	2.3	3.8
Corn, Soft, Mexican, Discovery*	1 Tortilla/40g	119	2.8	297	7.4	51.0	7.1	2.3
Corn, Soft, Old El Paso*	1 Tortilla/38g	129	2.6	343	10.0	60.0	7.0	0.0
Flour, American Style, Sainsbury's*	1 Tortilla/35g	108	2.4	313	8.6	53.9	7.0	2.5
Flour, Bakery, Asda*	1 Tortilla/43g	129	3.0	303	9.1	50.9	7.1	2.6
Flour, From Dinner Kit, Old El Paso*	1 Tortilla/42g	144	4.9	344	8.7	51.1	11.7	0.0
Flour, Mexican Style, Morrisons*	1 Tortilla/33g	103	2.3	313	8.6	53.9	7.0	2.5
Flour, Salsa, Old El Paso*	1 Tortilla/41g	132	3.7	323	9.0	52.0	9.0	0.0
Flour, Soft, Chilli & Jalapeno, Discovery*	1 Tortilla/40g	131	5.2	328	7.8	44.8	13.1	2.2
Flour, Soft, Discovery*	1 Tortilla/40g	119	2.8	298	8.0	49.6	7.1	2.4
Flour, Soft, Garlic & Coriander, Discovery*	1 Tortilla/40g	116	2.4	289	8.1	50.6	6.0	1.7
Flour, Wheat, Waitrose*	1 Tortilla/62g	203	6.1	327	8.5	51.5	9.8	0.0
Plain, Wheat, Waitrose*	1 Tortilla/43g	134	3.5	311	8.1	51.5	8.1	3.0
Wholemeal, Discovery*	1 Tortilla/40g	109	3.3	273	9.2	40.4	8.3	6.4
Wholewheat, Asda*	1 Tortilla/35g	88	2.7	252	9.8	35.7	7.8	7.1
Wholewheat, Magnifico*	1 Tortilla/34g	86	2.7	252	9.8	35.7	7.8	7.1
Wrap, 8 Pack, Asda*	1 Tortilla/50g	143	3.0	286	8.0	50.0	6.0	1.9
Wrap, 8 Pack, LC, Tesco*	1 Tortilla/50g	135	1.0	270	7.1	53.2	2.1	3.5

	Measure INFO/WEIGHT	per Measure KCAL	FAT	Nutrition Values per 100g / 100ml KCAL	PROT	CARB	FAT	FIBRE
TORTILLAS								
Wrap, Bueno*	1 Tortilla/63g	171	3.6	272	6.9	48.2	5.7	2.0
Wrap, Flour, Soft, Old El Paso*	1 Tortilla/58g	200	7.2	343	9.3	48.6	12.4	1.7
Wrap, Garlic & Parsley, Sainsbury's*	1 Tortilla/60g	166	3.7	277	7.2	48.0	6.2	1.8
Wrap, Low Carb, Tesco*	1 Tortilla/17g	77	1.5	453	39.4	53.5	8.8	23.5
Wrap, Low Fat, M & S*	1 Serving/180g	225	4.0	125	6.3	20.6	2.2	1.9
Wrap, Organic, Sainsbury's*	1 Tortilla/56g	167	4.3	298	8.6	48.8	7.7	2.1
Wrap, Plain, HL, Tesco*	1 Tortilla/67g	188	1.9	280	8.5	54.2	2.8	3.3
Wrap, Plain, Mini, Morrisons*	1 Tortilla/34g	91	1.4	267	8.1	48.9	4.0	2.8
Wrap, Plain, Nannak*	1 Tortilla/80g	134	3.5	167	8.9	62.2	4.4	0.0
Wrap, Plain, Ready to Eat, Sunnyhills, Aldi*	1 Tortilla/64g	181	2.2	283	7.1	54.5	3.4	3.0
Wrap, Plain, Tesco*	1 Tortilla/64g	192	3.8	300	8.4	52.2	5.9	2.7
Wrap, Spicy Tomato, Tesco*	1 Tortilla/63g	175	3.5	278	7.8	49.2	5.6	2.4
Wrap, Tomato & Herb, Tesco*	1 Tortilla/63g	165	3.5	262	7.9	45.1	5.5	2.1
Wrap, Weight Watchers*	1 Tortilla/42g	107	0.4	254	7.1	50.7	1.0	6.7
Wrap, White, M & S*	1 Tortilla/64g	170	2.4	265	7.9	49.0	3.8	1.6
Wrap, Whole & White, Mini, Kids, Sainsbury's*	1 Tortilla/26g	67	1.4	258	9.2	42.9	5.5	6.2
Wrap, Wholemeal, Morrisons*	1oz/28g	78	1.8	277	7.9	47.2	6.3	5.2
Wraps, Healthy 'n' White, Wrap 'n' Roll, Discovery*	1 Tortilla/40g	161	3.5	288	8.0	49.7	6.3	2.6
Wraps, Less Than 3% Fat, BGTY, Sainsbury's*	1 Tortilla/51g	128	1.1	250	7.8	50.1	2.2	2.9
Wraps, Mexican, Asda*	1 Tortilla/34g	100	2.8	295	7.9	47.2	8.3	3.9
Wraps, Multiseed, Discovery*	1 Tortilla/57g	160	2.8	280	8.7	50.1	5.0	3.6
Wraps, Plain, Sainsbury's*	1 Tortilla/56g	167	4.4	299	8.1	49.2	7.8	3.6
TREACLE								
Black, Average	***1 Tbsp/20g***	***51***	***0.0***	***257***	***1.2***	***67.2***	***0.0***	***0.0***
TRIFLE								
Average	1 Portion/170g	272	10.7	160	3.6	22.3	6.3	0.5
Banana & Mandarin, Co-Op*	¼ Trifle/125g	238	13.8	190	2.0	21.0	11.0	0.1
Blackforest, Asda*	1 Serving/100g	237	9.0	237	3.1	36.0	9.0	0.0
Blackforest, BGTY, Sainsbury's*	1 Pot/125g	171	5.6	137	2.1	21.9	4.5	1.6
Caramel, Galaxy, Mars*	1 Pot/100g	255	13.0	255	4.5	30.0	13.0	1.0
Cherry, Finest, Tesco*	¼ Trifle/163g	340	19.3	209	2.6	22.9	11.9	0.3
Chocolate, Asda*	1 Serving/125g	272	16.3	217	4.1	21.0	13.0	0.5
Chocolate, BGTY, Sainsbury's*	1 Pot/100g	137	2.7	137	4.8	23.4	2.7	1.6
Chocolate, Cadbury*	1 Pot/90g	234	13.8	260	4.8	22.5	15.3	0.0
Chocolate, Light, Cadbury*	1 Pot/93g	130	4.0	140	4.6	20.4	4.3	0.0
Chocolate, Tesco*	1 Serving/125g	312	19.0	250	4.3	24.0	15.2	0.7
Fruit, Sainsbury's*	1 Serving/125g	232	12.5	186	2.3	21.7	10.0	0.3
Fruit Cocktail, COU, M & S*	1 Trifle/140g	175	3.2	125	2.8	23.1	2.3	0.5
Fruit Cocktail, Individual, M & S*	1 Pot/135g	205	9.2	150	2.7	19.3	6.7	0.7
Fruit Cocktail, Individual, Shape, Danone*	1 Trifle/115g	136	3.1	118	3.2	19.6	2.7	1.6
Fruit Cocktail, Individual, Tesco*	1 Pot/113g	175	8.8	155	1.7	19.6	7.8	0.6
Fruit Cocktail, Low Fat, Danone*	1 Pot/115g	140	2.1	122	2.2	24.0	1.8	0.4
Fruit Cocktail, Luxury Devonshire, St Ivel*	1 Trifle/125g	211	9.9	169	1.9	22.6	7.9	0.2
Fruit Cocktail, M & S*	1 Serving/165g	272	13.7	165	2.4	19.6	8.3	0.9
Fruit Cocktail, Sainsbury's*	1 Trifle/150g	241	9.0	161	1.8	24.8	6.0	0.4
Mango, & Passion Fruit, Danone*	1oz/28g	50	1.4	177	2.6	30.7	4.9	0.4
Peach, & Zabaglione, COU, M & S*	1 Glass/130g	150	3.0	115	2.8	20.6	2.3	0.8
Raspberry, Asda*	1 Serving/100g	175	8.0	175	1.8	24.0	8.0	0.1
Raspberry, Sainsbury's*	1 Pot/135g	286	17.7	212	3.2	19.9	13.1	0.7
Raspberry, Tesco*	1 Pot/150g	210	9.8	140	1.7	18.5	6.5	1.0
Sherry, BGTY, Sainsbury's*	1 Pot/135g	146	2.3	108	3.0	20.2	1.7	0.5
Strawberry, BGTY, Sainsbury's*	1 Pot/125g	135	2.6	108	2.4	19.9	2.1	0.5
Strawberry, Co-Op*	1 Serving/120g	175	9.1	146	1.7	16.7	7.6	1.4

	Measure INFO/WEIGHT	per Measure KCAL	FAT	Nutrition Values per 100g / 100ml KCAL	PROT	CARB	FAT	FIBRE
TRIFLE								
Strawberry, Individual, Waitrose*	1 Pot/150g	206	8.6	137	1.8	19.7	5.7	1.0
Strawberry, Low Fat, Shape, Danone*	1oz/28g	38	0.9	137	3.8	22.8	3.1	1.8
Strawberry, Low Fat Goodies, Danone*	1 Pot/115g	148	2.1	129	2.2	26.0	1.8	0.3
Strawberry, Luxury Devonshire, St Ivel*	1 Trifle/125g	208	9.9	166	2.0	21.7	7.9	0.2
Strawberry, Sainsbury's*	¼ Tub/150g	261	15.4	174	2.2	18.1	10.3	1.0
Strawberry, St Ivel*	1 Trifle/113g	194	9.8	172	2.4	21.0	8.7	0.2
Strawberry, Tesco*	1 Trifle/605	998	55.7	165	1.5	19.1	9.2	0.8
Summerfruit, BGTY, Sainsbury's*	1 Trifle/125g	151	5.5	121	1.2	19.2	4.4	0.5
Triple Chocolate, Farmfoods*	¼ Trifle/86g	223	15.7	259	2.1	21.6	18.2	1.2
TRIFLE MIX								
Strawberry Flavour, Bird's*	1oz/28g	119	2.9	425	2.7	78.0	10.5	1.2
TRIFLE SPONGES								
Average	1 Sponge/24g	77	0.5	319	5.2	69.9	2.2	0.8
TRIPE &								
Onions, Stewed	1oz/28g	26	0.8	93	8.3	9.5	2.7	0.7
TROUT								
Brown, Steamed, Average	***1 Serving/120g***	***162***	***5.4***	***135***	***23.5***	***0.0***	***4.5***	***0.0***
Fillets, Scottish, Hot Smoked, TTD, Sainsbury's*	½ Pack/63g	85	3.4	136	20.8	1.0	5.4	0.5
Fillets, Skinless, Chunky, TTD, Sainsbury's*	½ Pack/123g	227	13.0	185	22.4	0.1	10.6	0.6
Grilled, Weighed with Bones & Skin	1 Serving/100g	98	3.9	98	15.7	0.0	3.9	0.0
Rainbow, Fillets, with Thyme & Lemon Butter, Asda*	1 Serving/147g	210	10.3	143	20.0	0.9	7.0	0.5
Rainbow, Grilled, Average	***1 Serving/120g***	***162***	***6.5***	***135***	***21.5***	***0.0***	***5.4***	***0.0***
Rainbow, Raw, Average	***1oz/28g***	***36***	***1.4***	***127***	***20.5***	***0.0***	***5.1***	***0.0***
Rainbow, Smoked, Average	***1 Pack/135g***	***190***	***7.6***	***140***	***21.7***	***0.8***	***5.6***	***0.0***
Raw, Average	***1 Serving/120g***	***159***	***6.5***	***132***	***20.6***	***0.0***	***5.4***	***0.0***
Smoked, Average	***2 Fillets/135g***	***187***	***7.1***	***138***	***22.7***	***0.3***	***5.2***	***0.1***
TUMS								
Extra 750, Sugar Free, Tums*	2 Tablets/2g	5	0.0	250	0.0	50.0	0.0	0.0
Extra 750, Tums*	2 Tablets/2g	10	0.0	500	0.0	100.0	0.0	0.0
Regular, Tums*	1 Tablet/2g	2	0.0	125	0.0	25.0	0.0	0.0
Smoothies, Extra Strength 750, Tums*	2 Tablets/2g	10	0.0	500	0.0	100.0	0.0	0.0
TUNA								
Albacore, in Olive Oil, TTD, Sainsbury's*	1 Serving/80g	162	8.7	203	26.1	0.0	10.9	0.0
Bluefin, Cooked, Dry Heat, Average	***1 Serving/100g***	***184***	***6.3***	***184***	***29.9***	***0.0***	***6.3***	***0.0***
Chunks, in Brine, Canned, Drained, Princes*	1oz/28g	29	0.1	105	25.0	0.0	0.5	0.0
Chunks, in Brine, Drained, Average	1 Can/130g	141	0.7	108	25.9	0.0	0.5	0.0
Chunks, in Spring Water, Drained, Average	***1 Can/130g***	***140***	***0.8***	***108***	***25.4***	***0.0***	***0.6***	***0.1***
Chunks, in Sunflower Oil, Drained, Average	***1 Can/138g***	***260***	***12.6***	***188***	***26.5***	***0.0***	***9.2***	***0.0***
Chunks, Skipjack, in Brine, Average	***1 Can/138g***	***141***	***0.8***	***102***	***24.3***	***0.0***	***0.6***	***0.0***
Chunks, with a Little Brine, No Drain, 120g, John West*	1 Can/120g	130	1.1	108	25.0	0.0	0.9	0.0
Chunks, with a Little Brine, No Drain, 60g, John West*	1 Can/60g	55	0.5	91	21.0	0.0	0.8	0.0
Coronation, BGTY, Sainsbury's*	1 Can/80g	90	2.1	112	16.5	5.7	2.6	1.0
Coronation Style, Canned, Average	1 Can/80g	122	7.6	152	10.2	6.5	9.5	0.6
Fillets, in Tomato Sauce, Princes*	1 Can/120g	131	3.0	109	19.0	2.5	2.5	0.0
Flakes, in Brine, Average	***1oz/28g***	***29***	***0.2***	***104***	***24.8***	***0.0***	***0.6***	***0.0***
Flakes, with Tomato & Onion, Canned, Mermaid Bay*	1 Can/85g	94	2.5	110	16.1	4.7	2.9	0.5
in Coronation Style Dressing, Weight Watchers*	1 Can/80g	75	2.0	94	9.3	8.7	2.5	0.4
in Light Lemon Mayonnaise, Slimming World, Princes*	1 Can/80g	99	3.8	124	16.8	3.5	4.8	0.0
in Light Mayonnaise, Slimming World, Princes*	1 Can/80g	96	3.3	120	17.3	3.6	4.1	0.0
in Red Chilli & Lime Dressing, Princes*	1 Sachet/85g	102	2.8	120	21.5	1.0	3.3	0.0
in Sweet & Sour Sauce, Yellowfin, Asda*	1 Pouch/250g	235	5.8	94	11.6	6.7	2.3	1.4
in Thousand Island Dressing, John West*	1 Can/185g	287	13.0	155	18.0	5.1	7.0	0.2
in Thousand Island Dressing, Weight Watchers*	1 Can/79g	67	1.7	85	8.3	7.8	2.2	0.4

	Measure INFO/WEIGHT	per Measure KCAL	FAT	Nutrition Values per 100g / 100ml KCAL	PROT	CARB	FAT	FIBRE
TUNA								
in Tikka Dressing, Slimming World, Princes*	1 Can/80g	108	4.6	135	16.8	4.0	5.7	0.0
in Tomato & Herb Dressing, Weight Watchers*	1 Can/80g	79	2.9	99	11.6	5.1	3.6	0.5
in Water, Average	***1 Serving/120g***	***126***	***1.0***	***105***	***24.0***	***0.1***	***0.8***	***0.0***
Light Lunch, Indian Style, John West*	1 Pack/240g	401	23.0	167	7.7	12.3	9.6	0.6
Light Lunch, Nicoise Style, John West*	1 Pack/250g	245	5.8	98	10.3	9.0	2.3	2.7
Lime & Black Pepper, John West*	1 Serving/85g	133	7.8	156	15.6	2.8	9.2	0.0
Puertorican Style, Tinned, Natura*	1 Can/185g	157	8.3	85	9.0	1.0	4.5	0.0
Steak, Control Chef, All About Weight*	1 Meal/270g	284	4.3	105	9.8	10.9	1.6	3.9
Steaks, Chargrilled, Italian, Sainsbury's*	1 Serving/125g	199	8.0	159	25.1	0.2	6.4	0.5
Steaks, in Brine, Average	***1 Sm Can/99g***	***106***	***0.5***	***107***	***25.6***	***0.0***	***0.6***	***0.0***
Steaks, in Cajun Marinade, Sainsbury's*	1 Steak/100g	141	2.4	141	29.8	0.0	2.4	0.0
Steaks, in Olive Oil, Average	***1 Serving/111g***	***211***	***10.7***	***190***	***25.8***	***0.0***	***9.6***	***0.0***
Steaks, in Oriental Sauce, Good Choice, Iceland*	1 Pack/260g	333	1.8	128	22.3	8.1	0.7	0.4
Steaks, in Sunflower Oil, Average	***1 Can/150g***	***276***	***12.9***	***184***	***26.7***	***0.0***	***8.6***	***0.0***
Steaks, in Water, Average	***1 Serving/200g***	***215***	***0.8***	***107***	***25.6***	***0.0***	***0.4***	***0.0***
Steaks, John West*	1 Can/130g	140	0.4	108	26.2	0.0	0.3	0.0
Steaks, Lemon & Herb Marinade, Seared, Sainsbury's*	½ Pack/119g	191	8.8	161	23.4	0.1	7.4	0.0
Steaks, Marinated, Sainsbury's*	1 Serving/100g	153	5.3	153	25.1	1.3	5.3	0.5
Steaks, Raw, Average	***1 Serving/140g***	***185***	***2.8***	***132***	***28.5***	***0.1***	***2.0***	***0.2***
Steaks, Skipjack, in Brine, Average	***½ Can/75g***	***73***	***0.4***	***98***	***23.2***	***0.0***	***0.6***	***0.0***
Steaks, Thai Style Butter, Tesco*	1 Serving/110g	191	9.1	174	24.7	0.0	8.3	0.0
Steaks, with a Little Brine, No Drain, John West*	1 Can/130g	140	0.4	108	26.2	0.0	0.3	0.0
Steaks, with a Little Olive Oil, No Drain, John West*	1 Can/130g	209	7.0	161	28.2	0.0	5.4	0.0
Steaks, with a Little Sunflower Oil, No Drain, John West*	1 Can/130g	209	7.0	161	28.2	0.0	5.4	0.0
Steaks, with Lime & Coriander Dressing, Tesco*	1 Serving/150g	156	0.6	104	21.6	3.6	0.4	0.6
Steaks, with Sweet Red Pepper Glaze, Sainsbury's*	1 Steak/100g	135	0.1	135	28.5	5.0	0.1	0.1
with a Twist, French Dressing, John West*	1 Pack/85g	135	8.2	159	15.2	2.8	9.7	0.1
TUNA MAYONNAISE								
& Sweetcorn, Canned, BGTY, Sainsbury's*	1 Can/80g	78	1.8	97	15.2	4.0	2.3	0.7
Garlic & Herb, John West*	½ Can/92g	243	20.4	264	12.0	4.0	22.2	0.2
Light, Slimming World*	1 Serving/80g	96	3.3	120	17.3	3.6	4.1	0.0
with Sweetcorn, From Heinz, Weight Watchers*	1 Can/80g	114	6.3	142	11.5	6.2	7.9	0.1
with Sweetcorn, John West*	½ Can/92g	231	19.0	251	12.0	4.5	20.6	0.2
with Sweetcorn & Green Peppers, GFY, Asda*	1 Pack/100g	103	3.0	103	14.0	5.0	3.0	0.8
TURBOT								
Grilled	***1oz/28g***	***34***	***1.0***	***122***	***22.7***	***0.0***	***3.5***	***0.0***
Raw	***1oz/28g***	***27***	***0.8***	***95***	***17.7***	***0.0***	***2.7***	***0.0***
TURKEY								
Breast, 3% Fat, Bernard Matthews*	1 Slice/20g	21	0.5	103	19.2	0.9	2.5	0.5
Breast, Butter Basted, Average	***1 Serving/75g***	***110***	***3.6***	***146***	***23.7***	***1.9***	***4.9***	***0.4***
Breast, Canned, Average	***1 Can/200g***	***194***	***4.7***	***97***	***18.3***	***0.7***	***2.4***	***0.0***
Breast, Chunks, Bernard Matthews*	1 Serving/55g	64	0.5	116	26.1	0.9	0.9	1.6
Breast, Diced, Healthy Range, Average	***1oz/28g***	***30***	***0.4***	***108***	***23.8***	***0.0***	***1.3***	***0.0***
Breast, Diced in a Hot & Spicy Marinade, Waitrose*	½ Pack/200g	286	7.0	143	24.1	3.5	3.5	0.5
Breast, Fillets, Marinated, Lidl*	1 Serving/250g	238	2.5	95	19.0	2.5	1.0	0.0
Breast, Honey Roast, Sliced, Average	***1 Serving/50g***	***57***	***0.7***	***114***	***24.0***	***1.6***	***1.4***	***0.2***
Breast, Joint, Butter Basted, Cooked, Braemoor, Lidl*	1 Serving/130g	220	9.9	169	21.0	4.0	7.6	0.5
Breast, Joint, Lemon & Pepper Basted, Tesco*	¼ Pack/132g	238	14.8	180	19.7	0.0	11.2	0.0
Breast, Joint, Raw, Average	***1 Serving/125g***	***134***	***2.6***	***108***	***21.3***	***0.7***	***2.1***	***0.6***
Breast, Joint, with Sage & Onion Stuffing, Waitrose*	1 Serving/325g	377	13.3	116	19.2	1.4	4.1	0.1
Breast, Raw, Average	***1oz/28g***	***33***	***0.6***	***117***	***24.1***	***0.5***	***2.0***	***0.1***
Breast, Roasted, Average	***1oz/28g***	***37***	***0.9***	***131***	***24.6***	***0.7***	***3.3***	***0.1***
Breast, Roll, Cooked, Average	***1 Slice/10g***	***9***	***0.1***	***92***	***17.6***	***3.5***	***0.8***	***0.0***

	Measure INFO/WEIGHT	per Measure KCAL	FAT	Nutrition Values per 100g / 100ml KCAL	PROT	CARB	FAT	FIBRE
TURKEY								
Breast, Slices, Cooked, Average	***1 Slice/20g***	***23***	***0.3***	***114***	***24.0***	***1.2***	***1.4***	***0.3***
Breast, Smoked, Sliced, Average	***1 Slice/20g***	***23***	***0.4***	***113***	***23.4***	***0.7***	***2.0***	***0.0***
Breast, Steaks, in Crumbs, Average	1 Steak/76g	217	14.1	286	13.7	16.4	18.5	0.2
Breast, Steaks, Raw, Average	***1oz/28g***	***30***	***0.3***	***107***	***24.3***	***0.0***	***1.1***	***0.0***
Breast, Steaks, Thai, Bernard Matthews*	1 Serving/175g	280	4.7	160	29.4	4.6	2.7	0.0
Breast, Strips, Chinese Style, Sainsbury's*	¼ Pack/163g	318	7.3	196	26.4	12.5	4.5	0.5
Breast, Strips, for Stir Fry, Average	***1 Serving/175g***	***205***	***2.7***	***117***	***25.6***	***0.1***	***1.6***	***0.0***
Breast, Stuffed, Just Roast, Sainsbury's*	1 Serving/100g	155	6.6	155	21.1	2.9	6.6	0.6
Breast, Wafer Thin, Chinese Style, Bernard Matthews*	1 Pack/100g	110	1.5	110	18.0	6.1	1.5	0.0
Breast Golden Norfolk, Bernard Matthews*	1 Slice/20g	22	0.2	109	23.8	0.9	1.1	0.8
Breast Slices, Bernard Matthews*	1 Slice/20g	21	0.5	103	19.2	0.9	2.5	0.5
Dark Meat, Raw, Average	***1oz/28g***	***29***	***0.7***	***104***	***20.4***	***0.0***	***2.5***	***0.0***
Drummers, Golden, Bernard Matthews*	1 Drummer/57g	147	10.3	258	13.1	11.0	18.0	1.1
Drummers, Golden, Grilled, Bernard Matthews*	1 Drummer/50g	147	10.6	294	15.6	10.0	21.2	1.0
Drumsticks, Tesco*	1 Serving/200g	272	12.6	136	19.9	0.0	6.3	0.0
Escalope, Average	***1 Escalope/138g***	***341***	***19.3***	***247***	***13.5***	***16.7***	***14.0***	***0.6***
Escalope, Creamy Pepper Topped, Tesco*	1 Escalope/165g	337	17.7	204	11.5	15.3	10.7	1.7
Escalope, Lemon & Pepper, Average	1 Escalope/143g	371	22.6	260	12.6	16.7	15.8	0.4
Escalope, Spicy Mango, Bernard Matthews*	1 Escalope/136g	354	17.4	260	11.6	24.6	12.8	0.0
Escalope, Tomato & Herb, Bernard Matthews*	1 Escalope/143g	336	19.2	236	10.5	18.0	13.5	0.0
Fillets, Chinese Marinated, Bernard Matthews*	1 Pack/200g	304	6.6	152	23.4	7.2	3.3	0.0
Goujons, Cooked, Bernard Matthews*	4 Goujons/128g	355	23.3	277	11.8	16.6	18.2	1.1
Leg, Roast, Uncooked, Bernard Matthews*	1 Serving/283g	317	15.3	112	15.4	0.5	5.4	0.0
Light Meat, Raw, Average	***1oz/28g***	***29***	***0.2***	***105***	***24.4***	***0.0***	***0.8***	***0.0***
Light Meat, Roasted	***1 Cup/140g***	***220***	***4.5***	***157***	***29.9***	***0.0***	***3.2***	***0.0***
Mince, Average	***1oz/28g***	***45***	***2.0***	***161***	***23.9***	***0.0***	***7.2***	***0.0***
Mince, Lean, Healthy Range, Average	***1oz/28g***	***33***	***1.1***	***118***	***20.3***	***0.0***	***4.1***	***0.0***
Rashers, Average	***1 Rasher/26g***	***26***	***0.4***	***101***	***19.1***	***2.3***	***1.6***	***0.0***
Rashers, Smoked, Average	***1 Serving/75g***	***76***	***1.4***	***101***	***19.8***	***1.5***	***1.8***	***0.0***
Ready to Roast, with Stuffing & Bacon, M & S*	1/3 Pack/169g	245	10.5	145	20.2	2.1	6.2	1.1
Roast, Meat & Skin, Average	***1oz/28g***	***48***	***1.8***	***171***	***28.0***	***0.0***	***6.5***	***0.0***
Roast, Meat Only, Average	***1 Serving/100g***	***157***	***3.2***	***157***	***29.9***	***0.0***	***3.2***	***0.0***
Roast, Sugar Marinade, Slices, M & S*	½ Pack/120g	156	1.9	130	29.0	0.2	1.6	0.5
Roast, Wafer Thin, Tesco*	1 Slice/8g	8	0.2	105	20.0	1.5	2.0	0.0
Roll, Dinosaur, Cooked, Bernard Matthews*	1 Slice/10g	17	1.0	170	13.6	6.0	10.2	1.1
Schnitzel, Lidl*	1 Schnitzel/115g	210	8.0	183	19.0	11.0	7.0	0.0
Steaks, Breaded, Bernard Matthews*	1 Steak/110g	319	20.0	290	11.0	20.5	18.2	1.5
Sticks, Honey Roast, Mini, Tesco*	1 Serving/90g	101	1.7	112	20.0	3.6	1.9	0.0
Strips, Stir-Fried, Average	1oz/28g	46	1.3	164	31.0	0.0	4.5	0.0
Thigh, Diced, Average	***1oz/28g***	***33***	***1.2***	***117***	***19.6***	***0.0***	***4.3***	***0.0***
Wafer Thin, Cooked, Average	1 Slice/10g	12	0.4	122	19.0	3.2	3.7	0.0
Wafer Thin, Honey Roast, Average	1 Slice/10g	11	0.2	109	19.2	4.2	1.7	0.2
Wafer Thin, Smoked, Average	1 Slice/10g	12	0.4	119	18.1	3.6	3.7	0.0
Whole, Raw, Weighed with Bone	1 Serving/100g	93	3.6	93	15.1	0.0	3.6	0.0
TURKEY DINNER								
Roast, Asda*	1 Pack/400g	344	6.4	86	7.0	11.0	1.6	2.0
Roast, Iceland*	1 Meal/400g	374	7.2	94	8.4	10.9	1.8	1.3
Roast, Meal for One, M & S*	1 Pack/370g	462	16.3	125	9.1	12.4	4.4	2.7
Roast, Sainsbury's*	1 Pack/450g	354	9.0	79	6.8	8.4	2.0	1.9
Roast Dinner, 105, Oakhouse Foods Ltd*	1 Dinner/430g	624	16.3	145	7.0	9.4	3.8	1.4
Traditional, Birds Eye*	1 Pack/340g	292	7.8	86	6.1	10.3	2.3	1.7
TURKEY HAM								
Average	***1 Serving/75g***	***81***	***2.9***	***108***	***15.6***	***2.8***	***3.9***	***0.0***

	Measure INFO/WEIGHT	per Measure KCAL	per Measure FAT	Nutrition Values per 100g / 100ml KCAL	PROT	CARB	FAT	FIBRE
TURKISH DELIGHT								
Assorted Flavours, Julian Graves*	1 Square/30g	110	0.0	366	0.5	91.1	0.1	0.0
Co-Op*	1 Bar/53g	207	4.2	390	2.0	78.0	8.0	0.1
Dark Chocolate Covered, Thorntons*	1 Chocolate/10g	39	1.1	390	2.7	69.0	11.0	2.0
Fry's*	1 Bar/51g	185	3.4	365	1.4	74.6	6.7	1.3
Milk Chocolate, M & S*	1 Pack/55g	220	4.7	400	1.6	79.0	8.5	0.0
Sultans*	1 Serving/16g	58	0.0	360	0.0	90.0	0.0	0.0
with Mixed Nuts, Hazer Baba*	1 Piece/12g	47	0.2	389	1.6	88.5	1.7	0.0
with Rose, Hazer Baba*	1 Square/18g	70	0.3	389	1.6	88.6	1.7	0.0
TURMERIC								
Powder	***1 Tsp/3g***	***11***	***0.3***	***354***	***7.8***	***58.2***	***9.9***	***0.0***
TURNIP								
Boiled, Average	***1oz/28g***	***3***	***0.1***	***12***	***0.6***	***2.0***	***0.2***	***1.9***
Greens, Leaves, Cooked	1 Serving/80g	16	0.2	20	1.1	4.4	0.2	3.5
Mash, Direct Foods*	½ Pack/190g	49	3.4	26	0.6	2.0	1.8	1.9
Mashed, Mash Direct*	1 Pack/400g	148	2.3	37	0.8	6.0	0.6	2.5
Raw, Unprepared, Average	***1oz/28g***	***6***	***0.1***	***23***	***0.9***	***4.7***	***0.3***	***2.4***
TURNOVER								
Apple, Bramley, Tesco*	1 Turnover/88g	304	22.8	346	2.7	25.4	25.9	0.9
Apple, Co-Op*	1 Turnover/77g	308	20.8	400	4.0	35.0	27.0	1.0
Apple, Dutch, Sainsbury's*	1 Serving/33g	130	5.5	393	3.6	56.9	16.8	1.4
Apple, Fresh Cream, Sainsbury's*	1 Turnover/84g	292	20.9	347	4.1	26.9	24.8	2.5
Apple, Tesco*	1 Turnover/88g	294	19.7	334	3.2	29.8	22.4	0.9
Mincemeat, Fresh Cream, Tesco*	1 Turnover/83g	334	22.2	405	3.1	37.5	26.9	1.1
Raspberry, Fresh Cream, Asda*	1 Turnover/100g	411	23.0	411	6.0	45.0	23.0	2.1
Raspberry, Tesco*	1 Turnover/84g	290	20.2	345	4.0	27.2	24.1	2.1
TWIGLETS								
Curry, Jacob's*	1 Bag/30g	134	6.4	448	8.0	55.7	21.5	6.0
Original, Jacob's*	1 Bag/30g	115	3.5	383	12.7	57.0	11.6	11.8
Tangy, Jacob's*	1 Bag/30g	136	6.6	454	8.1	55.9	22.0	5.4
TWIRL								
Cadbury*	1 Finger/22g	118	6.8	535	7.6	56.0	30.9	0.8
Treat Size, Cadbury*	1 Bar/21g	115	6.6	535	7.6	56.0	30.9	0.8
TWISTS								
Black Olive & Basil, Finest, Tesco*	¼ Pack/31g	151	7.9	483	11.3	53.1	25.1	3.9
Gruyere & Poppy Seed, TTD, Sainsbury's*	1 Serving/8g	41	2.3	509	13.7	50.5	28.0	2.6
Parmesan, All Butter, TTD, Sainsbury's*	1 Serving/8g	38	2.0	487	13.8	51.0	25.3	2.8
Strawberry, Sainsbury's*	1 Serving/10g	38	0.3	375	1.7	82.7	3.0	0.1
Tomato & Herb, Shapers, Boots*	1 Pack/20g	94	4.2	468	3.7	66.0	21.0	3.9
TWIX								
Fun Size, Mars*	1 Bar/20g	99	4.8	495	4.5	64.6	24.0	1.5
Standard, Mars*	1 Pack/58g	284	13.7	490	4.7	65.5	23.7	1.5
Top, Mars*	1 Bar/28g	143	7.8	511	5.2	60.2	27.7	0.0
Twixels, Mars*	1 Finger/6g	31	1.6	513	5.0	64.0	26.1	0.0
Xtra, Mars*	1 Pack/85g	416	20.1	490	4.7	65.5	23.7	1.5
TZATZIKI								
Average	1 Tbsp/15g	10	0.7	66	3.7	2.0	4.9	0.2
Fresh, Sainsbury's*	1 Serving/46g	59	4.8	129	4.4	4.4	10.4	0.2
Greek, Authentic, Total, Fage*	1 Serving/50g	50	3.5	99	4.9	4.1	7.0	1.0

T

	Measure INFO/WEIGHT	per Measure KCAL	FAT	Nutrition Values per 100g / 100ml KCAL	PROT	CARB	FAT	FIBRE
VANILLA								
Bean, Average	***1 Pod/2g***	***6***	***0.0***	***288***	***0.0***	***13.0***	***0.0***	***0.0***
Flavouring, Supercook*	1 Tsp/4g	2	0.0	50	6.2	0.0	0.0	0.0
VANILLA EXTRACT								
Average	***1 Tbsp/13g***	***37***	***0.0***	***288***	***0.1***	***12.6***	***0.1***	***0.0***
Pure, Nielsen Massey Vanillas*	1 Tsp/5ml	8	0.0	160	0.1	39.5	0.2	0.1
VEAL								
Chop, Loin, Raw, Weighed with Bone, Average	1 Chop/195g	495	27.8	254	29.5	0.0	14.3	0.0
Diced, Lean, British, Waitrose*	1 Pack/275g	300	7.4	109	21.1	0.0	2.7	0.0
Escalope, Fried, Average	1oz/28g	55	1.9	196	33.7	0.0	6.8	0.0
Escalopes, Breaded, M & S*	1 Escalope/130g	292	13.9	225	13.6	18.7	10.7	0.4
Mince, Raw, Average	***1oz/28g***	***40***	***2.0***	***144***	***20.3***	***0.0***	***7.0***	***0.0***
Shoulder, Lean & Fat, Roasted, Average	***1oz/28g***	***52***	***2.3***	***183***	***25.5***	***0.0***	***8.2***	***0.0***
Shoulder, Lean Only, Roasted, Average	***1oz/28g***	***46***	***1.6***	***164***	***26.1***	***0.0***	***5.8***	***0.0***
Sirloin, Lean & Fat, Roasted, Average	***1oz/28g***	***57***	***3.0***	***202***	***25.1***	***0.0***	***10.4***	***0.0***
Sirloin, Lean Only, Roasted, Average	***1oz/28g***	***48***	***1.8***	***168***	***26.3***	***0.0***	***6.2***	***0.0***
VEGEMITE								
Australian, Kraft*	1 Tsp/5g	9	0.0	173	23.5	19.7	0.0	0.0
VEGETABLE CHIPS								
Beetroot, Carrot & Parsnips, Hand Fried, Tyrrells*	½ Pack/25g	103	7.0	413	3.9	36.0	28.1	11.5
Cassava, Average	1oz/28g	99	0.1	353	1.8	91.4	0.4	4.0
Mixed Root, Tyrrells*	1oz/28g	133	8.3	476	5.7	35.4	29.8	12.8
Parsnip, Golden, Kettle Chips*	½ Pack/50g	258	18.8	515	4.6	39.5	37.6	8.4
Sweet Potato, Kettle Chips*	½ Pack/50g	242	16.4	483	2.4	44.4	32.8	9.3
VEGETABLE CRISPS								
Pan Fried, Glennans*	1 Bag/20g	98	6.7	490	5.0	42.5	33.5	11.0
VEGETABLE FAT								
Pure, Trex*	1 Tbsp/12g	108	12.0	900	0.0	0.0	100.0	0.0
VEGETABLE FINGERS								
Crispy, Birds Eye*	2 Fingers/60g	107	4.8	179	3.2	23.5	8.0	2.3
Crispy Crunchy, Dalepak*	1 Finger/28g	62	3.1	223	4.2	26.7	11.0	15.0
Sweetcorn, Tesco*	1 Finger/28g	66	3.5	236	7.7	23.0	12.6	3.0
VEGETABLE MEDLEY								
& New Potato, Asda*	½ Pack/175g	102	3.9	58	2.5	7.0	2.2	5.0
Asda*	1 Pack/300g	84	0.6	28	2.8	3.9	0.2	2.9
Asparagus Tips, Perfectly Balanced, Waitrose*	1 Serving/225g	122	7.6	54	1.3	4.6	3.4	1.4
Basil & Oregano Butter, Waitrose*	1 Serving/113g	59	3.8	52	1.7	3.7	3.4	1.9
Buttered, Sainsbury's*	½ Pack/175g	122	6.8	70	1.7	7.0	3.9	1.8
Carrot, Courgette, Fine Bean & Baby Corn, Tesco*	1 Serving/100g	36	2.4	36	1.1	2.4	2.4	3.0
Crunchy, M & S*	1 Pack/250g	75	2.0	30	3.1	2.8	0.8	2.5
Frozen, M & S*	1 Pack/500g	175	4.0	35	3.4	3.9	0.8	3.1
Green, HL, Tesco*	1 Serving/125g	59	2.2	47	3.7	4.1	1.8	4.1
Green, Sainsbury's*	1 Pack/220g	178	14.3	81	3.0	2.5	6.5	2.9
HL, Tesco*	1 Serving/100g	24	1.2	24	0.8	2.3	1.2	1.3
Roast, Four Seasons*	1 Pack/375g	202	12.0	54	2.8	3.5	3.2	2.7
Roasted, Waitrose*	½ Pack/200g	282	15.6	141	1.2	16.4	7.8	3.7
with Herby Butter, M & S*	1 Pack/300g	225	15.0	75	1.5	6.2	5.0	2.6
VEGETABLE SELECTION								
Chefs, M & S*	1 Pack/250g	88	1.2	35	2.6	4.5	0.5	2.9
Five, Sainsbury's*	½ Pack/125g	42	1.0	34	2.6	4.3	0.8	3.1
Fresh, Finest, Tesco*	1 Pack/250g	182	14.5	73	1.9	3.2	5.8	2.2
Garden, Tesco*	1 Pack/275g	124	9.1	45	1.2	2.7	3.3	1.2
Lightly Buttered & Seasoned, M & S*	1 Pack/300g	195	10.8	65	1.6	6.3	3.6	2.8
Oriental, with Soy Dressing, Sainsbury's*	1 Serving/80g	35	0.6	44	2.0	5.5	0.8	3.3

	Measure INFO/WEIGHT	per Measure KCAL	FAT	Nutrition Values per 100g / 100ml KCAL	PROT	CARB	FAT	FIBRE
VEGETABLE SELECTION								
Ready to Cook, Morrisons*	1 Serving/150g	51	0.9	34	2.4	4.8	0.6	2.3
Roast, COU, M & S*	1 Serving/250g	95	2.0	38	1.2	6.1	0.8	0.6
Winter, M & S*	1 Bag/400g	80	0.0	20	2.2	3.2	0.0	3.1
VEGETABLES								
Asparagus & Tenderstem Broccoli, Finest, Tesco*	½ Pack/95g	28	0.4	29	3.7	2.7	0.4	2.7
Baby, Frozen, Asda*	1 Serving/100g	25	0.3	25	1.9	3.7	0.3	1.9
Baby Mix, Freshly Frozen, Iceland*	1 Serving/100g	26	0.3	26	1.8	3.9	0.3	1.9
Broccoli, & Cauliflower, Layered, M & S*	½ Pack/135g	94	4.6	70	1.5	7.6	3.4	1.2
Broccoli, Leek & Cabbage, Fresh, Love Life, Waitrose*	1 Serving/100g	26	0.4	26	1.5	3.1	0.4	1.8
Butternut Squash, & Sweet Potato, Fresh Tastes, Asda*	½ Pack/225g	128	0.4	57	1.0	12.9	0.2	1.8
Butternut Squash, Broccoli & Spinach, Eat Well, M & S*	½ Pack/138g	55	0.7	40	2.3	5.0	0.5	2.3
Carrot, Broccoli & Cauliflower, Organic, Sainsbury's*	1 Serving/250g	62	1.5	25	1.9	3.0	0.6	2.2
Carrot & Sprouts, Microwaved, Fresh Tastes, Asda*	1 Pack/300g	150	0.9	50	1.9	8.7	0.3	2.3
Carrots, Peas & Sweetcorn, Steam, Tesco*	½ Pack/150g	150	4.2	100	3.4	15.0	2.8	3.2
Carrots, Sliced, & Broccoli Florets, Fresh, Morrisons*	1 Portion/100g	37	0.7	37	2.2	4.1	0.7	2.5
Casserole, Mixed, Co-Op*	1 Serving/100g	40	0.3	40	1.2	7.5	0.3	2.1
Chinese Inspired, Crisp, M & S*	1 Pack/250g	62	0.8	25	1.7	4.6	0.3	1.9
Crisp & Crunchy, Stir Fry, M & S*	½ Pack/115g	29	0.2	25	1.9	3.9	0.2	1.7
Crispy, Ready to Cook, Sainsbury's*	1 Serving/100g	24	0.3	24	1.8	3.6	0.3	2.2
Crush, Potato & Pea with Minted Butter, M & S*	½ Pack/200g	180	6.8	90	3.9	9.6	3.4	3.9
Farmhouse Mix, Frozen, Asda*	1 Serving/100g	25	0.8	25	2.5	2.2	0.8	0.0
Favourite Five Selection, M & S*	½ Pack/125g	25	0.8	20	1.8	2.4	0.6	2.9
Flower Sprout, M & S*	1 Portion/80g	36	1.2	45	3.0	8.7	1.5	2.5
for Roasting, M & S*	½ Pack/224g	190	12.5	85	1.2	7.7	5.6	2.4
Garden, Washed, Tesco*	1 Bag/250g	65	1.8	26	3.0	1.9	0.7	2.0
Green, Selection, Tender, Waitrose*	½ Pack/140g	66	1.1	47	3.9	3.8	0.8	3.8
Green Medley (Microwaved), Chosen By You, Asda*	1 Pack/220g	132	3.3	60	3.8	6.8	1.5	2.2
Italian, Roasted, M & S*	1 Serving/95g	218	20.0	230	1.8	7.1	21.0	1.7
Italiano Marinated, Roasted, Tesco*	½ Tub/100g	121	8.6	121	1.7	9.2	8.6	0.8
Julienne, Tesco*	1 Serving/100g	30	0.3	30	1.1	5.7	0.3	1.9
Kale, Spinach, Pak Choi & Jagallo Nero, Asda*	¼ Bag/45g	13	0.5	29	2.4	1.0	1.1	2.8
Layered, GFY, Asda*	½ Pack/150g	81	4.2	54	1.2	6.0	2.8	2.0
Layered, with Butter, Waitrose*	1 Pack/280g	207	16.2	74	1.7	3.6	5.8	2.4
Mediterranean, in Tomato Sauce, COU, M & S*	1 Pack/300g	105	2.1	35	2.5	4.3	0.7	2.2
Mediterranean, Ready to Roast, Waitrose*	1 Serving/200g	128	8.0	64	1.3	5.6	4.0	1.6
Mediterranean, Roasted, Tesco*	½ Pack/173g	95	3.1	55	1.3	7.6	1.8	2.0
Mediterranean, Sainsbury's*	1 Pack/400g	180	9.6	45	1.2	4.5	2.4	3.1
Mediterranean Style, Asda*	½ Pack/205g	113	3.7	55	1.7	7.9	1.8	1.3
Mediterranean Style, Finest, Tesco*	½ Pack/150g	155	12.2	103	1.5	5.5	8.1	3.0
Mediterranean Style, Roasting, Tesco*	1 Serving/200g	72	2.0	36	1.1	5.7	1.0	1.3
Moroccan, COU, M & S*	1 Pack/300g	165	4.5	55	2.4	8.2	1.5	1.7
Oriental, Waitrose*	1 Pack/300g	108	0.6	36	0.8	7.8	0.2	1.4
Oriental Inspired, M & S*	1 Pack/260g	78	1.3	30	1.9	4.6	0.5	2.7
Oriental Soup, TTD, Sainsbury's*	1 Pack/200g	64	0.6	32	1.9	4.3	0.3	2.0
Ribbon, Pan Stir Fry, Love Life, Waitrose*	½ Pack/134g	47	0.5	35	1.3	5.4	0.4	2.4
Roast, M & S*	1 Pack/420g	273	17.6	65	1.4	4.9	4.2	0.4
Roasting, Tesco*	1 Serving/350g	152	1.9	43	1.2	8.0	0.5	3.0
Root, for Mashing, Eat Fresh, Tesco*	1 Pack/600g	246	2.4	41	0.9	7.2	0.4	2.6
Root, Honey Roast, BGTY, Sainsbury's*	½ Pack/150g	174	2.2	116	2.5	23.1	1.5	5.5
Root, Honey Roast, Sainsbury's*	1 Pack/400g	748	34.8	187	0.0	25.8	8.7	5.2
Root, Ready to Roast, Sainsbury's*	½ Pack/200g	188	8.6	94	1.3	13.0	4.3	2.2
Root, Roasted, Extra Special, Asda*	½ Pack/205g	160	3.1	78	1.1	15.0	1.5	6.0
Sea, Dried, Average	1 Serving/15g	14	0.3	94	11.0	8.0	2.0	48.1

V

	Measure INFO/WEIGHT	per Measure KCAL	FAT	Nutrition Values per 100g / 100ml KCAL	PROT	CARB	FAT	FIBRE
VEGETABLES								
Seasonal, Pack, Sainsbury's*	1 Serving/261g	60	0.8	23	0.7	4.6	0.3	2.0
Selection, Roasted, COU, M & S*	1 Pack/250g	88	2.0	35	1.2	6.1	0.8	0.6
Soup Mix, Fresh, Classic, Prepared, Tesco*	1/3 Pack/163g	60	1.0	37	1.1	5.3	0.6	2.8
Soup Mix, Prepared & Washed, Morrisons*	½ Pack/300g	117	1.2	39	1.1	7.3	0.4	1.1
Summer, Rainbow, Roasting, Fresh Tastes, Asda*	½ Pack/175g	84	4.7	48	1.4	3.5	2.7	0.0
Summer, Roasted, TTD, Sainsbury's*	½ Pack/200g	160	2.2	80	1.8	14.5	1.1	2.6
Summer, Roasting, Tesco*	½ Pack/175g	105	6.6	60	1.0	5.1	3.8	1.6
Sweet & Crunchy, Tesco*	1 Serving/50g	22	0.3	43	2.3	7.0	0.6	2.4
Szechuan Style, Ready Prepared, Waitrose*	1 Pack/300g	132	3.9	44	2.3	5.7	1.3	1.9
Trivoglio, Peas, Potatoes & Carrots, Canned, Bonduelle*	½ Can/200g	114	1.0	57	3.3	7.5	0.5	4.8
Vietnamese, Wok, Findus*	1 Serving/100g	25	0.5	25	1.5	4.5	0.5	0.0
Winter, Crunchy, M & S*	½ Pack/125g	31	1.0	25	2.0	3.1	0.8	2.7
Winter, Fresh, Asda*	1 Bag/250g	75	2.5	30	3.0	2.2	1.0	2.3
Winter, Ready to Roast, Fresh, Sainsbury's*	1 Pack/272g	226	7.6	83	1.2	13.2	2.8	0.0
Winter, Roasted, HL, Tesco*	½ Pack/200g	160	5.0	80	1.9	12.7	2.5	3.6
Winter, Sainsbury's*	1 Serving/125g	38	1.0	30	2.0	3.6	0.8	2.2
Winter, Soup Mix, Sainsbury's*	1 Portion/149g	61	0.3	41	1.1	7.9	0.2	1.7
Wok, Chinese, Stir Fry, Classic, Findus*	1 Pack/500g	150	2.5	30	1.0	5.0	0.5	3.5
Wok, Sambal Oelek, Findus*	1 Serving/200g	170	0.8	85	3.0	17.0	0.4	0.0
Wok, Thai, Findus*	½ Pack/250g	88	0.8	35	1.5	7.0	0.3	0.0
Wok Mix, Stir Fry, Frozen, Essential, Waitrose*	1 Serving/200g	60	0.4	30	1.2	4.0	0.2	3.4
VEGETARIAN								
Chicken Style Pieces, Sainsbury's*	1 Pack/375g	754	26.2	201	25.5	9.0	7.0	0.6
Fingers, Fish Style, Breaded, The Redwood Co*	1 Finger/36g	94	5.2	262	16.5	16.0	14.5	0.0
Nut & Date Roast with Gravy, Asda*	1 Serving/196g	300	12.7	153	4.7	16.1	6.5	5.5
Pepperoni Style, Cheatin', The Redwood Co*	1 Slice/10g	28	1.8	282	25.3	5.2	17.7	0.2
Roast, Chicken Style, Vegeroast, Realeat*	4 Slices/114g	211	10.2	186	23.0	3.2	9.0	1.5
Roast, Linda McCartney*	¼ Roast/114g	222	10.2	196	19.4	9.4	9.0	1.5
Sausage & Mash, 617, Wiltshire Farm Foods*	1 Serving/400g	377	18.5	94	5.1	8.7	4.6	2.0
Slices, Sage & Onion, Vegi Deli, The Redwood Co*	1 Slice/10g	23	1.4	233	21.4	5.0	14.1	0.5
Slices, Vegetable, Tesco*	1 Slice/165g	452	30.5	274	5.6	21.4	18.5	3.3
VEGETARIAN MINCE								
Chicken Style Pieces, Realeat*	¼ Pack/88g	119	1.4	136	29.0	1.5	1.6	4.4
Easy Cook, Linda McCartney*	1oz/28g	35	0.1	126	21.4	9.3	0.4	1.7
Frozen, Meatfree, Improved Recipe, Sainsbury's*	1 Pack/454g	799	31.8	176	18.3	10.7	7.0	6.7
Meat Free, Boiled, Chosen By You, Asda*	1 Serving/75g	83	2.5	111	13.7	6.7	3.3	4.4
Vegemince, Realeat*	1 Serving/125g	218	12.5	174	18.0	3.0	10.0	3.0
VENISON								
Grill Steak, Average	***1 Grillsteak/150g***	***178***	***3.8***	***119***	***19.0***	***5.0***	***2.5***	***1.0***
in Red Wine & Port, Average	1oz/28g	21	0.7	76	9.8	3.5	2.6	0.4
Minced, Cooked, Average	***1 Serving/100g***	***187***	***8.2***	***187***	***26.4***	***0.0***	***8.2***	***0.0***
Minced, Raw, Average	***1 Serving/100g***	***157***	***7.1***	***157***	***21.8***	***0.0***	***7.1***	***0.0***
Raw, Haunch, Meat Only, Average	1 Serving/100g	103	1.6	103	22.2	0.0	1.6	0.0
Roasted, Average	***1oz/28g***	***46***	***0.7***	***165***	***35.6***	***0.0***	***2.5***	***0.0***
Steak, Raw, Average	***1oz/28g***	***30***	***0.5***	***108***	***22.8***	***0.0***	***1.9***	***0.0***
VERMICELLI								
Dry	***1oz/28g***	***99***	***0.1***	***355***	***8.7***	***78.3***	***0.4***	***0.0***
Egg, Cooked, Average	***1 Serving/185g***	***239***	***2.6***	***129***	***5.0***	***24.0***	***1.4***	***1.0***
VERMOUTH								
Dry	***1 Shot/50ml***	***54***	***0.0***	***109***	***0.1***	***3.0***	***0.0***	***0.0***
Sweet	***1 Shot/50ml***	***76***	***0.0***	***151***	***0.0***	***15.9***	***0.0***	***0.0***
VIMTO*								
Cordial, No Added Sugar, Diluted, Vimto Soft Drinks*	1 Glass/250ml	6	0.2	2	0.1	0.4	0.1	0.0

	Measure INFO/WEIGHT	per Measure KCAL	per Measure FAT	KCAL	PROT	CARB	FAT	FIBRE
				Nutrition Values per 100g / 100ml				
VIMTO*								
Cordial, No Added Sugar, Undiluted, Vimto Soft Drinks*	1 Serving/50ml	2	0.0	4	0.0	0.7	0.0	0.0
Cordial, Original, Diluted, Vimto Soft Drinks*	1 Serving/200ml	60	0.0	30	0.0	7.4	0.0	0.0
Cordial, Original, Undiluted, Vimto Soft Drinks*	1 Serving/50ml	49	0.0	98	0.0	23.6	0.0	0.0
VINAIGRETTE								
Balsamic, Hellmann's*	1 Tbsp/15ml	12	0.4	82	0.1	9.6	2.7	0.6
Balsamic Vinegar & Pistachio, Finest, Tesco*	1 Tbsp/15ml	56	5.9	370	0.2	2.8	39.2	0.0
Blush Wine, Briannas*	2 Tbsp/30ml	100	6.0	333	0.0	40.0	20.0	0.0
Fat Free, Hellmann's*	1 Serving/15ml	7	0.0	49	0.1	10.9	0.0	0.3
Frank Cooper*	1 Pot/28g	46	3.2	163	1.0	14.1	11.4	0.3
French, Real, Briannas*	2 Tbsp/30ml	150	17.0	500	0.0	0.0	56.7	0.0
French Style, Finest, Tesco*	1 Tbsp/15ml	93	9.8	620	0.6	6.3	65.3	0.2
Luxury French, Hellmann's*	1 Tsp/5ml	15	1.3	305	0.8	16.0	26.1	0.4
Olive Oil & Lemon, Amoy*	½ Sachet/15ml	38	3.6	250	0.3	3.0	24.0	0.0
Perfectly Balanced, Waitrose*	1 Tsp/5ml	4	0.0	89	0.4	20.9	0.4	0.5
Portuguese, Nando's*	1 Tbsp/15g	61	6.6	409	1.0	2.0	44.0	0.3
Waistline, 99% Fat Free, Crosse & Blackwell*	1 Tbsp/15ml	1	0.0	9	1.0	0.7	0.2	0.2
VINE LEAVES								
Preserved in Brine	***1oz/28g***	***4***	***0.0***	***15***	***3.6***	***0.2***	***0.0***	***0.0***
Stuffed, Mediterranean Deli, M & S*	1 Leaf/37g	39	1.5	105	2.6	14.2	4.1	1.2
Stuffed, Sainsbury's*	1 Parcel/38g	46	2.1	124	2.9	15.3	5.7	3.1
Stuffed with Rice	1oz/28g	73	5.0	262	2.8	23.8	18.0	0.0
Stuffed with Rice, Palirria*	½ Pack/140g	186	9.0	133	2.2	16.6	6.4	0.0
VINEGAR								
Apple Balsamic, Aspall*	1 Serving/100g	123	0.1	123	0.5	26.1	0.1	0.0
Balsamic, Average	***1 Tsp/5ml***	***6***	***0.0***	***115***	***0.9***	***26.0***	***0.0***	***0.0***
Balsamic Reduction, Secret Kitchen*	1 Tsp/5ml	15	0.0	309	0.4	50.0	0.1	0.0
Cider	***1 Tbsp/15ml***	***2***	***0.0***	***14***	***0.0***	***5.9***	***0.0***	***0.0***
Cyder, Aspall*	1 fl oz/30ml	5	0.0	18	0.0	0.1	0.0	0.0
Malt, Average	***1 Tbsp/15g***	***1***	***0.0***	***4***	***0.4***	***0.6***	***0.0***	***0.0***
Red Wine, Aspall*	1 Serving/100g	22	0.0	22	0.4	0.6	0.0	0.0
Red Wine, Average	1 Tbsp/15ml	3	0.0	19	0.0	0.3	0.0	0.0
Red Wine, Organic, Aspall*	1 Serving/100g	20	0.0	20	0.3	0.0	0.0	0.0
Rice, Mizkan*	1 Tbsp/15ml	4	0.0	26	0.2	2.6	0.0	0.0
Rice, White, Amoy*	1 Tsp/5ml	0	0.0	4	0.0	1.0	0.0	0.0
VODKA								
& Tonic, Ready Mixed, M & S*	1 Can/250ml	202	0.0	81	0.0	6.3	0.0	0.0
37.5% Volume	***1 Shot/35ml***	***72***	***0.0***	***207***	***0.0***	***0.0***	***0.0***	***0.0***
40% Volume	***1 Shot/35ml***	***78***	***0.0***	***222***	***0.0***	***0.0***	***0.0***	***0.0***
Bullett & Cola, Premixed, Canned, Diageo*	1 Can/250ml	218	0.0	87	0.0	10.6	0.0	0.0
Smirnoff & Cola, Premixed, canned, Diageo*	1 Can/250ml	178	0.0	71	0.0	8.9	0.0	0.0
Smirnoff & Cranberry, Premixed, Canned, Diageo*	1 Can/250ml	175	0.0	70	0.0	8.5	0.0	0.0
Smirnoff & Diet Cola, Premixed, Canned, Diageo*	1 Can/250ml	100	0.0	40	0.0	0.0	0.0	0.0
VOL AU VENTS								
Broccoli, M & S*	1oz/28g	105	7.4	375	6.8	28.5	26.4	1.0
Chicken & Mushroom, M & S*	1oz/28g	98	6.8	350	7.7	25.2	24.3	2.1
Garlic Mushroom, Mini, Asda*	1 Serving/17g	59	4.6	347	5.0	21.0	27.0	0.0
Ham & Cheese, M & S*	1oz/28g	106	7.5	380	8.8	25.7	26.7	1.8
Mushroom, Sainsbury's*	1 Serving/14g	49	3.1	350	6.9	30.8	22.1	1.4
Mushroom & Roast Garlic, M & S*	1 Serving/19g	65	4.6	345	6.2	25.2	24.3	1.9
Prawn, M & S*	1oz/28g	101	6.9	360	8.0	26.2	24.7	1.9
Seafood, Party, Youngs*	1 Serving/17g	60	4.2	354	8.3	26.0	24.8	1.0
Tomato, M & S*	1oz/28g	87	5.7	310	4.5	26.7	20.4	1.7

	Measure INFO/WEIGHT	per Measure KCAL	FAT	Nutrition Values per 100g / 100ml KCAL	PROT	CARB	FAT	FIBRE
WAFERS								
Cafe Curls, Rolled, Askeys*	1 Wafer/5g	21	0.4	422	5.8	80.3	8.6	0.0
Caramel, Dark Chocolate, Tunnock's*	1 Wafer/26g	128	6.6	492	5.2	60.7	25.4	0.0
Caramel, M & S*	1oz/28g	136	6.6	486	5.4	63.1	23.5	0.5
Caramel, Milk Chocolate, M & S*	1oz/28g	133	6.4	475	5.9	61.9	22.8	3.1
Caramel, Tunnock's*	1 Wafer/26g	116	4.5	448	3.6	69.2	17.4	2.5
Caramel Log, Tunnock's*	1 Wafer/32g	152	7.7	474	4.2	64.3	24.0	0.0
Caramel Mallow, Weight Watchers*	1 Mallow/17g	55	0.4	329	5.5	63.9	2.1	17.8
Cheese Footballs, Jacob's*	1 Serving/25g	139	9.2	556	11.8	43.9	36.7	1.5
Chocolate, Cadbury*	1oz/28g	147	8.3	526	7.0	61.2	29.8	0.0
Cream, Tunnock's*	1 Wafer/20g	103	5.6	513	6.6	63.2	28.0	0.0
Filled, Average	1oz/28g	150	8.4	535	4.7	66.0	29.9	0.0
for Ice Cream, Askeys*	1 Wafer/2g	6	0.0	388	11.4	79.0	2.9	0.0
Stilton, Fudges*	¼ Pack/25g	133	9.8	533	15.8	34.7	39.2	1.6
WAFFLES								
Belgian, TTD, Sainsbury's*	1 Waffle/25g	122	7.3	490	6.0	50.6	29.3	1.2
Caramel, Asda*	1 Waffle/8g	37	1.8	459	3.3	62.0	22.0	1.1
Chocolate, Milk, Tregroes*	1 Waffle/49g	220	20.5	450	4.5	57.0	42.0	0.5
Sweet, American Style, Sainsbury's*	1 Waffle/35g	160	8.9	457	7.2	50.6	25.3	1.1
Toasting, McVitie's*	1 Waffle/25g	118	6.3	474	6.0	52.6	25.5	0.6
WAGON WHEEL								
Chocolate, Burton's*	1 Biscuit/39g	165	5.7	424	5.3	67.4	14.6	1.9
Jammie, Burton's*	1 Biscuit/40g	168	5.6	420	5.1	67.7	14.1	1.9
WALNUT WHIP								
Nestle*	1 Whip/35g	173	8.8	494	5.3	61.3	25.2	0.7
The, Classics, M & S*	1 Whip/26g	127	7.1	490	7.2	54.9	27.4	1.1
Vanilla, Nestle*	1 Whip/34g	165	8.4	486	5.7	60.5	24.6	0.0
WALNUTS								
Average	***1 Nut/7g***	***48***	***4.8***	***691***	***15.6***	***3.2***	***68.5***	***3.5***
Cocoa Cream, Dusted, Julian Graves*	1 Bag/200g	1124	70.6	562	8.2	52.9	35.3	2.0
Halves, Average	***1 Half/3g***	***23***	***2.3***	***669***	***17.4***	***6.3***	***65.0***	***4.7***
Wholesome, Organic, Kernels, Love Life, Waitrose*	1 Serving/30g	207	20.6	689	14.7	3.3	68.5	6.8
WASABI								
Paste, Ready Mixed, Japanese, Yutaka*	1 Tsp/5g	14	0.4	286	2.7	53.0	7.0	0.0
WATER								
Apple & Elderflower, Mineral, Hedgerow*	1 Serving/250ml	85	0.0	34	0.0	8.2	0.0	0.0
Apple & Raspberry Flavour, Sparkling, Spar*	1 Glass/250ml	2	0.0	1	0.0	0.0	0.0	0.0
Apple & Strawberry Flavoured, Morrisons*	1 Serving/200ml	3	0.0	2	0.2	0.1	0.0	0.0
Berry Blast, Revive, Volvic*	1 Bottle/500ml	10	0.0	2	0.3	0.4	0.0	0.0
Blackberry & Strawberry, Sparkling, Strathmore*	1 Glass/250ml	45	0.0	18	0.0	4.3	0.0	0.0
Blackcurrant, Touch of Fruit, Volvic*	1 Serving/250ml	42	0.0	17	0.0	4.0	0.0	0.0
Blackcurrants, Juicy, Innocent*	1 Bottle/420ml	155	0.4	37	0.1	8.7	0.1	0.0
Cranberries & Raspberries, Juicy, Innocent*	1 Bottle/380ml	118	1.1	31	0.1	6.7	0.3	0.0
Cranberry & Blueberry, Lightly Sparkling, Waitrose*	1 Glass/250ml	10	0.0	4	0.0	0.7	0.0	0.0
Cranberry & Raspberry Still, MacB*	1 Bottle/500ml	4	0.0	1	0.1	0.0	0.0	0.0
Elderflower & Pear, Detox, V Water*	1 Bottle/500ml	40	0.0	8	0.0	1.9	0.0	0.0
Elderflower Presse, Bottle Green*	1 Serving/250ml	88	0.0	35	0.0	8.9	0.0	0.0
Grapefruit, Slightly Sparkling, Tesco*	1 Serving/200ml	4	0.0	2	0.0	0.2	0.0	0.0
Green Tea, De-Stress, V Water*	1 Bottle/500ml	40	0.0	8	0.0	1.9	0.0	0.0
Lemon, Vittel*	1 Bottle/500ml	6	0.0	1	0.0	0.0	0.0	0.0
Lemon & Lime, Shield, Sobe V Water*	1 Bottle/500ml	85	0.5	17	0.0	3.9	0.1	0.0
Lemon & Lime, Sparkling, M & S*	1 Bottle/500ml	15	0.0	3	0.0	0.4	0.0	0.0
Lemon & Lime, Still, M & S*	1 Bottle/500ml	5	0.0	1	0.0	0.2	0.0	0.0
Lemon & Lime, Sugar Free, Touch of Fruit, Volvic*	1 Bottle/150ml	2	0.0	1	0.0	0.0	0.0	0.0

	Measure INFO/WEIGHT	per Measure KCAL	FAT	Nutrition Values per 100g / 100ml KCAL	PROT	CARB	FAT	FIBRE
WATER								
Lemons & Limes, Spring Water, This Juicy Water*	1 Bottle/420ml	160	0.4	38	0.2	9.5	0.1	0.0
Life, Sparkling, Abokado*	1 Serving/500ml	0	0.0	0	0.0	0.0	0.0	0.0
Life, Still, Abokado*	1 Serving/500ml	0	0.0	0	0.0	0.0	0.0	0.0
Mandarin & Cranberry, Still, M & S*	1 Bottle/500ml	100	0.0	20	0.0	5.0	0.0	0.0
Mineral, Energy, Vittel*	1 fl oz/30ml	7	0.0	23	0.0	5.5	0.0	0.0
Mineral Or Tap	***1 Glass/200ml***	***0***	***0.0***	***0***	***0.0***	***0.0***	***0.0***	***0.0***
Orange & Passion Fruit, Vital V, V Water*	1 Bottle/500ml	45	0.0	9	0.0	2.1	0.0	0.0
Peach & Lemon, Still, M & S*	1 Bottle/500ml	100	0.0	20	0.0	5.0	0.0	0.0
Peach & Orange Flavoured, Morrisons*	1 Serving/200ml	3	0.0	2	0.2	0.1	0.0	0.0
Peach & Raspberry, Still, M & S*	1 Bottle/500ml	10	0.0	2	0.0	0.0	0.0	0.0
Pomegranate & Blueberry, Glow, V Water*	1 Bottle/500ml	40	0.0	8	0.0	2.0	0.0	0.0
Skinny, Bo-Synergy*	1 Bottle/500ml	9	0.0	2	0.0	0.3	0.0	0.0
Sparkling, Blueberry & Pomegranate, M & S*	1 Glass/250ml	5	0.0	2	0.0	0.4	0.0	0.0
Sparkling, Fruit, Aqua Libra*	1 Glass/200ml	54	0.0	27	0.0	5.1	0.0	0.0
Sparkling, San Pellegrino*	1 Glass/200ml	0	0.0	0	0.0	0.0	0.0	0.0
Spring, Apple & Blackcurrant, Hadrian*	1 Bottle/365ml	3	0.0	1	0.1	0.1	0.0	0.0
Spring, Apple & Raspberry, Shapers, Boots*	1 Bottle/500ml	10	0.0	2	0.0	0.2	0.0	0.0
Spring, Apple & Raspberry Flavoured, Sainsbury's*	1 fl oz/30ml	1	0.0	2	0.1	0.1	0.1	0.1
Spring, Blackberry & Blueberry Flavoured, Sainsbury's*	1 Serving/1000ml	20	1.0	2	0.1	0.2	0.1	0.1
Spring, Elderflower & Pear, Sainsbury's*	1 Glass/250g	5	0.2	2	0.1	0.2	0.1	0.1
Spring, Lemon & Lime, Slightly Sparkling, Tesco*	1 Serving/200ml	4	0.2	2	0.1	0.2	0.1	0.1
Spring, Orange & Passionfruit, Drench*	1 Serving/250ml	95	0.5	38	0.1	9.0	0.2	0.0
Spring, Raspberry & Cranberry, Shapers, Boots*	1 Bottle/500ml	10	0.0	2	0.0	0.5	0.0	0.0
Spring, Strawberry, Sparkling, Tesco*	1 Bottle/1000g	20	0.0	2	0.0	0.2	0.0	0.0
Spring, Strawberry & Kiwi, Still, Shapers, Boots*	1 Glass/250ml	2	0.0	1	0.0	0.1	0.0	0.9
Spring, Strawberry & Vanilla, Sainsbury's*	1 Glass/250ml	5	0.2	2	0.1	0.2	0.1	0.1
Spring, White Grape & Blackberry, Tesco*	1 Glass/200ml	4	0.0	2	0.0	0.5	0.0	0.0
Spring, with a Hint of Orange, Slightly Sparkling, Tesco*	1 Serving/250ml	5	0.0	2	0.0	0.2	0.0	0.0
Spring, with Grapefruit, Tesco*	1 Serving/200ml	4	0.0	2	0.0	0.2	0.0	0.0
Strawberry, Original, Touch of Fruit, Volvic*	1 Bottle/500ml	99	0.0	20	0.0	4.8	0.0	0.0
Strawberry, Sugar Free, Touch of Fruit, Volvic*	1 Bottle/500ml	7	0.0	1	0.0	0.1	0.0	0.0
Strawberry & Guava, Still, M & S*	1 Glass/250ml	5	0.0	2	0.0	0.1	0.0	0.0
Vitamin, Xxx, Triple Berry, Glaceau, Coca-Cola*	1 Bottle/500ml	95	0.0	19	0.0	4.6	0.0	0.0
WaterVit, Refresh & Revive, Shapers, Boots*	1 Bottle/500ml	10	0.0	2	0.0	0.2	0.0	0.0
WATER CHESTNUTS								
Raw, Average	***1oz/28g***	***10***	***0.0***	***34***	***1.0***	***7.8***	***0.0***	***0.1***
with Bamboo Shoots, Sainsbury's*	1 Serving/50g	29	0.1	58	2.0	12.0	0.2	1.1
WATER ICE								
Cubes	1 Serving/100g	0	0.0	0	0.0	0.0	0.0	0.0
Orange, Iceland*	1 Ice/75ml	73	0.0	98	0.2	24.4	0.0	0.2
Raspberry, Iceland*	1 Ice/75ml	67	0.0	89	0.0	22.2	0.0	0.2
WATERCRESS								
Baby, Steve's Leaves*	1 Bag/40g	10	0.2	25	2.6	2.5	0.5	2.1
Raw, Trimmed, Average	***1 Sprig/3g***	***1***	***0.0***	***22***	***3.0***	***0.4***	***1.0***	***1.5***
WATERMELON								
Flesh Only, Average	***1 Serving/250g***	***75***	***0.8***	***30***	***0.4***	***7.0***	***0.3***	***0.4***
Raw	***1 Wedge/286g***	***92***	***1.2***	***32***	***0.6***	***7.2***	***0.4***	***0.5***
Raw, Weighed with Skin, Average	1 Serving/100g	30	0.3	30	0.4	7.0	0.3	0.4
WHEAT								
Whole Grain, Split, Average	***1 Serving/60g***	***205***	***1.0***	***342***	***11.3***	***75.9***	***1.7***	***12.2***
WHEAT BRAN								
Average	***1 Tbsp/7g***	***14***	***0.4***	***206***	***14.1***	***26.8***	***5.5***	***36.4***
Coarse, Holland & Barrett*	1 Tbsp/4g	8	0.2	206	14.1	26.8	5.5	36.4

	Measure INFO/WEIGHT	per Measure KCAL	FAT	Nutrition Values per 100g / 100ml KCAL	PROT	CARB	FAT	FIBRE
WHEAT BRAN								
Natural, Jordans*	1 Tbsp/7g	13	0.4	188	16.3	17.4	5.9	44.5
WHEAT CRUNCHIES								
Golden Wonder*	1 Pack/35g	172	8.7	491	11.1	55.9	24.8	0.0
Salt & Vinegar, Golden Wonder*	1 Bag/34g	165	8.5	484	10.5	54.5	24.9	2.8
Worcester Sauce, Golden Wonder*	1 Bag/35g	172	8.9	492	9.3	56.4	25.5	3.9
WHEAT GERM								
Average	***1oz/28g***	***100***	***2.6***	***357***	***26.7***	***44.7***	***9.2***	***15.6***
Natural, Jordans*	2 Tbsp/16g	54	1.5	340	28.0	36.0	9.3	13.1
WHELKS								
Boiled, Weighed without Shell	***1oz/28g***	***25***	***0.3***	***89***	***19.5***	***0.0***	***1.2***	***0.0***
WHISKEY								
Irish, Jameson*	1 Shot/25ml	58	0.0	233	0.0	0.0	0.0	0.0
Jack Daniel's*	1 Shot/35ml	78	0.0	222	0.0	0.0	0.0	0.0
WHISKY								
37.5% Volume	***1 Shot/35ml***	***72***	***0.0***	***207***	***0.0***	***0.0***	***0.0***	***0.0***
40% Volume	***1 Shot/35ml***	***78***	***0.0***	***222***	***0.0***	***0.0***	***0.0***	***0.0***
Bells & Ginger Ale, Premixed, Canned, Diageo*	1 Can/250ml	170	0.0	68	0.0	7.6	0.0	0.0
Scots, 37.5% Volume	***1 Shot/35ml***	***72***	***0.0***	***207***	***0.0***	***0.0***	***0.0***	***0.0***
Scots, 40% Volume	***1 Shot/35ml***	***78***	***0.0***	***224***	***0.0***	***0.0***	***0.0***	***0.0***
Teacher's*	1 Shot/35ml	78	0.0	222	0.0	0.0	0.0	0.0
WHITE PUDDING								
Average	***1oz/28g***	***126***	***8.9***	***450***	***7.0***	***36.3***	***31.8***	***0.0***
WHITEBAIT								
in Flour, Fried	***1oz/28g***	***147***	***13.3***	***525***	***19.5***	***5.3***	***47.5***	***0.2***
Raw, Average	1 Serving/100g	172	11.0	172	18.3	0.0	11.0	0.0
WHITECURRANTS								
Raw, Average	***1oz/28g***	***7***	***0.0***	***26***	***1.3***	***5.6***	***0.0***	***3.4***
WHITING								
in Crumbs, Fried in Blended Oil	1 Serving/180g	344	18.5	191	18.1	7.0	10.3	0.2
Raw	***1oz/28g***	***23***	***0.2***	***81***	***18.7***	***0.0***	***0.7***	***0.0***
Steamed	***1 Serving/85g***	***78***	***0.8***	***92***	***20.9***	***0.0***	***0.9***	***0.0***
WIENER SCHNITZEL								
Average	1oz/28g	62	2.8	223	20.9	13.1	10.0	0.4
WINE								
Cherry, Lambrini*	1 Sm Glass/125ml	80	0.0	64	0.0	0.0	0.0	0.0
Diet, Lambrini*	1 Sm Glass/125ml	43	0.0	35	0.0	0.0	0.0	0.0
Fruit, Average	***1 Sm Glass/125ml***	***115***	***0.0***	***92***	***0.0***	***5.5***	***0.0***	***0.0***
Madeira, Henriques & Henriques*	1 Glass/100ml	130	0.0	130	0.0	0.0	0.0	0.0
Mulled, Homemade, Average	***1 Sm Glass/125ml***	***245***	***0.0***	***196***	***0.1***	***25.2***	***0.0***	***0.0***
Original, Lambrini*	1 Glass/125ml	88	0.0	70	0.0	0.0	0.0	0.0
Red, Amarone, Average*	1 Sm Glass/125ml	120	0.0	96	0.1	3.0	0.0	0.0
Red, Average	***1 Sm Glass/125ml***	***104***	***0.0***	***83***	***0.0***	***2.0***	***0.0***	***0.0***
Red, Burgundy, 12.9% Abv, Average	1 Sm Glass/125ml	110	0.0	88	0.1	3.7	0.0	0.0
Red, Cabernet Sauvignon, 13.1% Abv, Average	1 Sm Glass/125ml	105	0.0	84	0.1	2.6	0.0	0.0
Red, Cabernet Sauvigon, Non Alcoholic, Ariel*	1 Serving/240ml	50	0.0	21	0.0	4.8	0.0	0.0
Red, California, Blossom Hill*	1 Glass/175ml	132	0.0	75	0.0	0.9	0.0	0.0
Red, Claret, 12.8% Abv, Average	1 Sm Glass/125ml	105	0.0	84	0.1	3.0	0.0	0.0
Red, Gamay, 12.3% Abv, Average	1 Sm Glass/125ml	99	0.0	79	0.1	2.4	0.0	0.0
Red, Long Slim, Co-Op*	1 Glass/125ml	90	0.0	72	0.0	0.0	0.0	0.0
Red, Low Calorie, Asda*	1 Sm Glass/125ml	49	0.0	39	0.0	0.1	0.0	0.0
Red, Merlot, 13.3% Abv, Average	1 Sm Glass/125ml	105	0.0	84	0.1	2.5	0.0	0.0
Red, Non Alcoholic, Ame*	1 Sm Glass/125ml	42	0.0	34	0.0	5.7	0.0	0.0
Red, Petit Sirah, 13.5% Abv, Average	1 Sm Glass/125ml	108	0.0	86	0.1	2.7	0.0	0.0

	Measure INFO/WEIGHT	per Measure KCAL	FAT	Nutrition Values per 100g / 100ml KCAL	PROT	CARB	FAT	FIBRE
WINE								
Red, Pinot Noir, 13% Abv, Average	1 Sm Glass/125ml	104	0.0	83	0.1	2.3	0.0	0.0
Red, Sangiovese, 13.6% Abv, Average	1 Sm Glass/125ml	109	0.0	87	0.1	2.6	0.0	0.0
Red, Smooth, Weight Watchers*	1 Glass/125ml	75	0.1	60	0.1	1.4	0.1	0.1
Red, Syrah, 13.1% Abv, Average	1 Sm Glass/125ml	105	0.0	84	0.1	2.6	0.0	0.0
Red, Zinfandel, 13.9% Abv, Average	1 Sm Glass/125ml	111	0.0	89	0.1	2.9	0.0	0.0
Rose, Medium, Average	***1 Sm Glass/125ml***	***98***	***0.0***	***79***	***0.0***	***2.1***	***0.0***	***0.0***
Rose, Refreshing, Weight Watchers*	1 Glass/125ml	80	0.0	64	0.0	1.6	0.0	0.0
Rose, Sparkling, Average	1 Sm Glass/125ml	102	0.0	82	0.0	2.5	0.0	0.0
Rose, The Pink Chill, Co-Op*	1 Glass/125ml	85	0.0	68	0.0	0.0	0.0	0.0
Rose, Weight Watchers*	1 Bottle/187ml	112	0.2	60	0.1	1.8	0.1	0.1
Rose, White Grenache, Blossom Hill*	1 Glass/125ml	105	0.0	84	0.0	3.2	0.0	0.0
Rose, White Zinfandel, Ernest & Julio Gallo*	1 Glass/125ml	101	0.0	81	0.2	2.7	0.0	0.0
Sangria, Average	1 Glass/125ml	95	0.0	76	0.1	9.9	0.0	0.1
Vie, Rose, Low Alcohol, Blossom Hill*	1 Glass/175ml	93	0.0	53	0.0	3.9	0.0	0.0
White, Average	1 Sm Glass/125ml	95	0.0	76	0.0	2.4	0.0	0.0
White, Californian, Chardonnay, LC, Tesco*	1 Bottle/181ml	96	0.0	53	0.0	1.8	0.0	0.0
White, Chardonnay, Low Alcohol, McGuigan*	1 Glass/125ml	75	0.1	60	0.1	2.2	0.1	0.0
White, Chardonnay, Southern Australia, Kissing Tree*	1 Bottle/185ml	85	0.0	46	0.0	0.0	0.0	0.0
White, Chenin Blanc, 12% Abv, Average	1 Sm Glass/125ml	101	0.0	81	0.1	3.3	0.0	0.0
White, Dry, Average	***1 Glass/125ml***	***88***	***0.0***	***70***	***0.1***	***0.6***	***0.0***	***0.0***
White, Fume Blanc, 13.1% Abv, Average	1 Sm Glass/125ml	104	0.0	83	0.1	2.3	0.0	0.0
White, Gewurztraminer, 12.6% Abv, Average	1 Sm Glass/125ml	102	0.0	82	0.1	2.6	0.0	0.0
White, Late Harvest, 10.6% Abv, Average	1 Sm Glass/125ml	141	0.0	113	0.1	13.4	0.0	0.0
White, Medium, Average	***1 Sm Glass/125ml***	***92***	***0.0***	***74***	***0.1***	***3.0***	***0.0***	***0.0***
White, Muller-Thurgau, 11.3% Abv, Average	1 Sm Glass/125ml	96	0.0	77	0.1	3.5	0.0	0.0
White, Muscat, 11% Abv, Average	1 Sm Glass/125ml	104	0.0	83	0.1	5.2	0.0	0.0
White, Non Alcoholic, Ame*	1 Sm Glass/125ml	48	0.0	38	0.0	9.5	0.0	0.0
White, Pinot Blanc, 13.3% Abv, Average	1 Sm Glass/125ml	102	0.0	82	0.1	0.0	0.0	0.0
White, Pinot Grigio, 13.4% Abv, Average	1 Sm Glass/125ml	105	0.0	84	0.1	2.1	0.0	0.0
White, Riesling, 11.9% Abv, Average	1 Sm Glass/125ml	101	0.0	81	0.1	3.7	0.0	0.0
White, Sauvignon Blanc, 13.1% Abv, Average	1 Sm Glass/125ml	102	0.0	82	0.1	2.0	0.0	0.0
White, Semillon, 12.5% Abv, Average	1 Sm Glass/125ml	104	0.0	83	0.1	3.1	0.0	0.0
White, Sparkling, Average	***1 Sm Glass/125ml***	***92***	***0.0***	***74***	***0.3***	***5.1***	***0.0***	***0.0***
White, Sweet, Average	***1 Glass/120ml***	***113***	***0.0***	***94***	***0.2***	***5.9***	***0.0***	***0.0***
WINE GUMS								
Average	1 Sweet/6g	19	0.0	315	5.0	73.4	0.2	0.1
Haribo*	1 Pack/175g	609	0.4	348	0.1	86.4	0.2	0.4
Light, Maynards*	1 Pack/42g	90	0.1	215	4.6	48.0	0.2	27.9
Mini, Co-Op*	1 Sweet/2g	7	0.0	330	6.0	76.0	0.1	0.0
Mini, Rowntree's*	1 Sm Bag/36g	125	0.0	348	6.7	80.5	0.0	0.0
Sour, Bassett's*	¼ Bag/50g	160	0.0	319	3.7	78.0	0.0	0.0
WINKLES								
Boiled	***1oz/28g***	***20***	***0.3***	***72***	***15.4***	***0.0***	***1.2***	***0.0***
WISPA								
Bite, with Biscuit in Caramel, Cadbury*	1 Bar/47g	240	13.4	510	6.4	56.9	28.6	0.0
Cadbury*	1 Bar/40g	210	12.9	525	6.8	53.0	32.2	0.8
Gold, Cadbury*	1 Bar/52g	265	15.1	510	5.3	56.0	29.0	0.7
Mint, Cadbury*	1 Bar/50g	275	16.8	550	7.0	54.7	33.6	0.0
WONTON								
Prawn, Crispy from Selection, Modern Asian, M & S*	1 Wonton/25g	65	3.3	250	9.5	23.4	12.7	2.0
Prawn, Dim Sum Selection, Sainsbury's*	1 Wonton/10g	26	1.2	259	11.3	26.8	11.8	1.3
Prawn, Oriental Selection, Waitrose*	1 Wonton/18g	45	2.0	252	9.1	29.2	11.0	1.1
Prawn, Oriental Snack Selection, Sainsbury's*	1 Wonton/20g	53	2.7	265	10.6	25.6	13.4	2.0

	Measure INFO/WEIGHT	per Measure KCAL	FAT	Nutrition Values per 100g / 100ml KCAL	PROT	CARB	FAT	FIBRE
WOTSITS*								
Baked, Really Cheesy, Walkers*	1 Bag/23g	123	7.4	547	5.5	56.0	33.0	1.1
BBQ, Walkers*	1 Bag/21g	108	6.3	515	4.5	57.0	30.0	1.3
Flamin' Hot, Walkers*	1 Bag/19g	101	5.7	532	5.5	60.0	30.0	1.1
Prawn Cocktail, Walkers*	1 Bag/19g	99	5.7	522	4.5	58.0	30.0	1.1
Really Cheesy, Big Eat, Walkers*	1 Bag/36g	197	11.9	547	5.5	56.0	33.0	1.1
WRAP								
All Day Breakfast, M & S*	1 Pack/196g	529	31.4	270	10.8	21.2	16.0	1.4
American Deli, Shapers, Boots*	1 Pack/172g	249	4.5	145	9.5	21.0	2.6	2.0
BBQ Beef, Ginsters*	1 Pack/210g	404	12.2	192	6.7	28.4	5.8	1.8
Bean & Cheese, Average	1 Pack/200g	365	13.5	182	7.4	22.6	6.8	2.5
Beef, in Black Bean, M & S*	1 Pack/150g	338	17.1	225	10.2	20.5	11.4	1.6
Brie & Cranberry, M & S*	1 Pack/225g	550	27.8	245	6.1	27.3	12.4	1.7
Butternut Squash, COU, M & S*	1 Pack/182g	245	4.7	135	4.3	22.2	2.6	2.9
Caesar, Chicken, Tesco*	1 Pack/215g	516	24.3	240	11.6	23.0	11.3	1.2
Caesar, Chicken, Weight Watchers*	1 Pack/173g	298	4.7	172	11.2	24.5	2.7	1.3
Cajun, GFY, Asda*	1 Pack/176g	231	2.1	131	9.0	21.0	1.2	0.9
Cheese, Fiery, Ginsters*	1 Pack/210g	424	17.6	202	6.8	24.8	8.4	1.8
Cheese, Soft, & Spinach, to Go*	1 Serving/250g	278	6.7	111	4.5	17.4	2.7	0.0
Chicken, Barbecue, GFY, Asda*	1 Pack/176g	294	4.4	167	9.6	26.4	2.5	1.8
Chicken, Barbecue, Shapers, Boots*	1 Pack/181g	283	4.9	156	10.0	23.0	2.7	3.3
Chicken, Cajun, Sandwich King*	1 Pack/138g	386	19.9	279	12.3	25.0	14.4	0.0
Chicken, Cajun, Tesco*	1 Pack/184g	415	16.6	225	9.8	25.1	9.0	1.9
Chicken, Chargrilled, Perfectly Balanced, Waitrose*	1 Pack/230g	361	6.7	157	10.3	22.7	2.9	2.9
Chicken, Chilli, BGTY, Sainsbury's*	1 Pack/180g	313	4.3	174	10.2	28.0	2.4	0.0
Chicken, Chinese, M & S*	1 Pack/155g	239	1.6	154	14.0	22.3	1.0	2.0
Chicken, Italian, Sainsbury's*	½ Pack/211g	395	23.2	187	15.7	6.2	11.0	0.9
Chicken, M & S*	1 Pack/247g	530	24.9	215	8.2	23.4	10.1	1.6
Chicken, Mediterranean Style, Waitrose*	1 Pack/183g	296	11.0	162	8.3	18.6	6.0	2.3
Chicken, Mexican, M & S*	1 Serving/218g	447	22.5	205	8.6	19.7	10.3	1.3
Chicken, Moroccan, BGTY, Sainsbury's*	1 Pack/207g	315	3.1	152	9.4	25.3	1.5	0.0
Chicken, Moroccan, Shapers, Boots*	1 Serving/154g	251	2.3	163	10.0	27.0	1.5	1.9
Chicken, Nacho, No Mayo, Asda*	1 Pack/183g	392	13.9	214	12.0	24.3	7.6	3.1
Chicken, Red Thai, BGTY, Sainsbury's*	1 Pack/194g	384	7.6	198	11.3	29.3	3.9	1.0
Chicken, Red Thai, Shapers, Boots*	1 Pack/172g	234	3.6	136	9.5	20.0	2.1	2.4
Chicken, Salsa, LC, Tesco*	1 Pack/219g	340	5.9	155	9.7	22.6	2.7	1.9
Chicken, Southern Style, Ginsters*	1 Wrap/210g	491	22.0	234	6.4	28.3	10.5	1.8
Chicken, Sweet & Sour, Ginsters*	1 Pack/150g	378	5.8	252	13.4	40.8	3.9	2.4
Chicken, Tasties*	1 Pack/149g	324	10.6	218	11.7	26.5	7.1	0.0
Chicken, Thai, Spiced, Salad, Eat Well, M & S*	1 Pack/122g	92	1.5	75	5.2	9.5	1.2	1.5
Chicken, Thai Style, Boots*	1 Pack/156g	290	10.0	186	11.0	21.0	6.4	2.2
Chicken, with Stilton & Pear, Sainsbury's*	1 Serving/150g	264	11.0	176	25.4	2.1	7.3	0.1
Chicken & Bacon, Caesar, COU, M & S*	1 Pack/170g	260	4.2	153	10.6	22.0	2.5	2.1
Chicken & Bacon, Caesar Salad, Asda*	1 Pack/160g	565	35.2	353	18.0	20.8	22.0	0.9
Chicken & Bacon, Simple Solutions, Tesco*	1 Pack/300g	474	23.4	158	20.7	1.2	7.8	0.5
Chicken & Cous Cous, Moroccan Style, GFY, Asda*	1 Pack/164g	307	2.0	187	12.0	32.0	1.2	1.8
Chicken & Sweetfire Pepper, LC, Tesco*	1 Wrap/175g	350	7.9	200	10.2	28.5	4.5	1.4
Chicken Jalfrezi, Boots*	1 Pack/215g	456	15.7	212	8.6	28.0	7.3	1.7
Chicken Korma, Patak's*	1 Pack/150g	294	14.2	196	7.6	20.0	9.5	0.0
Chicken Nacho, HL, Tesco*	1 Pack/223g	390	10.0	175	12.3	21.2	4.5	2.6
Chicken Salad, Roast, Sainsbury's*	1 Pack/214g	443	19.9	207	10.0	20.9	9.3	2.5
Chicken Tikka, Average	1 Wrap/200g	403	15.1	202	9.5	23.6	7.6	4.4
Chicken Tikka Masala, Patak's*	1 Pack/150g	252	9.9	168	7.8	19.3	6.6	0.0
Chilli Bean & Cheese, Meat Free, Asda*	1 Wrap/151g	263	7.1	174	7.9	25.1	4.7	4.9

	Measure INFO/WEIGHT	per Measure KCAL	FAT	Nutrition Values per 100g / 100ml KCAL	PROT	CARB	FAT	FIBRE
WRAP								
Chilli Beef, Co-Op*	1 Pack/163g	310	9.8	190	10.0	26.0	6.0	2.0
Chilli Beef, COU, M & S*	1 Pack/179g	268	2.9	150	10.1	23.4	1.6	2.6
Cous Cous, Moroccan Style, Tesco*	1 Serving/240g	370	6.5	154	5.3	27.2	2.7	1.2
Crayfish, & Rocket, HL, Tesco*	1 Pack/164g	270	5.1	165	7.5	25.9	3.1	1.9
Crayfish, Lemon Dressing & Rocket, COU, M & S*	1 Pack/183g	274	4.9	150	9.5	22.5	2.7	1.2
Crunchy Lunch, Cranks*	1 Pack/212g	463	21.2	218	5.7	25.0	10.0	2.8
Duck, Food to Go, M & S*	1 Pack/257g	475	13.9	185	8.5	25.5	5.4	1.0
Duck, Hoi Sin, Delicious, Boots*	1 Pack/160g	295	4.3	184	11.0	28.0	2.7	2.0
Duck, Hoisin, M & S*	1 Pack/225g	405	8.3	180	8.4	27.7	3.7	1.5
Duck, Hoisin, No Mayo, Triple, Tesco*	1 Pack/270g	620	18.6	230	9.3	30.7	6.9	2.3
Egg Mayonnaise, Tomato & Cress, Sainsbury's*	1 Pack/255g	592	38.2	232	7.3	17.7	15.0	0.0
Fajita, Chicken, Asda*	1 Pack/180g	369	16.9	205	9.4	20.6	9.4	0.4
Fajita, Chicken, Daily Bread*	1 Pack/191g	392	10.5	205	9.4	29.4	5.5	0.0
Fajita, Chicken, Finest, Tesco*	1 Pack/213g	422	15.6	198	9.0	24.0	7.3	1.9
Fajita, Chicken, Perfectly Balanced, Waitrose*	1 Serving/218g	368	5.7	169	10.5	26.0	2.6	1.9
Fajita, Chicken, VLH Kitchens	1 Serving/170g	311	3.1	183	10.6	25.0	5.2	0.0
Fajita, Steak, Delicatessen, Waitrose*	1 Pack/232g	489	21.1	211	10.5	22.7	9.1	2.7
Feta Cheese, GFY, Asda*	1 Pack/165g	256	7.1	155	7.0	22.0	4.3	2.1
Goats Cheese, & Grilled Pepper, Asda*	1 Serving/75g	194	11.2	259	5.0	26.0	15.0	2.1
Greek Feta, Tortilla, Shapers, Boots*	1 Pack/169g	271	4.6	160	6.7	27.0	2.7	1.6
Greek Salad, COU, M & S*	1 Pack/180g	288	4.9	160	6.0	27.2	2.7	2.3
Greek Salad, Feta, Shapers, Boots*	1 Pack/158g	241	5.7	153	6.4	24.0	3.6	1.2
Greek Salad, M & S*	1 Pack/179g	250	4.5	140	8.1	21.5	2.5	1.0
Greek Salad, Sainsbury's*	1 Pack/167g	242	6.2	145	6.7	21.2	3.7	1.8
Ham, Cheese & Pickle Tortilla, Weight Watchers*	1 Pack/170g	296	4.8	174	10.9	26.4	2.8	1.2
Houmous, & Chargrilled Vegetables, Shapers, Boots*	1 Pack/186g	301	5.0	162	5.8	29.0	2.7	3.2
Houmous, Royal London Hospital*	1 Pack/200g	318	13.4	159	6.3	20.0	6.7	0.0
Houmous, Taste!*	1 Pack/170g	291	8.3	171	5.4	26.4	4.9	0.0
King Prawn, Shapers, Boots*	1 Pack/154g	227	2.2	147	9.2	24.0	1.4	2.1
Nacho Chicken, COU, M & S*	1 Pack/175g	280	4.2	160	10.2	24.4	2.4	2.0
Peking Duck, Average	1 Serving/183g	356	10.5	194	9.2	26.6	5.7	1.1
Prawn, & Rocket, Shapers, Boots*	1 Wrap/159g	218	4.1	137	7.6	19.0	2.6	3.0
Salmon, Smoked, & Prawn, Finest, Tesco*	1 Serving/59g	84	5.3	143	14.3	1.0	9.1	0.0
Salmon, Smoked, Finest, Tesco*	1 Pack/58g	113	8.4	194	15.5	0.6	14.4	0.3
Selection, Chicken, BBQ Steak, Hoisin Duck, M & S*	1 Pack/334g	685	23.7	205	10.9	24.3	7.1	1.7
Sunny Side Up, Cranks*	1 Pack/195g	423	18.9	217	7.8	23.3	9.7	1.7
Sushi Salmon & Cucumber, Waitrose*	1 Pack/180g	299	6.5	166	6.3	27.2	3.6	1.6
Sweet Chilli & King Prawn, COU, M & S*	1 Pack/155g	225	2.6	145	8.0	24.2	1.7	2.1
Sweet Chilli Chicken, Shapers, Boots*	1 Pack/195g	302	3.7	155	10.0	24.0	1.9	3.0
Sweet Chilli Chicken, Waitrose*	1 Pack/200g	390	14.7	195	10.2	22.0	7.4	2.4
Sweet Chilli King Prawn, M & S*	1 Pack/155g	225	3.1	145	8.0	24.2	2.0	2.1
Sweet Chilli Noodle, Sainsbury's*	1 Pack/210g	399	10.1	190	10.6	26.1	4.8	2.1
Three Bean, Mexican, M & S*	1 Pack/188g	405	19.2	215	6.9	24.3	10.2	2.2
Tortilla, BGTY, Sainsbury's*	1 Tortilla/50g	136	1.4	271	7.9	53.7	2.7	1.9
Tortilla, Chicken, Asda*	1 Pack/125g	252	2.2	202	9.6	36.9	1.8	3.3
Tortilla, Chicken Fajita, Sutherland*	1 Pack/158g	379	14.2	240	13.0	27.0	9.0	0.0
Tortilla, LC, Tesco*	1 Tortilla/64g	166	1.3	260	7.1	53.2	2.1	3.5
Tortilla, Mexican, Ainsley Harriott*	1 Pack/230g	421	17.2	183	7.1	22.4	7.5	0.0
Tortilla, Vegetable, Asda*	1 Pack/125g	245	2.8	196	6.8	37.2	2.2	0.8
Turkey, Bacon & Cranberry, COU, M & S*	1 Pack/144g	230	2.2	160	9.6	27.1	1.5	2.3
Vegetable, Roasted, & Feta, BGTY, Sainsbury's*	1 Serving/200g	318	8.0	159	5.8	25.0	4.0	0.0
Yellow Thai Prawn, COU, M & S*	1 Pack/171g	266	5.0	155	7.6	23.4	2.9	1.7

	Measure INFO/WEIGHT	per Measure KCAL	per Measure FAT	KCAL	PROT	CARB	FAT	FIBRE
				Nutrition Values per 100g / 100ml				
YAM								
Baked	***1oz/28g***	***43***	***0.1***	***153***	***2.1***	***37.5***	***0.4***	***1.7***
Boiled, Average	***1oz/28g***	***37***	***0.1***	***133***	***1.7***	***33.0***	***0.3***	***1.4***
Raw	***1oz/28g***	***32***	***0.1***	***114***	***1.5***	***28.2***	***0.3***	***1.3***
YEAST								
Dried, Average	***1 Tbsp/6g***	***10***	***0.1***	***169***	***35.6***	***3.5***	***1.5***	***0.0***
Extract	***1 Tsp/9g***	***16***	***0.0***	***180***	***40.7***	***3.5***	***0.4***	***0.0***
YOFU								
Natural, Alpro*	1 Pot/500g	230	11.5	46	4.0	2.1	2.3	1.0
YOGHURT								
0.1% Fat, Lidl*	1 Pot/150g	118	0.2	79	4.0	15.6	0.1	0.0
Activia, Danone*	1 Pot/132g	125	4.2	94	3.5	12.8	3.2	2.0
Apple, Light, Muller*	1 Pot/175g	94	0.2	54	4.4	9.0	0.1	0.0
Apple & Berry Pie, Dessert Recipe, Weight Watchers*	1 Pot/120g	58	0.1	49	4.1	6.8	0.1	0.3
Apple & Blackberry, Bio, Sainsbury's*	1 Pot/125g	134	3.4	107	4.1	16.6	2.7	0.2
Apple & Blackberry, Custard Style, Co-Op*	1 Pot/150g	195	8.0	130	3.7	15.9	5.3	0.1
Apple & Blackberry, Organic, Yeo Valley*	1 Pot/125g	121	4.1	97	4.3	12.5	3.3	0.1
Apple & Blackcurrant, Low Fat, Stapleton*	1 Pot/150g	106	0.8	71	3.2	13.9	0.5	1.2
Apple & Cinnamon, COU, M & S*	1 Pot/150g	68	0.2	45	4.2	6.1	0.1	0.2
Apple & Custard, Low Fat, Sainsbury's*	1 Pot/125g	116	1.9	93	4.3	15.5	1.5	0.2
Apple & Pear, Low Fat, Sainsbury's*	1 Pot/125g	115	1.9	92	4.3	15.2	1.5	0.2
Apple & Prune, Fat Free, Yeo Valley*	1 Pot/125g	98	0.1	78	5.1	14.1	0.1	0.2
Apricot, Bio, Low Fat, Benecol*	1 Pot/125g	98	0.8	78	3.9	14.3	0.6	0.0
Apricot, Bio Activia, Danone*	1 Pot/125g	121	4.0	97	3.7	13.3	3.2	1.7
Apricot, Fat Free, Activ8, Ski, Nestle*	1 Pot/120g	88	0.8	73	4.5	13.6	0.7	0.2
Apricot, Fat Free, Weight Watchers*	1 Pot/150g	62	0.2	42	4.1	4.9	0.1	0.2
Apricot, Fruity, Mullerlight, Muller*	1 Pot/175g	88	0.2	50	4.2	7.5	0.1	0.1
Apricot, Light, Fat Free, Muller*	1 Pot/190g	93	0.2	49	4.1	7.3	0.1	0.1
Apricot, Low Fat, Organic, Average	1 Serving/100g	84	1.0	84	5.8	13.3	1.0	0.6
Apricot, Pro Activ, Flora*	1 Pot/125ml	70	0.6	56	4.0	7.9	0.5	1.8
Apricot & Mango, Thick & Creamy, Sainsbury's*	1 Pot/150g	178	5.4	119	4.3	17.3	3.6	0.2
Apricot & Mango, Tropical Fruit, Activ8, Ski, Nestle*	1 Pot/120g	112	2.0	93	4.3	15.1	1.7	0.2
Apricot & Nectarine, Sunshine Selection, Sainsbury's*	1 Pot/125g	115	1.9	92	4.4	15.3	1.5	0.1
Banana, Custard Style, Asda*	1 Pot/150g	224	9.0	149	3.7	20.0	6.0	0.2
Banana, Low Fat, Average	1 Serving/100g	98	1.4	98	4.6	16.7	1.4	0.1
Banana, Smooth, M & S*	1 Pot/150g	165	2.6	110	4.8	19.3	1.7	0.2
Banoffee, Low Fat, Asda*	1 Pot/125g	126	1.5	101	4.6	18.2	1.2	1.0
Black Cherry, Average	1 Serving/100g	96	2.2	96	3.4	16.5	2.2	0.1
Black Cherry, Extremely Fruity, Bio, M & S*	1 Pot/150g	165	2.2	110	4.9	18.4	1.5	0.2
Black Cherry, Fat Free, Benecol*	1 Pot/120g	78	0.6	65	3.0	11.0	0.5	2.1
Black Cherry, Greek Style, Corner, Muller*	1 Pot/150g	172	4.5	115	5.0	16.2	3.0	0.1
Black Cherry, Live Bio, Perfeclty Balanced, Waitrose*	1 Pot/125g	115	0.1	92	4.6	18.3	0.1	0.1
Black Cherry, Low Fat, Average	1 Serving/100g	69	0.6	69	3.8	12.2	0.6	0.3
Black Cherry, Virtually Fat Free, Longley Farm Yoghurt*	1 Pot/150g	116	0.2	77	4.5	14.4	0.1	0.0
Black Cherry, VLH Kitchens	1 Serving/150g	188	2.5	125	3.7	19.6	3.7	1.0
Blackberry, Boysenberry & William Pear, M & S*	1 Pot/150g	188	9.8	125	4.0	13.6	6.5	2.4
Blackberry, Fat Free, Danone, Shape*	1 Pot/120g	74	0.2	62	6.7	8.4	0.2	2.4
Blackberry, Soya, Alpro Soya*	1 Pot/125g	91	2.6	73	3.7	9.2	2.1	1.2
Blackberry, Very Berry, Activ8, Ski, Nestle*	1 Pot/120g	114	2.0	95	4.4	15.5	1.7	0.7
Blackberry & Apple, BGTY, Sainsbury's*	1 Pot/122g	61	0.2	50	4.7	7.2	0.2	0.3
Blackberry & Raspberry, Fruit Corner, Muller*	1 Pot/150g	158	5.8	105	3.8	13.1	3.9	0.9
Blackberry & Raspberry Flip, Morrisons*	1 Pot/175g	206	8.0	118	3.4	15.8	4.6	0.5
Blackcurrant, BGTY, Sainsbury's*	1 Pot/200g	100	0.4	50	4.8	7.3	0.2	0.1
Blackcurrant, Fruity, Mullerlight, Muller*	1 Pot/175g	89	0.2	51	4.1	7.9	0.1	0.8

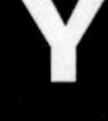

YOGHURT	Measure INFO/WEIGHT	per Measure KCAL	per Measure FAT	Nutrition Values per 100g / 100ml KCAL	PROT	CARB	FAT	FIBRE
Blackcurrant, Longley Farm*	1 Pot/150g	168	5.6	112	4.9	14.7	3.7	0.0
Blackcurrant, Munch Bunch, Nestle*	1 Pot/100g	107	3.1	107	4.4	15.3	3.1	0.5
Blackcurrant, Probiotic, Organic, Yeo Valley*	1 Pot/150g	152	5.8	101	4.1	12.4	3.9	0.2
Blackcurrant, Virtually Fat Free, Morrisons*	1 Pot/200g	114	0.4	57	5.4	8.4	0.2	0.2
Blueberry, Fruit Corner, Muller*	1 Pot/150g	156	5.7	104	3.8	12.9	3.8	0.4
Blueberry, Wholemilk, Organic, Sainsbury's*	1 Pot/150g	123	5.2	82	3.5	9.2	3.5	0.1
Blueberry, Wild, Finest, Tesco*	1 Pot/150g	212	10.2	141	3.4	16.6	6.8	0.5
Blueberry, Wild, Light, Fat Free, Muller*	1 Pot/175g	82	0.2	47	4.1	6.9	0.1	0.7
Blueberry & Elderberry, Bio, with Wholegrains, Optifit*	1 Pot/250g	150	3.5	60	4.9	7.0	1.4	1.6
Blueberry & Loganberry, Bio, Layered, Sainsbury's*	1 Pot/125g	134	3.4	107	4.0	16.6	2.7	0.2
Blueberry Bio, Co-Op*	1 Pot/125g	141	3.5	113	4.5	16.5	2.8	0.4
Boysenberry, Low Fat, Yoplait*	1 Pot/100g	49	0.1	49	5.3	6.7	0.1	0.0
Bramble & Apple, Virtually Fat Free, Longley Farm*	1 Pot/150g	118	0.2	79	5.5	13.9	0.1	0.0
Breakfast Crunch, Strawberry, Corner, Muller*	1 Pack/135g	163	3.5	121	5.5	0.0	2.6	0.0
Caramel, Organic, Onken*	1 Serving/50g	56	1.6	111	4.6	15.6	3.3	0.0
Cherry, 0.1% Fat, Shape, Danone*	1 Pot/120g	56	0.1	47	4.6	6.8	0.1	2.1
Cherry, Bio, Low Fat, Benecol*	1 Pot/150g	122	0.9	81	3.8	15.2	0.6	0.0
Cherry, Fat Free, Activia, Danone*	1 Pot/125g	76	0.1	61	4.8	9.8	0.1	0.9
Cherry, Fruit, Biopot, Onken*	1 Serving/100g	107	2.7	107	3.7	16.7	2.7	0.2
Cherry, Fruity, Mullerlight, Muller*	1 Pot/175g	86	0.2	49	4.3	7.0	0.1	0.2
Cherry, Greek Style, Shape, Danone*	1 Pot/125g	143	3.4	114	6.0	16.4	2.7	0.0
Cherry, Light, Fat Free, Muller*	1 Pot/175g	88	0.2	50	3.9	7.9	0.1	0.2
Cherry, Pots, Probiotic, Yeo Valley*	1 Pot/119g	124	4.4	104	4.9	12.8	3.7	0.1
Cherry & Vanilla Flavour, Light, Brooklea*	1 Pot/200g	138	0.2	69	5.5	11.4	0.1	0.6
Cherry Bakewell Tart Flavour, Muller*	1 Pot/175g	119	0.4	68	4.8	11.8	0.2	0.2
Cherry Bio, Co-Op*	1 Pot/125g	144	3.5	115	4.5	17.0	2.8	0.1
Chocolate, Orange, Crunch, Corner, Muller*	1 Pot/135g	204	6.5	151	3.4	23.1	4.8	0.7
Chocolate, Village Dairy*	1 Pot/125g	181	3.8	145	6.3	23.5	3.0	0.0
Chocolate, Vitaline*	1 Pot/125g	102	0.6	82	3.5	15.8	0.5	0.0
Chocolate, White & Milk, Puffed Rice, Nom Dairy UK*	1 Pot/150g	226	8.8	151	3.8	20.7	5.9	0.1
Chocolate Raisins, Naturally Creamy, Nom Dairy UK*	1 Pot/155g	245	9.5	158	3.4	22.4	6.1	0.2
Coconut, Biopot, Onken*	1 Pot/450g	562	23.4	125	3.9	15.6	5.2	0.9
Coconut, Malaysian, Thick & Creamy, Waitrose*	1 Pot/150g	242	15.9	161	3.9	12.6	10.6	0.3
Cranberry, Bio Activia, Danone*	1 Pot/125g	115	4.0	92	3.6	12.3	3.2	1.7
Cranberry & Raspberry, Creamy, Shapers, Boots*	1 Pot/150g	86	1.6	57	4.0	7.0	1.1	1.1
Eton Mess, British Classic, Corner, Muller*	1 Pot/135g	171	3.0	127	2.8	23.5	2.2	0.3
Exotic, Alpro*	1 Pot/125g	98	2.4	78	3.6	11.1	1.9	0.9
Fig, Bio, Activia, Danone*	1 Pot/125g	121	4.0	97	3.7	13.3	3.2	1.6
Fig, Date & Grape, Biopot, Lite, Wholegrain, Onken*	¼ Pot/120g	102	0.2	85	4.8	16.0	0.2	1.0
Forest Berries, Soya, Joya*	1 Pot/125g	108	2.8	86	3.8	12.1	2.2	1.3
Forest Fruits, 0.1% Fat, Shape, Danone*	1 Pot/120g	55	0.1	46	4.6	6.7	0.1	2.1
Forest Fruits, Bio, Fat Free, Activia, Danone*	1 Pot/125g	72	0.1	58	4.5	8.9	0.1	1.1
Forest Fruits, Farmhouse, Twekkelo, De Zuivelhoeve*	1 Pot/500g	555	16.5	111	4.2	16.0	3.3	0.5
Forest Fruits, M & S*	1 Pot/150g	148	2.4	99	4.7	16.8	1.6	0.5
French Set, Waitrose*	1 Pot/125g	120	3.9	96	3.5	13.4	3.1	0.0
French Style, Whole Milk, Smooth Set, Tesco*	1 Pot/125g	122	3.8	98	3.6	14.1	3.0	0.0
Fruit, Brooklea*	1 Pot/120g	97	0.1	81	2.7	15.0	0.1	0.0
Fruit, Garden, Wholemilk, Bio Live, Rachel's Organic*	1 Pot/125g	109	4.2	87	3.5	10.5	3.4	0.0
Fruit, Low Fat, Average	1 Pot/125g	112	0.9	90	4.1	17.9	0.7	0.0
Fruit, Whole Milk	1 Pot/150g	158	4.2	105	5.1	15.7	2.8	0.0
Fruits, with Cherries, Bio, 0% Fat, Danone*	1 Pot/125g	65	0.1	52	3.6	9.1	0.1	0.0
Fruity Favourites, Organic, Yeo Valley*	1 Pot/125g	126	4.9	101	4.1	12.4	3.9	0.2
Fudge, Devonshire, 0.06% Fat, TTD, Sainsbury's*	1 Pot/150g	219	9.0	146	3.5	19.5	6.0	0.0

	Measure INFO/WEIGHT	per Measure KCAL	FAT	Nutrition Values per 100g / 100ml KCAL	PROT	CARB	FAT	FIBRE
YOGHURT								
Fudge, Devonshire Style, Finest, Tesco*	1 Pot/150g	281	13.8	187	3.7	22.4	9.2	0.0
Fudge, Thick & Creamy, M & S*	1 Pot/150g	195	7.5	130	4.4	17.3	5.0	0.7
Fudge, Thick & Creamy, Waitrose*	1 Pot/150g	196	4.5	131	4.4	21.5	3.0	0.0
Ginger, Greek Style, Bio, Live, Rachel's Organic*	1 Serving/100g	134	7.1	134	3.2	14.3	7.1	0.0
Goats Whole Milk	***1 Carton/150g***	***94***	***5.7***	***63***	***3.5***	***3.9***	***3.8***	***0.0***
Gooseberry, Bio Live, Rachel's Organic*	1 Pot/450g	450	15.3	100	4.0	13.3	3.4	0.2
Gooseberry, Custard Style, Co-Op*	1 Pot/150g	216	8.0	144	3.7	19.3	5.3	0.3
Gooseberry, Custard Style, Shapers, Boots*	1 Pot/151g	106	1.1	70	3.9	12.0	0.7	0.2
Gooseberry, Low Fat, Average	1 Serving/100g	90	1.4	90	4.5	14.5	1.4	0.2
Gooseberry, Virtually Fat Free, Longley Farm*	1 Pot/150g	122	0.2	81	4.2	15.7	0.1	0.0
Greek, 0% Fat, Strained, Authentic, Total, Fage*	¼ Pot/125g	71	0.0	57	10.3	4.0	0.0	0.0
Greek, 2% Fat, Strained, Authentic, Total, Fage*	1 Pot/170g	124	3.4	73	9.9	3.8	2.0	0.0
Greek, Strained, Authentic, Original, Total, Fage*	1 Pot170g	163	8.5	96	9.0	3.8	5.0	0.0
Greek, with Honey, Strained, Authentic, Total, Fage*	1 Pot/150g	255	12.0	170	5.4	19.0	8.0	0.0
Greek, with Strawberry, 2% Fat, Total, Fage*	1 Pot/150g	140	2.4	93	6.7	12.9	1.6	0.0
Greek & Cranberry, Made Up, Easiyo*	1 Serving/100g	113	4.7	113	4.0	14.1	4.7	0.1
Greek 'n Coconut, Made Up, Easiyo*	1 Serving/100g	113	4.7	113	4.0	14.1	4.7	0.1
Greek Style, & Nectarines, Food to Go, M & S*	1 Pack/200g	100	4.2	50	2.9	6.3	2.1	1.0
Greek Style, with Black Cherry Compote, M & S*	1 Pot/241g	205	3.4	85	3.4	15.0	1.4	0.5
Greek Style, with Golden Honey, Activia, Danone*	1 Pack/126g	122	3.5	97	5.0	13.0	2.8	0.1
Greek Style, with Honey, Morrisons*	1/3 Pot/150g	236	14.3	157	4.1	13.5	9.5	0.7
Greek Style, with Strawberries, Asda*	1 Pot/125g	159	8.2	127	3.2	13.6	6.6	0.2
Greek Style, with Toffee & Hazelnuts, Asda*	1 Pot/125g	230	10.8	184	3.7	23.1	8.6	0.1
Greek Style, with Tropical Fruits, Asda*	1 Pot/125g	164	8.2	131	3.3	14.5	6.6	0.3
Guava & Orange, Fat Free, Organic, Yeo Valley*	1 Pot/125g	92	0.1	74	5.3	13.0	0.1	0.2
Guava & Passion Fruit, Virtualy Fat Free, Tesco*	1 Pot/125g	56	0.2	45	4.2	6.7	0.2	1.2
Hazelnut, Crunchy, Jordans*	1 Pot/150g	231	6.0	154	5.2	22.2	4.0	1.1
Hazelnut, Fabulously, Sainsbury's*	1 Pot/150g	194	8.4	130	4.4	15.3	5.6	0.2
Hazelnut, Longley Farm*	1 Pot/150g	201	8.5	134	5.5	16.0	5.7	0.0
Hazelnut, Low Fat, Average	1 Serving/100g	106	2.3	106	4.5	16.9	2.3	0.1
Hazelnut, Yoplait*	1 Pot/125g	166	5.0	133	4.6	19.6	4.0	0.0
Honey, & Muesli, Breakfast Break, Tesco*	1 Pot/170g	207	4.6	122	3.9	20.5	2.7	0.6
Honey, & Multigrain, Breakfast Selection, Sainsbury's*	1 Pot/125g	126	1.9	101	4.4	17.4	1.5	0.2
Honey, Breakfast Pot, Activia, Danone*	1 Pot/160g	192	4.2	120	4.9	18.8	2.6	0.7
Honey, Granola, Creamy, Nom Dairy UK*	1 Pot/150g	186	7.5	124	4.3	15.6	5.0	0.5
Honey, Greek Style,Co-Op*	1 Pot/150g	228	12.8	152	4.0	13.8	8.5	0.0
Honey, Layered, Greek Style, Shapers, Boots*	1 Pot/150g	136	3.0	91	4.2	14.0	2.0	0.0
Honey, Low Fat, Asda*	1 Pot/125g	130	1.4	104	4.6	19.0	1.1	0.0
Honey, Orange Blossom, Finest, Tesco*	1 Pot/150g	237	10.6	158	3.5	20.1	7.1	0.0
Honey & Ginger, Waitrose*	1 Pot/150g	240	12.9	160	3.8	16.8	8.6	0.1
Honeyed Peach, Greek Style, Mullerlight, Muller*	1 Pot/120g	85	0.2	71	6.3	10.3	0.2	0.2
Kiwi, Activia, Danone*	1 Pot/125g	119	4.1	95	3.6	12.7	3.3	0.3
Kiwi, Cereal, Fibre, Bio Activia, Danone*	1 Pot/120g	124	4.0	103	3.8	14.5	3.3	3.0
Kiwi, Made Up, Easiyo*	1 Serving/100g	97	2.6	97	5.3	14.6	2.6	0.0
Kiwi & Gooseberry, Naturally Creamy, Nom Dairy UK*	1 Pot/175g	189	6.6	108	3.1	15.3	3.8	0.1
Lemon, COU, M & S*	1 Pot/200g	90	0.2	45	4.2	6.6	0.1	0.4
Lemon, Fat Free, Nestle*	1 Pot/135g	105	0.1	78	3.1	16.2	0.1	0.0
Lemon, Greek Style, Shape, Danone*	1 Pot/125g	140	3.4	112	5.9	15.9	2.7	0.0
Lemon, Greek Style, Whipped, Bliss Corner, Muller*	1 Pack/110g	177	6.5	161	4.0	22.2	5.9	0.0
Lemon, Italian, Amore Luxury, Muller*	1 Pot/150g	219	11.7	146	2.8	16.2	7.8	0.1
Lemon, Longley Farm*	1 Pot/150g	159	5.6	106	5.0	13.4	3.7	0.0
Lemon, Low Fat, Average	1 Serving/100g	95	0.9	95	4.6	17.3	0.9	0.1
Lemon, Summer, Biopot, Onken*	1 Pot/150g	154	3.9	103	3.9	15.9	2.6	0.1

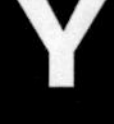

	Measure INFO/WEIGHT	per Measure KCAL	FAT	Nutrition Values per 100g / 100ml KCAL	PROT	CARB	FAT	FIBRE
YOGHURT								
Lemon, Thick & Fruity, Citrus Fruits, Weight Watchers*	1 Pot/120g	47	0.1	39	4.1	4.9	0.1	0.9
Lemon & Lime, BGTY, Sainsbury's*	1 Pot/125g	66	0.1	53	4.6	8.3	0.1	1.1
Lemon & Lime, Fat Free, Shape, Danone*	1 Pot/120g	61	0.1	51	4.5	7.3	0.1	0.1
Lemon Cheesecake, Average	1 Serving/100g	55	0.2	55	4.3	8.8	0.2	0.2
Lemon Curd, 0.06% Fat, TTD, Sainsbury's*	1 Pot/150g	224	9.0	149	3.8	20.0	6.0	0.2
Lemon Curd, Indulgent, Dessert, Waitrose*	1 Pot/150g	278	13.8	185	4.1	21.5	9.2	0.0
Lemon Curd, Thick & Creamy, Tesco*	1 Pot/150g	255	13.5	170	3.4	18.2	9.0	0.2
Lemon Curd, Very, Morrisons*	1 Pot/150g	262	13.6	175	4.1	19.2	9.1	0.0
Lemon Curd, West Country, TTD, Sainsbury's*	1 Pot/150g	243	10.0	162	3.7	21.6	6.7	0.5
Lemon Curd, with West Country Cream, Morrisons*	1 Pot/150g	244	12.7	163	3.4	17.9	8.5	0.5
Lemon Lime, Mousse, Shapers, Boots*	1 Pot/90g	89	3.8	99	4.2	11.0	4.2	0.1
Loganberry, 0.06% Fat, TTD, Sainsbury's*	1 Pot/150g	186	8.7	124	3.7	14.2	5.8	0.8
Loganberry, Low Fat, Sainsbury's*	1 Pot/125g	111	1.9	89	4.2	14.5	1.5	0.2
Loganberry, Sainsbury's*	1 Pot/150g	194	9.3	129	3.9	14.2	6.2	0.6
Low Calorie	1 Pot/120g	49	0.2	41	4.3	6.0	0.2	0.0
Mandarin, Fat Free, Mullerlight, Muller*	1 Pot/175g	95	0.2	54	4.2	8.5	0.1	0.0
Mandarin, Longley Farm*	1 Pot/150g	141	5.7	94	4.9	13.3	3.8	0.0
Mango, 0% Fat, Shape Delights*	1 Pot/120g	80	0.1	67	5.5	10.9	0.1	0.9
Mango, Bio Activia, Danone*	1 Pot/125g	121	4.0	97	3.7	13.4	3.2	1.6
Mango, Light, HL, Tesco*	1 Serving/125g	56	0.3	45	4.1	6.6	0.2	0.9
Mango, Light, Muller*	1 Pot/175g	96	0.2	55	4.3	9.2	0.1	0.0
Mango, Swiss, Emmi*	1 Serving/175g	184	4.4	105	3.5	17.0	2.5	0.3
Mango, Tropical Fruit, Thick & Fruity, Weight Watchers*	1 Pot/120g	49	0.1	41	3.9	6.0	0.1	1.1
Mango, Virtually Fat Free, Tesco*	1 Pot/125g	56	0.2	45	4.1	6.6	0.2	0.9
Mango, Zer0% Fat, No Added Sugar, Shape, Danone*	1 Pot/120g	72	0.1	60	6.0	8.8	0.1	0.9
Mango & Apple, Fat Free, Onken*	1 Serving/150g	132	0.2	88	4.4	16.0	0.1	0.2
Mango & Guava, Sunshine Selection, Sainsbury's*	1 Pot/125g	145	2.4	116	5.4	19.3	1.9	0.3
Mango & Passionfruit, Fruit Corner, Muller*	1 Yoghurt/150g	160	5.8	107	3.8	13.5	3.9	0.3
Mango & Passionfruit, Soya, Joya*	1 Serving/100g	61	1.9	61	3.3	7.3	1.9	1.1
Mango & Pineapple, BGTY, Sainsbury's*	1 Pot/124g	63	0.2	51	4.6	7.6	0.2	0.2
Maple & Cinnamon Granola, Low Fat, Natural, Asda*	1 Pot/140g	196	4.6	140	6.1	21.5	3.3	0.8
Melon, Berry & Granola, Crunch, Snack Pot, Terry's*	1 Pack/225g	185	3.2	82	3.1	13.9	1.4	1.2
Mississippi Mud Pie, Crunchable, Brooklea*	1 Pot/140g	237	6.3	169	4.0	28.0	4.5	0.3
Mixed Berries, Jogood, Imlek*	1 Pot/200g	172	4.4	86	2.9	13.4	2.2	0.0
Mixed Seeds, Probiotic, Yoplait*	1 Pot/125g	139	5.6	111	4.5	13.2	4.5	3.1
Morello Cherry, Amore Luxury, Muller*	1 Pot/150g	216	11.7	144	2.8	16.3	7.8	0.1
Morello Cherry, HL, Tesco*	1 Pot/125g	56	0.2	45	4.1	6.6	0.2	0.9
Natural, 0.1% Fat, Stirred, Biopot, Onken*	1 Serving/100g	48	0.1	48	5.4	6.4	0.1	0.0
Natural, Bio, Activia, Individual Pots, Danone*	1 Pot/125g	86	4.2	69	4.2	5.5	3.4	0.0
Natural, Bio, BFY, Morrisons*	1 Serving/100g	65	0.2	65	6.5	9.4	0.2	0.0
Natural, Bio, HL, Tesco*	1 Serving/100g	55	0.1	55	5.4	7.6	0.1	0.0
Natural, Bio, Life, Easiyo*	1 Pot/150g	95	2.7	63	5.0	6.7	1.8	0.0
Natural, Bio, Live, Very Low Fat, Ann Forshaw's*	1 Pot/125g	52	0.1	42	5.0	5.5	0.1	0.0
Natural, Bio, Set, Low Fat, Sainsbury's*	1 Pot/150g	78	2.2	52	3.9	5.7	1.5	0.0
Natural, Danone*	1 Pot/125g	71	3.6	57	3.2	3.8	2.9	0.0
Natural, Fat Free, Biopot, Dr Oetker*	¼ Pot/125g	60	0.1	48	5.4	6.4	0.1	0.0
Natural, Fat Free, Onken*	1 Serving/100g	46	0.1	46	5.4	4.3	0.1	0.0
Natural, Fat Free, Rachel's Organic*	1 Pot/500g	180	0.5	36	3.9	4.8	0.1	0.0
Natural, Greek Style, Average	1 Serving/100g	138	10.6	138	4.7	6.1	10.6	0.0
Natural, Greek Style, Fat Free, Tesco*	½ Pot/100g	55	0.2	55	7.5	4.8	0.2	0.4
Natural, Greek Style, Low Fat, Average	1 Serving/100g	77	2.7	77	6.1	7.3	2.7	0.2
Natural, Greek Style, Organic, Tesco*	1 Pot/500g	665	50.0	133	4.5	6.2	10.0	0.0
Natural, Greek Style, Probiotic, Unsweetened, M & S*	1 Serving/150g	195	15.2	130	5.5	4.6	10.1	0.1

Y

	Measure INFO/WEIGHT	per Measure KCAL	FAT	Nutrition Values per 100g / 100ml KCAL	PROT	CARB	FAT	FIBRE
YOGHURT								
Natural, Greek Style, with Cow's Milk, Tesco*	1 Pot/150g	214	16.4	143	4.5	6.6	10.9	0.0
Natural, Greek Style, with Honey Sauce, Sainsbury's*	1 Pot/140g	206	11.1	147	3.3	15.7	7.9	0.0
Natural, Longley Farm*	1 Pot/150g	118	5.2	79	4.8	7.0	3.5	0.0
Natural, Low Fat, Average	***1 Med Pot/125g***	***75***	***1.6***	***60***	***5.4***	***7.0***	***1.3***	***0.0***
Natural, Low Fat, Organic, Average	1 Serving/100g	87	1.2	87	5.7	7.7	1.2	0.0
Natural, Luxury, Bio Live, Jersey Dairy*	1 Pot/150g	225	12.0	150	4.6	8.2	8.0	0.0
Natural, Netto*	1 Serving/50g	40	1.8	80	4.8	6.9	3.7	0.0
Natural, Organic, Evernat*	1 Serving/100g	104	4.0	104	3.9	12.9	4.0	0.0
Natural, Organic, Yeo Valley*	1 Pot/150g	124	6.4	82	4.6	6.5	4.2	0.0
Natural, Pouring, Activia, Danone*	1 Carton/950g	484	16.2	51	4.1	4.9	1.7	0.0
Natural, Probiotic, 0.1% Fat, BGTY, Sainsbury's*	1 Serving/125g	69	0.1	55	5.6	8.0	0.1	0.0
Natural, Probiotic, 2% Fat, Sainsbury's*	¼ Pot/125g	76	1.9	61	4.9	7.0	1.5	0.0
Natural, Probiotic, Eat Smart, Morrisons*	¼ Pot/125g	76	0.4	61	6.3	8.3	0.3	0.0
Natural, Probiotic, Fat Free, Organic, Yeo Valley*	1 Pot/150g	87	0.2	58	5.9	8.4	0.1	0.0
Natural, Probiotic, Organic, Yeo Valley*	1 Pot/150g	124	6.4	82	4.5	6.6	4.2	0.0
Natural, Set, Low Fat, Waitrose*	1 Pot/150g	99	1.8	66	5.7	8.1	1.2	0.0
Natural, Simply More, M & S*	1 Serving/100g	85	3.4	85	5.3	7.9	3.4	0.5
Natural, Soya, Sojade*	1 Serving/100g	50	2.5	50	4.5	2.4	2.5	0.0
Natural, Whole Milk, Set, Biopot, Onken*	1 Serving/125g	85	4.4	68	4.5	4.1	3.5	0.0
Natural, Wholemilk, Live Bio, Organic, Waitrose*	1 Serving/100g	88	4.4	88	5.1	7.1	4.4	0.0
Nectarine, Fat Free, Weight Watchers*	1 Pot/120g	48	0.1	40	4.1	4.7	0.1	0.4
Nectarine & Orange, Best There Is, Yoplait*	1 Pot/122g	131	2.0	107	4.7	18.0	1.6	0.0
Nectarine & Orange, Channel Island, M & S*	1 Pot/150g	158	5.0	105	4.5	14.7	3.3	0.3
Nectarine & Orange, Fat Free, Average	1 Serving/100g	46	0.1	46	4.4	6.7	0.1	0.0
Nectarine & Orange, M & S*	1 Pot/150g	147	2.4	98	4.9	16.0	1.6	0.3
Nectarine & Passion Fruit, 0.1% Fat, Shape, Danone*	1 Pot/120g	55	0.1	46	4.6	6.7	0.1	2.1
Nectarine & Passion Fruit, BGTY, Sainsbury's*	1 Pot/151g	122	0.6	81	3.2	16.3	0.4	0.6
Nectarine & Passion Fruit, Low Fat, Stapleton Farm*	1 Pot/150g	120	0.8	80	3.2	16.3	0.5	0.6
Orange, Carrot & Mango, 0% Fat, Organic, Yeo Valley*	1 Serving/150g	110	0.0	73	4.9	13.1	0.0	0.0
Orange, Greek Style, Boots*	1 Pot/140g	207	12.0	148	3.7	14.0	8.6	0.2
Orange, Greek Style, Shape, Danone*	1 Pot/125g	140	3.4	112	6.0	16.0	2.7	0.1
Orange, Sprinkled with Dark Chocolate, Light, Muller*	1 Pot/165g	91	0.8	55	4.3	7.4	0.5	0.1
Orange, Valencia, Seriously Fruity, Low Fat, Waitrose*	1 Pot/150g	147	1.5	98	4.3	18.0	1.0	0.3
Orange & Pineapple, Tropical Fruit, Activ8, Ski, Nestle*	1 Pot/120g	112	2.0	93	4.4	15.1	1.7	0.2
Passion Fruit, with Elderflower Extract, Tesco*	1 Pot/150g	147	1.6	98	4.7	17.3	1.1	0.2
Peach, BGTY, Sainsbury's*	1 Pot/125g	61	0.2	49	4.7	7.2	0.2	0.2
Peach, Bio, Activia, Fat Free, Danone*	1 Sm Pot/125g	71	0.1	57	4.7	9.3	0.1	1.0
Peach, Bio, Fat Free, Snackpot, Activia, Danone*	1 Pot/165g	99	0.2	60	4.6	10.2	0.1	1.0
Peach, Biopot, Wholegrain, Onken*	1 Serving/100g	114	2.8	114	4.0	17.8	2.8	0.5
Peach, Custard Style, Low Fat, Sainsbury's*	1 Pot/125g	110	1.9	88	4.4	14.2	1.5	0.1
Peach, Dairy Free, Organic, Yofu, Soya, Provamel*	1 Serving/125g	100	2.8	80	3.9	10.3	2.2	0.8
Peach, Fat Free, Activ8, Ski, Nestle*	1 Yoghurt/120g	89	0.1	74	4.5	13.7	0.1	0.7
Peach, Forbidden Fruits, Rachel's Organic*	1 Pot/125g	156	7.6	125	3.4	14.0	6.1	0.0
Peach, Honeyed, Greek Style, Mullerlight, Muller*	1 Pot/120g	85	0.2	71	6.3	10.3	0.2	0.2
Peach, Low Fat, Average	1 Serving/100g	86	1.1	86	4.5	14.6	1.1	0.2
Peach, Low Fat, Probiotic, Tesco*	1 Pot/125g	106	1.8	85	3.9	14.3	1.4	0.3
Peach, Luscious, Low Fat, Rachel's Organic*	1 Pot/125g	112	2.0	90	4.0	14.9	1.6	0.2
Peach, Optimel, Campina*	1 Serving/200ml	70	0.0	35	4.0	4.5	0.0	0.0
Peach, Probiotic, Natural Balance, Asda*	1 Pot/125g	108	2.9	86	3.1	13.2	2.3	2.5
Peach, Smooth Style, Mullerlight, Muller*	1 Pot/125g	59	0.1	47	4.1	6.9	0.1	0.2
Peach, White, Seriously Fruity, Waitrose*	1 Pot/150g	152	2.6	101	4.8	16.5	1.7	0.2
Peach & Apricot, 0.1% Fat, Shape, Danone*	1 Pot/120g	55	0.1	46	4.6	6.7	0.1	2.1
Peach & Apricot, Fruit Corner, Muller*	1 Pot/150g	160	5.7	107	3.9	13.5	3.8	0.5

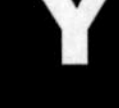

	Measure INFO/WEIGHT	per Measure KCAL	FAT	Nutrition Values per 100g / 100ml KCAL	PROT	CARB	FAT	FIBRE
YOGHURT								
Peach & Apricot, HL, Tesco*	1 Pot/92g	42	0.1	46	4.0	7.4	0.1	1.0
Peach & Apricot, Light, HL, Tesco*	1 Pot/200g	82	0.2	41	3.9	6.2	0.1	1.0
Peach & Lemon Balm, Biowild, Onken*	1 Pot/175g	158	2.6	90	4.3	14.9	1.5	0.1
Peach & Mango, 0.1% Actimel, Danone*	1 Serving/100g	29	0.1	29	2.7	3.6	0.1	0.1
Peach & Mango, Dairy Free, Organic, Yofu, Provamel*	1 Pot/125g	100	2.8	80	3.9	10.4	2.2	0.8
Peach & Mango, Juicy, Shapers, Boots*	1 Pot/150g	88	1.6	59	4.0	8.3	1.1	0.5
Peach & Mango, Thick & Creamy, Waitrose*	1 Pot/125g	136	3.1	109	3.7	17.8	2.5	0.3
Peach & Mango, Truly Fruity, Brooklea, Aldi*	1 Pot/200g	162	2.8	81	4.6	12.4	1.4	0.0
Peach & Maracuya, Mullerlight, Muller*	1 Pot/200g	102	0.2	51	4.5	8.1	0.1	0.0
Peach & Nectarine, Bio, Fat Free, Activia, Danone*	1 Pot/125g	70	0.1	56	4.5	9.3	0.1	1.0
Peach & Papaya, Fat Free, Yeo Valley*	1 Pot/125g	94	0.1	75	5.3	13.1	0.1	0.1
Peach & Papaya, Waitrose*	1 Pot/150g	129	0.2	86	4.2	17.1	0.1	0.2
Peach & Passion Fruit, Average	1 Serving/100g	66	0.7	66	4.5	10.6	0.7	0.4
Peach & Passion Fruit, BGTY, Sainsbury's*	1 Pot/125g	69	0.1	55	4.9	8.6	0.1	0.1
Peach & Passion Fruit, Fat Free, Shape, Danone*	1 Pot/120g	74	0.1	62	6.6	8.6	0.1	2.3
Peach & Passion Fruit, Fruit Layered, Bio, GFY, Asda*	1 Pot/126g	77	0.1	61	4.0	11.0	0.1	0.5
Peach & Passion Fruit, Layers, Mullerlight, Muller*	1 Pot/175g	94	0.2	54	3.1	9.7	0.1	0.2
Peach & Passion Fruit, Lite Biopot, Onken*	1/5 Pot/100g	45	0.2	45	4.6	6.0	0.2	0.2
Peach & Pear, Seriously Fruity, Low Fat, Waitrose*	1 Pot/125g	110	1.2	88	4.5	15.3	1.0	0.3
Peach & Pineapple, Fat Free, Mullerlight, Muller*	1 Pot/175g	89	0.2	51	4.3	7.7	0.1	0.2
Peach & Vanilla, Thick & Creamy, Co-Op*	1 Pot/150g	180	6.9	120	3.6	16.0	4.6	0.1
Peach & Vanilla Flip, Morrisons*	1 Pot/175g	212	8.0	121	3.4	16.5	4.6	0.6
Peach Apricot, Soya, Joya*	1 Serving/100g	86	2.0	86	3.6	12.9	2.0	1.0
Peach Melba, Low Fat, Average	1 Serving/100g	75	0.7	75	2.6	14.5	0.7	0.0
Peach Melba, Sveltesse, Nestle*	1 Pot/126g	70	0.1	56	4.7	9.1	0.1	0.2
Peach Melba, Value, Tesco*	1 Pot/125g	100	0.9	80	2.3	16.0	0.7	0.1
Peaches, Farmhouse, BGTY, Sainsbury's*	1 Pot/150g	134	0.6	89	3.2	17.8	0.4	0.3
Peaches & Cream, Intensely Creamy, Activia, Danone*	1 Pot/120g	118	3.6	98	4.8	13.0	3.0	0.3
Pear, Jubileum, Tine*	1 Carton/125g	168	6.5	134	3.2	18.6	5.2	0.0
Pear, Lidl*	1 Serving/125g	108	0.1	86	4.3	16.1	0.1	0.0
Pear & Butterscotch, Finest, Tesco*	1 Pot/150g	412	21.0	275	5.0	32.3	14.0	0.5
Pear & Vanilla, Thick & Creamy, Weight Watchers*	1 Pot/120g	54	0.6	45	4.2	5.8	0.5	0.2
Pineapple, Average	1 Serving/100g	73	1.1	73	4.4	11.3	1.1	0.5
Pineapple, Bio Activia, Fat Free, Danone*	1 Pot/125g	62	0.1	50	4.7	7.5	0.1	1.7
Pineapple, Channel Island, M & S*	1 Pot/150g	165	5.0	110	4.3	15.9	3.3	0.3
Pineapple, Low Fat, Average	1 Serving/100g	89	1.2	89	4.6	14.7	1.2	0.0
Pineapple, Virtually Fat Free, Tesco*	1 Pot/125g	55	0.2	44	4.1	6.5	0.2	0.9
Pineapple, Vitality, Low Fat, with Omega 3, Muller*	1 Pot/150g	138	2.8	92	4.2	13.8	1.9	0.7
Pineapple & Grapefruit, BGTY, Sainsbury's*	1 Pot/125g	68	0.1	54	4.4	8.8	0.1	0.1
Pineapple & Passion Fruit, Soya, Light, Alpro*	1 Pot/120g	94	2.3	78	3.6	10.3	1.9	0.8
Pineapple & Peach, Fruity, Mullerlight, Muller*	1 Pot/175g	89	0.2	51	4.2	7.7	0.1	0.2
Pink Grapefruit, Low Fat, Sainsbury's*	1 Pot/125g	116	1.8	93	4.2	15.9	1.4	0.1
Plain, Low Fat, Average	***1 Serving/100g***	***63***	***1.6***	***63***	***5.2***	***7.0***	***1.6***	***0.0***
Plain, Soya, Average	***1oz/28g***	***20***	***1.2***	***72***	***5.0***	***3.9***	***4.2***	***0.0***
Plain, Whole Milk, Average	***1oz/28g***	***22***	***0.8***	***79***	***5.7***	***7.8***	***3.0***	***0.0***
Plum, BGTY, Sainsbury's*	1 Pot/125g	69	0.1	55	4.8	8.8	0.1	0.1
Plum, Low Fat, Sainsbury's*	1 Pot/125g	118	2.1	94	4.5	15.2	1.7	0.1
Plum, Probiotic, Summer Selection, Yeo Valley*	1 Pot/125g	126	4.9	101	4.1	12.4	3.9	0.1
Plum, Soya, Dairy Free, Organic, with Fibre, Provamel*	1 Serving/125g	90	2.5	72	3.7	7.5	2.0	4.0
Probiotic, Aldi*	1 Serving/200g	178	2.8	89	4.1	14.2	1.4	0.0
Probiotic, Fat Free, Average	1 Tbsp/15g	8	0.0	56	5.4	7.7	0.3	0.6
Probiotic, Low Fat, Organic, Glenisk Organic Dairy Co*	1 Serving/150g	92	2.8	61	4.5	6.4	1.9	0.0
Prune, Bifidus, Activo, Mercadona*	1 Pot/125g	70	0.1	56	4.5	6.8	0.1	3.0

Y

	Measure INFO/WEIGHT	per Measure KCAL	FAT	Nutrition Values per 100g / 100ml KCAL	PROT	CARB	FAT	FIBRE
YOGHURT								
Prune, Bio Activia, Danone*	1 Pot/125g	110	3.5	88	3.5	12.2	2.8	0.2
Prune, Breakfast Selection, Sainsbury's*	1 Pot/125g	119	1.8	95	4.2	16.3	1.4	0.2
Prune, Probiotic, Natural Balance, Asda*	1 Pot/125g	105	2.9	84	2.1	13.8	2.3	0.8
Prune, Probiotic, Tesco*	1 Serving/170g	145	2.4	85	3.9	14.3	1.4	1.0
Prune, Vitality, Low Fat, with Omega 3, Muller*	1 Pot/150g	144	2.8	96	4.7	15.0	1.9	1.1
Raspberry, Bio, Activia, Danone*	1 Pot/125g	112	3.5	90	3.5	12.8	2.8	2.0
Raspberry, Bio, Activia, Fat Free, Danone*	1 Pot/125g	68	0.1	54	4.7	7.2	0.1	2.6
Raspberry, Bio, Fat Free, Snackpot, Activia, Danone*	1 Pot/165g	91	0.2	54	4.7	7.2	0.1	2.6
Raspberry, Bio, Low Fat, Benecol*	1 Pot/125g	99	0.8	79	3.8	14.5	0.6	0.0
Raspberry, Bio, Low Fat, Sainsbury's*	1 Pot/150g	146	1.6	97	4.7	17.0	1.1	0.7
Raspberry, Bio, Pur Natur*	1 Pot/150g	150	4.6	100	1.4	14.5	3.1	0.0
Raspberry, Bio Live, Low Fat, Rachel's Organic*	1 Pot/125g	114	2.0	91	4.1	15.1	1.6	0.1
Raspberry, Economy, Sainsbury's*	1 Pot/125g	85	1.2	68	3.0	11.9	1.0	0.0
Raspberry, Extremely Fruity, M & S*	1 Pot/200g	190	3.0	95	5.0	15.6	1.5	0.5
Raspberry, Fat Free, Average	1 Serving/100g	64	0.1	64	4.9	11.0	0.1	1.7
Raspberry, Fat Free, Probiotic, Organic, Yeo Valley*	1 Pot/125g	98	0.1	78	5.2	14.0	0.1	0.4
Raspberry, Forbidden Fruit, Rachel's Organic*	1 Pot/125g	155	7.6	124	3.4	13.8	6.1	0.1
Raspberry, French Set, Waitrose*	1 Pot/125g	120	3.9	96	3.5	13.4	3.1	2.0
Raspberry, Incredibly Fruity, Fat Free, Tesco*	1 Pot/150g	112	0.2	75	4.8	13.1	0.1	1.0
Raspberry, Jubileum, Tine*	1 Pot/135g	163	6.5	121	3.2	16.1	4.8	0.0
Raspberry, Juicy, Intensely Creamy, Activia, Danone*	1 Pot/110g	109	3.3	99	4.8	12.7	3.0	0.6
Raspberry, Lactose Free, Lactofree, Arla*	1 Pot/125g	130	3.4	104	3.3	16.5	2.7	0.7
Raspberry, Low Fat, Average	1 Serving/100g	83	1.1	83	4.1	14.1	1.1	0.8
Raspberry, Low Fat, Stapleton*	1 Serving/150g	105	0.8	70	3.3	13.6	0.5	2.0
Raspberry, Meadow Fresh, Lidl*	1 Sm Pot/125g	130	1.2	104	4.5	18.9	1.0	0.0
Raspberry, Naturally Light, Nom Dairy UK*	1 Pot/180g	133	0.2	74	4.3	13.9	0.1	0.2
Raspberry, Organic, Soya, Joya*	1 Serving/100g	83	2.1	83	3.7	11.6	2.1	1.3
Raspberry, Organic, Yeo Valley*	1 Pot/150g	152	5.8	101	4.2	12.3	3.9	0.4
Raspberry, Probiotic, Live, Yeo Valley*	1 Pot/125g	106	1.2	85	5.1	14.0	1.0	0.4
Raspberry, Probiotic, Low Fat, Organic, M & S*	1 Pot/170g	128	2.4	75	4.4	11.5	1.4	0.4
Raspberry, Probiotic, Low Fat, Tesco*	1 Pot/170g	144	2.4	85	3.9	14.3	1.4	0.3
Raspberry, Scottish, The Best, Morrisons*	1 Pot/150g	208	10.4	139	3.6	15.6	6.9	1.3
Raspberry, Smooth, Activ8, Ski, Nestle*	1 Pot/120g	113	2.0	94	4.6	14.8	1.7	0.7
Raspberry, Smooth, Mullerlight, Muller*	1 Pot/125g	64	0.1	51	4.2	7.8	0.1	0.6
Raspberry, Soya, Alpro*	1 Pot/125g	99	2.4	79	3.7	10.4	1.9	1.2
Raspberry, Summer, Biopot, Onken*	1/5 Pot/90g	91	2.4	101	3.8	15.0	2.7	0.6
Raspberry, Thick & Fruity, Probiotic, COU, M & S*	1 Pot/170g	76	0.2	45	4.2	6.9	0.1	0.6
Raspberry, Vitality, Low Fat, with Omega 3, Muller*	1 Pot/125g	115	2.5	92	4.3	13.4	2.0	1.3
Raspberry, with Fruit Layer, Bio Activia, Danone*	1 Pot/125g	116	3.5	93	3.4	12.5	2.8	2.0
Raspberry & Blackberry, Rich & Creamy, Spelga*	1 Serving/150g	188	7.0	125	3.7	17.2	4.7	0.1
Raspberry & Blackberry, Thick & Creamy, Co-Op*	1 Pot/150g	188	6.9	125	3.6	17.3	4.6	0.1
Raspberry & Cranberry, BGTY, Sainsbury's*	1 Pot/125g	65	0.1	52	4.4	8.4	0.1	0.5
Raspberry & Cranberry, Fat Free, Mullerlight, Muller*	1 Pot/175g	91	0.2	52	4.3	7.8	0.1	0.5
Raspberry & Cranberry, Light, HL, Tesco*	1 Pot/125g	55	0.2	44	4.2	6.3	0.2	1.1
Raspberry & Cranberry, Very Low Fat, Ann Forshaw's*	1 Pot/125g	91	0.1	73	4.6	14.2	0.1	0.2
Raspberry & Elderberry, Organic, Onken*	1 Serving/50g	53	1.6	106	3.8	15.0	3.1	0.0
Raspberry & Orange, Fat Free, Organic, Yeo Valley*	1 Serving/100g	77	0.1	77	5.1	13.7	0.1	0.1
Raspberry & Redcurrant, Low Fat, Morrisons*	1 Pot/125g	117	2.0	94	4.4	15.4	1.6	0.7
Raspberry & Redcurrant, Low Fat, Sainsbury's*	1 Pot/125g	109	1.8	87	4.2	14.5	1.4	0.5
Raspberry or Strawberry, Smooth, No Bits, Ski, Nestle*	1 Pot/120g	118	3.2	98	3.9	13.6	2.7	0.0
Red Berry, Healthy Balance, Corner, Muller*	1 Pot/150g	178	4.0	119	5.0	18.0	2.7	0.5
Red Berry, Vitality, Low Fat, with Omega 3, Muller*	1 Pot/150g	138	2.8	92	4.3	13.8	1.9	0.7
Red Cherry, Dairy Free, Organic, Yofu, Soya, Provamel*	1 Pot/125g	101	2.8	81	3.9	10.5	2.2	0.8

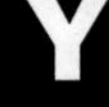

	Measure INFO/WEIGHT	per Measure KCAL	FAT	Nutrition Values per 100g / 100ml KCAL	PROT	CARB	FAT	FIBRE
YOGHURT								
Red Cherry, Fat Free, Ski, Nestle*	1 Pot 120g	97	0.1	81	4.5	15.6	0.1	0.1
Red Cherry, Fruit Corner, Muller*	1 Pot/150g	158	5.8	105	3.8	13.0	3.9	0.5
Red Cherry, Fruit Layered, GFY, Asda*	1 Pot/125g	75	0.1	60	3.7	11.0	0.1	0.0
Red Cherry, Very Cherry, Activ8, Ski, Nestle*	1 Pot/120g	115	2.0	96	4.5	15.7	1.7	0.1
Red Fruits, Crumble Style, Sveltesse, Nestle*	1 Pot/125g	100	0.2	80	4.9	14.6	0.2	0.4
Rhubarb, Bio Activia, Danone*	1 Pot/125g	112	4.0	90	3.5	11.8	3.2	2.2
Rhubarb, Country, Naturally Light, Nom Dairy UK*	1 Pot/180g	131	0.2	73	4.3	13.8	0.1	0.4
Rhubarb, Custard Style, Co-Op*	1 Pot/150g	202	8.0	135	3.7	17.2	5.3	0.3
Rhubarb, Eat Smart, Morrisons*	1 Pot/190g	79	0.2	42	4.1	6.1	0.1	1.4
Rhubarb, Extremely Fruity, Probiotic, Low Fat, M & S*	1 Pot/170g	153	1.7	90	4.4	15.5	1.0	0.7
Rhubarb, Fruity, Mullerlight, Muller*	1 Pot/175g	91	0.2	52	4.2	7.9	0.1	0.0
Rhubarb, Greek Style, Corner, Muller*	1 Pot/150g	170	4.5	113	5.0	15.8	3.0	0.1
Rhubarb, Longley Farm*	1 Pot/150g	165	5.6	110	4.9	14.3	3.7	0.0
Rhubarb, Low Fat, Average	1 Serving/100g	83	1.2	83	4.6	13.3	1.2	0.2
Rhubarb, M & S*	1 Pot/150g	148	2.1	99	4.4	17.4	1.4	0.3
Rhubarb, Spiced, Thick & Creamy, COU, M & S*	1 Pot/170g	68	0.2	40	4.3	5.8	0.1	0.5
Rhubarb & Champagne, Truly Irresistible, Co-Op*	1 Pot/150g	195	8.2	130	3.5	16.6	5.5	0.2
Rhubarb & Orange, Tesco*	1 Pot/150g	146	1.6	97	4.6	17.1	1.1	0.5
Rhubarb & Vanilla, Summer, Biopot, Onken*	1/5 Pot/90g	94	2.4	104	3.7	16.0	2.7	0.3
Rhubarb Crumble, Crunch Corner, Muller*	1 Pot/150g	238	8.4	159	3.6	23.5	5.6	0.5
Sheep's Milk, Total, Fage*	1 Pot/200g	180	12.0	90	4.8	4.3	6.0	0.0
Simply, Bio Lite, Ideal World*	1 Serving/100g	57	1.5	57	4.6	6.8	1.5	0.0
Simply, Lemon, Ideal World*	1 Serving/100g	108	4.0	108	4.6	19.4	4.0	0.0
Smooth Toffee, Fat Free, Mullerlight, Muller*	1 Pot/175g	89	0.2	51	4.1	7.9	0.1	0.0
Smooth Toffee & Apple, Low Fat, Co-Op*	1 Pot/125g	150	1.2	120	6.0	22.0	1.0	0.1
Strawberries & Cream, 0.06% Fat, TTD, Sainsbury's*	1 Pot/150g	183	8.2	122	3.5	14.7	5.5	0.4
Strawberries & Cream, Finest, Tesco*	1 Pot/150g	206	10.4	137	3.4	15.4	6.9	0.5
Strawberries & Jersey Cream, Rich & Creamy, Loseley*	1 Pot/150g	200	7.6	133	5.2	16.1	5.1	0.0
Strawberry, & Whole Grain, Bio Break, Tesco*	1 Pot/175g	175	1.9	100	4.7	17.8	1.1	0.2
Strawberry, Amore for Me, Muller*	1 Pot/150g	216	11.0	144	2.7	16.8	7.3	0.2
Strawberry, Balanced Lifestyle, Aldi*	1 Pot/150g	72	0.4	48	4.1	7.1	0.3	0.5
Strawberry, Bettabuy, Morrisons*	1 Pot/115g	91	1.5	79	4.4	12.8	1.3	0.3
Strawberry, BGTY, Sainsbury's*	1 Pot/125g	64	0.1	51	4.8	7.7	0.1	1.2
Strawberry, Bio, Co-Op*	1 Pot/125g	142	3.5	114	4.5	16.7	2.8	0.1
Strawberry, Bio, Fat Free, Snackpot, Activia, Danone*	1 Pot/165g	101	0.2	61	5.0	10.0	0.1	0.2
Strawberry, Bio, Granola, Corner, Muller*	1 Pot/135g	161	3.5	119	5.5	17.8	2.6	0.8
Strawberry, Bio, HE, Tesco*	1 Pot/125g	61	0.2	49	4.7	7.0	0.2	0.2
Strawberry, Bio, Low Fat, Dale Farm*	1 Pot/125g	125	2.1	100	3.9	17.0	1.7	0.2
Strawberry, Bio Activia, Danone*	1 Pot/125g	118	4.0	94	3.5	12.8	3.2	2.0
Strawberry, Biopot, Wholegrain, Onken*	1 Serving/100g	111	2.9	111	4.1	17.2	2.9	0.5
Strawberry, Cereals, Fibre, Bio Activia, Danone*	1 Pot/120g	113	3.8	94	3.7	12.7	3.2	3.0
Strawberry, Childrens, Co-Op*	1 Pot/125g	121	3.4	97	3.5	14.9	2.7	0.2
Strawberry, Custard Style, Shapers, Boots*	1 Pot/150g	117	1.0	78	3.9	14.0	0.7	0.5
Strawberry, Duo, Co-Op*	1 Pot/175g	219	8.8	125	3.0	17.0	5.0	0.7
Strawberry, Fat Free, Average	1 Serving/100g	66	0.1	66	4.9	11.1	0.1	0.6
Strawberry, Fat free, Greek Style, Brooklea, Aldi*	1 Pot/125g	72	0.3	57	4.9	8.8	0.2	0.2
Strawberry, Fat Free, Probiotic, Organic, Yeo Valley*	1 Pot/125g	108	1.2	86	5.1	14.1	1.0	0.1
Strawberry, Fruit Corner, Snack Size, Muller*	1 Pot/95g	108	3.8	114	3.9	15.6	4.0	0.4
Strawberry, Fruit 'n' Creamy, Ubley*	1 Pot/151g	167	4.4	111	4.3	16.9	2.9	0.3
Strawberry, Fruity, Mullerlight, Muller*	1 Pot/175g	89	0.2	51	4.1	7.9	0.1	0.0
Strawberry, Granose*	1 Pot/120g	108	1.9	90	4.5	15.5	1.6	0.0
Strawberry, Great Stuff, Asda*	1 Pot/60g	58	1.5	97	4.7	14.0	2.5	0.5
Strawberry, Healthy Balance, Corner, Muller*	1 Pot/135g	161	3.5	119	5.4	17.9	2.6	0.8

	Measure INFO/WEIGHT	per Measure KCAL	per Measure FAT	Nutrition Values per 100g / 100ml KCAL	PROT	CARB	FAT	FIBRE
YOGHURT								
Strawberry, Lactose Free, Lactofree, Arla*	1 Pot/125g	126	3.2	101	3.5	15.9	2.6	0.4
Strawberry, LC, Tesco*	1 Pot/200g	86	0.2	43	4.1	6.3	0.1	0.6
Strawberry, Light, HL, Tesco*	1 Pot/200g	80	0.2	40	3.5	6.4	0.1	0.8
Strawberry, Light & Refreshing, Campina*	1 Pot/125g	110	1.4	88	2.5	16.9	1.1	0.0
Strawberry, Little Town Dairy*	1 Pot/125g	82	2.0	66	2.9	9.9	1.6	0.0
Strawberry, Live, Turners Dairies*	1 Pot/125g	86	0.4	69	4.9	11.9	0.3	0.0
Strawberry, Low Fat, Average	1 Serving/100g	81	1.0	81	4.5	13.6	1.0	0.2
Strawberry, Low Fat, Probiotic, Organic, M & S*	1 Pot/170g	136	2.4	80	4.8	11.6	1.4	0.4
Strawberry, Luscious, Shapers, Boots*	1 Pot/150g	82	1.6	55	4.0	7.3	1.1	0.6
Strawberry, Luxury, Bio Live, Jersey Dairy*	1 Pot/150g	159	8.6	106	3.8	10.2	5.7	0.5
Strawberry, Mousse, Shapers, Boots*	1 Pot/91g	88	3.7	97	4.1	11.0	4.1	0.1
Strawberry, Naturally Creamy, Nom Dairy UK*	1 Pot/175g	186	6.6	106	3.1	15.0	3.8	0.3
Strawberry, Naturally Light, Nom Dairy UK*	1 Pot/180g	137	0.2	76	4.5	13.4	0.1	0.3
Strawberry, Orange Balls, Crunch Corner, Muller*	1 Pot/150g	222	8.1	148	4.0	20.8	5.4	0.2
Strawberry, Organic, Yeo Valley*	1 Pot/150g	159	5.7	106	4.7	13.2	3.8	0.1
Strawberry, Perfectly Balanced, Waitrose*	1 Pot/150g	136	0.2	91	4.6	17.8	0.1	0.1
Strawberry, Pouring, Activia, Danone*	1 Serving/100g	59	1.6	59	3.9	7.3	1.6	0.1
Strawberry, Probiotic, Natural Balance, Asda*	1 Pot/125g	109	3.0	87	3.1	13.3	2.4	2.4
Strawberry, Probiotic, Organic, Yeo Valley*	1 Pot/125g	125	5.0	100	4.4	11.7	4.0	0.1
Strawberry, Smooth, Activ8, Ski, Nestle*	1 Pot/120g	113	2.0	94	4.6	14.8	1.7	0.7
Strawberry, Smooth, Nom Dairy UK*	1 Yoghurt/125g	112	3.0	90	3.2	13.8	2.4	0.3
Strawberry, Smooth Set, French, Low Fat, Sainsbury's*	1 Pot/125g	112	4.0	90	3.7	11.8	3.2	0.0
Strawberry, Soya, Dairy Free, Organic, Yofu, Provamel*	1 Pot/125g	101	2.8	81	3.9	10.6	2.2	0.8
Strawberry, Soya, Joya*	1 Pot/125g	105	2.8	84	3.8	11.7	2.2	1.0
Strawberry, Soyage, GranoVita*	1 Pot/145g	112	0.6	77	1.8	16.5	0.4	0.0
Strawberry, Sveltesse, Nestle*	1 Serving/125g	61	0.1	49	4.8	7.1	0.1	0.2
Strawberry, Swiss, Emmi*	1 Pot/175g	177	4.4	101	3.5	16.0	2.5	0.3
Strawberry, Thick & Creamy, Co-Op*	1 Pot/150g	182	6.9	121	3.6	16.4	4.6	0.1
Strawberry, Thick & Creamy, Waitrose*	1 Pot/125g	135	3.1	108	3.7	17.6	2.5	0.4
Strawberry, Thick & Fruity, Probiotic, COU, M & S*	1 Pot/170g	76	0.2	45	4.1	7.3	0.1	0.4
Strawberry, Totally, Low Fat, Chosen By You, Asda*	1 Pot/125g	104	1.2	83	4.1	14.2	1.0	0.4
Strawberry, Very Berry, Activ8, Ski, Nestle*	1 Pot/120g	110	2.0	92	4.3	15.0	1.7	0.3
Strawberry, Virtually Fat Free, Average	1 Serving/100g	65	0.2	65	4.7	11.3	0.2	0.2
Strawberry, Vitality, Low Fat, with Omega 3, Muller*	1 Pot/150g	140	2.8	93	4.3	14.0	1.9	0.8
Strawberry, Wholemilk, Organic, Sainsbury's*	1 Pot/150g	123	5.2	82	3.5	9.2	3.5	0.1
Strawberry, Yoplait*	1 Pot/125g	61	0.2	49	4.2	7.6	0.2	0.9
Strawberry & Banana, Oatie Breakfast, Moma Foods*	1 Pot/235g	320	5.6	136	4.3	25.4	2.4	1.7
Strawberry & Clotted Cream, Luxury, Stapleton Farm*	1 Pot/150g	147	5.7	98	3.2	13.2	3.8	0.6
Strawberry & Cornish Clotted Cream, M & S*	1 Pot/150g	218	11.6	145	3.2	15.4	7.7	0.5
Strawberry & French Vanilla, Amore Luxury, Muller*	1 Pot/150g	225	11.7	150	2.9	17.0	7.8	0.1
Strawberry & Raspberry, HL, Tesco*	1 Pot/125g	58	0.1	46	4.2	7.0	0.1	0.0
Strawberry & Raspberry, Layered, Bio, GFY, Asda*	1 Pot/72g	43	0.1	60	3.8	11.0	0.1	0.4
Strawberry & Raspberry, Low Fat, Sainsbury's*	1 Pot/125g	109	1.8	87	4.2	14.3	1.4	0.2
Strawberry & Raspberry, Probiotic, Organic, Yeo Valley*	1 Pot/125g	125	4.9	100	4.2	12.0	3.9	0.1
Strawberry & Redcurrant, Bio Layered, Sainsbury's*	1 Serving/125g	134	3.4	107	4.1	16.5	2.7	0.2
Strawberry & Redcurrant, Farmhouse, Ann Forshaw's*	1 Pot/150g	194	7.4	129	3.8	17.4	4.9	0.2
Strawberry & Rhubarb, Channel Island, M & S*	1 Pot/150g	158	4.5	105	3.9	15.4	3.0	0.0
Strawberry & Rhubarb, Low Fat, Sainsbury's*	1 Pot/125g	108	1.8	86	4.2	14.1	1.4	0.2
Strawberry & Rhubarb, Onken*	1 Serving/100g	85	0.1	85	4.6	16.2	0.1	0.4
Summer Berries, Biopot, Lite, Wholegrain, Onken*	¼ Pot/120g	100	0.2	83	4.6	15.8	0.2	1.4
Summer Berries, Fat Free, Mullerlight, Muller*	1 Pot/175g	88	0.2	50	4.1	7.6	0.1	0.4
Summer Berries, Wholegrain, Biopot, Onken*	1 Portion/100g	110	2.9	110	4.1	16.9	2.9	0.7
Summer Fruits, Cool Country*	1 Serving/150g	136	2.2	91	3.0	16.3	1.5	0.0

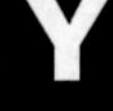

	Measure	per Measure		Nutrition Values per 100g / 100ml				
	INFO/WEIGHT	KCAL	FAT	KCAL	PROT	CARB	FAT	FIBRE
YOGHURT								
Summer Fruits, Greek Style, Corner, Muller*	1 Pot/150g	165	4.5	110	5.1	15.0	3.0	0.5
Summer Fruits, Light, Spelga*	1 Pot/175g	79	0.4	45	4.4	7.1	0.2	0.0
Summer Selection, Fat Free, Organic, Yeo Valley*	1 Pot/125g	89	0.1	71	5.2	12.3	0.1	0.2
Summer Selection, Thick & Fruity, COU, M & S*	1 Pot/145g	75	0.2	52	4.2	7.8	0.1	0.5
Summerfruits, Bio Live, Fat Free, Rachel's Organic*	1 Pot/125g	120	2.2	96	4.7	15.3	1.8	0.0
Summerfruits Bio, Boots*	1 Pot/150g	140	4.0	93	4.1	13.0	2.7	0.4
Sweet Treat, Low Fat, Tesco*	1 Pot/125g	131	2.9	105	3.1	18.0	2.3	0.3
Thick & Fruity Black Cherry, COU, M & S*	1 Pot/145g	72	0.1	50	4.2	7.8	0.1	0.5
Toffee, Benecol*	1 Pot/125g	124	0.9	99	3.8	19.3	0.7	0.0
Toffee, COU, M & S*	1 Pot/145g	65	0.3	45	4.2	7.7	0.2	0.0
Toffee, Devon, Low Fat, Sainsbury's*	1 Pot/126g	137	1.9	109	4.3	19.6	1.5	0.0
Toffee, Economy, Sainsbury's*	1 Pot/126g	91	1.3	72	3.0	12.8	1.0	0.0
Toffee, Greek Style, Tempting, Muller Light*	1 Pot/120g	84	0.1	70	6.3	10.1	0.1	0.0
Toffee, Live Bio, Perfectly Balanced, Waitrose*	1 Pot/150g	156	0.4	104	4.2	21.1	0.3	0.0
Toffee, Low Fat, Average	1 Pot/125g	136	3.1	109	4.3	19.5	2.4	0.1
Toffee, Probiotic, You Count, Love Life, Waitrose*	1 Pot/131g	85	0.1	65	4.4	11.5	0.1	0.5
Toffee, Smooth & Creamy, Fat Free, Weight Watchers*	1 Pot/120g	48	0.1	40	3.9	5.9	0.1	0.8
Toffee, Treacle, Dessert, Low Fat, Sainsbury's*	1 Pot/125g	149	2.4	119	4.3	21.2	1.9	0.0
Toffee, Vanilla, Low Fat, Sainsbury's*	1 Pot/125g	145	2.2	116	4.3	20.6	1.8	0.0
Toffee, Virtually Fat Free, Boots*	1 Pot/125g	69	0.1	55	5.1	8.3	0.1	0.0
Tropical, Low Fat, Luscious, Rachel's Organic*	1 Pot/125g	115	2.0	92	4.0	15.3	1.6	0.0
Tropical Crunch, Healthy Balance, Fruit Corner, Muller*	1 Pot/150g	170	3.2	113	4.7	18.2	2.1	0.5
Tropical Fruit, Bio, Granola, Corner, Muller*	1 Pot/135g	161	3.2	119	5.4	18.2	2.4	0.6
Tropical Fruit, Greek Style, Asda*	1 Pot/125g	170	8.8	136	3.3	15.0	7.0	0.0
Tropical Fruit, Greek Style, Shapers, Boots*	1 Pot/150g	100	2.2	67	3.6	9.8	1.5	0.8
Tropical Fruit, HL, Tesco*	1 Serving/125g	56	0.2	45	4.1	6.6	0.2	0.9
Vanilla, & Chocolate, Muller*	1 Pot/165g	86	0.8	52	4.0	7.2	0.5	0.1
Vanilla, Average	1 Serving/120g	100	5.4	83	4.5	12.4	4.5	0.8
Vanilla, Benecol*	1 Serving/125g	99	0.8	79	3.7	14.6	0.6	0.0
Vanilla, BGTY, Sainsbury's*	1 Pot/200g	98	0.2	49	4.5	7.5	0.1	0.0
Vanilla, Bio, BFY, Morrisons*	1 Pot/150g	82	0.4	55	5.7	8.4	0.3	0.0
Vanilla, Bio, Fat Free, Snackpot, Activia, Danone*	1 Pot/165g	87	0.2	53	5.0	8.1	0.1	0.9
Vanilla, Choco Balls, Crunch Corner, Muller*	1 Pot/135g	201	7.4	149	4.1	20.2	5.5	0.2
Vanilla, Chocolate, & Black Cherry, Mullerlight, Muller*	1 Pot/175g	103	0.7	59	3.1	10.3	0.4	0.3
Vanilla, Creamy, with Mini Smarties, Nestle*	1 Pot/120g	182	6.5	152	3.6	21.5	5.4	0.0
Vanilla, Delite, Yoplait*	1 Serving/125g	66	0.1	53	4.6	7.4	0.1	2.2
Vanilla, Fat Free, Onken*	½ Pot/225g	166	0.2	74	4.4	12.6	0.1	0.3
Vanilla, Lifestyle, Co-Op*	1 Pot/180g	81	0.2	45	5.0	6.0	0.1	0.0
Vanilla, Live, Bio, Bio Green Dairy*	1 Bottle/250ml	262	7.2	105	2.5	17.7	2.9	0.0
Vanilla, Live Bio, Low Fat, Perfectly Balanced, Waitrose*	1 Pot/150g	114	0.2	76	4.1	14.7	0.1	0.0
Vanilla, Low Fat, Bio, Sainsbury's*	1 Pot/150g	147	1.6	98	4.8	17.2	1.1	0.0
Vanilla, Low Fat, Probiotic, Organic, M & S*	1 Serving/100g	85	1.8	85	6.2	10.9	1.8	0.0
Vanilla, Low Fat, Tesco*	1 Pot/125g	125	2.1	100	4.9	16.3	1.7	0.0
Vanilla, Madagascan, 0.06% Fat, TTD, Sainsbury's*	1 Pot/150g	210	9.0	140	3.7	17.8	6.0	0.0
Vanilla, Madagascan, Indulgent, Dessert, Waitrose*	1 Pot/150g	240	11.4	160	3.7	19.2	7.6	0.0
Vanilla, Madagascan, West Country, TTD, Sainsbury's*	1 Pot/150g	192	8.4	128	3.9	15.5	5.6	0.0
Vanilla, Onken*	1 Serving/100g	100	2.7	100	3.1	15.9	2.7	0.0
Vanilla, Organic, Low Fat, Sainsbury's*	1 Pot/125g	114	1.2	91	5.3	15.3	1.0	0.0
Vanilla, Organic, Probiotic, Fat Free, Yeo Valley*	1 Pot/500g	400	0.5	80	5.4	14.2	0.1	0.0
Vanilla, Pouring, Activia, Danone*	1 Serving/100g	62	1.6	62	3.9	8.1	1.6	0.0
Vanilla, Smooth, Light, Fat Free, Muller*	1 Pot/175g	88	0.2	50	4.3	7.2	0.1	0.0
Vanilla, Smooth & Creamy, Fat Free, Weight Watchers*	1 Pot/120g	50	0.1	42	3.9	6.5	0.1	0.1
Vanilla, Soya, Dairy Free, Organic, Yofu, Provamel*	1 Pot/125g	114	2.8	91	3.8	13.3	2.2	0.7

	Measure INFO/WEIGHT	per Measure KCAL	per Measure FAT	Nutrition Values per 100g / 100ml KCAL	PROT	CARB	FAT	FIBRE
YOGHURT								
Vanilla, Thick & Creamy, Channel Island, M & S*	1 Pot/150g	188	6.6	125	4.5	17.5	4.4	1.0
Vanilla, Thick & Creamy, Probiotic, COU, M & S*	1 Pot/170g	76	0.2	45	4.2	6.9	0.1	0.6
Vanilla, Totally, Low Fat, Asda*	1 Pot/150g	134	1.6	89	4.7	15.1	1.1	0.0
Vanilla, Virtually Fat Free, Shapers, Boots*	1 Pot/125g	84	0.6	67	3.6	12.0	0.5	0.0
Vanilla, Virtually Fat Free, Yeo Valley*	1 Pot/150g	122	0.2	81	5.1	15.0	0.1	0.0
Vanilla, with Choc Flakes, Adore, Ehrmann*	1 Pot/150g	214	10.5	143	3.1	17.0	7.0	0.0
Vanilla, with Dark Chocolate Flakes, Light, Brooklea*	1 Pot/180g	104	1.8	58	4.9	7.0	1.0	0.5
Vanilla Flavour, Healthy Living, Light, Tesco*	1 Pot/200g	90	0.2	45	4.1	7.0	0.1	0.0
Vanilla Flavour, Organic, Low Fat, Tesco*	1 Pot/125g	114	1.2	91	5.3	15.3	1.0	0.0
Vanilla Flavour, Weight Watchers*	1 Pot/120g	47	0.1	39	4.2	5.2	0.1	0.2
YOGHURT DRINK								
Average	1fl oz/30ml	19	0.0	62	3.1	13.1	0.0	0.0
Ayran, Gazi*	1 Can/330ml	34	1.9	10	0.5	0.8	0.6	0.0
Banana & Honey, Ski Up & Go, Nestle*	1 Bottle/250g	215	2.2	86	0.0	16.0	0.9	0.0
Blueberry, Low Fat, Prebiotic & Probiotic, Muller*	1 Pot/100g	66	1.4	66	2.6	10.3	1.4	2.2
Blueberry & Blackcurrant, Orchard Maid*	1 Carton/250ml	148	0.1	59	1.6	13.6	0.0	0.0
Cholesterol Lowering, Asda*	1 Bottle/100g	76	1.4	76	2.9	13.0	1.4	1.0
Fristi*	1 Carton/330g	191	0.3	58	2.6	13.6	0.1	0.0
Fruit, Mixed, Actimel, Danone*	1 Bottle/100ml	88	1.5	88	2.7	16.0	1.5	0.0
Light, Benecol*	1 Bottle/68g	40	1.4	60	2.8	7.3	2.1	0.1
Light, Yakult*	1 Bottle/65ml	27	0.0	42	1.4	10.2	0.0	1.8
Mango, Probiotic, Mundella Foods*	1 Glass/250g	191	2.5	76	2.4	12.3	1.0	1.4
Mixed Berry, Up & Go, Ski, Nestle*	1 Bottle/250g	218	2.2	87	3.1	16.0	0.9	0.2
Multi Fruit, Actimel, Danone*	1 Bottle/100g	85	1.5	85	2.7	14.4	1.5	0.1
Multifruit, Natural Defences, Tesco*	1 Bottle/100g	70	1.1	70	3.2	11.8	1.1	0.7
Multifruit, Probiotic, Value, Tesco*	1 Serving/100g	75	1.1	75	2.8	12.5	1.1	0.3
Orange, Actimel, Danone*	1 Bottle/100g	74	1.5	74	2.9	11.5	1.5	0.0
Orange, Banana & Passion Fruit, One a Day, Muller*	1 Bottle/310ml	208	0.3	67	2.1	14.1	0.1	0.0
Orange, Pro Activ, Cholesterol, Flora*	1 Bottle/100g	45	1.5	45	3.2	5.6	1.5	1.1
Orange, Probiotic, Lidl*	1 Serving/125ml	105	2.0	84	2.5	14.7	1.6	0.0
Original, 0.1% Fat, Actimel, Danone*	1 Bottle/100g	28	0.1	28	2.8	3.3	0.1	1.9
Original, Actimel, Danone*	1 Bottle/100g	80	1.6	80	2.8	12.8	1.6	0.0
Original, Benecol*	1 Serving/70g	62	1.6	88	2.6	14.2	2.3	0.0
Original, Danacol, Danone*	1 Bottle/100ml	64	1.0	64	3.2	10.0	1.0	0.0
Peach & Apricot, Benecol*	1 Bottle/68g	38	1.5	56	2.8	6.2	2.2	0.0
Peach & Mango, Fristi*	1 Carton/330g	191	0.3	58	2.6	13.6	0.1	0.0
Pineapple, 0.1% Fat, Actimel, Danone*	1 Bottle/100g	33	0.0	33	2.7	5.5	0.0	1.8
Pomeganate & Raspberry Pro Active, Mini Drink, Flora*	1 Serving/100g	45	1.5	45	2.6	4.7	1.5	1.1
Raspberry, Pro Biotic, Omega 3 Plus, Flora*	1 Bottle/100g	58	1.6	58	2.6	8.5	1.6	0.0
Raspberry & Passion Fruit, Everybody, Yoplait*	1 Bottle/90g	60	0.8	67	2.6	12.2	0.9	0.0
Strawberry, Actimel, Danone*	1 Bottle/100g	74	1.5	74	2.9	11.5	1.5	0.0
Strawberry, Benecol*	1 Bottle/68g	38	1.4	56	3.2	6.2	2.0	0.0
Strawberry, Danacol, Danone*	1 Bottle/100g	68	1.2	68	3.2	11.2	1.2	0.0
Strawberry, Fristi*	1 Carton/250g	165	0.2	66	2.6	13.6	0.1	0.0
Strawberry, Low Fat, Pre & Probiotic, Muller*	1 Pot/100g	67	1.4	67	2.5	10.7	1.4	2.4
Strawberry, Pro Activ, Cholesterol, Flora*	1 Bottle/100g	45	1.5	45	2.6	4.7	1.5	0.0
Strawberry, Probiotic, Mundella Foods*	1 Glass/250g	191	2.5	76	2.4	12.3	1.0	1.4
Strawberry, Yop, Yoplait*	1 Bottle/330g	261	4.3	79	2.8	14.0	1.3	0.0
Sveltesse, 0%, Nestle*	1 Pot/125g	61	0.1	49	4.8	7.3	0.1	0.1
Vanilla, Activate, Probiotic, Little Town Dairy*	1 Bottle/265g	167	3.7	63	2.7	10.0	1.4	0.2
Vanilla, Probiotic, Mundella Foods*	1 Glass/250g	191	2.5	76	2.4	12.3	1.0	1.4
Yakult*	1 Pot/65ml	43	0.1	66	1.3	14.7	0.1	0.0

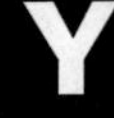

	Measure INFO/WEIGHT	per Measure KCAL	FAT	Nutrition Values per 100g / 100ml KCAL	PROT	CARB	FAT	FIBRE
YORK FRUITS								
Terry's*	1 Sweet/9g	29	0.0	320	0.0	78.5	0.0	0.5
YORKIE								
Honeycomb, Nestle*	1 Bar/65g	331	16.8	509	5.7	63.6	25.8	0.0
King Size, Nestle*	1 Bar/83g	445	26.1	537	6.1	57.3	31.5	0.0
Original, Nestle*	1 Bar/55g	302	17.4	546	6.2	57.9	31.5	1.9
Raisin & Biscuit, Nestle*	1 Bar/67g	331	17.4	497	5.5	59.7	26.2	0.9
YORKSHIRE PUDDING								
& Beef Dripping, M & S*	4 Puddings/100g	410	30.4	410	9.4	25.2	30.4	3.2
3", Baked, Aunt Bessie's*	1 Pudding/36g	91	2.8	252	9.0	36.4	7.9	1.7
4 Minute, Aunt Bessie's*	1 Pudding/18g	52	2.0	291	10.5	36.6	11.3	2.2
7", Baked, Aunt Bessie's*	1 Pudding/110g	290	9.9	264	8.5	37.4	9.0	2.0
Average	1 Pudding/30g	62	3.0	208	6.6	24.7	9.9	0.9
Batters, in Foils, Ready to Bake, Frozen, Aunt Bessie's*	1 Pudding/17g	47	1.8	276	9.1	32.6	10.8	1.4
Chicken & Vegetable, COU, M & S*	1 Pudding/150g	195	3.3	130	12.2	14.3	2.2	1.3
Filled, Chicken Casserole, Farmfoods*	1 Pack/280g	347	6.4	124	6.5	19.3	2.3	1.3
Filled, with Beef, Morrisons*	1 Serving/350g	514	21.0	147	7.4	15.7	6.0	0.5
Filled, with Beef, Tesco*	1 Pudding/300g	408	15.6	136	6.1	16.2	5.2	1.1
Filled, with Chicken, GFY, Asda*	1 Pack/381g	438	9.9	115	9.0	14.0	2.6	1.5
Filled, with Chicken, Tesco*	1 Pack/300g	366	8.7	122	6.5	17.4	2.9	1.3
Filled, with Chicken & Vegetable, GFY, Asda*	1 Pack/380g	376	9.9	99	6.0	13.0	2.6	1.1
Filled, with Sausage, Sainsbury's*	1 Pack/300g	576	31.2	192	6.9	17.5	10.4	0.9
Frozen, Ovenbaked, Iceland*	1 Pudding/12g	36	1.0	290	9.7	45.1	7.9	4.1
Fully Prepared, M & S*	1 Pudding/22g	63	2.9	285	9.4	31.6	13.2	1.2
Giant, Aunt Bessie's*	1 Pudding/110g	290	9.9	264	8.5	37.4	9.0	2.0
Giant, VLH Kitchens	1 Serving/110g	284	9.1	259	8.5	33.6	10.0	2.3
Heat & Serve, Waitrose*	1 Pudding/30g	86	3.5	288	9.5	35.3	11.7	1.7
Home Bake, Rise in 20 Minutes, Baked, Aunt Bessie's*	1 Pudding/25g	43	1.7	174	6.0	20.0	7.0	3.1
Large, Aunt Bessie's*	1 Pudding/40g	111	4.6	277	8.5	35.3	11.4	1.5
Large, The Real Yorkshire Pudding Co*	1 Pudding/34g	103	4.1	304	11.5	37.3	12.1	2.5
Made From Batter Mix, Sainsbury's*	1 Pudding/100g	248	5.3	248	9.9	40.1	5.3	4.0
Minced Beef Filled, Waitrose*	1 Serving/350g	525	24.8	150	7.5	14.1	7.1	1.0
Mini, Co-Op*	1 Serving/16g	50	2.0	312	6.2	43.8	12.5	2.5
Premium, Bisto*	1 Pudding/30g	74	3.3	248	7.3	30.3	10.9	2.1
Ready Baked, Smart Price, Asda*	1 Pudding/12g	36	1.1	297	10.0	44.0	9.0	2.8
Ready to Bake, Baked, Aunt Bessie's*	1 Pudding/17g	42	1.4	246	8.5	35.1	8.0	1.7
Ready to Bake, Sainsbury's*	1 Pudding/18g	48	1.6	263	9.9	35.9	8.9	1.3
Roast Chicken Filled, COU, M & S*	1 Pudding/150g	210	4.0	140	12.6	15.7	2.7	0.9
Roberts Bakery*	1 Pudding/18g	48	1.6	263	9.9	35.9	8.9	1.3
Sage & Onion, Tesco*	1 Pudding/19g	53	2.3	280	8.0	35.0	12.0	2.6
Sainsbury's*	1 Pudding/14g	43	2.0	309	7.9	37.5	14.1	2.9
Sausage Filled, Frozen, Tesco*	1 Pack/340g	510	19.7	150	6.6	17.8	5.8	1.8
Steak & Red Wine, Filled, COU, M & S*	1 Pack/162g	211	3.6	130	12.4	15.6	2.2	1.8
The Best, Morrisons*	1 Pudding/22g	60	1.8	271	8.3	43.0	8.0	1.6
Traditional, Giant, Asda*	1 Pudding/110g	310	11.0	282	10.0	38.0	10.0	2.3
Traditional Style, Medium, Asda*	1 Pudding/36g	86	3.2	241	9.0	31.0	9.0	2.4
Traditional Style, Small, Asda*	1 Pudding/20g	52	2.0	262	8.0	35.0	10.0	2.9
Unbaked, Iceland*	1 Serving/31g	81	2.7	263	9.9	35.9	8.9	1.3
Value, Tesco*	1 Pudding/16g	45	1.9	282	9.7	34.3	11.8	1.6
YULE LOG								
Chocolate, Sainsbury's*	1 Slice/35g	153	7.7	432	5.0	51.6	21.8	4.6
Christmas Range, Tesco*	1 Serving/30g	131	6.4	442	4.9	56.8	21.7	2.8
Mini, M & S*	1 Cake/36g	165	8.4	460	5.7	56.9	23.3	1.1

	Measure INFO/WEIGHT	per Measure KCAL	per Measure FAT	Nutrition Values per 100g / 100ml KCAL	PROT	CARB	FAT	FIBRE
ABOKADO								
BAGEL								
Bacon & Egg, Multigrain, Abokado*	1 Bagel/169g	473	15.6	280	12.4	37.3	9.2	4.1
Cream Cheese, Lite, Multigrain, Abokado*	1 Bagel/157g	387	12.9	246	10.6	32.7	8.2	3.7
Multigrain, Buttered, Abokado*	1 Bagel/122g	347	10.4	284	10.7	41.3	8.5	4.8
Multigrain, Toasted, Abokado*	1 Bagel/117g	310	6.2	265	11.2	43.1	5.3	5.0
Salmon, Smoked, Multigrain, Abokado*	1 Bagel/152g	389	11.7	256	13.7	33.0	7.7	3.8
BREAKFAST								
Granola, & Raspberry Compote, Bowl, Abokado*	1 Bowl/183g	175	4.1	96	4.8	14.9	2.2	1.3
Mango & Fig Bircher, Abokado*	1 Bowl/204g	240	4.1	117	4.0	20.0	2.0	2.3
Maple Syrup & Banana Bowl, Abokado*	1 Bowl/223g	249	4.2	112	4.1	20.4	1.9	1.2
BROWNIES								
Chocolate, Fairtrade, Abokado*	1 Serving/83g	341	17.6	411	5.1	50.5	21.2	2.2
CRACKERS								
Rice, Chilli, Abokado*	1 Serving/40g	236	15.4	590	4.0	7.0	38.5	0.5
CRISPS								
Popchips, Barbeque, Abokado*	1 Serving/23g	96	3.2	416	6.1	62.2	13.9	3.9
Popchips, Original, Abokado*	1 Serving/23g	95	3.2	413	6.1	61.7	13.9	4.4
Popchips, Sea Salt & Vinegar, Abokado*	1 Serving/23g	94	3.1	409	5.6	63.9	13.5	3.9
Popchips, Sour Cream & Onion, Abokado*	1 Serving/23g	95	3.2	414	6.5	62.6	13.9	3.9
DRINKS								
San Pellegrino Aranciata, Abokado*	1 Serving/330ml	142	0.0	43	0.1	10.3	0.0	0.0
Zico Coconut Water Mango, Abokado*	1 Serving/400ml	17	0.0	4	0.0	1.0	0.0	0.0
Zico Coconut Water Original, Abokado*	1 Serving/400ml	17	0.0	4	0.0	1.0	0.0	0.0
HOT POT								
Chicken, Thai, Fragrant, Red, Abokado*	1 Serving/540g	447	15.8	83	5.3	7.5	2.9	0.0
Shrimp, Thai, Fragrant, Red, Abokado*	1 Serving/510g	397	15.2	78	3.6	7.8	3.0	0.0
BURGER KING								
APPLES								
Fries, Burger King*	1 Serving/60g	28	0.1	47	0.1	12.0	0.1	2.0
BURGERS								
Angus, Bacon, Smoked, & Cheddar, Burger King*	1 Burger/270g	683	39.1	253	14.3	16.0	14.5	1.1
Angus, Classic, Burger King*	1 Burger/285g	571	36.6	200	13.0	14.8	12.8	0.8
Angus, Classic, Double, Burger King*	1 Burger/323g	829	61.6	257	20.3	13.1	19.1	0.7
Angus, Mini, Burger King*	1 Burger/97g	272	10.7	280	14.0	31.0	11.0	1.0
Angus, Mini, with Cheese, Burger King*	1 Burger/110g	321	15.4	292	15.0	27.0	14.0	1.0
Bacon, Double Cheese, Burger King*	1 Burger/181g	476	25.7	264	17.4	18.9	14.2	1.3
Bacon, Double Cheese, XL, Burger King*	1 Burger/302g	957	54.8	317	20.9	17.2	18.2	0.9
Bean Burger, Veggie, Kids, Burger King*	1 Burger/116g	293	10.4	253	6.9	39.0	9.0	2.9
Big King, Burger King*	1 Burger/190g	486	26.6	256	14.6	17.5	14.0	1.1
Big King, XL, Burger King*	1 Burger/338g	902	54.1	267	16.0	14.0	16.0	1.0
BK, Veggie Bean Burger, Burger King*	1 Burger/280g	625	26.7	223	6.5	26.9	9.5	2.4
Cheeseburger, Bacon Double, Burger King*	1 Burger/160g	478	25.6	299	19.0	19.0	16.0	1.0
Cheeseburger, Bacon Double, XL, Burger King*	1 Burger/302g	927	54.4	307	21.0	15.0	18.0	1.0
Cheeseburger, Burger King*	1 Burger/126g	316	13.2	251	13.7	25.7	10.5	1.4
Cheeseburger, Double, Burger King*	1 Burger/173g	460	13.8	266	16.8	19.1	8.0	1.2
Cheeseburger, Kids, Burger King*	1 Burger/113g	329	14.3	291	15.9	28.0	12.6	1.3
Chicken, Chargrilled, Mini, Burger King*	1 Burger/109g	214	3.3	196	15.0	28.0	3.0	1.0
Chicken, Spicy Tendercrisp, Burger King*	1 Burger/254g	621	32.7	245	11.0	20.1	12.9	1.2
Chicken Royale, Burger King*	1 Burger/210g	605	17.1	288	11.4	26.5	8.1	1.3
Chicken Royale, Sweet Chilli, Burger King*	1 Burger/210g	480	23.7	229	11.4	27.3	11.3	1.3
Chicken Royale, with Cheese, Burger King*	1 Burger/263g	688	39.5	261	11.0	20.2	15.0	1.1
Hamburger, Burger King*	1 Burger/114g	274	9.9	241	13.2	28.1	8.7	1.6
Hamburger, Kids, Burger King*	1 Burger/100g	272	9.7	272	14.8	31.8	9.7	1.7

	Measure INFO/WEIGHT	per Measure KCAL	FAT	Nutrition Values per 100g / 100ml KCAL	PROT	CARB	FAT	FIBRE
BURGER KING								
BURGERS								
Ocean Catch, Burger King*	1 Burger/196g	498	27.9	254	8.8	22.2	14.2	1.4
Steakhouse, Burger King*	1 Burger/239g	732	43.1	306	14.8	20.3	18.0	1.2
Whopper, Burger King*	1 Burger/292g	652	35.4	223	10.4	17.6	12.1	1.2
Whopper, Double, Burger King*	1 Burger/355g	894	52.8	252	14.5	14.6	14.9	1.1
Whopper, Double, with Cheese, Burger King*	1 Burger/380g	961	60.8	253	14.0	13.0	16.0	1.0
Whopper, Junior, Burger King*	1 Burger/152g	343	16.9	226	10.0	21.6	11.2	1.2
Whopper, with Cheese, Burger King*	1 Burger/299g	721	41.9	241	11.0	16.0	14.0	1.0
Whopper, with Cheese, Junior, Burger King*	1 Burger/161g	388	19.3	241	10.0	19.0	12.0	1.0
CHICKEN								
Bites, Burger King*	14 Bites/112g	317	15.0	283	16.1	25.0	13.4	0.9
Bites, Kids, Burger King*	1 Serving/56g	158	7.3	282	16.0	25.0	13.0	2.0
Nuggets, with Dip, Burger King*	6 Nuggets/138g	307	13.6	223	12.5	20.2	9.9	1.6
COFFEE								
Black, Large, Burger King*	1 Serving/284ml	6	0.0	2	0.0	0.0	0.0	0.0
Black, Regular, Burger King*	1 Serving/200ml	4	0.0	2	0.0	0.0	0.0	0.0
Cappuccino, Large, Burger King*	1 Serving/59g	81	3.0	137	10.0	15.0	5.0	0.0
Cappuccino, Regular, Burger King*	1 Serving/46g	64	1.8	139	9.0	15.0	4.0	0.0
Latte, Large, Burger King*	1 Serving/45g	60	1.8	133	11.0	13.0	4.0	0.0
Latte, Regular, Burger King*	1 Serving/62g	82	3.1	132	10.0	15.0	5.0	0.0
DIP								
Barbeque Sauce, Heinz, Pot, Burger King*	1 Pot/40g	48	0.0	120	0.1	28.0	0.1	0.1
Sweet Chilli, Heinz, Pot, Burger King*	1 Pot/40g	96	0.0	240	0.0	60.0	0.0	0.0
DRESSING								
French, Burger King*	1 Sachet/40g	7	0.0	18	0.0	2.5	0.0	0.0
Honey & Mustard, Burger King*	1 Sachet/40g	32	1.0	80	2.5	15.0	2.5	0.0
FRIES								
Medium, Burger King*	1 Serving/116g	277	12.4	238	3.1	31.4	10.7	2.2
HASH BROWNS								
Regular, Burger King*	1 Regular/102g	192	19.2	188	2.4	21.7	18.8	2.4
MAYONNAISE								
Heinz, Sachet, Burger King*	1 Sachet/12g	80	9.0	667	0.0	0.0	75.0	0.0
MILK								
Semi Skimmed, Kids, Burger King*	1 Carton/258g	117	3.9	47	3.5	4.6	1.6	0.0
MILK SHAKE								
Chocolate, Large, Burger King*	1 Serving/519g	612	10.4	118	3.0	22.0	2.0	0.0
Chocolate, Regular, Burger King*	1 Serving/401g	449	8.0	112	3.0	20.0	2.0	0.1
Chocolate, Small, Burger King*	1 Serving/276g	301	8.3	109	3.0	19.0	3.0	0.1
Strawberry, Large, Burger King*	1 Serving/519g	581	10.4	112	3.0	20.0	2.0	0.0
Strawberry, Regular, Burger King*	1 Serving/401g	433	8.0	108	3.0	19.0	2.0	0.0
Strawberry, Small, Burger King*	1 Serving/276g	293	8.3	106	3.0	18.0	3.0	0.0
Vanilla, Large, Burger King*	1 Shake/519g	460	11.5	89	2.7	14.2	2.2	0.0
Vanilla, Regular, Burger King*	1 Reg/401g	371	9.3	93	2.8	14.8	2.3	0.0
ONION RINGS								
Large, Burger King*	1 Serving/180g	535	26.5	297	5.1	34.2	14.7	3.7
Regular, Burger King*	1 Serving/120g	356	17.6	297	5.1	34.2	14.7	3.7
Super, Burger King*	1 Serving/240g	713	35.3	297	5.1	34.2	14.7	3.7
SALAD								
Chicken, Flame Grilled, Burger King*	1 Salad/240g	127	2.4	53	8.0	3.0	1.0	1.0
Garden, Burger King*	1 Serving/165g	33	1.6	20	1.0	4.0	1.0	1.0
SANDWICH								
Butty, Bacon, with Heinz Ketchup, Burger King*	1 Butty/77g	270	6.2	351	13.6	57.3	8.0	3.2
Butty, Bacon, with HP Sauce, Burger King*	1 Butty/77g	222	6.0	288	13.0	41.6	7.8	2.0

	Measure INFO/WEIGHT	per Measure KCAL	FAT	Nutrition Values per 100g / 100ml KCAL	PROT	CARB	FAT	FIBRE
BURGER KING								
SANDWICH								
Butty, Bacon & Egg, with Heinz Ketchup, Burger King*	1 Butty/140g	362	17.0	259	12.9	25.0	12.1	11.4
Butty, Bacon & Egg, with HP Sauce, Burger King*	1 Butty/140g	363	17.0	259	12.9	25.0	12.1	1.4
Butty, Big Breakfast, with Heinz Ketchup, Burger King*	1 Butty/297g	849	50.5	286	14.0	18.0	17.0	1.0
Butty, Egg & Cheese, with Heinz Ketchup, Burger King*	1 Butty/126g	346	12.4	275	12.9	32.9	9.8	1.8
Butty, Sausage, with Heinz Ketchup, Burger King*	1 Butty/119g	312	13.0	262	13.4	26.9	10.9	1.7
Butty, Sausage, with HP Sauce, Burger King*	1 Butty/119g	313	13.0	263	13.4	26.9	10.9	1.7
Butty, Sausage & Egg, with HP Sauce, Burger King*	1 Butty/182g	454	24.0	249	13.2	19.2	13.2	1.1
TEA								
Regular, White, No Sugar, Burger King*	1 Reg/200ml	22	4.0	11	1.0	1.0	2.0	0.0
WRAP								
Chicken, Sweet Chilli, Burger King*	1 Wrap/160g	298	6.9	186	14.4	22.1	4.3	1.3
Veggie, Burger King*	1 Wrap/231g	493	21.0	214	4.2	27.6	9.1	2.7
CAFFE NERO								
BARS								
Fruit & Seed, Caffe Nero*	1 Serving/65g	197	5.8	303	7.5	48.2	8.9	8.7
Granola, Organic, Caffe Nero*	1 Serving/64g	278	14.3	434	6.7	51.5	22.4	4.8
BISCOTTI								
Almond, Organic, Caffe Nero*	1 Serving/37g	147	5.9	397	9.0	54.6	15.9	2.7
Chocolate, Organic, Caffe Nero*	1 Serving/37g	136	4.3	369	7.0	59.1	11.6	2.7
BISCUITS								
Amaretti, Caffe Nero*	1 Biscuit/10g	40	1.2	401	3.9	70.1	11.7	10.6
Double Chocolate, Caffe Nero*	1 Biscuit/25g	126	6.8	505	5.5	57.4	27.3	3.7
Palmine, Caffe Nero*	1 Biscuit/14g	75	4.3	540	6.6	55.5	31.0	1.6
BREAD								
Ciabatta, Roll, Caffe Nero*	1 Roll/70g	180	2.7	257	8.7	46.9	3.9	1.7
BREAKFAST CEREAL								
Porridge, with Skimmed Milk, no Topping, Caffe Nero*	1 Serving/239g	210	3.8	88	4.8	14.0	1.6	1.5
Porridge, with Soya Milk, no Topping, Caffe Nero*	1 Serving/239g	232	7.7	97	4.9	12.1	3.2	2.0
BROWNIES								
Chocolate, Belgian, Caffe Nero*	1 Serving/75g	314	14.7	419	4.6	54.6	19.6	2.9
Chocolate, Double, GF, Organic, Caffe Nero*	1 Serving/75g	318	15.5	425	4.3	55.4	20.7	2.0
CAKE								
Cappuccino, Caffe Nero*	1 Serving/120g	486	22.7	405	3.7	56.2	18.9	0.5
Carrot, & Raisin, Organic, Wrapped, Caffe Nero*	1 Serving/70g	290	17.5	414	4.5	43.4	25.0	3.9
Carrot, & Raisin, Wheat Free, Organic, Caffe Nero*	1 Serving/70g	301	12.3	430	4.8	43.9	17.5	2.1
Chocolate Crunch, Caffe Nero*	1 Serving/65g	308	16.5	473	6.2	54.3	25.3	4.2
Chocolate Fudge, Caffe Nero*	1 Serving/124g	526	26.9	424	5.2	52.2	21.7	1.2
Lemon Drizzle, Organic, Caffe Nero*	1 Serving/73g	247	9.9	338	3.3	50.5	13.6	0.5
Lemon Drizzle, Slice, Organic, Wrapped, Caffe Nero*	1 Pack/70g	248	11.1	354	4.2	48.5	15.9	0.8
Red Velvet, Caffe Nero*	1 Slice/100g	414	19.9	414	4.2	54.7	19.9	0.9
CHEESECAKE								
Chocolate, White & Dark, Truffle, Caffe Nero*	1 Serving/131g	533	35.6	407	4.8	35.7	27.2	0.5
Sicilian Lemon, Caffe Nero*	1 Serving/107g	400	26.0	374	5.0	33.0	24.3	1.4
CHOCOLATE								
Bar, Dark, 50% Cocoa, Caffe Nero*	1 Bar/40g	213	12.4	534	6.4	53.6	31.1	7.0
Bar, Milk, Caffe Nero*	1 Bar/40g	223	13.5	561	8.0	55.0	34.0	1.5
Bar, Milk, with Hazelnuts, Caffe Nero*	1 Bar/40g	229	15.2	572	8.0	49.5	38.0	1.8
Coin, Caffe Nero*	1 Serving/25g	129	7.0	516	6.3	59.7	27.8	2.1
Penguin, Milk, Paolo Pinguino, Caffe Nero*	1 Serving/45g	246	14.8	547	6.6	55.5	32.8	1.8
COFFEE								
Cappuccino, Grande, Semi Skimmed, Caffe Nero*	1 Grande/263g	92	3.4	35	2.7	3.6	1.3	0.0
Cappuccino, Grande, Skimmed Milk, Caffe Nero*	1 Grande/262g	68	0.5	26	2.7	3.7	0.2	0.0

	Measure INFO/WEIGHT	per Measure KCAL	per Measure FAT	KCAL	PROT	CARB	FAT	FIBRE
				Nutrition Values per 100g / 100ml				
CAFFE NERO								
COFFEE								
Cappuccino, Grande, Soya Milk, Caffe Nero*	1 Grande/258g	90	4.4	35	2.8	1.9	1.7	0.5
Cappuccino, Regular, Semi Skimmed Milk, Caffe Nero*	1 Regular/142g	37	1.4	26	2.0	2.7	1.0	0.0
Cappuccino, Regular, Skimmed Milk, Caffe Nero*	1 Regular/142g	27	0.3	19	2.0	2.7	0.2	0.0
Cappuccino, Regular, Soya Milk, Caffe Nero*	1 Regular/138g	36	1.8	26	2.1	1.4	1.3	0.3
Caramelatte, Semi Skimmed Milk, Caffe Nero*	1 Serving/422g	485	25.3	115	2.3	12.3	6.0	0.0
Latte, Grande, Semi Skimmed Milk, Caffe Nero*	1 Grande/363g	138	5.1	38	2.9	3.9	1.4	0.0
Latte, Grande, Skimmed Milk, Caffe Nero*	1 Grande/364g	102	1.1	28	2.9	4.0	0.3	0.0
Latte, Grande, Soya Milk, Caffe Nero*	1 Grande/355g	135	6.4	38	3.1	2.1	1.8	1.8
Latte, Regular, Semi Skimmed Milk, Caffe Nero*	1 Regular/209g	69	2.5	33	2.5	3.4	1.2	0.0
Latte, Regular, Skimmed Milk, Caffe Nero*	1 Regular/212g	51	0.4	24	2.5	3.4	0.2	0.0
Latte, Regular, Soya Milk, Caffe Nero*	1 Regular/212g	68	3.4	32	2.6	1.8	1.6	0.4
Mocha, Regular, no Cream, Skimmed Milk, Caffe Nero*	1 Serving/232g	132	1.2	57	2.8	10.3	0.5	0.8
Mocha, Regular, no Cream, Soya, Caffe Nero*	1 Regular/231g	148	3.9	64	2.9	8.8	1.7	1.1
COFFEE BEANS								
Chocolate Coated, Caffe Nero*	1 Serving/25g	117	6.6	469	8.5	50.0	26.6	11.9
COOKIES								
Chocolate, Triple, Caffe Nero*	1 Serving/72g	333	17.5	463	5.6	55.6	24.3	3.3
Chocolate Chip, Organic, Caffe Nero*	1 Serving/60g	263	12.1	438	4.5	56.6	20.1	1.5
Chocolate Chunk, Milk, Caffe Nero*	1 Serving/72g	338	17.9	470	5.8	55.8	24.9	1.7
Oat & Raisin, Organic, Caffe Nero*	1 Serving/60g	282	14.0	470	4.4	60.5	23.4	2.6
CRISPS								
Mature Cheddar & Spring Onion, Caffe Nero*	1 Serving/40g	192	11.4	481	6.1	54.0	28.6	4.4
Sea Salt, Caffe Nero*	1 Serving/40g	197	10.8	493	7.0	54.0	27.1	4.5
Sea Salt & Balsamic Vinegar, Caffe Nero*	1 Serving/40g	192	11.0	482	7.0	54.1	27.5	4.0
CROISSANT								
Almond, Caffe Nero*	1 Serving/83g	350	19.8	422	10.0	41.7	23.9	2.6
Butter, Caffe Nero*	1 Serving/50g	204	11.6	408	8.5	40.9	23.3	1.7
Cheese Twist, Caffe Nero*	1 Serving/76g	316	18.4	416	13.4	36.1	24.2	2.6
Chocolate Twist, Caffe Nero*	1 Serving/79g	320	15.4	405	7.7	49.7	19.5	1.6
Pain au Chocolat, Caffe Nero*	1 Serving/65g	270	15.1	415	8.1	43.4	23.2	1.7
CUPCAKES								
Chocolate, Caffe Nero*	1 Serving/68g	311	19.1	457	3.1	48.7	28.1	0.5
Lemon, Caffe Nero*	1 Serving/72g	340	19.6	472	2.9	54.0	27.2	0.3
Raspberry, Caffe Nero*	1 Serving/67g	295	15.1	440	3.4	55.7	22.5	0.5
DANISH PASTRY								
Maple Pecan, Caffe Nero*	1 Pastry/82g	312	25.0	381	5.2	42.3	30.5	2.1
FRUIT SALAD								
Caffe Nero*	1 Serving/190g	103	0.2	54	0.6	12.1	0.1	1.5
HOT CHOCOLATE								
Milano, with Whipped Cream, Caffe Nero*	1 Serving/241g	424	22.6	176	3.5	19.3	9.4	2.0
Regular, No Cream, Skimmed Milk, Caffe Nero*	1 Serving/236g	217	1.9	92	3.3	17.6	0.8	1.5
Regular, No Cream, Soya Milk, Caffe Nero*	1 Serving/234g	229	4.4	98	3.4	15.9	1.9	1.9
JUICE								
Apple, Organic, Carton, Caffe Nero*	1 Carton/200g	94	0.0	47	0.5	11.2	0.0	0.0
Apple, Pressed, 100% Premium, Caffe Nero*	1 Bottle/250g	120	0.0	48	0.1	11.8	0.0	0.0
Apple & Mango Juice, Caffe Nero*	1 Serving/250g	125	0.0	50	0.2	12.3	0.0	0.1
Mango & Passion Fruit, Booster, Caffe Nero*	1 Serving/597g	191	0.6	32	0.4	7.8	0.1	0.6
Orange, 100% Squeezed, Fresh, Caffe Nero*	1 Serving/250g	95	0.0	38	0.5	8.8	0.0	0.1
Orange, Lemon & Lime, Booster, Caffe Nero*	1 Serving/591g	207	0.6	35	0.5	7.6	0.1	0.9
Strawberry & Raspberry, Booster, Caffe Nero*	1 Serving/589g	206	1.8	35	0.4	7.5	0.3	1.6
LEMONADE								
Italian, Sicilian, Still, Caffe Nero*	1 Serving/666g	320	0.7	48	0.1	11.3	0.1	0.3

	Measure INFO/WEIGHT	per Measure KCAL	FAT	Nutrition Values per 100g / 100ml KCAL	PROT	CARB	FAT	FIBRE
CAFFE NERO								
MILK SHAKE								
Frappe, Banana, Semi Skimmed, Caffe Nero*	1 Serving/420g	315	4.6	75	3.0	13.5	1.1	0.0
Frappe, Banana, Skimmed, Caffe Nero*	1 Serving/419g	285	1.3	68	3.0	13.6	0.3	0.0
Frappe, Banana, with Cream & Sprinkles, Caffe Nero*	1 Serving/347g	402	21.8	116	2.9	12.2	6.3	0.0
Frappe, Double Chocolate, Caffe Nero*	1 Shake/453g	317	4.5	70	2.9	12.3	1.0	0.5
Frappe, Double Chocolate, Skimmed Milk, Caffe Nero*	1 Shake/453g	290	1.4	64	2.9	12.3	0.3	0.5
Frappe, Latte, Cream, & Sprinkles, Caffe Nero*	1 Serving/344g	334	21.0	97	2.7	7.9	6.1	0.1
Frappe, Latte, Semi Skimmed Milk, Caffe Nero*	1 Serving/424g	225	3.8	53	2.8	8.5	0.9	0.1
Frappe, Latte, Skimmed Milk, Caffe Nero*	1 Frappe/430g	198	0.9	46	2.8	8.6	0.2	0.1
Frappe, Latte, Soya Milk, Caffe Nero*	1 Serving/388g	101	5.0	26	2.2	1.5	1.3	0.4
Frappe, Mint, Cream, & Sprinkles, Caffe Nero*	1 Serving/347g	399	21.9	115	2.9	12.0	6.3	0.0
Frappe, Mint, Semi Skimmed, Caffe Nero*	1 Frappe/419ml	310	4.6	74	3.0	13.3	1.1	0.0
Frappe, Mint, Semi Skimmed Milk, Caffe Nero*	1 Serving/419g	310	4.6	74	3.0	13.3	1.1	0.0
Frappe, Mocha Latte, Cream, & Sprinkles, Caffe Nero*	1 Serving/345g	386	21.4	112	2.8	11.2	6.2	0.5
Frappe, Mocha Latte, Semi Skimmed Milk, Caffe Nero*	1 Serving/459g	317	4.5	70	2.9	12.3	1.0	0.5
Frappe, Strawberry, Caffe Nero*	1 Serving/416g	316	4.6	76	3.0	13.6	1.1	0.0
Frappe, Vanilla, Caffe Nero*	1 Serving/420g	315	4.6	75	3.0	13.6	1.1	0.0
Frappe Cream, Banana & Caramel, Caffe Nero*	1 Frappe/446g	460	22.3	103	2.0	11.7	5.0	0.0
Frappe Creme, Coconut & Chocolate, Caffe Nero*	1 Frappe/473g	516	25.1	109	2.2	13.2	5.3	0.4
Frappe Creme, Strawberry & Vanilla, Caffe Nero*	1 Frappe/446g	469	21.4	105	2.0	13.7	4.8	0.0
Latte, Caramel, Semi Skimmed Milk, Caffe Nero*	1 Latte/428g	274	3.9	64	2.8	11.4	0.9	0.1
MUFFIN								
Apple, & Pecan, Spiced, Caffe Nero*	1 Muffin/120g	474	26.5	395	4.7	43.5	22.1	1.5
Bacon, & Tomato Sauce, English, Caffe Nero*	1 Muffin/106g	277	7.5	261	13.4	34.8	7.1	2.2
Blueberry, Caffe Nero*	1 Muffin/121g	463	24.6	382	5.0	44.1	20.3	1.3
Blueberry, Reduced Fat, Caffe Nero*	1 Muffin/115g	351	11.0	305	5.6	47.3	9.6	3.3
Chocolate, & Hazelnut, Filled, Caffe Nero*	1 Muffin/120g	528	27.8	440	5.6	51.5	23.2	1.5
Chocolate, Belgian, Triple, Caffe Nero*	1 Muffin/120g	530	28.1	441	6.2	49.5	23.4	2.2
Cranberry & Orange, Reduced Fat, Caffe Nero*	1 Muffin/120g	322	9.8	269	4.5	44.3	8.2	3.1
Ham, & Egg Mayo, with Cheese, English, Caffe Nero*	1 Muffin/134g	314	12.2	234	11.3	25.9	9.1	1.7
Lemon Poppy Seed, Caffe Nero*	1 Muffin/121g	478	24.1	394	6.3	46.7	19.9	1.2
Raspberry & White Chocolate, Caffe Nero*	1 Muffin/120g	493	25.4	411	5.1	48.1	21.2	1.0
PANINI								
All Day Breakfast, Caffe Nero*	1 Serving/196g	454	19.6	231	10.7	23.9	10.0	1.5
Bacon, & Tomato Sauce, Breakfast, Caffe Nero*	1 Serving/105g	263	9.7	251	11.1	30.6	9.3	1.4
Brie, Bacon, & Caramelised Onion, Caffe Nero*	1 Serving/185g	478	20.6	258	10.3	28.8	11.1	1.2
Cheddar, Mozzarella, & Tomato, Tostati, Caffe Nero*	1 Serving/88g	215	8.7	244	11.7	26.4	9.9	1.2
Chicken, Bacon, & Arrabbiata Sauce, Caffe Nero*	1 Serving/204g	363	6.5	178	12.3	24.4	3.2	1.4
Chicken Pesto, Caffe Nero*	1 Serving/210g	385	13.3	183	11.8	19.7	6.3	1.1
Ham, & Egg Mayo, Breakfast, Caffe Nero*	1 Serving/146g	326	16.4	223	10.8	19.9	11.2	1.2
Ham, Mozzarella & Emmental, Tostati, Caffe Nero*	1 Serving/93g	218	8.3	235	14.2	24.2	9.0	1.2
Il Genovese, Caffe Nero*	1 Panini/185g	424	16.8	229	14.1	22.1	9.1	1.3
Meatball, & Mozzarella, Napoletana, Caffe Nero*	1 Serving/213g	511	23.8	240	11.7	22.6	11.2	1.2
Mushroom, Mozzarella & Cheddar, Caffe Nero*	1 Serving/195g	348	11.9	178	8.4	21.8	6.1	1.3
Napoli Salami, & Mozzarella, Caffe Nero*	1 Serving/193g	404	17.8	209	10.1	21.5	9.2	1.2
Pepperoni, Mozzarella, & Tomato, Caffe Nero*	1 Serving/193g	472	23.4	244	11.1	22.1	12.1	1.1
Tomato, Vine, Mozzarella, & Basil, Caffe Nero*	1 Serving/212g	398	17.4	188	8.3	20.3	8.2	1.3
Tuna Melt, Caffe Nero*	1 Serving/201g	389	13.4	194	11.6	21.2	6.7	1.1
POPCORN								
Sea Salt, Caffe Nero*	1 Serving/23g	115	6.5	501	8.2	53.6	28.2	10.9
Sweet & Salt, Caffe Nero*	1 Serving/25g	123	6.2	492	7.1	60.0	24.6	9.5
SANDWICH								
BLT, Caffe Nero*	1 Sandwich/171g	471	27.2	275	10.4	21.6	15.9	2.0

	Measure INFO/WEIGHT	per Measure KCAL	FAT	Nutrition Values per 100g / 100ml KCAL	PROT	CARB	FAT	FIBRE
CAFFE NERO								
SANDWICH								
Chicken, Salad & Pesto, Roll, GF, Caffe Nero*	1 Roll/154g	357	19.2	232	9.7	18.4	12.5	3.4
Chicken Salad, Less than 300 Calories, Caffe Nero*	1 Serving/191g	272	4.2	142	9.8	19.9	2.2	1.6
Egg Mayonnaise, Free Range, Caffe Nero*	1 Serving/157g	323	13.7	205	9.4	21.2	8.7	2.5
Ham, & Cheddar, Caffe Nero*	1 Serving/179g	418	17.8	233	15.2	20.8	9.9	1.4
Mature Cheddar & Pickle, Caffe Nero*	1 Serving/191g	421	20.3	220	9.1	21.2	10.6	1.6
Tuna Salad, Caffe Nero*	1 Serving/147g	268	5.3	182	11.7	25.8	3.6	1.8
SAUCE								
Berry Compote, Topping, for Porridge, Caffe Nero*	1 Serving/40g	47	0.1	117	0.6	29.3	0.2	1.9
Maple, Topping, for Porridge, Caffe Nero*	1 Serving/40g	94	0.0	234	0.0	58.4	0.1	0.1
SCONE								
Fruit, Traditional, Caffe Nero*	1 Serving/99g	336	9.1	339	7.2	55.5	9.2	2.8
SHORTBREAD								
Buttery, Crunchy, Caffe Nero*	1 Pack/50g	245	14.4	490	5.0	52.9	28.7	1.2
SOUP								
Potato & Leek, Low Fat, Caffe Nero*	1 Serving/300g	114	4.2	38	1.0	4.9	1.4	0.6
Tomato, Sundried, & Basil, Organic, Caffe Nero*	1 Serving/300g	129	4.8	43	1.3	5.4	1.6	1.1
SYRUP								
Vanilla, Caffe Nero*	1 Shot/36g	122	0.0	339	0.0	84.2	0.0	0.0
Vanilla, Sugar Free, Caffe Nero*	1 Shot/38g	5	0.0	13	0.0	10.2	0.0	0.0
TART								
Apple & Blackcurrant, Caffe Nero*	1 Serving/101g	279	12.9	276	2.9	37.4	12.8	2.2
Custard, Portuguese, Caffe Nero*	1 Serving/69g	184	6.5	266	3.9	41.5	9.4	2.4
TEA								
Chai Latte, Semi Skimmed Milk, Caffe Nero*	1 Serving/401g	281	10.0	70	3.8	8.6	2.5	0.1
Chai Latte, Skimmed Milk, Caffe Nero*	1 Serving/405g	239	5.3	59	3.8	8.4	1.3	0.0
TIRAMISU								
Caffe Nero*	1 Serving/95g	311	20.6	327	3.9	28.4	21.7	1.0
WAFFLES								
Caramel, Caffe Nero*	1 Waffle/39g	177	8.2	453	3.5	62.0	21.0	1.0
WRAP								
Chicken Caesar, Caffe Nero*	1 Serving/165g	434	22.8	263	12.8	21.9	13.8	0.8
Falafel, Caffe Nero*	1 Serving/157g	424	21.8	270	8.7	29.4	13.9	1.8
YOGHURT								
Blackcurrant, Bio, Greek Style, Caffe Nero*	1 Serving/150g	235	12.9	157	5.3	14.2	8.6	0.2
Blueberry, Greek Style, Brunch Pot, Caffe Nero*	1 Serving/130g	198	6.1	152	6.2	20.8	4.7	1.2
Honey, Bio, Greek, Caffe Nero*	1 Serving/149g	231	13.0	155	5.0	14.0	8.7	0.0
Strawberry, Greek Style, Brunch Pot, Caffe Nero*	1 Serving/130g	197	6.1	151	6.2	20.6	4.7	1.1
COSTA								
BISCOTTI								
Almond, Costa*	1 Biscotti/50g	165	6.3	330	7.6	46.0	12.6	1.0
BISCUITS								
Almond, Mini, Bag, Costa*	1 Bag/78g	383	23.8	491	14.3	40.0	30.5	0.0
Bourbon, The Ultimate, Costa*	1 Biscuit/85g	427	22.8	502	6.0	57.3	26.8	3.7
Chocolate, Costa*	1 Serving/16g	76	5.0	448	4.9	41.1	29.3	0.0
Custard Cream, The Ultimate, Costa*	1 Biscuit/85g	410	18.2	482	4.4	67.2	21.4	1.4
Fruit & Oat, Costa*	1 Biscuit/30g	140	5.5	465	4.9	69.2	18.2	2.0
Garibaldi, Costa*	1 Biscuit/34g	158	8.1	464	5.3	57.3	23.8	2.9
BREAKFAST								
Bacon Roll, Costa*	1 Pack/130g	367	11.0	282	15.6	35.8	8.5	1.7
Egg & Mushroom Roll, Costa*	1 Pack/155g	354	12.3	228	8.4	30.9	7.9	1.8
BROWNIES								
Bites, Costa*	1 Serving/72g	342	22.1	475	5.4	44.3	30.7	0.0

	Measure INFO/WEIGHT	per Measure KCAL	FAT	Nutrition Values per 100g / 100ml KCAL	PROT	CARB	FAT	FIBRE
COSTA								
CAKE								
Belgian Chocolate, Jaffa, Costa*	1 Cake/100g	351	18.6	351	4.0	40.9	18.6	0.0
Carrot, Costa*	1 Slice/138g	514	23.4	374	5.1	48.6	17.0	0.0
Chocolate, Christmas, Costa*	1 Serving/162g	616	25.8	380	4.9	53.0	15.9	2.5
Chocolate, Costa*	1 Slice/150g	575	23.6	383	4.8	76.7	15.7	0.0
Lemon, Costa*	1 Slice/144g	576	25.4	399	3.6	56.0	17.6	0.0
Lemon Drizzle, Costa*	1 Serving/100g	374	20.7	374	4.9	41.4	20.7	1.2
Victoria Sandwich, Costa*	1 Slice/136g	546	25.6	401	3.5	54.0	18.8	0.0
Victoria Sponge, Mini, Costa*	1 Serving/100g	483	20.0	483	3.9	71.8	20.0	0.0
COFFEE								
Americano, Full Fat Milk, Massimo, Costa*	1 Massimo/600ml	44	2.2	7	0.4	0.7	0.4	0.0
Americano, Full Fat Milk, Medio, Costa*	1 Medio/480ml	40	2.1	8	0.5	0.7	0.4	0.0
Americano, Full Fat Milk, Primo, Costa*	1 Serving/380mlml	40	2.3	11	0.7	1.1	0.6	0.0
Americano, Massimo, Iced, Costa*	1 Massimo/600ml	62	0.4	10	0.1	2.4	0.1	0.0
Americano, no Added Milk, Massimo, Costa*	1 Massimo/600ml	12	0.4	2	0.1	0.3	0.1	0.0
Americano, no Added Milk, Medio, Costa*	1 Medio/480ml	8	0.3	2	0.1	0.2	0.1	0.0
Americano, no Added Milk, Primo, Costa*	1 Primo/360ml	6	0.2	2	0.1	0.2	0.1	0.0
Americano, Primo, Iced, Costa*	1 Primo/360ml	23	0.2	6	0.1	1.4	0.1	0.0
Americano, Skimmed Milk, Medio, Costa*	1 Medio/480ml	25	0.3	5	0.5	0.8	0.1	0.0
Americano, Skimmed Milk, Primo, Costa*	1 Primo/360ml	23	0.3	6	0.6	0.9	0.1	0.0
Americano, Soya Milk, Massimo, Costa*	1 Serving/600ml	31	1.3	5	0.4	0.5	0.2	0.0
Americano, Soya Milk, Medio, Costa*	1 Serving/480ml	27	1.2	6	0.4	0.5	0.2	0.0
Americano, Soya Milk, Primo, Costa*	1 Serving/200ml	14	0.6	7	0.5	0.6	0.3	0.0
Babyccino, Chocolate, Full Fat Milk, Costa*	1 Solo/30ml	138	5.0	460	16.0	60.7	16.7	0.0
Babyccino, Chocolate, Skimmed Milk, Solo, Costa*	1 Solo/30ml	102	0.8	340	16.7	62.0	2.7	0.0
Babyccino, Chocolate, Soya Milk, Solo, Costa*	1 Serving/30ml	107	2.8	357	15.0	51.0	9.3	0.0
Babyccino, Full Fat Milk, Solo, Costa*	1 Solo/30ml	109	4.4	363	14.3	43.3	14.7	0.0
Babyccino, Skimmed Milk, Solo, Costa*	1 Solo/30ml	73	0.2	243	14.7	44.7	0.7	0.0
Babyccino, Soya Milk, Solo, Costa*	1 Solo/30ml	78	2.3	260	13.3	34.0	7.7	0.0
Caffe Latte, Full Fat Milk, Massimo, Costa*	1 Massimo/600ml	260	14.4	43	2.2	3.2	2.4	0.0
Caffe Latte, Full Fat Milk, Medio, Costa*	1 Latte/480g	202	11.2	42	2.2	3.2	2.3	0.0
Caffe Latte, Full Fat Milk, Primo, Costa*	1 Primo/360ml	151	8.5	42	2.2	3.1	2.4	0.0
Caffe Latte, Skimmed Milk, Massimo, Costa*	1 Massimo/600ml	149	0.7	25	2.4	3.6	0.1	0.0
Caffe Latte, Skimmed Milk, Medio, Costa*	1 Medio/480ml	114	0.5	24	2.3	3.5	0.1	0.0
Caffe Latte, Skimmed Milk, Primo, Costa*	1 Primo/360ml	86	0.3	24	2.4	3.5	0.1	0.0
Caffe Latte, Soya Milk, Massimo, Costa*	1 Massimo/600ml	165	7.7	28	2.2	1.8	1.3	0.0
Caffe Latte, Soya Milk, Medio, Costa*	1 Medio/480ml	124	5.8	26	2.0	1.7	1.2	0.0
Caffe Latte, Soya Milk, Primo, Costa*	1 Primo/360ml	93	4.4	26	2.0	1.6	1.2	0.0
Cappuccino, Full Fat Milk, Massimo, Costa*	1 Massimo/655ml	223	7.7	34	1.1	1.6	1.2	0.0
Cappuccino, Full Fat Milk, Massimo, Iced, Costa*	1 Massimo/600ml	124	3.6	21	0.6	3.3	0.6	0.0
Cappuccino, Full Fat Milk, Medio, Costa*	1 Medio/480ml	167	8.9	35	1.8	2.8	1.8	0.0
Cappuccino, Full Fat Milk, Medio, Iced, Costa*	1 Medio/360ml	70	2.2	20	0.6	3.0	0.6	0.0
Cappuccino, Full Fat Milk, Primo, Costa*	1 Primo/360ml	101	5.2	28	1.4	2.4	1.4	0.0
Cappuccino, Full Fat Milk, Primo, Iced, Costa*	1 Primo/360ml	62	2.1	17	0.6	2.5	0.6	0.0
Cappuccino, Skimmed Milk, Massimo, Costa*	1 Massimo/600ml	121	0.8	20	1.8	3.0	0.1	0.0
Cappuccino, Skimmed Milk, Massimo, Iced, Costa*	1 Massimo/600ml	99	0.6	16	0.6	3.4	0.1	0.0
Cappuccino, Skimmed Milk, Medio, Costa*	1 Medio/480ml	99	0.6	21	1.8	3.1	0.1	0.0
Cappuccino, Skimmed Milk, Medio, Iced, Costa*	1 Medio/360ml	55	0.4	15	0.6	3.0	0.1	0.0
Cappuccino, Skimmed Milk, Primo, Costa*	1 Primo/360ml	64	0.5	18	1.5	2.7	0.1	0.0
Cappuccino, Skimmed Milk, Primo, Iced, Costa*	1 Primo/360ml	47	0.4	13	0.6	2.5	0.1	0.0
Cappuccino, Soya Milk, Massimo, Costa*	1 Massimo/600ml	134	5.9	22	1.6	1.7	1.0	0.0
Cappuccino, Soya Milk, Massimo, Iced, Costa*	1 Massimo/600ml	102	2.0	17	0.6	3.0	0.3	0.0
Cappuccino, Soya Milk, Medio, Costa*	1 Medio/480ml	108	4.7	22	1.6	1.7	1.0	0.0

	Measure INFO/WEIGHT	per Measure KCAL	FAT	Nutrition Values per 100g / 100ml KCAL	PROT	CARB	FAT	FIBRE
COSTA								
COFFEE								
Cappuccino, Soya Milk, Medio, Iced, Costa*	1 Medio/480ml	76	1.6	16	0.6	2.6	0.3	0.0
Cappuccino, Soya Milk, Primo, Costa*	1 Primo/360ml	69	3.0	19	1.4	1.6	0.8	0.0
Cappuccino, Soya Milk, Primo, Iced, Costa*	1 Primo/360ml	49	1.2	14	0.6	2.1	0.3	0.0
Cooler, Chocolate, Full Fat Milk, Medio, Creamy, Costa*	1 Medio/480ml	514	17.4	107	1.6	17.0	3.6	0.0
Cooler, Chocolate, Full Fat Milk, Primo, Creamy, Costa*	1 Primo/360ml	366	13.0	102	1.6	15.6	3.6	0.0
Cooler, Chocolate, Soya Milk, Medio, Creamy, Costa*	1 Medio/480ml	472	14.4	98	1.5	16.2	3.0	0.0
Cooler, Chocolate, Soya Milk, Primo, Creamy, Costa*	1 Primo/360ml	333	10.8	92	1.4	14.8	3.0	0.0
Cooler, Full Fat Milk, Massimo, Costa*	1 Massimo/568ml	297	4.4	52	0.8	10.5	0.8	0.0
Cooler, Full Fat Milk, Medio, Costa*	1 Medio/455ml	232	3.9	51	0.8	10.0	0.8	0.0
Cooler, Full Fat Milk, Primo, Costa*	1 Primo/341ml	170	2.2	50	1.0	9.2	0.6	0.0
Cooler, Mocha, Full Fat Milk, Massimo, Costa*	1 Massimo/600ml	481	6.7	80	1.1	16.4	1.1	0.0
Cooler, Mocha, Full Fat Milk, Medio, Costa*	1 Medio/480ml	370	5.5	77	1.1	15.5	1.2	0.0
Cooler, Mocha, Skimmed Milk, Massimo, Costa*	1 Massimo/600ml	445	2.5	74	1.1	16.4	0.4	0.0
Cooler, Mocha, Skimmed Milk, Medio, Costa*	1 Medio/480ml	339	1.9	71	1.1	15.6	0.4	0.0
Cooler, Mocha, Skimmed Milk, Primo, Costa*	1 Primo/360ml	233	1.2	65	1.2	14.2	0.3	0.0
Cooler, Mocha, Soya Milk, Massimo, Costa*	1 Massimo/600ml	450	4.5	75	1.0	15.9	0.8	0.0
Cooler, Mocha, Soya Milk, Medio, Costa*	1 Medio/480ml	343	3.7	71	1.0	15.0	0.8	0.0
Cooler, Mocha, Soya Milk, Primo, Costa*	1 Primo/360ml	237	2.9	66	1.1	13.4	0.8	0.0
Cooler, Skimmed Milk, Massimo, Costa*	1 Massimo/568ml	261	0.4	46	0.8	10.6	0.1	0.0
Cooler, Skimmed Milk, Medio, Costa*	1 Medio/455ml	201	0.3	44	0.9	10.1	0.1	0.0
Cooler, Skimmed Milk, Primo, Costa*	1 Primo/360ml	141	0.2	39	1.0	8.8	0.1	0.0
Cooler, Soya Milk, Massimo, Costa*	1 Massimo/568ml	266	2.4	47	0.7	10.0	0.4	0.0
Cooler, Soya Milk, Medio, Costa*	1 Medio/455ml	205	2.1	45	0.8	9.4	0.5	0.0
Cooler, Soya Milk, Primo, Costa*	1 Primo/341ml	145	1.9	43	0.9	8.5	0.6	0.0
Cooler, Strawberry, Full Fat Milk, Medio, Creamy, Costa*	1 Medio/480ml	489	15.8	102	1.3	16.8	3.3	0.0
Cooler, Strawberry, Full Fat Milk, Primo, Creamy, Costa*	1 Prino/360ml	348	11.9	97	1.3	15.5	3.3	0.0
Cooler, Strawberry, Soya Milk, Medio, Creamy, Costa*	1 Medio/480ml	446	12.8	93	1.2	16.0	2.7	0.0
Cooler, Strawberry, Soya Milk, Primo, Creamy, Costa*	1 Primo/360ml	315	9.6	88	1.2	14.7	2.7	0.0
Cooler, Toffee, Full Fat, Primo, Creamy, Costa*	1 Primo/360ml	420	16.6	117	1.4	17.4	4.6	0.0
Cooler, Toffee, Full Fat Milk, Medio, Creamy, Costa*	1 Medio/480ml	572	21.9	119	1.4	18.1	4.6	0.0
Cooler, Toffee, Skimmed Milk, Medio, Creamy, Costa*	1 Medio/480ml	522	16.2	109	1.4	18.2	3.4	0.0
Cooler, Toffee, Skimmed Milk, Primo, Creamy, Costa*	1 Primo/360ml	383	12.2	106	1.5	17.5	3.4	0.0
Cooler, Toffee, Soya Milk, Medio, Creamy, Costa*	1 Medio/480ml	529	19.0	110	1.3	17.3	4.0	0.0
Cooler, Toffee, Soya Milk, Primo, Creamy, Costa*	1 Primo/360ml	388	14.4	108	1.3	16.6	4.0	0.0
Cooler, Vanilla, Full Fat Milk, Medio, Creamy, Costa*	1 Medio/480ml	316	6.0	66	1.2	12.5	1.2	0.0
Cooler, Vanilla, Full Fat Milk, Primo, Creamy, Costa*	1 Primo/360ml	220	4.5	61	1.2	11.3	1.2	0.0
Cooler, Vanilla, Skimmed Milk, Medio, Creamy, Costa*	1 Medio/480ml	266	0.2	55	1.2	12.6	0.0	0.0
Cooler, Vanilla, Skimmed Milk, Primo, Creamy, Costa*	1 Primo/360ml	183	0.2	51	1.2	11.4	0.1	0.0
Cooler, Vanilla, Soya Milk, Medio, Creamy, Costa*	1 Medio/480ml	256	3.0	53	1.0	10.8	0.6	0.0
Cooler, Vanilla, Soya Milk, Primo, Creamy, Costa*	1 Primo/360ml	188	2.3	52	1.1	10.5	0.6	0.0
Cortado, Full Fat Milk, Solo, Costa*	1 Solo/30ml	74	4.1	247	13.0	18.7	13.7	0.0
Cortado, Skimmed Milk, Solo, Costa*	1 Serving/30ml	42	0.2	140	13.7	20.7	0.7	0.0
Cortado, Soya Milk, Solo, Costa*	1 Solo/30ml	46	2.2	153	12.0	10.0	7.3	0.0
Espresso, Ristretto, Doppio, Costa*	1 Doppio/60ml	6	0.2	10	0.7	1.3	0.3	0.0
Espresso, Ristretto, Solo, Costa*	1 Solo/30ml	3	0.1	10	0.7	1.3	0.3	0.0
Flat White, Full Fat Milk, Primo, Costa*	1 Primo/360ml	135	7.6	38	1.9	2.8	2.1	0.0
Flat White, Skimmed Milk, Primo, Costa*	1 Primo/360ml	77	0.3	21	2.1	3.1	0.1	0.0
Flat White, Soya Milk, Primo, Costa*	1 Primo/360ml	85	4.0	24	1.9	1.5	1.1	0.0
Latte, Caramel, Ful Fat, Medio, Costa*	1 Medio/480ml	251	11.2	52	2.2	5.7	2.3	0.0
Latte, Caramel, Full Fat Milk, Massimo, Costa*	1 Massimo/600ml	325	14.4	54	2.2	5.9	2.4	0.0
Latte, Caramel, Full Fat Milk, Primo, Costa*	1 Primo/360ml	184	8.5	51	2.2	5.4	2.4	0.0
Latte, Caramel, Skimmed Milk, Massimo, Costa*	1 Massimo/600ml	215	0.7	36	2.4	6.3	0.1	0.0

	Measure INFO/WEIGHT	per Measure KCAL	FAT	Nutrition Values per 100g / 100ml KCAL	PROT	CARB	FAT	FIBRE
COSTA								
COFFEE								
Latte, Caramel, Skimmed Milk, Medio, Costa*	1 Medio/480ml	164	0.5	34	2.3	6.0	0.1	0.0
Latte, Caramel, Skimmed Milk, Primo, Costa*	1 Primo/360ml	118	0.3	33	2.4	5.7	0.1	0.0
Latte, Caramel, Soya Milk, Massimo, Costa*	1 Massimo/600ml	231	7.7	38	2.2	4.4	1.3	0.0
Latte, Caramel, Soya Milk, Medio, Costa*	1 Medio/480ml	173	5.8	36	2.0	4.2	1.2	0.0
Latte, Caramel, Soya Milk, Primo, Costa*	1 Primo/360ml	126	4.4	35	2.0	3.9	1.2	0.0
Latte, Caramel, Sugar Free, Full Fat Milk, Medio, Costa*	1 Serving/480ml	205	11.2	43	2.2	3.5	2.3	0.0
Latte, Caramel, Sugar Free, Soya Milk, Medio, Costa*	1 Medio/480ml	127	5.8	26	2.0	2.0	1.2	0.0
Latte, Caramel, Sugar Free, Soya Milk, Primo, Costa*	1 Primo/360ml	95	4.4	26	2.0	1.9	1.2	0.0
Latte, Cinnamon, Full Fat Milk, Massimo, Costa*	1 Massimo/600ml	325	14.4	54	2.2	5.9	2.4	0.0
Latte, Cinnamon, Full Fat Milk, Medio, Costa*	1 Medio/480ml	173	9.7	36	2.0	4.2	2.0	0.0
Latte, Cinnamon, Full Fat Milk, Primo, Costa*	1 Primo/360ml	184	8.5	51	2.2	5.4	2.4	0.0
Latte, Cinnamon, Skimmed Milk, Massimo, Costa*	1 Massimo/600ml	215	0.7	36	2.4	6.3	0.1	0.0
Latte, Cinnamon, Skimmed Milk, Medio, Costa*	1 Medio/480ml	164	0.5	34	2.3	6.0	0.1	0.0
Latte, Cinnamon, Skimmed Milk, Primo, Costa*	1 Primo/360ml	121	0.3	34	2.4	5.7	0.1	0.0
Latte, Cinnamon, Soya Milk, Massimo, Costa*	1 Massimo/600ml	231	7.7	38	2.2	4.4	1.3	0.0
Latte, Cinnamon, Soya Milk, Primo, Costa*	1 Primo/360ml	126	4.4	35	2.0	3.9	1.2	0.0
Latte, Full Fat Milk, Massimo, Costa*	1 Massimo/600ml	240	10.5	40	1.6	4.5	1.8	0.0
Latte, Full Fat Milk, Medio, Iced, Costa*	1 Medio/480ml	184	8.3	38	1.6	4.2	1.7	0.0
Latte, Full Fat Milk, Primo, Iced, Costa*	1 Primo/360ml	132	6.3	37	1.7	3.6	1.8	0.0
Latte, Gingerbread, Full Fat Milk, Massimo, Costa*	1 Massimo/600ml	328	14.4	55	2.2	6.0	2.4	0.0
Latte, Gingerbread, Full Fat Milk, Medio, Costa*	1 Serving/480ml	253	11.2	53	2.2	5.8	2.3	0.0
Latte, Gingerbread, Full Fat Milk, Primo, Costa*	1 Serving/360ml	185	8.5	51	2.2	5.5	2.4	0.0
Latte, Gingerbread, Skimmed Milk, Massimo, Costa*	1 Serving/600ml	218	0.7	36	2.4	6.4	0.1	0.0
Latte, Gingerbread, Skimmed Milk, Medio, Costa*	1 Serving/480ml	166	0.5	35	2.3	6.1	0.1	0.0
Latte, Gingerbread, Skimmed Milk, Primo, Costa*	1 Serving/360ml	120	0.3	33	2.4	5.8	0.1	0.0
Latte, Gingerbread, Soya Milk, Medio, Costa*	1 Serving/480ml	175	5.8	36	2.0	4.3	1.2	0.0
Latte, Roasted Hazelnut, Full Fat Milk, Massimo, Costa*	1 Serving/600ml	323	14.4	54	2.2	5.9	2.4	0.0
Latte, Roasted Hazelnut, Full Fat Milk, Medio, Costa*	1 Serving/480ml	249	11.2	52	2.2	5.6	2.3	0.0
Latte, Roasted Hazelnut, Full Fat Milk, Primo, Costa*	1 Serving/360ml	183	8.5	51	2.2	5.3	2.4	0.0
Latte, Roasted Hazelnut, Skimmed Milk, Medio, Costa*	1 Serving/480ml	162	0.5	34	2.3	5.9	0.1	0.0
Latte, Roasted Hazelnut, Skimmed Milk, Primo, Costa*	1 Serving/360ml	117	0.3	32	2.4	5.7	0.1	0.0
Latte, Roasted Hazelnut, Soya Milk, Medio, Costa*	1 Serving/480ml	172	5.8	36	2.0	4.1	1.2	0.0
Latte, Roasted Hazelnut, Soya Milk, Primo, Costa*	1 Serving/360ml	125	4.4	35	2.0	3.8	1.2	0.0
Latte, Skimmed Milk, Massimo, Iced, Costa*	1 Massimo/600ml	155	0.6	26	1.7	4.7	0.1	0.0
Latte, Skimmed Milk, Medio, Iced, Costa*	1 Medio/480ml	116	0.4	24	1.7	4.2	0.1	0.0
Latte, Skimmed Milk, Primo, Iced, Costa*	1 Primo/360ml	81	0.4	22	1.7	3.8	0.1	0.0
Latte, Soya Milk, Massimo, Iced, Costa*	1 Massimo/600ml	166	5.4	28	1.5	3.4	0.9	0.0
Latte, Soya Milk, Medio, Iced, Costa*	1 Medio/480ml	125	4.3	26	1.5	3.0	0.9	0.0
Latte, Soya Milk, Primo, Iced, Costa*	1 Primo/360ml	87	3.3	24	1.5	2.5	0.9	0.0
Latte, Vanilla, Full Fat Milk, Medio, Costa*	1 Medio/480ml	253	11.2	53	2.2	5.8	2.3	0.0
Latte, Vanilla, Skimmed Milk, Massimo, Costa*	1 Massimo/600ml	217	0.7	36	2.4	6.4	0.1	0.0
Latte, Vanilla, Skimmed Milk, Medio, Costa*	1 Medio/480ml	165	0.5	34	2.3	6.1	0.1	0.0
Latte, Vanilla, Skimmed Milk, Primo, Costa*	1 Primo/360ml	120	0.3	33	2.4	5.8	0.1	0.0
Latte, Vanilla, Soya Milk, Massimo, Costa*	1 Serving/600ml	233	7.7	39	2.2	4.6	1.3	0.0
Latte, Vanilla, Soya Milk, Medio, Costa*	1 Serving/480ml	175	5.8	36	2.0	4.3	1.2	0.0
Latte, Vanilla, Soya Milk, Primo, Costa*	1 Primo/360ml	127	4.4	35	2.0	4.0	1.2	0.0
Light, Massimo, Costa*	1 Massimo/600ml	98	0.5	16	1.6	2.4	0.1	0.0
Light, Medio, Costa*	1 Medio/480ml	88	0.4	18	1.8	2.7	0.1	0.0
Light, Primo, Costa*	1 Primo/360ml	65	0.3	18	1.8	2.7	0.1	0.0
Mocha, Full Fat Milk, Massimo, Costa*	1 Massimo/600ml	381	15.8	64	2.5	7.3	2.6	0.0
Mocha, Full Fat Milk, Massimo, Iced, Costa*	1 Massimo/600ml	332	9.8	55	1.6	8.5	1.6	0.0
Mocha, Full Fat Milk, Medio, Costa*	1 Medio/480ml	324	12.7	68	2.5	8.2	2.6	0.0

	Measure INFO/WEIGHT	per Measure KCAL	FAT	Nutrition Values per 100g / 100ml KCAL	PROT	CARB	FAT	FIBRE
COSTA								
COFFEE								
Mocha, Full Fat Milk, Medio, Iced, Costa*	1 Medio/480ml	259	7.9	54	1.6	8.2	1.6	0.0
Mocha, Full Fat Milk, Primo, Costa*	1 Primo/360ml	213	8.5	59	2.2	7.0	2.4	0.0
Mocha, Full Fat Milk, Primo, Iced, Costa*	1 Primo/360ml	186	5.8	52	1.6	7.6	1.6	0.0
Mocha, Skimmed Milk, Massimo, Costa*	1 Massimo/600ml	272	3.4	45	2.5	7.4	0.6	0.0
Mocha, Skimmed Milk, Massimo, iced, Costa*	1 Serving/600ml	272	2.8	45	1.6	8.6	0.5	0.0
Mocha, Skimmed Milk, Medio, Costa*	1 Medio/480ml	250	3.2	52	2.7	8.6	0.7	0.0
Mocha, Skimmed Milk, Medio, Iced, Costa*	1 Massimo/480ml	210	2.1	44	1.6	8.3	0.4	0.0
Mocha, Skimmed Milk, Primo, Costa*	1 Primo/360ml	161	2.0	45	2.4	6.9	0.6	0.0
Mocha, Skimmed Milk, Primo, Iced, Costa*	1 Primo/360ml	148	1.5	41	1.6	7.8	0.4	0.0
Mocha, Soya Milk, Massimo, Costa*	1 Massimo/600g	293	9.7	49	2.4	5.9	1.6	0.0
Mocha, Soya Milk, Massimo, Iced, Costa*	1 Massimo/600ml	280	6.2	47	1.5	7.7	1.0	0.0
Mocha, Soya Milk, Medio, Costa*	1 Medio/480ml	265	8.4	55	2.5	6.9	1.8	0.0
Mocha, Soya Milk, Medio, Iced, Costa*	1 Medio/480ml	288	6.5	60	1.9	9.8	1.4	0.0
Mocha, Soya Milk, Primo, Costa*	1 Primo/360ml	172	5.5	48	2.2	5.9	1.5	0.0
Mocha, Soya Milk, Primo, Iced, Costa*	1 Primo/360ml	153	3.6	42	1.4	6.8	1.0	0.0
Mocha Cordato, Skimmed Milk, Solo, Costa*	1 Solo/30ml	78	0.8	260	16.0	42.3	2.7	0.0
Mocha Cortado, Full Fat Milk, Solo, Costa*	1 Solo/30ml	111	4.8	370	15.0	40.7	16.0	0.0
Mocha Cortado, Skimmed Milk, Solo, Costa*	1 Solo/30ml	78	0.8	260	16.0	42.3	2.7	0.0
Mocha Cortado, Soya Milk, Solo, Costa*	1 Solo/30g	82	2.8	273	14.3	31.7	9.3	0.0
Mocha Flake, Full Fat Milk, Massimo, Costa*	1 Massimo/600ml	552	29.8	92	2.8	8.8	5.0	0.0
Mocha Flake, Full Fat Milk, Medio, Costa*	1 Medio/480ml	495	26.8	103	2.8	10.2	5.6	0.0
Mocha Flake, Full Fat Milk, Primo, Costa*	1 Primo/360ml	360	20.1	100	2.7	9.6	5.6	0.0
Mocha Flake, Skimmed Milk, Massimo, Costa*	1 Massimo/600ml	443	17.4	74	2.8	9.0	2.9	0.0
Mocha Flake, Skimmed Milk, Medio, Costa*	1 Medio/480ml	421	17.3	88	3.0	10.5	3.6	0.0
Mocha Flake, Skimmed Milk, Primo, Costa*	1 Primo/360ml	308	13.6	85	2.8	9.9	3.8	0.0
Mocha Flake, Soya Milk, Massimo, Costa*	1 Massimo/600ml	464	23.7	77	2.6	7.5	4.0	0.0
Mocha Flake, Soya Milk, Medio, Costa*	1 Medio/480ml	436	22.4	91	2.8	8.9	4.7	0.0
Mocha Flake, Soya Milk, Primo, Costa*	1 Primo/360ml	319	17.1	89	2.6	8.4	4.8	0.0
Mocha Latte, Full Fat, Massimo, Costa*	1 Massimo/600ml	393	16.9	66	2.6	7.2	2.8	0.0
Mocha Latte, Full Fat Milk, Medio, Costa*	1 Medio/480ml	304	13.1	63	2.6	7.0	2.7	0.0
Mocha Latte, Full Fat Milk, Primo, Costa*	1 Primo/380ml	231	10.2	61	2.5	6.5	2.7	0.0
Mocha Latte, Skimmed Milk, Massimo, Costa*	1 Massimo/600ml	284	3.2	47	2.8	7.6	0.5	0.0
Mocha Latte, Skimmed Milk, Medio, Costa*	1 Medio/480ml	222	2.5	46	2.7	7.5	0.5	0.0
Mocha Latte, Skimmed Milk, Primo, Costa*	1 Primo/360ml	155	1.6	43	2.7	6.9	0.4	0.0
Mocha Latte, Soya Milk, Massimo, Costa*	1 Massimo/600ml	303	10.3	50	2.6	5.9	1.7	0.0
Mocha Latte, Soya Milk, Medio, Costa*	1 Medio/480ml	235	7.9	49	2.4	5.8	1.6	0.0
Mocha Latte, Soya Milk, Primo, Costa*	1 Primo/380ml	175	6.0	46	2.4	5.2	1.6	0.0
Strawberry, Skimmed Milk, Primo, Costa*	1 Primo/360ml	310	7.5	86	1.3	15.6	2.1	0.0
COOKIES								
Choc Chunk, Double, Costa*	1 Pack/60g	296	15.2	493	5.2	61.1	25.3	3.7
Fruit & Oat, Costa*	1 Pack/60g	283	12.7	472	5.1	65.2	21.2	2.0
CROISSANT								
Almond, Costa*	1 Croissant/88g	336	16.9	382	9.3	43.0	19.2	0.0
Butter, Costa*	1 Croissant/64g	276	16.7	431	8.3	40.6	26.1	0.0
Tomato & Emmental, Costa*	1 Croissant/98g	342	21.0	349	9.0	30.0	21.4	0.0
CUPCAKES								
Banoffee, Costa*	1 Cupcake/112g	431	17.7	385	3.7	56.7	15.8	0.0
Lemon, Costa*	1 Cupcake/97g	512	32.5	528	2.8	53.2	33.5	0.0
Rocky Road, Costa*	1 Cupcake/101g	427	17.7	421	5.1	58.9	17.5	0.0
FLAPJACK								
Fruity, Costa*	1 Serving/85g	353	12.1	415	4.9	67.0	14.2	12.5
Nutty, Costa*	1 Serving/85g	391	20.0	460	7.4	54.8	23.5	5.0

	Measure INFO/WEIGHT	per Measure KCAL	per Measure FAT	Nutrition Values per 100g / 100ml KCAL	PROT	CARB	FAT	FIBRE
COSTA								
FLATBREAD								
Cajun Chicken, Costa*	1 Pack/168g	310	5.1	184	12.7	26.6	3.0	0.0
Cheddar & Caramelised Onion Chutney, Costa*	1 Pack/118g	340	13.3	288	11.9	34.8	11.3	0.0
Chicken, Green Thai, Costa*	1 Pack/173g	325	6.4	188	12.2	26.6	3.7	0.0
Emmenthal & Mushroom, Costa*	1 Pack/158g	391	16.1	248	13.1	25.9	10.2	0.0
FLAVOURING FOR COFFEE								
Caramel, Massimo, Costa*	1 Massimo/600ml	66	0.0	11	0.0	2.7	0.0	0.0
Caramel, Medio, Costa*	1 Medio/480ml	49	0.0	10	0.0	2.5	0.0	0.0
Caramel, Primo, Costa*	1 Primo/360ml	33	0.0	9	0.0	2.2	0.0	0.0
Cinnamon, Massimo, Costa*	1 Massimo/600ml	66	0.0	11	0.0	2.7	0.0	0.0
Cinnamon, Medio, Costa*	1 Medio/480ml	49	0.0	10	0.0	2.5	0.0	0.0
Cinnamon, Primo, Costa*	1 Primo/360ml	33	0.0	9	0.0	2.2	0.0	0.0
Gingerbread, Massimo, Costa*	1 Massimo/600ml	68	0.0	11	0.0	2.8	0.0	0.0
Gingerbread, Medio, Costa*	1 Medio/480ml	51	0.0	11	0.0	2.6	0.0	0.0
Gingerbread, Primo, Costa*	1 Primo/360ml	34	0.0	9	0.0	2.3	0.0	0.0
Roasted Hazelnut, Massimo, Costa*	1 Massimo/600ml	63	0.0	10	0.0	2.6	0.0	0.0
Roasted Hazelnut, Medio, Costa*	1 Medio/480ml	48	0.0	10	0.0	2.4	0.0	0.0
Roasted Hazelnut, Primo, Costa*	1 Primo/360ml	32	0.0	9	0.0	2.2	0.0	0.0
Vanilla, Massimo, Costa*	1 Massimo/600ml	68	0.0	11	0.0	2.8	0.0	0.0
Vanilla, Medio, Costa*	1 Medio/480ml	51	0.0	11	0.0	2.6	0.0	0.0
Vanilla, Primo, Costa*	1 Primo/360ml	34	0.0	9	0.0	2.3	0.0	0.0
FRESCATO								
Coffee, Full Fat Milk, Primo, (Coffee Only), Costa*	1 Primo/340ml	302	5.6	89	1.4	17.1	1.6	0.0
Coffee, Skimmed Milk, Medio (Coffee Only), Costa*	1 Medio/454ml	359	0.5	79	1.6	18.0	0.1	0.0
Coffee, Skimmed Milk, Primo (Coffee Only), Costa*	1 Primo/340ml	256	0.5	75	1.5	17.2	0.2	0.0
Coffee, Soya Milk, Medio (Coffee Only), Costa*	1 Medio/454ml	375	3.9	83	1.5	17.1	0.9	0.0
Coffee, Soya Milk, Primo, (Coffee Only), Costa*	1 Primo/340ml	267	2.8	79	1.4	16.3	0.8	0.0
Coffee Caramel, Full Fat Milk, Medio, Costa*	1 Medio/454ml	488	7.9	107	1.5	21.5	1.7	0.0
Coffee Caramel, Skimmed Milk, Primo, Costa*	1 Primo/340ml	289	0.5	85	1.5	19.6	0.2	0.0
Coffee Caramel, Soya Milk, Primo, Costa*	1 Primo/340ml	300	2.8	88	1.4	18.6	0.8	0.0
Coffee Mocha, Full Fat Milk, Medio, Costa*	1 Medio/454ml	540	8.3	119	1.6	24.0	1.8	0.0
Coffee Mocha, Skimmed Milk, Medio, Costa*	1 Medio/454ml	477	1.2	105	1.7	24.1	0.3	0.0
Coffee Mocha, Skimmed Milk, Primo, Costa*	1 Primo/340ml	335	0.8	99	1.6	22.6	0.2	0.0
Coffee Vanilla, Full Fat Milk, Medio, Costa*	1 Medio/454ml	491	7.9	108	1.5	21.6	1.7	0.0
Coffee Vanilla, Full Fat Milk, Primo, Costa*	1 Primo/340ml	336	5.6	99	1.4	19.6	1.6	0.0
Coffee Vanilla, Skimmed Milk, Medio, Costa*	1 Medio/454ml	427	0.7	94	1.6	21.7	0.2	0.0
Coffee Vanilla, Skimmed Milk, Primo, Costa*	1 Primo/340ml	290	0.5	85	1.5	19.7	0.2	0.0
FRUIT COOLERS								
Mango & Passionfruit, Massimo, Costa*	1 Massimo/600ml	290	0.6	48	0.2	11.6	0.1	0.0
Mango & Passionfruit, Medio, Costa*	1 Medio/480ml	232	0.5	48	0.2	11.6	0.1	0.0
Mango & Passionfruit, Primo, Costa*	1 Primo/360ml	173	0.3	48	0.1	11.6	0.1	0.0
Peach, Massimo, Costa*	1 Massimo/600ml	406	0.3	68	0.2	16.3	0.0	0.0
Peach, Medio, Costa*	1 Medio/480ml	325	0.2	68	0.2	16.3	0.0	0.0
Peach, Primo, Costa*	1 Primo/360ml	243	0.2	68	0.2	16.3	0.1	0.0
Red Berry, Massimo, Costa*	1 Massimo/600ml	409	0.6	68	0.2	16.3	0.1	0.0
Red Berry, Medio, Costa*	1 Medio/480ml	327	0.5	68	0.2	16.3	0.1	0.0
Red Berry, Primo, Costa*	1 Primo/360ml	245	0.3	68	0.2	16.3	0.1	0.0
HOT CHOCOLATE								
Full Fat, Massimo, Costa*	1 Massimo/600ml	432	19.3	72	3.0	7.6	3.2	0.0
Full Fat, Medio, Costa*	1 Medio/480ml	327	14.6	68	2.8	7.2	3.0	0.0
Full Fat, Primo, Costa*	1 Primo/360ml	225	10.1	62	2.6	6.6	2.8	0.0
Skimmed, Massimo, Costa*	1 Massimo/600ml	296	3.0	49	3.1	7.9	0.5	0.0
Skimmed, Medio, Costa*	1 Medio/480ml	235	2.4	49	3.0	7.9	0.5	0.0

	Measure INFO/WEIGHT	per Measure KCAL	per Measure FAT	Nutrition Values per 100g / 100ml KCAL	PROT	CARB	FAT	FIBRE
COSTA								
HOT CHOCOLATE								
Skimmed, Primo, Costa*	1 Primo/360ml	156	1.5	43	2.8	7.0	0.4	0.0
Soya Milk, Massimo, Costa*	1 Massimo/600ml	323	11.3	54	2.8	6.0	1.9	0.0
Soya Milk, Medio, Costa*	1 Medio/480ml	256	9.0	53	2.8	6.0	1.9	0.0
Soya Milk, Primo, Costa*	1 Primo/360ml	172	6.1	48	1.5	5.3	1.7	0.0
with Marshmallows & Cream, Skim, Massimo, Costa*	1 Massimo/600ml	441	12.7	74	3.2	10.2	2.1	0.0
with Marshmallows & Cream, Skim, Medio, Costa*	1 Medio/480ml	380	12.1	79	3.2	10.7	2.5	0.0
with Marshmallows & Cream, Skim, Primo, Costa*	1 Primo/360ml	277	8.8	77	3.0	10.6	2.4	0.0
with Marshmallows & Cream, Soya Milk, Medio, Costa*	1 Medio/480ml	401	18.7	84	3.0	8.8	3.9	0.0
with Marshmallows & Cream, Soya Milk, Primo, Costa*	1 Primo/360ml	294	13.4	82	2.8	8.9	3.7	0.0
ICE DESSERTS								
Double Choc Flake, Full Fat Milk, Medio, Costa*	1 Medio/454ml	786	29.9	173	2.1	26.4	6.6	0.0
Simply Vanilla, Full Fat Milk, Medio, Costa*	1 Medio/454ml	421	7.8	93	1.4	17.9	1.7	0.0
Simply Vanilla, Full Fat Milk, Primo, Costa*	1 Primo/340ml	301	5.6	89	1.4	17.1	1.6	0.0
Simply Vanilla, Skimmed Milk, Primo, Costa*	1 Primo/340ml	255	0.5	75	1.5	17.2	0.2	0.0
Simply Vanilla, Soya Milk, Medio, Costa*	1 Medio/454ml	373	3.8	82	1.4	17.0	0.8	0.0
Simply Vanilla, Soya Milk, Primo, Costa*	1 Primo/340ml	267	2.7	79	1.4	16.2	0.8	0.0
Strawberry Shortcake, Full Fat Milk, Primo, Costa*	1 Primo/340ml	569	23.9	167	1.8	24.3	7.0	0.0
Strawberry Shortcake, Skimmed Milk, Medio, Costa*	1 Medio/454ml	694	19.0	153	1.9	27.2	4.2	0.0
JUICE DRINK								
Orange & Raspberry, Fruit Cooler, Medio, Costa*	1 Medio/480ml	320	0.2	67	0.2	15.9	0.0	0.0
Orange & Raspberry, Fruit Cooler, Primo, Costa*	1 Primo/360ml	241	0.2	67	0.2	16.1	0.1	0.0
Orange & Raspberry, Juice Drink, Massimo, Costa*	1 Massimo/600ml	403	0.3	67	0.2	16.1	0.0	0.0
Tropical Fruit, Fruit Cooler, Massimo, Costa*	1 Massimo/600ml	400	2.6	67	0.2	15.3	0.4	0.0
Tropical Fruit, Fruit Cooler, Medio, Costa*	1 Medio/480ml	317	2.0	66	0.2	15.2	0.4	0.0
Tropical Fruit, Fruit Cooler, Primo, Costa*	1 Primo/360ml	240	1.5	67	0.1	15.2	0.4	0.0
LEMONADE								
Iced, Massimo, Costa*	1 Massimo/600ml	196	0.0	33	0.0	7.9	0.0	0.0
Iced, Medio, Costa*	1 Medio/480ml	147	0.0	31	0.0	7.4	0.0	0.0
Iced, Primo, Costa*	1 Serving/360ml	98	0.0	27	0.0	6.6	0.0	0.0
Peach, Iced, Massimo, Costa*	1 Massimo/600ml	172	0.0	29	0.0	7.0	0.0	0.0
Peach, Iced, Medio, Costa*	1 Medio/480ml	129	0.0	27	0.0	6.6	0.0	0.0
Peach, Iced, Primo, Costa*	1 Primo/360ml	86	0.0	24	0.0	5.8	0.0	0.0
Raspberry & Cranberry, Iced, Massimo, Costa*	1 Massimo/600ml	179	0.0	30	0.0	7.3	0.0	0.0
Raspberry & Cranberry, Iced, Medio, Costa*	1 Medio/480ml	134	0.0	28	0.0	6.8	0.0	0.0
Raspberry & Cranberry, Iced, Primo, Costa*	1 Primo/360ml	89	0.0	25	0.0	6.1	0.0	0.0
Strawberry, Iced, Massimo, Costa*	1 Massimo/600ml	175	0.0	29	0.0	7.1	0.0	0.0
Strawberry, Iced, Medio, Costa*	1 Medio/480ml	131	0.0	27	0.0	6.7	0.0	0.0
Strawberry, Iced, Primo, Costa*	1 Primo/360ml	87	0.0	24	0.0	5.9	0.0	0.0
MUFFIN								
Banana & Pecan Breakfast Loaf, Costa*	1 Muffin/113g	442	23.4	391	5.1	44.0	20.7	0.0
Blueberry, Costa*	1 Muffin/132g	475	20.9	360	4.0	50.4	15.8	0.0
Chocolate, Mini, Costa*	1 Muffin/19g	73	3.9	383	4.3	44.5	20.5	0.0
Lemon & Orange, Low Fat, Costa*	1 Muffin/135g	319	3.1	236	4.6	49.4	2.3	1.1
Lemon & Poppyseed, Costa*	1 Muffin/131g	532	28.0	406	4.3	49.0	21.4	0.0
Lemon & White Chocolate, Costa*	1 Muffin/129g	472	20.4	366	5.4	52.3	15.8	0.0
Original Breakfast Loaf, Costa*	1 Muffin/128g	443	18.6	346	5.0	48.9	14.5	0.0
Raspberry & White Chocolate, Costa*	1 Muffin/135g	511	26.0	376	4.8	46.4	19.1	0.0
Raspberry & White Chocolate, Mini, Costa*	1 Muffin/19g	72	3.7	379	4.1	45.9	19.4	0.0
Triple Chocolate, Costa*	1 Muffin/130g	530	27.8	408	5.3	48.6	21.4	0.0
PAIN AU RAISIN								
Costa*	1 Pastry/119g	356	13.7	299	5.1	43.7	11.5	0.0

	Measure INFO/WEIGHT	per Measure KCAL	FAT	Nutrition Values per 100g / 100ml KCAL	PROT	CARB	FAT	FIBRE
COSTA								
PANINI								
Brie & Tomato Chutney, Costa*	1 Panini/177g	453	16.5	256	9.8	33.3	9.3	2.8
Chicken, & Pesto, Costa*	1 Serving/209g	419	21.4	200	22.5	57.9	10.2	0.0
Chicken, Roasted Pepper & Rocket, Costa*	1 Pack/185g	338	7.6	183	10.4	26.0	4.1	3.2
Goats Cheese, & Caramelised Onion Chutney, Costa*	1 Panini/172g	431	5.3	251	4.9	19.5	3.1	0.0
Goats Cheese, & Pepper, Costa*	1 Serving/197g	424	11.0	215	9.9	30.3	5.6	0.0
Ham & Cheese, Costa*	1 Panini/175g	461	21.2	263	12.5	26.2	12.1	0.0
Mozzarella, Tomato & Basil, Costa*	1 Panini/190g	400	11.0	211	8.3	29.8	5.8	0.0
Ragu Meatball, Costa*	1 Serving/190g	477	15.8	251	11.7	31.2	8.3	0.0
Steak & Cheese, Costa*	1 Serving/228g	492	16.4	216	11.3	25.7	7.2	0.0
Tuna Melt, Costa*	1 Panini/190g	462	14.3	243	14.4	29.5	7.5	0.0
SALAD								
Chargrilled Vegetable & Cous Cous, Costa*	1 Serving/291g	352	7.6	121	3.0	21.5	2.6	0.0
Chicken, Costa*	1 Serving/194g	297	4.1	153	12.4	21.2	2.1	0.0
Chicken & Pasta, Costa*	1 Serving/270g	427	11.1	158	8.4	21.9	4.1	0.0
Chicken & Pesto Pasta, Costa*	1 Pack/271g	420	11.4	155	7.8	21.3	4.2	1.7
Cous Cous, Moroccan Styles, Costa*	1 Pack/290g	392	7.3	135	3.6	24.6	2.5	2.2
Sunblush Tomato & Feta Pasta, Costa*	1 Pack/267g	360	13.6	135	4.4	17.1	5.1	2.2
Tuna, Costa*	1 Pack/181g	274	4.0	151	10.3	22.6	2.2	0.0
SANDWICH								
Bacon & Tomato Sauce, Tostato, Costa*	1 Tostato/132g	316	6.6	239	8.5	40.2	5.0	0.0
BLT, Costa*	1 Pack/169g	397	15.7	235	11.0	26.8	9.3	0.0
Brie, Apple & Grape, Costa*	1 Serving/225g	536	24.5	238	8.3	28.7	10.9	0.0
Chicken, Coronation, Costa*	1 Pack/258g	600	26.1	232	12.5	23.0	10.1	2.5
Chicken, Roast, Costa*	1 Pack/177g	325	7.1	184	13.0	23.8	4.0	0.0
Club, All Day Breakfast, Costa*	1 Pack/243g	592	20.9	244	11.0	30.6	8.6	0.0
Club, Chicken & Bacon, Costa*	1 Pack/213g	484	13.2	227	13.6	29.3	6.2	0.0
Egg, Free Range, Costa*	1 Pack/172g	377	14.6	219	9.7	25.9	8.5	0.0
Egg Mayonnaise & Tomato, Free Range, Costa*	1 Pack/174g	389	24.1	223	8.6	18.3	13.8	0.0
Ham Hock & Mustard Pickle, Roll, Costa*	1 Pack/163g	286	5.2	176	10.6	26.1	3.2	0.0
Houmous, Costa*	1 Pack/165g	263	4.7	160	6.4	25.9	2.8	0.0
Ploughmans, Cheese, Roll, Costa*	1 Pack/175g	431	21.3	247	9.4	25.0	12.2	0.0
Prawn, Tiger, with Lime & Chilli Dressing, Costa*	1 Pack/185g	367	19.0	198	8.2	21.2	10.2	0.0
Prawn Mayonnaise, on Wholemeal, Costa*	1 Pack/163g	291	7.7	178	9.0	23.6	4.7	0.0
Salmon, & Salad, Poached, Oatmeal, Costa*	1 Pack/151g	224	4.2	148	7.7	22.9	2.8	0.0
Sausage, Chorizo, & Vine Ripened Tomato, Costa*	1 Pack/181g	315	3.8	174	15.5	26.1	2.1	0.0
Scottish Smoked Salmon & Soft Cheese, Costa*	1 Pack/175g	372	10.7	213	12.9	25.5	6.1	1.9
Tuna, & Salad, Costa*	1 Pack/177g	289	4.1	163	11.9	25.7	2.3	0.0
SCONE								
Fruit, Costa*	1 Serving/110g	370	11.8	336	5.6	55.1	10.7	0.0
SHORTBREAD								
Mini, Bag, Costa*	1 Bag/65g	316	15.7	486	4.1	63.0	24.1	0.0
SHORTCAKE								
Raspberry, Costa*	1 Shortcake/45g	215	10.7	477	2.4	63.5	23.7	0.0
SLICES								
Cheese, Twist, Pastry, Costa*	1 Pastry/103g	346	20.4	336	11.1	29.5	19.8	0.0
Cinnamon Swirl, Pastry, Costa*	1 Pastry/92g	341	22.8	369	4.0	31.9	24.7	0.0
Pecan, Pastry, Costa*	1 Pastry/105g	465	29.9	443	5.6	42.1	28.5	3.0
TEA								
Iced, Lemon, Costa*	1 Bottle/275ml	91	0.0	33	0.0	8.0	0.0	0.0
Iced, Original, Massimo, Costa*	1 Massimo/600ml	179	0.0	30	0.0	9.1	0.0	0.0
Iced, Original, Medio, Costa*	1 Medio/480ml	135	0.0	28	0.0	6.9	0.0	0.0
Iced, Original, Primo, Costa*	1 Primo/360ml	88	0.0	24	0.0	6.0	0.0	0.0

	Measure INFO/WEIGHT	per Measure KCAL	per Measure FAT	Nutrition Values per 100g / 100ml KCAL	PROT	CARB	FAT	FIBRE
COSTA								
TEA								
Iced, Peach, Massimo, Costa*	1 Massimo/600ml	121	0.0	20	0.0	4.8	0.0	0.0
Iced, Peach, Medio, Costa*	1 Medio/480ml	91	0.0	19	0.0	4.5	0.0	0.0
Iced, Peach, Primo, Costa*	1 Primo/360ml	60	0.0	17	0.0	4.0	0.0	0.0
Iced, Raspberry, Massimo, Costa*	1 Massimo/600ml	133	0.0	22	0.0	5.4	0.0	0.0
Iced, Raspberry, Medio, Costa*	1 Medio/480ml	100	0.0	21	0.0	5.1	0.0	0.0
Iced, Raspberry, Primo, Costa*	1 Primo/360ml	67	0.0	19	0.0	4.5	0.0	0.0
Latte, Chai, Full Fat, Massimo, Costa*	1 Massimo/600ml	429	16.9	72	2.6	9.0	2.8	0.0
Latte, Chai, Full Fat, Medio, Costa*	1 Medio/480ml	325	12.7	68	2.5	8.6	2.6	0.0
Latte, Chai, Full Fat, Primo, Costa*	1 Primo/360ml	223	8.9	62	2.3	7.8	2.5	0.0
Latte, Chai, Skimmed, Massimo, Costa*	1 Massimo/600ml	293	0.6	49	2.8	9.4	0.1	0.0
Latte, Chai, Skimmed, Medio, Costa*	1 Medio/480ml	232	0.5	48	2.7	9.3	0.1	0.0
Latte, Chai, Skimmed, Primo, Costa*	1 Primo/360ml	154	0.3	43	2.5	8.2	0.1	0.0
Latte, Chai, Soya Milk, Massimo, Costa*	1 Massimo/600ml	320	8.9	53	2.5	7.5	1.5	0.0
Latte, Chai, Soya Milk, Medio, Costa*	1 Medio/480ml	254	7.0	53	2.5	7.4	1.5	0.0
Latte, Chai, Soya Milk, Primo, Costa*	1 Primo/360ml	170	4.8	47	2.3	6.6	1.3	0.0
TRAYBAKE								
Chocolate Tiffin Triangle, Costa*	1 Serving/85g	433	25.7	509	4.9	54.6	30.2	0.0
Fruit, Seed, Nut & Honey Bar, Costa*	1 Serving/75g	317	15.2	423	7.5	52.5	20.3	0.0
Granola Bar, Costa*	1 Bar/75g	317	15.2	423	7.5	52.5	20.3	0.0
Shortbread, Caramel, Costa*	1 Serving/77g	426	26.5	553	4.7	55.9	34.4	0.0
WRAP								
Chicken Caesar, Costa*	1 Pack/194g	420	15.6	216	11.8	24.1	8.0	1.4
Chicken Fajita, Costa*	1 Wrap/186g	416	12.9	223	12.1	28.0	6.9	0.0
Spicy Three Bean, Costa*	1 Pack/235g	456	14.3	194	7.1	27.7	6.1	0.0
YOGHURT								
Honey & Granola, Costa*	1 Pot/190g	303	6.1	159	5.3	27.3	3.2	0.0
Strawberry & Granola, Costa*	1 Pot/190g	253	7.4	133	5.4	19.0	3.9	0.0
DOMINO'S PIZZA								
PIZZA								
American Hot, BBQ Stuffed, Lge, Domino's Pizza*	1 Slice/404g	1052	41.3	260	10.6	30.7	10.2	1.9
American Hot, BBQ Stuffed, Med, Domino's Pizza*	1 Slice/376g	1031	42.1	274	13.0	29.4	11.2	2.0
American Hot, Classic, Large, Domino's Pizza*	1 Slice/315g	823	35.0	261	10.9	28.7	11.1	1.9
American Hot, Classic, Medium, Domino's Pizza*	1 Slice/288g	761	32.9	264	11.0	28.5	11.4	1.9
American Hot, Classic, Personal, Domino's Pizza*	1 Slice/204g	536	19.8	262	11.2	31.4	9.7	2.2
American Hot, Classic, Small, Domino's Pizza*	1 Slice/253g	669	28.1	264	12.2	27.7	11.1	1.9
American Hot, Dominator, Large, Domino's Pizza*	1 Slice/110g	307	12.1	279	13.2	31.7	11.0	1.9
American Hot, Domino's, Personal, Domino's Pizza*	1 Slice/61g	161	5.1	264	14.7	32.6	8.3	2.2
American Hot, GF, Delight, Small, Domino's Pizza*	1 Slice/53g	138	5.8	258	12.2	26.8	10.9	2.1
American Hot, GF, Small, Domino's Pizza*	1 Slice/53g	134	6.5	251	8.7	25.5	12.1	2.4
American Hot, Italian, Delight, Lge, Domino's Pizza*	1 Slice/66g	173	6.6	263	11.9	30.2	10.1	2.1
American Hot, Italian, Delight, Med, Domino's Pizza*	1 Slice/58g	155	6.2	266	12.0	29.7	10.6	2.1
American Hot, Stuffed, Delight, Med, Domino's Pizza*	1 Slice/86g	216	9.3	250	11.8	25.3	10.8	2.1
American Hot, Stuffed Crust, Large, Domino's Pizza*	1 Slice/92g	255	10.7	275	13.4	28.8	11.5	2.0
American Hot, Stuffed Crust, Medium, Domino's Pizza*	1 Slice/86g	240	10.1	278	13.5	28.8	11.7	20.0
American Hot, Thin & Crispy, Large, Domino's Pizza*	1 Slice/54g	149	7.6	277	11.6	25.2	14.1	1.7
American Hot, Thin & Crispy, Medium, Domino's Pizza*	1 Slice/50g	140	7.2	281	11.8	25.1	14.5	1.7
Americano, BBQ Stuffed, Delight, Med, Domino's Pizza*	1 Slice/88g	246	9.2	278	14.5	30.6	10.4	1.9
Americano, Classic, Delight, Medium, Domino's Pizza*	1 Slice/67g	197	6.3	292	15.1	35.8	9.4	2.1
Americano, Classic, Large, Domino's Pizza*	1 Slice/73g	221	8.1	301	14.3	35.3	11.0	2.4
Americano, Classic, Medium, Domino's Pizza*	1 Slice/68g	205	7.6	303	14.3	35.1	11.3	2.4
Americano, Classic, Personal, Domino's Pizza*	1 Slice/202g	609	20.8	301	15.1	36.0	10.3	2.4
Americano, Classic, Small, Domino's Pizza*	1 Slice/60g	183	7.3	305	15.5	32.4	12.1	2.5

	Measure INFO/WEIGHT	per Measure KCAL	per Measure FAT	KCAL	PROT	CARB	FAT	FIBRE
				Nutrition Values per 100g / 100ml				
DOMINO'S PIZZA								
PIZZA								
Americano, Double Decadence, Med, Domino's Pizza*	1 Slice/87g	264	11.5	302	13.2	31.5	13.1	2.6
Americano, GF, Small, Domino's Pizza*	1 Slice/52g	166	6.9	315	12.4	35.9	13.1	2.4
Americano, Italian, Delight, Med, Domino's Pizza*	1 Slice/57g	172	6.2	303	18.5	31.3	10.9	2.8
Americano, Italian Style, Large, Domino's Pizza*	1 Slice/64g	197	7.8	307	15.5	33.0	12.1	2.4
Americano, Italian Style, Small, Domino's Pizza*	1 Slice/50g	157	6.6	313	15.9	31.7	13.2	2.4
Americano, Personal Pizza, Domino's Pizza*	1 Slice/64g	184	4.9	287	19.4	35.0	7.7	2.5
Americano, Stuffed, Delight, Med, Domino's Pizza*	1 Slice/85g	240	9.3	282	15.1	30.0	10.9	1.9
Americano, Stuffed Crust, Large, Domino's Pizza*	1 Slice/91g	263	10.6	288	13.9	30.9	11.6	2.8
Americano, Stuffed Crust, Medium, Domino's Pizza*	1 Slice/85g	247	10.1	290	13.9	30.8	11.8	2.8
Americano, Thin & Crispy, Delight, Med, Domino's*	1 Slice/48g	152	5.8	315	17.2	33.3	12.1	2.3
Americao, Italian Style, Medium, Domino's Pizza*	1 Slice/57g	177	7.2	310	15.6	32.5	12.6	2.4
Bacon Dbl Cheese, BBQ, Delight, Med, Domino's*	1 Slice/97g	240	10.7	247	12.0	24.0	11.0	2.0
Bacon Dbl Cheese, Classic, Med, Domino's Pizza*	1 Slice/76g	200	9.2	262	12.0	25.6	12.1	1.8
Bacon Dbl Cheese, Dbl Decadence, Med, Domino's*	1 Slice/96g	261	13.1	272	12.2	24.1	13.7	1.8
Bacon Dbl Cheese, Italian, Delight, Med, Domino's*	1 Slice/66g	173	7.6	263	13.0	26.1	11.5	1.9
Bacon Dbl Cheese, Italian, Med, Domino's*	1 Slice/66g	156	7.6	237	11.9	20.9	11.6	1.7
Bacon Dbl Cheese, Stuffed, Delight, Med, Domino's*	1 Slice/94g	235	10.8	249	12.5	23.2	11.4	2.0
Bacon Dbl Cheese, Thin & Crispy, Med, Domino's*	1 Slice/57g	158	8.6	275	12.9	21.6	15.0	1.6
Carolina, BBQ Stuffed Crust, Large, Domino's Pizza*	1 Slice/100g	267	10.5	267	12.1	229.9	10.5	2.5
Carolina, BBQ Stuffed Crust, Medium, Domino's Pizza*	1 Slice/93g	249	9.8	268	12.1	19.9	10.6	2.5
Carolina, Classic, Delight, Large, Domino's Pizza*	1 Slice/79g	212	6.7	268	13.3	33.8	8.5	1.9
Carolina, Classic, Delight, Med, Domino's Pizza*	1 Slice/72g	194	6.2	269	13.4	33.7	8.6	1.9
Carolina, Classic, Delight, Small, Domino's Pizza*	1 Slice/64g	176	5.5	277	12.9	35.7	8.7	2.3
Carolina, Classic, Large, Domino's Pizza*	1 Slice/79g	220	8.2	278	12.6	33.0	10.3	2.1
Carolina, Classic, Medium, Domino's Pizza*	1 Slice/72g	201	7.5	280	12.6	33.0	10.4	2.1
Carolina, Classic, Personal, Domino's Pizza*	1 Slice/220g	624	23.4	283	13.3	32.9	10.6	2.0
Carolina, Classic, Small, Domino's Pizza*	1 Slice/63g	177	6.9	279	13.5	30.7	10.9	2.3
Carolina, Double Decadence, Large, Domino's Pizza*	1 Slice/101g	286	12.3	283	11.9	30.1	12.2	2.4
Carolina, Double Decadence, Medium, Domino's Pizza*	1 Slice/92g	260	11.3	284	12.0	30.1	12.3	2.4
Carolina, GF, Small, Domino's Pizza*	1 Slice/56g	160	6.6	284	10.3	33.7	11.7	2.1
Carolina, Italian Style, Delight, Med, Domino's Pizza*	1 Slice/61g	169	6.1	275	16.2	29.2	9.9	2.5
Carolina, Italian Style, Delight, Small, Domino's Pizza*	1 Slice/54g	147	5.5	274	16.1	28.6	10.2	2.4
Carolina, Italian Style, Large, Domino's Pizza*	1 Slice/69g	195	7.8	281	13.4	30.7	11.3	2.1
Carolina, Italian Style, Medium, Domino's Pizza*	1 Slice/61g	173	7.1	282	13.5	30.3	11.5	2.1
Carolina, Italian Style, Small, Domino's Pizza*	1 Slice/53g	150	6.2	281	13.5	29.6	11.7	2.1
Carolina, Stuffed Crust, Delight, Large, Domino's Pizza*	1 Slice/97g	254	9.8	263	13.7	28.5	10.1	1.8
Carolina, Stuffed Crust, Delight, Med, Domino's Pizza*	1 Slice/90g	237	9.2	264	13.7	28.6	10.2	1.8
Carolina, Stuffed Crust, Large, Domino's Pizza*	1 Slice/97g	262	10.6	271	12.5	29.3	11.0	2.6
Carolina, Thin & Crispy, Delight, Med, Domino's*	1 Slice/53g	149	5.7	282	14.7	30.6	10.8	2.0
Carolina, Thin & Crispy, Large, Domino's Pizza*	1 Slice/57g	170	7.4	296	13.3	31.0	12.9	1.7
Carolina, Thin & Crispy, Medium, Domino's Pizza*	1 Slice/53g	157	6.9	297	13.4	31.1	13.0	1.6
Cheese & Tom, BBQ Stuffed, Delight, Med, Domino's*	1 Slice/73g	184	6.1	251	11.7	31.0	8.3	2.3
Cheese & Tom, Classic, Delight, Med, Domino's Pizza*	1 Slice/53g	138	3.3	262	17.0	33.0	6.3	2.4
Cheese & Tomato, BBQ Stuffed Crust, Med, Domino's*	1 Slice/74g	208	6.8	283	13.7	35.1	9.3	2.2
Cheese & Tomato, Classic, Medium, Domino's Pizza*	1 Slice/53g	144	4.6	274	11.5	36.2	8.8	2.2
Cheese & Tomato, Classic, Personal, Domino's Pizza*	1 Slice/161g	435	11.3	270	11.6	38.9	7.0	2.5
Cheese & Tomato, Classic, Small, Domino's Pizza*	1 Slice/45g	122	3.5	269	12.9	35.8	7.7	2.3
Cheese & Tomato, GF, Small, Domino's Pizza*	1 Slice/73g	185	6.2	252	8.2	34.2	8.4	3.0
Cheese & Tomato, Italian Style, Large, Domino's Pizza*	1 Slice/48g	115	3.4	239	11.3	31.5	7.1	2.2
Cheese & Tomato, Italian Style, Med, Domino's Pizza*	1 Slice/42g	100	3.0	239	11.3	31.5	7.1	2.2
Cheese & Tomato, Italian Style, Small, Domino's Pizza*	1 Slice/35g	85	2.5	239	11.3	31.5	7.1	2.2
Cheese & Tomato, Stuffed Crust, Lge, Domino's Pizza*	1 Slice/76g	218	7.4	288	14.4	34.6	9.8	2.3

	Measure INFO/WEIGHT	per Measure KCAL	FAT	Nutrition Values per 100g / 100ml KCAL	PROT	CARB	FAT	FIBRE
DOMINO'S PIZZA								
PIZZA								
Cheese & Tomato, Stuffed Crust, Med, Domino's Pizza*	1 Slice/70g	203	6.9	288	14.4	34.6	9.8	2.3
Chicken Feast, Classic, Delight, Small, Domino's Pizza*	1 Slice/72g	165	3.7	228	16.5	29.0	5.1	2.3
Chicken Feast, Classic, Large, Domino's Pizza*	1 Slice/89g	201	5.6	226	14.6	27.8	6.3	2.1
Chicken Feast, Classic, Medium, Domino's Pizza*	1 Slice/81g	183	5.1	226	14.6	27.8	6.3	2.1
Chicken Feast, Classic, Small, Domino's Pizza*	1 Slice/72g	163	4.5	226	14.6	27.8	6.3	2.1
Chicken Feast, Dbl Decadence, Med, Domino's Pizza*	1 Slice/100g	232	6.6	232	14.3	28.9	6.6	2.1
Chicken Feast, Delight, Personal, Domino's Pizza*	1 Slice/62g	140	3.2	226	13.3	31.7	5.1	2.2
Chicken Feast, Dominator, Large, Domino's Pizza*	1 Slice/112g	289	9.2	258	13.9	32.3	8.2	2.0
Chicken Feast, Personal, Domino's Pizza*	1 Slice/62g	153	3.8	247	15.7	32.3	6.1	2.1
Chicken Feast, Thin Crust, Large, Domino's Pizza*	1 Slice/69g	195	8.0	283	16.5	28.1	11.6	2.4
Chicken Feast, Thin Crust, Medium, Domino's Pizza*	1 Slice/64g	181	7.4	283	16.5	28.1	11.6	2.4
Deluxe, Classic, Large, Domino's Pizza*	1 Slice/84g	209	7.9	250	13.2	26.9	9.4	2.1
Deluxe, Classic, Medium, Domino's Pizza*	1 Slice/76g	191	7.2	250	13.2	26.9	9.4	2.1
Deluxe, Classic, Small, Domino's Pizza*	1 Slice/70g	174	6.5	250	13.2	26.9	9.4	2.1
Deluxe, Personal, Domino's Pizza*	1 Slice/59g	159	5.4	270	14.4	31.4	9.1	2.1
Deluxe, Thin Crust, Large, Domino's Pizza*	1 Slice/65g	202	10.0	312	14.7	27.0	15.5	2.4
Deluxe, Thin Crust, Medium, Domino's Pizza*	1 Slice/60g	188	9.3	312	14.7	27.0	15.5	2.4
Extravaganzza, Classic, Large, Domino's Pizza*	1 Slice/104g	252	10.7	242	13.7	23.4	10.3	1.9
Extravaganzza, Classic, Medium, Domino's Pizza*	1 Slice/95g	230	9.8	242	13.7	23.4	10.3	1.9
Extravaganzza, Classic, Small, Domino's Pizza*	1 Slice/86g	209	8.9	242	13.7	23.4	10.3	1.9
Extravaganzza, Dominator, Large, Domino's Pizza*	1 Slice/127g	337	14.1	266	13.3	28.2	11.1	1.9
Extravaganzza, Double Decadence, Med, Domino's*	1 Slice/114g	328	17.7	287	13.1	23.7	15.5	2.1
Extravaganzza, Personal, Domino's Pizza*	1 Slice/75g	195	7.8	262	15.2	26.7	10.4	1.9
Extravaganzza, Thin Crust, Large, Domino's Pizza*	1 Slice/84g	235	12.8	280	15.0	20.7	15.2	2.2
Extravaganzza, Thin Crust, Medium, Domino's Pizza*	1 Slice/78g	227	12.1	291	15.1	22.6	15.5	2.1
Farmhouse, Classic, Large, Domino's Pizza*	1 Slice/88g	195	6.0	222	13.4	26.8	6.8	2.1
Farmhouse, Classic, Medium, Domino's Pizza*	1 Slice/81g	180	5.5	222	13.4	26.8	6.8	2.1
Farmhouse, Classic, Small, Domino's Pizza*	1 Slice/73g	162	5.0	222	13.4	26.8	6.8	2.1
Farmhouse, Dominator, Large, Domino's Pizza*	1 Slice/111g	283	9.4	255	13.0	31.7	8.5	2.0
Farmhouse, Double Decadence, Med, Domino's*	1 Slice/100g	277	13.4	277	12.7	26.5	13.4	2.3
Farmhouse, Personal, Domino's Pizza*	1 Slice/62g	151	4.0	244	14.8	31.5	6.5	2.1
Farmhouse, Thin Crust, Large, Domino's Pizza*	1 Slice/68g	180	8.1	265	14.8	24.6	11.9	2.5
Farmhouse, Thin Crust, Medium, Domino's Pizza*	1 Slice/63g	175	7.7	277	15.1	26.9	12.2	2.4
Firenze, Fresh Thin Crust, Large, Domino's Pizza*	1 Slice/60g	193	8.6	323	15.3	32.0	14.4	1.7
Firenze, Fresh Thin Crust, Medium, Domino's Pizza*	1 Slice/53g	172	7.7	323	15.3	32.0	14.4	1.7
Firenze, Fresh Thin Crust, Small, Domino's Pizza*	1 Slice/46g	149	6.6	323	15.3	32.0	14.4	1.7
Florentine, Fresh Thin Crust, Large, Domino's Pizza*	1 Slice/55g	152	5.5	277	12.6	33.3	10.0	1.7
Florentine, Fresh Thin Crust, Medium, Domino's Pizza*	1 Slice/48g	133	4.8	277	12.6	33.3	10.0	1.7
Florentine, Fresh Thin Crust, Small, Domino's Pizza*	1 Slice/41g	114	4.1	277	12.6	33.3	10.0	1.7
Four Seasons, Fresh Thin Crust, Large, Domino's Pizza*	1 Slice/71g	195	7.0	274	14.1	31.5	9.8	1.9
Four Seasons, Fresh Thin Crust, Medium, Domino's*	1 Slice/50g	137	4.9	274	14.1	31.5	9.8	1.9
Four Seasons, Fresh Thin Crust, Small, Domino's Pizza*	1 Slice/63g	173	6.2	274	14.1	31.5	9.8	1.9
Full House, Classic, Large, Domino's Pizza*	1 Slice/111g	268	9.9	241	13.2	27.0	8.9	2.1
Full House, Classic, Medium, Domino's Pizza*	1 Slice/102g	241	9.1	236	13.0	26.0	8.9	2.0
Full House, Classic, Small, Domino's Pizza*	1 Slice/94g	227	8.6	242	13.5	26.3	9.2	2.1
Full House, Dominator, Large, Domino's Pizza*	1 Slice/134g	351	13.0	262	12.6	31.0	9.7	2.0
Full House, Double Decadence, Medium, Domino's*	1 Slice/121g	346	17.8	286	12.4	25.9	14.7	2.2
Full House, Personal, Domino's Pizza*	1 Slice/70g	180	6.4	257	14.6	29.2	9.1	2.0
Full House, Thin Crust, Large, Domino's Pizza*	1 Slice/91g	251	12.6	276	14.0	23.7	13.9	2.4
Full House, Thin Crust, Medium, Domino's Pizza*	1 Slice/85g	247	12.2	290	14.3	25.9	14.3	2.3
Ham & Pineapple, Classic, Delight, Small, Domino's*	1 Slice/70g	163	4.0	233	15.7	29.7	5.7	2.3
Ham & Pineapple, Classic, Large, Domino's Pizza*	1 Slice/84g	194	5.9	231	13.7	28.5	7.0	2.0

	Measure INFO/WEIGHT	per Measure KCAL	FAT	Nutrition Values per 100g / 100ml KCAL	PROT	CARB	FAT	FIBRE
DOMINO'S PIZZA								
PIZZA								
Ham & Pineapple, Classic, Medium, Domino's Pizza*	1 Slice/77g	178	5.4	231	13.7	28.5	7.0	2.0
Ham & Pineapple, Classic, Small, Domino's Pizza*	1 Slice/70g	162	4.9	231	13.7	28.5	7.0	2.0
Ham & Pineapple, Delight, Personal, Domino's Pizza*	1 Slice/60g	137	3.4	229	12.4	32.3	5.6	2.2
Ham & Pineapple, Dominator, Large, Domino's Pizza*	1 Slice/107g	283	9.4	265	13.2	33.3	8.8	2.0
Ham & Pineapple, Double Decadence, Med, Domino's*	1 Slice/97g	278	13.4	287	12.9	27.8	13.8	2.2
Ham & Pineapple, Personal, Domino's Pizza*	1 Slice/60g	150	4.0	251	14.9	33.0	6.6	2.1
Ham & Pineapple, Thin Crust, Large, Domino's Pizza*	1 Slice/64g	181	8.1	283	15.4	26.8	12.7	2.5
Ham & Pineapple, Thin Crust, Medium, Domino's Pizza*	1 Slice/60g	175	7.6	292	15.4	29.0	12.7	2.3
Hawaiian, Classic, Delight, Small, Domino's Pizza*	1 Slice/79g	173	4.2	220	15.2	27.7	5.4	2.2
Hawaiian, Classic, Large, Domino's Pizza*	1 Slice/90g	203	6.0	226	13.4	27.9	6.7	2.0
Hawaiian, Classic, Medium, Domino's Pizza*	1 Slice/82g	180	5.4	219	13.1	26.8	6.6	2.0
Hawaiian, Classic, Small, Domino's Pizza*	1 Slice/75g	168	5.0	224	13.7	27.2	6.7	2.1
Hawaiian, Delight, Personal, Domino's Pizza*	1 Slice/66g	145	3.6	219	12.0	30.7	5.4	2.1
Hawaiian, Dominator, Large, Domino's Pizza*	1 Slice/113g	285	9.5	252	12.7	31.6	8.4	2.0
Hawaiian, Double Decadence, Medium, Domino's*	1 Slice/101g	277	13.3	274	12.5	26.6	13.2	2.2
Hawaiian, Pizza, Personal, Domino's Pizza*	1 Slice/63g	152	4.0	240	14.4	31.3	6.3	2.0
Hawaiian, Thin Crust, Large, Domino's Pizza*	1 Slice/70g	182	8.1	260	14.4	24.6	11.6	2.4
Hawaiian, Thin Crust, Medium, Domino's Pizza*	1 Slice/65g	177	7.7	273	14.6	26.9	11.9	2.3
Hot & Spicy, Classic, Large, Domino's Pizza*	1 Slice/85g	202	6.5	238	12.7	29.5	7.7	2.3
Hot & Spicy, Classic, Medium, Domino's Pizza*	1 Slice/77g	179	5.9	232	12.3	28.7	7.6	2.3
Hot & Spicy, Classic, Small, Domino's Pizza*	1 Slice/69g	164	5.3	237	12.8	29.3	7.7	2.3
Hot & Spicy, Dominator, Large, Domino's Pizza*	1 Slice/107g	282	9.8	264	12.2	33.0	9.2	2.2
Hot & Spicy, Double Decadence, Medium, Domino's*	1 Slice/96g	276	13.7	288	11.8	28.0	14.3	2.4
Hot & Spicy, Personal, Domino's Pizza*	1 Slice/59g	150	4.3	254	13.9	33.3	7.2	2.3
Hot & Spicy, Thin Crust, Large, Domino's Pizza*	1 Slice/65g	182	8.6	280	9.3	26.5	13.3	2.7
Hot & Spicy, Thin Crust, Medium, Domino's Pizza*	1 Slice/60g	176	8.1	294	13.7	29.2	13.6	2.6
House Special, Classic, Large, Domino's Pizza*	1 Slice/94g	232	8.8	247	15.8	23.8	9.4	1.9
House Special, Classic, Medium, Domino's Pizza*	1 Slice/86g	212	8.1	247	15.8	23.8	9.4	1.9
House Special, Classic, Small, Domino's Pizza*	1 Slice/77g	191	7.3	247	15.8	23.8	9.4	1.9
House Special, Pizza, Personal, Domino's Pizza*	1 Slice/65g	170	5.6	262	16.6	28.4	8.6	1.9
House Special, Thin Crust, Large, Domino's Pizza*	1 Slice/75g	226	11.0	300	17.8	23.1	14.6	2.1
House Special, Thin Crust, Medium, Domino's Pizza*	1 Slice/70g	209	10.2	300	17.8	23.1	14.6	2.1
Meat Lovers, Classic, Large, Domino's Pizza*	1 Slice/89g	235	9.3	264	16.1	26.5	10.4	1.9
Meat Lovers, Classic, Medium, Domino's Pizza*	1 Slice/81g	214	8.4	264	16.1	26.5	10.4	1.9
Meat Lovers, Classic, Small, Domino's Pizza*	1 Slice/74g	195	7.7	264	16.1	26.5	10.4	1.9
Meat Lovers, Dominator, Large, Domino's Pizza*	1 Slice/111g	320	12.6	288	15.1	31.4	11.3	1.9
Meat Lovers, Double Decadence, Medium, Domino's*	1 Slice/101g	314	16.5	311	14.9	26.3	16.3	2.1
Meat Lovers, Personal, Domino's Pizza*	1 Slice/61g	171	5.7	280	16.8	31.8	9.4	2.0
Meat Lovers, Thin Crust, Large, Domino's Pizza*	1 Slice/69g	219	11.4	318	18.3	24.2	16.5	2.3
Meat Lovers, Thin Crust, Medium, Domino's Pizza*	1 Slice/64g	211	10.7	330	18.5	26.5	16.7	2.2
Meateor, Classic, Large, Domino's Pizza*	1 Slice/87g	278	11.1	319	14.5	36.7	12.7	1.8
Meateor, Classic, Medium, Domino's Pizza*	1 Slice/80g	255	10.2	319	14.5	36.7	12.7	1.8
Meateor, Classic, Small, Domino's Pizza*	1 Slice/73g	233	9.3	319	14.5	36.7	12.7	1.8
Meateor, Dominator, Large, Domino's Pizza*	1 Slice/109g	341	13.8	313	13.3	36.6	12.7	1.8
Meateor, Double Decadence, Medium, Domino's Pizza*	1 Slice/99g	352	17.3	356	13.9	35.7	17.5	1.8
Meateor, Personal, Domino's Pizza*	1 Slice/66g	204	7.8	310	18.4	32.5	11.8	2.3
Meateor, Thin Crust, Large, Domino's Pizza*	1 Slice/67g	236	11.9	352	15.3	32.8	17.7	1.7
Meateor, Thin Crust, Medium, Domino's Pizza*	1 Slice/63g	247	12.2	392	16.0	38.6	19.3	2.0
Meatilicious, Stuffed Crust, Large, Domino's Pizza*	1 Slice/82g	235	9.4	286	16.1	28.5	11.5	1.9
Meatilicious, Stuffed Crust, Medium, Domino's Pizza*	1 Slice/76g	217	8.7	286	16.1	28.5	11.5	1.9
Meatzza, Classic, Large, Domino's Pizza*	1 Slice/87g	241	10.5	277	15.7	25.5	12.1	1.9
Meatzza, Classic, Medium, Domino's Pizza*	1 Slice/81g	223	9.7	277	15.7	25.5	12.1	1.9

	Measure INFO/WEIGHT	per Measure KCAL	FAT	Nutrition Values per 100g / 100ml KCAL	PROT	CARB	FAT	FIBRE
DOMINO'S PIZZA								
PIZZA								
Meatzza, Classic, Small, Domino's Pizza*	1 Slice/74g	205	9.0	277	15.7	25.5	12.1	1.9
Meatzza, Personal, Domino's Pizza*	1 Slice/59g	170	6.2	290	16.4	31.4	10.5	2.0
Meatzza, Thin Crust, Large, Domino's Pizza*	1 Slice/68g	234	12.6	343	17.7	25.2	18.5	2.1
Meatzza, Thin Crust, Medium, Domino's Pizza*	1 Slice/64g	221	11.9	343	17.7	25.2	18.5	2.1
Mexican Hot, Classic, Large, Domino's Pizza*	1 Slice/86g	213	7.8	247	13.7	26.4	9.1	2.1
Mexican Hot, Classic, Medium, Domino's Pizza*	1 Slice/79g	194	7.1	247	13.7	26.4	9.1	2.1
Mexican Hot, Classic, Small, Domino's Pizza*	1 Slice/71g	175	6.4	247	13.7	26.4	9.1	2.1
Mexican Hot, Personal, Domino's Pizza*	1 Slice/59g	157	4.9	264	14.9	31.3	8.3	2.2
Mexican Hot, Thin Crust, Large, Domino's Pizza*	1 Slice/67g	206	10.0	306	15.3	26.4	14.9	2.4
Mexican Hot, Thin Crust, Medium, Domino's Pizza*	1 Slice/62g	191	9.3	306	15.3	26.4	14.9	2.4
Mighty Meaty, Classic, Large, Domino's Pizza*	1 Slice/95g	243	9.7	256	15.0	26.1	10.2	2.0
Mighty Meaty, Classic, Medium, Domino's Pizza*	1 Slice/87g	218	8.9	251	14.7	25.0	10.3	1.9
Mighty Meaty, Classic, Small, Domino's Pizza*	1 Slice/80g	206	8.5	257	15.3	25.2	10.6	2.0
Mighty Meaty, Delight, Classic, Small, Domino's Pizza*	1 Slice/80g	202	7.3	253	16.5	26.1	9.1	2.2
Mighty Meaty, Delight, Personal, Domino's Pizza*	1 Slice/66g	166	5.9	250	13.3	29.1	8.9	2.1
Mighty Meaty, Dominator, Large, Domino's Pizza*	1 Slice/118g	326	13.1	276	14.0	30.0	11.1	1.9
Mighty Meaty, Double Decadence, Large, Domino's*	1 Slice/116g	350	18.2	302	13.7	25.3	15.7	2.1
Mighty Meaty, Double Decadence, Medium, Domino's*	1 Slice/107g	319	16.9	298	13.8	25.1	15.8	2.1
Mighty Meaty, Personal, Domino's Pizza*	1 Slice/66g	179	6.6	270	15.5	29.7	9.9	2.0
Mighty Meaty, Stuffed Crust, Domino's Pizza*	1 Slice/100g	274	11.6	274	15.2	26.5	11.6	1.9
Mighty Meaty, Stuffed Crust, Medium, Domino's Pizza*	1 Slice/94g	258	10.9	274	15.2	26.5	11.6	1.9
Mighty Meaty, Thin Crust, Large, Domino's Pizza*	1 Slice/75g	222	11.8	296	16.2	22.6	15.7	2.3
Mighty Meaty, Thin Crust, Medium, Domino's Pizza*	1 Slice/70g	216	11.2	309	16.5	24.6	16.0	2.1
Mixed Grill, Classic, Large, Domino's Pizza*	1 Slice/94g	244	10.6	259	13.5	25.0	11.2	2.0
Mixed Grill, Classic, Medium, Domino's Pizza*	1 Slice/86g	224	9.7	259	13.5	25.0	11.2	2.0
Mixed Grill, Classic, Small, Domino's Pizza*	1 Slice/79g	205	8.9	259	13.5	25.0	11.2	2.0
Mixed Grill, Personal, Domino's Pizza*	1 Slice/66g	182	6.9	275	14.8	29.6	10.4	2.0
Mixed Grill, Thin Crust, Large, Domino's Pizza*	1 Slice/74g	237	12.9	319	15.0	24.6	17.3	2.2
Mixed Grill, Thin Crust, Medium, Domino's Pizza*	1 Slice/70g	222	12.0	319	15.0	24.6	17.3	2.2
New Yorker, Classic, Delight, Large, Domino's Pizza*	1 Slice/87g	225	7.1	258	17.5	27.9	8.1	2.2
New Yorker, Classic, Delight, Medium, Domino's Pizza*	1 Slice/80g	207	6.5	258	17.5	27.9	8.1	2.2
New Yorker, Classic, Large, Domino's Pizza*	1 Slice/88g	225	8.2	257	15.5	26.7	9.4	2.0
New Yorker, Classic, Medium, Domino's Pizza*	1 Slice/80g	206	7.5	257	15.5	26.7	9.4	2.0
New Yorker, Classic, Small, Domino's Pizza*	1 Slice/73g	188	6.9	257	15.5	26.7	9.4	2.0
New Yorker, Delight, Classic, Small, Domino's Pizza*	1 Slice/73g	188	5.9	258	17.5	27.9	8.1	2.2
New Yorker, Delight, Personal, Domino's Pizza*	1 Slice/60g	151	4.5	252	13.7	31.4	7.5	2.2
New Yorker, Personal, Domino's Pizza*	1 Slice/60g	165	5.1	275	16.3	32.1	8.5	2.0
New Yorker, Thin Crust, Large, Domino's Pizza*	1 Slice/67g	217	10.4	322	17.6	26.7	15.5	2.2
New Yorker, Thin Crust, Medium, Domino's Pizza*	1 Slice/63g	203	9.8	322	17.6	26.7	15.5	2.2
Pepperoni Passion, Classic, Large, Domino's Pizza*	1 Slice/78g	228	9.1	292	16.7	28.7	11.6	2.0
Pepperoni Passion, Classic, Small, Domino's Pizza*	1 Slice/65g	190	7.5	292	16.7	28.7	11.6	2.0
Pepperoni Passion, Dbl Decadence, Med, Domino's*	1 Slice/91g	302	16.0	332	15.2	26.9	17.6	2.1
Pepperoni Passion, Dominator, Large, Domino's Pizza*	1 Slice/93g	310	16.4	332	15.2	26.9	17.6	2.1
Pepperoni Passion, Medium Classic, Domino's Pizza*	1 Slice/72g	210	8.3	292	16.7	28.7	11.6	2.0
Pepperoni Passion, Personal, Domino's Pizza*	1 Slice/59g	182	7.0	307	17.9	30.8	11.8	1.9
Pepperoni Passion, Stuffed Crust, Large, Domino's*	1 Slice/100g	305	13.0	305	16.9	29.0	13.0	1.9
Pepperoni Passion, Stuffed Crust, Medium, Domino's*	1 Slice/96g	293	12.5	305	16.9	29.0	13.0	1.9
Pepperoni Passion, Thin Crust, Medium, Domino's*	1 Slice/55g	199	10.3	362	19.0	27.5	18.8	2.2
Rustica, Fresh Thin Crust, Large, Domino's Pizza*	1 Slice/57g	164	5.0	287	15.4	35.7	8.8	2.1
Rustica, Fresh Thin Crust, Medium, Domino's Pizza*	1 Slice/50g	144	4.4	287	15.4	35.7	8.8	2.1
Rustica, Fresh Thin Crust, Small, Domino's Pizza*	1 Slice/43g	124	3.8	287	15.4	35.7	8.8	2.1
Scrummy, Classic, Large, Domino's Pizza*	1 Slice/92g	253	11.4	275	17.0	22.8	12.4	1.7

	Measure INFO/WEIGHT	per Measure KCAL	FAT	Nutrition Values per 100g / 100ml KCAL	PROT	CARB	FAT	FIBRE
DOMINO'S PIZZA								
PIZZA								
Scrummy, Classic, Medium, Domino's Pizza*	1 Slice/85g	233	10.5	275	17.0	22.8	12.4	1.7
Scrummy, Classic, Small, Domino's Pizza*	1 Slice/77g	213	9.6	275	17.0	22.8	12.4	1.7
Scrummy, Personal, Domino's Pizza*	1 Slice/69g	198	7.6	288	17.7	28.1	11.1	1.8
Scrummy, Thin Crust, Large, Domino's Pizza*	1 Slice/72g	237	12.9	328	19.1	21.9	17.8	1.9
Scrummy, Thin Crust, Medium, Domino's Pizza*	1 Slice/68g	222	12.0	328	19.1	21.9	17.8	1.9
Tandoori Hot, Classic, Delight, Small, Domino's Pizza*	1 Slice/73g	159	3.6	218	15.0	28.4	4.9	2.4
Tandoori Hot, Classic, Large, Domino's Pizza*	1 Slice/89g	198	5.6	223	13.4	28.1	6.3	2.2
Tandoori Hot, Classic, Medium, Domino's Pizza*	1 Slice/81g	176	5.0	217	13.0	27.2	6.2	2.2
Tandoori Hot, Classic, Small, Domino's Pizza*	1 Slice/73g	162	4.6	222	13.5	27.9	6.3	2.3
Tandoori Hot, Delight, Personal, Domino's Pizza*	1 Slice/62g	135	3.1	218	12.1	31.2	5.0	2.3
Tandoori Hot, Dominator, Large, Domino's Pizza*	1 Slice/112g	280	9.0	250	12.7	31.8	8.0	2.1
Tandoori Hot, Double Decadence, Medium, Domino's*	1 Slice/101g	276	13.0	273	12.4	26.9	12.9	2.3
Tandoori Hot, Personal, Domino's Pizza*	1 Slice/62g	149	3.7	240	14.5	31.9	6.0	2.2
Tandoori Hot, Thin Crust, Large, Domino's Pizza*	1 Slice/69g	177	7.6	257	14.3	24.9	11.1	2.6
Tandoori Hot, Thin Crust, Medium, Domino's Pizza*	1 Slice/64g	173	7.3	270	14.5	27.4	11.4	2.5
Texas BBQ, Classic, Delight, Small, Domino's Pizza*	1 Slice/71g	170	3.9	240	13.0	33.4	5.5	2.2
Texas BBQ, Classic, Large, Domino's Pizza*	1 Slice/87g	240	7.0	276	14.4	36.6	8.0	1.8
Texas BBQ, Classic, Medium, Domino's Pizza*	1 Slice/79g	218	6.3	276	14.4	36.6	8.0	1.8
Texas BBQ, Classic, Small, Domino's Pizza*	1 Slice/71g	196	5.7	276	14.4	36.6	8.0	1.8
Texas BBQ, Delight, Personal, Domino's Pizza*	1 Slice/61g	156	3.4	256	14.2	36.4	5.5	1.9
Texas BBQ, Dominator, Large, Domino's Pizza*	1 Slice/104g	293	9.5	283	12.9	37.3	9.2	1.8
Texas BBQ, Domino's Pizza*	1 Slice/93g	303	12.9	326	13.5	36.6	13.9	1.8
Texas BBQ, Personal, Domino's Pizza*	1 Slice/61g	171	4.0	280	18.4	35.6	6.6	2.5
Texas BBQ, Stuffed Crust, Large, Domino's Pizza*	1 Slice/97g	252	8.8	261	15.3	28.6	9.1	2.0
Texas BBQ, Stuffed Crust, Medium, Domino's Pizza*	1 Slice/90g	234	8.2	261	15.3	28.6	9.1	2.0
Texas BBQ, Thin Crust, Large, Domino's Pizza*	1 Slice/63g	183	7.3	289	15.3	30.8	11.6	1.7
Texas BBQ, Thin Crust, Medium, Domino's Pizza*	1 Slice/59g	206	8.0	351	15.6	40.3	13.7	2.1
The Sizzler, Classic, Large, Domino's Pizza*	1 Slice/95g	271	10.6	285	14.7	31.5	11.2	2.2
The Sizzler, Classic, Medium, Domino's Pizza*	1 Slice/87g	248	9.7	285	14.7	31.5	11.2	2.2
The Sizzler, Classic, Small, Domino's Pizza*	1 Slice/78g	222	8.7	285	14.7	31.5	11.2	2.2
The Sizzler, Dominator, Large, Domino's Pizza*	1 Slice/118g	346	13.5	293	13.7	34.1	11.4	2.1
The Sizzler, Double Decadence, Medium, Domino's*	1 Slice/106g	334	17.0	315	13.5	29.3	16.0	2.3
The Sizzler, Personal, Domino's Pizza*	1 Slice/65g	177	5.7	271	15.6	32.6	8.7	2.4
The Sizzler, Thin Crust, Large, Domino's Pizza*	1 Slice/75g	227	10.9	303	14.7	28.4	14.5	2.2
The Sizzler, Thin Crust, Medium, Domino's Pizza*	1 Slice/70g	243	12.0	347	16.1	32.1	17.1	2.4
Tuna Delight, Classic, Large, Domino's Pizza*	1 Slice/85g	203	5.9	238	13.1	29.6	6.9	2.2
Tuna Delight, Classic, Medium, Domino's Pizza*	1 Slice/77g	184	5.3	238	13.1	29.6	6.9	2.2
Tuna Delight, Classic, Small, Domino's Pizza*	1 Slice/69g	164	4.8	238	13.1	29.6	6.9	2.2
Tuna Delight, Personal, Domino's Pizza*	1 Slice/60g	155	3.9	259	14.5	34.1	6.6	2.2
Tuna Delight, Thin Crust, Large, Domino's Pizza*	1 Slice/65g	197	8.3	301	14.7	30.5	12.7	2.6
Tuna Delight, Thin Crust, Medium, Domino's Pizza*	1 Slice/60g	181	7.6	301	14.7	30.5	12.7	2.6
Veg-A-Roma, Classic, Delight, Small, Domino's Pizza*	1 Slice/70g	153	4.7	219	10.4	29.3	6.7	2.4
Veg-A-Roma, Classic, Large, Domino's Pizza*	1 Slice/86g	240	8.9	279	12.3	34.3	10.4	2.4
Veg-A-Roma, Classic, Medium, Domino's Pizza*	1 Slice/78g	218	8.1	279	12.3	34.3	10.4	2.4
Veg-A-Roma, Classic, Small, Domino's Pizza*	1 Slice/70g	195	7.3	279	12.3	34.3	10.4	2.4
Veg-A-Roma, Delight, Personal, Domino's Pizza*	1 Slice/61g	143	4.1	237	11.2	33.2	6.7	2.0
Veg-A-Roma, Personal, Domino's Pizza*	1 Slice/60g	160	4.8	265	13.7	34.7	8.0	2.5
Veg-A-Roma, Thin Crust, Large, Domino's Pizza*	1 Slice/66g	180	7.8	273	12.5	29.2	11.8	2.8
Veg-A-Roma, Thin Crust, Medium, Domino's Pizza*	1 Slice/61g	167	7.2	273	12.5	29.2	11.8	2.8
Vegetarian Supreme, Classic, Delight, Lge, Domino's*	1 Slice/88g	188	4.3	214	13.1	29.5	4.9	2.5
Vegetarian Supreme, Classic, Large, Domino's Pizza*	1 Slice/88g	192	5.5	218	11.5	29.1	6.3	2.3
Vegetarian Supreme, Classic, Medium, Domino's Pizza*	1 Slice/80g	170	4.9	213	11.0	28.3	6.1	2.3

	Measure INFO/WEIGHT	per Measure KCAL	FAT	Nutrition Values per 100g / 100ml KCAL	PROT	CARB	FAT	FIBRE
DOMINO'S PIZZA								
PIZZA								
Vegetarian Supreme, Classic, Small, Domino's Pizza*	1 Slice/72g	156	4.5	217	11.5	28.9	6.2	2.3
Vegetarian Supreme, Dbl Decadence, Med, Domino's*	1 Slice/99g	267	12.9	270	10.8	27.7	13.0	2.4
Vegetarian Supreme, Delight, Classic, Med, Domino's*	1 Slice/80g	171	3.9	214	13.1	29.5	4.9	2.5
Vegetarian Supreme, Delight, Classic, Small, Domino's*	1 Slice/72g	154	3.5	214	13.1	29.5	4.9	2.5
Vegetarian Supreme, Delight, Personal, Domino's Pizza*	1 Slice/61g	131	3.1	214	10.3	32.2	5.0	2.4
Vegetarian Supreme, Dominator, Large, Domino's*	1 Slice/111g	274	8.9	247	11.2	32.6	8.0	2.2
Vegetarian Supreme, Personal, Domino's Pizza*	1 Slice/61g	144	3.7	236	12.7	32.8	6.0	2.2
Vegetarian Supreme, Stuffed Crust, Large, Domino's*	1 Slice/93g	223	7.3	240	11.9	29.3	7.9	2.2
Vegetarian Supreme, Stuffed Crust, Medium, Domino's*	1 Slice/86g	206	6.8	240	11.9	29.3	7.9	2.2
Vegetarian Supreme, Thin Crust, Large, Domino's*	1 Slice/68g	171	7.5	252	11.8	26.1	11.1	2.7
Vegetarian Supreme, Thin Crust, Medium, Domino's*	1 Slice/63g	168	7.3	266	12.0	28.7	11.5	2.6
Vegi Lite, Classic, Large, Domino's Pizza*	1 Slice/80g	177	5.1	220	11.4	28.2	6.3	2.3
Vegi Lite, Classic, Medium, Domino's Pizza*	1 Slice/73g	160	4.6	220	11.4	28.2	6.3	2.3
Vegi Lite, Classic, Small, Domino's Pizza*	1 Slice/65g	143	4.1	220	11.4	28.2	6.3	2.3
Vegi Lite, Personal, Domino's Pizza*	1 Slice/56g	137	3.4	243	13.0	32.8	6.1	2.3
Vegi Lite, Thin Crust, Large, Domino's Pizza*	1 Slice/62g	171	7.3	277	12.5	28.6	11.9	2.7
Vegi Lite, Thin Crust, Medium, Domino's Pizza*	1 Slice/57g	157	6.7	277	12.5	28.6	11.9	2.7
Vegi Volcano, Classic, Large, Domino's Pizza*	1 Slice/91g	202	6.7	222	12.2	26.5	7.4	2.2
Vegi Volcano, Classic, Medium, Domino's Pizza*	1 Slice/83g	184	6.1	222	12.2	26.5	7.4	2.2
Vegi Volcano, Classic, Small, Domino's Pizza*	1 Slice/75g	167	5.6	222	12.2	26.5	7.4	2.2
Vegi Volcano, Delight, Classic, Small, Domino's Pizza*	1 Slice/75g	167	4.6	223	14.2	27.7	6.2	2.4
Vegi Volcano, Delight, Personal, Domino's Pizza*	1 Slice/64g	141	3.9	222	11.3	30.4	6.1	2.3
Vegi Volcano, Dominator, Large, Domino's Pizza*	1 Slice/114g	288	10.2	253	12.1	31.1	9.0	2.1
Vegi Volcano, Double Decadence, Medium, Domino's*	1 Slice/102g	282	14.0	276	11.7	26.3	13.7	2.3
Vegi Volcano, Personal, Domino's Pizza*	1 Slice/63g	154	4.5	243	13.7	31.0	7.1	2.2
Vegi Volcano, Thin Crust, Large, Domino's Pizza*	1 Slice/72g	189	9.0	262	13.3	23.9	12.5	2.6
Vegi Volcano, Thin Crust, Medium, Domino's Pizza*	1 Slice/66g	182	8.5	275	13.5	26.5	12.8	2.5
EAT								
BAGEL								
BLT, EAT*	1 Bagel/222g	567	20.5	255	14.7	28.8	9.2	1.8
Cheese & Chilli Jam, EAT*	1 Bagel/224g	583	21.1	260	11.1	33.5	9.4	1.8
Egg, Free Range & Chorizo, EAT*	1 Bagel/240g	561	24.0	234	10.7	25.9	10.0	1.6
Pastrami, New York, EAT*	1 Bagel/217g	468	11.7	216	13.6	29.1	5.4	1.5
Salmon, Smoked Scottish & Soft Cheese, EAT*	1 Bagel/199g	444	10.8	223	13.0	31.2	5.4	1.7
BAGUETTE								
Beef & Rocket, EAT*	1 Baguette/228g	556	18.2	244	13.2	29.2	8.0	1.8
Brie, Tomato & Basil, EAT*	1 Baguette/191g	455	17.2	238	9.2	29.1	9.0	1.9
Cheddar, Mature, & Sweet Chilli Jam, Eat*	1 Baguette/201g	577	25.1	287	10.4	33.1	12.5	1.7
Chicken, Bacon & Avocado, EAT*	1 Baguette/252g	552	19.9	219	13.2	23.8	7.9	1.9
Chicken, Thai, EAT*	1 Baguette/201g	432	12.3	215	11.9	28.4	6.1	1.8
Chicken Banh Mi, EAT*	1 Pack/282g	454	8.2	161	9.0	24.0	2.9	1.6
Egg & Bacon, Half, EAT*	1 Serving/112g	311	12.2	278	13.5	30.5	10.9	1.8
Egg & Tomato, EAT*	1 Serving/140g	304	12.2	217	9.0	24.8	8.7	1.7
Ham & Jarlsberg, EAT*	1 Pack/218g	566	23.3	260	15.4	24.9	10.7	1.4
Ham & Tomato, EAT*	1 Baguette/245g	422	10.3	172	9.6	23.2	4.2	1.6
Ham Brie & Cranberry, EAT*	1 Baguette/245g	583	25.1	239	11.0	25.8	10.3	1.4
Salmon, Smoked, & Soft Cheese, Half, EAT*	1 Pack/93g	218	6.7	235	11.0	30.2	7.2	1.7
Sticky BBQ Banh Mi, EAT*	1 Roll/269g	473	2.4	176	7.9	33.1	0.9	1.8
The Big Salami, EAT*	1 Baguette/254g	569	26.9	224	9.2	22.5	10.6	1.5
Tuna & Cucumber, EAT*	1 Baguette/208g	511	22.7	245	10.9	25.0	10.9	1.5
BREAD								
Brown, Chunk of Freshly Baked, EAT*	1 Serving/67g	141	1.3	211	7.4	44.0	1.9	2.7

	Measure INFO/WEIGHT	per Measure KCAL	FAT	Nutrition Values per 100g / 100ml KCAL	PROT	CARB	FAT	FIBRE
EAT								
BREAD								
Brown Roll, for Soup, EAT*	1 Roll/69g	187	3.5	271	8.5	47.4	5.1	2.0
Rye, Wheat Free Seeded, EAT*	1 Serving/144g	331	6.0	230	6.7	48.0	4.2	6.7
White, Chunk of Freshly Baked, EAT*	1 Serving/67g	162	2.9	242	7.3	46.4	4.3	1.9
White, Roll, for Soup, EAT*	1 Roll/69g	185	3.3	268	8.3	47.1	4.8	1.7
BREAKFAST CEREAL								
Bircher, Mango & Passionfruit, EAT*	1 Pot/225g	336	9.2	149	3.1	25.2	4.1	2.2
Granola, & Full Fat Milk, EAT*	1 Serving/230g	476	17.7	207	5.7	29.9	7.7	4.1
Granola, & Full Fat Milk, with Chocolate Syrup, EAT*	1 Serving/239g	509	18.4	213	5.7	31.2	7.7	4.4
Granola, & Skimmed Milk, EAT*	1 Serving/230g	435	13.3	189	5.7	30.0	5.8	4.1
Granola, & Skimmed Milk, with Chocolate Syrup, EAT*	1 Serving/239g	466	13.9	195	5.7	31.4	5.8	4.4
Granola, & Soya Milk, EAT*	1 Serving/230g	435	15.9	189	5.8	27.3	6.9	4.5
Granola, & Soya Milk, with Chocolate Syrup, EAT*	1 Serving/239g	468	16.7	196	5.9	28.7	7.0	4.7
Grapenuts, Banana & Honey, EAT*	1 Serving/228g	349	6.4	153	6.3	25.4	2.8	1.5
Muesli, Apple, Almond & Cinnamon, Bircher, EAT*	1 Serving/210g	361	12.2	172	6.1	23.3	5.8	2.3
Muesli, Swiss, Bircher, EAT*	1 Serving/205g	246	3.1	120	4.7	21.7	1.5	2.0
Porridge, Plain, Big, EAT*	1 Serving/280g	213	3.1	76	4.4	11.9	1.1	1.1
Porridge, Plain, Small, EAT*	1 Serving/180g	137	2.0	76	4.4	11.9	1.1	1.2
Porridge, Plain, Super, Small, EAT*	1 Serving/219g	136	3.5	62	2.4	9.0	1.6	1.8
Porridge, with Apple & Blackberry, Compote, Big, EAT*	1 Serving/331g	291	3.6	88	3.9	16.0	1.1	1.5
Porridge, with Banana, & Maple Syrup, Big, EAT*	1 Serving/315g	308	6.9	98	4.0	15.1	2.2	1.2
Porridge, with Banana, & Maple Syrup, Small, EAT*	1 Serving194g	177	1.9	91	4.1	16.0	1.0	1.0
Porridge, with Banana, & Maple Syrup, Super, Big, EAT*	1 Serving/364g	266	5.5	73	2.2	12.0	1.5	1.8
Porridge, with Banana, Big, EAT*	1 Serving/300g	234	0.9	78	4.1	12.8	0.3	1.2
Porridge, with Banana, Small, EAT*	1 Serving/200g	162	2.2	81	4.0	13.5	1.1	1.3
Porridge, with Banana, Super, Big, EAT*	1 Serving/350g	224	5.2	64	2.3	9.8	1.5	1.8
Porridge, with Banana, Super, Small, EAT*	1 Serving/240g	156	3.6	65	2.3	10.1	1.5	1.9
Porridge, with Berry Compote, Small, EAT*	1 Serving/230g	196	2.1	85	3.6	15.3	0.9	1.1
Porridge, with Berry Compote, Super, Big, EAT*	1 Serving/330g	284	3.3	86	3.8	15.5	1.0	1.2
Porridge, with Berry Compote, Super, Small, EAT*	1 Serving/30g	205	2.3	89	3.6	16.4	1.0	1.2
Porridge, with Maple Syrup, Big, EAT*	1 Serving/294g	253	3.2	86	4.2	14.6	1.1	1.0
Porridge, with Maple Syrup, Small, EAT*	1 Serving/195g	185	2.1	95	4.1	17.3	1.1	1.1
Porridge, with Maple Syrup, Super, EAT*	1 Serving/344g	244	5.5	71	2.3	11.4	1.6	1.7
Porridge, with Maple Syrup, Super, Small, EAT*	1 Serving/235g	176	3.5	75	2.3	12.6	1.5	1.7
BROWNIE								
Chocolate, Belgian, EAT*	1 Serving/73g	330	20.0	452	5.1	46.2	27.4	1.0
CAKE								
Banana Toffee & Pecan, EAT*	1 Serving/79g	247	10.8	313	3.3	45.1	13.7	0.9
Carrot, EAT*	1 Serving/100g	319	20.0	319	2.8	33.1	20.0	1.6
Chocolate, EAT*	1 Serving/63g	236	13.0	374	4.1	43.8	20.6	1.5
Lemon Drizzle, EAT*	1 Serving/70g	232	10.8	332	3.5	44.8	15.5	0.8
Millionares, EAT*	1 Cake/85g	396	21.2	466	3.5	57.6	25.0	0.8
Red Velvet, EAT*	1 Pack/128g	500	24.3	391	4.7	50.0	19.0	0.9
Victoria Sponge, EAT*	1 Serving/72g	166	7.9	230	2.5	30.5	10.9	0.6
CHEESECAKE								
Lemon, EAT*	1 Serving/114g	446	34.7	391	2.9	25.7	30.4	0.4
COFFEE								
Cappuccino, Skimmed Milk, EAT*	1 Tall/12oz	118	4.0	33	2.4	3.4	1.1	0.0
Cappuccino, Soya Milk, EAT*	1 Tall/12oz	131	4.9	37	3.2	3.5	1.4	0.9
Cappuccino, Whole Milk, Big, EAT*	1 Big/474ml	159	8.4	34	2.3	2.3	1.8	0.0
Cappuccino, Whole Milk, Small, EAT*	1 Tall/12oz	130	6.5	37	2.6	2.4	1.8	0.0
Espresso, Macchiato, Skimmed Milk, EAT*	1 Espresso/4oz	8	0.3	7	0.5	0.6	0.3	0.0
Espresso, Macchiato, Soya Milk, EAT*	1 Espresso/4oz	9	0.4	8	0.6	0.7	0.3	0.2

	Measure INFO/WEIGHT	per Measure KCAL	FAT	Nutrition Values per 100g / 100ml KCAL	PROT	CARB	FAT	FIBRE
EAT								
COFFEE								
Espresso, Macchiato, Whole Milk, Double, EAT*	1 Double/8oz	20	0.4	8	1.4	0.4	0.2	0.0
Espresso, Macchiato, Whole Milk, Single, EAT*	1 Single/4oz	13	0.3	11	1.5	0.6	0.2	0.0
Latte, Chai, Skimmed Milk, EAT*	1 Tall/12oz	305	1.0	86	3.2	17.7	0.3	0.0
Latte, Chai, Soya Milk, EAT*	1 Tall/12oz	279	5.3	79	2.4	13.9	1.5	0.5
Latte, Chai, Whole Milk, Big, EAT*	1 Big/16oz	332	12.8	70	2.7	9.0	2.7	0.0
Latte, Chai, Whole Milk, Small, EAT*	1 Small/12oz	262	10.2	74	2.9	9.3	2.9	0.0
Latte, Chiller, Skimmed Milk, EAT*	1 Tall/12oz	241	3.3	68	3.1	11.9	0.9	0.0
Latte, Chiller, Whole Milk, EAT*	1 Tall/12oz	412	14.8	116	1.8	17.8	4.2	0.2
Latte, Iced, Skimmed Milk, EAT*	1 Tall/12oz	95	3.2	27	1.9	2.7	0.9	0.0
Latte, Iced, Soya Milk, EAT*	1 Tall/12oz	105	3.9	30	2.5	2.8	1.1	0.7
Latte, Matcha, Skimmed Milk, EAT*	1 Tall/12oz	204	1.0	57	3.0	10.6	0.3	0.3
Latte, Matcha, Soya Milk, EAT*	1 Tall/12oz	201	5.8	57	3.0	7.4	1.6	0.3
Latte, Matcha, Whole Milk, EAT*	1 Tall/12oz	297	11.8	84	3.0	10.4	3.3	0.3
Latte, Skimmed Milk, EAT*	1 Small/12oz	99	3.4	42	3.0	4.2	1.4	0.0
Latte, Soya Milk, EAT*	1 Tall/12oz	157	5.9	46	4.0	4.3	1.7	1.1
Latte, Whole Milk, Big, EAT*	1 Big/16oz	224	11.6	47	3.1	3.2	2.4	0.0
Latte, Whole Milk, Small, EAT*	1 Small/12oz	173	9.0	49	3.3	3.2	2.5	0.0
Matcha, Chiller, Whole Milk, EAT*	1 Tall/12oz	418	14.9	118	1.9	18.2	4.2	0.3
Mocha, Chiller, Skimmed Milk, EAT*	1 Tall/12oz	243	3.4	68	2.5	12.6	1.0	0.0
Mocha, Chiller, Whole Milk, EAT*	1 Tall/12oz	283	7.5	80	2.5	12.6	2.1	0.0
Mocha, Skimmed Milk, EAT*	1 Tall/12oz	157	5.0	44	3.0	4.8	1.4	0.0
Mocha, Soya Milk, EAT*	1 Tall/12oz	173	6.1	49	4.0	5.0	1.7	1.2
Mocha, Whole Milk, EAT*	1 Tall/12oz	219	11.4	62	3.0	4.8	3.2	0.0
White, Flat, Skimmed Milk, EAT*	1 Tall/341ml	87	0.3	26	2.6	3.7	0.1	0.0
White, Flat, Soya Milk, EAT*	1 Tall/341ml	147	4.8	43	5.1	2.3	1.4	0.4
COOKIES								
Chocolate, EAT*	1 Serving/90g	401	16.8	446	6.6	61.4	18.7	2.7
Muesli, EAT*	1 Serving/90g	376	13.4	418	5.7	63.5	14.9	3.6
CROISSANT								
Almond, EAT*	1 Serving/83g	350	19.8	422	10.0	41.7	23.9	2.9
Chocolate, EAT*	1 Serving/81g	361	21.3	445	6.9	45.4	26.2	3.0
EAT*	1 Serving/71g	305	17.1	427	9.4	43.4	23.9	2.7
Egg, Cheese & Tomato, EAT*	1 Pack/149g	434	25.1	291	9.0	20.8	16.8	1.6
Egg & Bacon, EAT*	1 Pack/138g	497	31.8	361	13.2	24.8	23.1	1.7
Ham & Jarlsberg Croissant, EAT*	1 Serving/128g	339	21.1	265	15.6	20.8	16.5	0.0
Tomato & Jarlsberg, EAT*	1 Serving/123g	291	19.1	236	9.0	22.6	15.5	0.4
DANISH PASTRY								
Maple Pecan, Plait, EAT*	1 Serving/83g	377	26.0	454	4.7	38.4	31.3	5.2
FROZEN YOGHURT								
Brownie Sundae, EAT*	1 Serving/176g	308	6.0	175	3.6	34.1	3.4	2.0
Plain, EAT*	1 Serving/140g	169	0.3	121	3.5	29.0	0.2	2.0
with Fresh Berries, EAT*	1 Serving/200g	190	0.4	95	2.7	22.0	0.2	2.5
FRUIT SALAD								
Big, EAT*	1 Serving/279g	120	0.3	43	0.6	10.9	0.1	1.8
HOT CHOCOLATE								
Whole Milk, Big, EAT*	1 Big/16oz	380	15.6	80	3.1	9.7	3.3	1.2
HOT POT								
Chicken, Mexican, EAT*	1 Pot/315g	476	24.6	151	11.8	11.0	7.8	0.6
Chilli, Texan, EAT*	1 Pack/378g	386	9.5	102	5.8	13.6	2.5	1.9
Curry, Chicken, Burmese, EAT*	1 Bowl/385g	462	18.5	120	5.4	12.3	4.8	1.2
Curry, Chicken, Thai Green, EAT*	1 Pack/386g	491	22.0	127	5.9	11.3	5.7	0.9
Pork, BBQ, Pulled, EAT*	1 Pack/340g	510	15.0	150	9.7	17.3	4.4	0.8

	Measure INFO/WEIGHT	per Measure KCAL	per Measure FAT	KCAL	PROT	CARB	FAT	FIBRE
				Nutrition Values per 100g / 100ml				
EAT								
HOT POT								
Sausage, Cumberland, Mash & Onion Gravy, EAT*	1 Pack/470g	658	40.4	140	4.8	10.1	8.6	1.2
Sweet Potato, & Spinach Dal, EAT*	1 Pot/380g	380	6.1	100	3.6	17.0	1.6	1.8
JUICE DRINK								
Mango & Lime, Blast, EAT*	1 Tall/12oz	253	0.3	71	0.3	17.7	0.1	0.1
Peach & Mint, Blast, EAT*	1 Tall/12oz	216	0.2	61	0.2	15.1	0.1	0.0
Wild Berry, Blast, EAT*	1 Tall/12oz	330	0.2	93	0.2	23.5	0.1	0.5
MUFFIN								
Bacon Butty, Hot Toasted, EAT*	1 Serving/90g	291	10.9	324	17.1	36.1	12.1	0.8
Bacon Butty, Hot Toasted, Large, EAT*	1 Serving/190g	589	18.4	310	15.4	39.7	9.7	0.9
Blueberry, Low Fat, EAT*	1 Muffin/119g	383	13.4	322	5.8	47.9	11.3	2.5
Chocolate, Belgian, EAT*	1 Muffin/124g	511	26.4	412	5.0	48.9	21.3	2.1
Egg, Mushroom & Cheddar, Hot Toasted, EAT*	1 Serving/125g	240	6.9	192	9.1	26.2	5.5	1.0
Eggs Benedict, Hot Toasted, EAT*	1 Serving/120g	265	8.9	220	10.2	27.6	7.4	0.8
Fruit & Bran, EAT*	1 Muffin/124g	498	25.1	402	5.7	47.2	20.3	3.8
Full English Breakfast, EAT*	1 Serving/295g	687	24.5	233	10.7	28.4	8.3	0.7
Salmon, Smoked, & Egg, Hot Toasted, EAT*	1 Serving/126g	325	10.0	258	11.8	37.1	7.9	1.5
Sunshine, EAT*	1 Serving/124g	498	25.1	402	5.7	47.2	20.3	3.8
OLIVES								
Chilli & Herb, EAT*	1 Serving/75g	99	10.1	132	0.8	1.8	13.5	3.5
PAIN AU CHOCOLAT								
EAT*	1 Serving/78g	329	18.4	422	9.8	42.6	23.6	3.6
PANCAKE								
American Buttermilk, with Maple, EAT*	1 Serving/100g	239	2.2	238	3.6	55.5	2.2	1.0
American Buttermilk, with Maple & Bacon, EAT*	1 Serving/106g	292	4.9	275	8.5	50.0	4.6	0.8
American Buttermilk, with Maple & Banana, EAT*	1 Serving/113g	260	2.1	231	3.2	50.0	1.9	1.2
PEAS								
Wasabi, EAT*	1 Serving/38g	158	4.6	416	20.0	57.0	12.0	7.0
PIE								
Beef & Stilton, Pie Only, EAT*	1 Pie/270g	629	31.6	233	10.2	21.1	11.7	1.6
Beef & Stilton, with Mash & Gravy, EAT*	1 Pie/560g	885	40.3	158	5.9	15.9	7.2	1.9
Cheese & Onion, Pie Only, EAT*	1 Pie/270g	856	58.9	317	8.5	21.5	21.8	1.8
Cheese & Onion, with Mash & Gravy, EAT*	1 Pie/560g	1098	67.8	196	4.9	16.2	12.1	1.9
Chicken & Mushroom, with Mash & Gravy, EAT*	1 Pie/540g	929	47.0	172	6.1	16.5	8.7	1.7
Chicken & Mushroom Pie Only, EAT*	1 Pie/250g	685	37.8	274	11.3	22.6	15.1	1.4
Goats Cheese & Sweet Potato, Pie Only, EAT*	1 Pie/270g	694	36.7	257	6.6	26.2	13.6	1.9
Steak & Ale, Pie Only, EAT*	1 Pie/250g	670	37.8	268	10.4	22.1	15.1	1.5
Steak & Ale, with Mash & Gravy, EAT*	1 Pie/540g	913	47.0	169	5.7	16.3	8.7	1.7
SALAD								
Chicken, Simple, with Dressing, EAT*	1 Pack/366g	501	32.2	137	6.0	7.9	8.8	1.1
Chicken, Simple, without Dressing, EAT*	1 Pack/345g	376	19.0	109	6.4	7.8	5.5	1.2
Ham Hock & Egg, with Dressing, EAT*	1 Serving/166g	227	15.6	137	9.7	2.7	9.4	1.0
Ham Hock & Egg, without Dressing, EAT*	1 Serving/148g	142	7.1	96	10.7	1.9	4.8	1.1
Houmous & Falafel Mezze, without Dressing, EAT*	1 Box/353g	395	16.9	112	3.2	12.8	4.8	4.6
Houmous Detox Box, with Dressing, EAT*	1 Pack/254g	478	40.9	188	3.1	7.4	16.1	3.3
Houmous Detox Box, without Dressing, EAT*	1 Pack/262g	414	33.3	158	3.3	7.5	12.7	3.6
Mexican Bean Pot, Less Than 5% Fat, Vegetarian, EAT*	1 Salad/172g	192	4.0	111	5.2	17.1	2.3	4.1
Mezze, with Dressing, EAT*	1 Serving/306g	425	26.6	139	3.6	12.0	8.7	2.7
Mezze, without Dressing, EAT*	1 Serving/286g	349	20.3	122	3.8	11.0	7.1	2.9
Noodles, Chicken, Spicy, Less Than 5% Fat, EAT*	1 Serving/325g	419	9.1	129	8.9	16.8	2.8	1.6
Omega Booster, Salmon Box, with Dressing, EAT*	1 Pack/194g	392	34.9	202	6.6	2.3	18.0	1.9
Omega Booster, Salmon Box, without Dressing, EAT*	1 Pack/173g	281	23.6	162	7.4	1.3	13.6	2.1
Pea & Mint Pot, No Dressing, EAT*	1 Salad/106g	98	2.6	92	6.8	7.4	2.4	3.0

	Measure INFO/WEIGHT	per Measure KCAL	FAT	Nutrition Values per 100g / 100ml KCAL	PROT	CARB	FAT	FIBRE
EAT								
SALAD								
Pea & Mint Pot with Dressing, EAT*	1 Salad/125g	171	9.8	136	5.9	7.5	7.8	2.7
Prawn Cocktail Pot, EAT*	1 Salad/129g	218	17.2	169	9.9	2.1	13.3	0.6
Slaw, Vietnamese, Side, with Dressing, EAT*	1 Pack/156g	150	9.1	96	3.0	7.2	5.8	2.2
Slaw, Vietnamese, Side, without Dressing, EAT*	1 Pack/137g	81	2.9	59	2.4	7.4	2.1	2.3
Tuna, Simple, with Dressing, EAT*	1 Pack/322g	316	17.7	98	6.9	4.6	5.5	0.8
Tuna, Simple, without Dressing, EAT*	1 Pack/292g	193	5.8	66	7.4	4.3	2.0	0.9
SALADS								
Chicken Tandoori, Mango & Rice with dressing, EAT*	1 Serving/206g	251	5.6	122	8.3	15.6	2.7	1.6
Crayfish Noodles, Spicy, Less Than 5% Fat, EAT*	1 Serving/285g	348	8.0	122	6.6	18.2	2.8	1.6
Ham, Summer, & Potato, with dressing, EAT*	1 Serving/331g	480	36.7	145	6.0	4.9	11.1	0.8
Ham, Summer, & Potato, without dressing, EAT*	1 Serving/303g	370	26.4	122	6.4	4.3	8.7	0.9
Prawn Cocktail, Salad, EAT*	1 Serving/166g	345	29.4	208	9.4	2.4	17.7	0.7
Rainbow Superfood, with dressing, EAT*	1 Serving/340g	520	24.8	153	5.4	15.2	7.3	2.6
Rainbow Superfood, without Dressing, EAT*	1 Serving/340g	439	16.0	129	5.9	14.2	4.7	2.8
SANDWICH								
Bacon, Lettuce & Tomato, EAT*	1 Pack/204g	479	25.1	235	11.1	19.9	12.3	1.7
Bacon Butty, EAT*	1 Butty/170g	600	15.5	353	17.8	53.3	9.1	2.2
Bacon Butty, Small, EAT*	1 Butty/93g	330	9.2	355	18.6	51.0	9.9	2.2
Chicken, & Bacon, Very Small EAT*	1 Pack/114g	241	11.5	211	12.2	17.7	10.1	1.6
Chicken, Avocado & Basil, EAT*	1 Pack/233g	452	24.0	194	10.3	17.9	10.3	2.7
Chicken, Firecracker, Toastie, EAT*	1 Pack/252g	433	10.8	172	11.2	21.0	4.3	1.7
Chicken, Roast, Pork, Sage & Onion, Bloomer, EAT*	1 Pack/238g	569	25.9	239	11.8	24.7	10.9	1.8
Chicken, Smoked, & Basil, Toastie, EAT*	1 Pack/240g	550	24.7	229	12.1	22.3	10.3	1.2
Chicken, Smoked, Tomato & Pesto Bloomer, EAT*	1 Pack/244g	454	15.4	186	12.4	20.4	6.3	2.2
Chicken & Bacon, EAT*	1 Pack/229g	472	21.5	206	12.3	18.0	9.4	1.6
Chicken & Chipotle Salsa, Toastie, EAT*	1 Pack/284g	486	11.4	171	10.6	23.3	4.0	1.7
Chicken & Chorizo, EAT*	1 Pack/209g	416	17.4	199	12.3	19.7	8.3	1.7
Club, EAT*	1 Pack/296g	624	28.7	211	12.9	17.7	9.7	1.3
Crayfish, Lemon & Rocket, EAT*	1 Pack/188g	333	13.9	177	9.5	20.9	7.4	1.6
Crayfish, Lemon & Rocket, Very Small, EAT*	1 Pack/99g	174	6.8	176	9.4	19.9	6.9	1.4
Egg, Free Range & Roast Tomato, Bloomer, EAT*	1 Pack/215g	525	25.6	244	11.1	23.4	11.9	2.8
Egg Mayo, Free Range, & Tomato, Bloomer, EAT*	1 Pack/262g	627	38.8	239	7.3	19.1	14.8	1.5
Egg Mayonnaise, Free Range & Cress, Simple, EAT*	1 Pack/183g	410	20.9	224	8.7	21.6	11.4	1.8
Ham, & Cheese, Simply, Toastie, EAT*	1 Pack/240g	588	31.2	245	11.8	21.4	13.0	1.0
Ham, & Free Range Egg, Bloomer, EAT*	1 Pack/246g	573	28.5	233	13.0	19.4	11.6	2.0
Ham, Cheddar & Piccalilli, EAT*	1 Pack/246g	448	17.7	182	11.2	19.1	7.2	1.4
Ham, Simple, Kids, EAT*	1 Pack/121g	318	13.4	263	10.8	30.4	11.1	2.2
Ham, Tomato & Mustard, EAT*	1 Pack/203g	394	17.5	194	9.8	19.3	8.6	1.6
Houmous, Avocado & Harissa, EAT*	1 Pack/213g	396	15.1	186	6.1	25.2	7.1	3.8
Mozzarella, Tomato & Pesto, Toastie, EAT*	1 Pack/249g	545	26.9	219	9.6	20.8	10.8	1.2
Pastrami, New York, Bloomer, EAT*	1 Pack/240g	513	20.7	213	11.3	22.3	8.6	0.3
Pastrami, New York, EAT*	1 Pack/224g	358	11.4	160	9.9	18.6	5.1	1.3
Pork, Pulled, Brioche Bun, EAT*	1 Pack/235g	456	12.5	194	12.7	24.6	5.3	0.8
Salad, Cheddar, Mature, Simple, EAT*	1 Pack/188g	405	18.8	215	9.4	21.7	10.0	1.8
Salad, Chicken, Simple, less than 5% fat, EAT*	1 Pack/203g	327	9.7	161	10.1	19.3	4.8	1.9
Salmon, Smoked, Egg & Watercress, EAT*	1 Pack/211g	477	25.3	226	10.8	18.7	12.0	1.6
Salmon, Smoked, Scottish, & Soft Cheese, EAT*	1 Pack/165g	380	16.5	230	12.1	22.9	10.0	1.6
Steak & Cheese Melt,Toastie, EAT*	1 Pack/265g	552	24.9	208	10.8	21.2	9.4	1.3
The Hot Cubano, Toastie, EAT*	1 Pack/270g	521	22.4	193	10.8	20.0	8.3	0.9
Tuna, & Cheddar Melt, Toastie, EAT*	1 Pack/255g	594	28.6	233	13.9	20.7	11.2	1.0
Tuna, & Mayo, Simple, Kids, EAT*	1 Pack/138g	371	17.0	269	12.4	27.4	12.3	1.9
Tuna, & Rocket, EAT*	1 Pack/250g	577	29.9	230	11.1	19.8	11.9	2.3

	Measure INFO/WEIGHT	per Measure KCAL	FAT	Nutrition Values per 100g / 100ml KCAL	PROT	CARB	FAT	FIBRE
EAT								
SANDWICH								
Tuna, Skipjack, & Cucumber less than 5% fat, EAT*	1 Pack/187g	305	7.1	163	10.8	21.3	3.8	1.7
Tuna, Skipjack, Mayonnaise & Cucumber, Simple, EAT*	1 Pack/199g	338	11.1	170	9.6	20.1	5.6	1.6
Turkey, & Cranberry, Less Than 5% Fat, EAT*	1 Pack/223g	381	10.0	171	11.8	22.2	4.5	1.5
Turkey & Cranberry, Less Than 5% Fat, V Small, EAT*	1 Pack/109g	184	4.4	169	11.1	22.4	4.0	1.5
SLICES								
Cheese Twist, EAT*	1 Serving/74g	313	19.0	421	14.0	33.7	25.6	2.2
Cinnamon Swirl, EAT*	1 Serving/77g	360	24.5	470	5.1	40.4	32.0	4.4
Coconut & Raspberry, EAT*	1 Slice/75g	306	17.6	408	5.9	44.1	23.4	4.5
Oat & Fruit, EAT*	1 Serving/73g	292	11.7	400	4.1	61.2	16.0	3.3
SOUP								
Bacon & Lentil, Smokey, Small, Simple, EAT*	1 Small/300ml	249	3.9	83	5.9	11.4	1.3	1.2
Beef & Barley, with Garnish, Big, Bold, EAT*	1 Pack/400g	249	6.4	62	4.2	6.6	1.6	2.1
Beef & Barley, with Garnish, Small, Bold, EAT*	1 Pack/300g	187	4.8	62	4.2	6.6	1.6	2.1
Beef & Barley, with Garnish, Very Big, Bold, EAT*	1 Pack/600g	373	9.6	62	4.2	6.6	1.6	2.1
Beef & Barley, without Garnish, Big, Bold, EAT*	1 Pack/400g	248	6.4	62	4.2	6.6	1.6	2.1
Beef & Barley, without Garnish, Small, Bold, EAT*	1 Pack/300g	186	4.8	62	260.0	6.6	1.6	2.1
Beef & Barley, without Garnish, Very Big, Bold, EAT*	1 Pack/600g	372	9.6	62	4.2	6.6	1.6	2.1
Beef Rendang, Malaysian, with Garnish, Small, EAT*	1 Small/302g	263	12.7	87	4.2	7.5	4.2	1.1
Beef Rendang, Malaysian, without Garnish, Small, EAT*	1 Small/300g	261	12.6	87	4.2	7.5	4.2	1.1
Butternut Squash, Thai, Simple, EAT*	1 Small/300ml	168	6.6	56	1.0	6.9	2.2	1.5
Carrot, Cumin & Coriander, Small, Simple, EAT*	1 Pack/300g	135	3.0	45	1.1	7.2	1.0	1.9
Carrot, Cumin & Coriander, Very Big, Simple, EAT*	1 Pack/625g	281	6.2	45	1.1	7.2	1.0	1.9
Carrot, Parsnip & Ginger, Small, Simple, EAT*	1 Small/300g	150	4.2	50	1.0	7.8	1.4	1.8
Cauliflower Cheese, Small, Simple, EAT*	1 Small/300ml	216	13.8	72	2.5	5.1	4.6	1.0
Chana Dal, Super, Small, EAT*	1 Small/300g	198	3.6	66	3.9	10.0	1.2	3.0
Chicken, Creamy, Small, Simple, EAT*	1 Small/300ml	237	14.4	79	4.2	4.5	4.8	0.6
Chicken, Jerk, with Garnish, Big, Bold, EAT*	1 Pack/440g	436	18.1	99	4.9	11.1	4.1	1.1
Chicken, Jerk, with Garnish, Small, Bold, EAT*	1 Pack/340g	340	13.9	100	4.8	11.6	4.1	1.1
Chicken, Jerk, with Garnish, Very Big, Bold, EAT*	1 Pack/680g	680	27.9	100	4.8	11.6	4.1	1.1
Chicken, Jerk, without Garnish, Small, Bold, EAT*	1 Pack/300g	282	12.9	94	5.1	9.2	4.3	1.1
Chicken, Jerk, without Garnish, Very Big, Bold, EAT*	1 Pack/600g	564	25.8	94	5.1	9.2	4.3	1.1
Chicken, Leek & Bacon Risotto with garnish, EAT*	1 Serving/370ml	359	18.9	97	4.7	8.1	5.1	0.5
Chicken, Leek & Bacon Risotto without garnish, EAT*	1 Serving/400ml	344	23.2	86	5.2	3.0	5.8	0.4
Chicken & Garden Vegetable with Garnish, Small, EAT*	1 Small/319ml	131	1.6	41	4.5	4.5	0.5	0.7
Chicken & Rice Noodles, Pho, Pot, EAT*	1 Pot/875g	315	1.8	36	3.0	5.2	0.2	0.4
Chicken Chilli, Mexican, without garnish, EAT*	1 Serving/300ml	282	8.1	94	6.5	10.8	2.7	1.4
Chicken Chilli, with garnish, Mexican, EAT*	1 Serving/300ml	264	7.5	88	6.1	10.2	2.5	1.4
Chicken Curry, Green Thai, with Garnish, Small, EAT*	1 Small/340ml	309	14.3	91	4.4	8.1	4.2	0.6
Chicken Curry, Thai Green, no Garnish, Small, EAT*	1 Small/300ml	252	13.2	84	4.6	5.2	4.4	0.5
Chicken Harira, with Garnish, Bold, Small, EAT*	1 Small/310g	254	3.4	82	6.6	11.1	1.1	1.9
Chicken Harira, without Garnish, Bold, Small, EAT*	1 Small/300g	219	1.5	73	6.6	10.1	0.5	1.7
Chicken Laksa, without Garnish, Small, Bold, EAT*	1 Small/300g	273	15.0	91	5.0	5.1	5.0	0.1
Chicken Laksa with Garnish, Small, Bold, EAT*	1 Small/310ml	276	15.2	89	4.9	5.0	4.9	0.2
Chicken Laksa without garnish, Big, EAT*	1 Serving/625ml	569	31.3	91	5.0	5.1	5.0	0.1
Chicken Pho, EAT*	1 Serving/786ml	291	4.7	37	3.7	3.6	0.6	0.3
Chicken Pot Pie, with Garnish, Small, Bold, EAT*	1 Small/330ml	343	17.8	104	4.8	9.0	5.4	1.0
Chicken Pot Pie, without Garnish, Small, Bold, EAT*	1 Small/300g	216	9.0	72	4.6	6.8	3.0	1.0
Chicken Tortilla, Mexican, no Garnish, Simple, EAT*	1 Small/336g	138	2.7	41	4.2	3.6	0.8	1.0
Chicken Tortilla, Mexican, with Garnish, Simple, EAT*	1 Small/320g	176	6.1	55	4.2	4.7	1.9	1.2
Chorizo & Chickpea, EAT*	1 Serving/402ml	358	16.5	89	5.0	8.1	4.1	1.6
Chowder, Haddock, Smoked, with Garnish, Small, EAT*	1 Small/302g	236	10.9	78	3.8	7.1	3.6	0.8
Duck Gyoza Dumpling, & Egg Noodles Pho, Pot, EAT*	1 Pot/849g	382	5.1	45	2.1	7.8	0.6	0.6

	Measure INFO/WEIGHT	per Measure KCAL	FAT	Nutrition Values per 100g / 100ml KCAL	PROT	CARB	FAT	FIBRE
EAT								
SOUP								
Gazpacho, EAT*	1 Serving/279ml	78	1.4	28	1.0	4.5	0.5	1.0
Goan, Potato, Small, Simple, EAT*	1 Small/300g	246	13.2	82	2.0	6.9	4.4	1.2
Goulash, Hungarian, with Garnish, Big, EAT*	1 Serving/403ml	314	8.5	78	7.7	7.2	2.1	0.8
Goulash, Hungarian, with Garnish, Small, EAT*	1 Small/302g	995	6.4	329	7.7	7.2	2.1	0.8
Goulash, Hungarian, without Garnish, Big, EAT*	1 Serving/400ml	312	8.4	78	7.7	7.2	2.1	0.8
Goulash, Hungarian, without Garnish, Small, EAT*	1 Small/300g	234	6.3	78	7.7	7.2	2.1	0.8
Ham, Pea & Mint with garnish, EAT*	1 Serving/321ml	202	4.5	63	4.8	7.5	1.4	1.1
Ham, Pea & Mint without garnish, EAT*	1 Serving/626ml	388	8.8	62	4.7	7.4	1.4	0.6
Hoisin Duck Gyoza Dumpling, EAT*	1 Serving/847ml	432	7.6	51	2.3	8.4	0.9	0.5
Lobster Bisque, Simple, EAT*	1 Small/300g	267	21.6	89	1.5	4.1	7.2	1.1
Meatball, Italian, with Garnish, Small, EAT*	1 Small/310g	254	8.1	82	4.8	9.2	2.6	2.1
Meatball, Italian, without Garnish, Small, EAT*	1 Small/300g	225	6.0	75	4.1	9.5	2.0	2.2
Minestrone, with Pesto with Garnish, Chunky, EAT*	1 Small/319ml	188	7.6	59	2.1	7.0	2.4	1.4
Minestrone, with Pesto without garnish, Chunky, EAT*	1 Small/300ml	123	1.2	41	1.8	7.3	0.4	1.5
Mushroom, Wild, & Chestnut, Simple, EAT*	1 Small/300g	240	14.1	80	1.4	8.1	4.7	1.1
Mushroom, Wild Forest, EAT*	1 Serving/300ml	150	8.7	50	2.0	3.7	2.9	0.8
Onion, French, with Garnish, EAT*	1 Serving/316ml	136	3.8	43	1.6	6.2	1.2	0.5
Onion, French, without Garnish, EAT*	1 Serving/400ml	112	1.2	28	0.7	5.4	0.3	0.5
Prawn Tom Yum, EAT*	1 Serving/814ml	285	9.0	35	1.8	4.1	1.1	0.5
Prawn Tom Yum Pho, Pot, EAT*	1 Serving/839g	369	10.1	44	3.0	5.3	1.2	0.7
Squash & Maple, EAT*	1 Small/300g	198	9.0	66	0.9	8.4	3.0	1.1
Steak & Ale, Pot Pie, with garnish, EAT*	1 Serving/415ml	415	13.3	100	8.3	9.2	3.2	1.2
Steak & Ale, Pot Pie, without garnish, EAT*	1 Serving/625ml	550	13.8	88	8.4	8.3	2.2	1.2
Sweet Potato & Chilli, Simple, EAT*	1 Small/300ml	261	13.2	87	1.3	9.6	4.4	1.7
Sweetcorn, Creamy, Simple, EAT*	1 Small/300g	315	15.3	105	2.5	12.1	5.1	1.3
Tomato, Slow Roasted, Small, Simple, EAT*	1 Small/300ml	240	18.3	80	1.2	4.7	6.1	1.1
Tomato & Basil, Spicy, Simple, EAT*	1 Small/300ml	78	0.9	26	0.9	4.6	0.3	0.9
Vegetable, Garden, EAT*	1 Small/300ml	165	8.7	55	0.9	6.1	2.9	1.2
Vegetable, Spicy, Moroccan, Simple, EAT*	1 Small/300ml	138	2.1	46	1.7	7.8	0.7	1.9
Vegetarian, Gyoza Dumpling, EAT*	1 Serving/798ml	431	11.2	54	2.3	7.6	1.4	0.6
SUSHI								
Fish, without soy sauce, EAT*	1 Serving/289g	474	9.8	164	6.4	26.0	3.4	2.2
Vegetarian, without soy sauce, EAT*	1 Serving/165g	253	2.3	153	2.5	31.7	1.4	1.6
TEA								
Chai Latte, Soya, EAT*	1 Cup/355ml	208	6.4	59	4.2	7.1	1.8	0.0
TOAST								
Cheese & Marmite, EAT*	1 Pack/120g	344	13.4	287	13.1	33.5	11.2	2.2
Cheese & Tomato, EAT*	1 Toast/148g	305	10.4	206	10.0	25.6	7.0	2.1
Nutella & Banana, EAT*	1 Serving/153g	393	10.9	257	6.0	41.8	7.1	2.4
WAFFLES								
Toffee, EAT*	1 Serving/65g	301	11.7	463	3.5	71.7	18.0	2.2
WRAP								
Chicken, Mexican, EAT*	1 Pack/215g	396	13.6	184	9.9	22.1	6.3	2.0
Chicken, Mexican, Half, EAT*	1 Pack/108g	198	6.8	184	9.9	22.1	6.3	2.0
Chicken, Roast, Simple, EAT*	1 Wrap/185g	409	20.5	221	10.0	19.9	11.1	1.2
Houmous & Falafel, EAT*	1 Wrap/244g	471	21.2	193	5.9	22.9	8.7	3.7
Houmous & Falafel, Half, EAT*	1 Pack/122g	235	10.6	193	5.9	22.9	8.7	3.7
Houmous & Salad, Simple, EAT*	1 Wrap/202g	362	17.0	179	4.9	21.1	8.4	2.6
Peking Duck, EAT*	1 Wrap/208g	433	16.2	208	11.3	22.9	7.8	1.3
Tuna Nicoise, Naked, EAT*	1 Wrap/238g	457	19.0	192	10.6	19.2	8.0	1.8
YOGHURT								
& Granola, EAT*	1 Bowl/197g	313	11.4	159	7.7	19.6	5.8	1.9

	Measure INFO/WEIGHT	per Measure KCAL	per Measure FAT	Nutrition Values per 100g / 100ml KCAL	PROT	CARB	FAT	FIBRE
EAT								
YOGHURT								
Granola, & Mixed Red Berries, EAT*	1 Serving/180g	306	8.8	170	5.8	26.1	4.9	2.4
Mango & Passionfruit, EAT*	1 Serving/124g	145	3.6	117	5.6	17.1	2.9	0.2
GREGGS								
BAGUETTE								
Chicken, & Sweetcorn, Greggs*	1 Baguette/235g	480	11.0	204	10.2	29.8	4.7	0.0
Chicken, Chargrilled, Hot, Club, Greggs*	1 Baguette/167g	510	23.5	305	15.9	27.0	14.1	0.0
Chicken, Club, Greggs*	1 Baguette/265g	600	18.5	226	10.6	29.1	7.0	0.0
Chicken, Fajita, Hot, Greggs*	1 Baguette/165g	410	11.0	248	12.7	33.3	6.7	0.0
Chicken, Pesto, Greggs*	1 Baguette/214g	520	16.0	243	11.7	32.5	7.5	0.0
Chicken, Sweet Chilli, Greggs*	1 Baguette/237g	520	3.0	219	10.3	39.7	1.3	0.0
Chicken, Tandoori, Greggs*	1 Baguette/200g	490	16.0	245	10.5	36.0	8.0	0.0
Chicken, Tikka, Greggs*	1 Baguette/250g	490	10.5	196	10.2	29.0	4.2	0.0
Chicken Mayonnaise, Greggs*	1 Baguette/200g	510	16.0	255	10.5	33.8	8.0	0.0
Egg Mayonnaise, & Tomato, Free Range, Greggs*	1 Baguette/237g	480	13.0	203	8.2	29.3	5.5	0.0
Ham, & Cheese, Greggs*	1 Baguette/216g	580	19.0	269	14.4	32.2	8.8	0.0
Ham, & Cheese, Hot, Greggs*	1 Baguette/156g	430	17.5	276	16.4	26.9	11.2	0.0
Ham, & Coleslaw, Greggs*	1 Baguette/193g	450	10.5	233	9.3	35.8	5.4	0.0
Meatball Melt, Hot, Greggs*	1 Baguette/175g	390	12.5	223	9.4	29.1	7.1	0.0
Mexican Bandit, Greggs*	1 Baguette/265g	640	22.0	242	10.9	30.0	8.3	0.0
Mozzarella, & Tomato, Hot, Greggs*	1 Baguette/149g	460	20.5	309	12.8	31.2	13.8	0.0
Prawn Mayonnaise, Greggs*	1 Baguette/235g	500	15.0	213	8.7	4.5	6.4	0.0
Tuna Crunch, Greggs*	1 Baguette/235g	530	12.5	226	10.6	32.6	5.3	0.0
Tuna Crunch Melt, Hot, Greggs*	1 Baguette/187g	440	13.0	235	13.4	30.0	7.0	0.0
BAKE								
Chicken, Greggs*	1 Bake/138g	450	32.0	326	8.7	20.6	23.2	0.0
Chicken Curry, Greggs*	1 Bake/131g	400	25.5	305	7.6	21.4	19.5	0.0
Sausage, Bean & Cheese, Melt, Greggs*	1 Bake/140g	430	27.5	307	7.1	25.4	19.6	0.0
Steak, Greggs*	1 Bake/139g	430	27.5	309	12.2	20.5	19.8	0.0
The Spicy One, Fajita Flavour Chicken, Greggs*	1 Bake/143g	430	27.5	301	8.0	24.5	19.2	0.0
BISCUITS								
Jammy Heart, Greggs*	1 Serving/60g	305	16.0	508	5.2	61.7	26.7	0.0
Spikey Mikey, Greggs*	1 Biscuit/38g	201	10.0	536	5.3	69.3	26.7	0.0
BREAKFAST CEREAL								
Porridge, Golden Syrup, Greggs*	1 Pot/234g	260	3.5	111	3.6	19.7	1.5	0.0
Porridge, Plain Oats, Creamy, Greggs*	1 Pot/234g	260	5.0	111	3.6	20.1	2.1	0.0
Porridge, Sultana, Apple & Cinnamon, Greggs*	1 Pot/238g	270	4.5	113	4.0	21.2	1.9	0.0
BROWNIES								
Chocolate, Mini, Greggs*	1 Brownie/18g	90	5.0	500	8.3	58.3	27.8	0.0
BUNS								
Belgian, Greggs*	1 Bun/135g	420	5.0	311	4.8	64.1	3.7	0.0
Hot Cross, Greggs*	1 Bun/66g	176	1.5	265	7.1	54.1	2.3	0.0
Iced, Christmas Ring, Greggs*	1 Bun/60g	210	5.0	350	4.2	62.5	8.3	0.0
Iced, Finger, Greggs*	1 Bun/35g	111	3.0	316	7.0	52.4	8.7	1.6
CAKE								
Christmas Slice, Greggs*	1 Slice/86g	360	11.5	419	5.8	67.4	13.4	0.0
Gingerbread, Cupcake, Greggs*	1 Cake/97g	426	19.2	440	3.3	60.4	19.8	0.6
Sweet Lemon Cupcake, Greggs*	1 Cake/81g	380	16.0	469	0.0	71.6	19.8	0.0
COFFEE								
Black, Regular, Greggs*	1 Cup/455ml	20	0.6	4	0.3	0.3	0.1	0.0
White, Small, Greggs*	1 Small/340ml	30	0.9	9	0.6	0.7	0.3	0.0
COLD DRINKS								
Apple Juice, Fairtrade, Greggs*	1 Serving/500ml	220	0.0	44	0.0	11.0	0.0	0.0

	Measure INFO/WEIGHT	per Measure KCAL	FAT	Nutrition Values per 100g / 100ml KCAL	PROT	CARB	FAT	FIBRE
GREGGS								
COLD DRINKS								
Capri-Sun, Greggs*	1 Serving/330ml	143	0.0	43	0.0	10.5	0.0	0.0
Coca-Cola, Diet, Greggs*	1 Serving/330ml	2	0.0	1	0.0	0.0	0.0	0.0
Coca-Cola, Greggs*	1 Serving/500ml	210	0.0	42	0.0	10.6	0.0	0.0
Coke Zero, Greggs*	1 Serving/500ml	3	0.0	1	0.0	0.0	0.0	0.0
Cranberry/Raspberry Water, Greggs*	1 Serving/500ml	5	0.0	1	0.0	0.0	0.0	0.0
Dr Pepper, Greggs*	1 Serving/500ml	210	0.0	42	0.0	2.1	0.0	0.0
Fanta Orange, Greggs*	1 Serving/500ml	150	0.0	30	0.0	7.1	0.0	0.0
Irn-Bru, Diet, Greggs*	1 Serving/500ml	4	0.0	1	0.0	0.0	0.0	0.0
Irn-Bru, Greggs*	1 Serving/330ml	145	0.0	44	0.0	10.5	0.0	0.0
Lucozade Energy, Orange, Greggs*	1 Serving/500ml	350	0.0	70	0.0	17.2	0.0	0.0
Lucozade Sport, Greggs*	1 Serving/500ml	140	0.0	28	0.0	6.4	0.0	0.0
Oasis Citrus Punch, Greggs*	1 Serving/500ml	90	0.0	18	0.0	4.1	0.0	0.0
Oasis Summer Fruits, Greggs*	1 Serving/500ml	90	0.0	18	0.0	4.2	0.0	0.0
Orange Juice, Fairtrade, Greggs*	1 Serving/500ml	220	0.0	44	0.1	10.2	0.0	0.0
Ribena, Greggs*	1 Serving/288ml	124	0.0	43	0.0	10.5	0.0	0.0
Smoothie, Mango & Orange, Greggs*	1 Serving/250ml	145	0.0	58	0.6	13.2	0.0	0.0
Smoothie, Raspberry & Banana, Greggs*	1 Serving/250ml	135	0.0	54	0.6	12.2	0.0	0.0
Sprite, Greggs*	1 Serving/500ml	220	0.0	44	0.0	10.6	0.0	0.0
CROISSANT								
All Butter, Greggs*	1 Croissant/55g	250	14.5	455	9.1	45.4	26.4	0.0
DOUGHNUTS								
Blueberry Burst, Greggs*	1 Doughnut/96g	340	10.5	355	6.3	57.0	11.0	0.0
Chocolate, Triple, Vanilla Filled, Greggs*	1 Doughnut/91g	337	11.6	370	6.3	57.0	12.7	0.0
Cinnamon, Greggs*	1 Doughnut/96g	380	16.5	396	6.2	54.7	17.2	0.0
Finger, Creamed Filled, Topped with Jam, Greggs*	1 Finger/109g	390	26.5	358	5.5	27.5	24.3	0.0
Jaffa Cake, Greggs*	1 Doughnut/95g	320	8.5	337	5.3	58.4	9.0	0.0
Jam Filled, Greggs*	1 Doughnut/74g	250	7.5	338	7.4	53.4	10.1	0.0
Lemon Drizzle, Greggs*	1 Doughnut/105g	360	11.5	343	5.2	55.7	11.0	0.0
Strawberry Milkshake Filled, Greggs*	1 Doughnut/91g	360	15.0	396	6.3	53.8	16.5	0.0
Sugar, Mini, Greggs*	1 Doughnut/25g	59	3.2	236	0.0	28.0	12.8	0.0
Yum Yum, Greggs*	1 Yum Yum/79g	340	20.5	430	5.1	42.4	26.0	0.0
Yum Yum, Toffee Topping, Greggs*	1 Yum Yum/73g	290	16.5	397	5.5	43.2	22.6	0.0
ECLAIR								
Chocolate, with Cream, Greggs*	1 Eclair/93g	350	24.5	376	4.8	29.6	26.3	0.0
FLAPJACK								
Fruity, Mini, Greggs*	1 Flapjack/22g	110	5.0	500	6.8	59.1	22.7	0.0
FRUIT								
Tropical, Greggs*	1 Serving/150g	80	0.0	53	0.7	11.3	0.0	0.0
GINGERBREAD								
Man, with Chocolate Beans, Greggs*	1 Serving/47g	210	5.5	452	6.4	78.5	11.8	0.0
MUFFIN								
Chocolate, Rainbow, Greggs*	1 Muffin/92g	370	16.5	402	4.4	53.8	17.9	0.0
Chocolate, Triple, Greggs*	1 Muffin/139g	570	31.0	410	5.0	46.8	22.3	0.0
Lemon, Sicilian, Greggs*	1 Muffin/126g	500	24.5	397	5.2	48.8	19.4	0.0
Sticky Toffee, Greggs*	1 Muffin/128g	530	27.0	414	5.1	49.2	21.1	0.0
PAIN AU CHOCOLAT								
with Belgian Chocolate, Greggs*	1 Pain/81g	339	18.5	419	8.4	44.4	22.8	0.0
PASTA								
Cheese & Tomato, with Mixed Herbs, Pot, Greggs*	1 Pack/300g	380	11.0	127	5.2	18.0	3.7	0.0
Fajita Chicken, in Tomato Sauce, Spicy, Pot, Greggs*	1 Pack/300g	360	8.0	120	5.7	17.8	2.7	0.0
PASTY								
Cheese & Onion, Freshly Baked, Greggs*	1 Pasty/126g	390	26.0	310	6.0	23.4	20.6	0.0

	Measure INFO/WEIGHT	per Measure KCAL	FAT	Nutrition Values per 100g / 100ml KCAL	PROT	CARB	FAT	FIBRE
GREGGS								
PASTY								
Cornish, Greggs*	1 Pasty/190g	560	32.0	295	7.4	21.0	16.8	0.0
Ham & Cheese Past, Greggs*	1 Pasty/140g	420	28.0	300	7.0	22.0	20.0	0.0
PIE								
Mince, Sweet, Greggs*	1 Pie/70g	290	11.0	414	4.3	61.4	15.7	0.0
Mince, Sweet, Iced, Greggs*	1 Pie/63g	230	6.5	365	2.4	62.7	10.3	0.0
PIZZA								
Cheese & Tomato, Greggs*	1 Serving/111g	290	10.5	261	9.5	32.0	9.5	0.0
Chicken, Chargrilled, Greggs*	1 Serving/111g	340	11.5	306	14.9	36.5	10.4	0.0
Chicken, Spicy, Greggs*	1 Serving/183g	450	11.5	246	12.3	36.9	6.3	0.0
Pepperoni, Greggs*	1 Serving/121g	350	14.0	289	11.6	33.1	11.6	0.0
ROLL								
Bacon, Corn Topped Roll, Breakfast, Greggs*	1 Roll/124g	322	13.0	260	15.3	25.8	10.5	0.0
Sausage, Corn Topped Roll, Breakfast, Greggs*	1 Roll/164g	410	19.0	250	11.9	24.4	11.6	0.0
SALAD								
Chicken & Bacon, Layered, Greggs*	1 Pack/211g	250	9.5	118	6.9	10.9	4.5	0.0
SANDWICH								
BLT, Sweetcure, on Malted Brown, Classic, Greggs*	1 Serving/100g	258	13.2	258	8.9	24.2	13.2	0.0
Cheese, & Tom, Mature Cheddar, on Oatmeal, Greggs*	1 Sandwich/187g	490	23.0	262	9.9	26.7	12.3	0.0
Cheese, Savoury, on Seeded White, Greggs*	1 Pack/166g	480	22.0	289	10.8	31.0	13.2	0.0
Cheese Ploughman's, Oval Bite, Greggs*	1 Pack/201g	420	20.0	209	8.7	20.9	10.0	0.0
Chicken, & Mango, on Malted Brown, Bloomer, Greggs*	1 Bloomer/217g	510	18.5	235	11.3	28.3	8.5	0.0
Chicken, & Mango, on White, Bloomer, Greggs*	1 Bloomer/217g	510	19.5	235	11.3	26.7	9.0	0.0
Chicken, & Mayonnaise, on White, Sub, Greggs*	1 Sub/186g	400	15.0	215	11.6	22.3	8.1	0.0
Chicken, & Salsa, Chargrilled, on Oatmeal, Greggs*	1 Sandwich/216g	340	3.5	157	12.0	22.2	1.6	0.0
Chicken, BBQ, Oval Bite, Greggs*	1 Roll/204g	340	6.0	167	10.8	23.0	2.9	0.0
Chicken, Chargrilled, Oval Bite, Greggs*	1 Roll/211g	440	19.0	209	11.6	19.2	9.0	0.0
Chicken, Chilli, Double, Oval Bite, Greggs*	1 Roll/219g	390	9.5	178	11.0	22.4	4.3	0.0
Chicken, Mexican, Oval Bite, Greggs*	1 Roll/179g	420	15.0	235	14.2	24.0	8.4	0.0
Chicken, Southern Fried, Rustic, Greggs*	1 Pack/268g	563	16.0	210	11.2	27.2	6.0	0.0
Chicken, Sweet Chilli, on White, Bloomer, Greggs*	1 Sandwich/255g	460	3.0	180	10.8	31.0	1.2	0.0
Chicken Salad, Classic, on Malted Brown, Greggs*	1 Sandwich/248g	520	23.0	210	9.9	20.6	9.3	0.0
Christmas Dinner, Greggs*	1 Pack/205g	570	18.5	278	12.2	35.4	9.0	0.0
Egg Mayonnaise, on Seeded White, Greggs*	1 Pack/174g	420	17.5	241	11.2	26.7	10.1	0.0
Egg Mayonnaise, with Cracked Black Pepper, Greggs*	1 Sandwich/166g	420	12.0	253	9.9	35.5	7.2	0.0
Festive, Oval Bite, Greggs*	1 Sandwich/160g	410	18.0	256	13.4	23.8	11.2	0.0
Ham, & Egg, Honey Roast, Salad, on Oatmeal, Greggs*	1 Sandwich/243g	450	15.5	185	9.9	21.0	6.4	0.0
Ham, & Egg, with Salad, on White, Sub, Greggs*	1 Sub/220g	390	14.5	177	9.8	19.1	6.6	0.0
Ham, Cheese, & Pickle, On White, Bloomer, Greggs*	1 Bloomer/228g	510	18.0	224	11.2	27.4	7.9	0.0
Ham Salad, Oval Bite, Greggs*	1 Sandwich/175g	320	10.5	183	9.1	21.7	6.0	0.0
Prawn Mayonnaise, Reduced Fat, on Oatmeal, Greggs*	1 Sandwich/166g	300	7.5	181	10.2	23.8	4.5	0.0
Steak, & Cheese, Rustic, Greggs*	1 Pack/237g	512	16.0	216	13.5	24.9	6.8	0.0
Tuna, Sweet Chilli, & Red Pepper, on Oatmeal, Greggs*	1 Sandwich/206g	370	4.5	180	11.2	27.2	2.2	0.0
Tuna Crunch, on Brown, Bloomer, Greggs*	1 Sandwich/235g	520	15.0	221	11.1	28.9	6.4	0.0
Tuna Mayonnaise, & Cucumber, on Oatmeal, Greggs*	1 Sandwich/194g	400	11.0	206	12.1	25.5	5.7	0.0
Tuna Mayonnaise, On Malted Brown, Greggs*	1 Sandwich/203g	440	13.5	217	12.3	26.6	6.6	0.0
Tuna Mayonnaise, on Seeded White, Sub, Greggs*	1 Sub/222g	410	12.0	185	11.7	21.0	5.4	0.0
Tuna Mayonnaise, on White, Sub, Greggs*	1 Roll/202g	350	10.0	173	11.6	19.6	5.0	0.0
SAUSAGE ROLL								
Freshly Baked, Greggs*	1 Serving/103g	360	25.5	350	8.2	22.8	24.8	0.0
Mini, Greggs*	1 Roll/26g	81	6.5	310	8.5	21.5	25.0	0.0
SLICES								
Toffee Apple, Lattice, Greggs*	1 Slice/77g	277	15.0	360	4.0	41.0	19.5	0.0

	Measure INFO/WEIGHT	per Measure KCAL	FAT	Nutrition Values per 100g / 100ml KCAL	PROT	CARB	FAT	FIBRE
GREGGS								
SOUP								
Lentil & Bacon, Greggs*	1 Serving/300g	180	5.5	60	3.5	7.7	1.8	0.0
Tomato, Heinz, Greggs*	1 Pot/296g	200	7.4	68	0.9	10.5	2.5	0.0
TART								
Egg Custard, Greggs*	1 Tart/90g	257	13.0	286	5.5	33.2	14.5	0.0
Strawberry, Greggs*	1 Tart/65g	180	7.5	277	2.3	41.5	11.5	0.0
Strawberry, with Fresh Cream, Greggs*	1 Tart/94g	300	16.5	319	3.2	35.1	17.6	0.0
TEACAKES								
Bakery, Greggs*	1 Teacake/74g	210	3.5	284	7.4	52.0	4.7	0.0
TURNOVER								
Apple, Fresh Cream, Greggs*	1 Turnover/176g	540	32.5	307	2.8	34.1	18.5	0.0
WRAP								
Bacon & Cheese, Greggs*	1 Wrap/98g	410	31.0	421	14.4	19.0	31.8	0.0
Chicken, & Bacon, Caesar, Greggs*	1 Wrap/189g	450	23.5	238	10.8	20.4	12.4	0.0
Chicken, Chargrilled, Greggs*	1 Wrap/192g	410	18.5	214	10.2	20.8	9.6	0.0
YOGHURT								
Raspberry, & Granola, Natural, Greggs*	1 Pot/190g	228	4.8	120	5.0	18.5	2.5	0.0
J D WETHERSPOON								
BAGUETTE								
BLT, Malted Grain, J D Wetherspoon*	1 Baguette/399g	823	45.5	206	8.3	17.8	11.4	1.3
Club, Malted Grain, J D Wetherspoon*	1 Baguette/388g	768	36.8	198	9.8	18.5	9.5	1.4
Crayfish, Malted Grain, J D Wetherspoon*	1 Baguette/314g	594	25.5	189	6.1	23.2	8.1	1.7
Ham, Wiltshire, J D Wetherspoon*	1 Baguette/346g	536	13.1	155	9.9	20.4	3.8	1.5
Ploughmans, Lloyds, J D Wetherspoon*	1 Baguette/346g	778	34.3	225	8.6	25.5	9.9	2.2
Sausage, Hot, & Tomato Chutney, J D Wetherspoon*	1 Baguette/250g	839	33.4	336	14.1	40.7	13.4	3.8
Tuna Mayonnaise, Malted Grain, J D Wetherspoon*	1 Baguette/401g	710	31.3	177	8.9	18.1	7.8	1.3
BHAJI								
Onion, J D Wetherspoon*	1 Bhaji/30g	43	2.2	143	5.3	18.7	7.3	5.7
BIRYANI								
Chicken, without Naan, J D Wetherspoon*	1 Meal/614g	700	24.6	114	4.7	14.8	4.0	1.3
BREAD								
Garlic, Ciabatta, J D Wetherspoon*	1 Serving/142g	406	17.9	286	8.0	1.0	12.6	1.5
Naan, J D Wetherspoon*	1 Naan/90g	197	2.5	219	7.6	41.0	2.8	1.4
BREAKFAST								
Baguette, Quorn Sausage, J D Wetherspoon*	1 Baguette/285g	622	18.3	218	10.5	29.4	6.4	3.4
Bran, Fruit & Nut Muffin, J D Wetherspoon*	1 Serving/145g	571	31.7	394	7.2	43.0	21.9	1.1
Children's, J D Wetherspoon*	1 Serving/341g	613	37.1	180	10.4	10.8	10.9	2.3
Chocolate Muffin, J D Wetherspoon*	1 Muffin/125g	490	28.4	392	5.0	43.6	22.7	4.8
Eggs Benedict, J D Wetherspoon*	1 Serving/100g	573	30.9	573	38.7	33.6	30.9	2.4
Farmhouse, with Toast, J D Wetherspoon*	1 Serving/796g	1647	101.8	207	9.4	14.0	12.8	1.9
Morning Roll, with Bacon, J D Wetherspoon*	1 Roll/183g	546	34.6	298	11.1	21.7	18.9	1.1
Morning Roll, with Fried Egg, J D Wetherspoon*	1 Roll/143g	400	21.3	280	9.7	27.8	14.9	1.4
Morning Roll, with Quorn Sausage, J D Wetherspoon*	1 Roll/143g	367	16.1	257	10.1	29.5	11.3	2.6
Morning Roll, with Sausage, J D Wetherspoon*	1 Roll/158g	517	28.0	327	13.8	30.1	17.7	2.3
Muffin, Blueberry, J D Wetherspoon*	1 Muffin/124g	467	25.8	374	4.7	43.2	20.7	0.4
Scrambled Egg, on Toast, J D Wetherspoon*	1 Serving/265g	503	24.9	190	8.4	17.4	9.4	1.1
Toast & Preserves, J D Wetherspoon*	1 Serving/148g	420	15.2	284	5.7	41.8	10.3	3.2
Traditional, J D Wetherspoon*	1 Breakfast/523g	904	60.1	173	8.4	9.4	11.5	1.8
Vegetarian, J D Wetherspoon*	1 Breakfast/562g	984	57.1	175	6.7	14.3	10.2	2.1
BURGERS								
Beef, Double, & Chips, J D Wetherspoon*	1 Serving/598g	1382	81.6	231	16.8	11.4	13.6	0.5
Beef, Double, Cheese, & Chips, J D Wetherspoon*	1 Serving/654g	1565	91.4	239	17.2	10.7	14.0	0.5
Beef, with Bacon, Cheese & Chips, J D Wetherspoon*	1 Serving/531g	1295	78.9	244	15.2	12.6	14.8	0.5

	Measure INFO/WEIGHT	per Measure KCAL	per Measure FAT	Nutrition Values per 100g / 100ml KCAL	PROT	CARB	FAT	FIBRE
J D WETHERSPOON								
BURGERS								
Beef, with Cheese, & Chips, J D Wetherspoon*	1 Serving/456g	966	53.8	212	13.7	13.8	11.8	0.5
Beef, with Chips, J D Wetherspoon*	1 Serving/428g	881	46.4	206	12.8	15.7	10.8	0.6
Chicken, Fillet, with Chips, J D Wetherspoon*	1 Serving/465g	727	17.1	156	10.9	16.7	3.7	0.8
Lamb, Double, Minted, with Chips, J D Wetherspoon*	1 Serving/598g	1077	47.2	180	14.6	14.1	7.9	0.9
Lamb, Minted, with Chips, J D Wetherspoon*	1 Serving/428g	712	27.8	166	11.3	17.2	6.5	0.9
Vegetable, with Chips, J D Wetherspoon*	1 Serving/488g	839	25.9	172	4.7	27.2	5.3	2.0
BUTTY								
Bacon, Brown Bloomer, J D Wetherspoon*	1 Serving/309g	869	39.6	281	23.3	18.3	12.8	1.2
Bacon & Egg, Brown Bloomer, J D Wetherspoon*	1 Serving/269g	702	31.1	261	18.2	21.0	11.6	1.4
Bacon & Egg, White Bloomer, J D Wetherspoon*	1 Serving/269g	689	32.7	256	16.7	20.9	12.2	1.2
Chip, Brown Bloomer, J D Wetherspoon*	1 Serving/204g	478	14.7	234	7.6	35.7	7.2	1.9
Chip, White Bloomer, J D Wetherspoon*	1 Serving/204g	465	16.3	228	5.6	35.6	8.0	1.6
Chip & Cheese, Brown Bloomer, J D Wetherspoon*	1 Serving/232g	593	24.4	256	9.7	31.4	10.5	1.6
Chip & Cheese, White Bloomer, J D Wetherspoon*	1 Serving/232g	580	26.0	250	7.9	31.3	11.2	1.4
Sausage & Egg, Brown Bloomer, J D Wetherspoon*	1 Serving/331g	885	49.0	268	16.8	20.8	14.8	1.3
Sausage & Egg, White Bloomer, J D Wetherspoon*	1 Serving/331g	872	50.6	264	11.4	20.7	15.3	1.1
CAKE								
Chocolate Fudge, & Ice Cream, J D Wetherspoon*	1 Serving/239g	822	47.3	344	4.0	37.6	19.8	0.4
CAULIFLOWER CHEESE								
J D Wetherspoon*	1 Serving/220g	275	15.2	125	4.1	3.6	6.9	0.8
CHEESECAKE								
Chocolate Chip, J D Wetherspoon*	1 Serving/100g	270	11.5	270	4.9	36.8	11.5	0.5
White Chocolate & Raspberry, J D Wetherspoon*	1 Serving/175g	656	36.9	375	5.6	40.8	21.1	0.9
CHICKEN								
Wings, Buffalo, J D Wetherspoon*	1 Serving/328g	636	42.9	194	15.2	4.0	13.1	0.5
CHICKEN ALFREDO								
Pasta, with Dressed Side Salad, J D Wetherspoon*	1 Meal/576g	950	52.4	165	8.7	12.0	9.1	0.3
Pasta, with Garlic Bread, J D Wetherspoon*	1 Meal/501g	1007	47.6	201	10.8	13.0	9.5	0.3
Pasta, without Garlic Bread, J D Wetherspoon*	1 Meal/430g	804	38.7	187	11.3	15.0	9.0	0.1
CHICKEN FORESTIERRE								
J D Wetherspoon*	1 Serving/684g	626	26.0	92	7.7	8.7	3.8	1.0
CHICKEN ROAST								
with BBQ Sauce, J D Wetherspoon*	1 Meal/742g	948	37.5	128	11.3	9.2	5.0	0.6
with Chips & BBQ Sauce, J D Wetherspoon*	1 Meal/768g	1183	53.0	154	11.5	12.2	6.9	0.9
with Chips & Salad, J D Wetherspoon*	1 Meal/695g	983	52.1	141	13.1	5.9	7.5	0.6
with Jacket Potato, Salad, & Salsa, J D Wetherspoon*	1 Meal/785g	1193	57.3	152	12.2	10.2	7.3	1.3
with Piri Piri Sauce, J D Wetherspoon*	1 Serving/994g	994	47.1	100	8.4	5.8	4.7	0.8
CHICKEN VINDALOO								
J D Wetherspoon*	1 Meal/500g	704	19.0	141	6.4	21.0	3.8	1.3
CHIPS								
Bowl, J D Wetherspoon*	1 Serving/300g	750	30.4	250	3.5	36.5	10.1	2.9
with Cheese, J D Wetherspoon*	1 Serving/501g	1002	51.6	200	5.2	21.9	10.3	1.8
with Roast Gravy, J D Wetherspoon*	1 Serving/400g	392	12.4	98	2.5	17.6	3.1	0.0
CHUTNEY								
Mango, J D Wetherspoon*	1 Serving/25g	47	0.2	188	0.4	44.8	0.8	0.4
CIABATTA								
BBQ Chicken & Bacon Melt, J D Wetherspoon*	1 Ciabatta/333g	716	33.6	215	11.3	20.4	10.1	1.8
BLT, J D Wetherspoon*	1 Ciabatta/390g	789	47.3	202	8.2	15.4	12.1	1.5
Club, J D Wetherspoon*	1 Ciabatta/378g	734	38.6	194	9.7	16.1	10.2	1.6
Crayfish, J D Wetherspoon*	1 Ciabatta/305g	561	27.4	184	5.8	20.3	9.0	1.9
Mature Cheddar Cheese & Pickle, J D Wetherspoon*	1 Ciabatta/350g	662	31.5	189	7.8	19.4	9.0	1.7
Tuna Mayonnaise, J D Wetherspoon*	1 Ciabatta/391g	676	32.8	173	8.8	15.8	8.4	1.5

	Measure INFO/WEIGHT	per Measure KCAL	FAT	Nutrition Values per 100g / 100ml KCAL	PROT	CARB	FAT	FIBRE
J D WETHERSPOON								
CURRY								
Goan, Vegetable, without Naan, J D Wetherspoon*	1 Meal/748g	1017	41.9	136	3.1	18.3	5.6	1.3
Kashmiri, Lamb, with Naan, J D Wetherspoon*	1 Meal/704g	1021	33.1	145	7.2	19.5	4.7	1.2
Kashmiri, Lamb, without Naan, J D Wetherspoon*	1 Meal/615g	824	30.7	134	7.1	16.3	5.0	1.1
Kerala, Fish, with Naan, J D Wetherspoon*	1 Meal/706g	1066	36.0	151	7.0	20.0	5.1	1.0
Kerala, Fish, without Naan, J D Wetherspoon*	1 Meal/616g	869	33.3	141	6.9	16.9	5.4	0.9
Royal Thali, with Naan, J D Wetherspoon*	1 Meal/948g	1336	48.3	141	7.1	16.8	5.1	1.3
Thai, Green Chicken, without Naan, J D Wetherspoon*	1 Meal/617g	1037	46.9	168	7.5	17.6	7.6	0.5
Vegetable, Goan, with Naan Bread, J D Wetherspoon*	1 Meal/707g	1032	36.8	146	3.6	21.2	5.2	1.3
Vegetarian, Thali, with Naan, J D Wetherspoon*	1 Meal/950g	1320	42.7	139	5.3	20.3	4.5	2.4
DHANSAK								
Lamb, Meal, J D Wetherspoon*	1 Serving/720g	983	26.1	137	7.2	19.6	3.6	0.8
FISH & CHIPS								
Haddock, J D Wetherspoon*	1 Meal/496g	806	40.7	162	7.2	14.4	8.2	2.4
Plaice, Breaded, & Peas, J D Wetherspoon*	1 Serving/460g	550	15.6	120	6.8	15.0	3.4	1.7
Traditional, J D Wetherspoon*	1 Serving/495g	804	40.6	162	7.2	14.4	8.2	2.4
FISH CAKES								
Salmon & Lime, with Tartare Sauce, J D Wetherspoon*	1 Serving/355g	569	31.3	160	5.8	14.5	8.8	1.0
GAMMON								
Steak, 8oz, Eggs, Chips & Pineapple, J D Wetherspoon*	1 Meal/609g	1036	51.8	170	13.4	10.2	8.5	0.8
Steak, Egg, Chips & Side Salad, J D Wetherspoon*	1 Meal/593g	801	41.5	135	10.2	9.0	7.0	0.3
GAMMON &								
Chips, Peas, Tomato, & Egg, J D Wetherspoon*	1 Meal/564g	844	41.2	150	15.0	6.7	7.3	1.3
Chips, Peas, Tomato, & Pineapple, J D Wetherspoon*	1 Meal/575g	799	36.2	139	13.6	7.8	6.3	1.4
HAGGIS								
with Neeps & Tatties, J D Wetherspoon*	1 Meal/682g	982	52.5	144	4.6	15.0	7.7	1.9
HAM								
& Eggs, J D Wetherspoon*	1 Serving/396g	253	12.7	64	4.9	3.5	3.2	0.0
ICE CREAM								
Bombe, Mint Chocolate, J D Wetherspoon*	1 Serving/135g	300	13.4	222	2.6	30.6	9.9	0.8
Chocolate, Bomb, J D Wetherspoon*	1 Serving/100g	259	13.4	259	5.9	34.3	13.4	5.4
Neopolitan, Movenpick, J D Wetherspoon*	1 Bowl/100g	181	9.6	181	3.0	20.0	9.6	0.0
JALFREZI								
Chicken, Meal, with Naan Bread, J D Wetherspoon*	1 Meal/705g	916	19.7	130	6.8	19.9	2.8	1.3
Chicken, without Naan Bread, J D Wetherspoon*	1 Meal/615g	719	17.2	117	6.7	16.9	2.8	1.3
KORMA								
Chicken, Meal, without Naan, J D Wetherspoon*	1 Meal/617g	944	38.2	153	6.4	17.0	6.2	0.8
Chicken, with Naan, J D Wetherspoon*	1 Meal/704g	1141	40.8	162	6.6	20.1	5.8	0.9
LASAGNE								
Al Forno with Dressed Side Salad, J D Wetherspoon*	1 Meal/658g	823	40.8	125	5.5	11.4	6.2	0.8
MASALA								
Chicken, Hot, with Naan, J D Wetherspoon*	1 Meal/707g	1033	31.1	146	6.9	20.1	4.4	1.2
Chicken, Hot, without Naan, J D Wetherspoon*	1 Meal/614g	835	28.2	136	6.8	17.1	4.6	1.1
Vegetable, Tandoori, Meal, J D Wetherspoon*	1 Serving/720g	1020	36.0	142	3.4	20.7	5.0	2.3
MEATBALLS								
with Linguine Pasta, J D Wetherspoon*	1 Serving/512g	614	24.0	120	6.3	13.1	4.7	1.9
MELT								
BBQ Chicken, & Chips, & Salad, J D Wetherspoon*	1 Serving/643g	849	42.4	132	10.4	8.2	6.6	0.4
MIXED GRILL								
with Chips, & Dressed Side Salad, J D Wetherspoon*	1 Serving/784g	1324	87.0	169	12.0	5.6	11.1	0.3
MOUSSAKA								
Vegetarian, J D Wetherspoon*	1 Serving/555g	582	38.8	105	2.7	7.6	7.0	2.7

	Measure INFO/WEIGHT	per Measure KCAL	FAT	Nutrition Values per 100g / 100ml KCAL	PROT	CARB	FAT	FIBRE
J D WETHERSPOON								
NACHOS								
J D Wetherspoon*	1 Serving/366g	1139	67.3	311	7.0	29.2	18.4	3.2
with Chilli Con Carne, J D Wetherspoon*	1 Serving/570g	1505	88.9	264	8.6	22.2	15.6	1.8
with Fajita Chicken, J D Wetherspoon*	1 Serving/486g	1225	70.5	252	5.7	24.7	14.5	2.9
with Five Bean Chilli, J D Wetherspoon*	1 Serving/571g	1399	81.1	245	7.3	21.8	14.2	2.7
PANINI								
BBQ Chicken & Bacon, Melt, J D Wetherspoon*	1 Panini/337g	650	27.6	193	9.9	19.9	8.2	1.7
Cheese, Tomato, & Bacon, J D Wetherspoon*	1 Panini/261g	630	29.0	241	14.3	21.6	11.1	0.8
Cheese & Tuna, J D Wetherspoon*	1 Panini/221g	551	22.3	249	15.5	24.9	10.1	0.7
Club, J D Wetherspoon*	1 Panini/378g	734	38.6	194	9.7	16.1	10.2	1.6
Fajita Chicken, J D Wetherspoon*	1 Panini/235g	359	6.1	153	4.4	28.8	2.6	1.7
Mature, Cheddar Cheese & Tomato, J D Wetherspoon*	1 Panini/330g	750	27.1	227	10.4	18.0	8.2	1.7
Pepperoni & Mozzarella, J D Wetherspoon*	1 Panini/205g	617	33.4	301	11.6	27.5	16.3	1.0
Tomato, Mozzarella & Green Pesto, J D Wetherspoon*	1 Panini/245g	502	22.9	205	7.3	23.0	9.4	1.4
PASTA BAKE								
Mediterranean, J D Wetherspoon*	1 Serving/450g	577	22.1	128	4.3	16.4	4.9	0.9
PIE								
Cottage, with Chips & Peas, J D Wetherspoon*	1 Meal/682g	846	33.4	124	3.7	15.6	4.9	1.9
Scotch, J D Wetherspoon*	1 Serving/145g	302	15.4	208	13.1	7.8	10.6	0.9
Scotch, with Chips & Beans, J D Wetherspoon*	1 Serving/435g	603	22.2	139	6.8	14.9	5.1	1.5
PLATTER								
Italian Style, J D Wetherspoon*	1 Platter/1020g	1985	75.5	195	10.4	22.9	7.4	0.6
Mexican, Chilli, Sour Cream, J D Wetherspoon*	1 Platter/1062g	2560	141.2	241	7.5	22.6	13.3	2.8
Mexican, with Five Bean Chilli, J D Wetherspoon*	1 Platter/1002g	2358	123.2	235	6.2	25.6	12.3	3.6
Western, J D Wetherspoon*	1 Platter/1454g	2973	168.7	204	16.9	9.1	11.6	0.4
POPPADOMS								
& Dips, J D Wetherspoon*	1 Serving/134g	425	10.9	317	4.6	28.4	8.1	2.5
J D Wetherspoon*	1 Poppadom/12g	35	0.2	281	6.7	45.0	1.9	10.0
POTATO BOMBAY								
J D Wetherspoon*	1 Serving/300g	285	14.7	95	1.8	10.8	4.9	2.5
POTATO SKINS								
Cheese & Bacon, Loaded, J D Wetherspoon*	1 Serving/439g	949	58.4	216	8.9	15.2	13.3	1.5
Cheese & Red Onion, Loaded, J D Wetherspoon*	1 Serving/414g	835	51.3	202	6.0	16.5	12.4	1.6
Chilli Con Carne, Loaded, J D Wetherspoon*	1 Serving/503g	735	35.7	146	5.0	15.7	7.1	1.9
POTATO WEDGES								
Spicy, J D Wetherspoon*	1 Serving/270g	434	15.7	161	2.2	27.7	5.8	1.8
Spicy, with Sour Cream, J D Wetherspoon*	1 Serving/330g	558	27.4	169	2.3	23.4	8.3	1.5
POTATOES								
Baked, Jacket, Coleslaw, J D Wetherspoon*	1 Meal/596g	918	48.9	154	2.3	17.1	8.2	1.8
Mashed, Creamy, J D Wetherspoon*	1 Serving/279g	349	21.2	125	1.5	15.0	7.6	1.1
Roast, J D Wetherspoon*	1 Serving/200g	290	9.4	145	2.5	23.0	4.7	2.3
RIBS								
Double, J D Wetherspoon*	1 Serving/350g	767	40.9	219	16.7	11.9	11.7	0.4
Double, with Chips, J D Wetherspoon*	1 Serving/500g	949	46.5	190	12.5	14.9	9.3	0.3
Double, with Jacket Potato, J D Wetherspoon*	1 Serving/590g	1159	50.7	196	11.4	19.2	8.6	1.3
RICE								
Basmati, Yellow, J D Wetherspoon*	1 Serving/200g	286	1.2	143	3.4	31.1	0.6	0.2
J D Wetherspoon*	1 Serving/200g	274	0.4	137	2.9	30.9	0.2	0.2
ROGAN JOSH								
Lamb, Meal, without Naan, J D Wetherspoon*	1 Meal/617g	820	27.7	133	7.1	17.0	4.5	1.0
Lamb, with Naan, J D Wetherspoon*	1 Meal/706g	1017	30.4	144	7.2	20.1	4.3	1.1
SALAD								
Caesar, J D Wetherspoon*	1 Meal/211g	448	38.0	212	6.8	5.8	18.0	1.1

	Measure INFO/WEIGHT	per Measure KCAL	FAT	Nutrition Values per 100g / 100ml KCAL	PROT	CARB	FAT	FIBRE
J D WETHERSPOON								
SALAD								
Chicken, BBQ, Croutons & Dressing, J D Wetherspoon*	1 Serving/350g	315	8.4	90	9.4	7.5	2.4	0.8
Chicken & Bacon, Warm, J D Wetherspoon*	1 Serving/426g	600	41.3	141	9.8	3.8	9.7	0.6
Crayfish, J D Wetherspoon*	1 Serving/317g	247	18.0	78	4.4	2.7	5.7	0.6
Side, No Dressing, J D Wetherspoon*	1 Serving/195g	125	4.5	64	2.0	8.9	2.3	1.1
Side, with Dressing, J D Wetherspoon*	1 Serving/215g	263	19.6	122	2.2	8.1	9.1	1.0
Side, with Dressing & Croutons, J D Wetherspoon*	1 Serving/140g	221	18.3	158	2.1	8.6	13.1	1.1
Side, with Dressing & No Croutons, J D Wetherspoon*	1 Serving/129g	145	14.0	112	1.0	3.2	10.8	0.9
Side, without Croutons, J D Wetherspoon*	1 Serving/111g	157	10.8	141	9.8	3.8	9.7	0.6
Thai Noodle, J D Wetherspoon*	1 Serving/394g	433	21.3	110	2.7	12.7	5.4	1.4
Thai Noodle, with Chicken, J D Wetherspoon*	1 Serving/554g	637	27.7	115	9.2	9.6	5.0	1.4
Tiger Prawn, Dressing, & Chilli Jam, J D Wetherspoon*	1 Serving/340g	500	33.0	147	4.7	10.1	9.7	0.9
Tuna, with Eggs, Olives, & Croutons, J D Wetherspoon*	1 Serving/395g	679	51.7	172	10.3	3.2	13.1	0.7
SAMOSAS								
Lamb, J D Wetherspoon*	1 Samosa/90g	160	3.8	178	7.9	29.9	4.2	3.9
Vegetable, J D Wetherspoon*	1 Samosa/50g	92	3.1	184	5.4	28.4	6.2	2.2
SANDWICH								
Beef, Hot, Brown Bloomer, J D Wetherspoon*	1 Sandwich/299g	618	27.2	207	11.4	19.9	9.1	1.3
BLT, Brown Bloomer, J D Wetherspoon*	1 Sandwich/404g	885	39.6	219	18.0	14.6	9.8	1.2
BLT, White Bloomer, J D Wetherspoon*	1 Sandwich/404g	872	32.7	216	17.0	14.6	8.1	1.0
Cheddar, & Pickle, Brown Bloomer, J D Wetherspoon*	1 Sandwich/260g	665	31.9	256	11.0	25.4	12.3	1.9
Cheddar, & Pickle, White Bloomer, J D Wetherspoon*	1 Sandwich/260g	638	32.8	245	9.2	0.0	12.6	1.5
Chicken, Half Fat Mayo, Brown, Hot, J D Wetherspoon*	1 Sandwich/289g	628	28.3	217	11.8	20.7	9.8	1.7
Chicken, Half Fat Mayo, White, Hot, J D Wetherspoon*	1 Sandwich/289g	615	29.8	213	11.3	20.6	10.3	1.5
Egg Mayonnaise, Brown Bloomer, J D Wetherspoon*	1 Sandwich/295g	704	39.5	239	10.1	19.7	13.4	1.3
Egg Mayonnaise, White Bloomer, J D Wetherspoon*	1 Sandwich/295g	692	41.0	235	8.7	19.6	13.9	1.1
Ham, & Tomato, Brown Bloomer, J D Wetherspoon*	1 Sandwich/239g	514	17.2	215	11.4	24.4	7.2	1.8
Ham, & Tomato, White Bloomer, J D Wetherspoon*	1 Sandwich/239g	501	18.6	210	9.7	24.4	7.8	1.5
Prawn Mayonnaise, Brown Bloomer, J D Wetherspoon*	1 Sandwich/244g	579	26.6	237	11.0	23.8	10.9	1.6
Prawn Mayonnaise, White Bloomer, J D Wetherspoon*	1 Sandwich/244g	567	28.3	232	9.3	23.7	11.6	1.4
SAUSAGE								
with Bacon & Egg, J D Wetherspoon*	1 Serving/582g	1040	57.6	179	11.7	11.3	9.9	1.0
with Chips, & Beans, J D Wetherspoon*	1 Meal/554g	897	42.6	162	7.3	16.4	7.7	2.3
SAUSAGE & MASH								
with Red Wine Gravy, J D Wetherspoon*	1 Serving/677g	887	50.8	131	6.0	10.2	7.5	1.8
SCAMPI								
Breaded, Chips, Peas, Tartare, J D Wetherspoon*	1 Serving/561g	987	43.7	176	5.2	19.9	7.8	2.3
SORBET								
Mango & Passionfruit, J D Wetherspoon*	1 Serving/135g	115	0.1	85	0.2	20.0	0.1	0.2
SOUP								
Mushroom, No Bread, J D Wetherspoon*	1 Serving/305g	252	16.5	83	2.8	5.5	5.4	0.4
Mushroom, with Brown Bloomer, J D Wetherspoon*	1 Serving/429g	561	23.7	131	3.4	16.0	5.5	1.2
Mushroom, with White Bloomer, J D Wetherspoon*	1 Serving/429g	549	25.2	128	3.4	15.9	5.9	1.1
Tomato, No Bread, J D Wetherspoon*	1 Serving/305g	198	14.0	65	0.9	3.9	4.6	0.6
Tomato, with Brown Bloomer, J D Wetherspoon*	1 Serving/429g	576	25.8	134	3.7	15.7	6.0	1.3
Tomato, with White Bloomer, J D Wetherspoon*	1 Serving/429g	563	27.3	131	2.8	15.6	6.4	1.2
Tomato & Basil, Organic, J D Wetherspoon*	1 Serving/491g	584	23.1	119	2.9	15.8	4.7	1.2
SPONGE PUDDING								
Treacle, with Hot Custard, J D Wetherspoon*	1 Serving/515g	1267	71.1	246	2.3	41.8	13.8	0.2
SQUASH								
Butternut, Roast Dinner, J D Wetherspoon*	1 Meal/847g	1211	55.9	143	4.9	17.5	6.6	2.9
STEAK								
Ribeye, 8oz, Chips & Side Salad, J D Wetherspoon*	1 Meal/562g	1006	71.9	179	8.0	8.9	12.8	0.3

	Measure INFO/WEIGHT	per Measure KCAL	per Measure FAT	Nutrition Values per 100g / 100ml KCAL	PROT	CARB	FAT	FIBRE
J D WETHERSPOON								
STEAK &								
Breaded Scampi, Chips, & Peas, J D Wetherspoon*	1 Serving/816g	1369	72.6	168	10.1	11.3	8.9	1.2
STEAK WITH								
Chips, & Dressed Side Salad, Rump, J D Wetherspoon*	1 Meal/634g	922	60.2	145	9.5	6.3	9.5	0.3
Chips, & Dressed Side Salad, Sirloin, J D Wetherspoon*	1 Meal/577g	979	73.3	170	7.6	6.9	12.7	0.3
STEW								
Irish, J D Wetherspoon*	1 Serving/600g	516	23.4	86	7.3	5.6	3.9	0.9
STUFFING BALLS								
Sage & Onion, J D Wetherspoon*	1 Serving/70g	137	1.1	196	6.6	32.3	1.6	3.6
TART								
Apple, with Ice Cream, J D Wetherspoon*	1 Serving/235g	464	20.0	197	1.6	29.8	8.5	0.4
TIKKA								
Mixed Grill, Starter, J D Wetherspoon*	1 Serving/374g	460	23.9	123	13.4	3.2	6.4	0.9
WAFFLES								
Belgian, Ice Cream & Maple Syrup, J D Wetherspoon*	1 Serving/395g	934	33.6	236	13.8	28.4	8.5	0.8
WRAP								
Caesar Wetherwrap, J D Wetherspoon*	1 Wrap/159g	478	32.6	301	7.0	23.1	20.5	1.5
Caesar Wetherwrap, Tortillas & Salsa, J D Wetherspoon*	1 Serving/244g	624	38.8	256	5.7	23.4	15.9	1.6
Chicken, Cheese, & Potato Wedges, J D Wetherspoon*	1 Serving/401g	762	34.1	190	8.0	22.2	8.5	1.5
Chicken, Guacamole, Tortillas, Salsa, J D Wetherspoon*	1 Serving/273g	474	16.9	174	8.2	21.9	6.2	2.0
Chicken, with Chicken Breast, J D Wetherspoon*	1 Wrap/292g	450	21.6	154	9.4	14.5	7.4	1.5
Chicken, with Potato Wedges, J D Wetherspoon*	1 Serving/373g	647	24.2	174	6.7	23.9	6.5	1.7
Chicken, with Tortilla Chips & Salsa, J D Wetherspoon*	1 Serving/328g	584	23.0	178	7.5	22.3	7.0	1.6
Chicken & Cheese, J D Wetherspoon*	1 Wrap/271g	553	26.3	204	10.7	19.6	9.7	1.4
Fajita Chicken, J D Wetherspoon*	1 Wrap/228g	345	14.1	151	3.8	21.2	6.2	1.9
Fajita Chicken, Tortilla Chips, Salsa, J D Wetherspoon*	1 Serving/313g	491	20.3	157	3.5	21.9	6.5	1.9
Fajita Chicken, with Potato Wedges, J D Wetherspoon*	1 Serving/358g	554	21.8	155	3.2	23.5	6.1	1.9
Poached Salmon, Potato Wedges, J D Wetherspoon*	1 Serving/298g	656	34.3	220	7.1	24.2	11.5	1.5
Poached Salmon & Prawn Salad, J D Wetherspoon*	1 Serving/355g	512	34.1	144	9.8	4.5	9.6	0.5
YORKSHIRE PUDDING								
J D Wetherspoon*	2 Puddings/56g	132	4.6	236	8.2	32.9	8.2	1.1
KFC								
BEANS								
BBQ, Large, KFC*	1 Serving/292g	246	2.2	84	5.3	15.1	0.7	0.0
BBQ, Regular, KFC*	1 Serving/126g	106	0.9	84	5.3	15.1	0.7	6.9
BURGERS								
Fillet, KFC*	1 Burger/245g	479	19.8	196	11.1	19.6	8.1	0.0
Fillet, Mini, KFC*	1 Burger/114g	275	11.2	241	14.8	24.0	9.8	0.0
Fillet Tower Burger, KFC*	1 Burger/163g	617	21.0	378	24.3	41.4	12.9	0.0
Mini Fillet, Kids, KFC*	1 Burger/114g	253	6.4	222	15.8	27.0	5.6	0.0
Tower, KFC*	1 Burger/210g	628	20.8	299	15.9	30.0	9.9	0.0
Tower, Zinger, KFC*	1 Burger/264g	655	32.7	248	11.2	24.4	12.4	0.0
Zinger, Fillet, KFC*	1 Burger/185g	445	19.6	241	13.9	22.4	10.6	1.4
Zinger, KFC*	1 Burger/219g	481	20.8	220	12.2	22.0	9.5	0.0
CHEESECAKE								
Boysenberry, Chateau, KFC*	1 Serving/85g	196	9.4	230	4.0	30.0	11.0	0.0
Cookies & Cream, KFC*	1 Serving/80g	261	17.1	326	4.3	29.1	21.4	0.0
CHICKEN								
Breast, Original Recipe, KFC*	1 Breast/137g	285	13.3	207	24.9	5.6	9.7	0.0
Bucket, Bargain, 10 Piece, KFC*	1 Bucket/1.1kg	2425	139.2	220	20.7	6.3	12.6	0.0
Drumsticks, Original Recipe, KFC*	1 Drumstick/95g	162	9.5	170	11.9	9.1	10.0	0.0
Fillet, Mini, Not In a Bun, KFC*	1 Fillet/50g	116	4.0	232	26.6	14.0	8.0	0.0
Popcorn, Kids, KFC*	1 Serving/50g	137	7.6	274	20.2	14.6	15.2	0.0

	Measure INFO/WEIGHT	per Measure KCAL	FAT	Nutrition Values per 100g / 100ml KCAL	PROT	CARB	FAT	FIBRE
KFC								
CHICKEN								
Popcorn, Large, KFC*	1 Serving/170g	466	25.9	274	20.2	14.6	15.2	0.0
Ribs, Original Recipe, KFC*	1 Rib/126g	238	13.4	188	19.8	4.2	10.6	0.0
Strips, Crispy, KFC*	1 Strip/46g	112	5.4	243	15.4	20.4	11.7	0.0
Thighs, Original Recipe, KFC*	1 Thigh/134g	218	14.2	162	12.6	4.4	10.6	0.0
Wings, Hot, KFC*	1 Wing/58g	102	7.0	175	9.4	7.6	12.1	0.0
Wings, Original Recipe, KFC*	1 Wing/48g	126	3.8	262	25.0	8.3	8.0	0.0
COLESLAW								
Large, KFC*	1 Serving/200g	268	22.4	134	0.8	9.5	11.2	0.0
Regular, KFC*	1 Serving/100g	134	11.2	134	0.8	9.5	11.2	0.0
CORN								
Cobs, Cobette, KFC*	1 Serving/70g	141	8.5	201	4.3	20.1	12.1	0.0
DRESSING								
Caesar, KFC*	1 Sachet/35g	103	10.9	295	19.2	2.7	31.1	0.0
French, KFC*	1 Sachet/45g	30	1.3	66	0.2	2.9	2.9	0.0
Vinaigrette, Low Fat, KFC*	1 Sachet/35g	21	0.8	59	0.5	8.9	2.2	0.0
Yoghurt, Coriander & Chilli, KFC*	1 Sachet/45g	166	16.2	369	2.2	9.3	36.0	0.0
FRIES								
Large, KFC*	1 Serving/193g	448	23.0	232	3.1	32.4	11.9	0.0
Regular, KFC*	1 Serving/133g	308	15.8	232	3.1	32.4	11.9	0.0
GRAVY								
Large, KFC*	1 Serving/204g	144	8.0	71	2.4	7.4	3.9	0.0
Regular, KFC*	1 Serving/102g	72	4.0	71	2.4	7.4	3.9	0.0
ICE CREAM								
Avalanche, KFC*	1 Pot/28g	114	5.1	407	10.4	51.4	18.2	0.0
Soft, KFC*	1 Serving/110g	171	7.0	155	3.7	20.6	6.4	0.0
PIE								
Apple Slice, Colonel's Pies, KFC*	1 Slice/113g	310	13.9	274	1.7	38.9	12.3	0.0
Strawberry Creme, Slice, KFC*	1 Slice/78g	279	15.0	358	5.4	41.0	19.2	2.5
SALAD								
Chicken, Original Recipe, No Dressing, KFC*	1 Salad/292g	270	9.5	92	9.0	7.0	3.3	0.0
Chicken, Zinger, No Dressing, KFC*	1 Salad/285g	307	14.8	108	7.8	8.0	5.2	0.0
Potato, KFC*	1 Serving/160g	229	13.9	143	2.5	14.3	8.7	1.8
WRAP								
Twister, Pulled Chicken, KFC*	1 Wrap/250g	436	14.5	174	8.7	14.4	5.8	0.0
WRAP								
Twister, Salsa, Toasted, KFC*	1 Wrap/222g	516	24.9	232	8.7	24.6	11.2	0.0
Twister, Toasted, KFC*	1 Wrap/217g	509	24.8	235	8.9	24.6	11.5	0.0
Wrapstar, KFC*	1 Wrapstar/239g	642	36.6	269	11.4	25.9	15.3	0.0
KRISPY KREME								
DOUGHNUTS								
Apple Pie, Krispy Kreme*	1 Doughnut/80g	311	17.6	389	6.0	41.0	22.0	1.9
Blueberry, Powdered, Filled, Krispy Kreme*	1 Doughnut/86g	307	17.2	357	7.0	36.0	20.0	5.0
Butterscotch Fudge, Krispy Kreme*	1 Doughnut/93g	372	16.7	400	6.0	53.0	18.0	0.0
Chocolate, Glazed, Krispy Kreme*	1 Doughnut/80g	309	13.6	387	4.0	55.0	17.0	3.0
Chocolate Dreamcake, Krispy Kreme*	1 Doughnut/95g	390	19.0	411	6.0	51.0	20.0	3.0
Chocolate Iced, Creme Filled, Krispy Kreme*	1 Doughnut/87g	372	20.0	428	6.0	46.0	23.0	2.0
Chocolate Iced, Custard Filled, Krispy Kreme*	1 Doughnut/87g	318	16.5	366	5.0	41.0	19.0	1.8
Chocolate Iced, Ring, Glazed, Krispy Kreme*	1 Doughnut/66g	278	13.2	422	5.0	54.0	20.0	1.5
Chocolate Iced, with Creme Filling, Krispy Kreme*	1 Doughnut/87g	350	20.9	402	3.0	42.0	24.0	1.0
Chocolate Iced, with Sprinkles, Krispy Kreme*	1 Doughnut/71g	298	12.7	421	6.0	55.0	18.0	1.6
Chocolate Praline Fudge Cake, Krispy Kreme*	1 Doughnut/73g	346	21.2	474	6.0	43.0	29.0	5.6
Cinnamon Apple, Filled, Krispy Kreme*	1 Doughnut/81g	269	14.6	332	7.0	37.0	18.0	5.0

	Measure INFO/WEIGHT	per Measure KCAL	FAT	Nutrition Values per 100g / 100ml KCAL	PROT	CARB	FAT	FIBRE
KRISPY KREME								
DOUGHNUTS								
Cookie Crunch, Krispy Kreme*	1 Doughnut/73g	316	14.6	433	4.0	56.0	20.0	5.0
Cookies & Kreme, Krispy Kreme*	1 Doughnut/93g	379	16.7	408	4.0	57.0	18.0	0.0
Cruller, Glazed, Krispy Kreme*	1 Doughnut/54g	254	15.6	471	4.0	49.0	29.0	3.0
Glazed, with a Creme Filling, Krispy Kreme*	1 Doughnut/86g	309	15.5	359	5.0	44.0	18.0	4.0
Lemon Filled, Glazed, Krispy Kreme*	1 Doughnut/66g	218	10.5	331	5.0	41.0	16.0	4.0
Lemon Meringue Pie, Krispy Kreme*	1 Doughnut/83g	339	19.7	412	6.0	40.0	24.0	1.8
Maple Iced, Krispy Kreme*	1 Doughnut/66g	279	15.2	422	5.0	49.0	23.0	3.0
Orange Sundae Gloss, Krispy Kreme*	1 Doughnut/81g	338	17.0	418	5.0	50.0	21.0	3.0
Original, Glazed, Krispy Kreme*	1 Doughnut/52g	222	11.9	428	6.0	48.0	23.0	1.1
Raspberry, Glazed, Krispy Kreme*	1 Doughnut/86g	350	17.2	407	6.0	48.0	20.0	1.8
Sour Cream, Krispy Kreme*	1 Doughnut/80g	340	18.4	425	4.0	53.0	23.0	1.0
Strawberries & Kreme, Krispy Kreme*	1 Doughnut/91g	381	20.9	419	5.0	47.0	23.0	1.8
Strawberry Filled, Powdered, Krispy Kreme*	1 Doughnut/74g	248	13.3	335	7.0	36.0	18.0	5.0
Strawberry Gloss, Krispy Kreme*	1 Doughnut/62g	253	12.4	409	5.0	50.0	20.0	1.6
Vanilla, Krispy Kreme*	1 Doughnut/80g	315	13.7	391	4.0	57.0	17.0	2.0
White Chocolate & Almond, Krispy Kreme*	1 Doughnut/93g	421	24.2	453	8.0	45.0	26.0	1.9
MCDONALD'S								
BAGEL								
Toasted, with Strawberry Jam, McDonald's*	1 Bagel/105g	260	1.0	248	8.0	52.0	1.0	3.0
with Bacon, Egg & Cheese, McDonald's*	1 Bagel/173g	455	22.5	263	13.0	26.0	13.0	2.0
with Butter & Jam, McDonald's*	1 Bagel/122g	399	10.2	326	5.9	58.8	8.3	2.2
with Flora & Jam, McDonald's*	1 Bagel/120g	369	6.9	305	6.0	59.4	5.7	2.2
with Philadelphia, McDonald's*	1 Bagel/125g	318	5.9	254	7.7	47.5	4.7	2.1
with Sausage, Egg & Cheese, McDonald's*	1 Bagel/203g	540	28.4	266	14.0	22.0	14.0	2.0
with Sausage & Egg, McDonald's*	1 Bagel/207g	551	26.5	266	13.3	23.3	12.8	1.6
BREAD								
Bagel, Plain, Toasted, McDonald's*	1 Bagel/85g	210	0.8	248	9.0	50.0	1.0	3.0
BREAKFAST								
Big Breakfast, McDonald's*	1 Breakfast/264g	595	37.0	225	11.0	15.0	14.0	1.0
Big Breakfast Bun, McDonald's*	1 Bun/242g	571	32.2	236	13.0	15.1	13.3	0.9
BREAKFAST CEREAL								
Porridge, Oat So Simple, & Jam, McDonald's*	1 Serving/232g	246	5.3	106	4.0	17.0	2.3	0.9
Porridge, Oat So Simple, & Sugar, McDonald's*	1 Serving/215g	205	5.4	95	4.3	13.7	2.5	0.9
Porridge, Oat So Simple, Plain, McDonald's*	1 Serving/212g	195	4.2	92	5.0	13.0	2.0	1.0
BROWNIE								
Belgian Bliss, McDonald's*	1 Serving/85g	390	22.1	459	6.0	51.0	26.0	2.0
BURGERS								
1955 Burger, McDonald's*	1 Burger/281g	655	33.7	233	14.0	18.0	12.0	2.0
Bacon, Chicken & Onion, McDonald's*	1 Burger/255g	660	33.1	259	14.0	22.0	13.0	2.0
Big Mac, Bigger, McDonald's*	1 Burger/324g	714	34.0	220	12.9	18.5	10.5	1.6
Big Mac, McDonald's*	1 Burger/214g	491	25.7	229	13.0	19.0	12.0	2.0
Big Mac, No Sauce, No Cheese, McDonald's*	1 Burger/181g	400	16.0	221	12.2	23.8	8.8	1.1
Big Tasty, McDonald's*	1 Burger/346g	835	52.0	241	13.0	14.0	15.0	1.0
Big Tasty, with Bacon, McDonald's*	1 Burger/359g	890	57.4	248	14.0	14.0	16.0	1.0
Cheeseburger, Bacon, McDonald's*	1 Burger/127g	336	15.3	264	16.0	24.0	12.0	2.0
Cheeseburger, Double, McDonald's*	1 Burger/169g	440	23.7	260	17.0	19.0	14.0	1.0
Cheeseburger, McDonald's*	1 Burger/119g	300	12.0	253	14.4	26.2	10.1	2.5
Chicken & Cheddar Classic, Mcdonald's*	1 Burger/500g	640	32.0	128	7.0	10.6	6.4	0.5
Chicken Fiesta, McDonald's*	1 Burger/240g	610	26.4	254	14.0	24.0	11.0	2.0
Chicken Legend, with Bacon, Cool Mayo, McDonald's*	1 Burger/227g	590	22.7	260	15.0	27.0	10.0	2.0
Festive, Deluxe, McDonald's*	1 Burger/284g	770	45.5	271	16.0	17.0	16.0	1.0
Filet-O-Fish, McDonald's*	1 Burger/150g	350	18.1	232	10.0	24.0	12.0	1.0

	Measure	per Measure		Nutrition Values per 100g / 100ml				
	INFO/WEIGHT	KCAL	FAT	KCAL	PROT	CARB	FAT	FIBRE
MCDONALD'S								
BURGERS								
Filet-O-Fish, No Tartar Sauce, McDonald's*	1 Burger/124g	290	9.0	234	12.1	30.6	7.3	0.8
Hamburger, McDonald's*	1 Burger/104g	250	8.3	240	13.0	29.0	8.0	2.0
Mayo Chicken, McDonald's*	1 Burger/122g	310	13.4	254	10.0	30.0	11.0	2.0
McChicken Sandwich, McDonald's*	1 Sandwich/171g	385	17.2	224	9.0	26.0	10.0	2.0
Quarter Pounder, Bacon with Cheese, McDonald's*	1 Burger/230g	592	33.2	259	16.5	15.4	14.5	1.3
Quarter Pounder, Deluxe, McDonald's*	1 Burger/253g	521	26.8	206	11.4	16.1	10.6	1.7
Quarter Pounder, Double, with Cheese, McDonald's*	1 Burger/275g	710	40.3	259	19.5	12.2	14.7	1.1
Quarter Pounder, McDonald's*	1 Burger/178g	424	19.0	238	14.5	20.9	10.7	2.1
Quarter Pounder, with Cheese, McDonald's*	1 Burger/194g	490	25.3	252	16.0	19.0	13.0	2.0
Summer Chorizo, McDonald's*	1 Burger/238g	650	35.7	273	17.0	17.0	15.0	1.0
The M, McDonald's*	1 Serving/240g	580	28.8	242	16.0	18.0	12.0	1.0
The M, with Bacon, McDonald's*	1 Serving/249g	620	32.4	249	17.0	18.0	13.0	1.0
BURGERS VEGETARIAN								
Vegetable, Deluxe, McDonald's*	1 Burger/181g	411	16.3	227	6.0	30.0	9.0	6.0
BUTTER								
Country Life, McDonald's*	1 Pack/11g	85	9.0	752	0.0	0.0	80.0	0.0
CAKE								
Birthday, McDonald's*	1 Serving/158g	640	22.6	405	2.7	65.4	14.3	1.0
CARROTS								
Sticks, McDonald's*	1 Bag/80g	30	0.0	38	0.0	8.0	0.0	2.0
CHEESE								
Mozzarella, Dippers, McDonald's*	3 Dippers/85g	265	13.6	312	13.0	27.0	16.0	1.0
Soft, Philadelphia, Light, McDonald's*	1 Serving/35g	55	3.9	157	9.0	3.0	11.0	0.0
CHICKEN								
McNuggets, 4 Pieces, McDonald's*	4 Pieces/70g	170	9.3	238	13.0	19.0	13.0	1.0
McNuggets, 6 Pieces, McDonald's*	6 Pieces/105g	250	13.7	238	13.0	19.0	13.0	1.0
McNuggets, 9 Pieces, McDonald's*	9 Pieces/157g	375	20.5	238	13.0	19.0	13.0	1.0
Selects, 3 Pieces, McDonald's*	3 Pieces/130g	365	19.6	280	16.0	20.0	15.0	1.0
Selects, 5 Pieces, McDonald's*	5 Pieces/219g	612	32.8	280	16.0	20.0	15.0	1.0
COFFEE								
Black, Large, McDonald's*	1 Serving/428ml	0	0.0	0	0.0	0.0	0.0	0.0
Black, Regular, McDonald's*	1 Serving/312ml	0	0.0	0	0.0	0.0	0.0	0.0
Cappuccino, Large, McDonald's*	1 Serving/307ml	120	3.1	39	3.0	4.0	1.0	0.0
Cappuccino, Regular, McDonald's*	1 Serving/231ml	90	2.3	39	3.0	4.0	1.0	0.0
Caramel Frappe, Regular, McDonald's*	1 Serving/312ml	450	19.0	144	2.2	20.5	6.1	0.0
Espresso, Double Shot, McDonald's*	1 Double/60ml	0	0.0	0	0.0	0.0	0.0	0.0
Espresso, Single Shot, McDonald's*	1 Serving/30ml	0	0.0	0	0.0	0.0	0.0	0.0
Latte, Large, McDonald's*	1 Serving/451ml	185	4.5	41	3.0	4.0	1.0	0.0
Latte, Regular, McDonald's*	1 Serving/337ml	135	3.4	40	3.0	4.0	1.0	0.0
White, Large, McDonald's*	1 Serving/428ml	30	0.0	7	0.0	1.0	0.0	0.0
White, Regular, McDonald's*	1 Serving/313ml	25	0.0	8	1.0	1.0	0.0	0.0
COLA								
Coca-Cola, Diet, McDonald's*	1 Med/405ml	4	0.0	1	0.0	0.0	0.0	0.0
Coca-Cola, McDonald's*	1 Med/405ml	170	0.0	42	0.0	10.0	0.0	0.0
Coke, Zero, McDonald's*	1 Serving/200ml	2	0.0	1	0.0	0.0	0.0	0.0
CREAMER								
Uht, McDonald's*	1 Cup/14ml	17	1.4	123	4.2	4.2	10.0	0.0
CROUTONS								
McDonald's*	1 Sachet/14g	60	2.0	426	11.8	63.4	14.0	2.7
DIP								
BBQ, McDonald's*	1 Pot/50g	83	0.0	166	0.0	37.0	0.0	0.0
Caramelised Onion, McDonald's*	1 Dip/31g	45	1.9	144	3.0	19.0	6.0	3.0

	Measure INFO/WEIGHT	per Measure KCAL	FAT	Nutrition Values per 100g / 100ml KCAL	PROT	CARB	FAT	FIBRE
MCDONALD'S								
DIP								
Sour Cream & Chive, McDonald's*	1 Pot/50g	150	16.0	300	2.0	2.0	32.0	4.0
Sweet Chilli, McDonald's*	1 Pot/31g	80	0.9	256	0.0	58.0	3.0	0.0
DOUGHNUTS								
Chocolate Donut, McDonald's*	1 Donut/79g	345	16.2	437	5.7	43.8	20.5	1.0
Chocolate Donut, McMini, McDonald's*	1 Donut/17g	64	3.0	375	6.8	46.9	17.8	1.6
Cinnamon Donut, McDonald's*	1 Donut/72g	302	18.1	419	5.1	43.1	25.1	3.8
Sugared Donut, McDonald's*	1 Donut/49g	205	14.7	418	6.0	35.0	30.0	4.0
DRESSING								
Balsamic, Low Fat, McDonald's*	1 Sachet/33g	20	1.0	60	0.0	9.0	3.0	0.0
Caesar, Low Fat, McDonald's*	1 Sachet/80g	55	1.6	68	2.0	10.0	2.0	0.0
French, Low Fat, McDonald's*	1 Serving/22g	13	0.6	58	0.5	7.1	2.6	1.0
FANTA								
Orange, McDonald's*	1 Super/750ml	315	0.0	42	0.0	10.0	0.0	0.0
FISH FINGERS								
McDonald's*	3 Fingers/84g	195	9.2	232	15.0	19.0	11.0	1.0
FRIES								
French, Large, McDonald's*	1 Serving/160g	460	22.4	288	3.0	38.0	14.0	4.0
French, Medium, McDonald's*	1 Serving/114g	330	16.0	289	3.0	37.0	14.0	4.0
French, Small, McDonald's*	1 Serving/80g	230	11.2	288	2.0	38.0	14.0	4.0
FRUIT								
Bag, McDonald's*	1 Pack/80g	40	0.8	50	0.0	12.0	1.0	2.0
FRUIT DRINK								
Fruitizz, Sparkling, McDonald's*	1 Drink/250ml	160	0.0	64	0.4	15.6	0.0	0.0
FRUIT SHOOT								
Robinsons, McDonald's*	1 Bottle200ml	10	0.0	5	0.0	1.0	0.0	0.0
HASH BROWNS								
McDonald's*	1 Hash Brown/53g	140	9.0	264	2.0	26.0	17.0	2.0
HOT CHOCOLATE								
McDonald's*	1 Serving/330ml	164	3.6	50	0.7	8.8	1.1	0.0
HOT DOG								
& Ketchup, McDonald's*	1 Serving/116g	296	14.6	255	9.6	25.8	12.6	1.3
ICE CREAM								
Smartie, McDonald's*	1 Pot/120g	260	9.5	216	3.4	33.3	7.9	1.0
ICE CREAM CONE								
McDonald's*	1 Cone/90g	141	4.5	156	4.5	24.4	5.0	0.0
with Flake, McDonald's*	1 Cone/107g	204	7.7	191	4.8	27.0	7.2	0.0
JAM								
Strawberry, McDonald's*	1 Pack/20g	50	0.0	250	0.0	60.0	0.0	0.0
JUICE								
Tropicana, McDonald's*	1 Bottle/250ml	108	0.0	43	1.0	9.0	0.0	0.4
KETCHUP								
Tomato, McDonald's*	1 Serving/23g	25	0.0	109	0.0	26.0	0.0	0.0
LEMONADE								
Sprite, Z, McDonald's*	1 Lge/500ml	5	0.0	1	0.0	0.0	0.0	0.0
MARGARINE								
Flora, Original, McDonald's*	1 Serving/10g	55	6.0	550	0.0	0.0	60.0	0.0
MCFLURRY								
After Eight, McDonald's*	1 McFlurry/206g	400	16.5	194	3.0	27.0	8.0	1.0
Cadbury, Shortcake, Limited Edition, McDonald's*	1 McFlurry/206g	385	14.4	187	3.0	28.0	7.0	1.0
Chocolate, Cornetto, McDonald's*	1 McFlurry/207g	400	16.6	193	3.0	29.0	8.0	1.0
Cornetto, Mint Choc, McDonald's*	1 McFlurry/207g	400	16.6	193	3.0	29.0	8.0	1.0
Creme Egg, Cadbury's, McDonald's*	1 McFlurry/203g	381	12.9	188	2.9	29.8	6.3	0.5

	Measure INFO/WEIGHT	per Measure KCAL	FAT	Nutrition Values per 100g / 100ml KCAL	PROT	CARB	FAT	FIBRE
MCDONALD'S								
MCFLURRY								
Crunchie, McDonald's*	1 McFlurry/185g	330	11.1	178	3.0	28.0	6.0	1.0
Dairy Milk, McDonald's*	1 McFlurry/184g	340	12.9	184	3.0	28.0	7.0	1.0
Dairy Milk, with Caramel, McDonald's*	1 McFlurry/206g	385	13.0	187	2.9	29.1	6.3	0.0
Flake, Chocolate, McDonald's*	1 McFlurry/206ml	400	14.4	194	3.0	29.0	7.0	0.0
Flake, Raspberry, McDonald's*	1 McFlurry/205ml	370	12.3	180	3.0	27.0	6.0	0.0
Jammie Dodger, McDonald's*	1 McFlurry/128g	256	8.2	200	3.9	33.6	6.4	0.3
Raspberry, McDonald's*	1 McFlurry/206ml	370	12.3	180	3.0	27.0	6.0	0.0
Rolo, McDonald's*	1 McFlurry/205g	390	13.3	190	4.0	29.2	6.5	0.1
Smarties, McDonald's*	1 McFlurry/185g	330	11.1	178	3.0	28.0	6.0	1.0
Strawberry, Cornetto, McDonald's*	1 McFlurry/207g	375	12.4	181	3.0	29.0	6.0	0.0
Terry's Chocolate Orange, McDonald's*	1 McFlurry/204g	405	16.3	199	3.0	28.0	8.0	0.0
Toffee Swirl, Oreo Cookie, McDonald's*	1 McFlurry/206ml	400	12.4	194	3.0	31.0	6.0	1.0
Wispa Gold, McDonald's*	1 McFlurry/206g	395	14.0	192	2.9	29.1	6.8	0.5
Yorkie, McDonald's*	1 McFlurry/204g	379	14.9	186	3.4	27.0	7.3	0.8
MCMUFFIN								
Bacon & Egg, Double, McDonald's*	1 McMuffin/161g	395	21.0	244	15.0	16.0	13.0	1.0
Bacon & Egg, McDonald's*	1 McMuffin/146g	345	17.5	237	14.0	18.0	12.0	1.0
Sausage, No Egg, No Cheese, McDonald's*	1 McMuffin/96g	310	18.0	323	12.5	29.2	18.8	4.2
Sausage & Egg, Double, McDonald's*	1 McMuffin/222g	560	35.6	252	16.0	12.0	16.0	1.0
Sausage & Egg, McDonald's*	1 McMuffin/174g	420	24.3	242	14.0	16.0	14.0	1.0
Scrambled Egg, McDonald's*	1 McMuffin/147g	294	14.1	200	10.9	17.5	9.6	1.3
MELT								
Toasted Ham & Cheese, McDonald's*	1 Serving/100g	239	8.0	239	11.2	30.6	8.0	1.8
MILK								
Fresh, Serving, McDonald's*	1 Serving/14ml	10	0.0	69	0.0	7.0	0.0	0.0
Organic, McDonald's*	1 Bottle/250ml	118	5.0	47	4.0	5.0	2.0	0.0
MILK SHAKE								
Banana, Large, McDonald's*	1 Serving/432ml	545	13.0	126	3.0	21.0	3.0	0.0
Banana, Medium, McDonald's*	1 Serving/338ml	425	10.1	126	3.0	21.0	3.0	0.0
Banana, Small, McDonald's*	1 Serving/178ml	226	5.3	127	3.0	21.0	3.0	0.0
Cadburys Dairy Milk, Caramel, Medium, McDonald's*	1 Serving/394ml	480	15.8	122	3.0	19.0	4.0	1.0
Chocolate, Large, McDonald's*	1 Serving/431ml	530	12.9	123	3.0	20.0	3.0	0.0
Chocolate, Medium, McDonald's*	1 Serving/337ml	425	10.1	126	3.0	21.0	3.0	0.0
Chocolate, Small, McDonald's*	1 Serving/177ml	225	5.3	127	3.0	21.0	3.0	0.0
Starburst Mixed Berry Flavour, McDonald's*	1 Serving/177ml	200	4.0	113	2.8	20.3	2.3	0.0
Strawberry, Large, McDonald's*	1 Serving/432ml	540	13.0	125	3.0	21.0	3.0	0.0
Strawberry, Medium, McDonald's*	1 Serving/336ml	420	10.1	125	3.0	21.0	3.0	0.0
Strawberry, Small, McDonald's*	1 Serving/177ml	220	5.3	124	3.0	21.0	3.0	0.0
Vanilla, Large, McDonald's*	1 Serving/431ml	535	12.9	124	3.0	21.0	3.0	0.0
Vanilla, Medium, McDonald's*	1 Serving/336ml	420	10.1	125	3.0	21.0	3.0	0.0
Vanilla, Small, McDonald's*	1 Serving/177ml	220	5.3	124	3.0	21.0	3.0	0.0
MUFFIN								
Blueberry, Low Fat, McDonald's*	1 Muffin/126g	300	3.8	238	5.0	50.0	3.0	2.0
Double Chocolate, McDonald's*	1 Muffin/123g	515	28.3	419	6.0	46.0	23.0	2.0
ONION RINGS								
McDonald's*	1 Serving/99g	245	11.9	247	4.0	31.0	12.0	3.0
PANCAKE								
& Sausage, with Syrup, McDonald's*	1 Serving/223g	615	20.1	275	8.0	42.0	9.0	2.0
& Syrup, McDonald's*	1 Pack/175g	515	14.0	294	4.0	52.0	8.0	2.0
PIE								
Apple, McDonald's*	1 Pie/80g	231	12.8	289	2.0	35.0	16.0	0.0
Festive, McDonald's*	1 Pie/84g	310	17.6	369	4.0	42.0	21.0	1.0

	Measure INFO/WEIGHT	per Measure KCAL	FAT	Nutrition Values per 100g / 100ml KCAL	PROT	CARB	FAT	FIBRE
MCDONALD'S								
POTATO WEDGES								
McDonald's*	1 Serving/177g	349	17.7	197	3.3	23.3	10.0	2.8
QUORN*								
Burger, Premiere, McDonald's*	1 Burger/210g	311	6.1	148	9.1	24.2	2.9	2.7
ROLL								
Bacon, McBacon, McDonald's*	1 Roll/122g	349	14.0	286	13.5	30.5	11.5	1.7
Bacon, with Brown Sauce, McDonald's*	1 Roll/126g	350	8.8	278	15.0	37.0	7.0	2.0
Bacon, with Tomato Ketchup, McDonald's*	1 Roll/126g	345	8.8	273	15.0	36.0	7.0	2.0
SALAD								
Chicken, no Bacon, Grilled, McDonald's*	1 Salad/255g	115	2.6	45	7.0	2.0	1.0	1.0
Chicken, with Bacon, Grilled, McDonald's*	1 Salad/266g	164	5.3	62	9.0	2.0	2.0	1.0
Crispy Chicken, no Bacon, McDonald's*	1 Salad/281g	325	16.0	116	7.1	8.5	5.7	1.4
Crispy Chicken, with Bacon, McDonald's*	1 Salad/292g	326	14.6	111	10.0	7.0	5.0	1.0
Garden, Side, no Dressing, McDonald's*	1 Salad/91g	10	0.0	11	1.0	2.0	0.0	1.0
Garden, Side, with Balsamic Dressing, McDonald's*	1 Salad/128g	91	3.8	71	1.0	11.0	3.0	1.0
SANDWICH								
Deli, Chicken, Salad, McDonald's*	1 Sandwich/216g	350	8.6	162	7.0	24.0	4.0	2.0
Deli, Chicken, Sweet Chilli, McDonald's*	1 Sandwich/250g	570	22.5	228	12.0	28.0	9.0	2.0
Deli, Chicken & Bacon, McDonald's*	1 Sandwich/192g	405	13.4	211	10.0	27.0	7.0	2.0
Deli, Spicy Veggie, McDonald's*	1 Sandwich/216g	555	21.6	257	6.0	36.0	10.0	4.0
SAUCE								
Barbeque, McDonald's*	1 Serving/50g	85	1.0	170	0.0	38.0	2.0	0.0
Curry, Sweet, McDonald's*	1 Serving/29g	50	0.9	171	0.0	38.0	3.0	3.0
Mustard, Mild, McDonald's*	1 Serving/30g	64	3.6	212	1.0	24.8	12.1	0.0
Sweet & Sour, McDonald's*	1 Serving/29g	50	0.0	172	0.0	38.0	0.0	0.0
SUNDAE								
Hot Caramel, McDonald's*	1 Sundae/189g	357	8.3	189	3.8	33.9	4.4	0.0
Hot Fudge, McDonald's*	1 Sundae/187g	352	10.7	188	4.5	30.0	5.7	0.0
No Topping, McDonald's*	1 Sundae/149g	219	7.6	147	4.2	21.6	5.1	0.0
Strawberry, McDonald's*	1 Sundae/214g	360	8.6	168	2.0	33.0	4.0	0.0
Toffee, McDonald's*	1 Sundae/182g	350	9.1	192	3.0	34.0	5.0	1.0
SYRUP								
Pancake, McDonald's*	1 Pot/55g	190	0.0	345	0.0	84.0	0.0	0.0
TEA								
with Milk, McDonald's*	1 Serving/333ml	10	3.3	3	0.0	1.0	1.0	0.0
WRAP								
Breakfast, with Brown Sauce, McDonald's*	1 Wrap/229g	595	30.0	260	10.92358.0		13.1	1.7
Breakfast, with Tomato Ketchup, McDonald's*	1 Wrap/229g	595	30.0	260	10.9	23.6	13.1	1.7
Chicken, BBQ, Snack, McDonald's*	1 Wrap/115g	300	12.0	261	10.4	30.4	10.4	1.7
Chicken, Cajun, McDonald's*	1 Wrap/222g	585	33.4	263	9.0	22.0	15.0	2.0
Chicken, Cheese & Bacon Snack, McDonald's*	1 Wrap/100g	360	18.0	360	14.0	33.0	18.0	2.0
Chicken, Fajita, McDonald's*	1 Wrap/259g	647	31.1	250	8.9	26.7	12.0	1.2
Chicken, Grilled, Salad, McDonald's*	1 Wrap/221g	335	11.0	152	7.2	19.9	5.0	1.8
Chicken, Snack, McDonald's*	1 Wrap/112g	266	11.2	237	10.0	29.0	10.0	2.0
Garlic & Herb, Snack, McDonald's*	1 Wrap/121g	335	18.2	276	12.0	25.0	15.0	2.0
Oriental, Snack, McDonald's*	1 Wrap/127g	265	10.1	209	10.0	25.0	8.0	2.0
Vegetable, Spicy, McDonald's*	1 Wrap/203g	445	16.3	219	5.0	29.0	8.0	5.0
NANDO'S								
BREAD								
Garlic, Nando's*	1 Regular/100g	336	16.4	336	6.7	39.0	16.4	2.7
BURGERS								
Bean, Nando's*	1 Burger/265g	533	19.6	201	7.9	24.5	7.4	2.3
Chicken Breast Fillet, Nando's*	1 Burger/232g	368	6.3	159	15.1	17.9	2.7	1.3

	Measure INFO/WEIGHT	per Measure KCAL	FAT	Nutrition Values per 100g / 100ml KCAL	PROT	CARB	FAT	FIBRE
NANDO'S								
BURGERS								
Double Chicken Breast, Nando's*	1 Burger/309g	495	8.1	160	20.4	13.3	2.6	1.0
Veggie, Nando's*	1 Burger/265g	443	11.7	167	6.7	24.3	4.4	2.0
CHEESE								
Cheddar, Nando's*	1 Serving/20g	78	6.4	390	26.0	0.0	32.0	0.0
Halloumi, Grilled, Nando's*	1 Serving/54g	177	13.8	328	22.0	2.4	25.6	0.0
CHICKEN								
¼ Breast, Peri Peri, Nando's*	¼ Breast/193g	309	7.2	160	29.9	1.8	3.7	0.0
¼ Leg, Peri Peri, Nando's*	1 Serving/125g	314	19.6	251	27.1	0.3	15.7	0.0
½ Peri Peri, Nando's*	½ Chicken/318g	623	26.9	196	28.8	1.2	8.4	0.0
Breast, Fillet Strips, Nandinos, Nando's*	1 Serving/92g	130	1.8	141	30.6	0.2	2.0	0.0
Butterfly, Peri Peri, Flame Grilled, Nando's*	1 Serving/190g	310	8.9	163	30.1	0.1	4.7	0.5
Whole, Nando's*	1 Chicken/636g	1245	53.7	196	28.8	1.2	8.4	0.0
Wings, 10, Nando's*	10 Wings/236g	630	37.6	267	30.8	0.1	15.9	0.5
Wings, 3, Nando's*	3 Wings/71g	190	11.3	268	30.8	0.1	15.9	0.6
Wings, 5, Nando's*	5 Wings/118g	315	18.8	267	30.8	0.1	15.9	0.5
CHIPS								
Large, Nando's*	1 Serving/480g	1241	49.7	259	2.8	36.8	10.4	3.8
Regular, Nando's*	1 Serving/180g	465	18.6	258	2.8	36.8	10.3	3.8
COLESLAW								
Large, Nando's*	1 Serving/300g	528	48.0	176	0.8	8.0	16.0	1.7
Regular, Nando's*	1 Serving/150g	264	24.0	176	0.8	8.0	16.0	1.7
CORN								
On The Cob, Large, Nando's*	1 Lge/138g	138	3.7	100	5.7	22.0	2.7	4.6
CRISPS								
Hot Peri Peri, Nando's*	1 Bag/40g	206	10.8	514	5.1	57.4	27.0	3.4
Smoky Barbeque Peri Peri, Nando's*	½ Pack/75g	375	20.2	500	5.1	57.4	27.0	3.4
DESSERT								
Carrot Cake, Nando's*	1 Serving/215g	839	62.0	390	3.7	26.7	28.8	0.9
Choc-a-Lot Cake, Nando's*	1 Serving/182g	650	44.0	357	4.5	33.0	24.2	1.7
Chocolate Cheesecake, Nando's*	1 Serving/153g	565	40.8	369	5.3	28.0	26.7	0.8
Gooey Caramel Cheesecake, Nando's*	1 Serving/158g	582	41.9	368	5.3	28.9	26.5	0.8
Nata, Custard Tart, Nando's*	1 Serving/60g	168	6.5	280	5.5	40.3	10.8	2.0
FROZEN YOGHURT								
Banana, Nando's*	1 Serving/100g	87	0.1	87	3.3	18.2	0.1	0.1
Chocolate, Nando's*	1 Serving/100g	78	0.2	78	2.5	16.3	0.2	0.6
Strawberry, Nando's*	1 Serving/100g	71	0.2	71	2.5	15.2	0.2	0.1
Vanilla, Nando's*	1 Serving/100ml	70	0.1	70	2.5	15.0	0.1	0.1
HOUMOUS								
with Peri Peri Drizzle & Pitta, Nando's*	1 Serving/305g	825	34.3	270	7.2	34.1	11.2	3.2
ICE CREAM								
Chocolate, Nando's*	1 Serving/90g	191	10.0	212	2.2	24.0	11.1	1.0
Passion Fruit, Nando's*	1 Serving/90g	122	0.0	136	0.3	32.9	0.0	2.5
Strawberry, Nando's*	1 Serving/90g	164	6.3	182	2.4	24.8	7.0	0.5
Toffee, Nando's*	1 Serving/90g	178	7.3	198	3.9	20.8	8.1	1.0
Vanilla, Nando's*	1 Serving/90g	199	10.4	221	3.8	20.7	11.6	0.0
ICE LOLLY								
Chilly Billy, Nando's*	1 Lolly/70g	30	0.1	43	0.1	10.1	0.1	0.0
MASH								
Creamy, Large, Nando's*	1 Large/400g	540	31.6	135	1.7	13.0	7.9	2.5
Creamy, Regular, Nando's*	1 Regular/200g	270	15.8	135	1.7	13.0	7.9	2.5
Sweet Potato, Fino Side, Nando's*	1 Serving/200g	248	4.2	124	2.2	22.7	2.1	2.7

	Measure INFO/WEIGHT	per Measure KCAL	FAT	Nutrition Values per 100g / 100ml KCAL	PROT	CARB	FAT	FIBRE
NANDO'S								
NUTS								
Peri-Peri, Nando's*	1 Serving/100g	627	53.6	627	23.6	7.9	53.6	9.2
OLIVES								
Spicy, Mixed, Nando's*	1 Bowl/125g	133	13.0	106	0.9	0.6	10.4	3.0
PEAS								
Macho, Large, Nando's*	1 Serving/280g	336	20.7	120	4.7	7.0	7.4	4.2
Macho, Regular, Nando's*	1 Serving/140g	168	10.4	120	4.7	7.0	7.4	4.2
PITTA								
Bean, Nando's*	1 Pitta/240g	529	18.1	220	8.4	28.8	7.5	2.1
Chicken, Breast, Nando's*	1 Pitta/207g	364	4.8	176	16.7	22.0	2.3	1.0
Chicken, with Mayonnaise, Double, Nando's*	1 Pitta/275g	460	6.1	167	20.0	16.6	2.2	0.7
Veggie, Nando's*	1 Pitta/240g	439	10.2	183	7.1	28.5	4.2	1.8
RATATOUILLE								
Fino Side, Nando's*	1 Serving/180g	108	6.5	60	1.3	3.8	3.6	3.4
RICE								
Spicy, Large, Nando's*	1 Serving/300g	546	10.8	182	3.0	32.8	3.6	3.4
Spicy, Regular, Nando's*	1 Serving/150g	273	5.4	182	3.0	32.8	3.6	3.4
ROLL								
Portuguese, with Chicken Livers, Nando's*	1 Serving/220g	485	14.8	220	17.5	23.2	6.8	2.0
Prego Steak, Nando's*	1 Roll/220g	573	24.1	260	19.4	22.2	11.0	2.6
SALAD								
Avocado & Green Bean, Nando's*	1 Serving/245g	305	25.8	124	2.4	3.4	10.5	3.3
Caesar, No Chicken, Nando's*	1 Salad/226g	287	22.0	127	3.4	6.5	9.8	1.1
Mediterranean, Nando's*	1 Salad/290g	294	18.5	101	3.3	3.9	6.4	1.6
Mixed Leaf, Nando's*	1 Serving/115g	22	0.4	19	1.4	2.0	0.3	1.3
Side, Regular, Nando's*	1 Salad/53g	10	0.2	19	1.8	1.5	0.3	1.1
VEGETABLES								
Roasted, Saucy, Nando's*	1 Serving/103g	62	3.7	60	1.3	3.8	3.6	3.4
WRAP								
Beanie, Nando's*	1 Wrap/320g	716	30.1	224	7.2	26.2	9.4	2.1
Chicken, Breast, Fillet, Double, Nando's*	1 Wrap/360g	670	23.0	186	16.2	16.8	6.4	1.0
Chicken, Breast, Fillet, Nando's*	1 Wrap/280g	577	21.5	206	12.1	21.5	7.7	1.2
Portabello Mushroom & Halloumi Cheese, Nando's*	1 Wrap/344g	846	55.6	246	6.5	18.0	16.2	1.2
Veggie, Nando's*	1 Wrap/320g	677	26.1	212	7.0	26.9	8.2	2.5
PIZZA EXPRESS								
ANTIPASTO								
Italian, Classic, Sharing Starter, Pizza Express*	½ Serving/252g	562	29.7	223	11.1	19.1	11.8	2.1
AUBERGINE								
Parmigiana, Melanzane, Main, Pizza Express*	1 Serving/428g	728	56.1	170	4.9	7.9	13.1	0.8
BREAD								
Garlic, Starter, Pizza Express*	1 Serving/105g	239	4.9	228	7.8	39.8	4.7	2.5
Garlic, with Mozzarella, Starter, Pizza Express*	1 Serving/131g	304	9.3	232	11.2	32.1	7.1	2.0
BROWNIES								
GF, Dolcetti, Pizza Express*	1 Serving/55g	216	11.9	392	4.6	43.6	21.6	0.1
Piccolo, Pizza Express*	1 Serving/55g	216	11.9	392	4.6	43.6	21.6	0.1
BRUSCHETTA								
Con Funghi, Starter, Pizza Express*	1 Serving/272g	367	13.3	135	4.0	19.2	4.9	1.3
Starter, Pizza Express*	1 Serving/218g	392	19.6	180	4.5	21.2	9.0	1.6
CAKE								
Chocolate Fudge, & Ice Cream, Pizza Express*	1 Serving/161g	423	18.5	263	4.7	34.9	11.5	1.2
Chocolate Fudge, Mini, Dolcetti, Pizza Express*	1 Serving/85g	251	11.2	295	4.5	39.1	13.2	1.6
CALZONE								
Salami E Salsiccia, Main, Pizza Express*	1 Calzone/518g	984	50.8	190	8.7	17.5	9.8	1.4

	Measure INFO/WEIGHT	per Measure KCAL	FAT	Nutrition Values per 100g / 100ml KCAL	PROT	CARB	FAT	FIBRE
PIZZA EXPRESS								
CALZONE								
Verdure, Main, Pizza Express*	1 Calzone/564g	1280	80.7	227	6.4	19.0	14.3	1.4
CAVATAPPI								
Formaggi, Main, Pizza Express*	1 Serving/544g	1093	56.0	201	9.0	17.9	10.3	0.9
CHEESECAKE								
& Ice Cream, Pizza Express*	1 Serving/164g	464	28.9	283	4.8	26.6	17.6	0.5
CHIPS								
Polenta, Side, Pizza Express*	1 Serving/183g	441	23.4	241	3.7	27.4	12.8	1.2
DESSERT								
Caffe Reale, Dolcetti, Pizza Express*	1 Serving/65g	190	11.7	293	3.1	29.9	18.0	1.9
Chocolate Glory, Pizza Express*	1 Serving/309g	686	23.5	222	4.2	34.1	7.6	1.1
Semi Freddo Reale, Dolcetti, Pizza Express*	1 Serving/40g	134	8.8	336	2.6	29.0	22.1	0.3
Toffee Fudge Glory, Pizza Express*	1 Serving/295g	631	20.1	214	3.7	34.6	6.8	0.4
DOUGH BALLS								
& Garlic Butter, with Side Salad, Piccolo, Pizza Express*	1 Serving/158g	186	8.2	118	3.1	15.1	5.2	1.4
Doppio, Sharing Starter, Pizza Express*	½ Serving/130g	376	19.0	289	7.5	32.8	14.6	2.1
Starter, Pizza Express*	1 Serving/120g	347	16.8	289	7.0	35.0	14.0	2.2
GELATO								
Chocolate, Coppa, Pizza Express*	1 Serving/125g	252	10.5	202	4.5	27.6	8.4	1.8
Strawberry, Coppa, Pizza Express*	1 Serving/125g	215	3.4	172	0.7	35.8	2.7	0.3
Vanilla, Coppa, Pizza Express*	1 Serving/125g	245	9.1	196	4.7	28.1	7.3	0.5
Vanilla, Piccolo, Pizza Express*	1 Serving/60g	113	4.5	188	4.5	25.7	7.5	0.5
Vanilla, with Chocolate Sauce, Piccolo, Pizza Express*	1 Serving/70g	146	4.6	209	4.1	33.3	6.6	0.9
Vanilla, with Cone, Piccolo, Pizza Express*	1 Serving/62g	120	4.6	194	4.6	27.0	7.5	0.6
Vanilla, with Fresh Strawberry, Piccolo, Pizza Express*	1 Serving/62g	120	4.6	194	4.6	27.0	7.5	0.6
Vanilla, with Fruit Coulis, Piccolo, Pizza Express*	1 Serving/70g	125	4.6	178	3.9	26.3	6.5	0.7
Vanilla, with Fudge Cubes, Piccolo, Pizza Express*	1 Serving/70g	153	5.8	219	4.1	32.0	8.3	0.4
Vanilla, with Toffee Sauce, Piccolo, Pizza Express*	1 Serving/70g	143	4.5	204	3.9	32.7	6.4	0.4
LASAGNE								
Classica, Main, Pizza Express*	1 Serving/427g	623	32.9	146	9.0	10.4	7.7	0.1
Verde, Main, Pizza Express*	1 Serving/468g	744	52.4	159	4.4	9.7	11.2	0.2
PASTA								
Bianca, Piccolo, Main, Pizza Express*	1 Serving/219g	385	15.8	176	4.4	23.0	7.2	1.2
Bolognese, Piccolo, Main, Pizza Express*	1 Serving/256g	333	7.4	130	5.8	20.0	2.9	1.0
Burro, Piccolo, Main, Pizza Express*	1 Serving/115g	310	12.1	270	6.3	37.7	10.5	2.2
Napoletana, Piccolo, Main, Pizza Express*	1 Serving/219g	311	7.2	142	4.1	24.1	3.3	1.5
Pollo, Main, Pizza Express*	1 Serving/573g	923	47.0	161	7.9	14.0	8.2	0.8
PIE								
Banoffee, & Ice Cream, Pizza Express*	1 Serving/142g	524	38.9	369	2.1	28.4	27.4	2.6
PIZZA								
American, Classic, GF, Pizza Express*	1 Pizza/381g	1020	45.5	268	6.6	33.4	12.0	0.8
American, Classic, Main, Pizza Express*	1 Pizza/376g	805	33.5	214	10.3	24.2	8.9	1.6
American, Hot, Classic, GF, Pizza Express*	1 Pizza/401g	1023	45.6	255	6.3	31.7	11.4	0.8
American, Hot, Leggera, Main, Pizza Express*	1 Pizza/269g	395	15.6	147	8.1	16.5	5.8	1.3
American, Light Mozzarella, Piccolo, GF, Pizza Express*	1 Pizza/180g	408	14.8	227	7.0	31.2	8.2	0.8
American, Light Mozzarella, Piccolo, Pizza Express*	1 Pizza/190g	338	9.7	178	10.4	24.0	5.1	1.6
American, Piccolo, GF, Pizza Express*	1 Pizza/171g	424	23.0	248	6.3	32.8	13.5	0.8
American, Piccolo, Pizza Express*	1 Pizza/181g	355	11.9	196	9.9	25.3	6.6	1.7
American Hot, Classic, Main, Pizza Express*	1 Pizza/396g	808	33.3	204	9.8	23.2	8.4	1.6
American Hot, Romana, Main, Pizza Express*	1 Pizza/417g	863	37.5	207	10.4	22.1	9.0	1.5
Caprina Rossa, Romana, Main, Pizza Express*	1 Pizza/524g	901	39.3	172	7.7	19.4	7.5	1.5
Da Morire, Romana, Main, Pizza Express*	1 Pizza/537g	940	44.0	175	7.7	17.9	8.2	2.1
Diavolo, Romana, Main, Pizza Express*	1 Pizza/477g	978	42.9	205	11.0	20.2	9.0	1.6

	Measure INFO/WEIGHT	per Measure KCAL	FAT	Nutrition Values per 100g / 100ml KCAL	PROT	CARB	FAT	FIBRE
PIZZA EXPRESS								
PIZZA								
Etna, Romana, Main, Pizza Express*	1 Pizza/502g	1039	46.7	207	11.3	20.1	9.3	1.4
Fiorentina, Classic, GF, Pizza Express*	1 Pizza/493g	1045	45.1	212	6.2	26.2	9.1	0.7
Fiorentina, Classic, Main, Pizza Express*	1 Pizza/488g	830	32.7	170	9.0	19.1	6.7	1.4
Four Seasons, Classic, GF, Pizza Express*	1 Pizza/380g	894	35.0	235	4.3	33.4	9.2	1.0
Four Seasons, Classic, Main, Pizza Express*	1 Pizza/375g	679	22.9	181	8.0	24.4	6.1	1.9
Giardiniera, Classic, GF, Pizza Express*	1 Pizza/525g	1115	55.8	212	4.1	25.0	10.6	1.3
Giardiniera, Classic, Main, Pizza Express*	1 Pizza/520g	900	43.7	173	6.7	18.4	8.4	1.9
Il Padrino, Romana, Main, Pizza Express*	1 Pizza/532g	1123	59.1	211	9.7	18.6	11.1	1.4
La Reine, Classic, GF, Pizza Express*	1 Pizza/418g	954	38.2	228	6.0	30.4	9.1	0.9
La Reine, Classic, Main, Pizza Express*	1 Pizza/413g	739	26.0	179	9.4	22.1	6.3	1.7
La Reine, Light Mozzarella, Piccolo, GF, Pizza Express*	1 Pizza/203g	396	12.9	195	6.7	27.8	6.4	0.8
La Reine, Light Mozzarella, Piccolo, Pizza Express*	1 Pizza/213g	326	7.7	153	9.7	21.6	3.6	1.6
La Reine, Piccolo, GF, Pizza Express*	1 Pizza/193g	411	15.2	213	6.1	29.2	7.9	0.9
La Reine, Piccolo, Pizza Express*	1 Pizza/203g	341	9.9	168	9.3	22.6	4.9	1.7
Margherita, Classic, GF, Pizza Express*	1 Pizza/359g	899	45.5	250	5.5	35.1	12.7	0.8
Margherita, Classic, Main, Pizza Express*	1 Pizza/354g	683	22.7	193	9.4	25.7	6.4	1.7
Margherita, Light Mozzarella, Piccolo, Pizza Express*	1 Pizza/180g	290	5.4	161	9.6	25.3	3.0	1.6
Margherita, Piccolo, GF, Pizza Express*	1 Pizza/165g	388	14.0	235	5.9	33.8	8.5	0.8
Margherita, Piccolo, Pizza Express*	1 Pizza/175g	318	8.8	182	9.5	25.9	5.0	1.7
Margherita, Romana, Piccolo, GF, Pizza Express*	1 Pizza/220g	495	21.4	225	8.2	26.3	9.7	0.6
Margherita, Romana, Piccolo, Pizza Express*	1 Pizza/230g	426	16.1	185	10.9	20.6	7.0	1.4
Mushroom, Light Mozzarella, Piccolo, Pizza Express*	1 Pizza/201g	293	5.6	146	8.9	22.8	2.8	1.6
Mushroom, Piccolo, GF, Pizza Express*	1 Pizza/180g	377	13.0	210	4.9	31.0	7.2	0.8
Mushroom, Piccolo, Pizza Express*	1 Pizza/190g	308	7.8	162	8.4	23.2	4.1	1.7
Padana, Leggera, Main, Pizza Express*	1 Pizza/322g	415	10.0	129	4.1	21.6	3.1	1.4
Padana Romana, Main, Pizza Express*	1 Pizza/459g	831	27.1	181	7.4	25.4	5.9	1.5
Pollo, Light Mozzarella, Piccolo, GF, Pizza Express*	1 Pizza/190g	382	10.8	201	8.1	29.4	5.7	0.7
Pollo, Light Mozzarella, Piccolo, Pizza Express*	1 Pizza/200g	312	5.6	156	11.2	22.8	2.8	1.5
Pollo, Piccolo, GF, Pizza Express*	1 Pizza/180g	396	13.1	220	7.5	31.0	7.3	0.7
Pollo, Piccolo, Pizza Express*	1 Pizza/190g	327	7.8	172	10.8	23.9	4.1	1.6
Pollo Ad Astra, Leggera, Main, Pizza Express*	1 Pizza/367g	418	8.8	114	9.6	14.1	2.4	1.1
Pollo Ad Astra, Romana, Main, Pizza Express*	1 Pizza/491g	800	22.1	163	11.2	20.1	4.5	1.4
Polpette Bolognese, Romana, Main, Pizza Express*	1 Pizza/580g	1160	58.6	200	10.1	17.6	10.1	1.0
Pomodoro, Pesto, Leggera, Main, Pizza Express*	1 Pizza/316g	401	17.4	127	5.7	14.7	5.5	1.3
Pomodoro, Pesto, Romana, Main, Pizza Express*	1 Pizza/543g	1151	60.3	212	11.5	17.1	11.1	1.1
Quattro Formaggi, Romana, Main, Pizza Express*	1 Pizza/424g	886	39.0	209	10.9	21.6	9.2	1.4
Rustichella, Romana, Main, Pizza Express*	1 Pizza/511g	1022	46.5	200	9.8	20.5	9.1	1.8
Sloppy Giuseppe, Classic, Main, Pizza Express*	1 Pizza/469g	952	39.4	203	11.3	20.9	8.4	1.7
Sloppy Guiseppe, Classic, GF, Pizza Express*	1 Pizza/474g	1167	51.3	246	8.3	28.1	10.8	1.1
Toscana Romana, Main, Pizza Express*	1 Pizza/524g	1169	62.4	223	11.9	17.8	11.9	1.2
Veneziana, Romana, Main, Pizza Express*	1 Pizza/423g	795	30.0	188	9.1	23.0	7.1	1.7
RISOTTO								
Pollo Funghi, Starter, Pizza Express*	1 Serving/237g	367	21.8	155	6.4	11.3	9.2	0.4
SALAD								
Bosco, Main, Pizza Express*	1 Serving/362g	652	38.7	180	6.5	14.7	10.7	2.1
Caesar, Chicken, Grande, Main, Pizza Express*	1 Serving/350g	630	25.9	180	12.1	16.5	7.4	1.4
Caesar, Side, Pizza Express*	1 Serving/129g	313	25.4	243	8.1	8.1	19.7	0.9
Leggara, Superfood, Main, Pizza Express*	1 Serving/368g	294	19.9	80	4.1	4.2	5.4	1.4
Mixed Leaf, Side, Pizza Express*	1 Serving/411g	185	14.4	45	0.8	2.9	3.5	0.8
Mozzarella & Tomato, Starter, Pizza Express*	1 Serving/240g	458	38.8	191	9.5	2.0	16.2	0.4
Pollo Pancetta, Main, Pizza Express*	1 Serving/467g	425	8.4	91	6.2	12.2	1.8	1.0
Salmon, Leggera, Pizza Express*	1 Serving/407g	444	31.0	109	6.2	4.3	7.6	1.0

	Measure INFO/WEIGHT	per Measure KCAL	FAT	Nutrition Values per 100g / 100ml KCAL	PROT	CARB	FAT	FIBRE
PIZZA EXPRESS								
SORBET								
Raspberry, Dolcetti, Pizza Express*	1 Serving/65g	86	1.9	132	1.0	25.4	2.9	1.6
Raspberry, Piccolo, Pizza Express*	1 Serving/60g	61	0.2	101	0.6	23.7	0.4	1.1
Raspberry, Pizza Express*	1 Serving/130g	172	3.8	132	1.0	25.4	2.9	1.6
TALEGGIO								
Oven Baked, Sharing Starter, Pizza Express*	½ Serving/164g	377	16.6	230	11.3	24.0	10.1	1.6
TIRAMISU								
Dessert, Pizza Express*	1 Serving/199g	553	32.0	278	3.5	26.6	16.1	0.2
TORTA								
Double Chocolate Espresso, Dolcetti, Pizza Express*	1 Serving/81g	363	26.8	448	3.9	33.1	33.1	3.3
Lemon, & Mascarpone, Pizza Express*	1 Serving/167g	529	32.7	317	5.1	32.1	19.6	0.3
Lemon Meringue, Dolcetti, Pizza Express*	1 Serving/51g	185	10.0	362	5.9	40.6	19.6	0.9
PIZZA HUT								
BACON BITS								
Pizza Hut*	1 Serving/12g	60	3.6	496	8.3	48.7	29.8	0.0
BEANS								
Chocolate Coated, Ice Cream Factory, Pizza Hut*	1 Serving/30g	142	5.4	475	5.5	72.2	18.1	0.0
BEETROOT								
Pizza Hut*	1 Serving/25g	14	0.0	55	0.9	12.0	0.1	0.0
BREAD								
Garlic, Ciabatta, Pizza Hut*	2 Pieces/253g	820	32.1	324	9.1	43.4	12.7	0.0
Garlic, Dipsters, Pizza Hut*	1 Piece/90g	308	14.2	342	6.8	43.1	15.8	0.0
Garlic, Pizza Hut*	1 Slice/30g	95	4.6	318	6.8	38.1	15.4	0.0
Garlic, with Cheese, Pizza Hut*	4 Pieces/187g	568	34.0	304	15.9	19.0	18.2	0.0
BREADSTICKS								
Garlic, Pizza Hut*	1 Stick/50g	174	6.7	347	9.8	46.9	13.4	1.0
BROWNIES								
Fudge, Pizza Hut*	1 Serving/105g	418	16.4	398	4.3	60.1	15.6	0.0
BRUSCHETTA								
Light Lunch, Pizza Hut*	3 Pieces/211g	369	16.0	175	4.1	22.4	7.6	0.0
CAKE								
Chocolate Fudge, Dessert, Pizza Hut*	1 Piece/178g	684	31.9	384	4.2	51.4	17.9	0.0
CARBONARA								
Ham, Buffet, Pizza Hut*	1 Serving/200g	180	4.6	90	3.4	14.4	2.3	0.0
CHEESE								
4 & Vegetable, Buffet, Pizza Hut*	1 Serving/200g	210	8.6	105	4.0	12.6	4.3	0.0
Hard, Grated, Pizza Hut*	1 Serving/30g	121	9.0	404	33.0	0.1	30.0	0.0
Parmesan Reggiano, Grated at table, Pizza Hut*	1 Serving/5g	20	1.4	400	34.0	0.0	28.0	0.0
Three Cheese Melt, Starter, Pizza Hut*	3 Pieces/209g	546	38.1	261	11.2	12.3	18.2	0.0
CHEESECAKE								
Chocolate, Pizza Hut*	1 Serving/63g	228	11.1	360	5.6	44.9	17.5	0.0
Clotted Cream, Pizza Hut*	1 Serving/64g	205	10.4	323	4.6	39.3	16.4	0.0
Lemon & Ginger, Pizza Hut*	1 Serving/64g	205	9.7	323	4.2	42.4	15.2	0.0
New York Style, Baked, Pizza Hut*	1 Slice/113g	442	16.2	391	6.6	62.3	14.3	0.0
Vanilla, Madagascan, Dessert, Pizza Hut*	1 Serving/133g	397	18.1	298	4.8	39.2	13.6	0.0
CHICKEN								
Cheesy Jalapeno Poppers, Pizza Hut*	6 Pieces/150g	408	20.0	272	5.2	32.8	13.3	0.0
Dippin, Pizza Hut*	1 Serving/155g	332	14.4	214	15.7	17.1	9.3	0.0
Goujons, Pizza Hut*	5 Pieces/169g	311	13.5	184	17.0	11.0	8.0	1.5
Strips, Breaded, (Five Strips), Pizza Hut*	5 Pieces/175g	283	13.2	162	16.0	8.9	7.5	0.0
Strips, Breaded, with Wedges, 2, Kids, Pizza Hut*	1 Serving/231g	386	11.6	167	6.7	23.9	5.0	0.0
Strips, Breaded, with Wedges, 3, Kids, Pizza Hut*	1 Serving/265g	451	14.3	170	8.1	22.2	5.4	0.0
Strips, Breaded, Wrap Factory, 2, Kids, Pizza Hut*	1 Serving/247g	434	12.1	176	8.3	24.8	4.9	0.0

	Measure INFO/WEIGHT	per Measure KCAL	FAT	Nutrition Values per 100g / 100ml KCAL	PROT	CARB	FAT	FIBRE
PIZZA HUT								
CHICKEN								
Strips, Breaded, Wrap Factory, 3, Kids, Pizza Hut*	1 Serving/325g	617	17.9	190	9.2	25.9	5.5	0.0
Strips, Hot n Kicking, Pizza Hut*	7 Pieces/140g	276	12.6	197	17.0	12.0	9.0	0.0
Wings, BBQ, (Delivery Only), Pizza Hut*	6 Pieces/156g	303	14.4	194	23.2	4.6	9.2	0.0
Wings, BBQ, Pizza Hut*	6 Pieces/171g	306	14.5	179	21.4	4.4	8.5	0.0
Wings, BBQ, Saucy, Pizza Hut*	6 Wings/159g	355	21.8	223	21.4	3.6	13.7	0.0
Wings, Buffalo, Saucy, Pizza Hut*	6 Wings/181g	380	22.2	209	21.0	3.7	12.2	0.0
Wings, Spicy, Crunch, (Delivery Only), Pizza Hut*	1 Serving/218g	510	30.5	234	17.0	10.0	14.0	0.0
Wings, Texan BBQ Chicken, Pizza Hut*	6 Pieces/159g	355	21.8	223	21.4	3.6	13.7	0.0
Wings, with Sour Cream & Chive Dip, Pizza Hut*	1 Pack/178g	680	56.1	382	22.8	1.9	31.5	1.3
COLESLAW								
Pizza Hut*	1 Pot/38g	54	4.6	143	0.9	7.1	12.3	0.0
COUS COUS								
Pizza Hut*	1 Serving/100g	219	9.0	219	5.0	30.0	9.0	0.0
CREAM								
Single, Dessert, Pizza Hut*	1 Serving/40g	75	7.2	188	2.6	3.9	18.0	0.0
UHT, Serving, Pizza Hut*	1 Serving/12g	23	2.2	188	2.7	3.9	18.0	0.0
CROUTONS								
Pizza Flavoured, Pizza Hut*	1 Serving/12g	23	3.1	196	10.1	55.2	26.1	0.0
Salad, Large, Pizza Hut*	1 Serving/20g	94	4.2	470	11.0	59.1	21.1	0.0
DESSERT								
Cherries in Sauce, Pizza Hut*	1 Serving/20g	28	0.0	142	0.5	34.9	0.1	0.0
Chocolate Obsession, Pizza Hut*	1 Serving/100g	157	6.8	157	2.0	22.1	6.8	0.0
Toffee Apple Meltdown, Pizza Hut*	1 Serving/120g	325	11.0	271	3.3	43.7	9.2	0.0
DIP								
BBQ Sauce, in Restaurant, Pizza Hut*	1 Pot/28g	34	0.0	121	1.4	29.3	0.1	0.0
BBQ Tabasco, Pizza Hut*	1 Serving/25g	36	0.1	142	1.2	33.6	0.2	0.0
Garlic & Herb, Pizza Hut*	1 Serving/28g	93	9.2	331	1.4	7.6	32.6	0.0
Mayonnaise, Light, Restaurant Only, Pizza Hut*	1 Pot/50g	163	16.5	326	0.6	6.0	33.0	0.0
Sour Cream & Chive, Restaurant Only, Pizza Hut*	1 Serving/28g	83	8.7	296	0.7	3.6	31.1	0.0
Sweet Chilli Sauce, Restaurant Only, Pizza Hut*	1 Pot/28g	48	0.2	171	0.4	32.9	0.7	0.0
Tomato Ketchup, Restaurant Only, Pizza Hut*	1 Pot/28g	39	0.0	139	1.4	34.3	0.0	0.0
DRESSING								
1000 Island, Pizza Hut*	1 Serving/38g	107	9.7	280	0.7	11.5	25.5	0.0
Blue Cheese, Pizza Hut*	1 Serving/35g	91	8.0	258	1.7	11.5	22.7	0.0
Caesar, Pizza Hut*	1 Serving/40g	27	1.1	68	1.5	8.9	2.8	0.0
Ranch, Pizza Hut*	1 Serving/32g	163	18.0	510	1.2	1.5	56.4	0.0
Vinaigrette, Low Fat, Pizza Hut*	1 Serving/30ml	23	0.2	77	0.3	17.2	0.5	0.0
FISH								
Goujons (5 Strips), Pizza Hut*	5 Strips/210g	416	20.9	198	10.0	17.1	10.0	0.0
FRIES								
Seasoned, Savoury, Pizza Hut*	1 Serving/144g	238	11.5	165	2.4	20.8	8.0	0.0
FRUIT SALAD								
Apple & Grape, Fresh, Mix, Pizza Hut*	1 Serving/80g	39	0.8	49	0.4	12.0	1.0	0.0
ICE CREAM								
Coco Mango, Pizza Hut*	1 Serving/100g	88	1.8	88	0.6	17.3	1.8	0.0
Cookie Craving, Pizza Hut*	1 Serving/100g	149	6.9	149	1.6	20.1	6.9	0.0
Dairy, Dessert, Pizza Hut*	1 Serving/142g	272	12.6	192	4.6	23.3	8.9	0.2
Mix, Pizza Hut*	1 Serving/100g	147	6.2	147	4.0	18.8	6.2	0.0
Traditional, Dessert, Pizza Hut*	1 Serving/130g	251	13.5	193	2.6	22.4	10.4	0.0
Traditional, Kids, Pizza Hut*	1 Serving/89g	171	9.2	193	2.6	22.4	10.4	0.0
Traditional, Pizza Hut*	1 Serving/132g	254	13.7	193	2.6	22.4	10.4	0.0

	Measure INFO/WEIGHT	per Measure KCAL	FAT	Nutrition Values per 100g / 100ml KCAL	PROT	CARB	FAT	FIBRE
PIZZA HUT								
KETCHUP								
Heinz, Pizza Hut*	1 Serving/12g	14	0.0	119	0.5	28.4	0.1	0.0
LETTUCE								
Cos, Fresh, Pizza Hut*	1 Serving/80g	10	0.2	13	0.7	1.9	0.3	0.0
MACARONI CHEESE								
Pizza Hut*	1 Serving/41g	57	2.4	140	4.9	16.6	6.0	0.0
MARSHMALLOWS								
Mini, Ice Cream Factory, Pizza Hut*	1 Serving/30g	96	0.0	320	5.4	74.3	0.0	0.0
MAYONNAISE								
Sachet, Pizza Hut*	1 Sachet/12g	88	9.8	731	1.3	1.8	81.2	0.0
MEATBALLS								
in Pomodoro Sauce, Light Lunch, Pizza Hut*	1 Serving/253g	342	18.2	135	6.6	11.0	7.2	0.0
MELON								
Pieces, Fresh, Pizza Hut*	1 Serving/80g	27	0.0	34	0.8	8.2	0.0	0.0
MILK								
Half Fat, Servings, Millac Maid, Pizza Hut*	1 Serving/14g	6	0.2	45	6.0	5.1	1.6	0.0
MILK SHAKE								
Strawberry Cheesecake, Pizza Hut*	1 Serving/236g	371	14.1	157	3.4	22.3	6.0	0.0
The Chocoholic, Pizza Hut*	1 Serving/248g	442	20.4	178	3.6	22.8	8.2	0.0
Toffee Banoffee Shake, Pizza Hut*	1 Serving/404g	763	22.6	189	2.4	32.3	5.6	0.0
MUFFIN								
Cheesecake, Sicilian Lemon, Pizza Hut*	1 Muffin/130g	508	24.2	391	5.1	50.9	18.6	0.0
Fruity, Pizza Hut*	1 Muffin/115g	366	13.7	318	4.1	48.4	11.9	0.0
Mixed Berry, Pizza Hut*	1 Muffin/108g	402	22.6	372	4.4	41.6	20.9	0.0
Sicilian Lemon Cheesecake, Pizza Hut*	1 Muffin/130g	508	24.2	391	5.1	50.9	18.6	0.0
Strawberry & White Chocolate, Pizza Hut*	1 Muffin/108g	402	22.6	372	4.4	41.6	20.9	0.0
MUSHROOMS								
Blue Cheese, Pizza Hut*	1 Serving/256g	514	40.7	201	7.2	7.5	15.9	0.0
Breaded, Pizza Hut*	6 Pieces/180g	410	14.4	228	4.5	26.1	8.0	0.0
Garlic, 2, Pizza Hut*	1 Serving/230g	570	43.4	248	7.9	7.0	18.9	0.0
Garlic, Crispy Coated, Pizza Hut*	1 Serving/135g	240	10.1	178	4.1	23.4	7.5	0.0
Garlic, with BBQ Dip, Pizza Hut*	1 Serving/112g	263	11.2	234	6.2	30.5	10.0	3.4
Garlic, with Sour Cream & Chive Dip, Pizza Hut*	1 Serving/112g	426	34.6	380	6.4	20.0	30.8	3.4
NACHOS								
Chilli, Pizza Hut*	1 Serving/190g	550	33.1	289	8.8	27.2	17.4	0.0
Sharing Starters, Pizza Hut*	1 Serving/356g	1087	76.3	305	7.9	24.6	21.4	0.0
Side, Delivery Only, Pizza Hut*	1 Serving/222g	669	40.3	301	7.7	30.2	18.1	0.0
OLIVES								
Mixed, Pizza Hut*	1 Serving/70g	140	9.0	200	1.5	19.6	12.8	0.0
ONION RINGS								
Chilli, (Delivery Only), Pizza Hut*	1 Ring/13g	26	1.2	212	3.2	28.2	9.6	0.0
Chilli, Pizza Hut*	8 Rings/100g	212	9.6	212	3.2	28.2	9.6	0.0
ONIONS								
White, Pizza Hut*	1 Serving/24g	10	0.0	42	1.0	10.0	0.0	0.0
PANCAKE								
Fruity, Kids, Pizza Hut*	1 Serving/156g	227	3.3	146	1.9	30.6	2.1	0.0
PASTA								
3 Cheese & Vegetable, Pizza Hut*	1 Serving/300g	315	12.9	105	4.0	12.6	4.3	0.0
4 Cheese, Sharing, Pizza Hut*	1 Serving/1200g	1860	102.0	155	6.1	13.5	8.5	0.0
Adults, Pizza Hut*	1 Serving/100g	250	10.9	250	5.7	16.8	10.9	0.0
Alfredo, Chicken, Sharing, (Delivery Only), Pizza Hut*	1 Pack/1200g	1680	40.8	140	8.1	19.1	3.4	0.0
Alfredo, Light Lunch, Pizza Hut*	1 Serving/226g	294	5.0	130	4.1	23.3	2.2	0.0
Alfredo, Pizza Hut*	1 Serving/400g	520	8.8	130	4.1	23.3	2.2	0.0

	Measure INFO/WEIGHT	per Measure KCAL	FAT	Nutrition Values per 100g / 100ml KCAL	PROT	CARB	FAT	FIBRE
PIZZA HUT								
PASTA								
Arrabiata, Pizza Hut*	1 Serving/450g	441	13.0	98	2.9	15.0	2.9	0.0
Bolognese, Sharing, (Delivery Only), Pizza Hut*	1 Pack/1200g	1500	64.8	125	7.2	11.9	5.4	0.0
Bolognese, Sharing, Pizza Hut*	1 Pack/1200g	1500	64.8	125	7.2	11.9	5.4	0.0
Cannelloni, Spinach & Ricotta, Pizza Hut*	1 Serving/404g	566	27.5	140	6.2	13.1	6.8	0.0
Chicken Alfredo, Sharing, Pizza Hut*	1 Pack/1200g	1680	40.8	140	8.1	19.1	3.4	0.0
Gemelli, Pizza Hut*	1 Serving/100g	155	4.4	155	4.3	26.0	4.4	0.0
Ham & Mushroom, Pizza Hut*	1 Serving/450g	473	10.4	105	4.2	17.0	2.3	0.0
Kids, Pizza Hut*	1 Serving/100g	180	9.4	180	6.9	16.5	9.4	0.0
Lasagne, Traditional, Pizza Hut*	1 Serving/460g	589	26.7	128	5.9	13.0	5.8	0.0
Macaroni Cheese, Kids, Pizza Hut*	1 Serving/250g	332	16.2	133	4.0	14.8	6.5	0.0
Mezzaluna, Tomato & Mozzarella, Pizza Hut*	1 Serving/351g	340	10.2	97	3.1	14.7	2.9	0.0
Salmone Penne Al Forno, Pizza Hut*	1 Serving/496g	832	49.1	168	7.5	10.6	9.9	0.0
Spaghetti Bolognese, Kids, New, Pizza Hut*	1 Serving/234g	211	3.5	90	7.6	14.6	1.5	0.0
Tagliatelle, Alla Carbonara, Pizza Hut*	1 Serving/400g	548	32.4	137	5.6	10.4	8.1	0.0
Tagliatelle, Meatball, Italian Recipe, Pizza Hut*	1 Serving/240g	324	10.6	135	6.9	16.6	4.4	0.0
Tomato, Pizza Hut*	1 Serving/80g	149	7.4	186	3.7	21.8	9.3	0.0
Tomato & Pepperoni, Pizza Hut*	1 Serving/300g	312	8.1	104	3.6	16.3	2.7	0.0
PASTA BAKE								
Salmon, Pizza Hut*	1 Serving/400g	692	42.8	173	7.9	11.3	10.7	0.0
PASTA SALAD								
Sweetcorn & Pepper, Pizza Hut*	1 Serving/47g	75	2.5	159	4.6	23.1	5.3	0.0
Tomato, Dressed, Med, Pizza Hut*	1 Serving/100g	112	1.5	112	3.5	21.2	1.5	0.0
Tomato & Basil, Pizza Hut*	1 Serving/50g	50	0.8	100	3.7	17.8	1.5	0.0
PENNE								
Mediterranean Vegetable, Pizza Hut*	1 Serving/448g	592	19.7	132	3.7	18.3	4.4	0.0
PEPPERS								
Mixed, Fresh, Pizza Hut*	1 Serving/80g	12	0.2	15	0.8	2.6	0.3	0.0
Red & Green Wedges, Pizza Hut*	1 Serving/40g	6	0.1	15	0.8	2.6	0.3	0.0
Romano, Stuffed, Pizza Hut*	1 Serving/208g	250	13.3	120	2.7	13.3	6.4	0.0
PIE								
Banoffee, Dessert, Pizza Hut*	1 Serving/125g	428	25.3	340	2.5	37.3	20.1	0.0
Banoffee, Pizza Hut*	1 Serving/100g	350	21.5	350	4.2	34.9	21.5	0.0
PIZZA								
BBQ Deluxe, Cheesy Bites, Pizza Hut*	1 Slice/143g	358	11.6	251	11.7	34.4	8.1	0.0
BBQ Deluxe, Italian, Individual, Pizza Hut*	1 Slice/78g	185	6.1	238	10.9	34.3	7.9	0.0
BBQ Deluxe, Italian, Large, Pizza Hut*	1 Slice/95g	239	8.0	252	14.3	29.7	8.4	0.0
BBQ Deluxe, Italian, Medium, Pizza Hut*	1 Slice/105g	253	8.0	241	12.0	31.1	7.6	0.0
BBQ Deluxe, Pan, Individual, Pizza Hut*	1 Slice/79g	200	7.9	253	12.7	28.0	10.0	0.0
BBQ Deluxe, Pan, Large, Pizza Hut*	1 Slice/122g	306	12.1	251	11.8	28.6	9.9	0.0
BBQ Deluxe, Pan, Medium, Pizza Hut*	1 Slice/107g	276	11.3	257	11.7	28.8	10.5	0.0
BBQ Deluxe, Stuffed Crust, Pizza Hut*	1 Serving/155g	337	10.4	217	11.6	31.9	6.7	0.0
Cajun Chicken, Hot One, Italian, Medium, Pizza Hut*	1 Slice/100g	250	9.3	250	12.5	29.1	9.3	0.0
Cajun Chicken, Hot One, Pan, Large, Pizza Hut*	1 Slice/125g	321	14.7	257	12.9	24.7	11.8	0.0
Cajun Chicken, Hot One, Pan, Medium, Pizza Hut*	1 Slice/105g	273	12.3	259	12.7	25.6	11.7	0.0
Cajun Chicken, Hot One, Stuffed Crust, Pizza Hut*	1 Slice/135g	331	10.8	245	13.3	30.0	8.0	0.0
Cheese Feast, Italian, Medium, Pizza Hut*	1 Slice/96g	260	11.3	272	12.3	29.1	11.8	0.0
Cheese Feast, Pan, Medium, Pizza Hut*	1 Slice/106g	299	15.0	283	14.6	24.2	14.2	0.0
Cheese Feast, Stuffed Crust, Pizza Hut*	1 Slice/132g	361	13.8	273	14.3	30.5	10.4	0.0
Chicken, Hi Light, Medium, Pizza Hut*	1 Slice/83g	189	5.5	230	13.2	29.2	6.7	0.0
Chicken Feast, Italian, Medium, Pizza Hut*	1 Slice/100g	249	8.6	248	14.1	28.6	8.6	0.0
Chicken Feast, Pan, Medium, Pizza Hut*	1 Slice/109g	283	12.0	259	15.5	24.6	11.0	0.0
Chicken Feast, Stuffed Crust, Pizza Hut*	1 Slice/133g	337	12.6	254	14.8	27.3	9.5	0.0

	Measure INFO/WEIGHT	per Measure KCAL	FAT	Nutrition Values per 100g / 100ml KCAL	PROT	CARB	FAT	FIBRE
PIZZA HUT								
PIZZA								
Chicken Supreme, Cheesy Bites, Pizza Hut*	1 Slice/148g	322	10.0	218	11.8	29.5	6.8	0.0
Chicken Supreme, Express, Pizza Hut*	1 Slice/65g	143	5.8	221	10.1	28.1	9.0	0.0
Chicken Supreme, Italian, Individual, Pizza Hut*	1 Slice/74g	169	4.4	229	10.7	35.4	5.9	0.0
Chicken Supreme, Italian, Large, Pizza Hut*	1 Slice/111g	217	6.4	196	9.8	29.3	5.8	0.0
Chicken Supreme, Italian, Medium, Pizza Hut*	1 Slice/102g	220	6.3	215	10.3	31.9	6.2	0.0
Chicken Supreme, Pan, Individual, Pizza Hut*	1 Slice/81g	186	8.0	231	11.6	26.9	9.9	0.0
Chicken Supreme, Pan, Large, Pizza Hut*	1 Slice/124g	271	11.6	219	10.9	26.1	9.4	0.0
Chicken Supreme, Pan, Medium, Pizza Hut*	1 Slice/115g	251	9.9	219	11.2	26.6	8.6	0.0
Chicken Supreme, Stuffed Crust, Pizza Hut*	1 Slice/153g	367	11.0	240	11.6	34.8	7.2	0.0
Country Feast, Italian, Medium, Pizza Hut*	1 Slice/109g	252	9.6	232	9.7	28.6	8.8	0.0
Country Feast, Pan, Medium, Pizza Hut*	1 Slice/115g	279	12.1	243	11.4	25.8	10.5	0.0
Country Feast, Stuffed Crust, Pizza Hut*	1 Slice/144g	326	10.8	227	11.5	28.4	7.5	0.0
Express, Supreme, Pizza Hut*	1 Slice/68g	165	7.6	242	10.7	27.8	11.2	0.0
Farmhouse, Cheesy Bites, Pizza Hut*	1 Slice/133g	332	12.6	250	13.2	30.7	9.5	0.0
Farmhouse, Italian, Individual, Pizza Hut*	1 Slice/74g	188	6.0	253	11.8	33.1	8.1	0.0
Farmhouse, Italian, Large, Pizza Hut*	1 Slice/92g	206	6.7	224	10.2	34.0	7.3	0.0
Farmhouse, Italian, Medium, Pizza Hut*	1 Slice/84g	192	5.4	229	10.2	35.7	6.4	0.0
Farmhouse, Pan, Individual, Pizza Hut*	1 Slice/70g	179	7.4	256	11.3	31.6	10.6	0.0
Farmhouse, Pan, Large, Pizza Hut*	1 Slice/106g	257	11.0	242	11.4	29.7	10.4	0.0
Farmhouse, Pan, Medium, Delivery, Pizza Hut*	1 Slice/75g	182	7.8	242	11.3	28.6	10.4	0.0
Farmhouse, Pan, Medium, Pizza Hut*	1 Slice/100g	242	10.4	242	11.3	28.6	10.4	0.0
Farmhouse, Stuffed Crust, Pizza Hut*	1 Slice/132g	387	10.0	293	11.8	30.0	7.6	0.0
Ham, Hi Light, Medium, Pizza Hut*	1 Slice/82g	184	5.5	225	12.1	29.1	6.7	0.0
Happy Hour, Chicken & Mushroom, Pizza Hut*	1 Slice/80g	165	5.4	207	9.6	27.6	6.8	0.0
Happy Hour, Ham & Sweetcorn, Pizza Hut*	1 Slice/86g	174	5.6	202	9.4	27.0	6.5	0.0
Happy Hour, Pepper & Tomato, Pizza Hut*	1 Slice/86g	163	5.4	189	8.0	26.1	6.3	0.0
Happy Hour, Pepperoni & Onion, Pizza Hut*	1 Slice/80g	179	6.9	224	9.4	28.2	8.6	0.0
Hawaiian, Cheesy Bites, Pizza Hut*	1 Slice/136g	316	10.6	232	11.6	31.2	7.8	0.0
Hawaiian, Express, Pizza Hut*	1 Slice/60g	147	6.4	245	10.5	29.9	10.6	0.0
Hawaiian, Italian, Individual, Pizza Hut*	1 Slice/71g	164	4.2	229	9.8	37.9	5.8	0.0
Hawaiian, Italian, Large, Pizza Hut*	1 Slice/99g	221	7.0	223	10.0	33.2	7.1	0.0
Hawaiian, Italian, Medium, Pizza Hut*	1 Slice/92g	201	5.6	219	9.8	33.3	6.1	0.0
Hawaiian, Pan, Individual, Pizza Hut*	1 Slice/73g	175	6.5	240	10.9	32.2	8.9	0.0
Hawaiian, Pan, Large, Delivery, Pizza Hut*	1 Slice/89g	234	10.2	262	10.6	32.6	11.4	0.0
Hawaiian, Pan, Large, Pizza Hut*	1 Slice/112g	293	12.7	262	10.6	32.6	11.4	0.0
Hawaiian, Pan, Medium, Pizza Hut*	1 Slice/109g	245	9.7	224	10.1	28.5	8.9	0.0
Hawaiian, Stuffed Crust, Pizza Hut*	1 Slice/141g	306	10.3	217	11.0	30.7	7.3	0.0
Hot 'n' Spicy, Cheesy Bites, Pizza Hut*	1 Slice/127g	331	12.6	261	12.6	33.7	9.9	0.0
Hot 'n' Spicy, Italian, Individual, Pizza Hut*	1 Slice/66g	180	6.9	272	11.0	36.5	10.4	0.0
Hot 'n' Spicy, Italian, Large, Pizza Hut*	1 Slice/93g	236	9.4	254	11.2	32.7	10.1	0.0
Hot 'n' Spicy, Italian, Medium, Pizza Hut*	1 Slice/86g	222	8.4	259	11.0	34.5	9.8	0.0
Hot 'n' Spicy, Pan, Individual, Pizza Hut*	1 Slice/71g	183	7.9	259	10.9	30.4	11.2	0.0
Hot 'n' Spicy, Pan, Large, Pizza Hut*	1 Slice/105g	266	11.4	254	12.0	30.2	10.9	0.0
Hot 'n' Spicy, Pan, Medium, Pizza Hut*	1 Slice/93g	237	10.6	254	11.5	29.2	11.4	0.0
Hot 'n' Spicy, Stuffed Crust, Pizza Hut*	1 Slice/139g	329	11.0	236	11.8	33.1	7.9	0.0
Margherita, Cheesy Bites, Pizza Hut*	1 Slice/128g	337	12.9	263	12.8	33.1	10.1	0.0
Margherita, Fingers, Kids, Pizza Hut*	1 Slice/95g	258	12.1	273	11.0	28.4	12.8	0.0
Margherita, Italian, Individual, Pizza Hut*	1 Slice/67g	177	5.4	264	11.9	39.2	8.0	0.0
Margherita, Italian, Large, Pizza Hut*	1 Slice/91g	229	8.6	252	10.4	34.2	9.5	0.0
Margherita, Italian, Medium, Pizza Hut*	1 Slice/80g	205	7.0	256	11.0	35.7	8.8	0.0
Margherita, Pan, Individual, Pizza Hut*	1 Slice/71g	189	8.1	268	11.6	32.4	11.5	0.0
Margherita, Pan, Large, Pizza Hut*	1 Slice/105g	273	12.4	261	11.6	29.8	11.9	0.0

	Measure INFO/WEIGHT	per Measure KCAL	FAT	Nutrition Values per 100g / 100ml KCAL	PROT	CARB	FAT	FIBRE
PIZZA HUT								
PIZZA								
Margherita, Pan, Medium, Pizza Hut*	1 Slice/97g	256	11.4	265	11.6	30.6	11.8	0.0
Margherita, Stuffed Crust, Pizza Hut*	1 Slice/140g	349	12.4	248	14.0	31.6	8.8	0.0
Margherita, Thick, Kids, Pizza Hut*	1 Slice/202g	506	17.9	251	9.0	33.0	8.9	0.0
Meat Feast, Cheesy Bites, Pizza Hut*	1 Slice/142g	387	16.2	272	13.9	30.3	11.4	0.0
Meat Feast, Italian, Individual, Pizza Hut*	1 Slice/81g	220	8.8	270	13.9	32.3	10.8	0.0
Meat Feast, Italian, Large, Pizza Hut*	1 Slice/111g	279	12.7	251	12.9	27.3	11.4	0.0
Meat Feast, Italian, Medium, Pizza Hut*	1 Slice/100g	257	11.0	258	13.0	30.0	11.0	0.0
Meat Feast, Pan, Individual, Pizza Hut*	1 Slice/84g	220	9.9	262	13.3	27.6	11.8	0.0
Meat Feast, Pan, Large, Pizza Hut*	1 Slice/124g	344	16.4	277	12.6	29.1	13.2	0.0
Meat Feast, Pan, Medium, Pizza Hut*	1 Slice/112g	294	13.9	262	12.2	28.0	12.4	0.0
Meat Feast, Stuffed Crust, Pizza Hut*	1 Slice/152g	376	15.8	247	13.5	28.0	10.4	0.0
Meaty, The Edge, Medium, Pizza Hut*	1 Slice/36g	110	5.7	308	17.0	20.4	16.1	0.0
Meaty BBQ, Cheesy Bites, Delivery, Pizza Hut*	1 Slice/115g	282	10.8	245	11.3	31.1	9.4	0.0
Meaty BBQ, Italian, Medium, Delivery, Pizza Hut*	1 Slice/70g	154	5.0	220	10.9	30.0	7.2	0.0
Meaty BBQ, Pan, Medium, Delivery, Pizza Hut*	1 Slice/92g	215	8.7	234	11.1	25.9	9.5	0.0
Mediterranean Meat Deluxe, Italian, Medium, Pizza Hut*	1 Slice/91g	245	9.4	270	12.8	33.5	10.4	0.0
Mediterranean Meat Deluxe, Pan, Individual, Pizza Hut*	1 Slice/75g	212	10.4	284	13.5	29.5	13.9	0.0
Mediterranean Meat Deluxe, Pan, Medium, Pizza Hut*	1 Slice/98g	245	11.2	249	11.7	28.1	11.4	0.0
Mountain Fantastico, Italian, Individual, Pizza Hut*	1 Slice/75g	183	6.3	245	9.3	36.4	8.5	0.0
Pepperoni Feast, Cheesy Bites, Pizza Hut*	1 Slice/135g	382	16.7	284	15.8	29.6	12.4	0.0
Pepperoni Feast, Italian, Individual, Pizza Hut*	1 Slice/73g	205	8.4	282	11.4	36.3	11.6	0.0
Pepperoni Feast, Italian, Large, Delivery, Pizza Hut*	1 Slice/68g	195	9.5	286	12.0	30.8	14.0	0.0
Pepperoni Feast, Italian, Large, Pizza Hut*	1 Slice/103g	286	13.3	278	12.2	30.9	12.9	0.0
Pepperoni Feast, Italian, Medium, Pizza Hut*	1 Slice/93g	254	9.8	273	12.3	35.0	10.5	0.0
Pepperoni Feast, Pan, Individual, Pizza Hut*	1 Slice/79g	227	10.8	286	12.3	30.3	13.6	0.0
Pepperoni Feast, Pan, Large, Pizza Hut*	1 Slice/115g	347	20.2	302	12.0	26.4	17.6	0.0
Pepperoni Feast, Pan, Medium, Pizza Hut*	1 Slice/106g	297	15.9	279	12.6	26.2	14.9	0.0
Pepperoni Feast, Stuffed Crust, Pizza Hut*	1 Slice/143g	375	16.2	261	13.1	30.4	11.3	0.0
Seafood Fantastico, Italian, Individual, Pizza Hut*	1 Slice/81g	173	4.6	213	15.3	25.1	5.7	0.0
Seafood Fantastico, Italian, Large, Pizza Hut*	1 Slice/106g	228	6.6	215	15.1	24.6	6.2	0.0
Seafood Lovers, Italian, Individual, Pizza Hut*	1 Slice/66g	170	5.4	258	9.8	38.4	8.2	0.0
Seafood Lovers, Italian, Large, Pizza Hut*	1 Slice/90g	215	6.8	239	10.2	35.3	7.6	0.0
Seafood Lovers, Italian, Medium, Pizza Hut*	1 Slice/82g	202	6.6	245	10.1	35.3	8.0	0.0
Seafood Lovers, Pan, Individual, Pizza Hut*	1 Slice/69g	160	6.0	232	10.7	31.3	8.7	0.0
Seafood Lovers, Pan, Medium, Pizza Hut*	1 Slice/98g	233	10.4	237	9.7	28.3	10.6	0.0
Seafood Lovers, Stuffed Crust, Pizza Hut*	1 Slice/131g	314	10.9	239	12.3	31.8	8.3	0.0
Spicy, Hot One, Pan, Medium, Pizza Hut*	1 Slice/115g	274	13.0	239	11.2	23.1	11.3	0.0
Super Supreme, Cheesy Bites, Pizza Hut*	1 Slice/162g	393	16.2	242	12.4	26.9	10.0	0.0
Super Supreme, Italian, Individual, Pizza Hut*	1 Slice/97g	260	11.0	267	13.9	27.3	11.3	0.0
Super Supreme, Italian, Large, Pizza Hut*	1 Slice/128g	281	13.2	219	10.6	24.4	10.3	0.0
Super Supreme, Italian, Medium, Pizza Hut*	1 Slice/119g	267	11.5	225	11.1	26.3	9.7	0.0
Super Supreme, Pan, Individual, Pizza Hut*	1 Slice/96g	228	10.9	237	11.9	24.8	11.3	0.0
Super Supreme, Pan, Large, Pizza Hut*	1 Slice/148g	346	17.7	234	11.4	22.5	12.0	0.0
Super Supreme, Pan, Medium, Pizza Hut*	1 Slice/127g	323	18.5	255	11.4	22.8	14.6	0.0
Super Supreme, Stuffed Crust, Pizza Hut*	1 Slice/165g	397	14.3	241	11.7	29.0	8.7	0.0
Supreme, Italian, Individual, Pizza Hut*	1 Slice/81g	204	7.5	251	10.9	33.5	9.2	0.0
Supreme, Italian, Large, Pizza Hut*	1 Slice/113g	264	11.0	233	9.7	29.6	9.7	0.0
Supreme, Pan, Individual, Pizza Hut*	1 Slice/84g	209	9.6	248	11.0	28.0	11.4	0.0
Supreme, Stuffed Crust, Pizza Hut*	1 Slice/160g	371	13.8	232	11.9	29.7	8.6	0.0
The Sizzler, Cajun Chicken, Italian, Large, Pizza Hut*	1 Slice/83g	177	6.1	213	11.2	28.1	7.4	0.0
The Sizzler, Cajun Chicken, Italian, Medium, Pizza Hut*	1 Slice/67g	147	4.8	220	11.8	30.2	7.2	0.0
The Sizzler, Cajun Chicken, Pan, Large, Pizza Hut*	1 Slice/90g	215	7.9	238	10.8	27.2	8.8	0.0

	Measure INFO/WEIGHT	per Measure KCAL	FAT	Nutrition Values per 100g / 100ml KCAL	PROT	CARB	FAT	FIBRE
PIZZA HUT								
PIZZA								
The Sizzler, Cajun Chicken, Pan, Medium, Pizza Hut*	1 Slice/75g	166	7.0	221	10.3	27.3	9.3	0.0
The Sizzler, Cajun Chicken, Stuffed Crust, Pizza Hut*	1 Slice/114g	270	9.8	236	11.7	31.7	8.6	0.0
The Sizzler, Spicy Beef, Italian, Large, Pizza Hut*	1 Slice/80g	179	5.9	223	9.6	33.1	7.4	0.0
The Sizzler, Spicy Beef, Italian, Medium, Pizza Hut*	1 Slice/68g	163	6.1	240	10.9	31.6	9.0	0.0
The Sizzler, Spicy Beef, Pan, Large, Pizza Hut*	1 Slice/96g	240	11.0	250	10.5	29.1	11.5	0.0
The Sizzler, Spicy Beef, Pan, Medium, Pizza Hut*	1 Slice/76g	173	7.7	228	10.3	32.0	10.1	0.0
The Sizzler, Spicy Mushroom, Italian, Large, Pizza Hut*	1 Slice/79g	165	5.5	209	9.3	31.2	7.0	0.0
The Sizzler, Spicy Mushroom, Stuffed Crust, Pizza Hut*	1 Slice/116g	244	7.9	210	9.7	31.7	6.8	0.0
The Works, The Edge, Medium, Pizza Hut*	1 Slice/64g	150	6.7	235	12.7	19.5	10.4	0.0
Tortilla, Thin, Kids, Pizza Hut*	1 Slice/108g	264	14.4	245	9.1	20.9	13.4	0.0
Tuscani, Chicken & Mushroom, Pizza Hut*	1 Serving/491g	1032	55.0	210	10.5	16.9	11.2	0.0
Tuscani, Mediterranean Meat, Pizza Hut*	1 Pizza/379g	1065	56.8	281	13.6	21.8	15.0	0.0
Tuscani, Verde, Pizza Hut*	1 Serving/460g	878	42.3	191	8.0	18.6	9.2	0.0
Tuscani Caprina, Pizza Hut*	1 Pizza/474g	990	45.5	209	9.0	20.6	9.6	0.0
Vegetable Supreme, Cheesy Bites, Pizza Hut*	1 Slice/145g	312	10.0	215	10.0	30.7	6.9	0.0
Vegetable Supreme, Italian, Individual, Pizza Hut*	1 Slice/77g	160	4.7	207	8.7	32.4	6.1	0.0
Vegetable Supreme, Italian, Large, Pizza Hut*	1 Slice/111g	222	6.3	200	7.4	32.5	5.7	0.0
Vegetable Supreme, Italian, Medium, Pizza Hut*	1 Slice/99g	196	6.0	198	8.3	30.7	6.1	0.0
Vegetable Supreme, Pan, Individual, Pizza Hut*	1 Slice/84g	180	7.6	214	8.6	27.7	9.0	0.0
Vegetable Supreme, Pan, Large, Pizza Hut*	1 Slice/126g	258	11.6	204	8.1	25.7	9.2	0.0
Vegetable Supreme, Pan, Medium, Pizza Hut*	1 Slice/109g	263	11.2	241	9.9	30.0	10.3	0.0
Vegetable Supreme, Stuffed Crust, Pizza Hut*	1 Slice/156g	307	10.8	197	9.3	27.8	6.9	0.0
Vegetarian, Hi Light, Medium, Pizza Hut*	1 Slice/77g	170	5.1	221	10.3	30.0	6.6	0.0
Vegetarian Hot One, Cheesy Bites, Pizza Hut*	1 Slice/142g	302	10.1	212	9.8	30.3	7.1	0.0
Vegetarian Hot One, Italian, Individual, Pizza Hut*	1 Slice/78g	164	4.5	211	8.1	34.6	5.8	0.0
Vegetarian Hot One, Italian, Large, Pizza Hut*	1 Slice/114g	165	6.7	145	7.5	19.1	5.9	0.0
Vegetarian Hot One, Italian, Medium, Pizza Hut*	1 Slice/98g	188	5.4	192	9.3	29.5	5.5	0.0
Vegetarian Hot One, Pan, Individual, Pizza Hut*	1 Slice/82g	174	6.0	211	8.8	29.6	7.3	0.0
Vegetarian Hot One, Pan, Large, Pizza Hut*	1 Slice/126g	290	12.1	231	9.4	29.7	9.6	0.0
Vegetarian Hot One, Pan, Medium, Pizza Hut*	1 Slice/115g	234	9.9	204	8.4	26.6	8.6	0.0
Vegetarian Hot One, Stuffed Crust, Pizza Hut*	1 Slice/161g	334	11.1	208	10.1	30.2	6.9	0.0
Veggie, The Edge, Medium, Pizza Hut*	1 Slice/60g	136	5.4	227	11.2	22.2	9.0	0.0
PLATTER								
Favourites, Pizza Hut*	1 Platter/732g	1385	82.4	189	8.7	13.5	11.3	0.0
Tuscani, Pizza Hut*	1 Serving/462g	1223	89.5	265	8.8	13.2	19.4	0.0
POTATO SKINS								
Cheese & Bacon (6 Skins), Pizza Hut*	6 Skins/246g	408	17.8	166	6.4	20.1	7.2	0.0
Jacket, Loaded, with Cheese, Pizza Hut*	1 Serving/267g	571	34.2	214	13.6	11.2	12.8	0.0
Jacket, Pizza Hut*	1 Serving/224g	571	37.2	255	3.4	23.0	16.6	2.1
Jacket, with Sour Cream & Chive Dip, Pizza Hut*	1 Serving/224g	311	24.1	139	1.4	9.3	10.8	0.8
POTATO WEDGES								
without Dip, Pizza Hut*	1 Serving/390g	569	23.8	146	2.5	20.3	6.1	0.0
POTATOES								
Baby, Pizza Hut*	1 Serving/80g	63	1.4	79	1.2	14.6	1.8	0.0
PROFITEROLES								
Dessert, Pizza Hut*	1 Serving/100g	381	31.3	381	4.6	20.1	31.3	0.0
Pizza Hut*	1 Serving/100g	381	31.3	381	4.6	20.1	31.3	0.0
PUDDING								
Sticky Toffee, Pizza Hut*	1 Serving/105g	400	18.2	380	5.5	50.6	17.3	0.0
RAISINS								
Chocolate, Ice Cream Factory, Pizza Hut*	1 Serving/30g	122	4.3	405	5.4	63.3	14.2	0.0

	Measure INFO/WEIGHT	per Measure KCAL	FAT	Nutrition Values per 100g / 100ml KCAL	PROT	CARB	FAT	FIBRE
PIZZA HUT								
SALAD								
4 Leaf Mix, Pizza Hut*	1 Serving/100g	14	0.5	14	0.8	1.7	0.5	0.0
Beetroot & Carrot, with Balsamic Vinaigrette, Pizza Hut*	1 Serving/80g	24	0.2	30	1.1	5.7	0.3	0.0
Caesar, Chicken, Pizza Hut*	1 Sm/172g	263	12.7	153	14.1	7.4	7.4	0.0
Caesar, Classic, Pizza Hut*	1 Serving/194g	367	23.1	189	7.2	13.0	11.9	0.0
Caesar, Classic, Small, Pizza Hut*	1 Serving/97g	183	11.5	189	7.2	13.0	11.9	0.0
Caesar, Pizza Hut*	1 Salad/195g	344	20.2	177	6.0	14.8	10.4	0.0
Caesar, Prawn, Pizza Hut*	1 Serving/345g	459	24.2	133	9.6	7.6	7.0	0.0
Caesar, with Chicken & Bacon, Pizza Hut*	1 Serving/375g	588	29.6	157	14.4	6.8	7.9	0.0
Carrot Batons, Fresh, Pizza Hut*	1 Serving/80g	28	0.2	35	0.6	7.9	0.3	0.0
Cheese, Goats, Pizza Hut*	1 Serving/341g	525	40.2	154	7.5	4.4	11.8	0.0
Cheese, Hard, Grated, Pizza Hut*	1 Serving/50g	202	15.0	404	33.0	0.0	30.0	0.0
Chicken, Warm, Pizza Hut*	1 Salad/342g	403	17.4	118	11.0	6.8	5.1	0.0
Chicken & Bacon, Pizza Hut*	1 Serving/323g	514	32.0	159	10.3	6.9	9.9	0.0
Coleslaw, Pizza Hut*	1 Serving/80g	149	14.6	186	1.1	4.5	18.2	0.0
Dressed, Tabbouleh, Pizza Hut*	1 Serving/100g	189	8.1	189	4.2	24.9	8.1	0.0
Fresh, Carrot, Grated, Pizza Hut*	1 Serving/17g	5	0.1	30	0.7	6.0	0.5	0.0
Fresh, Cucumber, Slices, Pizza Hut*	1 Serving/80g	8	0.1	10	0.7	1.5	0.1	0.0
Fresh, Onion, Red, Slices, Pizza Hut*	1 Serving/80g	29	0.2	36	1.2	7.9	0.2	0.0
Fresh, Seasonal, Pizza Hut*	1 Serving/80g	12	0.5	15	0.7	1.8	0.6	0.0
Fresh, Tomatoes, Cherry, Pizza Hut*	1 Serving/80g	15	0.3	19	0.8	3.0	0.4	0.0
Leaf Mix, Pizza Hut*	1 Serving/41g	7	0.5	17	2.9	6.3	1.1	0.0
Mozzarella & Tomato, Light Lunch, Pizza Hut*	1 Serving/188g	387	30.6	206	12.3	2.4	16.3	0.0
Mozzarella & Tomato, Pizza Hut*	1 Salad/160g	234	19.0	146	7.8	2.1	11.9	0.0
Olive & Feta, Pizza Hut*	1 Serving/406g	345	26.0	85	3.8	3.6	6.4	0.0
Potato, Whole, Pizza Hut*	1 Serving/100g	154	10.1	154	1.6	13.5	10.1	0.0
Tuna, Pizza Hut*	1 Serving/461g	378	8.8	82	10.4	5.9	1.9	2.0
SAUCE								
Caramel, Ice Cream Factory, Pizza Hut*	1 Serving/25g	77	1.0	307	0.7	67.2	3.9	0.0
Chocolate, Ice Cream Factory, Pizza Hut*	1 Serving/25g	74	0.6	298	2.0	66.8	2.5	0.0
Strawberry, Ice Cream Factory, Pizza Hut*	1 Serving/25g	70	0.0	280	0.0	69.5	0.0	0.0
SMOOTHIE								
BananaBerry Split, Pizza Hut*	1 Serving/171g	258	0.4	151	1.5	33.6	0.2	0.0
Truly Tropical, Pizza Hut*	1 Serving/239g	234	0.3	98	0.6	24.0	0.1	0.0
Very Berry, Pizza Hut*	1 Serving/220g	189	0.3	86	0.6	20.4	0.1	0.0
SPAGHETTI BOLOGNESE								
Pizza Hut*	1 Serving/475g	745	31.3	157	6.2	17.8	6.6	0.0
SUNDAE								
Double Chocolate, Pizza Hut*	1 Sundae/145g	307	16.2	212	3.1	27.0	11.2	0.0
SWEETCORN								
Pizza Hut*	1 Serving/30g	24	0.2	79	1.8	16.8	0.8	0.0
TIRAMISU								
Delivery, Pizza Hut*	1 Serving/75g	223	10.3	297	3.9	39.5	13.7	0.0
Pizza Hut*	1 Serving/84g	248	11.4	297	3.9	39.5	13.7	0.0
TOMATOES								
Slices, Fresh, Pizza Hut*	1 Serving/80g	14	0.2	17	0.7	3.1	0.3	0.0
Spicy, & Red Pepper, Buffet, Pizza Hut*	1 Serving/200g	170	1.8	85	3.1	16.7	0.9	0.0
TOPPING								
Caramel Sauce, Pizza Hut*	1 Serving/100g	307	3.9	307	0.7	67.2	3.9	0.0
Chocolate Raisins, Pizza Hut*	1 Serving/100g	405	14.2	405	5.4	63.3	14.2	0.0
Chocolate Sauce, Pizza Hut*	1 Serving/100g	298	2.5	298	2.0	66.8	2.5	0.0
Coated Chocolate Beans, Pizza Hut*	1 Serving/100g	475	18.1	475	5.5	72.2	18.1	0.0
Lemon Sauce, Pizza Hut*	1 Serving/100g	280	0.0	280	0.1	69.0	0.0	0.0

	Measure INFO/WEIGHT	per Measure KCAL	FAT	Nutrition Values per 100g / 100ml KCAL	PROT	CARB	FAT	FIBRE
PIZZA HUT								
TOPPING								
Mini Marshmallows, Pizza Hut*	1 Serving/100g	320	0.0	320	5.4	74.3	0.0	0.0
Strawberry Sauce, Pizza Hut*	1 Serving/100g	280	0.0	280	0.0	69.5	0.0	0.0
PRET & MANGER								
MACARONI CHEESE								
Kale & Cauli, Pret*	1 Serving/360g	451	25.7	125	6.4	8.8	7.1	0.9
SALAD								
Salmon & Quinoa, Protein Pot, Pret & Manger*	1 Pack/140g	145	4.0	104	7.8	11.9	2.9	2.0
SOUP								
Asian Pepper, Pret*	1 Serving/370g	178	9.3	48	0.7	5.3	2.5	0.0
PRET A MANGER								
BAGUETTE								
Avocado & Basil, Pret a Manger*	1 Baguette/254g	163	7.2	163	4.6	19.8	7.2	2.8
Brie, Tomato & Basil, Pret a Manger*	1 Baguette/209g	418	17.3	200	8.2	23.2	8.3	1.6
Cheddar & Pickle, Posh, Artisan, Pret a Manger*	1 Baguette/243g	590	27.1	243	9.1	29.2	11.2	2.6
Chicken, Sweet Chilli, & Coriander, Pret a Manger*	1 Baguette/210g	390	11.4	186	10.2	23.8	5.4	1.5
Chicken Caesar & Bacon on Artisan, Pret a Manger*	1 Baguette/230g	584	25.8	254	13.5	24.3	11.2	1.8
Prawn,Thai, Pret a Manger*	1 Baguette/237g	374	9.6	158	7.8	22.5	4.0	1.6
Prosciutto, Italian, Artisan, Pret a Manger*	1 Baguette/246g	545	24.7	222	9.8	25.8	10.0	2.0
BARS								
Chocolate Brownie, Pret a Manger*	1 Bar/60g	320	19.1	500	6.2	49.3	29.8	4.7
Love Bar, Pret a Manger*	1 Bar/70g	324	18.3	463	6.1	50.6	26.1	3.6
Pret Bar, Pret a Manger*	1 Bar/65g	279	12.5	429	6.2	55.4	19.2	4.5
BISCUITS								
Fruit & Oat, Pret a Manger*	1 Pack/40g	187	9.8	468	8.2	50.0	24.5	6.2
BREAD								
Artisan Soup Bread, Pret a Manger*	1 Serving/80g	168	0.6	210	7.0	43.8	0.8	2.0
Baguette, White, for Soup, Pret a Manger*	1 Baguette/142g	336	1.7	237	8.3	48.3	1.2	2.7
BREAKFAST CEREAL								
Bircher Muesli Bowl, Pret a Manger*	1 Bowl/206g	304	9.7	148	6.3	20.2	4.7	1.4
Honey & Granola Pret Pot, Pret a Manger*	1 Serving/133g	263	7.8	198	7.3	28.8	5.9	1.3
Hot & Cold Granola, Pret a Manger*	1 Serving/226g	579	19.9	256	6.4	38.4	8.8	3.5
Porridge, No Topping, Pret a Manger*	1 Serving/300g	243	8.4	81	3.0	9.6	2.8	1.7
Porridge, with Compote, Pret a Manger*	1 Serving/332g	276	8.4	83	2.8	11.1	2.5	1.6
Porridge, with Honey, Pret a Manger*	1 Serving/335g	350	8.4	104	2.7	16.6	2.5	1.5
CAKE								
Apple, Slice, Pret a Manger*	1 Slice/100g	303	14.7	303	3.8	38.8	14.7	1.9
Banana, Slice, Pret a Manger*	1 Slice/82g	275	11.9	335	3.5	47.3	14.5	1.5
Carrot, Slice, Pret a Manger*	1 Slice/112g	400	22.2	357	3.9	40.6	19.8	2.4
Choc Bar, Pret a Manger*	1 Slice/70g	380	21.7	543	5.1	59.0	31.0	3.8
Chocolate, Slice, Pret a Manger*	1 Slice/88g	354	20.9	402	5.3	41.7	23.8	1.4
Lemon Cake Slice, Pret a Manger*	1 Slice/70g	257	10.6	367	4.1	52.4	15.1	2.1
CHEESECAKE								
Lemon, Pot, Pret a Manger*	1 Pot/120g	390	25.9	325	2.7	29.3	21.6	1.4
CHOCOLATE								
Dark, with Sea Salt, Pret a Manger*	1 Bar/25g	136	9.0	544	4.0	44.0	36.0	8.0
COFFEE								
Americano, Pret a Manger*	1 Serving/360ml	35	1.3	10	0.7	0.9	0.4	0.0
Americano, White, Semi Skimmed, Pret a Manger*	1 Cup/350g	14	0.5	4	0.3	0.4	0.1	0.0
Cappuccino, Pret a Manger*	1 Serving/231ml	88	3.1	38	2.7	3.8	1.3	0.0
Espresso, Pret a Manger*	1 Serving/137ml	0	0.0	0	0.0	0.0	0.0	0.0
Filter, Semi Skimmed Milk, Pret a Manger*	1 Serving/350ml	14	0.5	4	0.3	0.4	0.1	0.0
Flat White, Pret a Manger*	1 Serving/210ml	75	2.7	36	2.6	3.4	1.3	0.0

	Measure INFO/WEIGHT	per Measure KCAL	per Measure FAT	Nutrition Values per 100g / 100ml KCAL	PROT	CARB	FAT	FIBRE
PRET A MANGER								
COFFEE								
Latte, Merry, Very Berry, Pret a Manger*	1 Serving/295g	145	0.6	49	2.4	9.1	0.2	0.0
Latte, Skimmed Milk, Pret a Manger*	1 Serving/285ml	110	4.0	39	2.8	3.7	1.4	0.0
Macchiato, Pret a Manger*	1 Serving/60ml	5	0.2	8	0.5	0.8	0.3	0.0
Mocha, Semi Skimmed Milk, Pret a Manger*	1 Serving/293ml	175	5.0	60	3.0	8.0	1.7	0.0
Mocha, Skimmed Milk, Pret a Manger*	1 Regular/293ml	145	1.4	49	2.9	8.4	0.5	0.0
COOKIES								
Chocolate, White, & Orange, Pret a Manger*	1 Cookie/90g	365	11.6	406	5.4	65.7	12.9	2.4
Chocolate Chunk, Pret a Manger*	1 Cookie/90g	381	13.9	423	5.3	64.6	15.4	2.6
Oat, Apple & Raisin, Pret a Manger*	1 Cookie/90g	353	10.3	392	6.3	62.2	11.4	3.1
CRISPS								
Cheddar, Double, & Onion Topcorn, Pret a Manger*	1 Pack/25g	123	6.5	492	8.0	55.6	26.0	9.6
Cheese, Croxton Manor, & Red Onion, Pret a Manger*	1 Pack/40g	210	12.8	525	6.2	49.8	32.0	5.2
Maldon Sea Salt Crisps, Pret a Manger*	1 Pack/40g	218	14.3	545	5.2	48.0	35.8	5.5
CROISSANT								
Almond, Pret a Manger*	1 Croissant/95g	387	20.1	407	8.7	47.0	21.2	3.5
Chocolate, Pret a Manger*	1 Croissant/95g	420	23.2	442	7.7	46.5	24.4	2.9
French, Butter, Pret a Manger*	1 Croissant/80g	324	18.9	405	8.2	39.5	23.6	2.4
Ham, Bacon & Cheese, Pret a Manger*	1 Croissant/110g	351	22.7	319	12.2	19.8	20.6	1.2
Mozzarella & Tomato, Pret a Manger*	1 Croissant/110g	373	24.6	339	13.4	20.2	22.4	1.3
Pain au Raisin, Pret a Manger*	1 Croissant/110g	311	13.5	283	5.1	37.4	12.3	1.6
DRESSING								
for Crayfish & Avocado, Pret a Manger*	1 Serving/28g	144	14.8	514	0.7	8.2	52.9	0.0
for Greens & Grains, No Bread, Pret a Manger*	1 Pot/45g	41	3.0	91	4.0	3.8	6.7	0.2
for Pole & Line Caught Tuna Nicoise, Pret a Manger*	1 Pot/45g	231	23.8	513	0.7	8.0	52.9	0.0
for Roasted Vegetable & Feta, Pret a Manger*	1 Pot/45g	231	23.8	513	0.7	8.0	52.9	0.0
for Sesame Chicken & Noodle Salad, Pret a Manger*	1 Pot/45g	140	9.8	311	12.0	16.0	21.8	0.0
for Superfood Salad, Pret a Manger*	1 Pot/45g	231	23.8	513	0.7	8.0	52.9	0.0
DRIED FRUIT								
Mango, Pret a Manger*	1 Serving/35g	116	0.1	331	1.4	84.6	0.3	3.7
FRUIT								
British Berries, Pret a Manger*	1 Pot/130g	34	0.1	26	0.9	5.4	0.1	1.6
Five Berry Bowl, Pret a Manger*	1 Bowl/220g	379	12.4	172	6.7	23.3	5.6	1.7
Five Berry Pot, Pret a Manger*	1 Pot/148g	152	4.7	103	6.0	12.6	3.2	0.3
Fruit Salad, Pret's, Pret a Manger*	1 Serving/240g	113	0.4	47	0.6	9.7	0.2	1.8
Nectarine & Raspberries, Pret a Manger*	1 Serving/56g	24	0.1	43	1.4	7.8	0.2	2.7
Pomegranate & Orange, Pret a Manger*	1 Serving/116g	54	0.0	47	1.2	10.0	0.0	0.0
Seedless Grapes, Pret a Manger*	1 Serving/165g	109	0.0	66	0.4	15.4	0.0	1.0
GINGER BEER								
Pure Pret, Pret a Manger*	1 Serving/330ml	152	0.0	46	0.0	11.4	0.0	0.0
GINGERBREAD								
Godfrey, Pret's Gingerbread Man, Pret a Manger*	1 Serving/54g	195	7.3	361	4.6	55.4	13.5	1.7
HOT CHOCOLATE								
Pret a Manger*	1 Serving/285ml	237	5.9	83	3.4	12.7	2.1	0.0
JUICE								
Carrot, Pret a Manger*	1 Serving/250ml	60	0.3	24	0.5	5.7	0.1	0.0
Orange, Pret a Manger*	1 Serving/260ml	114	0.0	44	0.6	11.0	0.0	0.1
JUICE DRINK								
Apple, Pure Pret, Pret a Manger*	1 Serving/330ml	159	0.0	48	0.1	11.6	0.0	0.0
Orange, Pure Pret, Pret a Manger*	1 Serving/330ml	200	0.0	61	0.1	3.1	0.0	0.0
LEMONADE								
Still, Pure Pret, Pret a Manger*	1 Bottle/500ml	171	0.0	34	0.0	8.3	0.0	0.0

	Measure INFO/WEIGHT	per Measure KCAL	FAT	Nutrition Values per 100g / 100ml KCAL	PROT	CARB	FAT	FIBRE
PRET A MANGER								
MACARONI CHEESE								
Prosciutto, Pret a Manger*	1 Pack/360g	488	27.8	136	7.5	8.9	7.7	0.9
MACAROONS								
Coconut in Milk Chocolate, Pret a Manger*	1 Pack/108g	523	34.0	484	6.9	40.7	31.5	4.1
MOUSSE								
Chocolate, Pret a Manger*	1 Pack/306g	1170	117.4	382	3.8	22.2	38.4	1.6
MUFFIN								
Double Berry, Pret a Manger*	1 Muffin/145g	498	23.8	343	5.2	44.5	16.4	2.3
High Fibre, Pret a Manger*	1 Muffin/130g	442	24.4	340	8.0	28.6	18.8	9.0
NECTARINE								
Pret a Manger*	1 Fruit/1133g	53	0.1	40	1.4	9.0	0.1	1.1
POPCORN								
Rock Salt, Light, Pret a Manger*	1 Pack/29g	138	7.1	476	6.6	63.8	24.5	15.2
Sweet & Salt, Light, Pret a Manger*	1 Pack/30g	138	5.8	460	7.1	64.3	19.3	6.7
PRETZELS								
Pret a Manger*	1 Serving/105g	333	7.6	317	8.7	52.8	7.2	3.0
PROTEIN POT								
Chicken, & Humous, Pret a Manger*	1 Pack/217g	370	15.0	171	10.7	16.5	6.9	5.5
Salmon, Avocado & Quinoa, Pret a Manger*	1 Pack/163g	221	11.1	136	7.5	10.8	6.8	3.6
SALAD								
Beef, Asian, & Noodle, no Dressing, Pret a Manger*	1 Pack/266g	309	6.3	116	7.3	16.4	2.4	1.4
Ceasar, Chicken, Pret a Manger*	1 Pack/252g	370	16.0	147	11.9	9.1	6.4	0.8
Chicken, Chef's Italian, no Dressing, Pret a Manger*	1 Pack/282g	306	21.2	109	7.6	2.6	7.5	2.0
Chicken, Chipotle, Chefs, no Dressing, Pret a Manger*	1 Pack/308g	301	17.7	98	8.8	2.5	5.7	1.6
Chicken, Chipotle, Chefs, with Dressing, Pret a Manger*	1 Pack/329g	436	32.5	132	8.3	3.0	9.9	1.5
Crayfish & Quinoa, Protein Pot, Pret a Manger*	1 Pack/168g	210	7.4	125	9.4	12.0	4.4	2.0
Duck, Hoisin, No Bread, Pret a Manger*	1 Pack/202g	138	10.6	68	7.5	7.5	5.2	1.7
Edamame Bowl, Pret a Manger*	1 Pack/125g	94	4.2	76	6.3	4.9	3.4	0.0
Salmon, Smoked, & Sweet Pickle, Pret a Manger*	1 Pack/271g	481	22.5	177	8.2	16.8	8.3	2.0
Superfood, No Dressing, Pret a Manger*	1 Pack/337g	375	17.8	111	4.3	11.9	5.3	4.2
SANDWICH								
BLT, Beech Smoked, Pret a Manger*	1 Pack/232g	444	20.0	191	8.4	20.0	8.6	1.9
Cheddar, Mature, & Pret Pickle, Pret a Manger*	1 Pack/246g	479	24.3	195	7.6	18.4	9.9	1.7
Cheese, Kid's, Pret a Manger*	1 Pack/127g	399	20.2	314	13.9	28.9	15.9	2.2
Chicken, & Pesto, Bloomer, Pret a Manger*	1 Pack/273g	477	17.1	175	10.2	18.0	6.3	1.9
Chicken Avocado, Pret a Manger*	1 Pack/246g	469	23.4	191	9.7	16.1	9.5	2.7
Classic, Super Club, Pret a Manger*	1 Pack/255g	505	24.8	198	11.1	15.7	9.7	1.5
Corned Beef, Bloomer, Pret a Manger*	1 Pack/289g	536	21.4	185	10.7	18.5	7.4	1.9
Crayfish, Sweet Chilli, & Mango, Bloomer, Pret*	1 Pack/215g	401	12.2	187	9.3	24.6	5.7	2.3
Crayfish, Wild, & Rocket, Pret a Manger*	1 Pack/194g	374	15.0	193	10.6	19.4	7.7	1.5
Egg Mayo, Free-Range, Pret a Manger*	1 Pack/189g	426	23.5	225	8.9	19.6	12.4	1.6
Eggs Florentine, Bloomer, Pret a Manger*	1 Pack/254g	545	26.8	215	9.8	19.4	10.6	2.1
Falafel & Humous, Moroccan, Pret a Manger*	1 Pack/285g	525	17.6	184	5.8	23.0	6.2	3.3
Ham, Kid's, Pret a Manger*	1 Pack/127g	289	8.2	228	13.4	28.9	6.5	2.2
Ham & Eggs, Bloomer, Classic, Pret a Manger*	1 Pack/225g	547	25.2	243	14.7	20.9	11.2	1.9
Humous, Crunchy, Bloomer, Pret a Manger*	1 Pack/224g	511	17.5	228	10.1	30.1	7.8	7.0
Jambon Beurre, Pret a Manger*	1 Pack/144g	359	13.1	249	11.3	29.6	9.1	1.9
Salad, Cheese, Emmental, Pret a Manger*	1 Pack/239g	494	28.2	207	8.3	16.9	11.8	1.8
Salad, Edam, Pret a Manger*	1 Pack/212g	473	26.6	223	8.8	18.7	12.6	1.8
Salad, Egg, Cracking, Pret a Manger*	1 Pack/241g	430	23.1	178	7.0	16.2	9.6	1.5
Salad, Falafel, Moroccan, Pret a Manger*	1 Pack/278g	417	8.8	150	5.5	21.2	3.2	1.4
Salmon, Smoked, Scottish, Pret a Manger*	1 Pack/156g	366	14.2	235	14.5	23.6	9.1	1.8
The New York, Bloomer, Pret a Manger*	1 Pack/227g	507	22.0	223	13.0	22.0	9.7	2.2

	Measure INFO/WEIGHT	per Measure KCAL	FAT	Nutrition Values per 100g / 100ml KCAL	PROT	CARB	FAT	FIBRE
PRET A MANGER								
SANDWICH								
Tuna Mayo, Kid's, Pret a Manger*	1 Pack/150g	372	17.3	248	10.9	24.9	11.5	1.9
SMOOTHIE								
Mango, Pret a Manger*	1 Serving/250ml	143	0.5	57	0.6	13.7	0.2	3.0
Strawberry, Pret a Manger*	1 Serving/250ml	128	0.8	51	0.9	11.2	0.3	0.0
Vitamin Volcano, Pret a Manger*	1 Serving/250ml	138	0.8	55	0.6	12.4	0.3	1.3
SOUP								
Broccoli & Italian Cheese, Pret a Manger*	1 Pack/370g	226	14.1	61	2.2	3.8	3.8	1.3
Butternut Squash, & Sage, Pret a Manger*	1 Pot/370g	104	3.0	28	0.9	3.9	0.8	0.0
Cashew, Butternut, & Spice Soup, Pret a Manger*	1 Pack/370g	266	14.4	72	1.9	7.0	3.9	1.4
Chicken, & Roasted Corn, Chowder, Pret a Manger*	1 Soup/370g	259	8.9	70	3.5	7.6	2.4	1.0
Chicken, Broccoli, & Brown Rice, Pret a Manger*	1 Serving/370g	134	2.2	36	2.7	4.6	0.6	0.0
Chicken, Moroccan, Pret a Manger*	1 Serving/370g	304	9.9	82	4.5	8.8	2.7	2.4
Chilli, Mexican, with a Hint of Chocolate, Pret*	1 Pack/370g	344	8.9	93	3.8	12.4	2.4	3.2
Curry, Chicken, Malaysian, Pret a Manger*	1 Serving/370g	270	14.8	73	2.7	5.5	4.0	2.0
Curry, Lentil & Coconut, Pret a Manger*	1 Pack/370g	403	15.9	109	5.4	11.5	4.3	1.5
Ham, Hock, Pret a Manger*	1 Serving/370g	410	18.9	111	6.0	8.9	5.1	2.6
Meatball, Italian, Pret a Manger*	1 Serving/370g	263	15.5	71	2.4	5.8	4.2	1.0
Minestrone, Pret a Manger*	1 Pack/370g	218	10.7	59	2.0	5.3	2.9	1.5
Miso, Pret a Manger*	1 Serving/20g	32	1.0	160	10.0	0.0	5.0	0.0
Mushroom, Cream of, Pret a Manger*	1 Pack/370g	159	8.9	43	1.3	3.2	2.4	0.6
Mushroom Risotto, Pret a Manger*	1 Serving/370g	259	13.7	70	2.4	6.4	3.7	0.0
Pea, Garden, & Mint, Pret a Manger*	1 Pack320g	253	17.6	79	2.4	4.0	5.5	0.0
Pea & Ham, Pret a Manger*	1 Pack/370g	233	10.7	63	4.5	3.8	2.9	2.0
Pork, BBQ, Pulled, & Bean, Pret a Manger*	1 Pack/370g	341	7.4	92	6.4	10.8	2.0	2.4
Red Pepper, & Creme Fraiche, Pret a Manger*	1 Pack/370g	215	15.2	58	1.1	3.7	4.1	0.9
Root Veg & Bean, Smoky, Pret a Manger*	1 Serving/370g	192	3.0	52	2.3	7.4	0.8	3.2
Sausage, Hot Pot, Pret a Manger*	1 Serving/370g	230	13.0	62	4.0	2.6	3.5	2.0
Sweet Tomato & Saffron, Pret a Manger*	1 Pack/370g	255	14.8	69	1.7	5.9	4.0	0.7
Tomato, Classic, Pret a Manger*	1 Serving/370g	218	10.7	59	1.8	6.0	2.9	0.8
SUSHI								
Bento Box, Deluxe, Pret a Manger*	1 Serving/256g	353	10.0	138	6.4	19.5	3.9	1.7
California Rolls, Pret a Manger*	1 Pack/206g	354	9.3	172	5.1	27.5	4.5	1.4
Deluxe, Pret a Manger*	1 Pack/232g	382	9.3	165	6.2	25.8	4.0	1.3
Maki & Nigiri, Pret a Manger*	1 Serving/200g	314	8.4	157	5.4	23.4	4.2	1.0
Salmon & Prawn, Pret a Manger*	1 Serving/232g	382	9.3	165	6.2	25.8	4.0	1.3
Veggie, Pret a Manger*	1 Pack/226g	333	5.8	147	3.6	27.7	2.6	2.0
TART								
Bakewell Tart, Pret a Manger*	1 Serving/68g	318	18.1	468	7.6	49.7	26.6	2.5
TEA								
Ceylon, Breakfast, Pret a Manger*	1 Serving/360ml	14	0.5	4	0.3	0.4	0.1	0.0
Chai, Vanilla, Pret a Manger*	1 Serving/360ml	14	0.5	4	0.3	0.4	0.1	0.0
Green, Tropical, Pret a Manger*	1 Serving/60ml	0	0.0	0	0.0	0.0	0.0	0.0
Iced, Peach, Pure, Still, Pret a Manger*	1 Serving/500ml	78	0.0	16	0.0	3.8	0.0	0.0
Red Berries, Pret a Manger*	1 Serving/60ml	0	0.0	0	0.0	0.0	0.0	0.0
TOASTIE								
Chicken & Bacon, Pret a Manger*	1 Pack/254g	533	21.2	210	14.2	19.1	8.4	2.0
Halloumi & Red Pepper, Pret a Manger*	1 Pack/233g	543	25.5	233	11.7	21.6	10.9	2.9
Ham, Cheese & Mustard Toastie, Pret a Manger*	1 Serving/215g	588	27.6	273	17.8	21.8	12.8	2.0
Mozzarella & Pesto, Italian, Pret a Manger*	1 Serving/234g	511	24.3	218	10.3	20.8	10.4	2.2
Tuna Melt, Pret a Manger*	1 Serving/219g	555	24.0	253	16.8	21.5	11.0	2.4
WRAP								
Avocado, & Herb Salad, Pret a Manger*	1 Wrap/246g	460	30.5	187	4.8	13.6	12.4	2.6

	Measure INFO/WEIGHT	per Measure KCAL	FAT	Nutrition Values per 100g / 100ml KCAL	PROT	CARB	FAT	FIBRE
PRET A MANGER								
WRAP								
Beef Samosa, Hot, Pret a Manger*	1 Wrap/235g	531	29.1	226	8.3	20.2	12.4	2.3
Chicken, Jalapeno, Hot, Pret a Manger*	1 Wrap/262g	430	14.5	164	12.7	15.1	5.5	1.9
Chicken, Sesame, Sushi, Pret a Manger*	1 Wrap/227g	400	16.2	176	10.8	16.9	7.1	2.4
Chicken Raita, with Salad, Pret a Manger*	1 Wrap/233g	314	7.1	135	9.7	16.3	3.0	2.2
Chunky Humous, Salad, Pret a Manger*	1 Wrap/209g	446	20.9	213	7.2	24.0	10.0	5.8
Duck, Hoisin, Pret a Manger*	1 Wrap/212g	341	19.5	161	8.4	19.8	9.2	1.5
Falafel & Halloumi, Hot, Pret a Manger*	1 Wrap/244g	578	22.8	237	7.4	24.8	9.3	1.7
Guacamole, GF, Mexican, Pret a Manger*	1 Wrap/234g	389	20.1	166	2.9	17.4	8.6	4.3
Meatball, Swedish, Hot, Pret a Manger*	1 Wrap/233g	674	41.3	289	14.1	17.9	17.7	1.8
Nori, Super Veg, Pret a Manger*	1 Wrap/187g	347	13.5	186	5.6	23.5	7.2	0.0
Pizza, Italian, Hot, Pret a Manger*	1 Wrap/200g	391	17.2	196	8.7	20.8	8.6	2.4
Salmon, O'mega, Salad, Pret a Manger*	1 Wrap/200g	319	13.2	160	9.2	15.8	6.6	1.6
YOGHURT								
Yoghurt Nuts, Pret a Manger*	1 Pack/75g	430	33.2	573	6.9	29.7	44.3	6.9
YOGHURT DRINK								
Blueberry, Probiotic, Pret a Manger*	1 Serving/250ml	185	4.3	74	2.3	12.4	1.7	0.0
Vanilla, Probiotic, Pret a Manger*	1 Serving/250ml	203	6.3	81	2.9	9.7	2.5	0.0
STARBUCKS								
BAGEL								
Salmon, Smoked, with Cream Cheese, Starbucks*	1 Bagel/165g	370	11.1	224	12.7	27.2	6.7	1.7
BARS								
Chocolate, Dark, Fairtrade, Starbucks*	1 Bar/45g	259	20.8	575	6.7	27.6	46.3	10.7
Chocolate, Milk, Fairtrade, Starbucks*	1 Bar/45g	242	17.4	537	6.4	49.0	38.6	2.2
Granola, Starbucks*	1 Bar/85g	398	22.0	468	7.2	48.9	25.9	5.1
BISCUITS								
Ginger Snaps, Starbucks*	1 Biscuit/30g	134	4.6	445	4.8	71.9	15.4	1.5
BREAD								
Fruit, Starbucks*	1 Serving/145g	481	11.6	332	7.5	55.7	8.0	3.4
Pumpkin, Starbucks*	1 Serving/100g	322	11.6	322	5.0	50.4	11.6	1.6
BREAKFAST CEREAL								
Granola, Maple & Honey, Topping, Starbucks*	1 Serving/25g	112	4.0	448	9.0	64.5	15.9	5.6
Porridge, Dairy, Starbucks*	1 Serving/230g	244	6.2	106	4.1	17.4	2.7	1.8
Porridge, Soy, Starbucks*	1 Serving/230g	205	4.8	89	4.6	13.9	2.1	2.2
Sauce, Maple & Honey, Topping, Starbucks*	1 Serving/40g	120	0.0	300	0.1	74.8	0.1	0.2
Very Berry Compote, Topping, Starbucks*	1 Serving/50g	59	0.1	119	0.6	29.7	0.2	2.1
BROWNIES								
Chocolate, Belgian, GF, Fairtrade, Starbucks*	1 Cake/72g	370	22.8	514	4.1	51.9	31.7	2.6
BUTTIE								
Bacon, Starbucks*	1 Buttie/118g	414	18.2	351	19.1	33.3	15.4	1.4
CAKE								
Chocolate Chilli, Petite, Starbucks*	1 Cake/38g	170	8.7	448	5.3	57.6	22.8	4.4
Chocolate Chilli, Starbucks*	1 Cake/38g	170	8.7	448	5.3	57.6	22.8	4.4
Loaf, Banana Nut, Starbucks*	1 Cake/103g	431	25.8	418	6.5	40.5	25.0	2.8
Loaf, Lemon, Starbucks*	1 Cake/86g	365	20.2	424	5.0	47.3	23.5	1.6
Loaf, Raspberry & Coconut, Starbucks*	1 Cake/89g	402	22.8	452	4.5	49.9	25.6	2.1
Loaf Cake, Chocolate Hazelnut, Starbucks*	1 Cake/85g	331	20.8	389	4.0	38.4	24.5	3.2
Marshmallow Twizzle, Chocolate, Starbucks*	1 Cake/40g	193	8.6	483	4.4	66.9	21.6	1.8
Marshmallow Twizzle, Red White & Blue, Starbucks*	1 Cake/35g	147	4.9	421	4.4	68.8	13.9	1.6
Rocky Road, Starbucks*	1 Cake/78g	423	27.1	542	4.3	51.5	34.8	2.7
CHEWING GUM								
Sugar Free, Starbucks*	1 Chew/3g	5	0.0	166	0.0	80.0	0.0	0.0

	Measure INFO/WEIGHT	per Measure KCAL	FAT	Nutrition Values per 100g / 100ml KCAL	PROT	CARB	FAT	FIBRE
STARBUCKS								
COFFEE								
Caffe Americano, Grande, Starbucks*	1 Grande/473ml	17	0.0	4	0.2	0.6	0.0	0.0
Caffe Americano, Short, Starbucks*	1 Short/236ml	6	0.0	2	0.2	0.4	0.0	0.0
Caffe Americano, Tall, Starbucks*	1 Tall/355ml	11	0.0	3	0.2	0.6	0.0	0.0
Caffe Americano, Venti, Starbucks*	1 Venti/591ml	23	0.0	4	0.2	0.7	0.0	0.0
Caffe Latte, Grande, Semi Skimmed Milk, Starbucks*	1 Grande/473ml	188	7.0	40	2.6	3.9	1.5	0.0
Caffe Latte, Grande, Skimmed Milk, Starbucks*	1 Grande/473ml	131	0.3	28	2.7	4.1	0.1	0.0
Caffe Latte, Grande, Soy, Starbucks*	1 Grande/473ml	148	5.3	31	2.2	2.7	1.1	0.3
Caffe Latte, Grande, Whole Milk, Starbucks*	1 Grande/473ml	223	11.5	47	2.6	3.8	2.4	0.0
Caffe Latte, Short, Semi Skimmed Milk, Starbucks*	1 Short/236ml	95	3.5	40	2.7	4.0	1.5	0.0
Caffe Latte, Short, Skimmed Milk, Starbucks*	1 Short/236ml	67	0.1	28	2.7	4.2	0.0	0.0
Caffe Latte, Short, Soy, Starbucks*	1 Short/236ml	75	2.7	32	2.2	2.8	1.1	0.3
Caffe Latte, Short, Whole Milk, Starbucks*	1 Short/236ml	113	5.8	48	2.6	3.9	2.5	0.0
Caffe Latte, Skimmed Milk, Tall, Starbucks*	1 Tall/355ml	102	0.2	29	2.7	4.3	0.1	0.0
Caffe Latte, Soy, Tall, Starbucks*	1 Tall/355ml	110	4.0	31	2.2	2.8	1.1	0.3
Caffe Latte, Tall, Semi Skimmed Milk, Starbucks*	1 Tall/355ml	143	5.1	40	2.7	4.2	1.4	0.0
Caffe Latte, Tall, Whole Milk, Starbucks*	1 Tall/355ml	172	8.4	48	2.6	4.2	2.4	0.0
Caffe Latte, Venti, Semi Skimmed Milk, Starbucks*	1 Venti/591ml	248	9.2	42	2.8	4.2	1.6	0.0
Caffe Latte, Venti, Skimmed Milk, Starbucks*	1 Venti/591ml	174	0.4	29	2.8	4.4	0.1	0.0
Caffe Latte, Venti, Soy, Starbucks*	1 Venti/591ml	185	6.7	31	2.2	2.8	1.1	0.3
Caffe Latte, Venti, Whole Milk, Starbucks*	1 Venti/591ml	299	15.0	51	2.6	4.2	2.5	0.0
Caffe Misto, Grande, Semi Skimmed Milk, Starbucks*	1 Grande/473ml	106	4.1	22	1.5	2.0	0.9	0.0
Caffe Misto, Grande, Skimmed Milk, Starbucks*	1 Grande/473ml	73	0.2	15	1.5	2.2	0.0	0.0
Caffe Misto, Grande, Soy, Starbucks*	1 Grande/473ml	82	3.2	17	1.2	1.4	0.7	0.2
Caffe Misto, Grande, Whole Milk, Starbucks*	1 Grande/473ml	126	6.8	27	1.5	2.0	1.4	0.0
Caffe Misto, Short, Semi Skimmed Milk, Starbucks*	1 Short/236ml	54	2.1	23	1.5	2.1	0.9	0.0
Caffe Misto, Short, Skimmed Milk, Starbucks*	1 Short/236ml	37	0.1	16	1.6	2.2	0.0	0.0
Caffe Misto, Short, Soy, Starbucks*	1 Short/236ml	42	1.6	18	1.3	1.4	0.7	0.2
Caffe Misto, Short, Whole Milk, Starbucks*	1 Short/236ml	65	3.5	28	1.5	2.0	1.5	0.0
Caffe Misto, Tall, Semi Skimmed Milk, Starbucks*	1 Tall/355ml	81	3.2	23	1.6	2.1	0.9	0.0
Caffe Misto, Tall, Skimmed Milk, Starbucks*	1 Tall/355ml	56	0.2	16	1.6	2.2	0.1	0.0
Caffe Misto, Tall, Soy, Starbucks*	1 Tall/355ml	63	2.4	18	1.3	1.4	0.7	0.2
Caffe Misto, Tall, Whole Milk, Starbucks*	1 Tall/355ml	97	5.2	27	1.5	2.0	1.5	0.0
Caffe Misto, Venti, Semi Skimmed Milk, Starbucks*	1 Venti/591ml	134	5.2	23	1.5	2.1	0.9	0.0
Caffe Misto, Venti, Skimmed Milk, Starbucks*	1 Venti/591ml	92	0.3	16	1.6	2.2	0.0	0.0
Caffe Misto, Venti, Soy, Starbucks*	1 Venti/591ml	104	4.0	18	1.3	1.4	0.7	0.2
Caffe Misto, Venti, Whole Milk, Starbucks*	1 Venti/591ml	160	8.6	27	1.5	2.0	1.5	0.0
Caffe Mocha, & Whip, Grande, Soy, Starbucks*	1 Grande/473ml	302	13.7	64	2.4	8.1	2.9	0.6
Caffe Mocha, & Whip, Grande, Whole Milk, Starbucks*	1 Grande/473ml	364	18.7	77	2.8	9.0	4.0	0.4
Caffe Mocha, & Whip, Short, Semi Skim, Starbucks*	1 Short/236ml	184	9.1	78	2.8	9.3	3.9	0.4
Caffe Mocha, & Whip, Short, Skim Milk, Starbucks*	1 Short/236ml	161	6.4	68	2.9	9.5	2.7	0.4
Caffe Mocha, & Whip, Short, Whole Milk, Starbucks*	1 Short/236ml	198	11.0	84	2.8	9.2	4.7	0.4
Caffe Mocha, & Whip, Tall, Semi Skim Milk, Starbucks*	1 Tall/355ml	273	12.7	77	2.8	9.4	3.6	0.4
Caffe Mocha, & Whip, Tall, Skim Milk, Starbucks*	1 Tall/355ml	238	8.5	67	2.8	9.5	2.4	0.4
Caffe Mocha, & Whip, Tall, Whole Milk, Starbucks*	1 Tall/355ml	297	15.5	84	2.7	9.4	4.4	0.4
Caffe Mocha, & Whip, Venti, Semi Skim Milk, Starbucks*	1 Venti/591ml	417	17.7	70	2.7	9.2	3.0	0.4
Caffe Mocha, & Whip, Venti, Skim Milk, Starbucks*	1 Venti/591ml	359	10.9	61	2.8	9.3	1.8	0.4
Caffe Mocha, & Whip, Venti, Soy, Starbucks*	1 Venti/591ml	373	15.8	63	2.5	8.4	2.7	0.7
Caffe Mocha, & Whip, Venti, Whole Milk, Starbucks*	1 Venti/591ml	456	22.3	77	2.7	9.2	3.8	0.4
Caffe Mocha, & Whip Cream, Short, Soy, Starbucks*	1 Short/236ml	167	8.5	71	2.5	8.4	3.6	0.6
Caffe Mocha, & Whip Cream, Tall, Soy, Starbucks*	1 Tall/355ml	247	11.8	70	2.5	8.4	3.3	0.7
Caffe Mocha, Whip, Grande, Semi Skim, Starbucks*	1 Grande/473ml	335	15.0	71	2.8	9.1	3.2	0.4
Caffe Mocha, Whip, Grande, Skim Milk, Starbucks*	1 Grande/473ml	288	9.5	61	2.8	9.3	2.0	0.4

	Measure INFO/WEIGHT	per Measure KCAL	FAT	Nutrition Values per 100g / 100ml KCAL	PROT	CARB	FAT	FIBRE
STARBUCKS								
COFFEE								
Cappuccino, Grande, Semi Skimmed Milk, Starbucks*	1 Grande/473ml	115	4.1	24	1.6	2.5	0.9	0.0
Cappuccino, Grande, Skimmed Milk, Starbucks*	1 Grande/473ml	82	0.2	17	1.6	2.6	0.0	0.0
Cappuccino, Grande, Soy, Starbucks*	1 Grande/473ml	92	3.2	19	1.4	1.8	0.7	0.2
Cappuccino, Grande, Whole Milk, Starbucks*	1 Grande/473ml	136	6.8	29	1.6	2.4	1.4	0.0
Cappuccino, Short, Semi Skimmed Milk, Starbucks*	1 Short/236ml	78	2.8	33	2.2	3.3	1.2	0.0
Cappuccino, Short, Skimmed Milk, Starbucks*	1 Short/236ml	55	0.1	23	2.2	3.4	0.0	0.0
Cappuccino, Short, Soy, Starbucks*	1 Short/236ml	62	2.2	26	1.8	2.3	0.9	0.2
Cappuccino, Short, Whole Milk, Starbucks*	1 Short/236ml	92	4.7	39	2.1	3.2	2.0	0.0
Cappuccino, Tall, Semi Skimmed Milk, Starbucks*	1 Tall/355ml	97	3.4	27	1.8	2.9	1.0	0.0
Cappuccino, Tall, Skimmed Milk, Starbucks*	1 Tall/355ml	70	0.1	20	1.8	3.0	0.0	0.0
Cappuccino, Tall, Soy, Starbucks*	1 Tall/355ml	74	2.5	21	1.4	2.0	0.7	0.2
Cappuccino, Tall, Whole Milk, Starbucks*	1 Tall/355ml	116	5.6	33	1.7	2.9	1.6	0.0
Cappuccino, Venti, Semi Skimmed Milk, Starbucks*	1 Venti/591ml	161	5.7	27	1.8	2.8	1.0	0.0
Cappuccino, Venti, Skimmed Milk, Starbucks*	1 Venti/591ml	115	0.2	19	1.8	2.9	0.0	0.0
Cappuccino, Venti, Soy, Starbucks*	1 Venti/591ml	123	4.2	21	1.4	2.0	0.7	0.2
Cappuccino, Venti, Whole Milk, Starbucks*	1 Venti/591ml	192	9.3	33	1.7	2.8	1.6	0.0
Espresso, Con Panna, Doppio, Starbucks*	1 Doppio/60ml	36	2.5	61	1.5	4.5	4.2	0.0
Espresso, Con Panna, Solo, Starbucks*	1 Solo/30ml	31	2.5	103	1.7	5.7	8.3	0.0
Espresso, Doppio, Starbucks*	1 Doppio/60ml	11	0.0	19	1.2	3.3	0.0	0.0
Espresso, Solo, Starbucks*	1 Solo/30ml	6	0.0	19	1.3	3.3	0.0	0.0
Espresso Macchhiato, Doppio, Soy, Starbucks*	1 Doppio/60ml	14	0.1	22	1.5	3.3	0.2	0.0
Espresso Macchhiato, Doppio, Whole Milk, Starbucks*	1 Doppio/60ml	15	0.2	24	1.5	3.8	0.3	0.0
Espresso Macchiato, Doppio, Semi Skim, Starbucks*	1 Doppio/60ml	14	0.1	24	1.5	3.8	0.2	0.0
Espresso Macchiato, Doppio, Skimmed Milk, Starbucks*	1 Doppio/60ml	13	0.0	22	1.7	4.0	0.0	0.0
Espresso Macchiato, Solo, Semi Skim Milk, Starbucks*	1 Solo/30ml	8	0.1	27	1.7	4.0	0.3	0.0
Espresso Macchiato, Solo, Skimmed Milk, Starbucks*	1 Solo/30ml	7	0.0	24	1.7	4.0	0.0	0.0
Espresso Macchiato, Solo, Soy, Starbucks*	1 Solo/30ml	7	0.1	25	1.7	3.7	0.3	0.0
Espresso Macchiato, Solo, Whole Milk, Starbucks*	1 Solo/30ml	8	0.2	28	1.7	4.0	0.7	0.0
Filter, Grande, Starbucks*	1 Grande/473ml	5	0.1	1	0.1	0.0	0.0	0.0
Filter, Short, Starbucks*	1 Short/236ml	3	0.1	1	0.1	0.0	0.0	0.0
Filter, Tall, Starbucks*	1 Tall/355ml	4	0.1	1	0.1	0.0	0.0	0.0
Filter, Venti, Starbucks*	1 Venti/591ml	6	0.1	1	0.1	0.0	0.0	0.0
Flat White, Short, Whole Milk, Starbucks*	1 Short/236ml	119	5.8	50	2.8	4.3	2.5	0.0
Iced, Caffe Americano, Grande, Starbucks*	1 Grande/473ml	17	0.0	4	0.2	0.6	0.0	0.0
Iced, Caffe Americano, Tall, Starbucks*	1 Tall/335ml	11	0.0	3	0.2	0.6	0.0	0.0
Iced, Caffe Americano, Venti, Starbucks*	1 Venti/591ml	23	0.0	4	0.2	0.7	0.0	0.0
Iced, Caffe Mocha, & Whip, Grande, Soy, Starbucks*	1 Grande/473ml	300	16.1	63	1.8	7.6	3.4	0.6
Iced, Caffe Mocha, & Whip, Tall, Semi Skim, Starbucks*	1 Tall/335ml	225	11.8	67	1.9	8.4	3.5	0.4
Iced, Caffe Mocha, & Whip, Tall, Skim Milk, Starbucks*	1 Tall/335ml	208	9.8	62	2.0	8.5	2.9	0.4
Iced, Caffe Mocha, & Whip, Tall, Soy, Starbucks*	1 Tall/335ml	214	11.3	64	1.8	7.9	3.4	0.5
Iced, Caffe Mocha, & Whip, Tall, Whole Milk, Starbucks*	1 Tall/335ml	236	13.1	71	1.9	8.4	3.9	0.4
Iced, Caffe Mocha, & Whip, Venti, Skim Milk, Starbucks*	1 Venti/591ml	315	14.1	53	1.7	7.7	2.4	0.4
Iced, Caffe Mocha, & Whip, Venti, Soy, Starbucks*	1 Venti/591ml	325	16.4	55	1.5	7.2	2.8	0.5
Iced, Caramel Macchiato, Grande, Soy, Starbucks*	1 Grande/473ml	206	5.3	43	1.8	6.3	1.1	0.2
Iced, Caramel Macchiato, Semi Skim, Starbucks*	1 Tall/335ml	146	3.7	43	1.6	6.8	1.1	0.0
Iced, Caramel Macchiato, Skim, Starbucks*	1 Venti/591ml	189	1.2	32	1.3	6.2	0.2	0.0
Iced, Caramel Macchiato, Skimmed Milk, Starbucks*	1 Tall/335ml	124	1.1	37	1.6	6.8	0.3	0.0
Iced, Caramel Macchiato, Tall, Soy, Starbucks*	1 Tall/335ml	134	3.3	40	1.4	6.2	1.0	0.2
Iced, Caramel Macchiato, Tall, Whole Milk, Starbucks*	1 Tall/335ml	161	5.5	48	1.5	6.8	1.6	0.0
Iced, Caramel Macchiato, Venti, Soy, Starbucks*	1 Venti/591ml	201	4.2	34	1.1	5.6	0.7	0.1
Iced, Caramel Macchiato, Venti, Whole Milk, Starbucks*	1 Venti/591ml	243	7.5	41	1.2	6.1	1.3	0.0
Iced, Caramel Macchiato, Whole Milk, Starbucks*	1 Grande/473ml	257	9.8	54	2.0	7.0	2.1	0.0

	Measure INFO/WEIGHT	per Measure KCAL	FAT	Nutrition Values per 100g / 100ml KCAL	PROT	CARB	FAT	FIBRE
STARBUCKS								
COFFEE								
Iced, Grande, Starbucks*	1 Grande/473ml	4	0.1	1	0.1	0.0	0.0	0.0
Iced, Tall, Starbucks*	1 Tall/335ml	3	0.1	1	0.1	0.0	0.0	0.0
Iced, Venti, Starbucks*	1 Venti/591ml	5	0.1	1	0.1	0.0	0.0	0.0
Iced Caffe Latte, Grande, Semi Skim, Starbucks*	1 Grande/473ml	126	4.5	27	1.8	2.7	1.0	0.0
Iced Caffe Latte, Grande, Skimmed Milk, Starbucks*	1 Grande/473ml	90	0.2	19	1.8	2.8	0.0	0.0
Iced Caffe Latte, Grande, Soy, Starbucks*	1 Grande/473ml	104	3.6	22	1.5	2.0	0.8	0.2
Iced Caffe Latte, Grande, Whole Milk, Starbucks*	1 Grande/473ml	149	7.5	32	1.7	2.6	1.6	0.0
Iced Caffe Latte, Tall, Semi Skimmed Milk, Starbucks*	1 Tall/335ml	87	3.0	26	1.7	2.8	0.9	0.0
Iced Caffe Latte, Tall, Skimmed Milk, Starbucks*	1 Tall/335ml	63	0.1	19	1.7	2.8	0.0	0.0
Iced Caffe Latte, Tall, Soy, Starbucks*	1 Tall/335ml	71	2.4	21	1.5	2.0	0.7	0.2
Iced Caffe Latte, Tall, Whole Milk, Starbucks*	1 Tall/335ml	104	4.9	31	1.6	2.8	1.5	0.0
Iced Caffe Latte, Venti, Semi Skimmed Milk, Starbucks*	1 Venti/591ml	132	4.6	22	1.5	2.4	0.8	0.0
Iced Caffe Latte, Venti, Skimmed Milk, Starbucks*	1 Venti/591ml	95	0.2	16	1.5	2.4	0.0	0.0
Iced Caffe Latte, Venti, Soy, Starbucks*	1 Venti/591ml	109	3.7	18	1.3	1.7	0.6	0.2
Iced Caffe Latte, Venti, Whole Milk, Starbucks*	1 Venti/591ml	158	7.5	27	1.4	2.4	1.3	0.0
Iced Cappuccino, Grande, Semi Skim, Starbucks*	1 Grande/473ml	135	4.9	29	1.9	2.9	1.0	0.0
Iced Cappuccino, Grande, Skimmed Milk, Starbucks*	1 Grande/473ml	96	0.2	20	1.9	3.0	0.0	0.0
Iced Cappuccino, Grande, Soy, Starbucks*	1 Grande/473ml	111	4.0	23	1.6	2.1	0.8	0.2
Iced Cappuccino, Grande, Whole Milk, Starbucks*	1 Grande/473ml	163	8.1	34	1.8	2.9	1.7	0.0
Iced Cappuccino, Tall, Semi Skimmed Milk, Starbucks*	1 Tall/335ml	94	3.3	28	1.8	3.0	1.0	0.0
Iced Cappuccino, Tall, Skimmed Milk, Starbucks*	1 Tall/335ml	68	0.1	20	1.9	3.0	0.0	0.0
Iced Cappuccino, Tall, Soy, Starbucks*	1 Tall/335ml	78	2.7	23	1.6	2.2	0.8	0.2
Iced Cappuccino, Tall, Whole Milk, Starbucks*	1 Tall/335ml	113	5.4	34	1.8	3.0	1.6	0.0
Iced Cappuccino, Venti, Semi Skim, Starbucks*	1 Venti/591ml	141	4.9	24	1.6	2.5	0.8	0.0
Iced Cappuccino, Venti, Skimmed Milk, Starbucks*	1 Venti/591ml	101	0.2	17	1.6	2.6	0.0	0.0
Iced Cappuccino, Venti, Soy, Starbucks*	1 Venti/591ml	116	3.9	20	1.4	1.8	0.7	0.2
Iced Cappuccino, Venti, Whole Milk, Starbucks*	1 Venti/591ml	168	8.1	28	1.5	2.5	1.4	0.0
Macchiato, Caramel, Grande, Semi Skim, Starbucks*	1 Grande/473ml	240	6.7	51	2.2	7.2	1.4	0.0
Macchiato, Caramel, Grande, Skim, Starbucks*	1 Grande/473ml	193	1.1	41	2.3	7.4	0.2	0.0
Macchiato, Caramel, Grande, Soy, Starbucks*	1 Grande/473ml	207	5.3	44	1.9	6.2	1.1	0.2
Macchiato, Caramel, Grande, Whole Milk, Starbucks*	1 Grande/473ml	269	10.5	57	2.2	7.1	2.2	0.0
Macchiato, Caramel, Short, Semi Skim, Starbucks*	1 Short/236ml	122	3.8	52	2.3	6.9	1.6	0.0
Macchiato, Caramel, Short, Skimmed, Starbucks*	1 Short/236ml	97	0.9	41	2.4	7.1	0.4	0.0
Macchiato, Caramel, Short, Soy, Starbucks*	1 Short/236ml	104	3.0	44	1.9	5.9	1.3	0.2
Macchiato, Caramel, Short, Whole Milk, Starbucks*	1 Short/236ml	137	5.7	58	2.2	6.8	2.4	0.0
Macchiato, Caramel, Tall, Semi Skimmed, Starbucks*	1 Tall/355ml	209	6.3	59	2.8	7.9	1.8	0.0
Macchiato, Caramel, Tall, Skimmed Milk, Starbucks*	1 Tall/355ml	165	1.0	46	2.9	8.1	0.3	0.0
Macchiato, Caramel, Tall, Soy, Starbucks*	1 Tall/355ml	167	4.6	47	2.1	6.5	1.3	0.2
Macchiato, Caramel, Tall, Whole Milk, Starbucks*	1 Tall/355ml	240	9.8	68	2.7	7.9	2.8	0.0
Macchiato, Caramel, Venti, Semi Skim, Starbucks*	1 Venti/591ml	329	9.3	56	2.6	7.8	1.6	0.0
Macchiato, Caramel, Venti, Skimmed Milk, Starbucks*	1 Venti/591ml	261	1.2	44	2.6	8.0	0.2	0.0
Macchiato, Caramel, Venti, Soy, Starbucks*	1 Venti/591ml	280	7.4	47	2.1	6.6	1.2	0.3
Macchiato, Caramel, Venti, Whole Milk, Starbucks*	1 Venti/591ml	376	14.6	64	2.4	7.8	2.5	0.0
Mocha, White Choc, Whip, Grande, Soy, Starbucks*	1 Grande/473ml	439	17.0	93	2.8	12.3	3.6	0.2
Mocha, White Choc, Whip, Semi Skim, Starbucks*	1 Grande/473ml	471	18.4	100	3.2	13.3	3.9	0.0
Mocha, White Choc, Whip, Short, Skimmed, Starbucks*	1 Short/236ml	229	8.0	97	3.3	13.7	3.4	0.0
Mocha, White Choc, Whip, Short, Soy, Starbucks*	1 Short/355ml	236	10.1	66	1.9	8.3	2.8	0.2
Mocha, White Choc, Whip, Skimmed, Starbucks*	1 Grande/473ml	425	12.9	90	3.2	13.4	2.7	0.0
Mocha, White Choc, Whip, Tall, Semi Skim, Starbucks*	1 Tall/355ml	323	14.5	91	3.2	13.4	4.1	0.0
Mocha, White Choc, Whip, Tall, Skimmed, Starbucks*	1 Tall/355ml	327	10.4	92	3.2	13.6	2.9	0.0
Mocha, White Choc, Whip, Tall, Soy, Starbucks*	1 Tall/355ml	465	20.4	131	4.7	15.3	5.8	0.2
Mocha, White Choc, Whip, Tall, Whole Milk, Starbucks*	1 Tall/355ml	385	17.1	108	3.1	13.4	4.8	0.0

	Measure INFO/WEIGHT	per Measure KCAL	FAT	Nutrition Values per 100g / 100ml KCAL	PROT	CARB	FAT	FIBRE
STARBUCKS								
COFFEE								
Mocha, White Choc, Whip, Venti, Skimmed, Starbucks*	1 Venti/591ml	515	14.3	87	3.2	13.4	2.4	0.0
Mocha, White Choc, Whip, Venti, Soy, Starbucks*	1 Venti/591ml	530	19.5	90	2.8	12.2	3.3	0.2
Mocha, White Choc, Whip, Whole Milk, Starbucks*	1 Grande/473ml	500	22.1	106	3.1	13.2	4.7	0.0
Refresha, Cool Lime, Grande, Starbucks*	1 Grande/475ml	50	0.0	11	0.0	13.0	0.0	0.0
Refresha, Cool Lime, Tall, Starbucks*	1 Tall/355ml	40	0.0	11	0.0	2.9	0.0	0.0
Refresha, Cool Lime, Trenta, Starbucks*	1 Trenta/918ml	100	0.0	11	0.0	2.7	0.0	0.0
Refresha, Cool Lime, Venti, Starbucks*	1 Venti/710ml	80	0.0	11	0.0	2.8	0.0	0.0
Refresha, Valencia Orange, Grande, Starbucks*	1 Grande/473ml	71	0.0	15	0.0	3.8	0.0	0.0
Refresha, Valencia Orange, Short, Starbucks*	1 Short/236ml	63	0.0	27	0.0	5.9	0.0	0.0
Refresha, Valencia Orange, Tall, Starbucks*	1 Tall/254ml	93	0.0	37	0.0	7.9	0.0	0.0
Refresha, Valencia Orange, Venti, Starbucks*	1 Venti/200ml	51	0.0	26	0.0	5.6	0.0	0.0
COOKIES								
Chocolate Chunk, Starbucks*	1 Cookie/107g	499	20.5	466	7.4	65.0	19.2	1.7
Fruit & Oat, Starbucks*	1 Cookie/50g	216	8.8	433	4.4	64.3	17.6	3.1
CRISPS								
Pepperoni, Potato Chips, Starbucks*	1 Pack/50g	239	14.1	478	6.0	53.6	28.2	4.9
Sea Salt, Potato Chips, Starbucks*	1 Pack/50g	244	15.0	488	5.6	53.3	30.0	4.5
Sea Salt & Cider Vinegar, Potato Chips, Starbucks*	1 Pack/50g	248	14.2	496	6.2	54.2	28.3	4.3
CROISSANT								
Almond, Starbucks*	1 Croissant/104g	433	21.8	416	6.4	50.1	21.0	2.0
Butter Croissant, Starbucks*	1 Croissant/70g	267	15.8	381	5.8	38.2	22.5	1.3
Cinnamon Swirl, Starbucks*	1 Croissant/115g	371	11.7	323	7.4	49.1	10.2	2.6
Ham & Emmental Croissant, Starbucks*	1 Croissant/120g	378	21.0	315	13.8	25.2	17.5	0.9
DOUGHNUTS								
Apple Fritter, Starbucks*	1 Doughnut/115g	473	24.3	411	6.0	47.5	21.1	3.1
DRIED FRUIT								
Starbucks*	1 Serving/30g	90	0.1	299	1.9	73.0	0.4	2.0
FRAPPUCCINO								
Caramel, No Whip, Grande, Skimmed Milk, Starbucks*	1 Grande/473ml	134	0.1	28	0.7	6.3	0.0	0.0
Caramel, No Whip, Tall, Skimmed Milk, Starbucks*	1 Tall/335ml	96	0.1	29	0.7	6.3	0.0	0.1
Caramel, No Whip, Venti, Skimmed Milk, Starbucks*	1 Venti/591ml	165	0.1	28	0.7	6.2	0.0	0.1
Caramel, with Whip, Grande, Semi Skim, Starbucks*	1 Grande/473ml	390	13.7	82	0.9	13.3	2.9	0.0
Caramel, with Whip, Grande, Skimmed Milk, Starbucks*	1 Grande/473ml	375	11.9	79	0.9	13.4	2.5	0.0
Caramel, with Whip, Grande, Soy, Starbucks*	1 Grande/473ml	380	13.4	80	0.8	13.0	2.8	0.1
Caramel, with Whip, Grande, Whole Milk, Starbucks*	1 Grande/473ml	400	15.0	85	0.8	13.3	3.2	0.0
Caramel, with Whip, Tall, Semi Skimmed, Starbucks*	1 Tall/335ml	286	10.2	85	1.0	13.6	3.0	0.0
Caramel, with Whip, Tall, Skimmed Milk, Starbucks*	1 Tall/335ml	273	8.7	82	1.0	13.7	2.6	0.0
Caramel, with Whip, Tall, Soy, Starbucks*	1 Tall/335ml	278	9.9	83	0.9	13.3	3.0	0.1
Caramel, with Whip, Tall, Whole Milk, Starbucks*	1 Tall/335ml	294	11.2	88	1.0	13.6	3.3	0.0
Caramel, with Whip, Venti, Semi Skimmed, Starbucks*	1 Venti/591ml	444	13.0	75	0.8	13.2	2.2	0.0
Caramel, with Whip, Venti, Skimmed Milk, Starbucks*	1 Venti/591ml	427	10.9	72	0.8	13.2	1.8	0.0
Caramel, with Whip, Venti, Soy, Starbucks*	1 Venti/591ml	433	12.6	73	0.7	12.9	2.1	0.1
Caramel, with Whip, Venti, Whole Milk, Starbucks*	1 Venti/591ml	455	14.3	77	0.7	13.1	2.4	0.0
Chocolate Cream, & Whip, Grande, Soy, Starbucks*	1 Grande/473ml	322	14.2	68	1.1	9.8	3.0	0.3
Chocolate Cream, & Whip, Semi Skim, Starbucks*	1 Venti/591ml	386	14.4	65	1.2	10.3	2.4	0.2
Chocolate Cream, & Whip, Tall, Semi Skim, Starbucks*	1 Tall/335ml	243	10.7	72	1.3	10.3	3.2	0.2
Chocolate Cream, & Whip, Tall, Skimmed, Starbucks*	1 Tall/335ml	226	8.7	67	1.4	10.4	2.6	0.2
Chocolate Cream, & Whip, Tall, Soy, Starbucks*	1 Tall/335ml	232	10.3	69	1.2	9.9	3.1	0.3
Chocolate Cream, & Whip, Tall, Whole Milk, Starbucks*	1 Tall/335ml	253	12.0	75	1.3	10.3	3.6	0.2
Chocolate Cream, & Whip, Venti, Skim Milk, Starbucks*	1 Venti/591ml	361	11.5	61	1.2	10.4	2.0	0.2
Chocolate Cream, & Whip, Venti, Soy, Starbucks*	1 Venti/591ml	370	13.8	63	1.0	9.9	2.3	0.3
Chocolate Cream, & Whip, Whole Milk, Starbucks*	1 Venti/591ml	401	16.4	68	1.2	10.3	2.8	0.2

	Measure INFO/WEIGHT	per Measure KCAL	FAT	Nutrition Values per 100g / 100ml KCAL	PROT	CARB	FAT	FIBRE
STARBUCKS								
FRAPPUCCINO								
Coffee, No Whip, Grande, Semi Skim, Starbucks*	1 Grande/473ml	232	1.9	49	0.7	10.6	0.4	0.0
Coffee, No Whip, Grande, Skimmed Milk, Starbucks*	1 Grande/473ml	216	0.1	46	0.7	10.6	0.0	0.0
Coffee, No Whip, Grande, Soy, Starbucks*	1 Grande/473ml	222	1.6	47	0.6	10.3	0.3	0.1
Coffee, No Whip, Grande, Whole Milk, Starbucks*	1 Grande/473ml	242	3.2	51	0.7	10.6	0.7	0.0
Coffee, No Whip, Tall, Semi Skimmed Milk, Starbucks*	1 Tall/335ml	170	1.6	51	0.8	10.7	0.5	0.0
Coffee, No Whip, Tall, Skimmed Milk, Starbucks*	1 Tall/335ml	157	0.1	47	0.9	10.8	0.0	0.0
Coffee, No Whip, Tall, Soy, Starbucks*	1 Tall/335ml	162	1.3	48	0.7	10.4	0.4	0.1
Coffee, No Whip, Tall, Whole Milk, Starbucks*	1 Tall/335ml	178	2.6	53	0.8	10.7	0.8	0.0
Coffee, No Whip, Venti, Semi Skimmed Milk, Starbucks*	1 Venti/591ml	286	2.1	48	0.6	10.6	0.4	0.0
Coffee, No Whip, Venti, Skimmed Milk, Starbucks*	1 Venti/591ml	268	0.1	45	0.7	10.7	0.0	0.0
Coffee, No Whip, Venti, Soy, Starbucks*	1 Venti/591ml	275	1.7	46	0.6	10.3	0.3	0.1
Coffee, No Whip, Venti, Whole Milk, Starbucks*	1 Venti/591ml	296	3.5	50	0.6	10.6	0.6	0.0
Espresso, No Whip, Grande, Semi Skim Milk, Starbucks*	1 Grande/473ml	210	1.3	44	0.6	9.9	0.3	0.0
Espresso, No Whip, Grande, Skimmed Milk, Starbucks*	1 Grande/473ml	200	0.1	42	0.6	9.9	0.0	0.0
Espresso, No Whip, Grande, Soy, Starbucks*	1 Grande/473ml	204	1.1	43	0.5	9.7	0.2	0.1
Espresso, No Whip, Grande, Whole Milk, Starbucks*	1 Grande/473ml	217	2.1	46	0.6	9.9	0.4	0.0
Espresso, No Whip, Tall, Semi Skim, Starbucks*	1 Tall/335ml	143	0.9	43	0.6	9.5	0.3	0.0
Espresso, No Whip, Tall, Skimmed Milk, Starbucks*	1 Tall/335ml	136	0.0	41	0.6	9.5	0.0	0.0
Espresso, No Whip, Tall, Soy, Starbucks*	1 Tall/335ml	139	0.7	41	0.5	9.3	0.2	0.1
Espresso, No Whip, Tall, Whole Milk, Starbucks*	1 Tall/335ml	148	1.5	44	0.6	9.4	0.4	0.0
Espresso, No Whip, Venti, Semi Skim, Starbucks*	1 Venti/591ml	262	1.5	44	0.5	9.9	0.3	0.0
Espresso, No Whip, Venti, Skimmed Milk, Starbucks*	1 Venti/591ml	250	0.1	42	0.5	10.0	0.0	0.0
Espresso, No Whip, Venti, Soy, Starbucks*	1 Venti/591ml	254	1.2	43	0.5	9.8	0.2	0.1
Espresso, No Whip, Venti, Whole Milk, Starbucks*	1 Venti/591ml	270	2.5	46	0.5	9.9	0.4	0.0
Light, No Whip, Grande, Skimmed Milk, Starbucks*	1 Grande/473ml	118	0.1	25	0.7	5.4	0.0	0.1
Light, No Whip, Tall, Skimmed Milk, Starbucks*	1 Tall/335ml	83	0.1	25	0.8	5.3	0.0	0.1
Light, No Whip, Venti, Skimmed Milk, Starbucks*	1 Venti/591ml	139	0.1	24	0.7	5.0	0.0	0.1
Mango Passion, Tea, Grande, Starbucks*	1 Grande/473ml	191	0.3	40	0.2	9.8	0.1	0.3
Mango Passion, Tea, Tall, Starbucks*	1 Tall/335ml	157	0.2	47	0.2	11.4	0.1	0.3
Mango Passion, Tea, Venti, Starbucks*	1 Venti/591ml	228	0.3	39	0.2	9.4	0.0	0.2
Mocha, No Whip, Grande, Skimmed Milk, Starbucks*	1 Grande/473ml	143	0.8	30	0.8	6.7	0.2	0.2
Mocha, No Whip, Tall, Skimmed Milk, Starbucks*	1 Tall/335ml	96	0.5	29	0.9	6.3	0.1	0.1
Mocha, No Whip, Venti, Skimmed Milk, Starbucks*	1 Venti/591ml	179	0.9	30	0.9	6.7	0.2	0.2
Mocha, with Whip, Grande, Semi Skim, Starbucks*	1 Grande/473ml	361	13.7	76	1.0	12.2	2.9	0.1
Mocha, with Whip, Grande, Skimmed Milk, Starbucks*	1 Grande/473ml	346	12.0	73	1.0	12.2	2.5	0.1
Mocha, with Whip, Grande, Soy, Starbucks*	1 Grande/473ml	352	13.3	74	0.9	11.9	2.8	0.2
Mocha, with Whip, Grande, Whole Milk, Starbucks*	1 Grande/473ml	370	14.8	78	1.0	12.1	3.1	0.1
Mocha, with Whip, Tall, Semi Skimmed Milk, Starbucks*	1 Tall/335ml	266	10.0	79	1.1	12.6	3.0	0.1
Mocha, with Whip, Tall, Skimmed Milk, Starbucks*	1 Tall/335ml	254	8.6	76	1.1	12.7	2.6	0.1
Mocha, with Whip, Tall, Soy, Starbucks*	1 Tall/335ml	258	9.7	77	1.0	12.3	2.9	0.2
Mocha, with Whip, Tall, Whole Milk, Starbucks*	1 Tall/335ml	274	11.0	82	1.1	12.6	3.3	0.1
Mocha, with Whip, Venti, Semi Skim, Starbucks*	1 Venti/591ml	427	13.2	72	0.9	12.7	2.2	0.2
Mocha, with Whip, Venti, Skimmed Milk, Starbucks*	1 Venti/591ml	410	11.3	69	0.9	12.7	1.9	0.2
Mocha, with Whip, Venti, Soy, Starbucks*	1 Venti/591ml	416	12.8	70	0.8	12.4	2.2	0.2
Mocha, with Whip, Venti, Whole Milk, Starbucks*	1 Venti/591ml	437	14.6	74	0.9	12.7	2.5	0.2
Raspberry, Tea, Grande, Starbucks*	1 Grande/473ml	192	0.1	41	0.1	10.0	0.0	0.2
Raspberry, Tea, Venti, Starbucks*	1 Venti/591ml	229	0.1	39	0.1	9.5	0.0	0.1
Raspberry, Tea,Tall, Starbucks*	1 Tall/335ml	158	0.1	47	0.1	11.6	0.0	0.2
Strawberries & Cream, & Whip, Grande, Soy, Starbucks*	1 Grande/473ml	391	13.1	83	0.9	13.7	2.8	0.2
Strawberries & Cream, & Whip, Semi Skim, Starbucks*	1 Grande/473ml	404	13.6	85	1.0	14.1	2.9	0.1
Strawberries & Cream, & Whip, Skim Milk, Starbucks*	1 Tall/335ml	300	8.1	90	1.2	16.1	2.4	0.1
Strawberries & Cream, & Whip, Tall, Soy, Starbucks*	1 Tall/335ml	306	9.6	91	1.0	15.6	2.9	0.2

	Measure INFO/WEIGHT	per Measure KCAL	per Measure FAT	Nutrition Values per 100g / 100ml KCAL	PROT	CARB	FAT	FIBRE
STARBUCKS								
FRAPPUCCINO								
Strawberries & Cream, & Whip, Venti, Soy, Starbucks*	1 Venti/591ml	431	12.5	73	0.8	12.8	2.1	0.2
Strawberries & Cream, & Whip, Whole Milk, Starbucks*	1 Grande/473ml	415	15.1	88	1.0	14.1	3.2	0.1
Vanilla, with Whip, Grande, Semi Skim, Starbucks*	1 Grande/473ml	327	13.9	69	1.1	9.7	2.9	0.0
Vanilla, with Whip, Grande, Skimmed Milk, Starbucks*	1 Grande/473ml	305	11.3	65	1.1	9.8	2.4	0.0
Vanilla, with Whip, Grande, Soy, Starbucks*	1 Grande/473ml	313	13.4	66	0.9	9.3	2.8	0.1
Vanilla, with Whip, Grande, Whole Milk, Starbucks*	1 Grande/473ml	341	15.6	72	1.1	9.7	3.3	0.0
Vanilla, with Whip, Tall, Semi Skimmed Milk, Starbucks*	1 Tall/335ml	233	10.0	69	1.2	9.6	3.0	0.0
Vanilla, with Whip, Tall, Skimmed Milk, Starbucks*	1 Tall/335ml	216	8.1	64	1.2	9.6	2.4	0.0
Vanilla, with Whip, Tall, Soy, Starbucks*	1 Tall/335ml	222	9.7	66	1.0	9.1	2.9	0.1
Vanilla, with Whip, Tall, Whole Milk, Starbucks*	1 Tall/335ml	243	11.4	73	1.1	9.5	3.4	0.0
Vanilla, with Whip, Venti, Semi Skim, Starbucks*	1 Venti/591ml	372	13.4	63	1.0	9.7	2.3	0.0
Vanilla, with Whip, Venti, Skimmed Milk, Starbucks*	1 Venti/591ml	347	10.4	59	1.0	9.8	1.8	0.0
Vanilla, with Whip, Venti, Soy, Starbucks*	1 Venti/591ml	346	12.4	59	0.7	9.2	2.1	0.1
Vanilla, with Whip, Venti, Whole Milk, Starbucks*	1 Venti/591ml	388	15.4	66	1.0	9.7	2.6	0.0
FRUIT								
Fairtrade Banana, Starbucks*	1 Banana/120g	108	0.5	90	0.8	22.6	0.4	2.7
FRUIT SALAD								
Starbucks*	1 Pot/183g	95	0.4	52	0.6	11.1	0.2	1.6
HOT CHOCOLATE								
Classic, with Whip, Grande, Semi Skim, Starbucks*	1 Grande/473ml	323	15.0	68	2.6	8.7	3.2	0.4
Classic, with Whip, Grande, Skimmed Milk, Starbucks*	1 Grande/473ml	277	9.5	58	2.7	8.8	2.0	0.4
Classic, with Whip, Grande, Soy, Starbucks*	1 Grande/473ml	291	13.7	62	2.3	7.7	2.9	0.6
Classic, with Whip, Grande, Whole Milk, Starbucks*	1 Grande/473ml	352	18.7	74	2.6	8.6	4.0	0.4
Classic, with Whip, Short, Semi Skim, Starbucks*	1 Short/236ml	178	9.1	75	2.7	8.9	3.9	0.4
Classic, with Whip, Short, Skimmed Milk, Starbucks*	1 Short/236ml	155	6.4	66	2.8	9.1	2.7	0.4
Classic, with Whip, Short, Soy, Starbucks*	1 Short/236ml	162	8.5	69	2.3	7.9	3.6	0.6
Classic, with Whip, Short, Whole Milk, Starbucks*	1 Short/236ml	193	11.0	82	2.6	8.8	4.7	0.4
Classic, with Whip, Tall, Semi Skimmed Milk, Starbucks*	1 Tall/335ml	260	12.5	78	3.0	9.5	3.7	0.4
Classic, with Whip, Tall, Skimmed Milk, Starbucks*	1 Tall/335ml	222	8.0	66	3.0	9.7	2.4	0.4
Classic, with Whip, Tall, Soy, Starbucks*	1 Tall/335ml	234	11.4	70	2.6	8.4	3.4	0.7
Classic, with Whip, Tall, Whole Milk, Starbucks*	1 Tall/335ml	284	15.5	85	3.0	9.4	4.6	0.4
Classic, with Whip, Venti, Semi Skim, Starbucks*	1 Venti/591ml	398	17.5	67	2.8	8.7	3.0	0.4
Classic, with Whip, Venti, Skimmed Milk, Starbucks*	1 Venti/591ml	336	10.2	57	2.8	8.9	1.7	0.4
Classic, with Whip, Venti, Soy, Starbucks*	1 Venti/591ml	355	15.7	60	2.4	7.7	2.7	0.6
Classic, with Whip, Venti, Whole Milk, Starbucks*	1 Venti/591ml	437	22.5	74	2.7	8.6	3.8	0.4
Signature, with Whip, Grande, Semi Skim, Starbucks*	1 Grande/473ml	537	30.7	113	3.2	12.4	6.5	1.4
Signature, with Whip, Grande, Skimmed, Starbucks*	1 Grande/473ml	505	27.0	107	3.3	12.6	5.7	1.4
Signature, with Whip, Grande, Soy, Starbucks*	1 Grande/473ml	515	29.8	109	3.0	11.8	6.3	1.6
Signature, with Whip, Grande, Whole Milk, Starbucks*	1 Grande/473ml	556	33.5	118	3.2	12.5	7.1	1.4
Signature, with Whip, Short, Semi Skim, Starbucks*	1 Short/236ml	283	16.9	120	3.3	12.6	7.2	1.4
Signature, with Whip, Short, Skimmed Milk, Starbucks*	1 Short/236ml	267	15.0	113	3.3	12.7	6.4	1.4
Signature, with Whip, Short, Soy, Starbucks*	1 Short/236ml	272	16.4	115	3.1	11.9	6.9	1.6
Signature, with Whip, Short, Whole Milk, Starbucks*	1 Short/236ml	293	18.1	124	3.2	12.5	7.7	1.4
Signature, with Whip, Tall, Semi Skim, Starbucks*	1 Tall/335ml	418	24.2	125	3.5	13.5	7.2	1.5
Signature, with Whip, Tall, Skimmed Milk, Starbucks*	1 Tall/335ml	393	21.3	117	3.6	13.6	6.4	1.5
Signature, with Whip, Tall, Soy, Starbucks*	1 Tall/335ml	401	23.5	120	3.3	12.8	7.0	1.7
Signature, with Whip, Tall, Whole Milk, Starbucks*	1 Tall/335ml	433	26.1	129	3.5	13.4	7.8	1.5
Signature, with Whip, Venti, Semi Skim, Starbucks*	1 Venti/591ml	665	37.2	113	3.3	12.7	6.3	1.4
Signature, with Whip, Venti, Skimmed Milk, Starbucks*	1 Venti/591ml	624	32.4	106	3.3	12.7	5.5	1.4
Signature, with Whip, Venti, Soy, Starbucks*	1 Venti/591ml	637	36.0	108	3.0	12.0	6.1	1.6
Signature, with Whip, Venti, Whole Milk, Starbucks*	1 Venti/591ml	690	40.4	117	3.2	12.5	6.8	1.4

	Measure INFO/WEIGHT	per Measure KCAL	FAT	Nutrition Values per 100g / 100ml KCAL	PROT	CARB	FAT	FIBRE
STARBUCKS								
MILK								
Steamed, Grande, Semi Skimmed Milk, Starbucks*	1 Grande/473ml	203	8.0	43	2.8	4.0	1.7	0.0
Steamed, Grande, Skimmed Milk, Starbucks*	1 Grande/473ml	138	0.3	29	2.9	4.2	0.1	0.0
Steamed, Grande, Soy, Starbucks*	1 Grande/473ml	157	6.1	33	2.3	2.7	1.3	0.3
Steamed, Grande, Whole Milk, Starbucks*	1 Grande/473ml	244	13.2	52	2.8	3.9	2.8	0.0
Steamed, Short, Semi Skimmed Milk, Starbucks*	1 Short/236ml	102	4.0	43	2.9	4.1	1.7	0.0
Steamed, Short, Skimmed Milk, Starbucks*	1 Short/236ml	70	0.2	30	2.9	4.3	0.1	0.0
Steamed, Short, Soy, Starbucks*	1 Short/236ml	79	3.1	34	2.4	2.7	1.3	0.3
Steamed, Short, Whole Milk, Starbucks*	1 Short/236ml	123	6.7	52	2.8	3.9	2.8	0.0
Steamed, Tall, Semi Skimmed Milk, Starbucks*	1 Tall/335ml	155	6.1	46	3.1	4.4	1.8	0.0
Steamed, Tall, Skimmed Milk, Starbucks*	1 Tall/335ml	106	0.3	32	3.1	4.6	0.1	0.0
Steamed, Tall, Soy, Starbucks*	1 Tall/335ml	120	4.7	36	2.5	2.9	1.4	0.4
Steamed, Tall, Whole Milk, Starbucks*	1 Tall/335ml	187	10.1	56	3.0	4.2	3.0	0.0
Steamed, Venti, Semi Skimmed Milk, Starbucks*	1 Venti/591ml	258	10.2	44	2.9	4.1	1.7	0.0
Steamed, Venti, Skimmed Milk, Starbucks*	1 Venti/591ml	175	0.4	30	2.9	4.3	0.1	0.0
Steamed, Venti, Soy, Starbucks*	1 Venti/591ml	199	7.8	34	2.4	2.7	1.3	0.3
Steamed, Venti, Whole Milk, Starbucks*	1 Venti/591ml	309	16.7	52	2.8	3.9	2.8	0.0
MINTS								
After Coffee, Starbucks*	1 Mint/2g	5	0.0	250	0.0	100.0	0.0	0.0
MUFFIN								
Blueberry, Skinny, Starbucks*	1 Muffin/118g	306	1.9	259	5.7	54.5	1.6	1.9
Chocolate & Belgian Choc Sauce, Starbucks*	1 Muffin/119g	430	17.8	361	6.6	48.7	15.0	2.6
Classic Blueberry, Starbucks*	1 Muffin/110g	481	18.6	437	5.6	47.4	16.9	1.6
Lemon & Poppy Seed, Skinny, Starbucks*	1 Muffin/122g	338	2.3	277	5.4	58.5	1.9	2.2
Lemon & Poppyseed Iced, Skinny, Starbucks*	1 Muffin/139g	399	6.1	287	3.9	56.6	4.4	2.6
Peach & Raspberry, Skinny, Starbucks*	1 Muffin/136g	369	3.9	271	6.2	53.9	2.9	2.3
Rise & Shine, Starbucks*	1 Muffin/124g	448	18.8	361	7.1	47.8	15.2	2.3
NUTS								
Mixed, Starbucks*	1 Pack/75g	401	25.2	535	17.7	41.1	33.6	6.7
Roasted Almonds, Starbucks*	1 Pack/75g	484	41.4	646	21.2	17.7	55.2	10.5
PAIN AU CHOCOLAT								
Starbucks*	1 Pastry/65g	269	15.9	414	5.7	42.2	24.4	2.6
PAIN AU RAISIN								
Starbucks*	1 Pastry/110g	373	19.2	339	4.7	40.3	17.5	1.4
PANCAKE								
Buttermilk, Starbucks*	1 Pack/90g	227	2.4	252	4.6	51.9	2.7	1.2
PANINI								
All Day Breakfast, Starbucks*	1 Panini/158g	338	15.2	214	11.5	19.7	9.6	1.4
Cheese & Marmite, Starbucks*	1 Panini/130g	373	17.8	287	14.3	26.0	13.7	1.1
Chicken, Roast, & Tomato, Starbucks*	1 Panini/223g	375	8.0	168	10.2	23.1	3.6	1.4
Croque Monisieur, Starbucks*	1 Panini/190g	456	17.7	240	12.8	25.9	9.3	0.9
Italian Mozzarella & Slow Roast Tomato, Starbucks*	1 Panini/178g	470	20.5	264	11.2	28.0	11.5	1.5
Meatball, Starbucks*	1 Panini/216g	521	22.5	241	11.2	25.0	10.4	1.4
Steak, Cheese & Caramelised Onion, Starbucks*	1 Panini/210g	525	20.4	250	14.9	25.3	9.7	1.0
Tuna Melt & Mature Cheddar, Starbucks*	1 Panini/200g	492	21.0	246	13.3	24.2	10.5	0.9
SALAD								
Chicken, & Red Pesto, Bistro Box, Starbucks*	1 Salad/296g	275	13.9	93	5.1	7.1	4.7	1.1
Falafel Mezze, Bistro Box, Starbucks*	1 Salad/329g	494	14.5	150	5.0	20.9	4.4	3.6
Guacamole, Holy, Starbucks*	1 Pack/290g	374	11.3	129	7.3	15.0	3.9	2.6
Ham, Cured, Hock, Bistro Box, Starbucks*	1 Salad/302g	387	20.5	128	7.9	8.2	6.8	1.3
Tuna, Potato & Pea, Bistro Box, Starbucks*	1 Salad/286g	320	14.6	112	6.3	9.5	5.1	1.7
SANDWICH								
Cheese & Pickle, GF, Starbucks*	1 Sandwich/197g	552	32.5	280	7.5	23.9	16.5	2.9

	Measure INFO/WEIGHT	per Measure KCAL	FAT	Nutrition Values per 100g / 100ml KCAL	PROT	CARB	FAT	FIBRE
STARBUCKS								
SANDWICH								
Chicken, with Herb Mayonnaise, Roasted, Starbucks*	1 Sandwich/201g	314	7.2	156	10.6	19.2	3.6	2.1
Egg Mayonnaise, Free Range, Starbucks*	1 Sandwich/191g	365	15.3	191	10.3	18.6	8.0	1.9
SHORTBREAD								
Chocolate Chunk, Fairtrade, Starbucks*	1 Shortbread/96g	497	29.0	518	6.2	53.5	30.2	3.1
SYRUP								
1 Pump - 1/4 fl oz 10g, Starbucks*	1 Pump/10g	20	0.0	202	0.0	50.0	0.0	0.0
2 Pumps - 1/2 fl oz - 20 g, Starbucks*	2 Pumps/20g	40	0.0	202	0.0	50.5	0.0	0.0
3 Pumps - 3/4 fl oz - 30 g, Starbucks*	3 Pumps/30g	61	0.0	202	0.0	50.3	0.0	0.0
4 Pumps - 1 fl oz - 40 g, Starbucks*	4 Pumps/40g	81	0.0	202	0.0	50.2	0.0	0.0
5 Pumps - 1 1/4 fl oz - 50 g, Starbucks*	5 Pumps/50g	101	0.0	202	0.0	50.2	0.0	0.0
Bar Mocha, 1 Pump - 1/2 fl oz - 17 g, Starbucks*	1 Pump/17g	26	0.6	156	3.5	37.6	3.5	5.9
Bar Mocha, 2 Pumps - 1 fl oz - 34 g, Starbucks*	2 Pumps/34g	53	1.1	156	3.8	37.6	3.2	5.9
Bar Mocha, 3 Pumps - 1 1/2 fl oz - 51 g, Starbucks*	3 Pumps/51g	79	1.7	156	3.7	37.5	3.3	5.9
Bar Mocha, 4 Pumps - 2 fl oz - 68 g, Starbucks*	4 Pumps/68g	106	2.3	156	3.7	37.5	3.4	5.7
Bar Mocha, 5 Pumps - 2 1/2 fl oz - 85 g, Starbucks*	5 Pumps/85g	132	2.8	156	3.6	37.5	3.3	5.8
TEA								
Brewed, Grande, Starbucks*	1 Grande/473ml	0	0.0	0	0.0	0.0	0.0	0.0
Brewed, Short, Starbucks*	1 Short/236ml	0	0.0	0	0.0	0.0	0.0	0.0
Brewed, Tall, Starbucks*	1 Tall/335ml	0	0.0	0	0.0	0.0	0.0	0.0
Brewed, Venti, Starbucks*	1 Venti/591ml	0	0.0	0	0.0	0.0	0.0	0.0
Chai, Latte, Grande, Semi Skimmed Milk, Starbucks*	1 Grande/473ml	236	4.0	50	1.6	9.3	0.8	0.0
Chai, Latte, Grande, Skimmed Milk, Starbucks*	1 Grande/473ml	204	0.2	43	1.6	9.4	0.0	0.0
Chai, Latte, Grande, Soy, Starbucks*	1 Grande/473ml	213	3.2	45	1.3	8.6	0.7	0.2
Chai, Latte, Grande, Whole Milk, Starbucks*	1 Grande/473ml	255	6.5	54	1.5	9.2	1.4	0.0
Chai, Latte, Short, Semi Skimmed Milk, Starbucks*	1 Short/236ml	119	2.0	50	1.6	9.3	0.8	0.0
Chai, Latte, Short, Skimmed Milk, Starbucks*	1 Short/236ml	103	0.1	44	1.6	9.4	0.0	0.0
Chai, Latte, Short, Soy, Starbucks*	1 Short/236ml	108	1.6	46	1.4	8.6	0.7	0.2
Chai, Latte, Short, Whole Milk, Starbucks*	1 Short/236ml	129	3.3	55	1.6	9.3	1.4	0.0
Chai, Latte, Tall, Semi Skimmed Milk, Starbucks*	1 Tall/335ml	179	3.0	53	1.7	9.8	0.9	0.0
Chai, Latte, Tall, Skimmed Milk, Starbucks*	1 Tall/335ml	154	0.2	46	1.7	10.0	0.1	0.0
Chai, Latte, Tall, Soy, Starbucks*	1 Tall/335ml	162	2.4	48	1.4	9.1	0.7	0.2
Chai, Latte, Tall, Whole Milk, Starbucks*	1 Tall/335ml	194	5.0	58	1.6	9.8	1.5	0.0
Chai, Latte, Venti, Semi Skimmed Milk, Starbucks*	1 Venti/591ml	297	5.0	50	1.6	9.3	0.8	0.0
Chai, Latte, Venti, Skimmed Milk, Starbucks*	1 Venti/591ml	256	0.3	43	1.6	9.4	0.0	0.0
Chai, Latte, Venti, Soy, Starbucks*	1 Venti/591ml	268	4.0	45	1.3	8.6	0.7	0.2
Chai, Latte, Venti, Whole Milk, Starbucks*	1 Venti/591ml	322	8.3	54	1.5	9.2	1.4	0.0
Iced, Chai, Latte, Grande, Skimmed Milk, Starbucks*	1 Grande/473ml	205	0.2	43	1.6	9.4	0.0	0.0
Iced, Chai, Latte, Grande, Soy, Starbucks*	1 Grande/473ml	219	3.4	46	1.4	8.6	0.7	0.2
Iced, Chai, Latte, Grande, Whole Milk, Starbucks*	1 Grande/473ml	259	6.9	55	1.5	9.2	1.5	0.0
Iced, Chai, Latte, Tall, Semi Skimmed Milk, Starbucks*	1 Tall/335ml	176	3.0	52	1.6	9.7	0.9	0.0
Iced, Chai, Latte, Tall, Skimmed Milk, Starbucks*	1 Tall/335ml	152	0.2	45	1.6	9.9	0.1	0.0
Iced, Chai, Latte, Tall, Soy, Starbucks*	1 Tall/335ml	162	2.4	48	1.4	9.1	0.7	0.2
Iced, Chai, Latte, Tall, Whole Milk, Starbucks*	1 Tall/335ml	191	5.0	57	1.6	9.7	1.5	0.0
Iced, Chai, Latte, Venti, Semi Skimmed Milk, Starbucks*	1 Venti/591ml	277	4.4	47	1.3	9.0	0.7	0.0
Iced, Chai, Latte, Venti, Skimmed Milk, Starbucks*	1 Venti/591ml	242	0.3	41	1.4	9.0	0.0	0.0
Iced, Chai, Latte, Venti, Soy, Starbucks*	1 Venti/591ml	256	3.5	43	1.2	8.5	0.6	0.2
Iced, Chai, Latte, Venti, Whole Milk, Starbucks*	1 Venti/591ml	299	7.2	51	1.3	9.0	1.2	0.0
TOPPING								
Caramel - 4 g, Starbucks*	1 Serving/4ml	15	0.6	372	0.0	62.5	15.0	0.0
Chocolate - 4 g, Starbucks*	1 Serving/4ml	6	0.1	152	2.5	37.5	2.5	2.5
Sprinkles - 1 g, Starbucks*	1 Serving/1g	4	0.0	380	0.0	100.0	0.0	0.0
Whipped Cream, Cold, Grande, Starbucks*	1 Grande/32g	114	11.2	356	1.9	9.4	35.0	0.0

	Measure INFO/WEIGHT	per Measure KCAL	FAT	Nutrition Values per 100g / 100ml KCAL	PROT	CARB	FAT	FIBRE
STARBUCKS								
TOPPING								
Whipped Cream, Cold, Tall, Starbucks*	1 Tall/25g	81	8.0	324	1.6	8.0	32.0	0.0
Whipped Cream, Cold, Venti, Starbucks*	1 Venti/35g	104	10.2	297	1.7	8.6	29.1	0.0
Whipped Cream, Hot, Short, Starbucks*	1 Short/16g	52	5.1	325	1.9	6.2	31.9	0.0
Whipped Cream, Hot, Tall Beverage - 19g, Starbucks*	1 Tall/19g	62	6.1	326	1.6	10.5	32.1	0.0
WAFFLES								
Caramel, Large, Starbucks*	1 Waffle/80g	354	16.2	443	3.2	62.2	20.3	1.1
YOGHURT								
Apple, Oats & Berries, Breakfast Pot, Starbucks*	1 Pot/180g	319	11.9	177	4.1	24.3	6.6	2.1
Natural, Creamy, Starbucks*	1 Serving/140g	132	6.4	94	5.5	7.5	4.6	0.0
SUBWAY								
BACON								
2 Strips, Subway*	2 Strips/9g	40	2.9	444	33.3	0.0	32.2	0.0
BREAD								
Flatbread, Subway*	1 Flatbread/85g	203	2.5	239	9.4	42.4	2.9	3.1
Rolls, Sub, Honey Oat, 9 Grain, 6 Inch, Subway*	1 Sub/78g	198	1.5	254	11.5	44.9	1.9	6.7
Rolls, Sub, Italian, Hearty, 6 Inch, Subway*	1 Sub/75g	201	1.5	268	10.7	50.7	2.0	2.8
Rolls, Sub, Italian, Herbs & Cheese, 6 Inch, Subway*	1 Sub/82g	234	4.3	285	12.2	46.3	5.2	2.3
Rolls, Sub, Wheat, 9 Grain, 6 Inch, Subway*	1 Sub/78g	198	1.5	254	11.5	44.9	1.9	6.7
Rolls, Sub, White, Italian, 6 Inch, Subway*	1 Sub/71g	190	1.3	268	9.9	50.7	1.8	2.2
CANDY								
Chocolate Chip, Subway*	1 Serving/45g	211	9.7	469	4.4	66.7	21.6	2.0
CHEESE								
American, Subway*	1 Serving/11g	40	3.4	364	18.2	9.1	30.9	0.0
Cheddar, Monterey, Subway*	1 Serving/14g	57	4.4	407	25.0	0.0	31.4	0.0
Peppered, Subway*	1 Serving/11g	39	3.1	355	18.2	0.0	28.2	0.0
COOKIES								
Choc Chip, Double, Subway*	1 Cookie/45g	221	11.7	491	4.4	60.0	26.0	2.7
Chocolate Chip, Subway*	1 Cookie/45g	218	10.3	484	4.4	64.4	22.9	2.4
Chocolate Chunk, Subway*	1 Cookie/45g	214	10.2	476	4.4	66.7	22.7	2.0
Oatmeal Raisin, Subway*	1 Cookie/45g	196	8.1	436	6.7	66.7	18.0	1.1
Rainbow, Subway*	1 Cookie/45g	211	9.7	469	4.4	66.7	21.6	2.0
White Chip, Mac Nut, Subway*	1 Cookie/45g	218	11.0	484	4.4	62.2	24.4	1.1
DOUGHNUTS								
Chocolate, Subway*	1 Doughnut/55g	243	15.5	442	7.3	38.2	28.2	2.2
Sugared, Subway*	1 Doughnut/49g	207	11.6	422	6.1	42.9	23.7	1.0
DRESSING								
Ranch, Subway*	1 Serving/21g	44	4.5	210	0.0	4.8	21.4	0.0
FLATBREAD								
Bacon, Breakfast, Subway*	1 Flatbread/113g	276	7.3	244	13.7	31.9	6.5	2.3
Bacon, Egg, & Cheese, Breakfast, Subway*	1 Flatbread/145g	335	12.4	231	11.7	25.9	8.6	1.9
Beef, Melt, Big, Subway*	1 Flatbread/247g	418	17.9	169	8.5	16.4	7.2	2.0
Beef, Subway*	1 Flatbread/226g	287	4.0	127	9.9	17.2	1.8	1.6
Chicken, & Bacon, Ranch, Melt, Subway*	1 Flatbread/299g	508	20.2	170	12.4	13.8	6.8	1.2
Chicken, Breast, Subway*	1 Flatbread/240g	309	4.0	129	11.0	16.7	1.7	1.5
Chicken, Tandoori, Subway*	1 Flatbread/261g	320	4.7	123	10.3	14.9	1.8	1.4
Chicken, Temptation, Subway*	1 Flatbread/269g	411	9.7	153	9.8	19.8	3.6	1.3
Chicken, Teriyaki, & Sweet Onion, Subway*	1 Flatbread/283g	359	4.2	127	9.6	18.2	1.5	1.4
Chicken, Tikka, Subway*	1 Flatbread/240g	128	1.7	128	11.0	16.4	1.7	1.5
Club, Subway*	1 Flatbread/259g	315	4.4	122	10.9	15.2	1.7	1.4
Egg, & Cheese, Breakfast, Subway*	1 Flatbread/131g	299	10.0	228	10.0	28.6	7.6	2.1
Ham, Subway*	1 Flatbread/226g	274	4.5	121	8.3	17.6	2.0	1.6
Italian, BMT, Subway*	1 Flatbread/233g	401	17.7	172	8.8	16.9	7.6	1.6

	Measure INFO/WEIGHT	per Measure KCAL	FAT	Nutrition Values per 100g / 100ml KCAL	PROT	CARB	FAT	FIBRE
SUBWAY								
FLATBREAD								
Italian, Spicy, Subway*	1 Flatbread/229g	476	26.3	208	8.9	17.0	11.5	1.6
Meatball, Marinara, Subway*	1 Flatbread/307g	440	16.5	143	7.5	16.4	5.4	2.2
Mega Melt, Breakfast, Subway*	1 Flatbread/221g	512	23.5	232	12.8	20.4	10.6	1.6
Sausage, Breakfast, Subway*	1 Flatbread/161g	379	13.6	235	12.1	27.1	8.4	2.1
Sausage, Egg, & Cheese, Breakfast, Subway*	1 Flatbread/207g	475	21.1	229	11.9	21.8	10.2	1.7
Steak, & Cheese, Subway*	1 Flatbread/252g	348	9.5	138	9.9	16.4	3.8	1.6
Subway Melt, with Cheese, Subway*	1 Flatbread/256g	364	10.2	142	10.6	15.6	4.0	1.4
Tuna, Subway*	1 Flatbread/240g	364	13.6	152	8.4	16.9	5.7	1.5
Turkey, & Ham, Subway*	1 Flatbread/235g	283	4.0	120	9.2	16.7	1.7	1.5
Turkey, Breast, Subway*	1 Flatbread/226g	274	3.2	121	9.2	17.2	1.4	1.6
Veggie Delite, Subway*	1 Flatbread/169g	218	2.6	129	5.2	22.7	1.5	2.1
Veggie Patty, Subway*	1 Flatbread/254g	385	9.7	152	8.2	18.6	3.8	1.4
MAYONNAISE								
Light, Subway*	1 Serving/15g	56	6.0	373	0.0	6.7	40.0	0.0
MEATBALLS								
Bowl, Subway*	1 Bowl/206g	317	19.1	154	9.2	9.2	9.3	2.0
MUFFIN								
Blueberry, Subway*	1 Muffin/111g	352	20.6	317	4.5	36.0	18.6	2.7
Chocolate Chunk, Subway*	1 Muffin/111g	394	22.9	355	5.4	39.6	20.6	2.6
Double Chocolate Chunk, Subway*	1 Muffin/111g	389	22.0	350	5.4	40.5	19.8	2.8
NACHOS								
Cheese, Melted, Subway*	1 Serving/126g	415	24.3	329	8.7	28.6	19.3	2.1
SALAD								
Beef, Subway*	1 Salad/328g	118	2.4	36	4.9	1.8	0.7	1.1
Chicken, Breast, Subway*	1 Salad/342g	139	2.4	41	5.8	2.0	0.7	1.0
Chicken, Teriyaki, & Sweet Onion, Subway*	1 Salad/385g	189	2.6	49	5.4	4.9	0.7	1.0
Chicken, Tikka, Subway*	1 Salad/342g	137	2.4	40	5.8	1.8	0.7	1.0
Club, Subway*	1 Salad/361g	145	2.8	40	6.1	1.9	0.8	1.0
Garden, Side, Subway*	1 Salad/135g	21	0.2	16	0.7	2.2	0.2	1.3
Ham, Subway*	1 Salad/328g	104	2.9	32	3.7	2.1	0.9	1.1
Turkey, & Ham, Subway*	1 Salad/338g	113	2.3	33	4.7	1.8	0.7	1.1
Turkey, Breast, Subway*	1 Salad/328g	104	1.6	32	4.6	1.8	0.5	1.1
Veggie Delite, Subway*	1 Salad/271g	49	1.0	18	1.1	1.8	0.4	1.3
SAUCE								
BBQ, Low Fat, Subway*	1 Serving/21g	37	0.1	176	0.0	42.9	0.5	1.0
Chipotle Southwest, Subway*	1 Serving/21g	90	9.2	429	0.0	9.5	43.8	0.5
Honey Mustard,Low Fat, Subway*	1 Serving/21g	32	0.2	152	0.0	33.3	1.0	0.5
Sweet Onion, Low Fat, Subway*	1 Serving/21g	34	0.1	162	0.0	38.1	0.5	0.5
SOUP								
Beef Goulash, Subway*	1 Serving/250g	199	11.8	80	3.3	6.0	4.7	0.9
Carrot and Coriander, Subway*	1 Serving/250g	81	1.8	32	0.9	5.6	0.7	1.1
Chicken, Cream of, Subway*	1 Serving/250g	160	11.3	64	2.7	3.1	4.5	0.0
Chicken & Vegetable, Country, Subway*	1 Serving/250g	168	11.0	67	2.7	4.2	4.4	0.2
Leek & Potato, Subway*	1 Serving/250g	124	3.0	50	1.7	8.0	1.2	1.1
Lentil, & Potato, Subway*	1 Serving/250g	182	5.0	73	4.4	9.3	2.0	1.1
Lentil & Bacon, Subway*	1 Serving/250g	182	5.0	73	4.4	9.3	2.0	1.1
Minestrone, Subway*	1 Serving/250g	125	3.0	50	1.7	7.8	1.2	1.0
Mushroom, Cream of, Subway*	1 Serving/250g	150	10.8	60	1.0	4.4	4.3	0.3
Mushroom, Wild, Subway*	1 Serving/250g	101	5.5	40	1.0	4.1	2.2	0.3
Red Pepper, & Tomato, Subway*	1 Serving/250g	100	4.0	40	1.4	6.0	1.6	0.9
Tomato, Subway*	1 Serving/250g	103	3.8	41	0.8	6.1	1.5	0.3
Vegetable, Highland, Subway*	1 Serving/250g	73	0.3	29	1.5	5.5	0.1	0.9

	Measure INFO/WEIGHT	per Measure KCAL	per Measure FAT	Nutrition Values per 100g / 100ml KCAL	PROT	CARB	FAT	FIBRE
SUBWAY								
SOUP								
Vegetable, Thai Style, Subway*	1 Serving/250g	87	1.0	35	1.1	6.7	0.4	0.8
SUBS								
Bacon, Breakfast, Subway*	1 Sub/106g	271	6.3	256	15.1	33.0	5.9	4.9
Bacon, Egg, & Cheese, Breakfast, Subway*	1 Sub/138g	330	11.4	239	13.0	26.1	8.3	3.9
Beef, Kids Pak, Subway*	1 Sub/156g	210	2.2	135	10.3	18.6	1.4	3.1
Beef, Low Fat, Subway*	1 Sub/219g	282	3.0	129	10.5	17.4	1.4	2.9
Chicken, & Bacon, Ranch Melt, Subway*	1 Sub/292g	503	19.2	172	13.0	13.7	6.6	2.2
Chicken, & Jalapeño, Melt, Subway*	1 Sub/249g	345	6.4	139	11.7	15.7	2.6	2.6
Chicken, Breast, Low Fat, Subway*	1 Sub/233g	304	3.0	130	11.6	16.7	1.3	2.7
Chicken, Tandoori, Low Fat, Subway*	1 Sub/254g	315	3.7	124	11.0	15.0	1.5	2.5
Chicken, Temptation, Subway*	1 Sub/262g	406	8.7	155	10.3	19.8	3.3	2.4
Chicken, Teriyaki, Sweet Onion, Low Fat, Subway*	1 Sub/276g	354	3.3	128	10.1	18.1	1.2	2.4
Chicken, Tikka, Low Fat, Subway*	1 Sub/233g	302	3.0	130	11.6	16.3	1.3	2.7
Club, Low Fat, Subway*	1 Sub/252g	310	3.4	123	11.5	15.1	1.4	2.5
Egg, & Cheese, Breakfast, Subway*	1 Sub/124g	294	9.0	237	11.3	29.0	7.3	4.4
Ham, Kids Pak, Subway*	1 Sub/147g	192	2.2	131	8.2	19.7	1.5	3.3
Ham, Low Fat, Subway*	1 Sub/219g	269	3.5	123	8.7	17.4	1.6	2.9
Italian, Spicy, Subway*	1 Sub/222g	471	25.3	212	9.5	17.1	11.4	2.8
Italian BMT, Subway*	1 Sub/226g	396	16.8	175	9.3	16.8	7.4	2.8
Meatball Marinara, Subway*	1 Sub/300g	435	15.5	145	8.0	16.3	5.2	3.1
Mega Melt, Breakfast, Subway*	1 Sub/214g	507	22.5	237	13.6	20.6	10.5	2.9
Sausage, Breakfast, Subway*	1 Sub/154g	374	12.6	243	13.0	27.3	8.2	4.0
Sausage, Egg, & Cheese, Breakfast, Subway*	1 Sub/200g	470	20.1	235	12.5	22.0	10.0	3.1
Steak & Cheese, Subway*	1 Sub/245g	343	8.5	140	10.6	16.3	3.5	2.7
Subway Melt, Includes Cheese, Subway*	1 Sub/249g	359	9.3	144	11.2	15.7	3.7	2.5
Tuna, Subway*	1 Sub/233g	359	12.6	154	9.0	16.7	5.4	2.7
Turkey, & Ham, Low Fat, Subway*	1 Sub/228g	278	3.0	122	9.6	16.7	1.3	2.8
Turkey, Breast, Kids Pak, Subway*	1 Sub/156g	201	1.6	129	9.6	18.6	1.0	3.1
Turkey, Breast, Low Fat, Subway*	1 Sub/219g	269	2.2	123	10.0	17.4	1.0	2.9
Veggie Delite, Kids Pak, Subway*	1 Sub/118g	164	1.2	139	5.9	24.6	1.0	4.1
Veggie Delite, Low Fat, Subway*	1 Sub/162g	213	1.6	131	5.6	22.8	1.0	3.9
Veggie Patty, Subway*	1 Sub/247g	380	8.7	154	8.9	18.6	3.5	2.6
TOASTIE								
Cheese, Subway*	1 Toastie/64g	210	9.5	328	17.2	29.7	14.8	1.2
Pepperoni Pizza, Subway*	1 Toastie/93g	247	12.4	266	11.8	23.7	13.3	1.4
WRAP								
Beef, Subway*	1 Wrap/242g	412	8.1	170	9.1	25.6	3.4	1.3
Chicken, Breast, Subway*	1 Wrap/256g	434	8.1	170	10.2	24.6	3.2	1.2
Chicken, Temptation, Subway*	1 Wrap/285g	536	13.8	188	9.1	27.0	4.8	1.1
Chicken & Bacon Ranch Melt, Subway*	1 Wrap/315g	633	24.3	201	11.8	20.6	7.7	1.0
Chicken Tikka, Subway*	1 Wrap/256g	432	8.1	169	10.2	24.6	3.2	1.2
Ham, Subway*	1 Wrap/242g	399	8.6	165	7.8	26.0	3.6	1.3
Italian, Spicy, Subway*	1 Wrap/245g	602	30.4	246	8.2	25.3	12.4	1.3
Italian B.M.T., Subway*	1 Wrap/249g	526	21.8	211	8.4	25.3	8.8	1.2
Meatball Marinara, Subway*	1 Wrap/323g	561	20.2	174	7.1	22.9	6.2	1.9
Onion, Sweet & Chicken Teriyaki, Subway*	1 Wrap/299g	484	8.3	162	9.0	25.1	2.8	1.2
Steak & Cheese, with Peppers & Onions, Subway*	1 Wrap/268g	473	13.6	176	9.3	24.2	5.1	1.3
Subway Club, Subway*	1 Wrap/275g	440	8.5	160	10.2	22.9	3.1	1.1
Subway Melt with Cheese, Subway*	1 Wrap/272g	489	14.3	180	9.9	23.2	5.3	1.1
Tuna, Subway*	1 Wrap/256g	489	17.7	191	7.8	25.0	6.9	1.2
Turkey, Breast, & Ham, Subway*	1 Wrap/251g	408	8.1	163	8.8	25.1	3.2	1.2
Turkey, Breast, Subway*	1 Wrap/242g	399	7.3	165	8.7	25.6	3.0	1.3

	Measure INFO/WEIGHT	per Measure KCAL	FAT	Nutrition Values per 100g / 100ml KCAL	PROT	CARB	FAT	FIBRE
SUBWAY								
WRAP								
Veggie Delite, Subway*	1 Wrap/185g	343	6.7	185	4.9	33.5	3.6	1.7
Veggie Patty, Subway*	1 Wrap/270g	510	13.8	189	7.8	26.3	5.1	1.2
WAGAMAMA								
BEANS								
Edamame with Salt, Wagamama*	1 Serving/202g	179	6.3	89	6.6	3.7	3.1	9.9
BEEF								
Teriyaki Soba, Wagamama*	1 Serving/607g	829	38.5	137	8.1	11.2	6.3	1.0
CAKE								
Chocolate Fudge, with Vanilla Ice Cream, Wagamama*	1 Serving/203g	671	36.9	331	4.0	37.6	18.2	0.4
CHA HAN								
Chicken & Prawn, Rice, Wagamama*	1 Dinner/778g	972	24.9	125	5.1	18.6	3.2	0.8
CHEESECAKE								
Chocolate, White, Ginger, Wagamama*	1 Serving/142g	460	22.2	324	5.2	40.3	15.6	0.6
CHICKEN								
Firecracker, Stir Fried with Vegetables, Wagamama*	1 Serving/720g	1056	27.4	147	7.7	20.1	3.8	0.6
Grilled, Katsu Curry, Wagamama*	1 Serving/569g	871	30.2	153	6.0	20.1	5.3	0.5
Itame, & Noodles in Green Coconut Soup, Wagamama*	1 Serving/829g	850	51.4	103	4.5	6.6	6.2	1.1
Mini, with Sauce & Rice, Wagamama*	1 Serving/295g	484	13.9	164	8.0	22.2	4.7	0.5
Raisukaree, in Coconut Curry Sauce, Wagamama*	1 Serving/774g	1276	58.0	165	5.7	18.4	7.5	0.5
Tama Rice, Wagamama*	1 Serving/810g	917	25.9	113	4.5	16.4	3.2	0.5
Tebasaki, Wagamama*	1 Serving/105g	274	15.5	261	21.7	9.8	14.8	1.3
Teriyaki Donburi, Wagamama*	1 Serving/580g	934	17.0	161	9.1	24.2	2.9	0.6
Tori Kara Age, Wagamama*	1 Serving/171g	494	30.4	289	25.9	6.3	17.8	0.1
CURRY								
Chicken, Chu Chee, Wagamama*	1 Serving/824g	1350	61.7	164	4.9	18.8	7.5	0.7
Chicken, Kastu, Wagamama*	1 Serving/619g	1103	45.2	178	7.5	20.5	7.3	0.5
FROZEN YOGHURT								
Chocolate, Chilli & Ginger, Wagamama*	1 Serving/195g	300	3.7	154	5.0	28.7	1.9	1.4
Citrus Yuzu, Wagamama*	1 Serving/133g	196	2.8	147	4.7	27.3	2.1	0.2
Strawberry & Five Spices, Wagamama*	1 Serving/133g	224	2.5	168	4.5	33.2	1.9	0.2
GYOZA								
Chicken & Vegetable, Dumplings, Wagamama*	1 Serving/149g	236	10.6	158	7.6	15.0	7.1	2.0
Duck Dumplings, with Hoi Sin Sauce, Wagamama*	1 Serving/115g	299	12.3	260	10.4	29.2	10.7	2.8
Ebi, Prawn & Vegetable Dumplings, Wagamama*	1 Serving/112g	219	8.4	196	8.3	22.0	7.5	3.2
Sweet Ginger & Apple, Dumplings, Wagamama*	5 Dumplings/135g	358	9.6	265	3.3	46.4	7.1	1.2
Yasai, Vegetable Dumplings, Wagamama*	1 Serving/150g	301	19.0	201	3.1	17.5	12.7	2.3
ICE CREAM								
Coconut Reika, Wagamama*	1 Serving/195g	417	21.4	214	3.5	25.0	11.0	0.7
ITAME								
Prawn, Wagamama*	1 Bowl/769g	746	49.2	94	2.0	6.9	6.2	1.1
JUICE								
Apple, Mint, Celery & Lime, Wagamama*	1 Serving/273g	153	0.3	56	0.2	13.8	0.1	0.3
Apple & Orange, Wagamama*	1 Serving/271g	129	0.3	48	0.4	11.2	0.1	0.6
Blueberry, Apple & Ginger, Wagamama*	1 Serving/359g	183	0.4	51	0.4	11.2	0.1	2.0
Carrot, with a Hint of Ginger, Wagamama*	1 Serving/312g	72	0.0	23	0.2	5.0	0.0	1.1
Fruit, Refreshing Cleansing Blend, Wagamama*	1 Serving/311g	128	0.0	41	0.4	9.9	0.0	0.3
Tropical, Wagamama*	1 Serving/210g	100	0.0	48	0.4	10.4	0.0	1.6
KUSHIYAKI								
Lollipop Prawn, Wagamama*	1 Serving/122g	228	16.6	187	10.4	5.6	13.6	0.4
NOODLES								
Amai Udon, Teppan Fried, Wagamama*	1 Serving/676g	865	35.1	128	5.5	13.9	5.2	1.7
Chicken, Ginger, Udon, Wagamama*	1 Serving/605g	752	28.4	124	7.0	12.6	4.7	1.6

	Measure INFO/WEIGHT	per Measure KCAL	FAT	Nutrition Values per 100g / 100ml KCAL	PROT	CARB	FAT	FIBRE
WAGAMAMA								
NOODLES								
Chicken & Prawn, Pad Thai, Wagamama*	1 Serving/648g	794	31.0	123	5.4	13.8	4.8	1.4
Chicken Ramen with Vegetables in Soup, Wagamama*	1 Serving/810g	519	13.0	64	5.1	7.0	1.6	0.4
Fish, Grilled, Mini, & Vegetables, Wagamama*	1 Serving/248g	309	6.7	125	7.5	17.4	2.7	0.5
Yaki Udon, Wagamama*	1 Serviing/619g	716	26.0	116	5.8	12.8	4.2	1.8
Yasai Chilli Men, Wagamama*	1 Serving/673g	923	44.2	137	3.6	15.4	6.6	1.1
Yasai Pad Thai, Wagamama*	1 Serving/632g	820	36.7	130	4.4	14.3	5.8	1.4
PRAWNS								
Firecracker, Stir fried with Vegetables, Wagamama*	1 Serving/659g	906	24.4	138	3.8	21.9	3.7	0.7
RAMEN								
Beef, Chilli, Wagamama*	1 Serving/989g	680	22.7	69	5.1	6.7	2.3	0.6
Chicken, Chilli, Wagamama*	1 Serving/949g	597	16.1	63	4.6	6.9	1.7	0.6
Fish, Grilled, Seafood & Noodles, Wagamama*	1 Serving/685g	463	4.8	68	5.6	9.5	0.7	0.4
SALAD								
Beef, Ginger, & Coriander, Wagamama*	1 Serving/433g	686	54.6	158	8.4	2.5	12.6	1.0
Chicken Mandarin, & Sesame, Wagamama*	1 Serving/393g	790	54.2	201	11.0	7.7	13.8	1.1
SOUP								
Salmon, Teriyaki, Ramen, Wagamama*	1 Serving/913g	711	22.9	78	5.6	7.8	2.5	0.8
Yasai Itame, Wagamama*	1 Serving/799g	845	58.8	106	2.3	7.0	7.4	1.2
SQUID								
Deep Fried, with Shichimi & Chilli Sauce, Wagamama*	1 Serving/208g	493	33.3	237	8.7	14.3	16.0	0.4
SUSHI								
California Roll, Inside Out with Surimi, Wagamama*	1 Serving/93g	132	3.3	142	2.0	25.1	3.5	0.8
Cucumber Hosomaki, Wagamama*	1 Serving/108g	138	0.6	129	1.5	29.2	0.6	0.5
Hosomaki, Avocado, Wagamama*	1 Serving/113g	176	4.5	157	1.7	28.0	4.0	1.0
Tuna Hosomaki, Wagamama*	1 Serving/118g	171	0.9	145	8.0	26.5	0.8	0.0
Tuna Nigiri, Wagamama*	1 Serving/72g	102	0.7	142	10.1	23.1	1.0	0.0
Uramaki, Mango, Avocado & Cucumber, Wagamama*	1 Serving/84g	114	2.4	136	1.7	25.2	2.9	0.9
Uramaki, Salmon Skin with Avocado, Wagamama*	1 Serving/95g	169	6.3	178	6.0	23.3	6.7	0.7
Yasai Selection, Wagamama*	1 Serving/249g	345	6.3	139	1.7	26.8	2.5	0.9
TUNA								
Sashimi, Raw, Wagamama*	1 Serving/91g	109	1.9	120	21.6	3.7	2.1	0.0
Tataki, Wagamama*	1 Serving/98g	95	1.1	96	17.4	3.6	1.1	1.4
WIMPY								
BACON								
Extras, Wimpy*	1 Serving/91g	267	22.0	294	24.2	0.0	24.2	0.0
BEANS								
Baked, Heinz, Wimpy*	1 Serving/110g	85	0.2	77	4.4	12.6	0.2	3.6
BREAKFAST								
Hashbrown, Wimpy*	1 Serving/424g	545	41.1	129	4.1	8.7	9.7	1.9
Roll, Bacon, Breakfast, Wimpy*	1 Roll/144g	278	5.1	193	13.3	24.7	3.5	0.0
Roll, Bacon & Egg, Breakfast, Wimpy*	1 Roll/194g	368	12.1	190	13.4	18.3	6.2	0.0
Roll, Sausage, Breakfast, Wimpy*	1 Roll/161g	437	21.5	271	11.3	26.6	13.4	0.0
Roll, Sausage & Egg, Wimpy*	1 Roll/211g	527	28.4	250	11.8	20.3	13.5	0.0
The Country Breakfast, Wimpy*	1 Serving/271g	392	23.1	145	9.4	6.9	8.5	1.7
The Great Wimpy Breakfast, Wimpy*	1 Serving/459g	910	53.6	198	10.7	12.7	11.7	1.2
Wimpy Club, Wimpy*	1 Serving/330g	767	38.6	232	14.7	18.2	11.7	0.8
BURGERS								
BBQ, Wimpy*	1 Burger/236g	644	30.5	273	14.2	24.6	12.9	1.6
Bean, Spicy, Wimpy*	1 Burger/233g	611	29.4	262	5.9	30.5	12.6	2.7
Bean, Spicy, with Cheese, Wimpy*	1 Burger/245g	1459	98.3	596	24.2	35.5	40.1	2.7
Bender, with Cheese, in a Bun, Wimpy*	1 Burger/170g	424	23.4	249	10.2	20.8	13.8	1.2
Cheeseburger, Bacon, Classic,,Wimpy*	1 Burger/192g	405	19.0	211	13.6	16.8	9.9	0.0

	Measure INFO/WEIGHT	per Measure KCAL	per Measure FAT	KCAL	PROT	CARB	FAT	FIBRE
WIMPY								
BURGERS								
Cheeseburger, with Chips, Junior, Kids Meal, Wimpy*	1 Burger/191g	497	23.5	260	10.0	27.8	12.3	2.1
Chicken, & Bacon, Melt, Wimpy*	1 Burger/172g	443	20.2	258	12.6	25.4	11.7	0.0
Chicken, Fillet, in a Bun, Hot & Spicy, Wimpy*	1 Burger/193g	398	18.5	206	10.6	19.1	9.6	1.8
Chicken, Fillet, in a Bun, Savoury, Wimpy*	1 Burger/218g	356	13.8	163	10.4	16.1	6.3	1.1
Chicken, Fillet, Wimpy*	1 Burger/327g	380	16.8	116	6.7	11.1	5.1	0.0
Chicken, in a Bun, Wimpy*	1 Burger/191g	449	21.4	235	10.4	22.7	11.2	1.3
Classic, Kingsize, Wimpy*	1 Burger/227g	551	31.1	243	16.2	14.2	13.7	0.0
Classic, Wimpy*	1 Burger/159g	337	15.1	212	12.4	19.9	9.5	0.0
Classic, with Cheese, Wimpy*	1 Burger/175g	379	18.5	217	12.7	17.3	10.6	1.1
Halfpounder, with Bacon & Cheese, Wimpy*	1 Burger/312g	892	50.5	286	19.2	15.5	16.2	0.8
Mega Burger, Wimpy*	1 Burger/206g	594	36.0	288	15.3	18.0	17.5	0.0
Quarterpounder, Wimpy*	1 Burger/200g	538	31.3	269	15.0	18.0	15.6	0.0
Quarterpounder, with Bacon & Cheese, Wimpy*	1 Burger/237g	658	33.4	278	16.8	20.5	14.1	1.1
Quarterpounder, with Cheese, Wimpy*	1 Burger/213g	578	34.6	271	15.1	17.2	16.2	0.0
CHEESE								
Mozzarella, Meltz 3, Extras, Wimpy*	3 Meltz/79g	253	15.4	320	15.4	25.7	19.5	2.5
Mozzarella, Meltz 6, Extras, Wimpy*	6 Meltz/157g	506	30.8	322	15.6	25.9	19.6	2.5
Slices, Extras, Wimpy*	1 Slice/12g	40	3.3	333	18.3	5.0	27.5	0.0
CHICKEN								
Chunks, with Chips, Kids, Wimpy*	1 Serving/172g	440	26.1	256	8.4	22.2	15.2	1.8
Chunks, with Chips, Wimpy*	1 Serving/333g	779	46.8	234	8.3	19.0	14.0	1.5
Chunks, with Salad, Kids Meal, Wimpy*	1 Serving/187g	265	16.8	142	6.8	8.4	9.0	0.8
CHIPS								
Large Serving, Extras, Wimpy*	1 Serving/143g	333	17.1	233	3.0	30.4	12.0	3.0
Standard Serving, Extras, Wimpy*	1 Serving/114g	267	13.7	234	3.0	30.5	12.0	3.0
CHOCOLATE								
Crushed Flake (for desserts), Wimpy*	1 Serving/20g	104	6.1	520	7.5	57.0	30.5	1.0
COLESLAW								
Extras, Wimpy*	1 Serving/50g	49	3.8	98	1.4	6.2	7.6	0.8
DESSERT								
Brown Derby, with Dairy Ice Cream, Wimpy*	1 Serving/180g	431	20.6	239	4.5	31.3	11.4	1.4
Brownie Sundae, Wimpy*	1 Sundae/252g	574	21.8	228	3.8	34.7	8.6	0.6
Cheese Cake, Wimpy*	1 Serving/144g	412	18.3	286	4.5	38.5	12.7	0.0
Chocolate Fudge Cake, Wimpy*	1 Serving/100g	371	12.4	371	4.7	60.2	12.4	0.0
Ice Cream Sundae, Plain, Wimpy*	1 Sundae/170g	190	8.8	112	3.1	15.0	5.2	0.0
Knickerbocker Glory, Mini, with Ice Cream, Wimpy*	1 Serving/194g	190	8.5	98	1.6	13.2	4.4	0.0
EGGS								
Extras, Wimpy*	1 Egg/50g	90	7.0	180	13.6	0.0	14.0	0.0
FISH								
Bites, with Chips, Kids Meal, Wimpy*	1 Serving/160g	380	20.9	238	6.7	24.7	13.1	2.1
Bites, with Salad, Kids Meal, Wimpy*	1 Serving/175g	205	11.6	117	5.2	9.8	6.6	0.9
Haddock, Peas & Chips, Wimpy*	1 Serving/314g	674	37.9	215	6.6	21.2	12.1	2.4
Scampi & Chips with Peas, Wimpy*	1 Serving/303g	577	29.8	190	5.2	22.7	9.8	2.3
GRILL								
All-Day Breakfast, Wimpy*	1 Serving/410g	731	39.7	178	8.3	14.5	9.7	0.0
BBQ Rib Rack, Platter, Wimpy*	1 Serving/439g	713	35.2	162	5.6	17.5	8.0	1.4
Chicken, Platter, Gourmet, Wimpy*	1 Serving/392g	525	21.4	134	11.4	10.0	5.5	1.4
Classic Bacon, Wimpy*	1 Serving/321g	722	45.3	225	11.5	14.0	14.1	0.0
Sausage, Egg & Chips, Wimpy*	1 Serving/244g	597	38.8	245	9.0	17.4	15.9	1.7
Steak, Platter, Wimpy*	1 Serving/424g	719	38.0	170	9.9	12.9	9.0	0.0
The International, Wimpy*	1 Serving/416g	1010	71.3	243	13.9	10.0	17.1	0.9

(KCAL, PROT, CARB, FAT, FIBRE: Nutrition Values per 100g / 100ml)

	Measure INFO/WEIGHT	per Measure KCAL	per Measure FAT	KCAL	PROT	CARB	FAT	FIBRE
				Nutrition Values per 100g / 100ml				
WIMPY								
HAMBURGER								
with Chips, Kids Meal, Wimpy*	1 Serving/184g	457	20.0	248	9.0	29.9	10.9	0.0
with Salad, Kids Meal, Wimpy*	1 Serving/199g	283	10.7	142	7.5	16.4	5.4	0.0
HASH BROWNS								
Extras, Wimpy*	1 Serving/55g	93	7.8	169	2.2	19.6	14.2	1.8
HOT DOG								
with Salad, Kids, Wimpy*	1 Serving/241g	425	21.1	176	7.0	17.3	8.8	0.0
ICE CREAM								
Banana Longboat with Soft Ice Cream, Wimpy*	1 Serving/209g	260	6.0	124	2.3	23.9	2.9	0.0
Brown Derby with Dairy Ice Cream, Wimpy*	1 Serving/125g	397	19.7	318	5.6	38.9	15.8	0.0
Choc Nut Sundae, Wimpy*	1 Serving/83g	196	6.2	236	4.6	38.4	7.5	0.0
Dairy, with Chocolate Sauce, Wimpy*	1 Serving/88g	200	8.1	227	3.4	32.5	9.2	0.0
Dairy, with Strawberry Sauce, Wimpy*	1 Serving/88g	199	7.9	226	3.0	34.3	9.0	0.0
Fruit & Nut Sundae, Wimpy*	1 Serving/83g	138	5.8	166	4.2	23.2	7.0	0.0
Knickerbockerglory, with Soft Ice Cream, Wimpy*	1 Serving/138g	196	6.0	142	2.7	24.7	4.4	0.0
Soft, with Chocolate Sauce, Wimpy*	1 Serving/71g	137	3.2	193	2.8	36.1	4.5	0.0
Soft, with Strawberry Sauce, Wimpy*	1 Serving/71g	137	3.0	193	2.4	38.3	4.2	0.0
Strawberry Sundae, Triple, with Soft Ice Cream, Wimpy*	1 Serving/170g	123	3.3	72	1.4	13.1	1.9	0.0
ONION RINGS								
Large (12), Extras, Wimpy*	1 Serving/180g	401	23.2	223	3.2	23.6	12.9	0.0
Standard (6), Extras, Wimpy*	1 Serving/90g	201	11.6	223	3.2	23.6	12.9	3.0
PANINI								
Cheese, with Red Onion, Wimpy*	1 Panini/205g	673	22.8	329	14.6	42.7	11.1	1.9
Cheese & Tomato, Wimpy*	1 Panini/225g	694	25.1	309	14.6	37.4	11.1	2.2
Ham, Tomato & Cheese, Wimpy*	1 Panini/275g	1145	39.0	417	33.0	38.4	14.2	2.2
Ham & Cheese, Wimpy*	1 Panini/235g	944	33.3	402	32.0	35.7	14.2	1.4
Steak, Cheese & Onion, Wimpy*	1 Panini/305g	688	28.6	226	13.8	21.4	9.4	1.0
POTATOES								
Baked, Jacket, Plain, with Butter, Wimpy*	1 Serving/327g	453	7.6	139	3.5	27.7	2.3	2.4
Baked, Jacket, with Baked Beans, Wimpy*	1 Serving/452g	549	7.9	121	3.4	23.5	1.8	2.7
Baked, Jacket, with Beans & Cheese, Wimpy*	1 Serving/577g	1069	51.5	185	8.4	18.4	8.9	2.1
Baked, Jacket, with Coleslaw, Wimpy*	1 Serving/452g	576	17.1	127	2.9	21.7	3.8	2.0
Baked, Jacket, with Grated Cheese, Wimpy*	1 Serving/452g	973	51.2	215	9.6	20.0	11.3	1.8
Baked, Jacket, with Tuna Mayo, Wimpy*	1 Serving/452g	764	34.2	169	5.9	20.6	7.6	1.8
RIBS								
Pork, Wimpy*	1 Rib/189g	463	22.4	245	13.0	21.6	11.9	0.0
ROLL								
Bacon, in a Bun, Wimpy*	1 Roll/125g	341	16.1	273	16.0	22.6	12.9	1.4
Bacon & Egg, in a Bun, Wimpy*	1 Roll/155g	702	41.7	453	29.6	22.6	26.9	1.4
SALAD								
Chicken, Gourmet, Wimpy*	1 Serving/358g	251	4.3	70	11.9	2.7	1.2	0.4
Chicken, Hot & Spicy, Wimpy*	1 Serving/290g	283	15.2	98	6.1	6.7	5.2	0.9
Fish, Wimpy*	1 Serving/356g	389	21.3	109	4.6	9.9	6.0	0.0
Scampi, Wimpy*	1 Serving/356g	376	19.1	106	4.2	10.7	5.4	0.0
Side, Extras, Wimpy*	1 Serving/145g	44	0.3	30	1.4	6.1	0.2	0.8
Steak, Wimpy*	1 Serving/355g	329	16.9	93	10.0	2.7	4.8	0.4
SAUCE								
Chocolate (for sundae), Wimpy*	1 Serving/28g	80	0.4	286	1.4	66.1	1.4	1.1
Maple Flavoured Syrup (for dessert), Wimpy*	1 Serving/28g	74	0.1	264	0.0	67.9	0.4	0.0
Strawberry (for dessert), Wimpy*	1 Serving/28g	78	0.0	279	0.0	69.6	0.0	0.4
SAUSAGE								
with Chips, Kids Meal, Wimpy*	1 Serving/160g	428	27.7	268	8.9	19.9	17.3	1.9

	Measure INFO/WEIGHT	per Measure KCAL	per Measure FAT	Nutrition Values per 100g / 100ml KCAL	PROT	CARB	FAT	FIBRE
WIMPY								
SPONGE PUDDING								
Treacle, Wimpy*	1 Serving/130g	504	21.3	388	3.9	56.1	16.4	0.0
SPOTTED DICK								
Wimpy*	1 Serving/130g	400	16.5	308	4.1	44.2	12.7	0.0
SUNDAE								
Toffee, Wimpy*	1 Sundae/239g	537	23.6	225	3.8	30.8	9.9	0.8
SWEETS								
Mini Marshmallows (for desserts), Wimpy*	1 Serving/10g	33	0.0	330	4.0	83.0	0.0	0.0
TEACAKES								
Toasted, with Butter, Wimpy*	1 Teacake/66g	227	2.3	344	1.7	10.4	3.4	0.4
TOAST								
with Jam, Extras, Wimpy*	1 Serving/89g	276	8.3	310	7.3	52.6	9.3	1.7
TOASTIE								
Cheese, with Salad, Kids, Wimpy*	1 Serving/250g	367	8.8	147	5.9	24.2	3.5	1.2
WAFFLES								
Chocolate, Half, with Dairy Ice Cream, Wimpy*	1 Serving/116g	395	18.8	341	4.0	44.7	16.2	0.0
Chocolate, with Dairy Ice Cream, Wimpy*	1 Serving/178g	691	37.0	388	5.1	45.3	20.8	0.0
Eskimo, Wimpy*	1 Serving/228g	694	30.2	304	4.6	42.7	13.2	1.3
WAFLES								
Chocolate, with Squirty Cream, Wimpy*	1 Serving/158g	667	36.9	422	5.1	47.7	23.4	0.0

Useful Resources

Weight Loss
Weight Loss Resources is home to the UK's largest calorie and nutrition database along with diaries, tools and expert advice for weight loss and health.
Tel: 01733 345592 Email: helpteam@weightlossresources.co.uk
Website: www.weightlossresources.co.uk

Exercise Equipment for Home
Diet and Fitness Resources has a range of equipment for exercise at home, from pedometers to treadmills and fitballs to weights. As well as diet tools such as food diaries, a weight loss kit and diet plates.
Tel: 01733 345592 Email: helpteam@dietandfitnessresources.co.uk
Website: www.dietandfitnessresources.co.uk

Dietary Advice
The British Dietetic Association has helpful food fact leaflets and information on how to contact a registered dietitian.
Tel: 0121 200 8080 Email: info@bda.uk.com
Website: www.bda.uk.com

Healthy Eating
The British Nutrition Foundation has lots of in depth scientifically based nutritional information, knowledge and advice on healthy eating for all ages.
Tel: 0207 7557 7930 Email: postbox@nutrition.org.uk
Website: www.nutrition.org.uk

Healthy Heart
The British Heart Foundation provides advice and information for all on all heart aspects from being healthy, to living with heart conditions, research and fundraising.
Tel: 0207 554 000 Email: via their website
Website: www.bhf.org.uk

Cancer Research
Cancer Research UK is the leading UK charity dedicated to research, education and fundraising for all forms of cancer.
Tel: 0300 123 1022 Email: via their website
Website: www.cancerresearchuk.org

Diabetes Advice
Diabetes UK is the leading charity working for people with diabetes. Their mission is to improve the lives of people with diabetes and to work towards a future without diabetes
Tel : 0345 123 2399 Email: info@diabetes.org.uk
Website: www.diabetes.org.uk

Beating Bowel Cancer
Beating Bowel Cancer is a leading UK charity for bowel cancer patients, working to raise awareness of symptoms, promote early diagnosis and encourage open access to treatment choice for those affected by bowel cancer.Tel: 08450 719301 Email: nurse@beatingbowelcancer.org
Website: www.beatingbowelcancer.org

Safety and Standards
The Food Standards Agency is an independent watchdog, set up to protect the public's health and consumer interests in relation to food.
Tel: 0207 276 8829 Email: helpline@foodstandards.gsi.gov.uk
Website: www.food.gov.uk

Feedback

If you have any comments or suggestions about The Calorie, Carb & Fat Bible, or would like further information on Weight Loss Resources, please call, email, or write to us:

Tel: 01733 345592
Email: helpteam@weightlossresources.co.uk
Address: Laurence Beeken,
Weight Loss Resources Ltd,
2C Flag Business Exchange,
Vicarage Farm Road,
Peterborough,
PE1 5TX.

Reviews for The Calorie Carb & Fat Bible

'What a brilliant book. I know I'll be sinking my teeth into it.'
GMTV Nutritionist Amanda Ursell, BSc RD

'To help you make low-cal choices everyday, invest in a copy.'
ZEST magazine

'There is no doubt that the food listings are extremely helpful for anyone wishing to control their calorie intake in order to lose pounds or maintain a healthy weight.'
Women's Fitness magazine

'Useful if you don't want to exclude any overall food groups.'
Easy Living magazine

'Quite simply an astonishing achievement by the authors.'
Evening Post, Nottingham

'The book gives you all the basic information so you can work out your daily calorie needs.'
Woman magazine

'This is a welcome resource in view of the 'national epidemic of obesity.'

Bryony Philip, Bowel Cancer UK

'The authors seem to understand the problems of slimming.'

Dr John Campion

'Jam-packed with info on dieting, and full to bursting point with the calorie, carbohydrate and fat values of thousands of different foods, it's the perfect weight loss tool.'

Evening Express, Aberdeen

'Excellent resource tool - used by myself in my role as a Practice Nurse.'

Pam Boal, Sunderland

'I recently bought your book called the Calorie, Carb & Fat Bible and would love to tell you what a brilliant book it is. I have recently started a weight management programme and I honestly don't know where I'd be without your book. It has helped me a lot and given me some really good advice.'

Rachel Mitchell

About Weight Loss Resources

weightlossresources.co.uk

"What this does is put you in control with no guilt, no awful groups and no negativity! Fill in your food diary, get support on the boards and watch it fall off!"

LINDAB, Weight Loss Resources Member

How Does It Work?

Weight Loss Resources is home to the UK's biggest online calorie and nutrition database. You simply tap in your height, weight, age and basic activity level - set a weight loss goal, and the programme does all the necessary calculations.

What Does It Do?

The site enables you to keep a food diary which keeps running totals of calories, fat, fibre, carbs, proteins and portions of fruit and veg. You can also keep an exercise diary which adds the calories you use during exercise. At the end of a week, you update your weight and get reports and graphs on your progress.

How Will It Help?

You'll learn a great deal about how your eating and drinking habits affect your weight and how healthy they are. Using the diaries and other tools you'll be able to make changes that suit your tastes and your lifestyle. The result is weight loss totally tailored to your needs and preferences. A method you can stick with that will help you learn how to eat well for life!

Try It Free!

Go to **www.weightlossresources.co.uk** and take a completely free, no obligation, 24 hour trial. If you like what you see you can sign up for membership from £6.95 per month.